Surgical Pathology of the Ovaries

For Churchill Livingstone

Commissioning Editor: Gavin Smith
Copy Editor: Julie Gorman
Project Controller: Anita Sekhri
Indexer: Nina Boyd
Cover Design: Jeannette Jacobs

Surgical Pathology of the Ovaries

Peter Russell MD BSc (Med) MB BS FRCPA
Professor of Pathology, The University of Sydney;
Head, Department of Anatomical Pathology, Royal Prince Alfred Hospital and
King George V Memorial Hospital for Mothers and Babies, Camperdown, Australia;
Director of Pathology, Sydney IVF;
Deputy Chairman and Director of Pathology, Institute for Magnetic Resonance Research,
Sydney, Australia

Annabelle Farnsworth MB BS FRCPA MIAC Dip Cytopath
Director of Cytology, Gynaecological Pathologist, Douglass Hanly Moir Laboratories,
North Ryde, New South Wales, Australia

SECOND EDITION

CHURCHILL
LIVINGSTONE

NEW YORK EDINBURGH LONDON MADRID MELBOURNE SAN FRANCISCO TOKYO 1997

Distributed in the United States of America by Churchill Livingstone Inc., 650 Avenue of the Americas, New York, N.Y. 10011, and by associated companies, branches and representatives throughout the world.

First published 1989
Second edition 1997

ISBN 0 443 05384 7

British Library Cataloguing in Publication Data
A catalogue record for this book is available from the British Library.

Library of Congress Cataloging in Publication Data
A catalog record for this book is available from the Library of Congress.

The publisher's policy is to use **paper manufactured from sustainable forests**

Produced by Longman Singapore Publishers (Pte) Ltd
Printed in Singapore

Preface

Since the compilation and publication of the first edition, very significant changes have taken place in the "landscape" of ovarian surgical pathology. In the intervening eight short years, several dozen new entities have been described, and as many old ones redefined or dispensed with. We see differently, and perhaps more clearly, the relationships between certain pathological processes, while others remain as enigmatic and controversial as before. As in the first edition, the framework of tumor classification is that of the World Health Organization and its modification, completed but not yet published, by the International Society of Gynecological Pathologists.

Much effort has been put into presenting what we perceive to be current thinking in this edition, rather than recapitulating or building upon the established "historical foundation". Historical reference and description are given only where critical to our current understanding. The most useful of the information about immunohistochemical profiles, cytogenetic and molecular genetic studies on various tumor types is summarised in each chapter. Ultrastructural features are again noted only in passing, and only as they offer specific diagnostic assistance or insight. Controversial issues in the major subtypes of surface epithelial-stromal tumors are addressed and illustrated in detail. These include, specifically, the nature of proliferating serous tumors and the accompanying extra-ovarian lesions (i.e. "implants"), and the splitting of ovarian mucinous tumors into "mullerian" and "intestinal" subtypes with their vastly different clinical correlates (e.g. endometriosis, pseudomyxoma peritonei). Recently described entities such as ovarian fibromatosis, small cell desmoplastic tumor, undifferentiated small cell carcinoma of pulmonary type, to mention just a few, are presented in particular detail.

As a consequence of the importance we place on clinicopathologic correlation in the diagnosis of ovarian pathology, several chapters have been completely rewritten, this time by clinicians, to enhance their relevance for specialist gynecologic pathologist and clinician alike. These include the chapters on intersex, laboratory investigation of ovarian function and polycystic ovary syndrome. Clinically relevant introductory chapters to all the major tumor groups have been added. A new chapter has been added on medical imaging of the ovaries with the same objective in mind. Finally, a new chapter has been added, in the form of a color atlas, to address intraoperative cytologic diagnosis, a technique of increasing usefulness in our laboratory.

As before, this monograph is specifically aimed at meeting the particular needs of our clinical colleagues for accurate tissue diagnosis of the ovarian surgical specimen. Our thanks to them for their support and stimulation and also to the various technical and laboratory staff of the Royal Prince Alfred Hospital who have enabled its completion.

P.R.
A.F.

Preface to the first edition

Few, if any, organs exhibit the diversity of pathological entities to be found in the human ovaries. It was this diversity which initially excited our interest and led to an appreciation, over the years, of some of the diagnostic difficulties encountered in the histological assessment of surgical ovarian biopsies.

This book is aimed at addressing these difficulties in as practical a fashion as possible, using a traditional morphological approach. We have taken the decision to exclude many of the theoretical aspects of ovarian disease from this text, except where they impact upon practical clinicopathological correlation (e.g. the concept of 'mullerian neoplasia'). Immunohistochemical techniques found to be useful, in our experience, are discussed. Ultrastructural examination, while contributing significantly to an understanding of many of the entities covered here, plays only a minor role in routine laboratory diagnosis and has therefore been mentioned only when it can resolve specific problems in differential diagnosis. Clinicopathological correlation has been emphasized throughout, since we believe it is central to arriving at a correct pathological diagnosis. The framework for discussing ovarian neoplasms is that of the World Health Organization, currently being modified by the International Society of Gynecological Pathologists.

We acknowledge the guidance and intellectual stimulation of our friends and colleagues in pathology and clinical practice and the challenges of the difficult consultation cases referred by them. We are indebted to the staff of the Audiovisual Services Department of Royal Prince Alfred Hospital for their assistance in the preparation of the illustrations.

1989

P.R.
P.B.

Contributors

John A Eden MB BS MD MRCOG FRACOG CREI
Senior Lecturer in Reproductive Medicine, Royal Hospital for Women, Paddington, New South Wales, Australia

Annabelle Farnsworth MB BS FRCPA MIAC Dip Cytopath
Director of Cytology, Gynaecological Pathologist, Douglass Hanly Moir Laboratories, North Ryde, New South Wales, Australia

Alan J Ferrier MB BS MSc FRACOG MRCOG
Senior Lecturer, Department of Obstetrics and Gynaecology, Gynaecological Oncology Unit, University of Sydney Royal North Shore Hospital, St Leonards, New South Wales, Australia

Ian S Fraser MD BSc(Hons) MBChB FRCOG FRACOG CREI DUa
Professor of Reproductive Medicine, Department of Obstetrics and Gynaecology, University of Sydney; Visiting Medical Officer, King George V and Royal Prince Alfred Hospitals, New South Wales, Australia

Robert P S Jansen MD(Syd) FRACP FRACOG CREI
Clinical Professor in Gynaecology, Royal Prince Alfred Hospital and the University of Sydney, Sydney, Australia

Kathryn A Occhipinti MD
Diagnostic Radiologist, Women's Imaging – MRI of the Pelvis, Plantation General Hospital, Florida, USA

Jeanette Philips MB BCh(Rand) FRCPA FIAC
Clinical Associate Professor of Pathology, University of Sydney; Senior Staff Specialist, Department of Anatomical Pathology, Royal North Shore Hospital, Sydney; Consultant Pathologist, Sydney Surgical Pathology (A Division of Hampton Pathology), Australia

Peter Russell MD BSc(Med) MB BS FRCPA
Professor of Pathology, The University of Sydney; Head, Department of Anatomical Pathology, Royal Prince Alfred Hospital and King George V Memorial Hospital for Mothers and Babies, Camperdown, Australia; Director of Pathology, Sydney IVF; Deputy Chairman and Director of Pathology, Institute for Magnetic Resonance Research, Sydney, Australia

Contents

Dedication

To Gail, Robert, Mark, Trent, Robert Jr and James

"As philosophers constantly tell us, and we keep finding out the hard way, science is tentative; existing perceptions are constantly replaced by new ones. And so it will be in the future, because this is the way of scientific progress. But I hope, too, that fifteen years experience have helped me to be less inclined than I once was vigorously to defend conclusions, to insist that what we think we know is the Truth. Absolute truth is like a mirage: it tends to disappear when you approach it. One of the most important lessons for me during these years is my learning that, passionately though I may seek certain answers, some will remain, like the mirage, forever beyond my reach."

(Reproduced with permission from Richard Leakey, *Origins Reconsidered*, published by Abacus, a division of Little, Brown & Company (UK) Limited)

SECTION 1

The fundamentals

1

Embryology

P. Russell A. Farnsworth

GONADAL DEVELOPMENT

Gonadal development in the earliest stages is the same in both male and female embryos. The developing gonad appears about 1 month after fertilization in embryos of 4–5 mm crown–rump length as multilayered ridges of mesodermally derived coelomic epithelium (mesothelium) on the medial border of the urogenital ridge (Fig. 1.1A). As these genital ridges differentiate, the basement membrane between the coelomic epithelium and the underlying mesenchyme disappears and cell cords grow down from the surface epithelium to form the predominant component of the gonad. Primordial germ cells migrate from the yolk sac to these developing gonads via the hindgut, the migration commencing approximately 3 weeks after fertilization. The primitive germ cells are spherical and distinctly larger than the surrounding mesenchymal cells, with large vesicular nuclei and amphophilic cytoplasm.

At this stage the gonad is termed 'indifferent', meaning it is not histologically distinguishable as male or female (Fig. 1.2). Whether the gonad then goes on to differentiate as testis or ovary depends on the presence of *testicular determining factor* (TDF). Without TDF, ovaries develop and the embryo then assumes a female phenotype by 'default', regardless of genetic sex (Fig. 1.1). Recent work suggests that TDF is coded for by a gene called SRY (sex-determining region Y) located in region 1A1 at the distal end of the short arm of the Y chromosome (Sinclair et al 1990). This gene is absent from the normal X chromosome and genetic engineering of this gene into chromosomally female embryos causes development as a male (Koopman et al 1991). Further details are given in Chapter 9.

If TDF is present, the proliferating cell cords, which have grown down from the surface epithelium, differentiate into testicular tubules, the epithelial cells becoming Sertoli cells and the gonadal stroma giving rise to interstitial or Leydig cells. Some of this early epithelial proliferation contributes to the connection between the sex cords and the mesonephric tubules which will eventually form the testis and duct of the epididymis. In testicular development, the germ cells are then incorporated into the tubules. The surface epithelium gives rise to the surrounding capsule or tunica albuginea. The gonad is histologically distinguishable as a testis by day 14 with early tubule formation and immature Sertoli cells.

When TDF is absent, i.e. normal 46,XX females, the surface epithelial cells also form sex cords but these subsequently break up into isolated masses (Fig. 1.1C,D). The sex cords are not as well formed or distinctly cord-like as in the testis and have been termed the 'cortical lobules'. This may represent the first recognizable difference between the developing male and female gonad. These cells aggregate to form primordial follicles by encapsulating ova and it is possible that they become pregranulosa cells. The development of primordial follicles begins at about week 12 of gestation. The primitive germ cells proliferate and divide into oogonia and primary oocytes. The greatest complement of oogonia in the ovary (approximately 6 000 000) is formed by about the sixth month of fetal life, at which time proliferation ceases and the inexorable process of atresia commences. The cells remain quiescent at the primary oocyte stage in prophase of the first meiotic division with DNA synthesis resuming only in the event of fertilization. In the ovary the prolifer-

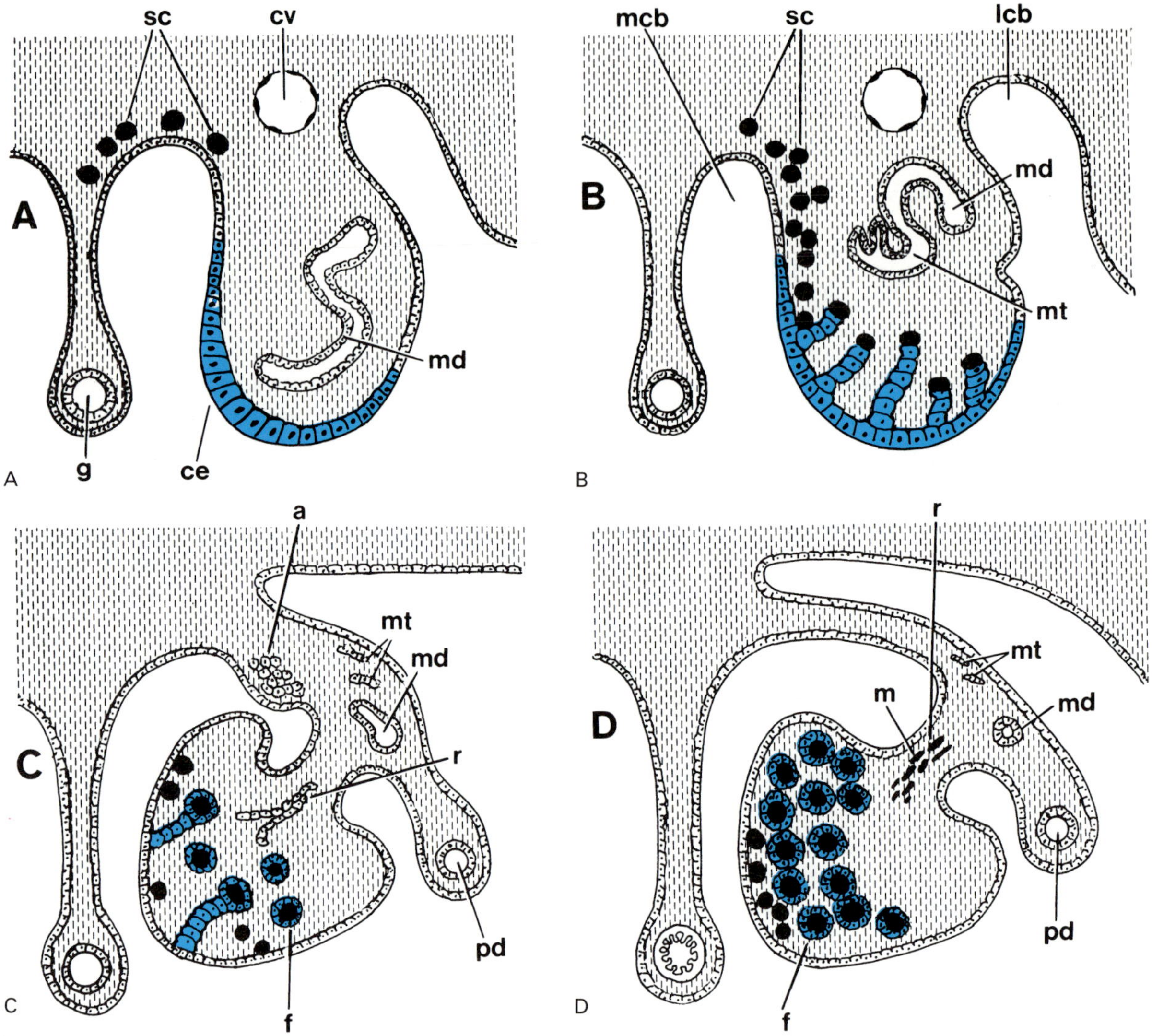

Fig. 1.1 Schema of early embryonic and fetal development of the ovary. (A) Indifferent gonad of 25–30 somite embryo. Primitive germ cells migrate to the urogenital ridge via the hindgut mesentery. (B) Indifferent gonad of 25–30 somite embryo. Germ cells and invaginating coelomic epithelial cells proliferate in the urogenital ridge. (C) Ovary of 12 mm embryo with poorly formed rete in mesovarium and adjacent development of paramesonephric (mullerian) duct. (D) Ovary of 14-week fetus (menstrual age). Primordial follicles are aggregated in the cortex. Rete and mesonephric structures are regressing. a, Developing adrenal cortex; ce, coelomic epithelium; cv, posterior cardinal vein; f, primordial follicles; g, gut; lcb, lateral coelomic bay; m, mesovarium; mcb, medial coelomic bay; md, mesonephric duct; mt, mesonephric tubule; pd, paramesonephric duct; r, rete ovarii; sc, primitive sex cells

ating sex cords degenerate in the ovarian hilum, not connecting with the wolffian duct, as in the testis. The few tubular remnants are left as the rete ovarii. Interstitial (Leydig) cells develop extensively in the stromal tissue of the second trimester female gonad but degenerate in most cases by term.

Continuing development of the ovary and its attached mesentery takes place as deep grooves arise on the lateral and medial aspects of the enlarging gonad, partly separating it from the regressing mesonephros laterally and the supra-renal anlage dorsomedially. The grooves deepen, resulting in the formation of the gonadal mesen-

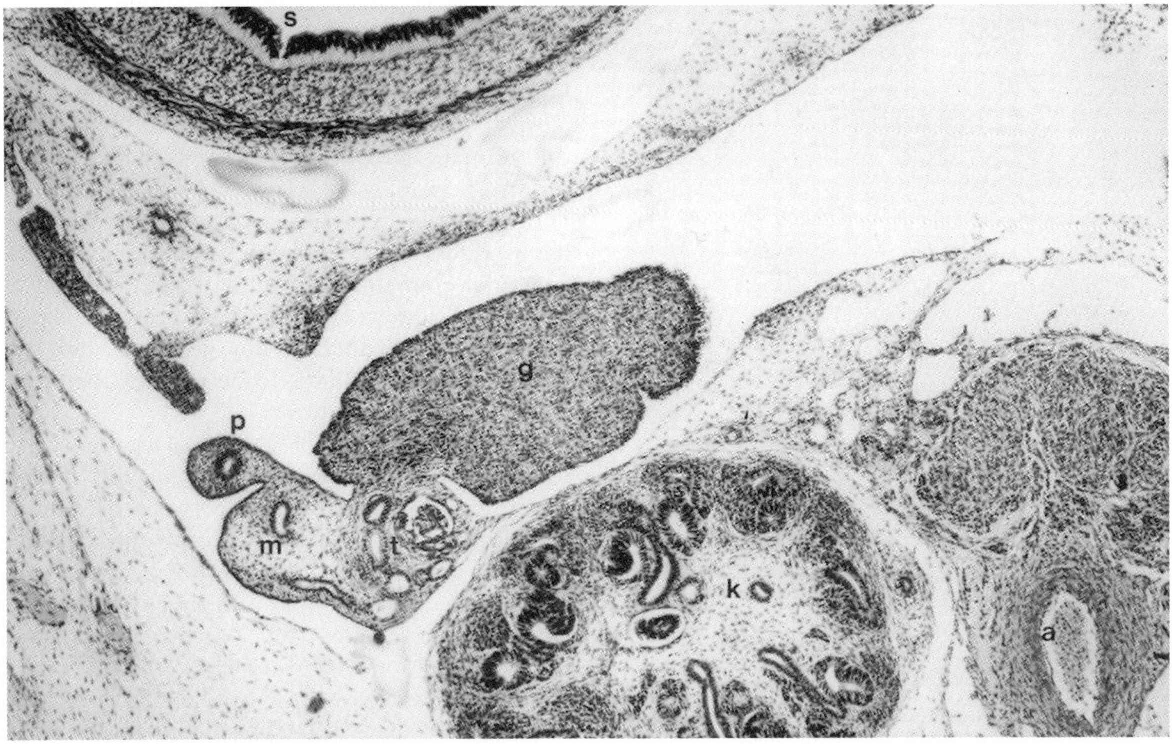

Fig. 1.2 Indifferent gonad (g) at 20 mm stage of embryonic development. Adjacent structures are the paramesonephric duct (p), mesonephric duct (m), mesonephric tubules and glomeruli (t), metanephros (k), aorta (a), and stomach (s). H + E ×50

tery (mesovarium), and the urogenital mesentery attenuates. As the tubal portion of the urogenital ridge traverses the pelvic brim it is connected to the anterior abdominal wall by a mesodermal thickening, the inguinal fold or plica inguinalis in which the gubernaculum of the ovary later develops.

At the fifth or sixth month, mesenchymal cells invade the ovary via the mesovarium (Fig. 1.3). These spindle-shaped cells ultimately provide the bulk of the ovarian stroma or parenchyma – both cortex and medulla. There is no evidence at any stage in fetal ovarian development, that granulosa cells of sex-cord origin differentiate into stromal cells, or vice versa. The primitive cell clusters containing the oogonia become dispersed. The germ cells with an investment of granulosa cells survive, while those without undergo atresia and disappear.

During descent of the ovary into the pelvis, the gubernaculum acquires an additional attachment to the lateral margin of the uterine fundus to produce, on either side of this attachment, the round ligament of the uterus and the ligament of the ovary. This is intended to prevent the further descent of the ovary into the inguinal canal (see Ch. 6).

DEVELOPMENT OF REPRODUCTIVE ORGANS

Subsequent development of the male or female phenotype is dependent on two hormones produced by the fetal testis, *antimullerian hormone* (AMH) and testosterone. AMH is produced by normal testicular Sertoli cells during fetal life. In the female, in the absence of testes, AMH is produced in insignificant amounts. AMH secretion in the male commences from about day 56 to day 62 after fertilization. Its main function is to inhibit development of the mullerian ducts which is completed by about day 77. AMH has a local action

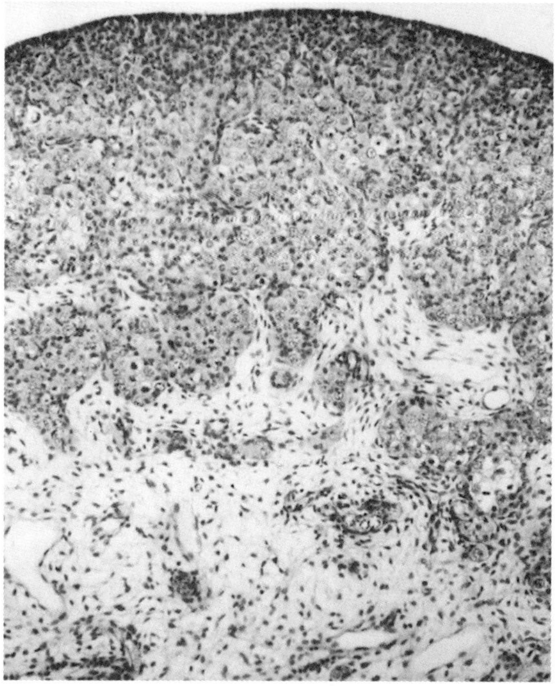

Fig. 1.3 Ovary of a normal 20-week fetus showing aggregation of primordial follicles in the superficial (cortical) portion of the ovary with the deeper (medullary) stroma composed predominantly of spindle-shaped mesenchymal cells. H + E ×75

and inhibits development of the ipsilateral fallopian tube. AMH continues to be produced even after complete regression of mullerian structures takes place. Expression in the testes remains high after birth, then decreases thereafter to the low levels found at puberty (Lee & Donahoe 1993). Testosterone is necessary for the wolffian duct to differentiate into epididymis, vas deferens, and seminal vesicle.

In the absence of these two hormones, the mullerian ducts develop from invaginations of the coelomic epithelium on the lateral surface of the urogenital ridge at about 6 weeks gestation, lateral to the wolffian ducts. They grow caudally and need the wolffian ducts to be present for proper caudal migration to occur.

Median inclination of the caudal segment of the urogenital ridges allows fusion in the midline forming a urogenital septum between the bladder and hindgut. Subsequent fusion of the mullerian ducts in the midline form the uterovaginal canal which is the primordium of the uterus and vagina. The fallopian tubes develop from the lateral unfused portions of mullerian ducts. In the absence of testosterone the wolffian ducts involute. Remnants of these ducts are the epoophoron, the paroophoron, and Gartner ducts.

AMH is produced by the ovaries postnatally. It is produced by the granulosa cells and the highest levels are found in the pubertal and adult ovary. Its function may be to inhibit meiosis in the developing follicle in normal ovaries (Lee & Donahoe 1993).

REFERENCES

Koopman P, Gubbay J, Vivian N, Goodfellow P, Lovell-Badge R 1991 Male development of chromosomally female mice transgenic for Sry. Nature 351: 117–121

Lee M M, Donahoe P K 1993 Mullerian inhibiting substance: a gonadal hormone with multiple functions. Endocrine Reviews 14: 152–164

Sinclair A H, Beta P, Palmer M S et al 1990 A gene for the human sex determining region encodes a protein with homology to a conserved DNA binding motif. Nature 346: 240–244

2

Surgical anatomy

P. Russell   A. Farnsworth

The human ovaries are symmetrical ovoid paired organs normally measuring approximately 2 × 0.5 × 0.5 cm in term infants (Fig. 2.1) and 3 × 2 × 1 cm in adults. They enlarge during pregnancy, and shrink somewhat in the postmenopausal period (Fig. 2.2). They are smooth

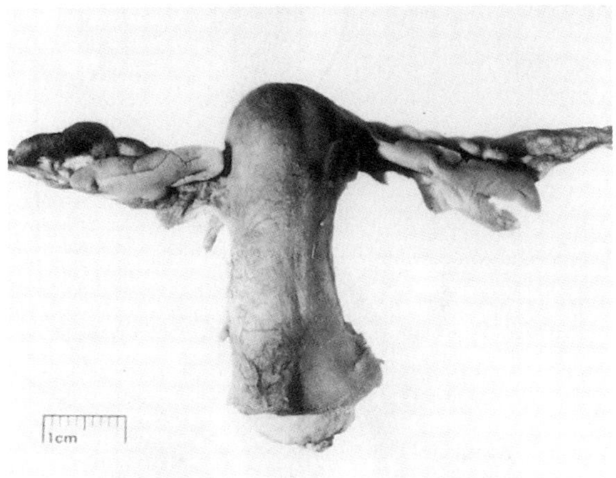

Fig. 2.1 Term newborn infant. Posterior aspect of the uterine corpus and cervix with attached fallopian tubes and ovaries. Note the elongated 'roe-like' shape of the ovaries and the relative size of the structures

Fig. 2.2 Postmenopausal woman. Posterior aspect of uterine corpus and cervix (removed by extrafascial hysterectomy) with attached fallopian tubes and ovaries. Note the smooth peritoneal reflection between these latter structures readily facilitating orientation of the specimen

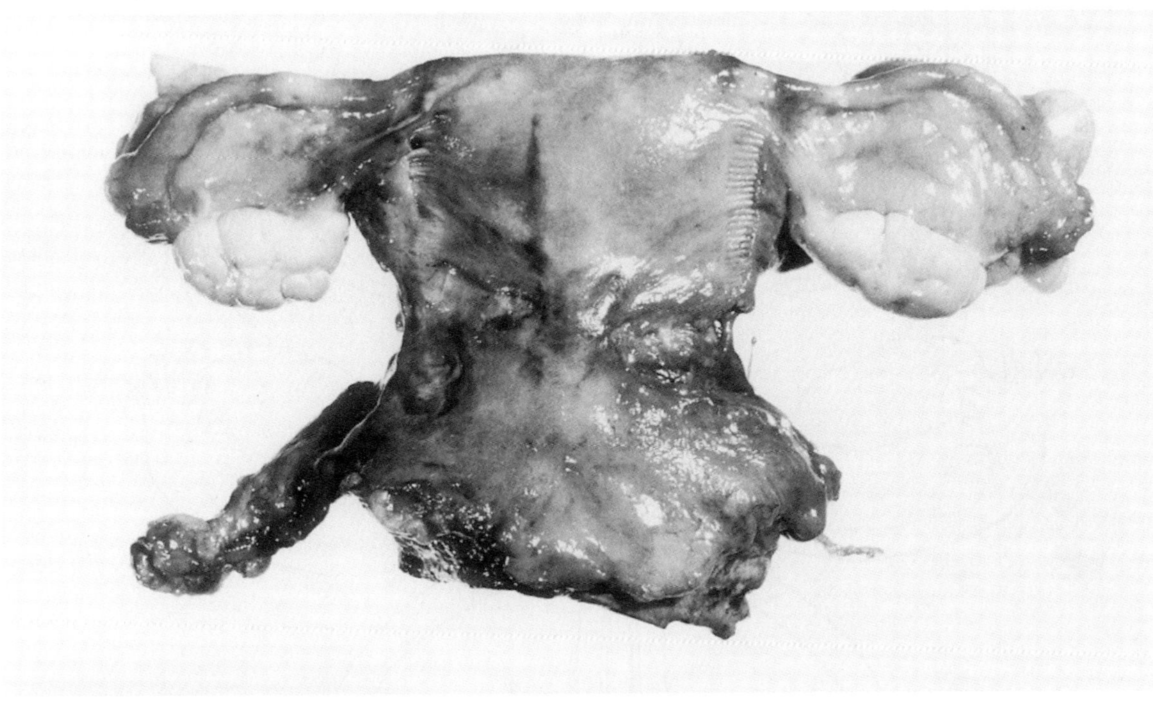

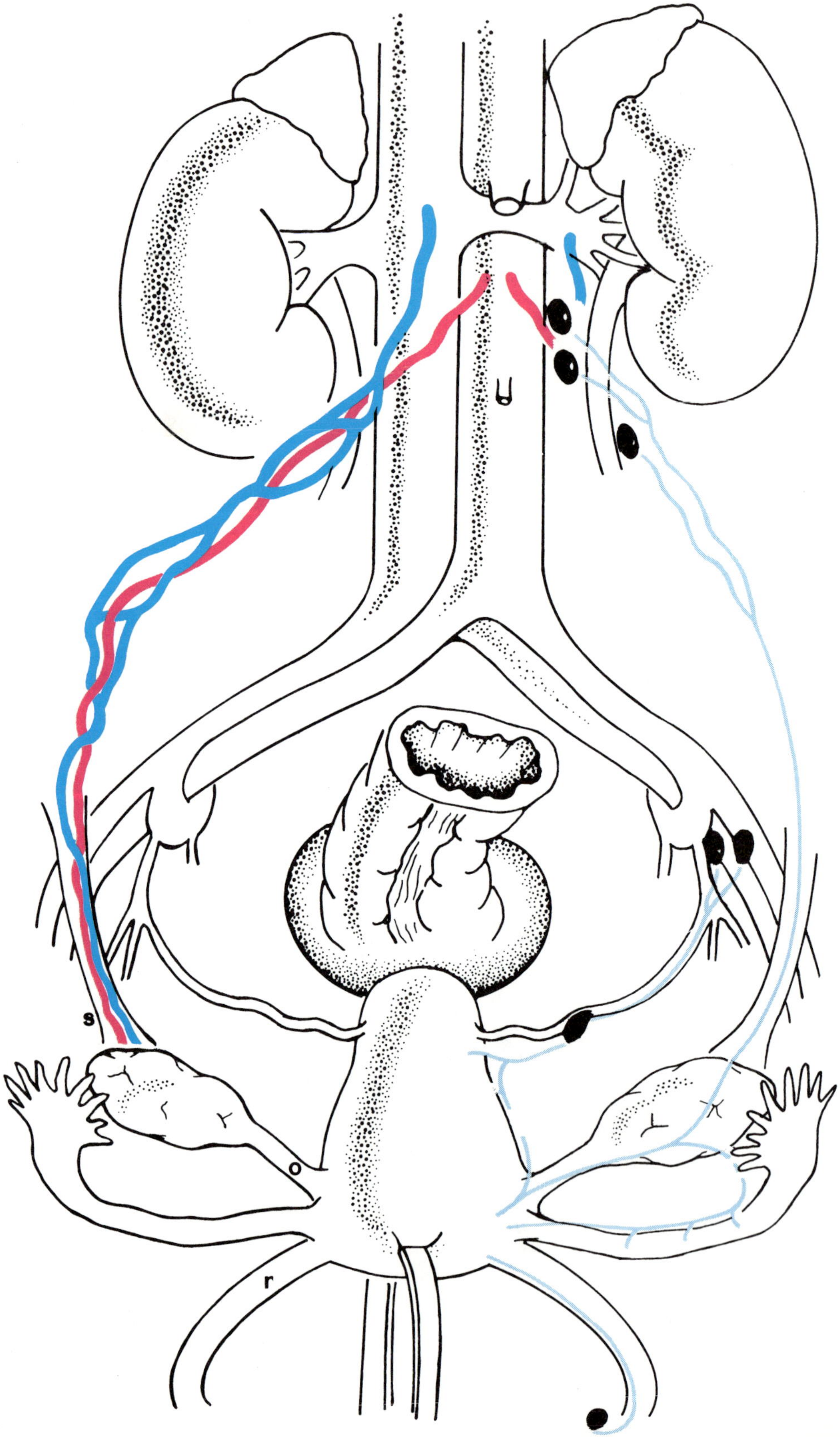
s
o
r

surfaced, but irregularly contoured due to the presence of developing follicles, ovulatory stigmata, and corpora lutea. In the nonparous adult woman, each lies in a depression at the side wall of the lesser pelvis in the angle between the internal and external iliac vessels, attached to the posterosuperior surface of the broad ligament by a double fold of peritoneum which is called the mesovarium. The mesovarium is attached equatorially around the ovary, but does not envelop it. The ovary sometimes lies flush with the posterior leaf of the broad ligament, in which case there is no mesovarium. Laterality of adnexal structures, even if detached, is easily determined by noting this smooth posterior peritoneal reflection between the fallopian tube and subjacent ovary (Fig. 2.2).

Each ovary is slung medially to the cornu of the uterus by the ligament of the ovary. This is a cord of fibrous tissue and smooth muscle enveloped by the broad ligament, and is continuous with the round ligament. It represents the remnant of the gubernaculum. Laterally there is a second fold of peritoneum, the suspensory ligament, which contains the ovarian vessels, lymphatics, and nerves, and which crosses the external iliac vessels to become continuous with the peritoneum on the psoas muscle. The ovary in its normal position can just be palpated through the vagina by the tip of the examining finger. It is overlaid by the loops of the sigmoid colon and small bowel that lie in the pelvis. During pregnancy, the enlarging uterus lifts the ovaries out of the true pelvis; this process is facilitated by softening of ligaments and the uncoiling of the ovarian blood vessels. The ovary feels softer owing to increased vascularity and edema, and one potential complication of this physiological relocation of the adnexae is an increased risk of torsion of the ovary and tube (see Ch. 17).

The principal vascular supply to the ovary is the ovarian artery, arising from the abdominal aorta immediately below the renal artery (Fig. 2.3). This vessel runs retroperitoneally to cross the ureter obliquely, on the psoas muscle. It intersects the pelvic brim and enters the infundibulopelvic fold at the lateral extremity of the uterine broad ligament. It gives off a branch to the fallopian tube which runs medially between the layers of the broad ligament to anastomose with the uterine artery. Large tortuous (helicine) vessels from the region of this anastomosis enter the ovarian hilus and branch profusely as they course through the medulla. Their tortuosity is thought to be an adaptation for potential pregnancy. At the corticomedullary junction they form a plexus from which smaller arterioles penetrate radially, between the follicles, into the cortex.

Veins accompany the arteries within the ovary. In the medulla they are also large and tortuous. A venous plexus is formed in the mesovarium and the infundibulopelvic fold (the pampiniform plexus) and drains into a pair of ovarian veins. These accompany the ovarian artery and usually fuse before their termination. The right ovarian vein joins the inferior vena cava; that on the left enters the left renal vein (Fig. 2.3).

The ovarian lymphatics drain principally to para-aortic nodes alongside the origin of the ovarian vessels, just below the level of the kidneys (Fig. 2.3). Minor branches drain via the broad ligament to the external, internal, and common iliac groups of nodes.

The autonomic nerve supply of the ovary derives from the renal, aortic, and hypogastric plexuses, and accompanies the ovarian vessels. However, because the ovary lies against the obturator nerve in the pelvis, ovarian pain is often referred along the cutaneous distribution of this nerve (the inner side of the thigh down to the knee).

Fig. 2.3 Schematic diagram of the arterial supply and venous drainage (left side) and lymphatic drainage (right side) of the ovaries. Ovarian ligaments are shown: s, suspensory ligament; r, round ligament; o, ovarian ligament

3

Histology

P. Russell   A. Farnsworth

The ovaries are covered by a single layer of modified mesothelial cells (which are cuboidal in young females (Fig. 3.1) and tend to become flattened in later life). The layer of cells is directly continuous, at the ovarian hilus, with the flat mesothelium of the peritoneal cavity. These surface epithelial cells are poorly preserved in routine histological sections (except within small invaginations and clefts) and therefore easily missed on cursory examination of the ovary.

The surface epithelial cells do have unique properties compared to the extraovarian mesothelial cells. They have 17β-hydroxysteroid dehydrogenase activity and estrogen, progesterone, and epidermal growth factor receptors. Immunoreactivity for cytokeratin, vimentin and desmoplakin, but not desmin, has been demonstrated.

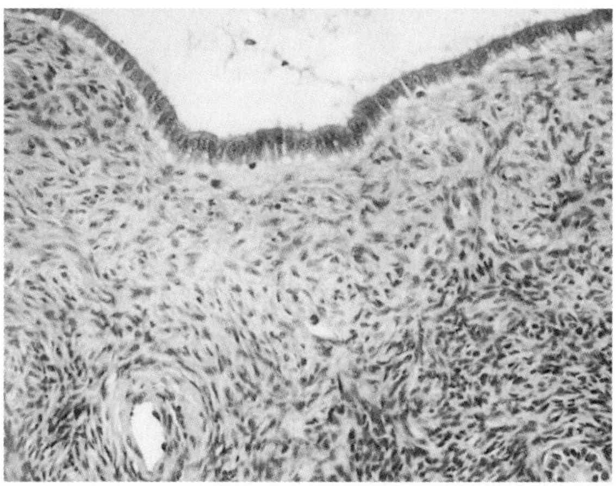

Fig. 3.1 Cuboidal surface epithelial cells covering the ovary and separated from the cellular cortex by the narrow tunica albuginea. H + E ×125

The antigens CA-125 and CA19-9, usually associated with ovarian tumors of surface epithelial–stromal origin have been demonstrated with variable frequency.

Immediately beneath the surface epithelium, there is a thin layer of fibrous, relatively acellular, connective tissue, known as the tunica albuginea (Fig. 3.1). This tunica thickens somewhat with age but still remains poorly developed compared with its homolog in the testis. The ovarian parenchyma is composed of an outer, highly cellular zone or cortex which contains the ovarian organelles (developing and involuting follicles, corpora lutea, etc.), and an inner medulla or zona vasculosa (Fig. 3.2). The ovarian cortical stroma consists of uniform spindle-shaped cells, sometimes arranged in bundles or storiform whorls, and a meshwork of reticulin fibers. These cells give rise to ovarian stromal or interstitial lutein cells and, in pregnancy, are capable of decidualization. They also give rise to the sheath (or theca) of specialized cells enveloping the follicles. Occasional neuroendocrine cells (Hidvegi et al 1982) and smooth muscle cells are present in the ovarian cortex.

The interface between cortex and medulla is less well defined before (Fig. 3.2) than after the menopause (Fig. 3.3). The medulla is composed of connective tissue, less dense than that in the cortex, and a number of thick-walled coiled blood vessels, sometimes almost angioma-like in their prominence (Fig. 3.4). Fibroblasts, mast cells, elastic fibers, and strands of smooth muscle cells accompany the blood vessels. In the ovarian hilus and adjacent mesovarium, single or grouped large epithelioid cells with small round nuclei may be found closely associated with small blood

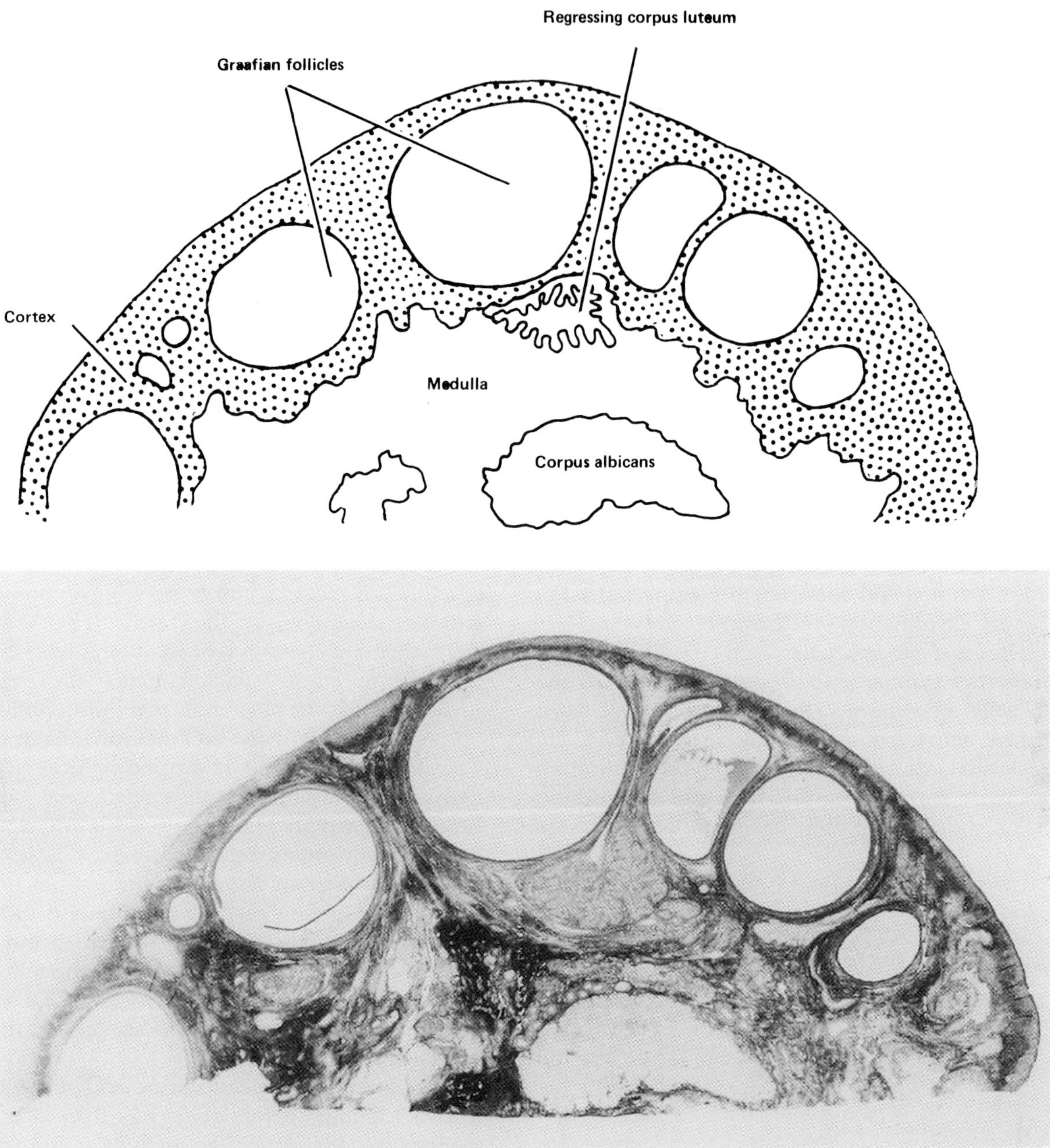

Fig. 3.2 Coronal section of normal ovary from a 32-year-old woman showing various stages of follicular development in the deep cortex and corpora albicantes and vascular structures in the medulla. H + E ×5

vessels and nonmyelinated nerve fibers. These hilus cell clusters are seen in 83% of ovaries (Boss et al 1965) and are more prominent during pregnancy and at menopause. They are indistinguishable from Leydig cells of the testis, being oval or polygonal, 15–25 μm in diameter with brightly eosinophilic or finely granular cytoplasm (Fig. 3.5A), rich in lipid, containing cholesterol esters and lipochrome pigment, and even having spherical cytoplasmic hyaline bodies and Reinke's crystals. These crystals are typically eosinophilic rod-like structures with rounded, blunt or tapered

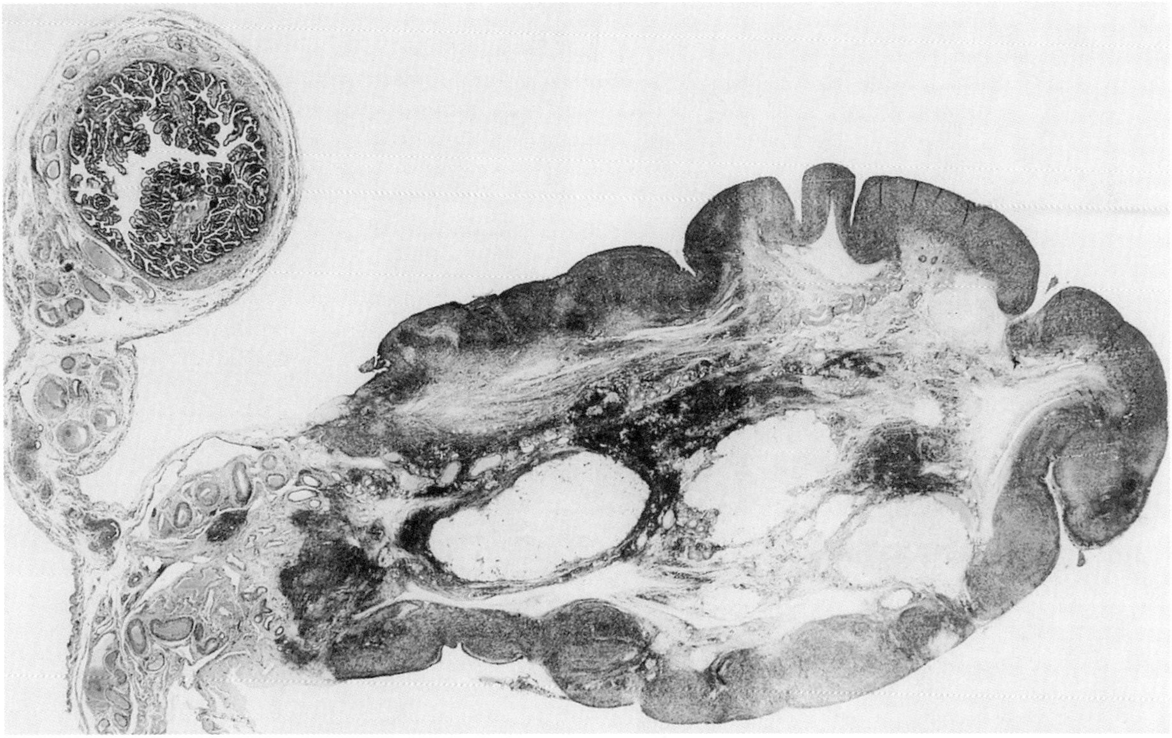

Fig. 3.3 Coronal section of postmenopausal ovary. H + E ×5

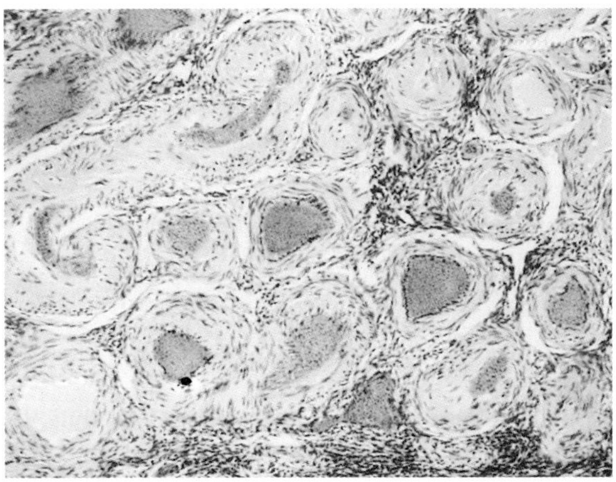

Fig. 3.4 Prominent thick-walled coiled vessels in the ovarian medulla. H + E ×60

ends, and measure 10–30 μm in length. They are located intracytoplasmically but may protrude beyond the cell margins. They usually have a definite halo around them and they stain strongly with Mallory's trichrome and Phosphotungstic Acid Haematoxylin (PTAH) methods (Fig. 3.5B).

The cortical stroma, which comprises about one-half or more of the ovary in women of reproductive age, contains follicles in which are found the female sex cells, the primary oocytes. The follicles vary considerably in size, representing different stages of development. The vast majority are unilaminar or primordial follicles (Fig. 3.6), and are mainly in the superficial cortex where they form a discontinuous layer immediately beneath the tunica albuginea, often in small focal aggregates. The younger the individual, the more numerous they are – the ovaries of newborn females contain 1–2 million follicles and at puberty there is a complement of about 380 000 (Hammond & Ory 1985). Their number decreases progressively with time; about 8000 are present in women in their early forties and at the menopause they are extremely difficult to find, although a few may persist into old age. Their complete (or almost complete) absence, a relative

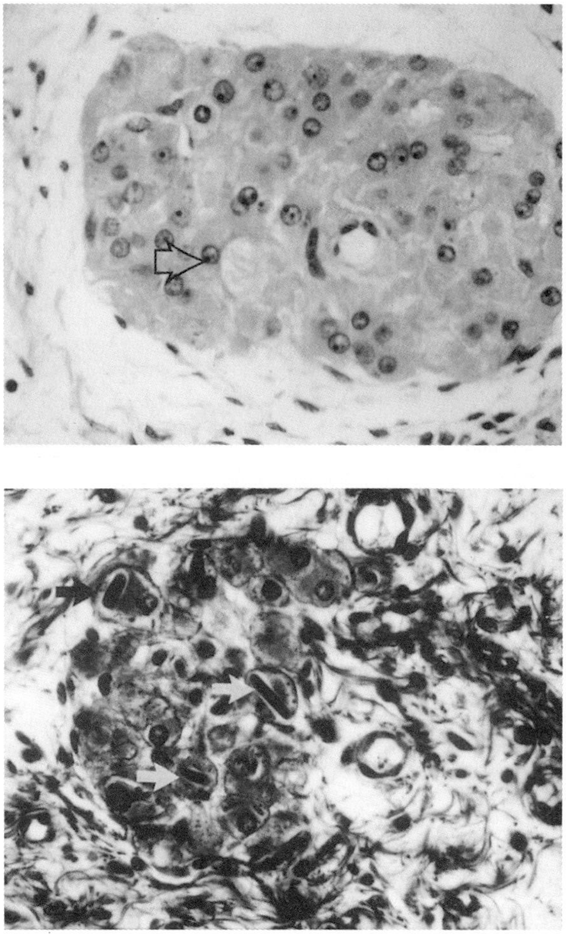

A

B

Fig. 3.5 Normal hilus (Leydig) cells. (A) Surrounding a small blood vessel and peripheral nerve (arrow) in the ovarian hilus. H + E ×250. (B) Reinke's crystals (arrows). PTAH ×250

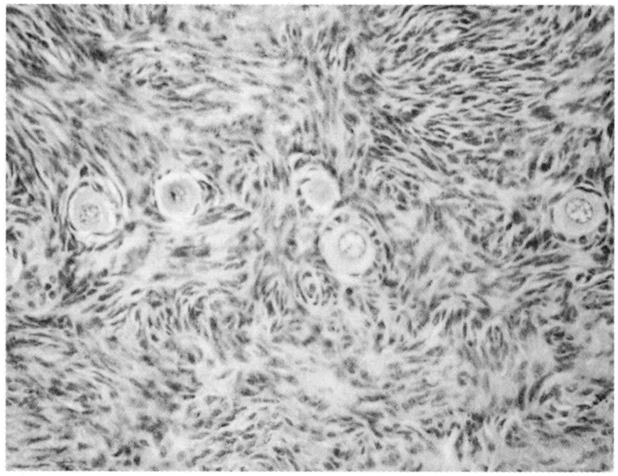

Fig. 3.6 Cellular superficial cortex containing a number of primordial follicles. H + E ×125

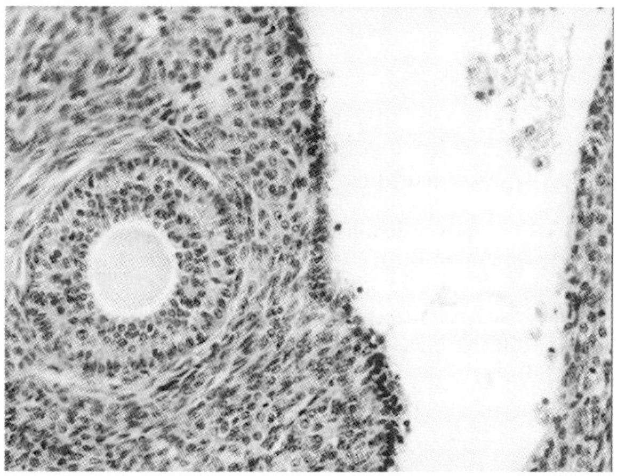

Fig. 3.7 A late primary or preantral follicle with a prominent zona pellucida surrounding the ovum and an occasional Call–Exner body within the developing granulosa cell layer (to the right of ovum). The spindle-shaped cells of the emerging theca are apparent. A regressing cystic follicle is in the right half of the field. H + E ×125

diminution in the size of the cortex, and a clearer distinction between cortex and medulla (Fig. 3.3) form the most readily appreciable histological correlates of the menopause, although other minor changes may also be evident (Nicosia 1987). Each primordial follicle consists of a large round oocyte surrounded by a single layer of flattened follicular or granulosa cells. The oocyte has a large, eccentric vesicular nucleus with a fine chromatin pattern and a large nucleolus. Primordial follicles may rarely contain more than one oocyte.

Folliculogenesis

The stimulation of inactive primordial follicles in response to pituitary gonadotrophins (chiefly follicle-stimulating hormone (FSH)) leads initially to oocyte enlargement (up to 120 μm in diameter). At the same time, the single layer of follicular cells become first cuboidal or low columnar, and then multilayered through conspicuous cell division. In such primary follicles (Fig. 3.7) the oocyte is surrounded by a refractile, filamentous, eosinophilic layer rich in acid mucopolysaccharide, the zona pellucida. The growing follicles increase in size

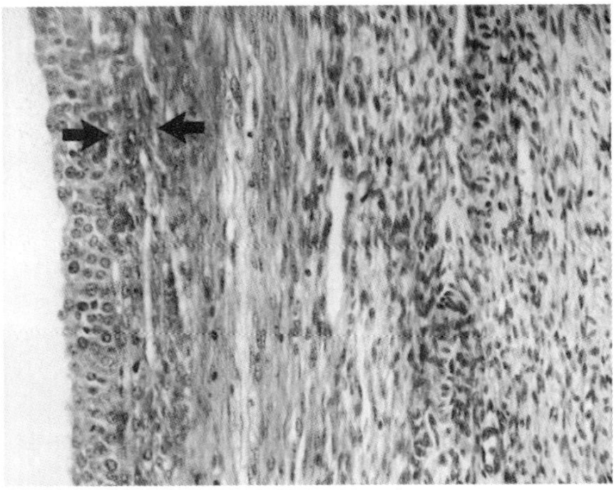

Fig. 3.8 Developing follicle showing the granulosa cell (left), theca interna (between arrows) and theca externa layers. H + E ×125

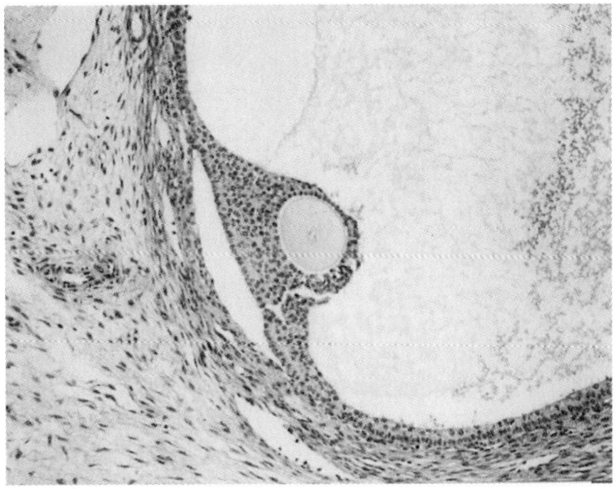

Fig. 3.9 Secondary or Graafian follicle with an eccentric cumulus oophorus containing the oocyte. H + E ×60

and gradually move deeper into the cortex. With the proliferation of the granulosa cell layer, the theca develops from the cortical stroma around each follicle. This layer subsequently differentiates into a highly vascular, inner layer of polyhedral, endocrinologically active cells, the theca interna, and an outer connective tissue layer of spindle cells, the theca externa (Fig. 3.8). Small vessels traverse the theca externa to supply a rich capillary plexus in the theca interna, but the granulosa remains avascular and poor in reticulin fibres during the preovulatory phase of development.

Under continuing FSH stimulation, the growing follicle assumes an oval shape and the oocyte becomes eccentric in position. When the follicle reaches about 0.2 mm in diameter, intercellular spaces containing clear liquid appear among the granulosa cells and these coalesce to form a single crescentic cavity, the antrum. The fluid stains with the Periodic Acid Schiff (PAS) technique consonant with its neutral or weakly acid mucopolysaccharide and glycogen content. The follicle is then described as a secondary or Graafian follicle (Fig. 3.9), and it continues to enlarge, occasionally reaching a diameter of 15–20 mm. The granulosa cell layer is now stratified (up to 4–6 cells thick) and exhibits a local thickening on one side called the cumulus oophorus which harbors the oocyte in its center (Fig. 3.9). The granulosa is limited on the outside by a prominent Periodic Acid Schiff (PAS)-positive basal lamina that separates it from the theca interna. Small accumulations of densely staining material may appear among the granulosa cells. Whether they are intra- or extracellular is arguable, but they appear to be delimited from the surrounding granulosa cells by a basal lamina. These so-called Call–Exner bodies also stain positively with PAS and probably represent sequestered basal lamina material and cellular debris.

Approaching follicular maturity, mitotic activity in the granulosa cells gradually subsides. The oocyte becomes detached from the granulosa cell layer by the development of liquid-filled intercellular spaces in the cumulus oophorus; but one or two layers of radially disposed granulosa cells remain attached to form the corona radiata. This loose cellular investment persists even after ovulation and transport of the oocyte to the fallopian tube. Clusters of granulosa cells are also shed into the follicular fluid and, in an aspirated cytological preparation, give a characteristic pattern (Fig. 3.10). The theca interna of the mature follicle consists of large somewhat spindle-shaped or polygonal cells with oval nuclei and fine cytoplasmic sudanophilic droplets. Unlike the granulosa, they have a network of fine reticulin fibers surrounding individual cells, which are continuous with those of the theca externa and the rest of the ovarian stroma. The theca interna cells have cytological characteristics similar to other steroid-

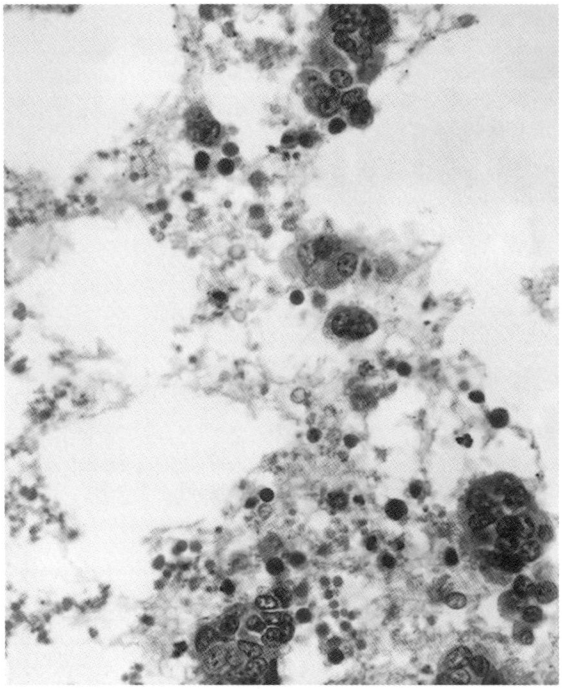

Fig. 3.10 Shed clusters of granulosa cells in the fluid of a preovulatory follicle. Degenerate nuclei and proteinaceous fluid form the background and suggest early atresia. A not uncommon pitfall for the novice is to misinterpret the cellularity and high Nuclear Cytoplasmic ratio of the aspirated cells as suggestive of epithelial malignancy (see Ch. 12). H + E ×300

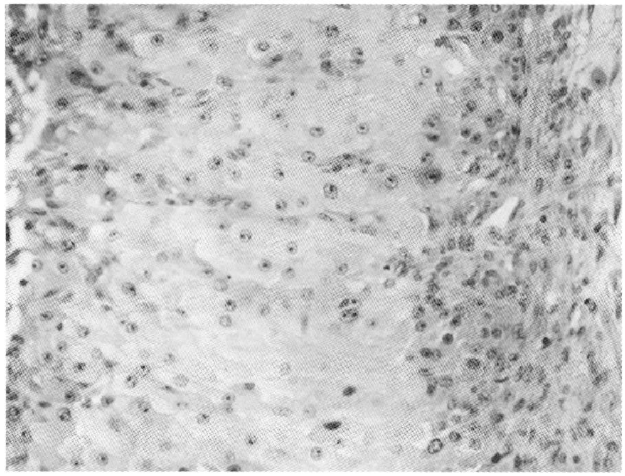

Fig. 3.11 Early corpus luteum with antrum to the left, granulosa lutein layer in the center, and the theca to the right, but no vascularization of the granulosa. H + E ×125

secreting endocrine cells and, consistent with this endocrine function, are supplied by a rich capillary plexus. The theca externa consists of concentrically arranged fibers and fusiform cells that do not have any secretory function. The larger blood vessels of the theca externa supply the capillaries of the theca interna.

Ovulation and postovulatory changes

As maturity proceeds, the follicle comes once again to lie closer to the cortical surface of the ovary. Immediately prior to ovulation, the follicular fluid accumulates more quickly, in response to the pituitary midcycle luteinizing hormone (LH) surge, and the part of the follicular wall that bulges on the ovarian surface becomes progressively thinner and may be recognized laparoscopically by a local change in color and translucency of the follicular wall due to ischemic changes. The germinal epithelium overlying this area disaggregates and the intervening stroma greatly attenuates. At this stage the mature oocyte completes the first meiotic or reduction division, giving rise to the first polar body, and is now termed a secondary oocyte.

Ovulation and discharge of the follicular fluid through the stigma lead to collapse of the follicle and plication of the granulosa cell lining, while bleeding from the vasculature of the theca interna results in the formation of a central coagulum. The granulosa and theca interna cells alter dramatically – enlarging, accumulating lipid, and becoming plump, pale-staining granulosa lutein and theca lutein cells (Fig. 3.11). This accumulation of lipid will later impart a yellow color to the follicle which is thus known as a corpus luteum. The granulosa lutein cells (fully transformed by the fourth day after ovulation) form the bulk of the luteal tissue, while those at the periphery, derived from the theca interna, are slightly smaller and more deeply staining (Fig. 3.11). Identification of the two types of lutein cell, however, may be very difficult late in the stages of development of a corpus luteum. The lipid in these lutein cells is dissolved in routine histological preparations, leaving numerous cytoplasmic vacuoles. The small capillaries of the theca interna proliferate and invade the granulosa layer, accompanied by fibroblasts which form a delicate reticulum around the lutein cells

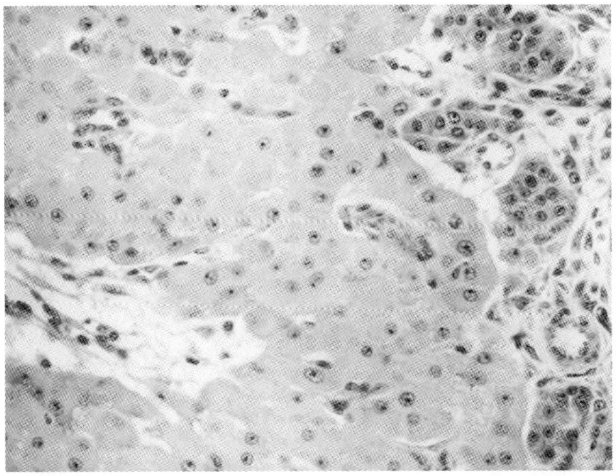

Fig. 3.12 Mature corpus luteum with well vascularized granulosa and immature granulation tissue organizing the central coagulum (left). H + E ×125

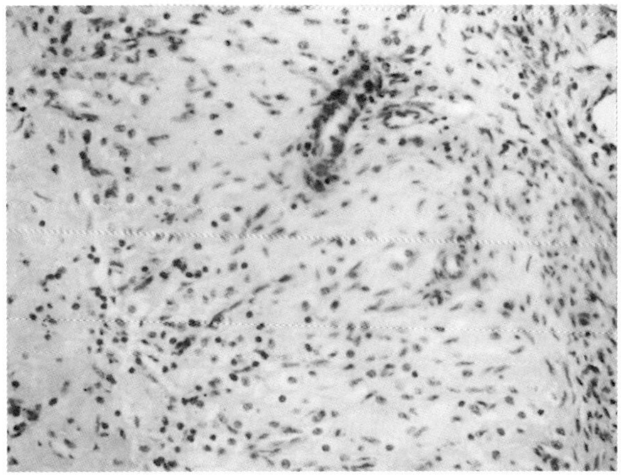

Fig. 3.13 Regressing corpus luteum, showing considerable diminution in size of luteal cells, complete vascularization of the granulosa, and collagenization of the antral clot (left). H + E ×125

and commence the organization of the central hematoma (Fig. 3.12). The luteal cells are arranged more or less radially around the central hematoma separated into cords by vascular septa. Theca lutein cells may accompany the vessels in these septa, further accentuating this pseudolobular appearance of the granulosa.

In the absence of fertilization, the corpus luteum lasts for about 14 days. In response to local prostaglandin release ($PGF_{2\alpha}$) it then undergoes involution, manifest by gross accumulation of sudanophilic lipid and lipofuscin by the lutein cells and subsequent degeneration (Fig. 3.13). Mesenchymal cell nuclei become pyknotic, hyaline intercellular material accumulates, and the corpus luteum is reduced to a convoluted white scar, the corpus albicans (Fig. 3.14). This comes to lie deeper within the medulla of the ovary (see Fig. 3.2) and gradually disappears over a period of many months or years. Occasionally, regression of the corpus luteum, especially if cystic, is retarded and functionally active cells may persist beyond the normal 2 week period. Such corpora lutea are identifiable by a change in the character (maturation) of the fibrous tissue in the organized central antrum (Fig. 3.15).

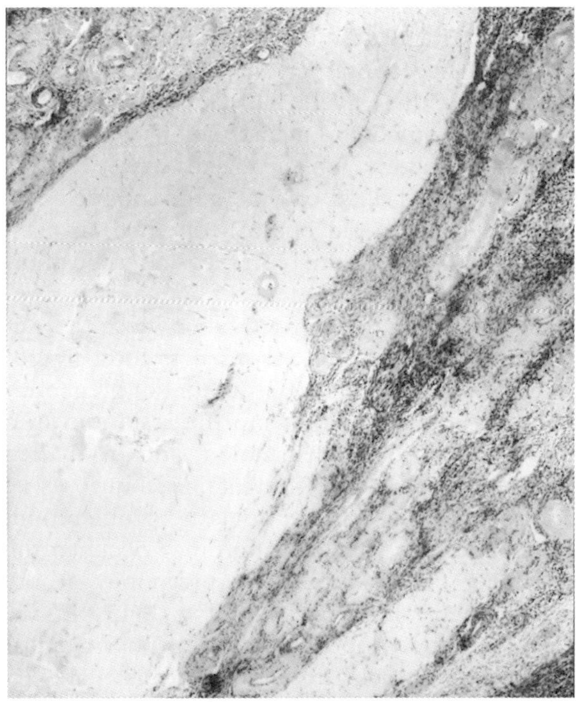

Fig. 3.14 Corpus albicans with an adjacent smaller atretic follicle (right). H + E ×30

Corpus luteum of pregnancy

If fertilization occurs, the corpus luteum enlarges further and becomes a corpus luteum of pregnancy, which persists morphologically for about 6–8 weeks and then regresses slowly in the second and third trimesters. The fully formed corpus

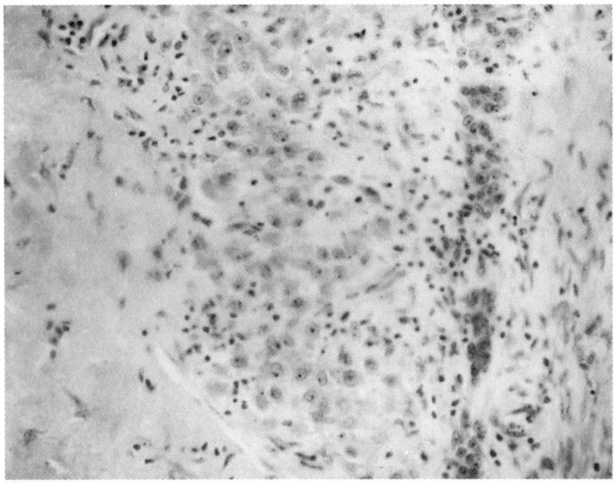

Fig. 3.15 A persistent corpus luteum. Dense acellular fibrous connective tissue of 3 weeks' duration lines the antral space (left), while viable granulosa lutein (center) and small theca lutein (right) cells persist at the periphery. H + E ×125

luteum of pregnancy (Fig. 3.16) is larger than its nonpregnant counterpart (up to 3 cm across compared with an average of 2 cm for the developed corpus luteum of menstruation), and has an obviously mature collagenized center which encloses a fluid-filled cavity. Large rounded colloid droplets (colloid bodies), often in clusters, are readily found in the plump eosinophilic granulosa lutein cells. These cells are arranged in sheets broken up by delicate blood vessels; reticulin fibers are scanty. Scattered mitotic figures may be present. The corpus luteum of pregnancy involutes to a scar similar to the residuum of a corpus luteum of menstruation, and from then until term it is passively maintained but loses its central cavity to dense fibroblastic proliferation. Microspherules of calcification may occur in the regressing corpus luteum of pregnancy at the sites of the colloid droplets (Fig. 3.17) in the third trimester. Another feature of physiological corpus luteum degeneration are the stellate 'K' cells found scattered amongst the granulosa cells (see Fig. 3.16B). These cells have darker staining cytoplasm than their neighbors and a pyknotic nucleus, features consistent with cells undergoing apoptosis. After delivery or intrauterine death of the fetus, involution of the corpus luteum of pregnancy is accelerated and may, on rare occasions, be hyperacute, appearing histologically as

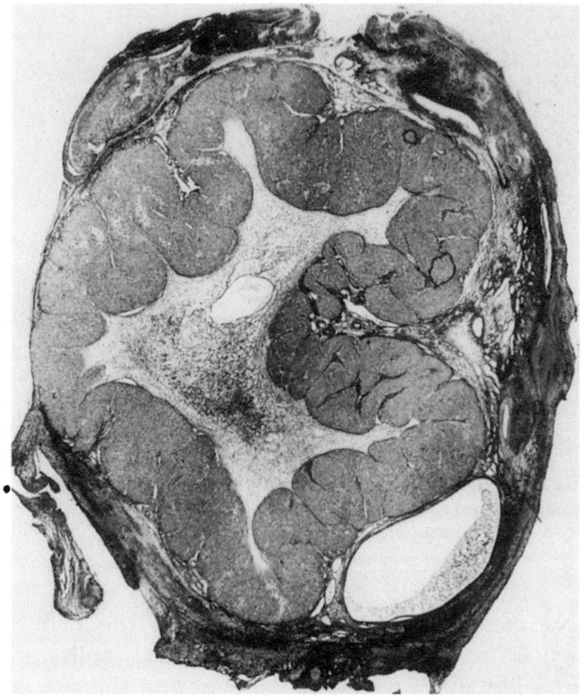

A

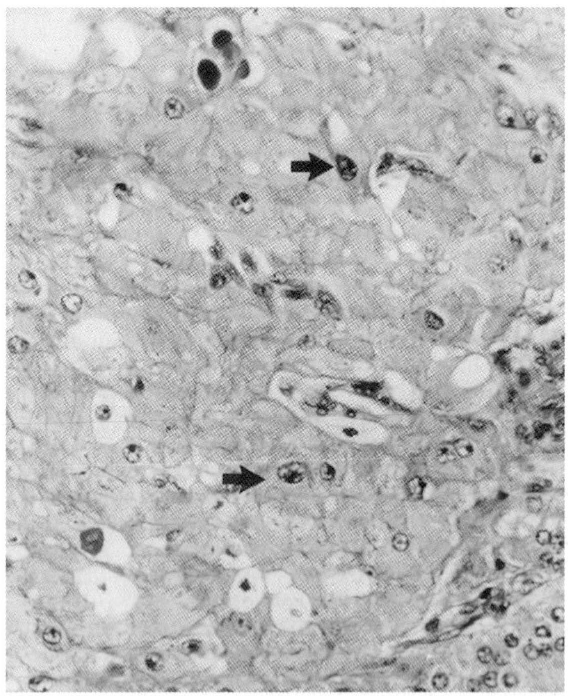

B

Fig. 3.16 Established corpus luteum of pregnancy. (A) Scan. H + E ×5. (B) Large pale granulosa lutein cells, theca lutein cells (lower right), occasional 'K' cells with pyknotic nuclei and darker cytoplasm (arrows), and 'colloid bodies' (top center) within some cells. H + E ×150

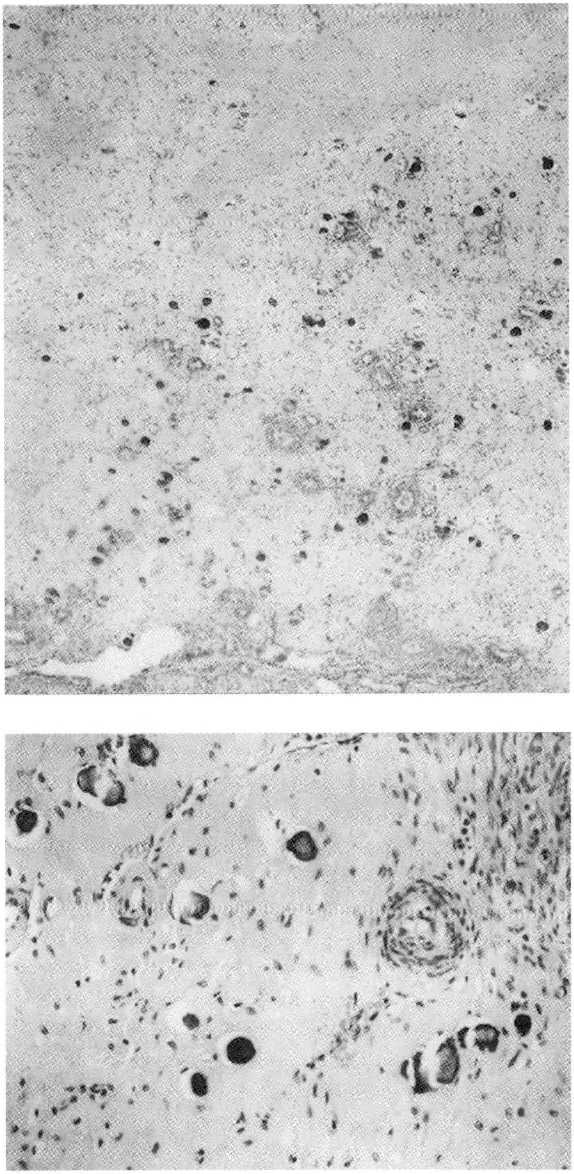

A

B

Fig. 3.17 Regressing corpus luteum of pregnancy, showing microcalcification at the sites of previous 'colloid bodies'. (A) H + E ×30. (B) Higher power showing microcalcispherules, resembling psammoma bodies. H + E ×125

frank necrosis (Fig. 3.18). The puerperium is generally a period of relative quiescence for the ovary. Ovulation and, to a lesser extent, follicular development are suppressed. The changes noted during this period are indistinguishable from those seen in association with pathological hyper-

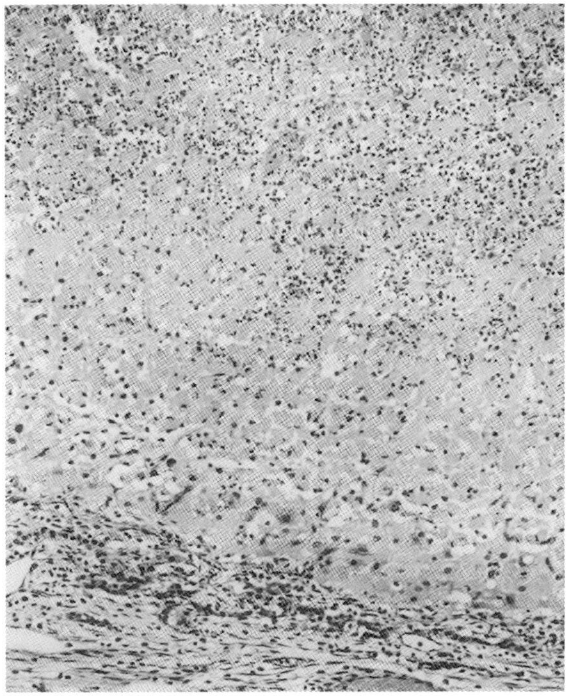

Fig. 3.18 Hyperacute regression of a corpus luteum of pregnancy after death in utero of the fetus. H + E ×75 (Tissue courtesy of Dr Andrew Östör, Melbourne)

prolactinemia or the use of some forms of oral contraceptive agent.

Follicular atresia

The number of follicles that begin to develop in each cycle greatly exceeds those which reach maturity. Degeneration or involution (termed atresia) may occur at any stage of development from primordial follicle onward. Every normal ovary, therefore, contains follicles in different stages of atresia. This process is observed not only in the adult but also throughout childhood, the ovary even then containing simultaneously primordial, developing, and atretic follicles (Peters 1979). As a rule, one follicle undergoes the LH-induced preovulatory swelling and rupture in each cycle; only occasionally does more than one follicle undergo this process. The remainder of the follicles undergo atresia, although some may persist into the postovulatory period in coexistence with the corpus luteum (Bomsel-Helmreich et al 1979). It is calculated that all but a fraction of 1%

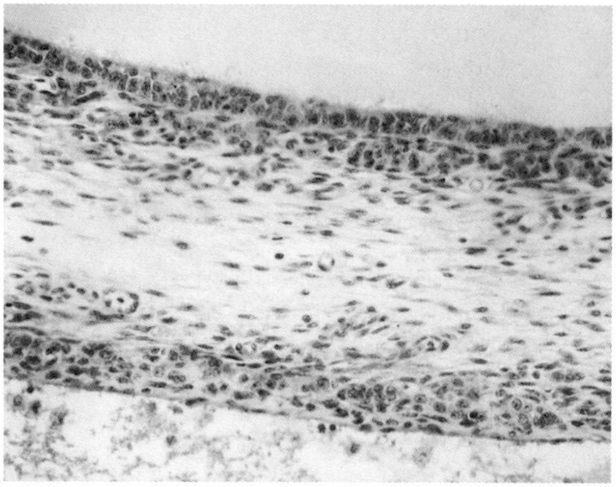

Fig. 3.19 Adjacent cystic follicles with early atresia in the lower follicle. The granulosa is degenerate and has been partly shed into the antrum. H + E ×125

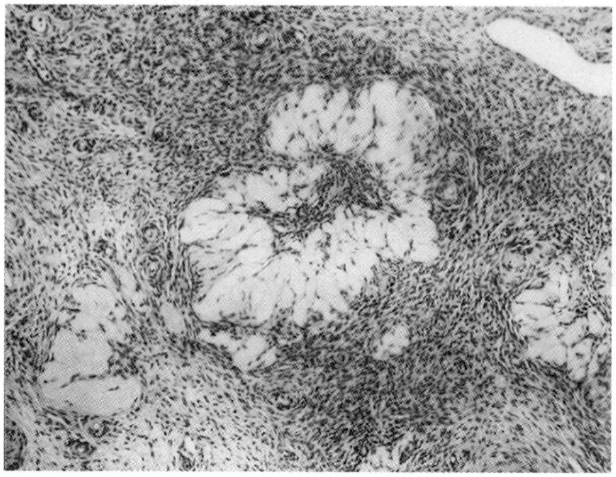

Fig. 3.20 Small follicles showing advanced atresia with typical festooned contour and fibroblastic tissue occupying the site of the original antrum. H + E ×60

of oocytes present in the ovaries at birth are destined to involute and disappear by the process of atresia. In primary and small secondary follicles the earliest sign of atresia is the eccentric position of the oocyte nucleus, which develops a coarse granularity and finally becomes pyknotic. In larger follicles atresia is more complex and variable, with the process being initiated in the granulosa cell layer (Fig. 3.19) and secondarily affecting the oocyte. Invasion of the granulosa layer by small blood vessels is followed by shedding of the degenerate granulosa cells into the antrum and a hypertrophy of the theca interna. The follicular fluid inspissates, the follicle collapses, its outline convolutes, and the cavity fills with a large number of fibroblasts, histiocytes, and small vessels. The residua of the degenerated follicular epithelium are resorbed, while the folded zona pellucida may remain. The basal lamina that separates the theca interna from the granulosa often increases in thickness, and is transformed into a thick layer of hyaline substance, the 'glassy membrane', characteristic of follicles in advanced atresia (Fig. 3.20). The thecal cells may be resorbed and replaced by fibrosis or, depending on the presence of a luteinizing influence (such as pregnancy), may enlarge further and be disposed in radial groups or strands, separated by smaller fusiform cells and fibres (Fig. 3.21). The thecal cells in this circumstance acquire an epithelioid appearance due to

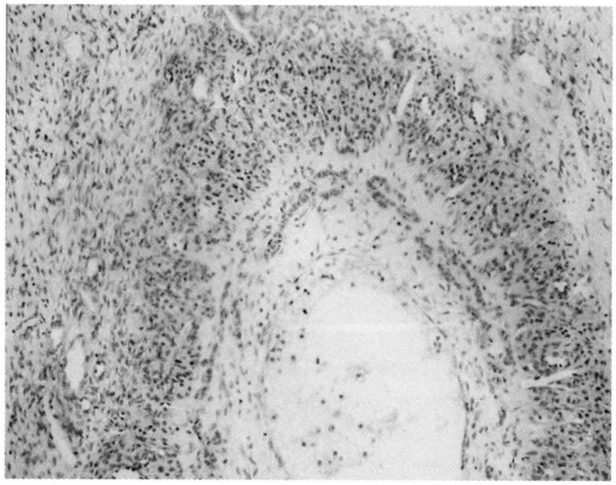

Fig. 3.21 Atretic follicle showing secondary thecal hyperplasia in pregnancy. H + E ×60

accumulation of lipid, giving an histological appearance of such an atretic follicle not dissimilar to that of an old corpus luteum. The main differences are a smaller size and, of course, the presence of the glassy membrane, degenerate granulosa cells, and a zona pellucida in the center of the atretic follicle. Connective tissue elements and blood vessels ultimately penetrate the glassy membrane and complete the organization process. The resulting scar with its hyaline streaks sometimes resembles a corpus albicans, but is smaller and sooner or later disappears. 'Cystic atresia' affects larger Graafian follicles, giving rise to cystic cavities with a fibrous connective tissue wall (Fig. 3.22). The cuff of hypertrophied theca cells surrounding the cavity of the atretic follicle is broken up by the invading fibrous tissue into separate cell nests of various sizes, yet these may persist for some time as luteinized interstitial or stromal cells, which are found most readily during the first year of life when atretic follicles are most numerous. The ovarian cortical stroma of prepubertal girls contains conspicuous clusters and cords of such cells, while in the adult ovary they are widely scattered but sparse in the stroma. They become more easily identifiable again in the medulla of postmenopausal women. It is doubtful whether, in aggregate, they can be considered to represent true interstitial tissue or the so-called 'interstitial gland' (Balboni 1976).

Connective tissue elements

Networks of lymphatic capillaries arise in the cortex, especially in the theca externa of the large follicles. The nerves of the ovary are derived from the ovarian plexus and from the uterine nerves. They enter the organ through the hilus accompanying the blood vessels. They consist, for the most part, of nonmyelinated fibers, but thin myelinated fibers are also present and most supply the muscularis of blood vessels. Many fibers are identifiable (using special stains) in the cortex and form plexuses around the follicles and under the germinal epithelium. It seems doubtful that they penetrate through the basal lamina into the granulosa of the follicles. Sensory fibers ending in corpuscles of Pacini have been described in the ovarian stroma. Small accumulations of subcapsular fat cells are found in the ovarian cortex of about 2% of ovaries (Hart & Abell 1970, Honore & O'Hara 1980); patients are usually perimenopausal and obese (Fig. 3.23). The groups of adipocytes are thought to be metaplastic. Endometrial stromal-type cells (ovarian stromatosis) may also be present.

In the broad ligament and mesovarium, fallopian tube wall, and mesosalpinx, but separated from the ovary itself, small rests of adrenal-cortex-like tissue (Fig. 3.24) have also been described in 28% of cases (Scully 1979). As far as we can determine, such an adrenal rest has only once been recorded within the ovary (Symonds & Driscoll 1973).

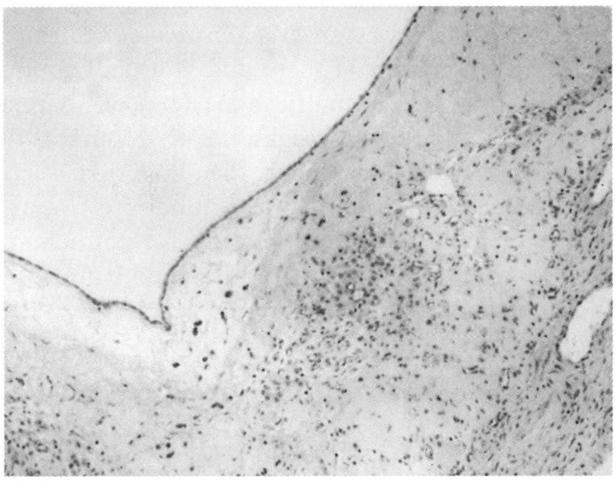

Fig. 3.22 Cystic atresia. A fibrous connective tissue wall is subtended by a layer of residual lutein cells. An unusual finding is an epithelial-like lining which was present in part of this cystic follicular remnant. H + E ×60

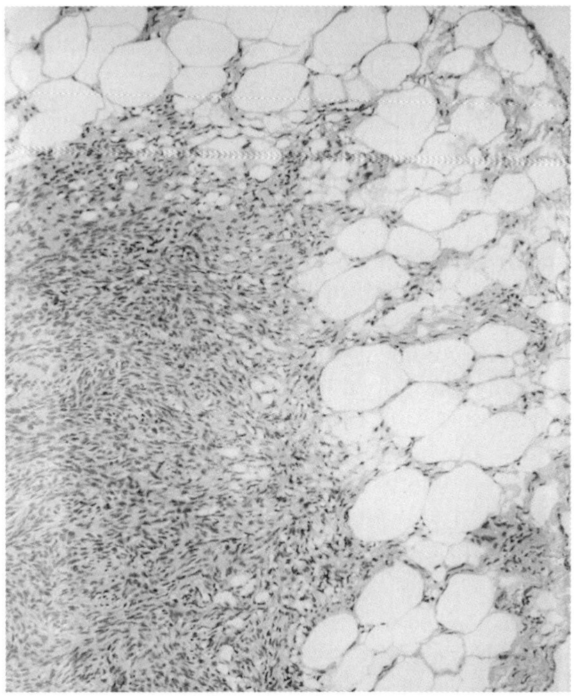

Fig. 3.23 So-called adipocytic prosoplasia. Accumulations of variously sized adipose cells beneath the ovarian surface (top right) and infiltrating the cortical stroma. H + E ×75

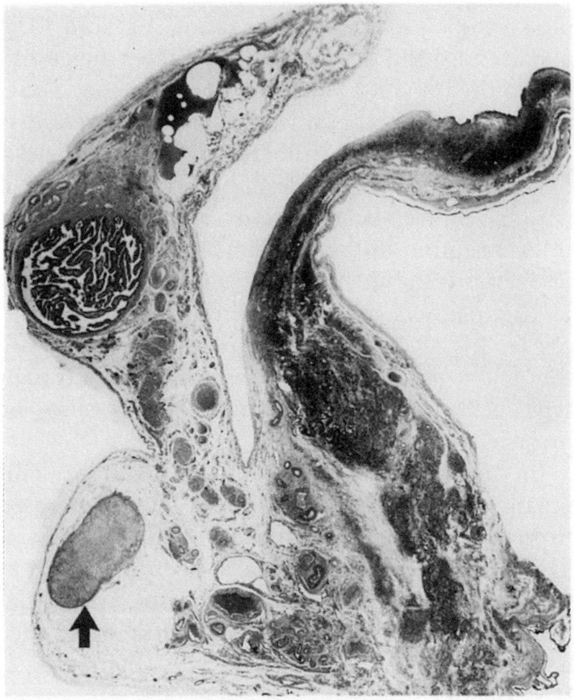

Fig. 3.24 Adrenal rest (arrow) in mesovarium. The adjacent ovary is enlarged by a benign serous cyst. H + E ×5

Normal vestigial remnants

The epoophoron

These are small parallel or divergent extraovarian tubules which are the nonfunctional remnants of the embryonic, mesonephros. In the normal male the mesonephros develops into the epididymis, but in the absence of testosterone this structure simply regresses (see Ch. 1). Varying amounts of this embryological structure will remain in the normally developed ovary. When present they are usually found running from the ovarian hilus toward the fallopian tube. They are lined by low cuboidal to columnar, sometimes ciliated, epithelium and are surrounded by a connective tissue layer containing abundant smooth muscle fibers.

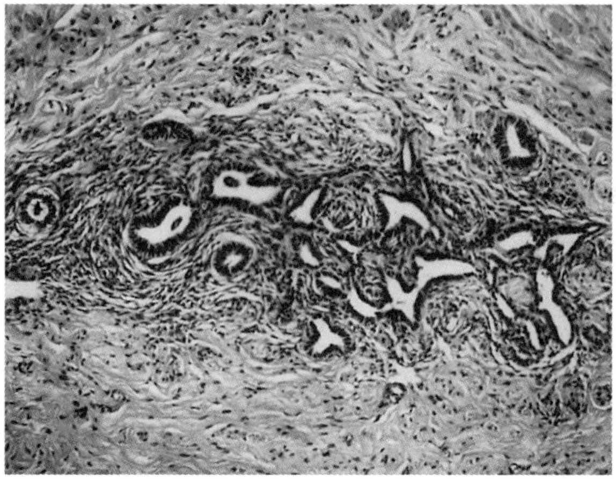

Fig. 3.25 Normal rete ovarii. Slit-like tubular spaces lined by low-cuboidal epithelium. H + E ×60

The rete ovarii

These are the intraovarian remnants of the embryonic mesonephric tubules. They represent ducts which in the male develop to join the seminiferous tubules to the epididymis but which, in the absence of testosterone, regress in the developing ovary (Fig. 3.25). They are seen as a mass of anastomosing slit-like tubules within the hilus of the normal ovary. These spaces are lined by an attenuated nondescript epithelium and lack the smooth muscle coat of the epoophoron.

Mullerian (paramesonephric) duct remnants These may be located in the mesosalpinx and broad ligament. They may form *paraovarian, paratubal,* or *fimbrial cysts.* The *hydatid of Morgagni* is the most common of these and is usually found dangling from one of the fimbria. They all share a common embryological origin, i.e. are remnants of the most cephalic portion of the mullerian ducts which form the normal fallopian tube (see Ch. 1). They are lined by endosalpingeal-like epithelium and are surrounded by a cuff of smooth muscle. The appearances of the lining epithelium may be modified by compression and atrophy of the lining cells.

REFERENCES

Balboni G C 1976 Histology of the ovary. In: James V H T, Serio M, Giusti G (eds) The endocrine function of the human ovary. Academic Press, London, p 1–24

Bomsel-Helmreich O, Gougeon A, Thebault A et al 1979 Healthy and atretic human follicles in the preovulatory phase: differences in evolution of follicular morphology and steroid content of follicular fluid. Journal of Clinical Endocrinology and Metabolism 48: 686–694

Boss J H, Scully R E, Wegner K H, Cohen R B 1965 Structural variations in the adult ovary – clinical considerations. Obstetrics and Gynecology 25: 747–764
Hammond C B, Ory S J 1985 Endocrine aspects of menopause. In: Shearman R P S (ed) Clinical reproductive endocrinology. Churchill Livingstone, Edinburgh, p 185–208
Hart W R, Abell M R 1970 Adipose prosoplasia of ovary. American Journal of Obstetrics and Gynecology 106: 929–931
Hidvegi D, Cibils L A, Sorenson K, Hidvegi I 1982 Ultrastructural and histochemical observations of neuroendocrine granules in nonneoplastic ovaries. American Journal of Obstetrics and Gynecology 143: 590–594
Honore L H, O'Hara K E 1980 Subcapsular adipocytic infiltration of the human ovary: a clinicopathologic study of eight cases. European Journal of Obstetrics, Gynecology and Reproductive Biology 10: 13–20
Nicosia S V 1987 The aging ovary. Medical Clinics of North America 71: 1–11
Peters H 1979 The human ovary in childhood and early maturity. European Journal of Obstetrics Gynecology and Reproductive Biology 9: 137–144
Scully R E 1979 Tumors of the ovary and maldeveloped gonads. AFIP Fascicle 16, Second Series. Armed Forces Institute of Pathology, Washington, p 9–24
Symonds D A, Driscoll S G 1973 An adrenal cortical rest within the fetal ovary. American Journal of Clinical Pathology 60: 562–564

4

Examination of the ovarian specimen

P. Russell   A. Farnsworth

Pathologists are physicians and human beings. They have as great a capacity for error and susceptibility to subjective distractions as other practitioners of the art of medicine. Because of certain nineteenth century dogmas and because the teaching of pathology used to be relegated primarily to the long-forgotten pre-clinical phase, pathologists traditionally have been regarded to be more scientific than many of their colleagues. A mystic perversion of this assumption prevails among those clinicians who believe that the pathologist, given only a piece of a patient's tissue, has all of the other ingredients necessary to produce a statement of absolute truth at the end of his report. More dangerous to mankind is a pathologist with the same concept . . .

Oscar Rambo 1962

The pathologist may receive ovarian tissue from patients in a variety of clinical circumstances which determine different specimen handling. The surgeon may perform an oophorectomy in association with a hysterectomy with no expectation or realization of ovarian pathology and a simple 'routine' pathological examination will suffice. By contrast, ovaries excised for suspected or proven neoplasms may require several different specialized analyses in addition to histological assessment. In some circumstances, e.g. ovarian failure, it may be appropriate to have a preoperative consultation to discuss the appropriate site and size of the biopsy and its immediate handling in the theater in order to optimize resolution of the clinical problem.

FRESH SPECIMENS

Ideally, if physical proximity of the surgical pathology department to the operating theaters permits, all specimens should be presented to the pathologist immediately upon removal in the fresh unfixed state so that all relevant examinations can be initiated as soon as possible. However, because of time constraints, the logistics of transport and the possibility of out-of-hours emergency surgery, this system may not always be possible or appropriate. The surgical pathology department should therefore provide the operating theater staff with the necessary materials and instructions for the proper handling and fixation of specimens. The accompanying request for histopathological examination should include basic patient identification data, pertinent clinical history and reference to relevant previous biopsies. The specific anatomical site from which the material comes (if not self-evident) should be indicated (diagrams are helpful).

On receipt of a fresh unfixed specimen, the surgical pathologist must decide immediately, before fixation, whether tissue is required for:

- microbiological culture
- cytogenetic studies
- imprints for cytological examination
- electron microscopy
- immunohistochemistry requiring frozen sections
- DNA flow cytometry
- nuclear magnetic resonance spectroscopy
- specimen radiography
- photography.

Microbiological culture. Sterile instruments, swabs and containers should be available for the collection of samples for bacteriological or fungal culture. Specimens for chlamydial and viral culture should be placed in tissue culture or viral transport medium.

Cytogenetic studies. A piece of viable tissue (approximately 0.5 cm^3) should be collected under sterile conditions and placed in tissue culture medium or buffered salt solution and despatched to the cytogenetics laboratory as soon as possible. For this and the other tests listed below, beware not to give away vital diagnostic material!

Imprints and scrapes. It is desirable to take imprints from fresh tumor tissue for cytological examination. These are a useful adjunct to histology as well as providing comparative material for the cytological assessment of ascitic fluid or peritoneal washings from the patient and also provide a permanent reference source. In our department, they provide the substrate for an alternative to intraoperative frozen section diagnosis (see Ch. 57).

Electron microscopy. If the need for electron microscopic examination is anticipated, 1 mm cubes of tissue from viable and potential diagnostic areas should be fixed in cold, freshly prepared 4% glutaraldehyde solution. Although adequate material for electron microscopy can also be retrieved from specimens already well fixed in buffered 10% formalin solution, ultrastructural detail is not as well preserved. A compromise approach is the use of McDowell's solution (phosphate buffered 1% glutaraldehyde combined with 4% formaldehyde solution), which is suitable for both light and electron microscopy work. It is our practice to fix samples for electron microscopy from all tumors at the time of receipt of the specimen in the department. Further processing of this material, in selected cases, is dictated by the light microscopic features (see also Special Techniques below).

Immunohistochemistry. A block of tissue may be frozen in liquid nitrogen or in the 'cryostat' (refrigerated microtome) and sections cut immediately or later for some immunohistochemical techniques such as immunotyping of lymphocytic infiltrates. The remainder of the block may be stored frozen or thawed and fixed for routine histology (see also Special Techniques below).

DNA flow cytometry. Approximately 1 cm^3 of fresh tissue (not necessarily sterile) is required; this may be stored in the refrigerator until processed (up to 24 h) (see also Special Techniques below).

Nuclear magnetic resonance spectroscopy. This examination requires about 0.5 cm^3 of fresh tumor tissue kept at 37°C in tissue culture medium or physiological phosphate-buffered saline (for up to 2 h) (see also Special Techniques below).

Specimen radiography. Radiography of the fresh or fixed specimen can facilitate identification of teratomatous elements (teeth, bone) in germ cell tumors and pre-existing calcified gonadoblastomas associated with dysgerminomas.

Photography. Specimen photography for teaching or record purposes may be most appropriate at this point, but may need to be repeated after fixation and further dissection.

FROZEN SECTION EXAMINATION

The surgical pathology department's frozen section service should include intraoperative assessment of excised ovarian tissues. Some ovarian lesions, e.g. mature cystic teratomas, are sufficiently characteristic that the experienced surgical pathologist can offer a provisional diagnosis on the macroscopic appearance alone. Similarly, cystic ovaries, in which the locules all have entirely smooth linings and lack mural nodules, do not warrant frozen section in most clinical situations. Tumors requiring frozen section should be sliced and blocks selected from solid non-necrotic portions or from indurated areas or papillary excrescences in cyst walls. Sectioning of more than one block may be necessary to exclude invasive malignancy in a large complex ovarian tumor. Scraping of cells by scalpel blade from the cut surface of an ovarian mass, smearing of the resultant cells on a slide and staining with hematoxylin and eosin is a very quick and useful alternative to frozen section diagnosis (see Ch. 57). Frozen sections are necessary for some immunocytochemical techniques (see below) and can also be used to select appropriate tissue to be submitted for other specialized examinations.

SPECIMEN FIXATION

There is no preferred fixative for ovarian tissue.

Buffered 10% formaldehyde solution is a suitable all-purpose fixative which is compatible with subsequent electron microscopy and most immunohistochemical techniques. We use acetic alcoholic formalin (FAA, Tellyesniczky's solution – see Appendix E) for all gynecological specimens, principally because of its rapid fixation, with good penetration, of large dense specimens (such as uteri) and for lysis of blood in endometrial curettage specimens. Its further advantages are excellent preservation of nuclear and cytological detail and suitability for subsequent immunohistochemical work. Its disadvantage is damage to intracellular organelles, which effectively precludes subsequent electron microscopic examination. This drawback is circumvented by receiving tumor specimens (or others for which electron microscopy is anticipated) fresh within the department.

More important than the type of fixative is probably the adequacy of its volume. Fixative equivalent to 10 times the volume of tissue should be used and care must be taken that the specimen is not distorted by its container. Normal sized or moderately enlarged ovaries (up to 6 cm in diameter) may be fixed intact. Larger ovaries should be sliced (see the section on blocktaking below) to assist penetration of fixative. Large cysts should be opened, but remember to measure the ovary first. Note the consistency and color of fluid released and make sure that no mural or detached tumor is discarded with the fluid. The shape of the ovary can be preserved by packing the cyst(s) with cotton wool soaked in fixative.

MACROSCOPIC ASSESSMENT AND SAMPLING (BLOCKTAKING)

Ovaries should be measured in three dimensions. Weighing large ovarian tumors and cysts may provide a more readily appreciable assessment of the size of the lesion. If a tubo-ovarian mass is submitted, careful dissection may be necessary to identify its components. In pelvic inflammatory disease the ovary is relatively spared and should be readily recognized once the surrounding adhesions have been teased away. The course of the fallopian tubes should be identified and the condition of the fimbriae noted. A hydrosalpinx or parovarian cyst, especially if associated with adhesions, may cause confusion if diligent efforts are not made to establish the anatomical relationships. In cases of suspected neoplasia, identify the surgical margins and their proximity to apparent tumor; relevant margins can be identified with Indian ink. Initial careful dissection may resolve whether a tumor is arising in the ovary or fallopian tube. Examine the ovarian capsule and other serosal surfaces, noting the presence and nature of adhesions, tumor nodules, or rupture.

Blocktaking from small or moderately enlarged non-neoplastic ovaries

The ovary should be incised by parallel transverse cuts. Note the presence of a corpus luteum, cystic follicles (if excessive in number), cysts, or hemorrhage. One block is sufficient from a macroscopically normal ovary, but this should include cortex, medulla, and hilus – conveniently sampled by a single section through the middle of the ovary. Additional blocks of possible pathological structures will be required. Sample any adhesions, since these may provide evidence of endometriosis, previous surgery, or pelvic inflammatory disease. A small postmenopausal ovary may be bisected longitudinally and one-half submitted for processing. Wedge resections (from patients with polycystic ovary syndrome) usually display multiple small cystic follicles beneath a smooth thick capsule. Take two blocks from each wedge.

Blocktaking from large cystic or neoplastic ovaries

Fresh tissue will have already been taken for electron microscopy, DNA flow cytometry, etc. Pay attention to the capsule as indicated above and then slice the ovary at 1 cm intervals. Many ovarian tumors are cystic and all locules should be opened with scissors or sliced through with a sharp long-bladed knife. Note the character of the fluid in the cyst (serous (i.e. watery), mucoid, blood stained, oily, gelatinous) and the smoothness or otherwise of its lining. A smooth shiny lining usually indicates a benign lesion. Large thin-walled cysts can be sampled very effectively by making a 'jam-roll' from a strip of cyst wall (Fig. 4.1). Ragged hemorrhagic cysts are sugges-

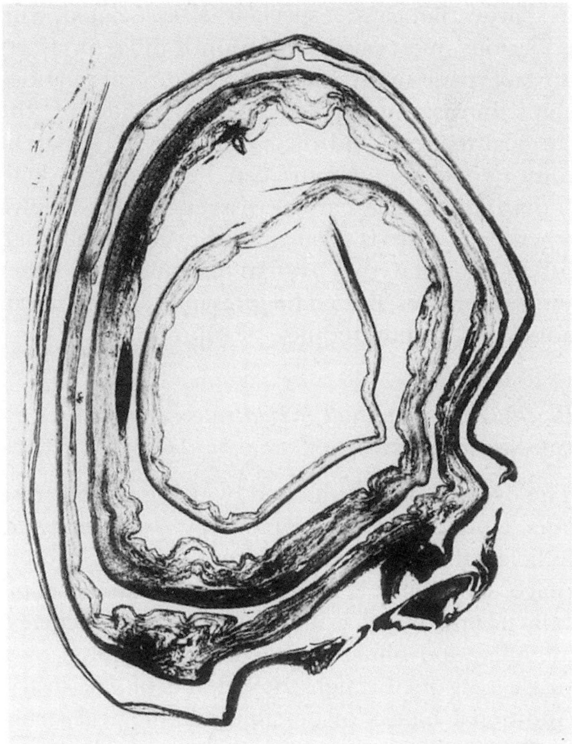

Fig. 4.1 'Jam-roll' made from thin-walled ovarian cyst. H + E ×10

tive of endometriosis, but several blocks may be necessary in order to identify the diagnostic portion of the lining. Mature cystic teratomas (dermoid cysts) should be emptied as completely as possible of enclosed hair and sebaceous material. The mural nodule (Rokitansky's tubercle) will usually become evident and this will be the most rewarding source of diagnostic material (see Ch. 46). Granularity, fine friable papillary excrescences, or soft fleshy nodules arising from cyst walls should arouse suspicions of malignancy and be thoroughly sampled. If the tumor has a variegated appearance, sample as many apparently different areas as possible. Take blocks from areas where the tumor comes closest to the capsule or resection margin, and particularly from the surface adhesions if tumor is close to the capsule at these points. A minimum of four blocks is suggested for an apparently benign cyst/tumor and eight for a malignant one. A good rule of thumb is to take one block per 1 cm of solid tumor diameter. In addition, look for and sample residual nontumorous ovarian tissue. Look for the fallopian tube, which may be incorporated in or stretched over the tumor mass/cyst. We like to take multiple tubal sections (as many as 12 transverse sections in two blocks) in cases of ovarian carcinoma (especially serous) because of the possibility of identifying coexistent tubal mucosal neoplasia. Early invasive carcinoma may be found in macroscopically normal tubes. An example of blocktaking from a complex ovarian mass is provided in Figure 4.2.

If the ovary has undergone torsion, the tissues may be extremely hemorrhagic and edematous or even necrotic. Slice the ovary finely, looking for any viable tissue or residua of a cyst or solid tumor that may have precipitated the torsion. Reticulin stains on suspicious areas may help to highlight the underlying pathology (see Fig. 17.3). The accompanying fallopian tube, if also involved, should be closely examined because it may be, albeit rarely, the site of the inciting lesion. However, in children, torsion of normal adnexa is not uncommon (see Ch. 17).

SPECIAL SITUATIONS

Staging operations for ovarian carcinoma

There is need for close cooperation between surgeon and pathologist in the staging operations for assessment of ovarian carcinomas. These may involve intraoperative assessment of excised tissues, including frozen section, as well as the histological examination of multiple specimens and cytological assessment of peritoneal washings and ascitic fluid. The extent to which the pathologist is involved in this area is reflected in the recommendations to surgeons for definitive exploration in ovarian cancer (Richardson et al 1985):

1. Perform midline incision extending above umbilicus
2. Evaluate ovarian mass with help of pathologist
   - rule out benign cyst

Fig. 4.2 Blocktaking from a complex ovarian mass, external surface (above) and cut surface (below). Bar equals 1 cm. Blocks required to sample all important features. a, Fallopian tube – multiple transverse sections; b, papillary surface nodule; c, adhesions; d, l, small cysts; e, locule with papillary lining; f, locule with granular lining; g, large thin-walled cysts; h, resection margin; j, possible capsular invasion; k, solid area

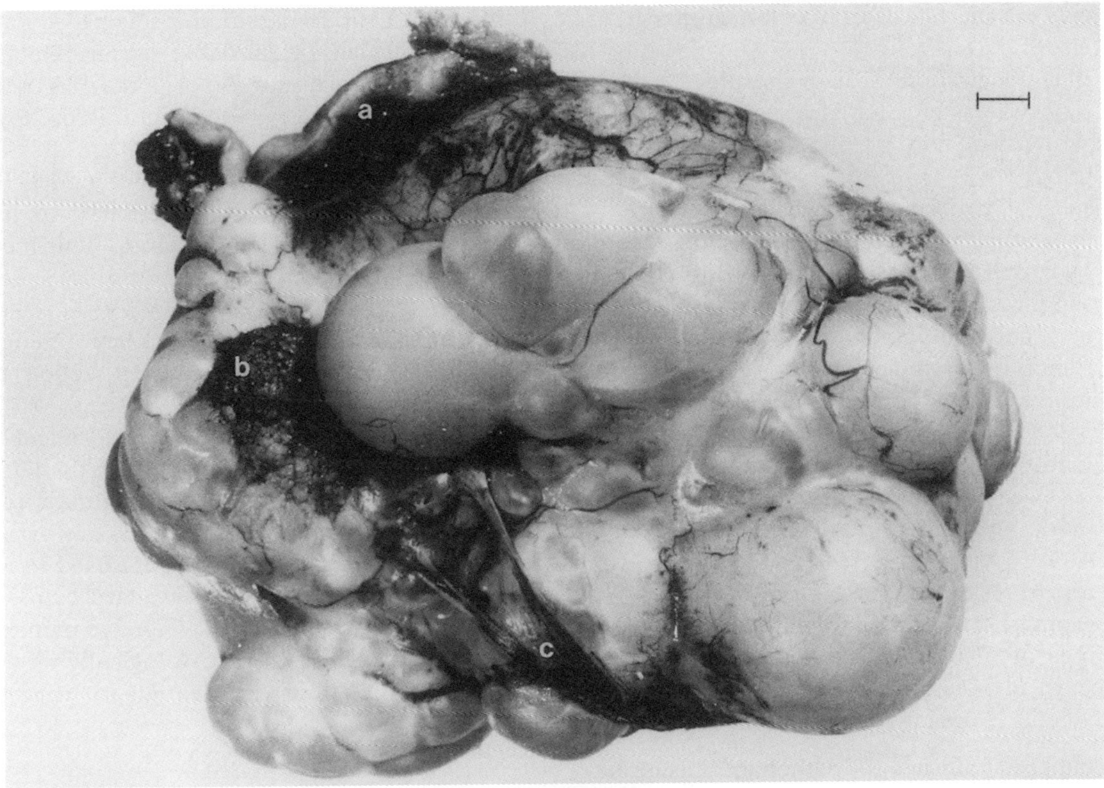

a

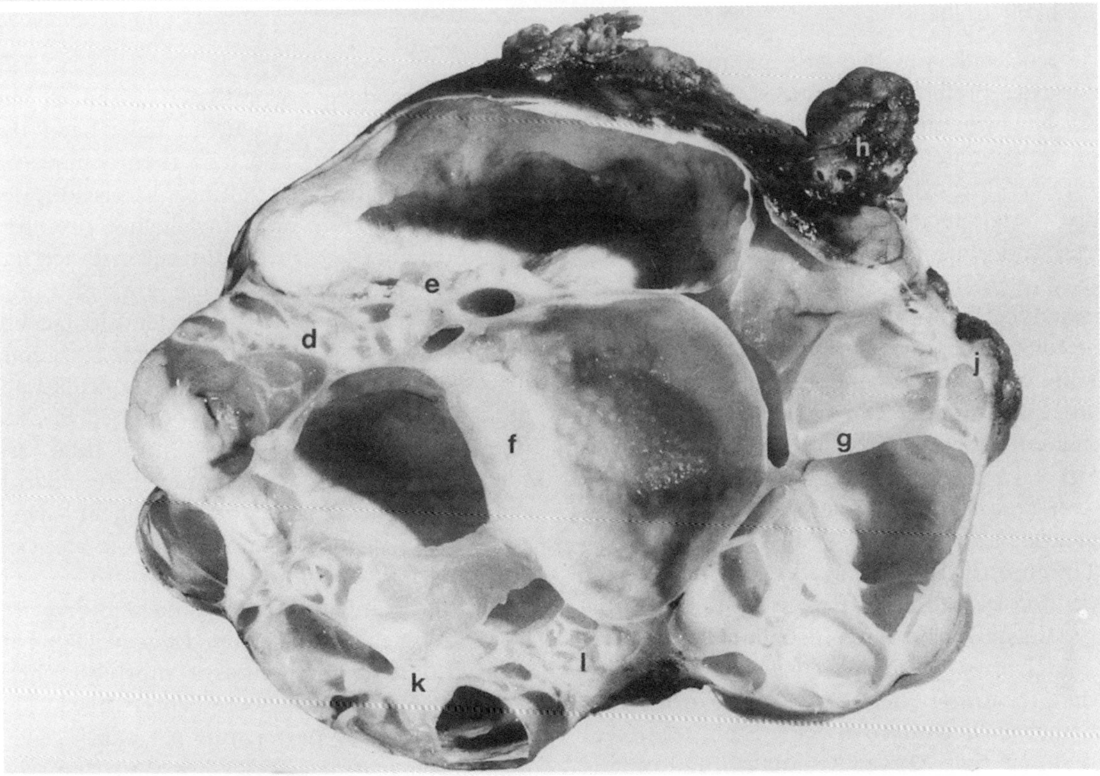

b

- rule out metastasis from colon, stomach, or elsewhere
- note penetration through capsule
- biopsy areas of adherence

3. Obtain ascitic fluid or saline washings for cytology
4. Inspect all peritoneal surfaces
   - prove that apparent implants are malignant by frozen section, or submit multiple samples for permanent section, or both
   - inspect diaphragm, with biopsy of visible lesions or scrapings for cytology
5. Confirm stage of apparent stage 1 or 2 disease by generous omental biopsy and biopsy of palpable pelvic and para-aortic nodes
6. After excision
   - mark specimen for pathologist – site(s) of rupture and/or area(s) of adherence
   - record residual disease – location and estimation of number or extent, and measurement of largest lesion.
7. Record FIGO staging (see Appendix C) and all details in operative note.

Specimens submitted for pathological examination are likely to include:

1. Uterus with attached or separately submitted adnexa, preferably delivered fresh to the pathologist immediately after excision. Before taking fresh tissue samples for electron microscopy, DNA flow cytometry, etc., carefully examine the whole specimen noting clearance of the tumor(s) and mark the excision margins if necessary. Complete the assessment of the ovaries as recommended above. Before fixation, open the uterine cavity, keeping in mind the possibility of a coexisting endometrial carcinoma or hyperplasia. Scrutinize the uterine serosal surface for tumor deposits and remember to section later any adhesions to exclude microscopic metastases (since these will alter the FIGO staging from 1 to at least 2a (see Appendix C)).

2. Omentum. Slice finely, looking for tumor deposits and block these. If none are found, sample any unusually firm areas (usually fibrous adhesions which may or may not be associated with microscopic tumor deposits) or, if none are found, take two random blocks. Steinberg et al (1986) found that 22% of grossly normal omentums from ovarian carcinoma staging operations had histologically identifiable tumor. Note that any extraovarian tumor deposits may be used for DNA flow cytometry, electron microscopy, or other special analyses.

3. Pelvic and/or para-aortic lymph nodes. Block all lymphoid tissue and step-section at six levels, unless obviously involved by tumor. This method maximizes the chance of finding microscopic metastases.

4. Peritoneal biopsies. These are often very small and our practice is to step-section these unless an obvious tumor nodule is seen.

5. Peritoneal washings. These are collected by the surgeon by saline irrigation from the left and right paracolic gutters, subdiaphragmatic region and pouch of Douglas. The fluids are cytocentrifuged and the spun deposits are used to make direct smears, according to standard cytological techniques (see Fig. 23.44). The remainder of the deposit is processed histologically as a cell block. Ascitic fluid is treated in the same manner.

Secondary cytoreductive surgery and 'second-look laparotomy'

These procedure are still performed in women with ovarian carcinoma who have been treated with chemotherapy and who then achieve partial or apparently complete clinical remission, despite evidence that they probably do not prolong survival (see Ch. 22). In the former instance laparotomy is performed with the aim of removing previously unresectable tumor deposits (secondary cytoreductive surgery). In the latter situation, the gynecological oncologist needs confirmation that complete tumor ablation has occurred in order to discontinue chemotherapy (and thus reduce further morbidity from treatment). At laparotomy the surgeon examines the peritoneal cavity for evidence of residual tumor (which is biopsied for confirmation – sometimes with frozen section assessment) and takes free fluid and/or washings for cytological assessment. Because laparotomy itself can lead to significant morbidity or even mortality, surgeons in some centers have attempted to avoid it by performing a laparoscopy, with the option of proceeding directly to laparotomy if no evidence of residual tumor is found. Laparoscopic biopsies can be examined immediately by frozen section and the fluids are processed immediately by cytocentrifugation and stained using a modified Papanicolaou method. Results can be available within 30 min. The combined results of three series (62 women) which used this protocol showed that 32.2% of women were found to have laparoscopic evidence of residual ovarian carcinoma and were spared laparotomy at that time (Piver et al 1980).

Investigation of ovarian failure and disordered sex differentiation

Ovarian biopsy is not necessary to confirm premature ovarian failure but is required to distinguish between true premature menopause and the resistant ovary syndrome, which cannot be separated on clinical and endocrinological grounds.

Laparoscopic biopsies are generally not adequate for assessment of follicular activity and do not provide sufficient material for the necessary supplementary investigations detailed below. The surgeon should be advised to take a longitudinal wedge of ovarian tissue (preferably bilaterally) 5 mm thick at the capsular surface and extending into the medulla. The biopsies should be submitted fresh to the surgical pathology laboratory and portions allocated for cytogenetic analysis (fresh tissue for fibroblast culture) and routine histology (all tissue remaining after the above should be embedded). Blocks may require step-sectioning if no follicles are found in the initial slides.

Gonadal biopsies from patients with disordered sex differentiation should be treated similarly, but immunohistochemical studies are not necessary.

Bilateral oophorectomy for endocrine ablation

This surgical method of endocrine ablation is still sometimes used in the treatment of advanced breast carcinoma. Slice the ovaries finely, looking for tumor deposits. Block suspicious areas or, if no nodules can be found, take two blocks from each ovary to identify possible microscopic deposits.

SPECIAL TECHNIQUES

Cytology

Cytological assessment of ovarian lesions may be of benefit in a number of clinical situations. Caution, however, does need to be exercised and both the clinician and pathologist should be aware of the technical pitfalls. The use of *intraoperative cytological examination* in diagnosis rather than frozen section is proving to be increasingly beneficial and is discussed extensively in Chapter 57.

Cytological examination of ovarian lesions by *fine needle aspiration biopsy* (FNAB) is still controversial. The problems and benefits of this technique are discussed in Chapter 12. Although usually contraindicated, FNAB of solid or semisolid ovarian lesions may be the diagnostic method of choice when:

- The patient is medically unfit for laparotomy
- The patient has inoperable ovarian carcinoma but confirmation of malignancy and histological typing may be beneficial
- After tumor resection when a secondary mass occurs either intra-abdominally or elsewhere
- As an adjunct to staging of ovarian carcinoma. Extraovarian masses in the liver, omentum and retroperitoneal lymph nodes may be aspirated.

Cytological examination of ascitic fluid and peritoneal washings is done routinely at staging laparotomies. All the fluid sent to the laboratory should be examined. It is routine to prepare both air-dried and wet-fixed specimens for examination.

Cytological examination may also be requested of *fluid from the pouch of Douglas*. This should be prepared as for other fluids.

Immunohistochemistry

Since the first edition of this textbook, immunohistochemistry has become a standard laboratory technique that has largely replaced special stains and electron microscopy as aids to the differential diagnosis of tumors. This technique can be applied to sections of paraffin-embedded tissues, examined by simple light microscopy, and result in permanent colorimetric representations of antigens in sections which can also be counterstained to allow localization of the reactions to specific cells.

Table 4.1 Immunohistochemical techniques useful in differential diagnosis of ovarian disease

Disease	Immunohistochemical reactions
Germ cell tumor	AFP, β-hCG, PlAP, cytokeratins, Leu-MI
Sex cord-stromal tumor, polycystic ovary syndrome	Estradiol, progesterone, testosterone, vimentin
Carcinoid tumor	NSE, chromogranin, specific peptide hormones
Malignant lymphoma	LCA, immunoglobulins, light chains
Mesothelioma	Cytokeratins, B72.3. S-100 protein
Struma ovarii	Thyroglobulin
Malignant melanoma	S-100 protein, NKI-C3, HMB-45
Mixed mullerian tumor, mesenchymal tumor	Myoglobin, desmin, vimentin
Undifferentiated tumor	EMA, LCA, NSE, desmin, vimentin, keratins, CEA, CA-125
Epithelial–stromal tumor	EMA, cytokeratins, CEA, CA-125, GFAP

Antigens that can be identified by immunohistochemical techniques and are valuable in the differential diagnosis of ovarian disease are listed in Table 4.1. Their application and interpretation with regard to the identification of specific tumor types are described in most of the relevant chapters of Sections 5–8. However, to make optimum use of this technique, pathologists need to be aware of the problems and pitfalls that may arise.

Antigens in tissue are not morphologically identifiable. They are usually proteins, although they can be carbohydrates expressed within or on the surface of cells. Visualization of these antigens involves two major components: a primary antibody and a detection system to identify the resulting antigen–antibody complex.

Fixation considerations are important to optimize preservation of the tissue antigens. Formalin fixation, by far the most common method, does not destroy most antigens, but there is inevitable loss of antigenicity, particularly if tissues are left in formalin for a long time. Pretreatment by proteolytic enzymes (enzyme digestion) such as trypsin, pepsin and pronase may be necessary to recover some antigens e.g. keratin, factor VIII, laminin, collagen type IV, neurofilament, desmin estrogen receptors, and CA-125. Acid fixatives such as Bouin's solution and FAA (see Appendix E) are less destructive than buffered formalin, while gluteraldehyde and Zenker-like fixatives are more damaging (Crum & Fenoglio 1980, Kurman 1984). Fortunately, there appears to be no loss of antigenicity after paraffin embedding so that old blocks can be processed in parallel with current material. Some monoclonal antibodies must be applied to frozen sections.

There are available a number of *detection system* methods, including the following:

- peroxidase–antiperoxidase (PAP) technique
- alkaline phosphatase and antialkaline phosphatase (APAAP) technique
- avidin biotin complex (ABC) technique
- biotin–streptavidin amplified technique.

In large laboratories performing large numbers of immunohistochemical tests, the particular method (or methods) most suitable will have been set up. It is beyond the scope of this book to describe each of these methods or to discuss their relative merits. Readers are referred to suitable texts that describe the methodology in detail. Commercial immunohistochemical kits are also available, which should be carefully assessed by individual laboratories. Positive and negative controls must always be used for proper interpretation, whichever technique is used. A file of control antigen-positive tissues should be maintained. Convenient positive controls may sometimes be present in the test section.

In smaller laboratories where immunohistochemical stains are required infrequently, referral of tissue or sections to a reference laboratory may be preferable. This may be especially so in cases of difficult differential diagnoses and where commercial kits have been untested, or appropriate positive and negative controls are unavailable.

DNA flow cytometry

Flow cytometers provide a rapid, reliable, and reproducible assessment of the physical characteristics of cell constituents and can also be used for cell sorting. Their facility for DNA measurement and cell cycle analysis is now being used by diagnostic pathologists for assessment of tumors. Methods and applications are reviewed by Quirke & Dyson (1986). A cell suspension is prepared from fresh or frozen unfixed tissue or, if this is no longer available, from a paraffin block (Hedley et al 1983). Care must be taken in sampling the tumor in order to minimize nontumorous components such as connective tissue. After DNA staining, the cell suspension is passed through a light beam and the patterns of electrical signals generated by the light scattering of the individual cells (10 000–100 000 cells) are then analyzed by a computer. DNA quantification is relative and requires an internal standard, usually chicken erythrocytes. Normal (nontumor) cells forming part of the study sample provide an additional internal standard. The computer generates DNA histograms with separately identified G_0/G_1, S and $G_2 + M$ phase components for normal diploid cells. Additional G_0/G_1 peaks indicate abnormal multiploid or aneuploid cell lines (Fig. 4.3).

Flow cytometric DNA analysis has been used extensively in studies of epithelial carcinomas of the ovary. In particular, they analyze the DNA ploidy and S-phase fraction of these tumors in relationship to their prognosis.

Friedlander et al (1983) demonstrated that ovarian cancers are commonly aneuploid and that there is a close association between stage and ploidy, with earlier stage tumors (stage 1–2) tending to be diploid whereas advanced tumors (stage 3–4) are aneuploid. Patients with diploid tumors had a significantly longer survival (60 months) than those with aneuploid tumors (13 months). Multivariate analysis revealed that tumor ploidy was an independent prognostic variable and the most important predictor of survival (Freidlander et al 1988).

Although there is no clear relationship between DNA ploidy and histological type, most serous and undifferentiated carcinomas are DNA aneuploid. The frequency of aneuploidy in the other cell types is highly variable.

DNA ploidy analysis of proliferating serous tumors shows that, although the great majority were DNA diploid, aneuploid proliferating tumors do occur (Bell et al 1988). The literature is divided as to the relationship of ploidy to outcome. Some studies have shown aneuploidy to be associated with an adverse outcome (Friedlander et al 1984, Kaerns et al 1990). Others have failed to confirm this (Bell 1992). Further studies are

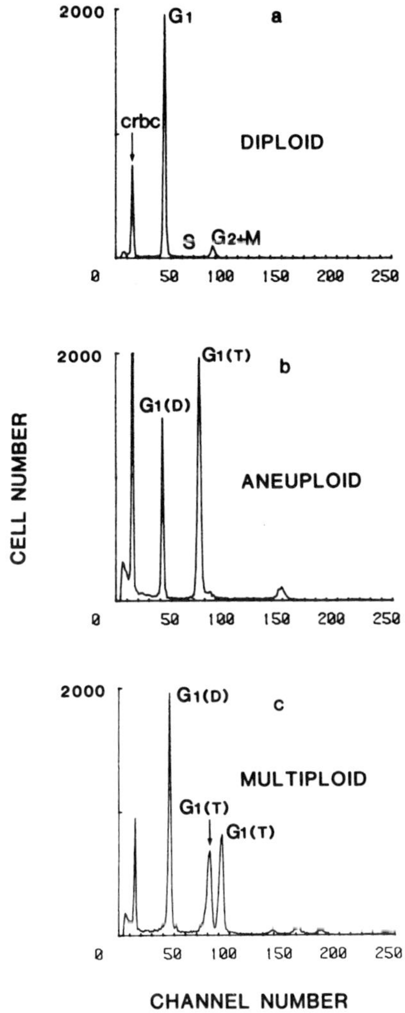

Fig. 4.3 DNA flow cytometry. Sample histograms from (a) diploid, (b) aneuploid, and (c) multiploid ovarian tumors. Channel number represents relative fluorescence intensity which is proportional to DNA content. G_{1D}, diploid peak; G_{1T}, additional G_1 peak of tumor cell population; crbc, internal biological standard

required and the prognostic significance of DNA aneuploidy in proliferating tumors has yet to be definitely established. Although rare, DNA aneuploidy may be found in benign tumors (Klemi et al 1988, Lage et al 1992).

Apart from determining tumor ploidy, flow cytometric analysis also provides information on cell cycle distribution. The proliferative fraction (S phase) determined flow cytometrically correlates with thymidine labeling index, and there is some suggestion that this may be of prognostic significance in ovarian cancer (Kallioniemi et al 1988). This has not been shown in all studies (Conte et al 1989). De Souza & Friedlander (1992) point out that technical problems exist and better methods are required before it is truly suitable for clinical application.

Estrogen/progesterone receptors

The presence of estrogen and progesterone receptors in ovarian tumors is well documented and occurs in 40–70% of patients (Creasman et al 1981, Quinn et al 1982, Bizzi et al 1988). Some investigators have demonstrated a correlation between steroid receptor level and a number of tumor/patient characteristics such as tumor stage and histological type and grade (de Souza & Friedlander 1992). Conclusions regarding the prognostic significance of steroid receptors are conflicting. Some studies have demonstrated that steroid receptors have independent prognostic significance (Slotman et al 1990, Sevelda et al 1990), whereas others have not.

Cytogenetic and molecular genetic studies

There has been extensive work undertaken on the molecular biology of ovarian cancer. The primary aim of these studies has been to elucidate the molecular events involved in the development of ovarian cancer (Boente et al 1993). Other studies have attempted to associate these molecular events with prognosis. These are addressed in several of the relevant tumor chapters.

Various oncogenes and tumor suppressor genes are activated in ovarian cancer. As with all cancer, tumors from different patients will have different activation patterns of the cancer-causing genes (Berchuk et al 1992). The genes that have been associated with ovarian carcinoma to date are HER-2/neu, an oncogene of the tyrosine kinase class; Ki-ras a G-protein oncogene, C-myc a nuclear transcription oncogene and p53 a tumor suppressor gene (Berchurck et al 1992). The oncogene C-erb B2 has also recently been identified (Meden et al 1994) in some cases of ovarian cancer. A study of oncogene expression in mixed-mullerian tumors identified a SIS PDGF-B chain (Kacinski et al 1989).

Although the surgical pathologist may supply (fresh) tissue for these studies, most authors agree that in terms of clinical significance and prognostic indicators much more work needs to be done (de Souza & Friedlander 1992). For every oncogene that has been studied in ovarian cancer there are at least half a dozen which remain unexplored (Berchuck et al 1992, Cliby et al 1993). Chromosome studies have also shown loss of heterozygosity on chromosomes 6 and 17 (Foulkes et al 1993). Genetic studies into other types of ovarian malignancy are rare. There has been one report of a genetic analysis of germ cell tumors that identified i (12p) as a specific cytogenetic abnormality as well as other chromosomal abnormalities in more than 80% of germ cell tumors (Ilson et al 1991).

Nuclear magnetic resonance spectroscopy

Excised tumors, including some of ovarian origin, have been examined by nuclear (proton) magnetic resonance spectroscopy (MRS). This is to be distinguished from magnetic resonance imaging (MRI) (see Ch. 58), although the technologies are closely related. Malignant tumors yield a characteristic high-resolution magnetic resonance spectrum with a long transverse (T_2) relaxation time which is thought to originate in the proteolipids of the plasma membranes of the malignant cells. Five of six ovarian epithelial tumors with atypical proliferation yielded spectra similar to those of malignant tumors, while one produced a featureless spectrum typical of a benign lesion (Mountford et al 1986). Similar proteolipid complexes have been identified by MRS and biochemical analysis in the serum of cancer patients (Wieczorek et al 1985, Mountford et al 1986). MRS may become an important adjunct in the biological characterization of tumors, and may be capable of identifying tumors with invasive or metastatic potential. It is our view that the chemical markers of malignancy identified by MRS could well form the substrate for preoperative *chemical shift imaging* by whole-body MRI techniques of patients suspected of having ovarian neoplasms, a fusion of MRS and MRI (Mountford et al 1993).

Electron microscopy

Ultrastructural studies have been important in determining the histogenesis of various ovarian neoplasms (e.g. mucinous tumors, strumal carcinoids, and adenomatoid tumors), and have thereby assisted in their classification. Many ovarian tumors have distinctive electron microscopic features e.g. the various subtypes of epithelial–stromal tumors, adenomatoid tumors, carcinoid tumors, steroid-producing stromal tumors (especially granulosa cell, Sertoli and Leydig cell tumors), dysgerminomas, endodermal sinus tumor, heterologous sarcomas, lymphomas, Krukenberg tumors, and melanomas. Electron microscopy can be used to confirm or exclude a provisional histological diagnosis. However, the sample preparation and examination are expensive and time consuming, and there is always the problem of inappropriate tissue sampling. In addition, the characteristic ultrastructural features of most tumors are likely to be considerably less readily recognizable, or absent, in the problematic poorly differentiated lesions. Many of the differential diagnoses previously resolved by electron microscopic examination can now be made by immunohistochemical methods, which are relatively cheap and fast, although not always reliable.

The distinctive electron microscopic appearances of ovarian lesions are presented in review articles, monographs and in studies of individual entities as indicated in the relevant chapters (Ferenczy 1979, Ferenczy & Richart 1974, Ferenczy & Fenoglio 1979, Salazar & Gonzalez-Angulo 1984, Ferenczy & Roth 1985), but are not examined in any great detail in this text. The ultrastructural features of normal ovarian tissues are illustrated by Ferenczy & Richart (1974).

Histomorphometry

This is the quantitative or semiquantitative assessment of morphological features in histological material (Aherne & Dunnill 1982, Baak & Oort 1983). Morphometric principles can be applied to the assessment of single variables (such as tumor size, mitotic activity, and DNA content) or to multiple morphological variables, the latter generally requiring statistical analysis by a computer. Volumes or ratios of tissue components can be deduced from the two-dimensional images of histological sections. Electronic image analyzers can be used to assist in quantitating morphological features such as nuclear shape. The mass of collected data can then be analyzed according to the principles of multivariate analysis. Surgical pathologists have used these techniques to attempt to refine and standardize the diagnosis of conditions that form a morphological continuum, e.g. proliferative endometrial lesions (hyperplasia – carcinoma) and epithelial–stromal tumors of the ovary (Baak et al 1981, Langley & Baak 1984).

More recently, the technique of image analysis has been used to measure DNA content. Proliferating epithelial–stromal tumors showing an aneuploid DNA content by these techniques have been shown to have a significant increased risk of recurrence (Drescher et al 1993) and death (Padberg et al 1993).

Although only small in number, studies using computerized morphometric analysis have been able to distinguish between proliferating and malignant ovarian tumors (Komitowski et al 1989, Hytiroglou et al 1992). Much of this work remains highly specialized and may not be applicable in the context of general surgical pathology, although it is of interest and potential benefit (Baak 1988).

REFERENCES

Aherne W A, Dunnill M S 1982 Morphometry. Arnold, London

Baak J P A, Oort J 1983 A manual of morphometry in diagnostic pathology. Springer-Verlag, Berlin

Baak J P 1988 Possibilities and progress of quantitative pathological examination of ovarian tumours. European Journal of Obstetrics Gynecology and Reproductive Biology 29: 183–189

Baak J P A, Agrafojo Blanco A, Kurver P H J et al 1981 Quantitation of borderline and malignant mucinous ovarian tumours. Histopathology 5: 353–360

Bell D A 1992 Flow cytometry of ovarian neoplasms. Current Topics in Pathology 85: 337–356

Bell D A, Pastel-Levy C, Flotte T J 1988 DNA content in serous borderline tumors [abstract]. Laboratory Investigation 58: 8A

Berchuck A, Kohler M F, Bast R C 1992 Oncogenes in ovarian cancer. Haematologic Oncology Clinics of North America 6: 813–827

Bizzi A, Codegoni A N, Landoni F 1988 Steroid receptors in epithelial ovarian carcinoma. Relation to clinical parameters to survival. Cancer Research 48: 6222–6226

Boente M P, Hurteau J, Rodriguez G G, Bast R C, Berchuck A 1993 The biology of ovarian cancer. Current Opinion in Oncology 5: 900–907

Cliby W, Ritland S, Hartman L et al 1993 Human epithelial ovarian cancer allelotype. Cancer Research 53(10 suppl) 2393–2398

Conte P F, Alama A, Rubagotte A 1989 Cell kinetics in ovarian cancer. Relationship to clinicopathologic features responsiveness to chemotherapy and survival. Cancer 64: 1189–1191

Creasman W T, Sasso R A, Weed J C, McCarty K S 1981 Ovarian carcinoma histologic and clinical correlation of cytoplasmic oestrogen and progesterone study. Gynecologic Oncology 12: 319–327

Crum C P, Fenoglio C M 1980 The immunoperoxidase technique. A review of its application to diseases of the female genital tract. Diagnostic Gynecology and Obstetrics 2: 103–115

De Souza P L, Friedlander M L 1992 Prognostic factors in ovarian cancer. Haematologic Oncology Clinics of North America 6: 761–789

Drescher C W, Flint A, Hopkins M P, Roberts J A 1993 Prognostic significance of DNA content and nuclear morphology in borderline tumours. Gynecologic Oncology 48: 242–246

Ferenczy A 1979 Diagnostic electron microscopy in gynecologic pathology. Pathology Annual 1: 353–381

Ferenczy A, Fenoglio C M 1979 Female genital tract. In: Johannessen J V (ed) Electron microscopy in human medicine, vol 9 (Urogenital system and breast). McGraw-Hill, New York, p 297–384

Ferenczy A, Roth L M 1985 The ultrastructure of ovarian neoplasms. In: Roth L M, Czernobilsky B (eds) Tumors and tumorlike conditions of the ovary. Churchill Livingstone, New York, p 175–205

Foulkes W D, Ragoussis J, Stamp G W, Allan G J, Trowsdale J 1993a Frequent loss of heterozygosity in chromosome 6 in human ovarian carcinoma. British Journal of Cancer 67: 551–559

Foulkes W D, Black D M, Stamp G W, Solomon E, Trowsdale J 1993b Very frequent loss of heterozygosity throughout chromosome 7 in sporadic ovarian cancer. International Journal of Cancer 54: 220–225

Friedlander M L, Taylor I W, Russell P 1983 Ploidy as a prognostic factor in ovarian cancer. International Journal of Gynecological Pathology 1: 55–62

Friedlander M L, Russell P, Taylor I W, Hedley D W, Tattersall M H N 1984 Flow cytometric analysis of cellular DNA content as an adjunct to the diagnosis of ovarian tumours of borderline malignancy. Pathology 16: 301–306

Friedlander M L, Hedley D W, Swansee C, Russell P 1988 Prediction of long-term survival by flow cytometric analysis of cellular DNA content in patients with advanced ovarian cancer. Journal of Clinical Oncology 6: 282–290

Hedley D W, Friedlander M L, Taylor I W, Rugg C A, Musgrove E A 1983 Method for analysis of cellular DNA content of paraffin-embedded pathological material usung flow cytometry. Journal of Histochemistry and Cytochemistry 31: 1333–1335

Hytiroglou P, Harpa Z N, Heller D S, Liu Z Y, Deligdisch L, Gil J 1992 Differential diagnosis of borderline and invasive serous cystadenocarcinoma of the ovary by computerized interactive morphometric analyses of nuclear features. Cancer 69: 988–992

Ilson D H, Bosl G J, Motzer R, Dmitrovsky E, Chaganti R S 1991 Genetic analysis of germ cell tumours: current progress and future prospects. Haematologic Oncology Clinics of North America 5: 1271–1283

Kacinski B M, Carter D, Kohorn E I, Mitta K, Bloodgood G S, Donahue J 1989 Oncogene expression in vivo by ovarian adenocarcinomas and mixed mullerian tumours. Yale Journal of Biological Medicine 62: 379–392

Kaerns J, Trope C, Kjorstad K E, Abeler V, Petterson E O 1990 Cellular DNA content as a new prognostic tool in patients with borderline tumours of the ovary. Gynecologic Oncology 38: 452–457

Kaloniemi O P, Punnonen R, Mattila J 1988 Prognostic significance of DNA index multiploidy and S-phase traction in ovarian cancer. Cancer 61: 334–339

Klemi P J, Jaensuu H, Kiiholme P, Maenpaa J 1988 Clinical significance of abnormal nurclear DNA content in serous ovarian tumours. Cancer 62: 2005–2010

Komitowski D, Janson C, Szamaboiski J, Czernobilsky B 1989 Quantitative nuclear morphology in the diagnosis of ovarian tumours of low malignant potential. Cancer 64: 905–910

Kurman R J, Ganjei P, Nadji M 1984 Contributions of immunocytochemistry to the diagnosis and study of ovarian neoplasms. International Journal of Gynecological Pathology 3: 3–26

Lage J M, Weiberg D S, Huettner P C, Mark S D 1992 Flow cytometric analysis of nuclear DNA content in ovarian tumors. Association of ploidy with tumor type histological grade and clinical stage. Cancer 69: 2668–2675

Langley F A, Baak J P A 1984 Quantitative methods in diagnostic gynaecological pathology. Clinics in Obstetrics and Gynaecology 11: 79–92

Meden H, Marx D, Rath W et al 1994 Overexpression of the oncogene c-erb B2 in primary ovarian cancer evaluation of the prognosis value in a Cox proportional hazards multiple regression. International Journal of Gynecological Pathology 13: 45–53

Mountford C E, Saunders J K, May G L et al 1986 Classification of human tumours by high-resolution magnetic resonance spectroscopy. Lancet i: 651–653

Mountford C E, Lean C L, Mackinnon W B, Russell P 1993 The use of proton MR in cancer pathology. In: Webb G A (ed) Annual reports on NMR spectroscopy, vol 27. Academic Press, London, p 173–216

Padberg B C, Arp H, Frank U et al 1992 DNA cytomorphometry and prognosis in ovarian tumours of borderline malignancy. A clinicomorphological study of 80 cases. Cancer 69: 2510–2514

Piver M S, Lele S B, Barlow J J, Gamarra M 1980 Second-look laparoscopy prior to proposed second-look laparotomy. Obstetrics and Gynecology 55: 571–573

Quinn M A, Pearce P, Rome R 1982 Cytoplasmic steroid receptors in ovarian tumour. British Journal of Obstetrics and Gynaecology 89: 754–759

Quirke P, Dyson J E D 1986 Flow cytometry: methodology and applications in pathology. Journal of Pathology 149: 79–87

Richardson G S, Scully R E, Nikrui N, Nelson J H 1985 Common epithelial cancer of the ovary. New England Journal of Medicine 312: 415–424

Salazar H, Gonzalez-Angulo A 1984 Ultrastructural diagnosis in gynaecological pathology. Clinics in Obstetrics and Gynaecology 11: 25–77

Sevelda P, Denison U, Schempe M 1990 Oestrogen and progesterone receptor content as a prognostic factor in advanced epithelial ovarian carcinoma. British Journal of Obstetrics and Gynaecology 97: 706–712

Slotman B J, Narta J J P, Rao B R 1990 Survival of patients with ovarian cancer. Apart from stage and grade, tumour progesterone receptor content is a prognostic indicator. Cancer 66: 740–744

Steinberg J J, Demopoulos R I, Bigelow B 1986 The evaluation of the omentum in ovarian cancer. Gynecologic Oncology 24: 327–330

Wieczorek A J, Rhyner C, Block L H 1985 Isolation and characterization of an RNA–proteolipid complex associated with the malignant state in humans. Proceedings of the National Academy of Sciences of the United States of America 82: 3455–3459

5

Ovarian function and its laboratory assessment

I. S. Fraser

NORMAL OVARIAN FUNCTION

The reproductive years

The main function of the ovary is to produce mature and fertilizable oocytes, and to coordinate the processes of ovulation, fertilization, and implantation by precise hormonal changes so that successful pregnancy is possible. Knowledge of the details of ovarian function is continuing to increase rapidly through animal studies and research in in-vitro fertilization.

Hypothalamic–pituitary function

Ovarian function is controlled directly by hormones secreted by the hypothalamic–pituitary unit, and in turn has complex feedback relationships through effects of its own hormonal secretions on higher brain centers, hypothalamic centers, and the anterior pituitary. Gonadotrophin-releasing hormone (GnRH) is a decapeptide, synthesized in cell bodies in the hypothalamus, from where it is transported in vesicles down the axons to neuronal terminals which abut capillaries in the median eminence of the hypothalamus. GnRH is secreted from the neuronal terminals in small pulsatile bursts approximately once every 1–2 h, the frequency and amplitude of secretory pulses being influenced greatly by the reproductive state and the stage of the menstrual cycle. It is now recognized that a large number of neurotransmitters and neuromodulator substances in the brain may directly or indirectly influence GnRH secretion. The complexity of this system allows for multiple and subtle effects of environmental factors and higher centers to influence ovarian function.

GnRH is secreted into median eminence capillaries and then passes down portal vessels in the pituitary stalk to the anterior pituitary where it stimulates secretion of both glycoprotein gonadotrophins, follicle stimulating hormone (FSH), and luteinizing hormone (LH) from the same gonadotroph cells. Hence, simultaneous episodic peaks of LH and FSH can be detected by frequent blood sampling.

FSH stimulates cell proliferation and metabolism within ovarian antral follicles, and stimulates aromatase enzyme activity within the granulosa cells allowing steroid precursors to be converted into estrogens. LH is necessary to stimulate enzymes in the early part of the ovarian synthesis pathways. LH also has a number of functions, which are most obvious at midcycle when it stimulates the sequence of events leading to ovulation. LH stimulates resumption of the first meiotic division in the oocyte, and causes changes in enzyme function leading to the process of luteinization. It also increases ovarian blood flow, and small amounts of LH are necessary during the luteal phase to maintain normal corpus luteum function.

Follicular function

Ovarian follicle function is extremely complex. Steroids are synthesized in both granulosa and theca cells, with the theca secreting mainly androgenic precursors and the granulosa predominantly secreting oestradiol. It should be remembered that the theca interna is a very vascular tissue, while the granulosa is surrounded by a basement membrane and is therefore not directly supplied by blood vessels. Some of the steroids secreted by granulosa cells pass in high concentration into follicular fluid where estradiol is bound to protein, and the remainder pass across the basement membrane into the general circulation.

Granulosa cells also secrete a variety of putative intrafollicular paracrine and autocrine regulatory molecules which have a variety of effects, including oocyte meiosis inhibition, luteinization inhibition, inhibition of FSH binding, and in situ modulation of the vascularity, growth and function of the follicle. Strong evidence now exists to indicate that inhibin is secreted into the general circulation under physiological circumstances and has a direct inhibitory effect on pituitary gonadotroph secretion of FSH. This is one mechanism by which FSH and LH secretion can be controlled independently.

Ovulation

The process of ovulation is the release of a mature oocyte surrounded by a cumulus of granulosa cells from the Graafian follicle. This is preceded by a precisely timed sequence of endocrine events (Fig. 5.1). The follicular estradiol rise usually reflects normal maturation of the growing follicle, and the estradiol peak usually precedes ovulation by about 48 h. This peak is followed within 24 h by the LH (and FSH) peak, which in turn is followed within 18–24 h by ovulation.

One of the major functions of the LH surge is to trigger a sequence of events within the mature follicle, which leads to weakening of the follicle wall and subsequent rupture. The changes are mediated by the release within the follicle of various enzymes, such as plasminogen activator and collagenase, and prostaglandins. Changes also occur within the granulosa cells, leading to changes in proteoglycans and to loosening of intercellular bonds, especially around the cumulus oophorus, so that the oocyte and its surrounding cumulus can be released after follicle rupture. The oocyte needs to be surrounded by its cumulus in order to facilitate pick up by the ciliated processes of the tubal fimbriae. A further important function of the LH surge is to trigger the resumption of the first meiotic division in the oocyte. The second meiotic division is only completed if fertilization occurs.

Luteal function

Following ovulation the follicle cells luteinize, again under the influence of the LH surge, and gain the enzymatic capability to secrete progesterone as well as estradiol. This process is associated with parenchymal cell hypertrophy and matrix remodeling, probably under the influence of insulin-like growth factors and androgens. New blood vessels grow in under the influence of basic fibroblast growth factor to form the highly vascular corpus luteum. Granulosa cells form large luteal cells that have a relatively fixed lifespan limited by their inability to generate new LH receptors. Theca cells form somewhat smaller luteal cells that require LH (or chorionic gonadotrophin (hCG) from the implanting blastocyst) to continue to secrete progesterone and estradiol. If implantation does not occur, hCG is not secreted and the corpus luteum undergoes luteolysis by a process which is not well understood in humans. Human corpus luteum function is probably limited by a combination of intrinsic lifespan effects, need for increasing amounts of LH or hCG, and a local release of luteolytic prostaglandins. Morphological details of these processes are given in Chapter 3.

Summary of menstrual cycle endocrinology

Changes in secretion and peripheral blood (plasma or serum) concentration of FSH, LH, estradiol, and progesterone during the menstrual cycle are summarized in Fig. 5.1. The perimenstrual surge

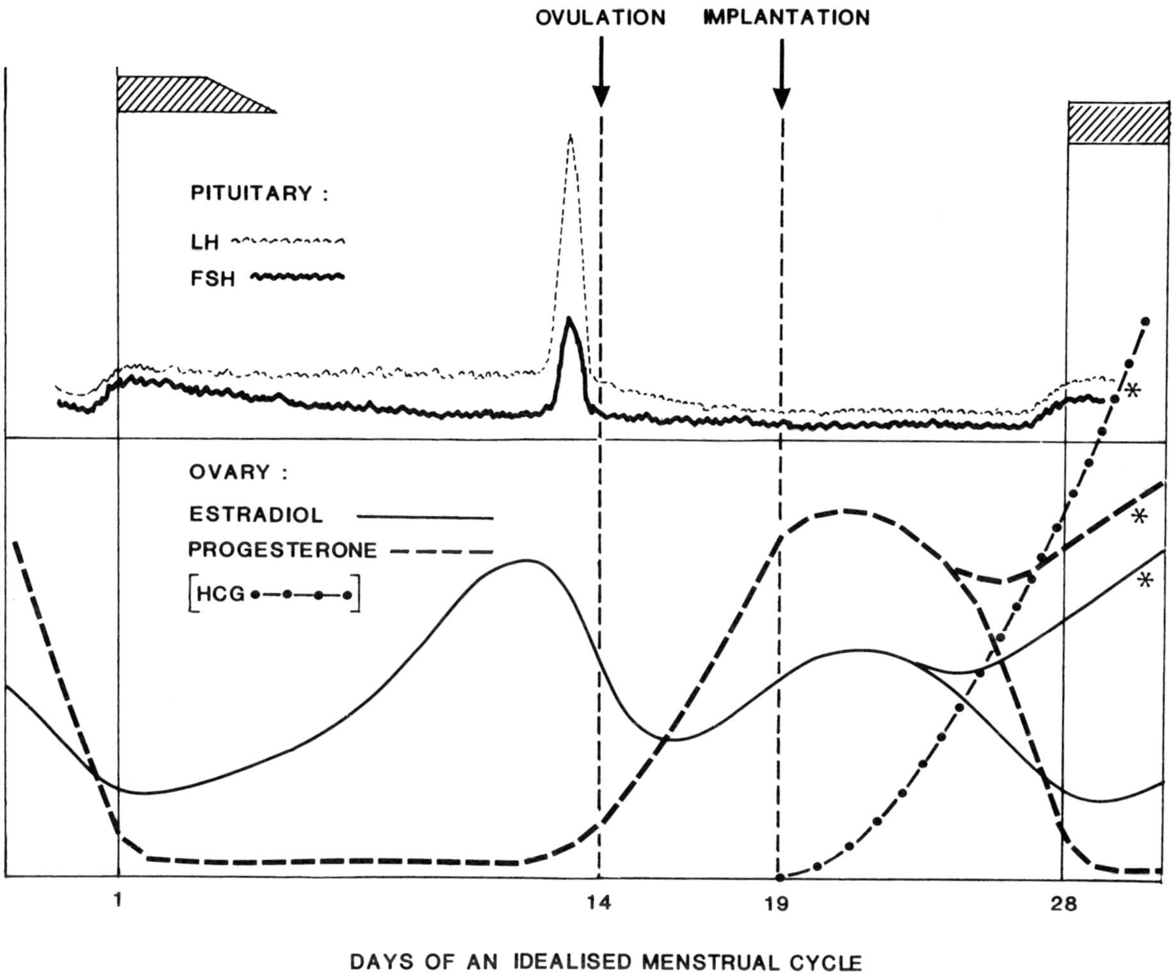

Fig. 5.1 Schematic illustration of serum levels of the main pituitary and ovarian hormones during an idealized 28 day menstrual cycle. (▨) Menstruation. *Late luteal phase elevations in estradiol, progesterone, and hCG which occur after successful implantation

of FSH stimulates further development of a crop of antral follicles (thought to be around 20). The small LH surge assists in stimulating steroidogenesis resulting in a rise in estradiol secretion. This leads to suppression of FSH by the negative feedback mechanism, and the fall in FSH is partly responsible for the majority of follicles failing to grow further and eventually undergoing atresia. Usually one, or perhaps two, follicles have generated sufficient FSH receptors to maintain their growth and secretion of estradiol and to become preovulatory or Graafian follicles. Sufficient estradiol is now being secreted to trigger the midcycle LH and FSH surges via the positive feedback mechanism. The LH surge then triggers ovulation and initiates the enzyme changes leading to luteinization.

Estradiol secretion temporarily drops during this period and then increases again after formation of the corpus luteum. Progesterone secretion begins to increase coincident with the LH surge and rises to high levels during the luteal phase. Secretion and feedback pathways are indicated in Figure 5.2.

If blastocyst implantation does not occur the corpus luteum undergoes the process of luteolysis, by poorly understood mechanisms (probably involving prostaglandins, cytokines, reactive

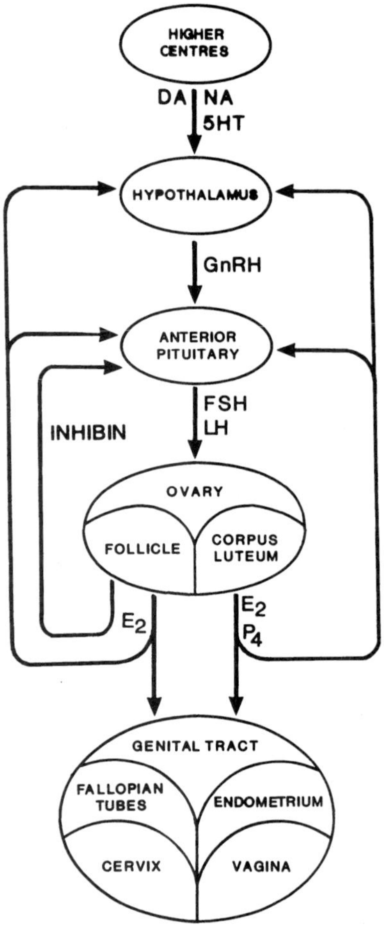

Fig. 5.2 Schematic illustration of the pathways of biological activity and feedback activity of reproductive hormones in women. DA, Dopamine; NA, noradrenaline; 5HT, 5-hydroxytryptamine (serotonin); GnRH, gonadotrophin-releasing hormone; FSH, follicle stimulating hormone; LH, luteinizing hormone; E_2, estradiol; P_4, progesterone

oxygen, and withdrawal of LH support), and ultimately forms a corpus albicans. During this time estradiol and progesterone secretion fall. The endometrium consequently breaks down and menstruation occurs. This fall in ovarian steroid secretion triggers the perimenstrual rise in FSH and LH secretion which starts the next cycle. It is postulated that repeated exposure of the ovary to free oxygen radicals at the time of luteolysis may lead to an increased risk of ovarian cancer in later life.

If implantation occurs the blastocyst begins to secrete hCG, which passes into the general circulation and has a luteotrophic effect to maintain corpus luteum function and secretion of estradiol and progesterone until the placenta takes over these functions at 6–8 weeks gestation (4–6 weeks after fertilization).

Ovarian function at puberty

The ovary remains relatively quiescent during most of childhood, although small antral follicles may sometimes be seen and follicular atresia is a continual process. Only tiny amounts of estradiol are secreted until puberty begins. The basic mechanism triggering puberty is unknown, but the first clinical signs can be detected between the ages of 6 and 9 years. The very first sign of puberty is usually the appearance of small amounts of pubic hair, initially on the labia majora, followed shortly after by breast bud development. The breasts will eventually reach their maximal development 5–10 years later after passing through five continuous and somewhat arbitrary stages, as described by Tanner (1962). Other clinical events that occur during the course of pubertal development include an obvious growth spurt and maturation of the genital tract. These are followed some time later by the menarche, the first menstrual period that a girl experiences. This usually occurs somewhere in the middle of the continuum of pubertal development. The first few menstrual cycles are usually anovulatory and may then pass through a phase of deficient luteal function before reaching adequate ovulation within 6–24 months following the menarche.

At the menarche it has been calculated that around 300 000 to 400 000 oocytes are present in the two ovaries. This is a great deal less than the maximal number of oocytes present (about 6 000 000) at about 6 months of in utero age and the 1 500 000 which are probably present at birth (Baker 1963). This indicates that oocytes and follicles undergo relatively rapid atresia from late fetal life onwards. This process continues through until the menopause. It is surprising and apparently very wasteful that only about 400 oocytes are destined to ovulate during a woman's life out of the very large number theoretically available.

The factor, or factors, which initiate puberty are still unknown. However, details of the hormone changes associated with puberty are now fairly well understood. The very first change in hormone levels is in circulating androgens of adrenal origin. This is followed by a gradual increase in secretion of FSH and LH, and finally an increase in ovarian estradiol. During childhood the hypothalamus is extremely sensitive to suppression by the relatively small concentrations of estradiol produced by the ovaries. This sensitivity steadily decreases through puberty until the adult stage is reached. This allows increasing secretion of GnRH, and hence FSH and LH with a consequent rise in ovarian follicle activity and estradiol secretion. During puberty most of these hormones fluctuate in an erratic manner, but the first rise in LH secretion is noticed as episodic bursts which are only detectable during sleep. A degree of inhibition may be exerted on the hypothalamus during childhood by the pineal gland (and melatonin secretion) and the limbic system of the brain, including the amygdala, the cingulate gyrus, and the hippocampus. As the menarche approaches, the fluctuations of estradiol in peripheral blood gradually increase until they reach a stage where they cause stimulation of endometrial growth to such a level that some breakdown of tissue and hence menstruation occurs when the estrogen levels subsequently fall. At this stage the negative-feedback control system on hypothalamic pituitary function is fully developed, but the positive-feedback system, which is associated with midcycle LH release, only develops in the second half of puberty.

There is clear evidence that the average age of puberty has gradually decreased over the past century in many countries. The reason for this is unclear, but there is some concern that the age of emotional and intellectual maturity has not decreased at the same rate as the physical change.

Menopause

This is the last menstrual period which a woman experiences and is associated with the loss of active follicles and oocytes from the ovaries. The menopause is but one event in a continuum of declining ovarian function which lasts 5–10 years and is usually known as the climacteric. The menopause is a diagnosis which can only be made in retrospect and is usually said to have occurred when a woman has had no periods for 6–12 months and is in the appropriate age group. In most societies the mean age of menopause is 50–52 years, but menopause can be regarded as normal even if it occurs as early as the age of 40 years. There is a difference of opinion about the age below which menopause should be regarded as 'premature', hence meriting investigation. Most investigators agree that this lies somewhere between the ages of 35 and 40 years, and cases should be managed on an individual basis.

The climacteric is preceded by a decline in fertility which can be detected as early as the mid-thirties. This decline in fertility may be associated with disturbances of hypothalamic–pituitary function, aging changes within the ovaries and genital tract, and an increase in the incidence of gynecological disorders such as endometriosis and leiomyomas. Pregnancy is uncommon in women in the mid- to late forties and is very rare in women over the age of 50 years.

The menopause does not always occur with the sudden cessation of previously regular periods, but is more often associated with increasing irregularity of menstrual cycles for 1–5 years. During this time a rise in serum plasma levels of FSH can often be detected. This is probably related to a decline in sensitivity of the residual ovarian follicles. Anovulatory cycles and dysfunctional uterine bleeding are common during this time.

At the time of menopause a small number of oocytes are still recognizable within the ovaries, but most of these appear to be chromosomally or morphologically abnormal or are in some other way resistant to stimulation by normal levels of pituitary FSH. The menopause occurs because the ovaries are no longer able to secrete estradiol and the concentration of this hormone falls to very low levels in the bloodstream. These changes are followed by a relatively rapid rise in serum levels of FSH and LH. Mean serum concentrations of FSH continue to rise for 2–5 years following the menopause and then gradually decline into old age. Serum hormone levels are summarized in Table 5.1.

Serum levels of total testosterone also decline after the menopause, but this is mainly due to a fall in the levels of sex hormone binding globulin

Table 5.1 Normal serum hormone levels before and after menopause

	Premenopause	Postmenopause
Estradiol (pmol/l)	75–1500	30–60
Estrone (pmol/l)	60–650	100–200
Estriol (pmol/l)	20–50	15–25
Testosterone (nmol/l)	1–4	0.5–1.0
Androstenedione (nmol/l)	4–7	1–4
LH (iu/l)	2–16	30–80
midcycle peak (iu/l)	50–120	30–80
FSH (iu/l)	0–7	40–80
Prolactin (iu/l)	100–600	50–400
Pregnenolone (nmol/l)	2	1
DHA (nmol/l)	14*	6*
Cortisol (nmol/l)	400	400

*Mean level.

(secretion of which is estrogen dependent). Serum levels of free testosterone do not change substantially. After the menopause the main circulating estrogen is estrone and most of this circulates as estrone sulfate. Serum levels of several adrenal androgenic steroids, such as pregnenolone and dehydroepiandrosterone (DHA), also decline in parallel with the fall in estrogen, indicating a direct effect of ovarian estrogen on the adrenal secretion of some androgens.

A spectrum of specific problems may develop during the climacteric and after the menopause. These are mainly related to estrogen deficiency. These effects fall into five broad groups: hot flushes and night sweats; genital tract and lower urinary tract atrophy; osteoporosis; cardiovascular changes leading to arterial wall damage; and a complex of symptoms known as the 'menopausal syndrome', including such subjective but often troublesome feelings as depression, agitation, loss of concentration, poor memory, loss of libido, and lethargy.

ASSESSMENT OF NORMAL OVARIAN FUNCTION

Most tests utilize direct or indirect endocrine assays, although other techniques may provide ancillary information. The aim of most assays is to confirm the occurrence of ovulation, although it should be recognized that the only absolute confirmation of ovulation is pregnancy or, in very recent years, the collection of an ovum from the uterine cavity by a flushing technique. Strong presumptive evidence of adequate ovulation can be obtained from a clear biphasic basal body temperature chart, serial midluteal serum progesterones, and a premenstrual endometrial biopsy (Fig. 5.3) or serial ovarian ultrasound scans around midcycle.

The basal body temperature chart should be recorded every morning before rising using a special 'fertility thermometer' inserted vaginally or rectally for the full recommended time (2–3 min).

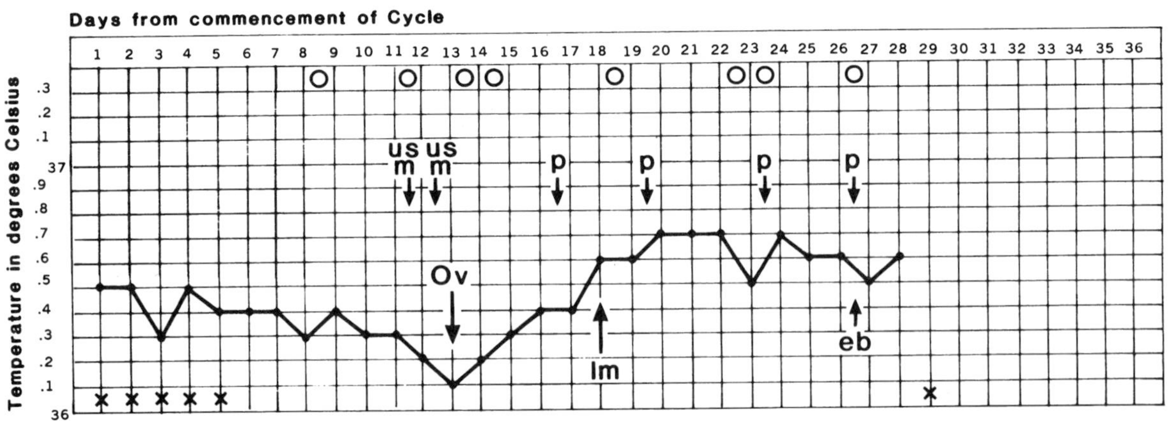

Fig. 5.3 An idealized basal body temperature chart indicating the approximate timing of physiological events such as ovulation (Ov), implantation (Im), menstruation (×) and sexual intercourse (○). The timing of helpful investigations such as follicle ultrasound scanning (us), preovulatory cervical mucus sampling (m), serum progesterone sampling (p), and a premenstrual endometrial biopsy (eb) is also shown.

The chart can also be used to record the presence of preovulatory cervical mucus (an end-organ effect of the preovulatory estradiol surge), the occurrence of midcycle 'periovulatory' lower abdominal pain (Mittelschmerz), and the timing of blood samples and a premenstrual endometrial biopsy (Fig. 5.3). The basal body temperature rise is due to a minor resetting of the hypothalamic 'thermostat' by circulating progesterone. The typical histological appearances of a well-timed premenstrual endometrial biopsy are due to an integrated effect of unopposed follicular phase estradiol followed by a combination of luteal phase estradiol and progesterone in appropriate amounts for the optimum length of time. A normal appearance also confirms the appropriate endometrial response to these precise hormone changes. Abnormal appearances require very careful assessment before a diagnosis of luteal phase defect can be made.

In recent years very detailed endocrine information on follicle development has been obtained by daily, or more frequent, blood sampling (for FSH, LH, estradiol, progesterone, and sometimes other steroids) during induction of ovulation in amenorrheic women, during stimulated and unstimulated cycles for in vitro fertilization, as well as in women with apparently normal ovarian function. Normal patterns are summarised in Figure 5.1 and Table 5.1. These have been complemented by ovarian ultrasound scanning of follicle growth and the process of ovulation. Modern ultrasound, especially using a transvaginal probe, can accurately demonstrate daily changes in size of the growing follicle(s), and collapse of the follicle at ovulation. This technique indicates that the symptom of Mittelschmerz usually precedes follicle collapse. Clinicians should beware ultrasound reports of ovarian 'cysts', since these are frequently merely growing or atretic follicles. In general, simple unilocular 'cysts' should only be considered pathological if they are larger than 5 cm in diameter and have not disappeared on repeat scanning 2–3 weeks later.

Reproductive potential declines steadily with increasing age over 35 years, and extensive recent data indicate that this is due mainly to changes within the ovary. This correlates with processes of follicular depletion and diminished oocyte quality, and may be termed 'diminished ovarian reserve'. A number of tests have been developed which have high predictive value for failure to conceive (Scott & Hoffman 1995).

DISTURBANCES OF OVARIAN FUNCTION AND THEIR ASSESSMENT

Normal ovarian function has been discussed in detail in the previous section. In this section those factors that may disturb ovarian function and the conditions that accompany them are considered in moderate detail, with recommendations for investigation of each condition. Those readers who wish to obtain greater detail are referred to the end section on further reading.

Factors interfering with ovarian function

Hypothalamic factors

Numerous factors have the possibility of influencing ovarian function through higher centers, with the hypothalamus as the final common pathway. These include substantial weight loss, excessive exercise, acute psychological stress, and a variety of medications. Rare conditions such as organic hypothalamic disease, malnutrition, severe illness, or cachexia may have the same effect. These usually result in amenorrhea through suppression of GnRH secretion or stimulation of prolactin secretion.

Pituitary factors

Any pituitary disease which interferes with FSH and LH secretion will interfere with ovarian function. These include panhypopituitarism, postpartum pituitary necrosis (Sheehan's syndrome), craniopharyngioma, prolactinoma, mixed growth hormone and prolactin secreting adenomas, and, rarely, other pituitary adenomas or granulomas. Pituitary tumors secreting excessive amounts of FSH or LH have not been recorded in women.

Ovarian factors

Numerous primary ovarian diseases may interfere with normal ovarian function, and these are discussed in detail below. They include causes of premature ovarian failure, as well as a range of benign and malignant tumors.

Pelvic factors

Pelvic factors such as periovarian adhesions and endometriosis may temporarily disturb ovarian function. Adhesions have occasionally been demonstrated to cause luteal phase defect and often interfere mechanically with ovum transfer to the tubal fimbria. Some women with endometriosis may exhibit the luteinized unruptured follicle syndrome where the ovum remains entrapped in the follicle in spite of luteinization and other endocrine changes suggestive of ovulation.

Secondary amenorrhea

This can be defined in several ways, but is usually accepted as a condition where a woman has previously had fairly regular menstrual periods, but then becomes significantly overdue with her next period. It is usually due to insufficient cyclical secretion of ovarian estradiol to cause endometrial proliferation and, later, endometrial breakdown and bleeding as estradiol (± progesterone) levels fall. It does not usually require investigation until 6–12 months have elapsed.

Oligomenorrhea is a condition where menstruation occurs less frequently than normal and is usually classified broadly into mild (5–8 weekly cycles), moderate (8–12 weekly cycles) and severe oligomenorrhea (less than four menstrual periods per year). The causes are very similar to those for secondary amenorrhea (Table 5.2), and oligomenorrhea can be regarded as a spectrum of menstrual cycle frequency and regularity from normal cycles through to complete amenorrhea. Women with moderate or severe oligomenorrhea should generally undergo simple endocrine investigations to elucidate the cause. The majority of women with oligomenorrhea will be found to have polycystic ovarian disease.

The commonest physiological causes of amenorrhea are, of course, pregnancy and subsequent lactation. In most developed countries the frequency of different pathological types of secondary amenorrhea is approximately as follows: hypothalamic (50%); hyperprolactinemia (20%); polycystic ovarian disease (20%); true premature menopause (5%); and other causes, including resistant ovary syndrome, thyroid disease, and intrauterine adhesions (5%). Associated symptoms may often serve to suggest the underlying cause, but further investigations are usually mandatory (Table 5.3).

Table 5.2 Causes of amenorrhea

Hypothalamic
Excessive weight loss
Excessive exercise
Psychological 'stress'
'Post-pill' amenorrhea
Psychiatric conditions
Severe chronic illness
Rare tumors and granulomas
Hyperprolactinemia
No detectable pituitary lesion
Pituitary prolactinoma (micro-/macroadenoma)
Other pituitary tumor
Hypothyroidism
Drugs (e.g. phenothiazines)
Rare causes, such as renal failure
Hypopituitarism
Panhypopituitarism
Sheehan's syndrome
Rare causes, such as trauma, surgery, irradiation, infections, and granulomas
Polycystic ovarian disease
True premature menopause
Resistant ovary syndrome
Genital tract causes
Intrauterine adhesions
Cervical stenosis
Hysterectomy
Other (rare)
Hypo- and hyperfunction of thyroid or adrenal cortex
Androgen-secreting tumor
Chronic active hepatitis
Chronic renal failure
Cushing's syndrome

Table 5.3 Investigations for secondary amenorrhea

- Height and weight estimations (body mass index)
- Serum prolactin – to detect hyperprolactinemia
- Serum FSH – to detect ovarian failure
- Serum LH – to detect polycystic ovarian disease and confirm ovarian failure
- Serum estradiol – to assess risk of osteoporosis
- Serum TSH and thyroid function tests – to detect hypo- and hyperthyroidism
- Pituitary fossa CT scan (if hyperprolactinemia is present) to assess presence of an adenoma
- Other, if indicated (consider pregnancy test)

'Hypothalamic' amenorrhea is that form of amenorrhea associated with a decreased frequency and amplitude of GnRH secretion in the presence of normal prolactin secretion. A variety of different conditions may act through this common pathway, and these include: very low body weight and substantial weight loss (in extreme cases this includes anorexia nervosa); excessive exercise; some psychological stresses (e.g. grief reactions); some psychiatric conditions; and, occasionally, following cessation of oral contraceptives ('post-pill amenorrhea', which is statistically more common in women with a history of preceding oligomenorrhea). Severe physical illnesses such as conditions causing cachexia and severe malnutrition probably act via this pathway. The substantial depression in GnRH secretion results in a significant depression in FSH and LH secretion and hence low serum levels of these hormones. This, in turn, leads to reduced ovarian follicle stimulation with low serum levels of estradiol, no ovulation, and very low serum levels of progesterone. Serum levels of prolactin, androgens, thyrotrophin (TSH), and thyroid function tests usually remain within the normal range. The main concerns about long-term amenorrhea associated with low estrogen secretion are those of osteoporosis, vaginal atrophy, and sometimes reduced libido (see the section on menopause, above).

Increased secretion of prolactin causes a suppression of GnRH secretion in proportion to the degree of hyperprolactinemia resulting in depressed FSH and LH secretion, and hence depressed ovarian stimulation (and therefore oligo- or amenorrhea). Hyperprolactinemia can be caused by a number of factors (Table 5.2) and levels greater than twice the upper limit of normal on repeated testing should always be investigated further. It should be remembered that prolactin is a stress hormone and levels may be transiently elevated by many factors. Levels are also influenced by the time of day and are markedly elevated during sleep. The major concern is the possibility of a pituitary tumor (prolactin-secreting micro- or macroadenoma), and a high resolution computed tomography (CT) scan or magnetic resonance imaging (MRI) scan is the most effective means of evaluating this. Prolactin can be released by thyrotrophin-releasing hormone (TRH), and hence hyperprolactinemia may sometimes be caused by primary hypothyroidism where TRH and TSH secretion are increased.

Both hypothyroidism (elevated serum TSH levels and depressed T3 and T4) and hyperthyroidism (low levels of TSH and elevated T3 and T4) can cause depression of ovarian function and hence amenorrhea. Abnormalities of adrenal cortical function may also cause amenorrhea.

Intrauterine or cervical adhesions (Asherman's syndrome), endometrial fibrosis, and endometrial tuberculosis are the only conditions which are likely to cause secondary amenorrhea by a direct effect on the genital tract. In these conditions cyclical ovarian function usually continues normally.

Investigations initially recommended (Table 5.3) include those detailed below.

Serum prolactin is the most important single investigation in women with secondary amenorrhea to exclude hyperprolactinemia and a risk of pituitary adenoma. If prolactin is elevated on two occasions to more than twice the upper limit of normal (usually about 2–20 ng/ml or 100–600 iu/l), the pituitary should be evaluated for the presence of an adenoma by a high resolution CT or MRI scan. Prolactin may be mildly elevated in women with polycystic ovaries, or those taking certain drugs.

Serum FSH will be greatly elevated if premature ovarian failure or resistant ovary syndrome is present. Levels will be in the normal range (Table 5.1) or low, with hypothalamic amenorrhea, hyperprolactinemia, or polycystic ovarian disease.

Serum LH will be elevated with premature ovarian failure, resistant ovary syndrome, or polycystic ovarian disease. Levels will be normal (Table 5.1) or low, with hypothalamic amenorrhea or hyperprolactinemia.

Serum estradiol (Table 5.1) will be low or very low in cases of hypothalamic amenorrhea, hyperprolactinemia, or ovarian failure. The importance of this assay is to assess the risk of long-term osteoporosis which increases progressively as the mean estradiol concentration falls below 150 pmol/l.

Serum thyrotrophin (TSH) and thyroid function tests are necessary to exclude hypo- and hyperthyroidism.

Height and weight should always be recorded,

and the body mass index (BMI) can be calculated (weight in kilograms divided by height in meters squared) to give an indication of the degree of obesity or thinness (normal range 20–25).

Other investigations are only indicated if there is suspicion of a less usual cause of amenorrhea, for example, a hysterosalpingogram, hysteroscopy, or attempted dilatation and curettage may confirm cervical stenosis or intrauterine adhesions (Asherman's syndrome). Curettage may also remove tissue from the rare case of missed abortion, where retained products of conception cause amenorrhea.

Transvaginal ovarian ultrasound scan may demonstrate unilocular thin-walled cystic structures within the ovary in some women with different types of amenorrhea. These cystic structures are usually follicles (immature or atretic) which show episodic changes in size. They do not require laparotomy and removal, or even assessment by laparoscopy, unless they are persistent or greater than 5 cm in diameter.

Primary amenorrhea

This condition is usually defined as the failure of menstruation to occur on any occasion by the age of 17 years. It is important to distinguish those women in whom other signs of puberty have occurred at the normal age from those in whom amenorrhea is but one feature of the complete absence of pubertal changes (delayed puberty). It is reasonable to initiate investigations at the age of 15 years in the girl with delayed puberty. It should be recognized that primary amenorrhea is a relatively uncommon condition, while secondary amenorrhea is common. In some cases the pathogenesis of primary and secondary amenorrhea is similar, but there are important differences.

Delayed puberty

- Premature ovarian failure – including chromosome anomalies such as Turner's syndrome, ovarian agenesis with normal chromosomes, autoimmune, galactosemia, and some cases of 46,XY gonadal dysgenesis.
- Physiological delay.
- Hypothalamic amenorrhea due to weight loss, heavy exercise, or anorexia nervosa.
- Isolated GnRH deficiency (hypogonadotrophic hypogonadism) is probably due to a functional lesion higher in the brain interrupting the normal mechanisms which trigger puberty. An important subgroup is associated with congenital anosmia (Kallmann's syndrome), where there is a genetically determined failure of migration of GnRH neurons from their embryonic origins in the olfactory region of the brain.
- Organic central nervous system defects. These are very rare and include craniopharyngioma, other intracranial tumors, trauma, and panhypopituitarism.
- Primary hypothyroidism.

Primary amenorrhea with normal onset of puberty

- Mullerian agenesis
- Imperforate hymen
- Polycystic ovarian disease
- Hyperprolactinemia (with or without pituitary adenoma)
- Testicular feminization (46,XY).

Primary amenorrhoea with virilization at onset of puberty.

- Adrenal hyperplasia
- True hermaphrodite

A number of other rare conditions have been described which can occasionally cause primary amenorrhea or delayed puberty.

The priorities for investigation of delayed puberty and primary amenorrhea are different from those of secondary amenorrhea, but the principles are the same (Table 5.4). Initial investigations should look to distinguish premature ovarian failure, hypogonadotrophic hypogonadism (including isolated GnRH deficiency), polycystic ovarian disease, hyperprolactinemia, and mullerian agenesis. Rarer causes should only be investigated when these commoner causes have been excluded. The main investigations are serum measurements of FSH, LH, prolactin, TSH, and thyroid function tests. Pelvic ultrasound and cranial CT scanning may provide useful imaging of ovary, uterus, and intracranial structures. Chromosome studies may be helpful in ovarian failure or if an intersex condition is suspected.

Table 5.4 Investigations for primary amenorrhea

- Height and weight estimations (body mass index)
- Serum FSH – to detect ovarian failure
- Serum LH – to detect polycystic ovarian disease and confirm ovarian failure
- Serum prolactin – to detect hyperprolactinemia
- Serum estraidol – to assess risk of osteoporosis
- Serum TSH and thyroid function tests
- Chromosomes – to detect chromosomal anomalies in ovarian failure and intersex conditions
- Transvaginal ultrasound scan – to assess uterine and ovarian size and follicular activity
- Examination under anesthesia – to exclude mullerian agenesis or 'imperforate hymen'
- Pituitary CT scan – to exclude pituitary and hypothalamic tumors, including craniopharyngioma
- Other, if indicated

Table 5.5 Investigation of premature ovarian failure

- Serum FSH – greatly elevated
- Serum LH – elevated
- Serum estradiol – low; mean levels below 150 pmol/l may be associated with risk of osteoporosis
- Tissue antibody screen – to identify individual with autoimmune ovarian failure and other autoimmune conditions
- Chromosomes – to detect karyotype abnormalities
- Galactose 1-phosphate and galactose assay – to exclude galactosemia
- Bilateral ovarian wedge biopsy – to distinguish resistant ovary syndrome from true premature menopause

Premature ovarian failure

Ovarian failure may be caused at an early age by several recognized mechanisms, although many cases remain of unknown cause. Ovarian failure before the age of 40 years is usually designated as premature menopause and should be investigated. True premature menopause should be distinguished from resistant ovary syndrome (see Ch. 8). Established causes include genetic mechanisms, immunological factors leading to the development of ovarian autoantibodies (usually to antigens on the follicular apparatus), galactosemia, some mucopolysaccaridoses, mumps oophoritis, and some types of chemotherapy. Genetic mechanisms may act through gross errors such as major chromosome deletions (e.g. 45,X, Turner's syndrome), or in a more subtle manner in those families with a strong family history of premature ovarian failure, but no obvious chromosome anomaly or families with blepharophimosis. Increasing numbers of case reports are appearing with descriptions of X-chromosome microdeletions.

Endocrine findings with true premature menopause are identical to those with natural menopause. In women with resistant ovary syndrome serum levels of FSH and LH are markedly elevated, but usually to a lesser degree than in true menopause. Investigations are summarized in Table 5.5.

Serum FSH is always greatly elevated above the upper limit of the normal range during the reproductive years. There is no overlap between the postovarian failure range and the reproductive range. Women with resistant ovary syndrome also have elevated levels, but usually somewhat less than true ovarian failure. If these women are treated with estrogen, serum FSH levels fall.

Serum LH is also elevated, but markedly pulsatile fluctuations allow an overlap with the normal range in the reproductive years.

Serum estradiol is usually very low, and levels below 150 pmol/l correlate with a progressively increasing long-term risk of osteoporosis.

Autoimmune screen may identify those individuals with an immunological basis for their premature ovarian failure. As well as looking for serum ovarian autoantibodies, the patient should have a more detailed screen, looking particularly for antibodies to adrenal cortical, thyroid, parathyroid, and gastric parietal tissues. Autoimmune failure of one or more of these organs may precede or follow autoimmune ovarian failure.

Karyotyping should always be carried out if the patient is in the younger reproductive years because of the possibility of detecting women with some X-chromosome anomalies (especially Turner's syndrome 45,X or Turner mosaics). Karotyping is normally performed on white blood cells, but skin fibroblasts (or even ovarian tissue, if possible) should also be tested if mosaicism is suspected.

Screening for galactose-1-phosphatase activity should be carried out to exclude cases of galactosemia that have remained undiagnosed through childhood and adolescence. This can be done by measuring blood levels of galactose and galactose 1-phosphate.

Bilateral ovarian wedge biopsy is sometimes

advised to distinguish between true ovarian failure, with complete or almost complete depletion of oocytes, and resistant ovary syndrome in which histologically normal oocytes (usually primordial follicles only) are still present. It is usually advised that a deep wedge should be excised through a small laparotomy incision with use of a uterine elevator to bring the ovaries close to the incision. Precautions of the type used in pelvic microsurgery should be utilized to minimize the risk of postoperative adhesion formation. Biopsies obtained through the laparoscope may be too small for definitive diagnosis. Recently, the value of ovarian biopsy has been questioned because of the occasional pregnancy which has occurred in women in whom biopsy had not demonstrated any oocytes. Even bilateral ovarian wedge biopsies collected at laparotomy may not be entirely representative of all areas of each ovary, but the information obtained is often helpful in counseling. Ovarian biopsy may also demonstrate white cell infiltrates in cases with an autoimmune basis.

Polycystic ovarian disease

This is a complex condition which is discussed in fuller detail in Chapter 13. Most women exhibit enlarged ovaries which contain an increased number of variable sized follicles (generally 1–10 mm in diameter) which vary through immature stages to atresia. It is uncommon to find mature Graafian follicles and ovulation. Many variants are found in terms of clinical presentation, hormone patterns and ovarian appearances.

The endocrinology of this condition is just as complex as the clinical features (Table 5.6). Most women demonstrate a substantially increased pulsatile release of LH and a low, or low to normal, circulating level of FSH. This gives an LH/FSH ratio of greater than 3 in typical cases. However, several separate serum measurements may be required to demonstrate this convincingly because of the pulsatile nature of the LH release. Recent studies have demonstrated an increase in circulating levels of inhibin, but this assay is only available in a small number of research centers. The relatively unfluctuating level of FSH means that few, if any, follicles are stimulated to reach full maturity and ovulate, however many immature antral follicles are present which are capable of being stimulated by the increased levels of LH. Since immature follicles tend to produce mainly androgenic steroids, including androstenedione and testosterone, circulating levels of these hormones are often clearly elevated. Serum levels of free testosterone are usually well above the normal range. Dehydroepiandrosterone sulfate (DHAS) may be marginally elevated, suggesting a subtle adrenal androgenic involvement. Serum levels of prolactin may also be mildly elevated and these can be capable of stimulating an increase in adrenal androgen secretion. Many women with polycystic ovarian disease are obese and the increased amount of adipose tissue may be capable of peripheral aromatization of circulating androgens into estrogens, particularly estrone. In view of this conversion there may be an increase in the serum ratio of estrone to estradiol (a reversal of the ratio found in most women in the reproductive age group). Although estrone is less biologically active than estradiol, it has sufficient activity to stimulate estrogen receptors, thus interfering with estrogen feedback mechanisms in the hypothalamus and pituitary. This may also cause endometrial stimulation, resulting in cystic glandular hyperplasia, abnormal bleeding and, if prolonged over many years, occasionally endometrial adenocarcinoma at a young age.

Table 5.6 Investigation of polycystic ovarian disease

- Height and weight measurements (body mass index)
- Serum LH – usually elevated
- Serum FSH – usually low
- Serum LH to FSH ratio – often >3
- Serum testosterone (preferably free testosterone) – usually elevated
- Serum estrone to estradiol ratio – usually elevated
- Serum prolactin – often mildly elevated
- Dilatation and curettage – to exclude those women with hyperestrogenism and endometrial hyperplasia
- Transvaginal pelvic ultrasound – to assess ovaries
- Short ACTH stimulation test – to distinguish polycystic ovarian disease from late-onset congenital adrenal hyperplasia
- Glucose tolerance test – to detect carbohydrate intolerance

Polycystic ovarian disease (PCOS) has recently been investigated in greater detail than previously with the use of transvaginal ultrasound scanning. This has resulted in the recent widely accepted definition that polycystic ovarian disease is the typical ultrasound appearance combined with one or more symptoms. It needs to be recognized that ultrasound appearances consistent with PCOS may be found in 20% of women with regular cycles, which probably defines an 'at-risk' population. The typical appearance demonstrated on ultrasound is of a 'necklace' of small follicles around the periphery of both ovaries. Ideally, at least 10 follicles should be seen in each ovary.

Polycystic ovarian disease should be distinguished from the adolescent-onset type of congenital adrenal hyperplasia due to incomplete 21-hydroxylase deficiency (preferably by a short adrenocorticotrophic hormone (ACTH) stimulation test following low dose dexamethasone suppression). The association between polycystic ovarian disease and the condition sometimes called ovarian hyperthecosis is not at all clear, but it seems most likely that the majority of cases are a late stage or a variant of polycystic ovarian disease. They are usually associated with substantially increased ovarian androgen secretion and a moderately elevated LH/FSH ratio.

Hirsutism

Hirsutism is the excessive growth of terminal hair, in a male distribution, in women and it is frequently associated with an excessive secretion of androgens from the ovaries. Hirsutism is generally a benign condition and is frequently associated with a greater or lesser degree of acne on the face, chest, and back. The most important clinical need is to look for signs of virilization, including clitoromegaly, frontal balding, deepening of the voice, and increased muscle mass. These signs make the presence of a rare androgen-secreting tumor much more likely. The extent of the hirsutism should be assessed objectively and recorded using a scoring system such as that proposed by Ferriman & Galwey (1969).

Clinical associations with hirsutism (Table 5.7) include: polycystic ovarian disease; ovarian stromal hyperplasia; adolescent-onset congenital adrenal hyperplasia; androgen-secreting tumors of ovarian and adrenal origin; the ingestion of drugs such as danazol, norethisterone, levonorgestrel, androgens, and occasionally others; and, rarely, such diseases as Cushing's syndrome, acromegaly, hypothyroidism, and porphyria. Very rarely, hirsutism and virilization may occur in pregnancy because of the development of an androgen-secreting luteoma of pregnancy, hyperreactio sex cord-stromal tumor.

Table 5.7 Causes of hirsutism

- Racial and constitutional factors
- Polycystic ovarian disease (70–80% of cases)
- Idiopathic benign hirsutism (usually mild ovarian hyperandrogenism)
- Late onset congenital adrenal hyperplasia (typically familial and in certain racial groups, such as Ashkenazy Jews)
- Drugs (especially danazol and certain progestogens)
- Androgen-secreting ovarian or adrenal tumors
- Cushing's syndrome
- Acromegaly
- Hypothyroidism
- Porphyria
- Pregnancy-associated ovarian luteoma

Table 5.8 Investigations for hirsutism

- Hirsutism scoring (Ferriman and Galwey score)
- Serum testosterone (preferably serum free testosterone, which can only be assayed in a few centers)
- Nil else required (in mild cases with regular menstrual cycles)
- Other androgens including dehydroepiandrosterone sulfate (DHAS) – to assess a possible adrenal component
- Serum LH and FSH – to assess the presence of PCOS
- Serum sex hormone binding globulin (SHBG) – may sometimes be depressed by hyperandrogenism
- Serum prolactin – sometimes mildly elevated in hirsute women with PCOS
- Transvaginal ultrasound – to assess presence of PCOS
- 24-h urinary free cortisol – to exclude Cushing's disease
- Short-ACTH stimulation test – to detect late-onset congenital adrenal hyperplasia
- Other investigations if specifically indicated, e.g. pelvic and abdominal CT scan, laparoscopy, or laparotomy to exclude tumor

Most women with benign hirsutism have a mild to moderate degree of hyperandrogenism (Table 5.8). This is most easily demonstrated by an increase in the serum concentration of *free* testosterone. The majority of circulating testosterone is bound to sex hormone binding globulin which may often be suppressed in women with hyperandrogenism. For this reason the level of *total* circulating testosterone is often only slightly increased. There is also a significant increase in the secretion rate of testosterone. The hyperandrogenism is usually associated with an increase in local hair follicle sensitivity to androgens through an increase in 5a-reductase enzyme activity. Local variations in hair follicle sensitivity at different sites on the body presumably account for the very variable distribution of excessive hair growth in different individuals with hirsutism.

In some women there is an increase in the circulating levels of 17-hydroxyprogesterone and DHAS, and this usually indicates an adrenal component in the increased androgen secretion. A short ACTH stimulation test with low dose dexamethasone suppression and the measurement of 17-hydroxyprogesterone and DHAS will demonstrate the presence of an adrenal component (especially late-onset congenital adrenal hyperplasia). Measurement of 24-h urinary free cortisol will usually demonstrate the presence of Cushing's syndrome. A substantially elevated ratio of plasma LH/FSH will usually confirm or exclude the presence of polycystic ovarian disease. Sometimes this condition is also associated with mild hyperprolactinemia.

If the total serum testosterone level is greater than twice the upper limit of the normal range, an androgen secreting tumor becomes a much more likely cause and should be excluded. The most likely site is in the ovary and this may be investigated further by high resolution transvaginal ultrasound scan, high resolution pelvic CT, laparoscopy, or even laparotomy with incision of both ovaries. It should be remembered than androgen-secreting tumors may be quite small. Most clinical investigators now feel that venous catheterization studies, and stimulation and suppression tests with measurement of local androgen concentrations should rarely be used. These are difficult techniques and there are problems in interpreting the results. The presence of an adrenal tumor is nowadays best excluded by high resolution CT scan or MRI.

Ovarian neoplasms may secrete a range of estrogenic and androgenic steroids and it is not usually possible to predict the type of tumor from the pattern of circulating androgens and estrogens. Ovarian tumors which may secrete androgens include hilus cell tumors, thecomas, stromal luteomas, androblastomas, gynandroblastomas, granulosa cell tumors, gonadoblastomas and, occasionally, adenocarcinomas metastatic to the ovaries.

Finally, it should be recognized that women with mild to moderate benign hirsutism and regular menstrual cycles probably do not need any specific investigations apart from total serum testosterone and a hirsutism score before therapy is instituted. However, if the woman exhibits irregular menstrual cycles or signs of virilization, then further investigation is mandatory and the extent of the investigations pursued will depend upon the clinical features and the degree of hyperandrogenism.

Precocious puberty

Precocious puberty is a rare clinical problem. This usually includes the obvious occurrence of breast or pubic hair changes before the age of 8 years, or the menarche before the age of 9 years. This can occur at almost any age and menarche has even been recorded in a child before the age of 1 year. This should be distinguished from the occasional occurrence of menstrual bleeding soon after birth, which is associated with transient ovarian or endometrial stimulation by maternal hormones. In girls, isosexual precocity is usually of the 'constitutional' type (true precocious puberty), in that the cause appears to be an early triggering of the normal mechanisms of puberty (Table 5.9). However, occasionally tumors or other causes may be found to be the cause of isosexual pseudoprecocity.

Feminizing ovarian tumors are uncommonly seen, and the commonest of these are granulosa cell tumors (see Ch. 33).

A range of different investigations may be helpful in determining the cause of apparent precocious puberty, and these are summarized in Table 5.10.

Intersex conditions

A useful working definition of intersex is an individual who demonstrates conflict between

Table 5.9 Causes of precocious puberty

- Constitutional
- Central nervous system causes, tumors, granulomas
- Ovarian tumors
- Adrenal tumors
- Gonadotrophin-secreting tumors
- Other, including McCune–Albright syndrome

Table 5.10 Investigations for precocious puberty

- Serum estradiol – if very high may indicate tumor
- Serum FSH and LH – of limited value; usually within adult range
- Serum androgens – usually in adult female range; may be elevated with virilizing tumor or tumor secreting both estrogens and androgens
- X-ray of hands and wrists – for bone age
- X-ray of long bones – to exclude McCune Albright syndrome
- CT scan or MRI of head – to exclude CNS disease
- Abdominal ultrasound scan of pelvis – to detect ovarian tumors, including follicular cysts secondary to ovarian stimulation, and to assess size of uterus
- CT scan or MRI of upper abdomen may be used to assess adrenals

chromosomal sex, gonadal sex, internal genital sex, and external genital or phenotypic sex. This is usually manifest at one or two times in life: first in the infant with ambiguous genitalia at the time of birth; and, secondly, at the time of puberty when a female child virilizes. This rare and complex situation is beginning to be evaluated by molecular biological techniques and is discussed thoroughly in Chapter 9.

Hormone-secreting neoplasms

The morphological characteristics of these tumors are described elsewhere, but they are briefly described here from a clinical viewpoint.

Ovarian tumors may sometimes secrete estrogens, androgens, a range of unusual steroids, chorionic gonadotrophin and, rarely, almost any other known type of hormone.

Localization of suspected ovarian tumors can be assisted by the use of transvaginal pelvic ultrasound, high resolution CT scanning or MRI. Sometimes laparoscopy or laparotomy (in difficult cases the ovaries may even need to be bivalved) may be required to diagnose or accurately assess the presence or extent of a tumor. Venous catheterization studies and specific stimulation or suppression tests are fraught with difficulties in interpretation and are not nowadays usually regarded as being particularly helpful. A number of nonhormonal circulating tumor markers such as inhibin, α-fetoprotein (AFP), and carcinoembryonic antigen (CEA) may have value in assessing and monitoring some tumors.

It should be noted that tumors in other parts of the genital tract, and even adrenal tumors, can sometimes secrete hormones that will mimic a functional ovarian tumor. Interestingly, it appears that steroid secretion requires a considerable degree of cellular specialization, and ectopic steroid secretion as a paraneoplastic phenomenon has not been encountered. The tumors which produce steroids arise in tissues that physiologically secrete steroids.

FURTHER READING

A great deal of ground has been covered only superficially in this chapter, and those who wish a more detailed review of individual aspects are referred to specialized texts such as:

Yen S Sc, Jaffe R B (eds) 1991 Reproductive endocrinology, W B Saunders, Philadelphia

REFERENCES

Baker T G 1963 A quantitative and cytological study of germ cells in human ovaries. Proceedings of the Royal Society 158: 417–429

Ferriman D, Galwey J D 1969 Clinical assessment of body hair growth in women. Journal of Clinical Endocrinology and Metabolism 21: 1440–1445

Scott R T, Hofmann G E 1995 Prognostic assessment of ovarian reserve. Fertility and Sterility 63: 1–11

Tanner J M 1962 Growth at adolescence. Blackwell Scientific, Oxford

SECTION 2

Dysgenesis, dystopia, and dysfunction

6

Anomalies of ovarian development and descent

P. Russell   A. Farnsworth

SUPERNUMERARY AND ACCESSORY OVARIES

Anomalies of ovarian development and descent are only rarely encountered. Ectopic ovarian tissue may occur in the presence or absence of normally sited ovaries. Where this occurs with normally sited ovaries they can be divided into (a) 'accessory' and (b) 'supernumerary' ovaries, as suggested by Wharton (1959), although the distinction is not always clear in the subsequent literature. Such anomalies are either isolated or occur with other congenital genitourinary malformations (such as unicornuate or bicornuate uterus, vaginal aplasia, accessory adrenal glands, lobulated liver). The additional ovarian tissue possesses functional potential.

Accessory ovarian tissue (the more common of the two variants) is typically seen as small nodules up to 1 cm across situated near a normally placed ovary, either within or suspended from the posterior leaf of the broad ligament, and physically connected to that normal ovary. In the past, these small pieces of tissue have been mistaken for lymph nodes at operation and only diagnosed upon histological examination (Schultze & Fenger 1986). They are mostly solitary.

Supernumerary ovaries (Printz et al 1973, Kosasa et al 1976, Cruikshank & van Drie 1982, Hahn-Pedersen & Larsen 1984, Lee & Gore 1984) are located at some distance from the eutopic ovary. They have been reported in the pelvis (in relation to the uterus, bladder, or pelvic wall) and the abdomen (retroperitoneum, omentum, or mesentery of the colon), and are not connected to the normal ovary. They may be single or multiple. They range in size from a few millimeters across to the dimensions of a normal ovary and may contain grossly visible follicular structures. The vast majority are incidental findings at autopsy, laparoscopy, or surgery. The documented sites of accessory and supernumerary ovarian tissue may possibly explain the origin of nonmullerian ovarian-type tumors in extraovarian sites such as the broad ligament and retroperitoneum, as well as accounting for persistent menstruation after bilateral oophorectomy (Kosasa et al 1976).

DYSTOPIC OVARIES

One or both ovaries, structurally and functionally normal, may be found in abnormal positions due to aberrant descent into the pelvis. They have been identified as high as the lower pole of the kidney, close to their embryological site of origin and as low as the inguinal canal (Goske et al 1984, Bradshaw & Carr 1986). There is one reported case of bilateral retroperitoneal ovaries (Campbell & Julian 1988). In some instances, malposition (dystopia) or maldescent of the ovaries is associated with ipsilateral anomalies of the mullerian duct derivatives (Rock et al 1986). In other patients, displacement of the ovary may be due to torsion, detachment, or parasitic attachment to the omentum or other intraperitoneal structures (Lachman & Berman 1991).

OVARIAN AGENESIS

Confusion exists concerning the terms agenesis and dysgenesis (see Ch. 7), and many of the reports in the early literature undoubtedly were examples of streak gonads rather than true agenesis. Rare cases of truly agonadal individuals have been reported usually with a karyotype 46,XY, and rarely with 46,XX (Peer et al 1981, Penney & Betz 1977).

Rarely, one ovary may be absent in an otherwise normal woman. Associated findings include agenesis or malformation of the ipsilateral fallopian tube, round ligament, kidney, and ureter, either alone or in combination. This may be due to dysgenesis of the urogenital ridge in early embryonic development (Ashley & Mostofi 1960). Most reported cases of absent ovaries, however, are probably due to antenatal torsion of an otherwise normal fallopian tube and ovary with necrosis and resorption of the adnexal structures (Best et al 1991) (see Ch. 17).

OVARIAN HYPOPLASIA

As a concept, this overlaps with both ovarian dysgenesis and premature ovarian failure, depending on the pathogenesis of the particular abnormality observed. The ovaries in patients with Turner's syndrome (with typical 45,X or mosaic karyotype) may have greatly reduced numbers of primordial follicles and little evidence of follicular activity at any stage of childhood or adult life. In most adult patients with Turner's syndrome, the end result of this ovarian 'hypoplasia' is a typical fibrous streak (see Ch. 7).

SPLENOGONADAL FUSION

This is a rare developmental abnormality in which, during an early phase of intrauterine development, there is an admixture of splenic and gonadal tissues resulting in the presence of splenic tissue in proximity to the ovary and hilar ductules (Watson 1968, Heinemann 1973). Splenogonadal fusion may be continuous, in which case a fibrous cord connects the splenic tissue in the pelvis with the spleen; or discontinuous, where no cord is present and nodules of splenic tissue are present along its presumed path. Putchar & Manion (1956) summarized the world literature to that date and recognized that a significant number of patients with splenogonadal fusion had severe congenital malformations of the extremities such as phocomelia. The coexistence of these abnormalities suggests that both were induced sometime between week 5 and 8 of gestation, possibly by administration of drugs or by intercurrent viral disease while the patient was in utero (Lenz & Knapp 1962, Mellin & Katzenstein 1962).

'UTERUS-LIKE MASS' REPLACING OVARY

In this rare condition the ovary is replaced by a mass characterized by a central cavity lined by endometrial tissue and surrounded by a thick smooth muscle wall (Cozzutto 1981, Pueblitz-Peredo et al 1985, Rahilly & Al-Nafussi 1991). The origin of this lesion may be an acquired tumor-like lesion, i.e. an ovarian endometriotic cyst with smooth muscle metaplasia (Cozzutto 1981), or it may be a congenital malformation of mullerian duct origin, with no normal ovarian development having taken place. The latter interpretation is supported by the presence of congenital abnormalities of the urinary tract in two cases (Rosai 1982, Pueblitz-Peredo et al 1985).

REFERENCES

Ashley D J B, Mostofi F K 1960 Renal agenesis and dysgenesis. Journal of Urology 83: 211–230

Best C L, Feldmann D B, Sobenes J R, Sueldo C E 1991 Unexplained displacement of ipsilateral ovary and fallopian tube. Obstetrics and Gynecology 78: 558–560

Bradshaw K D, Carr B R 1986 Ovarian and tubal inguinal hernia. Obstetrics and Gynecology 68: 50s–52s

Campbell B F, Julian T M 1988 Bilateral retroperitoneal ovaries. A case report. Journal of Reproductive Medicine 33: 839–842

Cozzutto C 1981 Uterus-like mass replacing ovary. Report of a new entity. Archives of Pathology and Laboratory Medicine 105: 508–511

Cruikshank S H, van Drie D M 1982 Supernumerary ovaries: update and review. Obstetrics and Gynecology 60: 126–129

Goske M J, Emmens R W, Rabinowitz R 1984 Inguinal

ovaries in children demonstrated by high resolution real-time ultrasound. Radiology 151: 635–636
Hahn-Pedersen J, Larsen P M 1984 Supernumerary ovary. Acta Obstetricia et Gynecologica Scandinavica 63: 365–366
Heinemann S 1973 Spleno-gonadal fusion. Urology 6: 686–687
Kosasa T S, Griffiths C T, Shane J M, Leventhal J M, Naftolin F 1976 Diagnosis of a supernumerary ovary with human chorionic gonadotropin. Obstetrics and Gynecology 47: 236–238
Lachman M F, Berman M M 1991 The ectopic ovary. A case report and review of the literature. Archives of Pathology and Laboratory Medicine 115: 233–235
Lee B, Gore B Z 1984 A case of supernumerary ovary. Obstetrics and Gynecology 64: 738–740
Lenz W, Knapp K 1962 Thalidomide embryopathy. Archives of Environmental Health 5: 100–105
Mellin G, Katzenstein M 1962 The saga of thalidomide. New England Journal of Medicine 267: 1184–1193
Peer E, Peretz B A, Makler A, Paldi E 1981 Bilateral adnexal agenesis with an ectopic ovary – case report and review of the literature. European Journal of Obstetrics Gynecology and Reproductive Biology 12: 37–42
Penny L L, Betz G 1977 Agonadism. Case report and review. American Journal of Obstetrics and Gynecology 127: 299–301
Printz J L, Choate J W, Townes P L, Harper R C 1973 The embryology of supernumerary ovaries. Obstetrics and Gynecology 41: 246–252
Pueblitz-Peredo S, Luevano-Flores E, Rincon-Taracena R, Ochoa-Carillo F J 1985 Uteruslike mass of the ovary: endomyometriosis or congenital malformation? Archives of Pathology and Laboratory Medicine 109: 361–364
Putchar W G, Manion W C 1956 Splenic–gonadal fusion. American Journal of Pathology 32: 15–33
Rahilly M A, Al-Nafussi A 1991 Uterus-like mass of the ovary associated with endometrioid carcinoma. Histopathology 18: 549–551
Rock J A, Parmley T, Murphy A A, Jones H W Jr 1986 Malposition of the ovary associated with uterine anomalies. Fertility and Sterility 45: 561–563
Rosai J 1982 Uterus-like mass replacing ovary (Letter). Archives of Pathology and Laboratory Medicine 106: 364–365
Schultze H, Fenger C 1986 Accessory ovary. Acta Obstetricia et Gynecologica Scandinavica 65: 503–504
Watson R J 1968 Splenogonadal fusion. Surgery 63: 853–858
Wharton L R 1959 Two cases of supernumerary ovary and one of accessory ovary with an analysis of previously reported cases. American Journal of Obstetrics and Gynecology 78: 1101–1118

7

Dysgenesis

P. Russell   A. Farnsworth

This chapter briefly describes a miscellany of histological appearances representing aberrant growth patterns or dysgenesis – some with known chromosomal and clinical associations, but others of unknown cause and significance. While 'dysplasia', in the strict sense of the word, may be an equally appropriate term, it has in recent times acquired certain connotations of premalignant atypia (Deligdisch & Gil 1989, Deligdisch et al 1993) entirely inappropriate to this discussion.

GONADAL DYSGENESIS (STREAK GONADS)

Dysgenetic or absent gonads may frequently be found in phenotypic females with 45,X karyotype, Turner's mosaic, 45,X/46,XY mosaic, trisomy 13, trisomy 18, structural X-aberrations, X/X-rearrangements and Y-aberrations, partial deletions of chromosome 2q (Davis et al 1991), and occasionally in association with 46,XX, 46,XY, trisomy 13, and triploidy (Cunniff et al 1991). The entity encompasses phenotypic females who are both SRY gene positive and negative, and is not therefore to be construed as indicating either testicular or ovarian dysgenesis (see below). In patients exhibiting chromosomal mosaicism, the gonadal development will reflect the relative proportions of normal and abnormal cells, and the resulting gonads will show features intermediate between normal ovaries and typical rudimentary streaks. Gonadal dysgenesis, therefore, extends beyond the clinically descriptive entity of 'streak gonad syndrome' of Bosze & Laszlo (1979). The term 'pure' gonadal dysgenesis has been applied to phenotypic females with bilateral streak gonads, a normal height (i.e. not Turner's phenotype), and a variety of karyotypes similar to those noted above. The term 'mixed' gonadal dysgenesis refers to comparable phenotypic and genotypic individuals who exhibit: (a) a dysgenetic gonad on one side and a testis, ovary or a gonadal tumor on the contralateral side; or (b) a gonad absent on one side and a testis, ovary, or gonadal tumor on the other side (the presence of ovary in these combinations is extremely rare (Schellhas 1974)). For example, in individuals with 46,XY pure gonadal dysgenesis, absence of testicular tissue suggests a mutation in the initial steps of the male-sex-determining pathway (Vilain et al 1993). Recent studies show this to produce a complete ('pure') or an incomplete ('mixed') form, the former with typical streaks and normal Mullerian ducts and female external genitalia, and the latter with ambiguous external genitalia and partial development of Mullerian and Wolffian structures (Berkovitz et al 1991). These patients showed a mixture of dysgenetic testes, streak gonads with ovarian stroma, occasional primitive sex cords and even rare primordial follicles, and ovotestes. Dysgenetic gonads are usually identified during the course of investigation for amenorrhea (usually primary but occasionally secondary) (McClure et al 1992), primary ovarian failure (see Ch. 8), and intersex states (see Ch. 9). Cardinal features observed in such individuals include infantile breasts, sparse pubic and axillary hair, infantile external genitalia and vagina, retarded ossification, and osteoporosis. High serum follicle stimulating hormone (FSH) levels and low estradiol levels confirm hypergonadotrophic hypogonadism.

A major consideration, however, is the known preneoplastic potential which has been shown to depend on the presence of Y-chromosomal elements in the karyotype (an intact Y chromosome or fragments) (Shah et al 1988, Krasna et al 1992). An overall risk of malignancy of approximately 25% in young phenotypic females with gonadal dysgenesis (higher with 'pure' dysgenesis and lower with 'mixed' forms) and a karyotype which includes Y-chromosomal material argues strongly for early prophylactic gonadectomy in these individuals (Olsen et al 1988, Muller et al 1992, Gourlay et al 1994). About 75% of tumors occurring in such individuals are gonadoblastomas (see Ch. 51), either alone or complicated by the supervention of a malignant germ cell tumor (Petersen et al 1992). The remainder are mostly pure dysgerminomas (Schellhas 1974, Scully 1979, Deligdisch et al 1988). The association of rare hematological malignancies (leukemia with a mixed germ cell tumor in a patient with 46,XY/47,XY+8 karyotype (Kaplan et al 1991), and true histiocytic malignancy with a malignant teratoma in a patient with 46,XY karyotype (Koo et al 1992)) in phenotypic female patients with XY gonadal dysgenesis also appears to be other than coincidental.

Macroscopic features

Typical dysgenetic or streak gonads exhibit a variable but usually conspicuous reduction in size, but a preservation of the normal anatomical relationships to adjacent pelvic ligaments and mullerian duct derivatives. They may measure up to 2–3 cm in length, but are frequently only a few millimeters thick.

Microscopic features

Dysgenetic gonads, in the adult, are composed almost exclusively of dense but inactive and relatively hypercellular ovarian-type stroma with no clear subdivision into cortex and medulla (Fig. 7.1). Typically, follicular structures or remnants are absent (Fig. 7.2), although a few may rarely persist in those individuals who are Turner's mosaics (it should be noted that, in early fetal life, these gonads are indistinguishable from normal and it is only progressive loss of oogonia and oocytes, as a result of faulty meiotic pairing – usually complete by puberty – which determines their ultimate histological appearances). Cortical inclusions may be present and these should not be mistaken for follicles. The rete ovarii and meso-

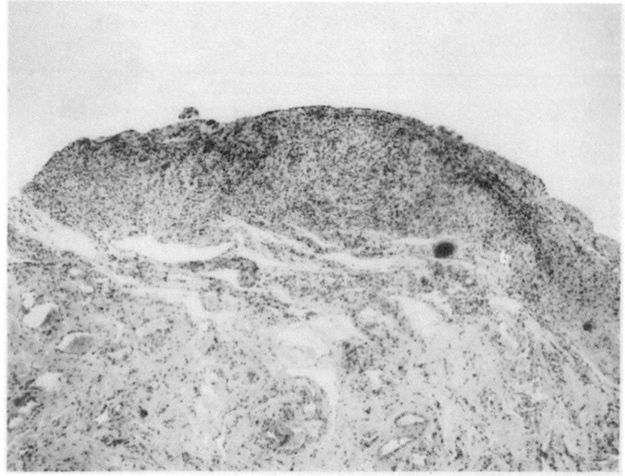

Fig. 7.1 Dysgenetic or streak gonad in a case of XY mixed gonadal dysgenesis. The rudimentary gonad is only a few millimeters across and is composed of ovarian-type stroma. H + E ×25

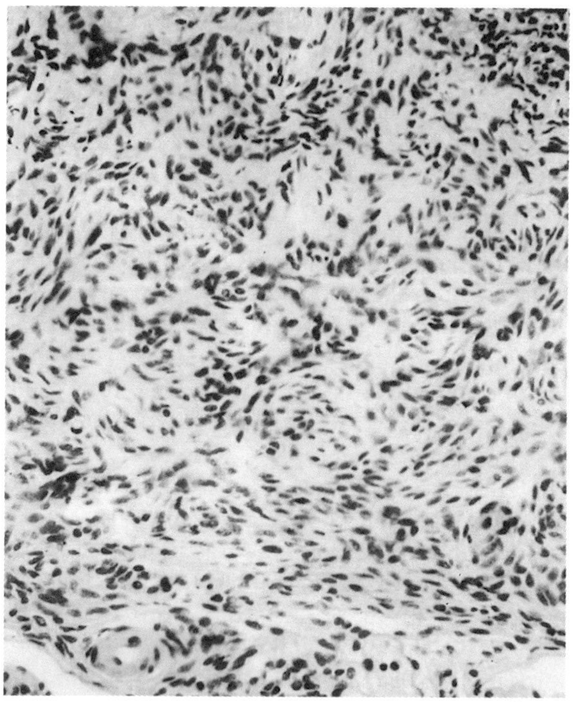

Fig. 7.2 Higher power image of Figure 7.1, showing typical dense hypercellular cortical stroma devoid of follicular structures or oocytes. H + E ×150

nephric tubular remnants are usually readily identifiable in the hilus, and Leydig cells may be seen in normal or somewhat increased numbers (Parmley 1983). Scattered lutein-like or Leydig-like cells may be present in the stroma but these do not aggregate to form consistently identifiable structures.

OVARIAN DYSGENESIS

A high percentage of live newborn babies with trisomy 18 are female, probably because male fetuses with this chromosomal anomaly selectively abort early in pregnancy. In a review of the literature, Warkany (1971) described 'ovarian hypoplasia' in 7 of 84 cases examined at autopsy. In most cases, the ovaries were small and either stated to be histologically normal or were not examined microscopically. However, the cases reported by Alexiou et al (1971) and our own studies (Russell & Altshuler 1975) showed microscopic abnormalities in most cases and severe ovarian dysgenesis in many, characterized by:

- Reduction in the numbers of both oocytes and primordial follicles; 'naked' oocytes in cortical stroma.
- Persistent plexiform cortical (secondary) sex cords in the gonadal stroma (Figs 7.3 and 7.4), containing pregranulosa cells and oocyte clusters.

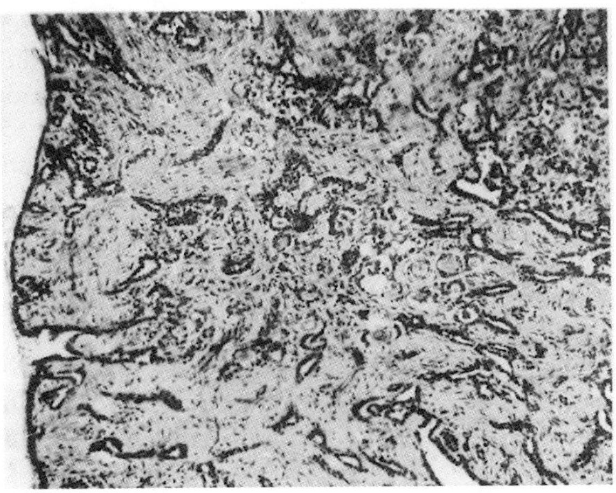

Fig. 7.3 Dysgenetic ovary in trisomy 18. Irregular cleft-like invaginations of surface coelomic epithelium into the ovarian cortex with disruption of normal architecture. H + E ×60

- Binucleate ova.
- Unilateral cystic follicles, up to 2 cm in diameter, and atretic follicles, some of which are dysplastic (see below).

A similar spectrum of anomalies has been found in cases of trisomy 13 (Moerman et al 1988) and an XXX karyotype with and without an associated trisomy 18 (Uchida et al 1962, Alexiou et al 1971, Spear & Porto 1988, Hood et al 1990). Fetal 'ovarian dysplasia' has been commented upon following induction of ovulation in the mother by clomiphene (Ford & Little 1981), but details were not given of histological findings.

FOLLICULAR DYSGENESIS (DYSPLASIA)

Dysplastic primary (pre-antral) and secondary (antral) follicles are occasionally encountered in otherwise normally functioning ovaries. The term 'follicular dysgenesis' has also been applied to polyovular primordial follicles (i.e. containing two

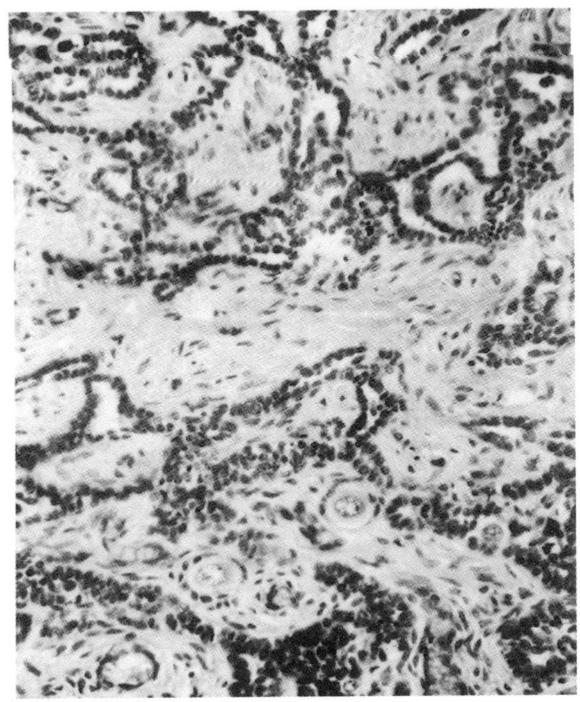

Fig. 7.4 Ovarian dysgenesis. Anastomosing cords and tubules of small granulosa-like cells, some incorporating oocytes. The intervening stroma is dense and fibrotic. H + E ×150

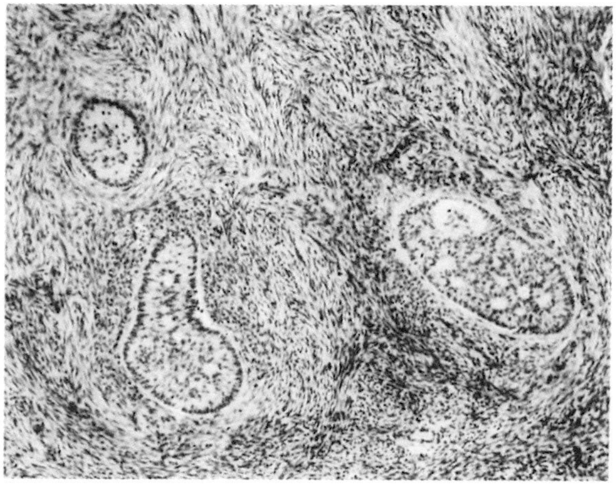

Fig. 7.5 Follicular dysgenesis. Three adjacent developing but dysgenetic or dysplastic follicles. Oocytes are absent. The cuff of theca interna cells is most obvious around the follicle to the lower left. H + E ×60

oocytes) by Parmley (1983), but it is the changes in developing follicles to which we believe the term is appropriate. Dysgenetic follicles differ morphologically from normal follicles by disorganization of the proliferated granulosa, frequently without an antrum despite the follicular size, and containing multiple Call–Exner bodies (Fig. 7.5). Some authors have likened these lesions to microscopic gonadoblastomas and have noted their frequent occurrence (25%) in pediatric ovaries (Manivel et al 1988). The follicular outline is also distorted with irregular extensions into the adjacent stroma (see Figs 8.5 and 8.6). Sometimes, follicular fragmentation produces small nests or cords of granulosa cells. Mitoses are reduced in these cells. Rarely, they contain cytoplasmic lipid. About one-third of dysplastic follicles are surrounded by a prominent cuff of theca interna cells (see Fig. 8.6) which are focally or partially luteinized. Atresia of the dysplastic follicles is generally accompanied by persistence of the granulosa – a phenomenon which is only occasionally observed in normal ovaries. Occasional dysplastic follicles show convoluted and rounded deposits of hyaline PAS-positive material similar to, and continuous with, the basement membrane (glassy membrane) of the regressing follicles. These deposits are interposed between the cords of granulosa cells in a manner resembling sex-cord tumors

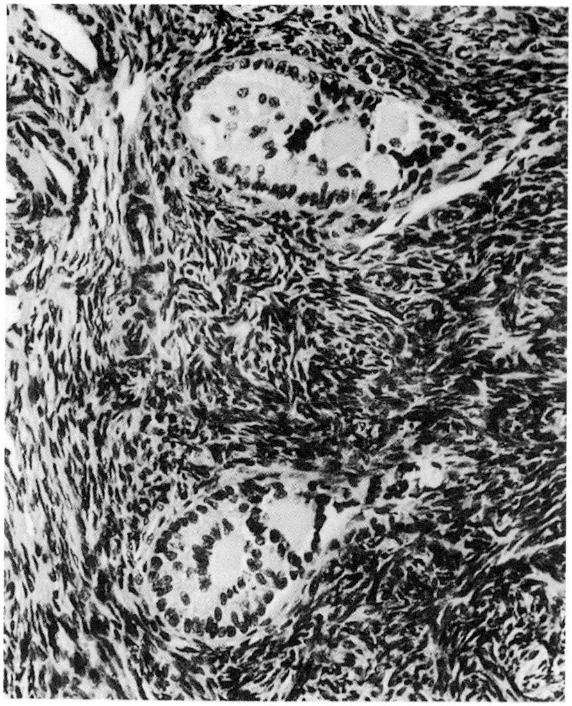

Fig. 7.6 Follicular dysgenesis. Markedly dysplastic primary follicles with a partly bilaminar arrangement of granulosa cells and interposition of eosinophilic hyaline material. The resultant appearance is similar to that found in sex-cord tumors with annular tubules (SCTAT) associated with Peutz–Jegher's syndrome (see Ch. 37). H + E ×150

with annular tubules (Fig. 7.6), a resemblance also commented upon by others (Safneck & de Sa 1986, Manivel et al 1988, Byrne et al 1989).

Hughesdon & Anderson (1985) have reported two and reviewed an additional two cases of follicular dysplasia which they interpret as representing a variant of polycystic ovarian disease. Their cases were associated with enlarged ovaries ('giant nodular ovaries'), and there was clinical and laboratory evidence suggestive of polycystic ovarian disease (gonadotrophin levels were not recorded). We have seen a similar morphological pattern in association with documented hypergonadotrophic premature ovarian failure (see Figs 8.5 and 8.6), but the relationship of the follicular changes to altered hypothalamic–pituitary–ovarian function remains unclear. Dysplastic follicles have been seen in some cases of autoimmune oophoritis (see Fig. 19.16), and in a case of ovarian fibromatosis (Byrne et al 1989).

REFERENCES

Alexiou D, Chrysostonidou O, Vlahos I, Deligeorgis D 1971 Trisomy 18 with ovarian dysgenesis. Acta Pediatrica Scandinavica 60: 93–97

Berkovitz G D, Fechner P Y, Zacur H W et al 1991 Clinical and pathologic spectrum of 46,XY gonadal dysgenesis: its relevance to the understanding of sex differentiation. Medicine Baltimore 70: 375–383

Bosze P, Laszlo J 1979 The streak gonad syndrome. Obstetrics and Gynecology 54: 544–548

Byrne P, Vella E J, Rollason T, Frampton J 1989 Ovarian fibromatosis with minor sex cord elements. Case report. British Journal of Obstetrics and Gynaecology 96: 245–248

Cunniff C, Jones K L, Benirschke K 1991 Ovarian dysgenesis in individuals with chromosomal abnormalities. Human Genetics 86: 552–556

Davis E, Grafe M, Cunniff C, Jones K L, Bogart M 1991 Interstitial deletion of chromosome 2q associated with ovarian dysgenesis. Clinical Genetics 39: 386–390

Deligdisch L, Gil J 1989 Characterization of ovarian dysplasia by interactive morphometry. Cancer 63: 748–755

Deligdisch L, Richards C J, Reyniak V J 1988 Pure gonadal dysgenesis and gonadal tumors: report of three cases and review of literature. Mount Sinai Journal of Medicine 55: 313–317

Deligdisch L, Miranda C, Barba J, Gil J 1993 Ovarian dysplasia: nuclear texture analysis. Cancer 72: 3253–3257

Ford W D A, Little K E T 1981 Fetal ovarian dysplasia possibly associated with clomiphene. Lancet i: 1107

Gourlay W A, Johnson H W, Pantzar J T, McGillivray B, Crawford R, Nielsen W R 1994 Gonadal tumors in disorders of sexual differentiation. Urology 43: 537–540

Hood O J, Hartwell E A, Shattuck K E, Rosenberg H S 1990 Multiple congenital anomalies associated with a 47,XXX chromosome constitution. American Journal of Medical Genetics 36: 73–75

Hughesdon P E, Anderson M C 1985 Giant nodular ovaries with aberrant follicles. Histopathology 9: 51–62

Kaplan S S, Bornstein S G, Christopherson W A, Surti U 1991 Associated leukemia and mixed germ cell tumor in a patient with gonadal dysgenesis. International Journal of Gynaecology and Obstetrics 35: 83–88

Koo C H, Reifel J, Kogut N, Cove J K, Rappaport H 1992 True histiocytic malignancy associated with a malignant teratoma in a patient with 46XY gonadal dysgenesis. American Journal of Surgical Pathology 16: 175–183

Krasna I H, Lee M L, Smilow P, Sciorra L, Eierman L 1992 Risk of malignancy in bilateral streak gonads: the role of the Y chromosome. Journal of Pediatric Surgery 27: 1376–1380

McClure N, Henry O, Harley J M 1992 Pure XY gonadal dysgenesis presenting as secondary amenorrhea. A case report. Journal of Reproductive Medicine 37: 291–292

Manivel J C, Dehner L P, Burke B 1988 Ovarian tumorlike structures, biovular follicles, and binucleate oocytes in children: their frequency and possible pathological significance. Pediatric Pathology 8: 283–292

Moerman P, Fryns J P, van der Steen K, Kleczkowska A, Lauweryns J 1988 The pathology of trisomy 13 syndrome. A study of 12 cases. Human Genetics 80: 349–356

Muller J, Visfeldt J, Philip J, Skakkebaek N E 1992 Carcinoma in situ, gonadoblastoma, and early invasive neoplasia in a nine-year-old girl with 46,XY gonadal dysgenesis. Acta Pathologica Microbiologica et Immunologica Scandinavica 100: 170–174

Olsen M M, Caldamone A A, Jackson C L, Zinn A 1988 Gonadoblastoma in infancy: indications for early gonadectomy in 46XY gonadal dysgenesis. Journal of Pediatric Surgery 23: 270–271

Parmley T 1983 The histologic morphology of gonadal dysgenesis: Early premature gonadal failure. Seminars in Reproductive Endocrinology 1: 121–127

Petersen L, Kock K, Jacobsen B B 1992 Germ cell neoplasms in three intersex patients with 46,XY karyotype. International Urology and Nephrology 24: 633–639

Phansey S A, Satterfield R, Jorgensen R I, Salinas C F, Yoder F E, Mathur R S, Williamson H O 1980 XY gonadal dysgenesis in three siblings. American Journal of Obstetrics and Gynecology 138: 133–138

Russell P, Altshuler G 1975 The ovarian dysgenesis of trisomy 18. Pathology 7: 149–155

Safneck J R, de Sa D J 1986 Structures mimicking sex cord-stromal tumors and gonadoblastomas in the ovaries of normal infants and children. Histopathology 10: 909–920

Schellhas H F 1974 Malignant potential of the dysgenetic gonad. Part I. Obstetrics and Gynecology 44: 298–309

Scully R E 1979 Tumors of the ovary and maldeveloped gonads. AFIP Fascicle 16, 2nd Series. Armed Forces Institute of Pathology, Washington, DC, p 300–310

Shah K D, Kaffe S, Gilbert F, Dolgin S, Gertner M 1988 Unilateral microscopic gonadoblastoma in a prepubertal Turner mosaic with Y chromosome material identified by restriction fragment analysis. American Journal of Clinical Pathology 90: 622–627

Spear G S, Porto M 1988 47,XXX chromosome constitution, ovarian dysgenesis, and genito-urinary malformation. American Journal of Medical Genetics 29: 511–515

Uchida I A, Lewis A J, Bowman J M, Wang H C 1962 A case of double trisomy: trisomy no. 18 and triplo-X. Journal of Pediatrics 60: 498–502

Vilain E, Jaubert F, Fellous M, McElreavey K 1993 Pathology of 46,XY pure gonadal dysgenesis: absence of testis differentiation associated with mutations in the testis-determining factor. Differentiation 52: 151–159

Warkany J 1971 Congenital malformations. Year Book, Chicago, IL, p 303–310

8

Ovarian failure

P. Russell   A. Farnsworth

Failure of ovarian steroidogenesis and ovulation may be associated with either elevated or depressed gonadotrophin levels Hypergonadotrophic hypogonadism (ovarian failure) is due to a congenital or acquired intrinsic ovarian defect, or failure of the ovaries to respond to pituitary gonadotrophins, despite the presence of follicles. Hypogonadotrophic hypogonadism is due to failure of the pituitary gland to secrete gonadotrophins (follicle stimulating hormone (FSH) and leutenizing hormone (LH)) in sufficient amounts to stimulate the ovaries.

Both ovarian failure and hypogonadotrophic hypogonadism can present as primary or secondary amenorrhea. Some patients with the former will qualify as having a premature menopause which is defined, in our institution, as secondary amenorrhea (with well developed secondary sex characteristics and a history of normal menarche) with continuously raised gonadotrophin levels, where the last menstrual period occurs prior to 35 years of age (i.e. 2 SD below the mean age of menopause of 51 years). The laboratory assessment of apparent ovarian failure is discussed in Chapter 5.

OVARIAN FAILURE (HYPERGONADOTROPHIC HYPOGONADISM)

Ovarian failure may be divided clinically into premature follicular depletion ('true premature menopause'), irreversible ovarian failure due to depletion of follicles (afollicular ovarian failure), and the resistant ovary syndrome ('gonadotrophin insensitivity syndrome'), in which primordial follicles are present but fail to respond appropriately to gonadotrophin stimulation (follicular ovarian failure) (Kinch et al 1965). Patients with apparent ovarian failure associated with chronic (autoimmune) oophoritis fit best into the latter category on therapeutic grounds – namely the possibility, in practice very slight, of recovery of ovarian function and reproductive capability. This separation into follicular and afollicular forms is somewhat artificial, since it is likely that many of the latter cases are end-stages of the former, but is critical clinically, since premature follicular depletion signifies permanent loss of reproductive function. Although ovarian biopsy is not necessary for the diagnosis of ovarian failure, and is argued against by some (Fox 1992, Khastgir et al 1994), it is the only means of distinguishing between follicular and afollicular types and is therefore recommended in patients desiring pregnancy (Gandar 1988, Fujii et al 1993), but one should bear in mind the possible surgical morbidity of the procedure and sampling problems, even in open biopsies. Bilateral wedge biopsies including medulla are required (Rebar et al 1982, Russell et al 1982), unless initial investigations have demonstrated a Y chromosome in the patient's karyotype, in which case bilateral total gonadectomy is indicated because of the risk of development of a germ cell tumor (see Ch. 7). The technical aspects of ovarian biopsies for the investigation of ovarian failure are discussed fully in Chapter 4. Clinical guidelines for the investigation and management of these patients are given by Tulandi & Kinch (1981), Coulam (1982), Rebar et al (1982), Friedman et al (1983), Alper et al (1986), Gandar (1988), Santoro & Schmidt (1990) and Rebar & Connolly (1990). Recent developments in physiological estradiol/proges-

Table 8.1 Ovarian failure: pathological and etiological classification

Afollicular
Exogenous (iatrogenic):
Surgery
Irradiation
Chemotherapeutic and other drugs
Environmental toxins
Endogenous (spontaneous):
Chromosomal, maldeveloped gonads
Familial
Autoimmune
Galactosaemia
Mucopolysaccharidosis
Infection (mumps, others)
Hemorrhage
Malignant infiltration
Blepharophimosis
Malouf syndrome
Perrault syndrome
Roberts-SC phocomelia syndrome
Idiopathic
Follicular
Idiopathic resistant ovary syndrome
Chronic (autoimmune) oophoritis
Galactosemia
Blepharophimosis

terone replacement cycles in such women (Massai et al 1993), and cryopreservation of oocytes from unstimulated follicles (Toth et al 1994), provide potential alternatives to oocyte donation programs (Devroey et al 1988).

A combined pathological and etiological classification of ovarian failure is given in Table 8.1.

Afollicular ovarian failure (premature follicular depletion, true premature menopause)

Sometimes the cause of ovarian failure is obvious from the patient's history, e.g. bilateral oophorectomy for endocrine ablation, or removal of neoplastic or non-neoplastic disease. Prior irradiation or chemotherapy may be implicated, or the more subtle damage caused by environmental toxins. These exogenous or iatrogenic factors are discussed in Chapter 11.

Chromosomal abnormalities are an important cause of endogenous or spontaneous ovarian failure, more commonly present with primary rather than secondary amenorrhea. Gonadal dysgenesis, in which cases the ovaries are typically but not always gonadal streaks, includes Turner's syndrome (45,X) (Jacquemyn et al 1989), Swyer's syndrome (46,XY) and so-called pure gonadal dysgenesis (46,XX). There is some doubt as to the validity of this last-mentioned entity, which frequently has a familial incidence and which overlaps clinically with cases of idiopathic premature follicular depletion (Friedman et al 1983). The pathology of gonadal dysgenesis is discussed in detail in Chapter 7. Primary ovarian failure has also been reported in association with 47,XXX (Michalak et al 1983, Villanueva & Rebar 1983), 45,X/46,XX mosaicism, and structurally abnormal X chromosomes (Bates & Howard 1990, Therman & Susman 1990). Cytogenetic analysis of ovarian tissue and skin is an important investigation in patients with ovarian failure in whom the preoperative work-up does not reveal an abnormal karyotype in peripheral blood leucocytes, since analysis of cells from multiple sites is the only way to detect chromosomal mosaicism (Portuondo et al 1984, Abdel Gadir & Ramadan 1990).

About 10% of patients with premature ovarian failure have a family member with the same condition (Russell et al 1982, Friedman et al 1983). Several pedigrees of familial cases have been published (Coulam et al 1983, Mattison et al 1984) in addition to those associated with a known specific genetic abnormality such as galactosemia (see below). Analysis of the apparently idiopathic cases has suggested an autosomal dominant sex-linked inheritance (Smith et al 1979, Coulam et al 1983, Mattison et al 1984). The pathogenetic basis of these cases is not clear, but possibilities include a decrease in the number of primordial germ cells or an increase in the rate of attrition of an initially normal complement of primordial follicles (Coulam et al 1983, Speed 1988). Mathematical models suggest that the latter is the more important mechanism (Mattison et al 1984).

There is a documented association between premature ovarian failure and a variety of autoimmune disorders, e.g. Addison's and Hashimoto's diseases, rheumatoid arthritis, myasthenia gravis, diabetes mellitus and pernicious anemia, hypoparathyroidism, and systemic lupus erythematosus (Irvine et al 1968, de Moraes-Ruehsen et al 1972, Edmonds et al 1973, Vasquez & Kenny 1973, Irvine & Barnes 1975, Collen et al 1979, Friedman et al 1983, Case Records of the Massachusetts General Hospital 1986, Muir & Maclaren 1991). Some investigators (Coulam 1983, Alper & Garner 1985, Damewood et al 1986) have found that 20–40% of patients with premature ovarian failure have associated autoimmune disease, although this is certainly not our experience nor that of some other observers (Board et al 1979, Ho et al 1988). Irvine & Barnes (1975) found that 25% of patients with Addison's disease had primary or secondary amenorrhea, and suggested that the ovarian damage might also be due to autoimmunity. Further support lies in the demonstration of antiovarian antibodies in many premature ovarian failure patients, both with and without associated autoimmune disorders (Irvine et al 1969, de Moraes-Ruehsen et al 1972, Coulam & Ryan 1979, Damewood et al 1986), and reports of response to corticosteroid therapy (Coulam et al 1981a). Antibodies in patients' serum have reacted against theca interna (Irvine et al 1968) and to oocytes and granulosa of normal ovarian tissue (Damewood et al 1986), as well as producing a cytotoxic effect on granulosa cells in culture (McNatty et al 1975).

Clinical gonadal failure has been reported in both type I and type II familial polyendocrine deficiency syndromes, which are considered to be autoimmune in nature (Loriaux 1985). Hypogonadism in these patients may be hypo- or hypergonadotrophic, reflecting damage either to the pituitary gland or the ovary itself. There is an association with HLA antigens DR3 and B8 (Alper & Garner 1985, Loriaux 1985, Case Records of the Massachusetts General Hospital 1986). Premature follicular depletion has been recognized in women with ataxia telangectasia, but the mechanism is unclear (Bowden et al 1963, Miller & Chatten 1967, Friedman et al 1984). It is postulated that low neonatal gonadotrophins in athymic mice with resultant disorganized folliculogenesis may have a parallel in athymic women with ataxia telangectasia (Friedman et al 1984).

Kaufman et al (1979, 1981) were the first to draw attention to the high incidence of premature ovarian failure in patients with galactosemia. The few reports of laparoscopic appearances and ovarian biopsy findings in such patients have described small ovaries with follicular depletion or only sparse follicles (Beauvais & Guilhaume 1984, Robinson et al 1984). Two galactosemic sisters, reviewed at our institution, had open ovarian biopsies at ages 26 and 31 years which demonstrated resistant ovary syndrome and premature follicular depletion, respectively, suggesting that a phase of 'follicular resistance' may precede follicular depletion (Fraser et al 1986). The mechanism of ovarian damage in galactosemia is unknown, but most investigators favor a toxic effect of galactose or its metabolites on germ cells/follicular structures, possibly beginning in utero and probably continuing in the postnatal period (Levy et al 1984, Fraser et al 1986). The correlation between the occurrence of ovarian failure and age of commencement and rigorousness of dietary management of galactosemia is poor. In mucopolysaccharidosis, another hereditary metabolic disorder, premature follicular depletion, secondary to destruction from the accumulation of toxic substances within the ovary, has been reported (McDonough 1980).

Females with the blepharophimosis syndrome have been noted to have a high incidence of menstrual irregularities and amenorrhea; hypergonadotrophic hypogonadism has been documented in one case (Jones & Collin 1984). Two women with premature ovarian failure and the blepharophimosis syndrome, reviewed at our institution, have had open ovarian biopsies which showed premature follicular depletion in one case and resistant ovary syndrome in the other (Fraser et al 1988). Rare cases of afollicular ovarian failure have been documented in association with the Malouf syndrome (Narahara et al 1992), the Perrault syndrome (Pallister et al 1979) and the Roberts-SC phocomelia syndrome (Robins et al 1989).

The contribution of infections to premature ovarian failure is not known. As indicated in Chapter 18, the ovaries are relatively resistant to suppurative inflammation and are often spared parenchymal involvement, despite florid pelvic inflammatory disease. The frequency of involvement of the ovaries in the common viral diseases is not known. Mumps oophoritis is clinically but not pathologically documented (see Ch. 18), and has been claimed to be a cause of some cases of premature ovarian failure (Morrison et al 1975, Aleem 1981, Taparelli et al 1988).

Isolated spontaneous bilateral ovarian hemorrhages have been documented by Coulam et al (1981b) as a cause of premature ovarian failure. Torsion is a possible cause of such an event (although this would rarely be bilateral). There is also the possibility that anticoagulants could precipitate destructive ovarian hemorrhage.

Metastatic tumor infiltration could theoretically cause premature ovarian failure, but this is unlikely to be a significant clinical problem. Patients with previously treated non-ovarian malignant disease are more likely to present with premature ovarian failure as a result of ovarian damage incidental to chemotherapy or radiotherapy (see Ch. 11).

In the majority of patients with premature follicular depletion none of the above etiological factors can be demonstrated clinically or histologically. Such unexplained cases may be due to an as yet undefined genetic defect resulting in congenitally small ovaries with reduced numbers of primordial follicles (Tulandi & Kinch 1981), or increased utilization of follicles or rapid follicular atresia (Emperaire et al 1970, Friedman et al 1983).

Macroscopic features

The appearance of the ovaries in premature follicular depletion probably represents end-stage disease and hence is common to the many conditions which lead to follicle depletion. The ovaries are usually described as being small and scarred, without macroscopically evident follicles.

Microscopic features

The cortical stroma is dense and hypercellular and notable for a complete absence of primordial and antral follicles, although it has been said that a rare primordial follicle does not exclude the diagnosis (Starup & Sele 1973). Serosal inclusions are common, and care is needed to avoid confusing the smaller ones with primordial or pre-antral follicles. Atretic follicles (usually at corpus fibrosum stage) may be present, indicating previous follicular activity (Fig. 8.1). In the deeper cortex and medulla, there is often evidence of previous ovulation, most commonly in the form of corpora albicantes, but occasionally regressing corpora lutea. If there is absolutely no evidence of past or present follicular activity and if there is no apparent corticomedullary differentiation, it may be difficult, especially in small laparoscopic biopsies, confidently to differentiate such an ovary from a streak (see Ch. 7). Minor stromal changes may be present, such as small clusters of luteinized stromal cells. We have observed minor inflammatory foci in occasional cases which, in serial sections, exhibited no relationship to follicular remnants and their significance was not obvious (Fig. 8.2). It is reasonable to speculate, however, that such infiltrates represent the end result of a chronic autoimmune oophoritis.

Most patients with premature ovarian failure considered to be of autoimmune origin on clinical and/or serological grounds show follicle depletion (as described above) which probably represents, in this situation, the end-result of an autoimmune oophoritis (see below). This latter may be a transient phase, rarely detected histologically (Gloor & Hurlimann 1984; see Ch. 19).

The ovaries in the familial candida endocrinopathy syndrome have shown appearances ranging from small follicle-depleted gonads to normal sized ovaries with lymphoplasmacytic infiltrates around plentiful follicles (Dempster et al 1981), the latter appearance being consistent with autoimmune oophoritis.

In galactosemic women, follicular depletion is the most likely picture to be encountered, but small ovaries with occasional follicles may be seen or, rarely, normal-sized ovaries with the features of the resistant ovary syndrome.

In women with premature ovarian failure secondary to infection, obvious features of pelvic inflammatory disease, such as florid adhesions, chronic oophoritis with scarring, and chronic interstitial salpingitis, will be present.

The case report of premature ovarian failure secondary to bilateral ovarian hemorrhages describes abundant stromal hemosiderin in addition to follicular depletion (Coulam et al 1981b).

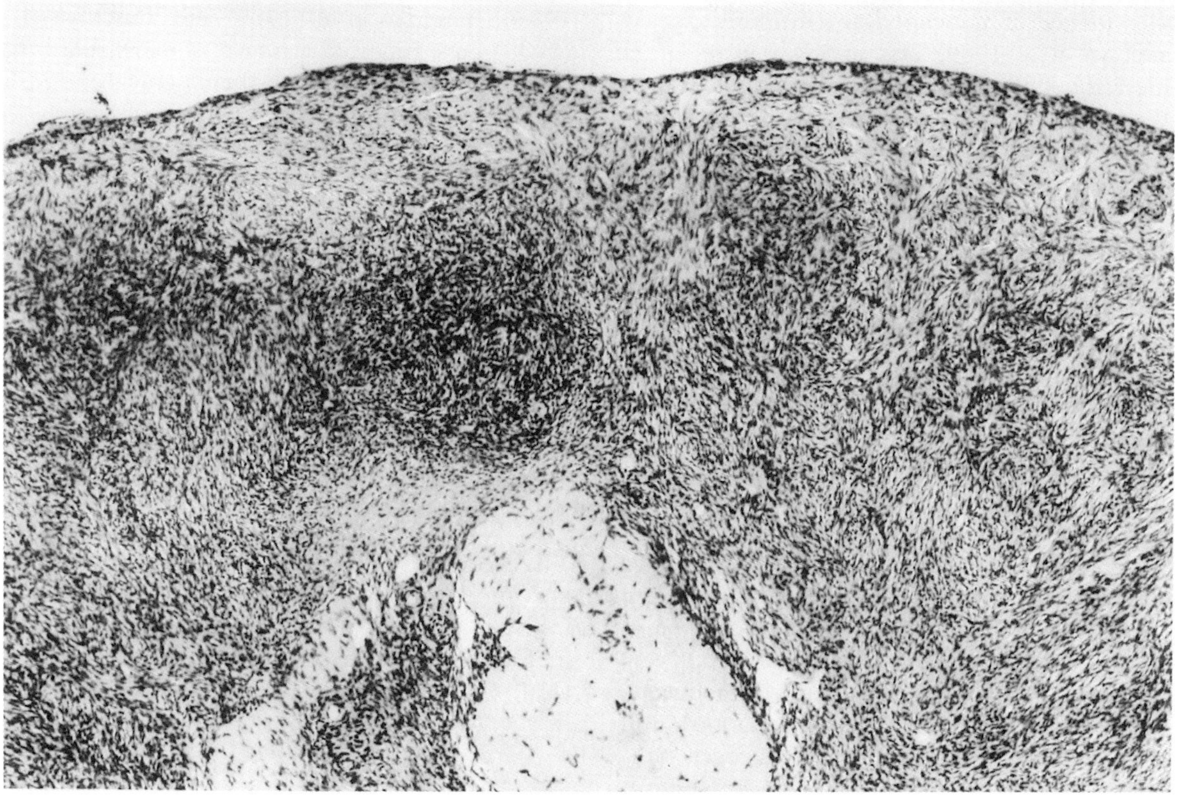

Fig. 8.1 Premature follicular depletion. Dense cortical stroma devoid of primordial or developing follicles. Corpus fibrosum in the deep cortex. H + E ×80

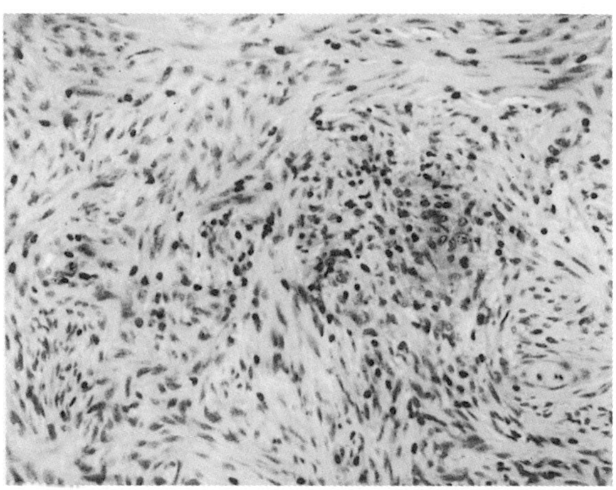

Fig. 8.2 Premature follicular depletion. A small focus of stromal inflammatory cells; no follicular structures were noted nearby. H + E ×125. (Reproduced, with permission, from International Journal of Gynaecological Pathology, 1982)

Follicular ovarian failure

Resistant ovary syndrome (Savage syndrome, gonadotrophin insensitivity syndrome)

This has been defined by van Campenhout et al (1972) as continuous hypersecretion of pituitary gonadotrophins, normal follicles in an ovarian biopsy, and insensitivity of the ovaries to exogenous stimulation by human gonadotrophins, even in massive doses. The proportion of cases of ovarian failure which fall into this group is approximately 15–20%. Paradoxically, high endogenous production of gonadotrophins by pituitary tumors may also be associated with reversible suppression of follicular function (Okuda et al 1989). Patients with this syndrome are distinguished from others with premature ovarian failure by the presence of ovarian follicles some of which show early and abortive development, but without evidence of recent ovulation. There is a low incidence of associated autoimmune disease (Tsuchiya et al 1989) and antiovarian or other tissue antibodies (Friedman et al 1983, Maxson & Wentz 1983). Some patients suffer from galactosemia or blepharophimosis (Fraser et al 1986). There is a single case report of the syndrome occurring in a patient with Wilson's disease, but the authors do not claim a causal relationship (Hartemann et al 1983).

The history of apparently normal menstrual activity prior to the onset of symptoms and a resistance to exogenous gonadotrophins suggests that the resistant ovary syndrome is usually an acquired disorder not related to any intrinsic abnormality of FSH. The absence of identified antibodies to FSH supports the concept of a gonadotrophin receptor-related defect (Verhoeven & Wilson 1979, Talbert et al 1984). Antibodies to FSH receptors have been identified in a few patients, including some who also have myasthenia gravis (Kuki et al 1981, Escobar et al 1982) or systemic lupus erythematosus (Case Records of the Massachusetts General Hospital 1986). Since gonadotrophin receptors are modulated by local estrogen production, an abnormality in estrogen metabolism has also been put forward as a possible cause of the syndrome (Evers & Rolland 1981). It should also be noted that, in the physiological perimenopausal period, the last remaining follicles are relatively resistant to gonadotrophin stimulation and that, by analogy, the picture of resistant ovary syndrome in women with premature ovarian failure may merely reflect a stage of premature perimenopause preceding total follicular depletion (Maxson & Wentz 1983).

Ovarian resistance to gonadotrophins may be relative (Koninkcx & Brosens 1977, Verhoeven & Wilson 1979) rather than absolute, and even temporary or episodic (Dewhurst et al 1975, Shangold et al 1977). The significance of these observations is that ovarian function and reproductive capacity is not necessarily irrevocably lost in such patients and, in fact, there are several reports of return of the menses and, rarely, pregnancies following a diagnosis of resistant ovary syndrome. Ovarian 'resistance' has been overcome by estrogen therapy (Evers & Rolland 1981, Lim et al 1984, Alper et al 1986) and high dose gonadotrophin therapy (Friedman et al 1983). Bateman et al (1983) and Tsuchiya et al (1989) have reported a return of menstrual function in a woman with myasthenia gravis and resistant ovary syndrome after plasmapheresis. A response to corticosteroid therapy has been reported by Meldrum et al (1980).

Macroscopic features

The appearance of the ovaries is within the range expected for normally functioning ovaries, including the presence of small cystic follicles. However, corpora lutea and ovulation stigmas are absent. The capsule may appear sclerotic.

Microscopic features

The cortical stroma appears uniformly dense and superficially sclerotic (Fig. 8.3). Primordial follicles are variable in number and, as in normal ovaries, there is a tendency to clustering (Fig. 8.4). Adequately sized biopsies and step-

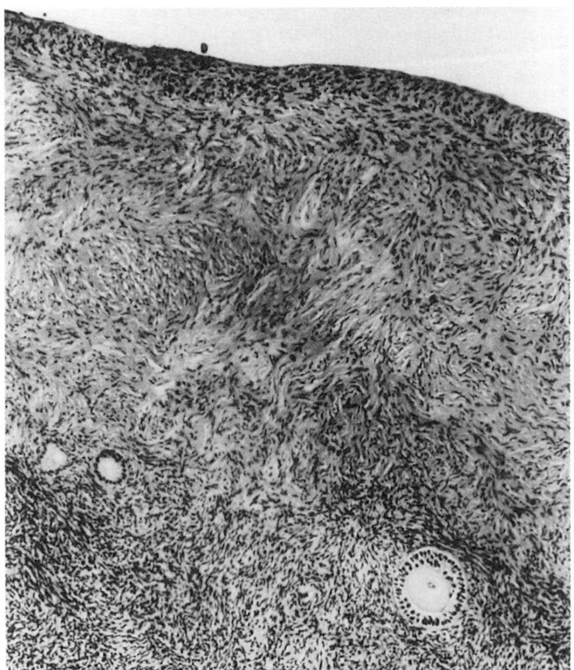

Fig. 8.3 Resistant ovary syndrome. Sclerotic cortical stroma with two primary follicles in more cellular stroma below. H + E ×200

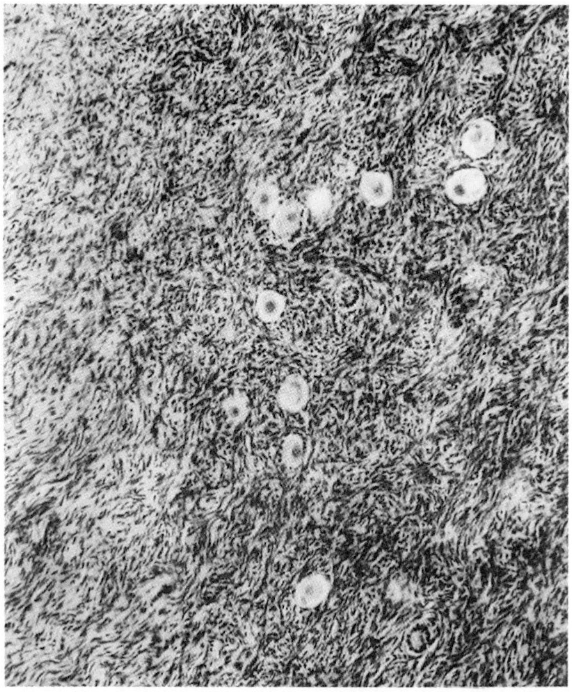

Fig. 8.4 Resistant ovary syndrome in patient with galactosemia. Clusters of primordial and primary follicles in dense cortical stroma. No inflammatory infiltrate present. H + E ×90. (Reproduced, with permission, from International Society of Gynaecological Pathology).

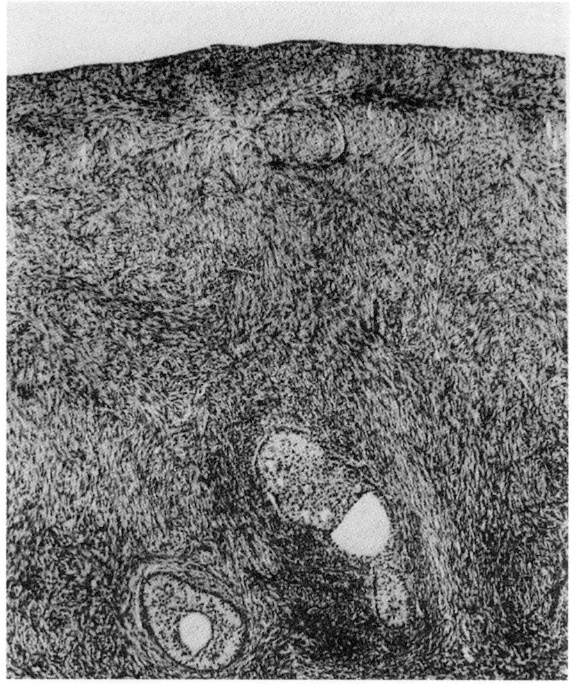

Fig. 8.5 Partial resistant ovary syndrome. Dense cortical stroma displaying two large dysplastic follicles with abnormal profiles, abundant granulosa and numerous Call–Exner bodies (in early antral follicle at right). H + E ×50

sectioning of these assumes some importance in this context. Ova are histologically viable. In cases of partial ovarian resistance, i.e. those with some follicular development, dysplastic primary follicles (see Ch. 7) are commonly observed. These are often enlarged and have rounded or irregular profiles outlined by thickened basement membranes; Call–Exner bodies may be numerous (Figs 8.5, 8.6). Sometimes the granulosa cells are broken up by hyaline material forming small round nodules and ribbons in a pattern resembling that seen in sex-cord tumors with annular tubules (see Ch. 37; Figs. 7.5, 7.6). Some follicles are almost totally replaced by the hyaline material (Fig. 8.6C). Comparable changes have been observed by Scully (Case Records of the Massachusetts General Hospital 1986). It is of interest that morphologically similar follicles have been noted in the ovaries of stillborn fetuses, infants, and children, and were most commonly identified in fetuses of 30–41 weeks gestation, a period when a massive physiological reduction of oocytes occurs (Safneck & de Sa 1986). In occasional extraordinary cases, oocytes are replaced by nonlaminated granular basophilic material which may or may not be calcium (Gloor et al 1982, Biberoglu et al 1988). Rare early antral follicles may be present, and evidence of previous ovulation, e.g. corpora albicantes, is not unexpected. Follicular atresia, when present, appears to be normal, with disappearance of the granulosa. Some biopsies show the expected complement of primordial follicles, but absolutely no evidence of developing or atretic follicles, and these cases are histologically indistinguishable from those of hypogonadotrophic hypogonadism. No inflammatory infiltrate is present. Foci of stromal luteinisation are seen in about one-third of cases (Fig. 8.6D).

Autoimmune oophoritis. While the presence of antiovarian antibodies or the association of ovarian failure in a patient with a variety of disor-

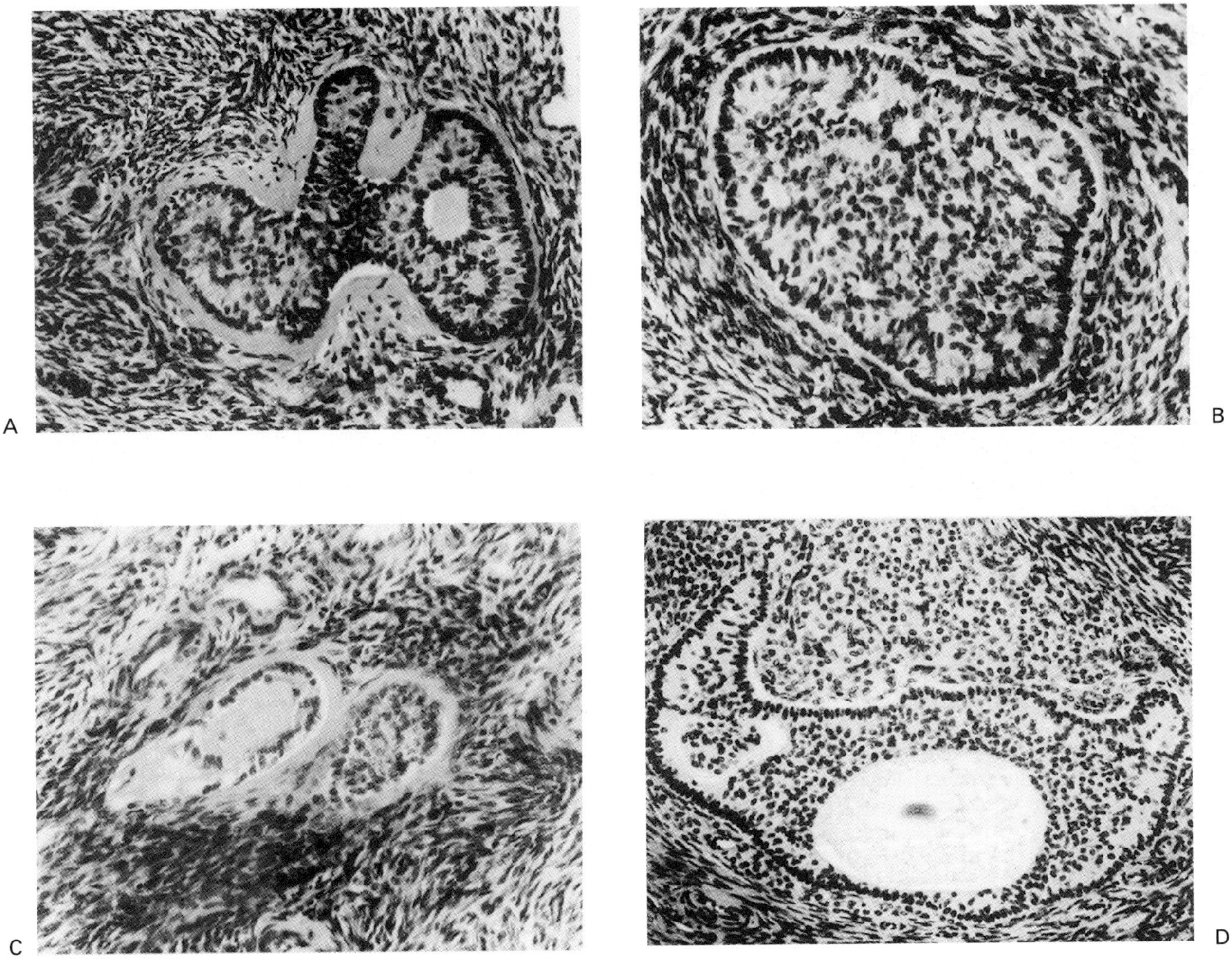

Fig. 8.6 Dysplastic follicles in partial resistant ovary syndrome. (a) Bizarre-shaped follicle with grossly thickened basement membrane. Note ribbon-like arrangement of granulosa cells. H + E ×160. (b) Large preantral follicle with numerous Call–Exner bodies, slight thickening of basement membrane. H + E ×200. (c) Dysplastic follicle, apparently bilobed in this section, with obliterative fibrosis of much of the granulosa. H + E ×200. (d) Large bizarre early antral follicle with perifollicular stromal luteinization (best seen above). H + E ×125

ders of autoimmune type may be taken as *prima facie* evidence of autoimmune oophoritis, such observations are far from conclusive (Fox 1992) and have, in the past, led to an overemphasis on this mechanism as a cause for secondary amenorrhea. Some patients, however, who fall into the clinicopathological category of follicular ovarian failure as defined above have a florid chronic oophoritis, the histological characteristics of which (see Ch. 19) leave no doubt as to its autoimmune basis, although antiovarian antibodies are rarely reported (Irvine et al 1968, Irvine 1980, Coulam et al 1981a, Russell et al 1982, Gloor & Hurlimann 1984, Rabinowe et al 1986, Case Records of the Massachusetts General Hospital 1987, Friedman et al 1987, Sedmak et al 1987, Wolfe & Stirling 1988, Biscotti et al 1989, Bannatyne et al 1990, Lonsdale et al 1991). Experimental models in thymectomized mice (Miyake et al 1988) and human studies (Moncayo & Moncayo 1992) provide valuable insight into this process of autoimmune destruc-

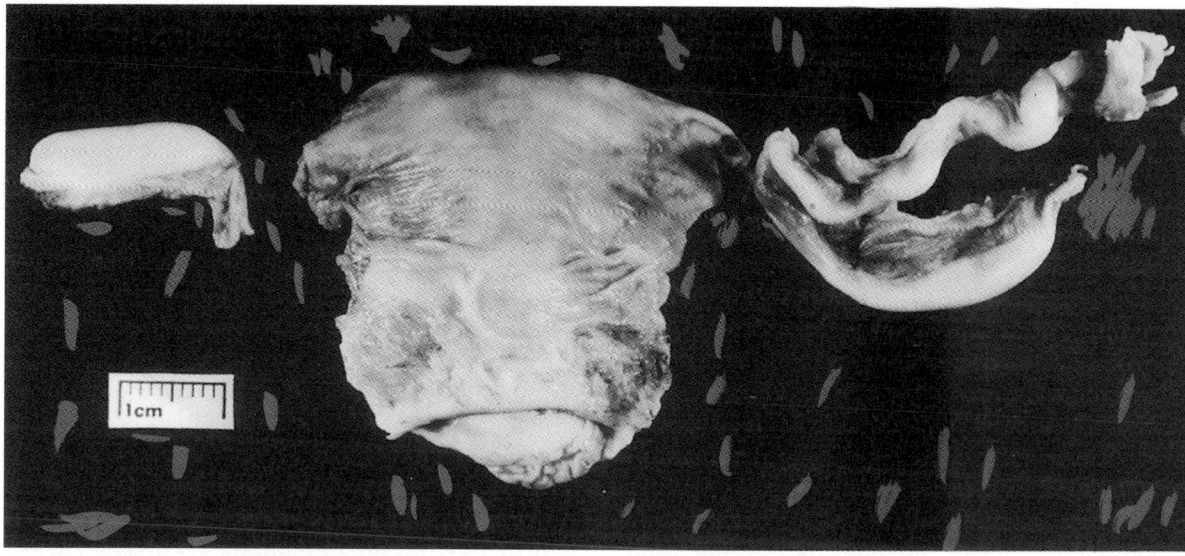

Fig. 8.7 Hypogonadotrophic hypogonadism. Uterus, fallopian tube, and ovaries from a 32-year-old woman who died from complications of craniopharyngioma partially removed at 6 years of age. Infantile cord-like unscarred ovaries and immature uterus.

tion of ovarian follicles, identifying circulating antibodies to ooplasm, zona pellucida, and steroid-producing cells. Autoimmune oophoritis presents as either primary or secondary amenorrhea, preceded by progressive oligomenorrhea and hypomenorrhea. Although uncommon, autoimmune oophoritis is important to recognize as it represents a definable, potentially treatable process (Muir & Maclaren 1991), leading to premature ovarian failure, and also indicates that the patient is at increased risk of having or developing other endocrine or nonendocrine autoimmune disease (which may develop even several years after onset of amenorrhea). Adrenal antibodies may be a useful predictor of the subsequent development of adrenal failure (Irvine 1980), not only in this group but also in any patient with ovarian failure.

There would appear to be potential for treating autoimmune oophoritis with corticosteroids, as suggested by Irvine et al (1968), or by plasmapheresis (Rebar et al 1982). Coulam et al (1981a) treated a patient with autoimmune oophoritis and premature ovarian failure with corticosteroids and there was a transient return of menses. Adrenal failure subsequently devel-

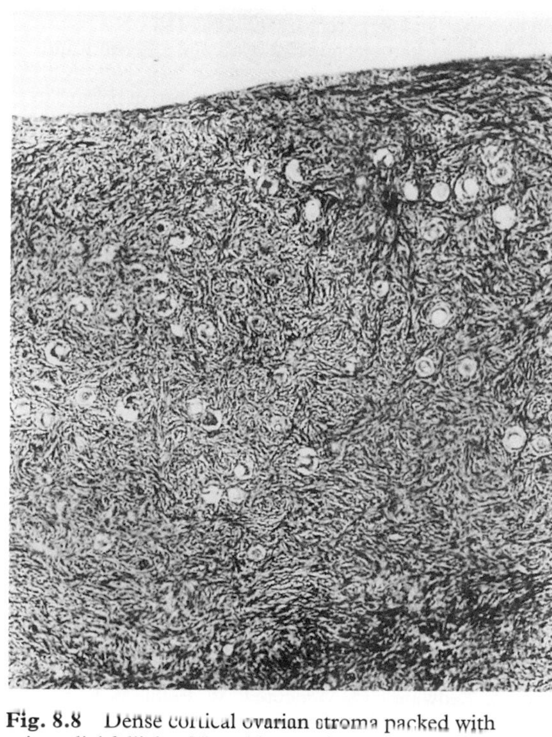

Fig. 8.8 Dense cortical ovarian stroma packed with primordial follicles. No evidence of current or past follicular activity (same case as in Fig. 8.7). H + E ×50

oped (antiadrenal antibodies were present at initial presentation). A similar response has been reported by Sedmak et al (1987). The challenge is to identify cases of autoimmune oophoritis before irreparable damage to the ovarian parenchyma occurs.

HYPOGONADOTROPHIC HYPOGONADISM

This is due to intrinsic disorders of the hypothalamus or hypophysis, or to local anatomical alterations or infiltrations, which interfere with secretion of releasing factors or gonadotrophins. Acquired causes are more common and include tumors, infections, granulomas, anorexia nervosa, irradiation, surgery, and head trauma. Congenital or hereditary causes include dysmorphic and polyglandular syndromes, isolated gonadotrophin deficiency and Kallman's syndrome (hypothalamic hypogonadism and anosmia). Further clinical details are given by Shearman (1985).

Macroscopic features

The ovaries are normal or small, depending on the duration of the precipitating condition and age of onset, i.e. pre- or postpubertal. Scarring may be present if onset was after the menarche (Fig. 8.7).

Microscopic features

Primordial follicles are plentiful but no follicular development is evident (Goldenberg et al 1976). If the onset of failure was after the menarche, corpora fibrosa or albicantes may be evident. The cortical and medullary stroma are unremarkable and there is no inflammation. To this extent the picture may be indistinguishable from some cases of the resistant ovary syndrome (Fig. 8.8).

REFERENCES

Abdel Gadir A, Ramadan A A 1990 Abnormal ovarian cell line: a cause for ovarian failure. Case report. British Journal of Obstetrics and Gynaecology 97: 446–448

Aleem F A 1981 Familial gonadal dysgenesis. Fertility and Sterility 35: 317–320

Alper M M, Garner P R 1985 Premature ovarian failure: Its relationship to autoimmune disease. Obstetrics and Gynecology 66: 27–30

Alper M M, Jolly E E, Garner P R 1986 Pregnancies after premature ovarian failure. Obstetrics and Gynecology 67: 59S–62S

Bannatyne P, Russell P, Shearman R P 1990 Autoimmune oophoritis. A clinicopathologic assessment of 12 cases. International Journal of Gynecological Pathology 9: 191–207

Bateman B G, Nunley W C, Kitchin J D 1983 Reversal of apparent premature ovarian failure in a patient with myasthenia gravis. Fertility and Sterility 39: 108–110

Bates A, Howard P J 1990 Distal long arm deletion of the X chromosome and ovarian failure. Journal of Medical Genetics 27: 722–723

Beauvais P, Guilhaume A 1984 L'insuffisance ovarienne de la galactosémie congénitale. La Presse Médicale 13: 2685–2687

Biberoglu K O, Damewood M D, Parmley T, Rock J A 1988 Insensitive ovary syndrome with a unique process of follicular degeneration. Fertility and Sterility 49: 367–369

Biscotti C V, Hart W R, Lucas J G 1989 Cystic ovarian enlargement resulting from autoimmune oophoritis. Obstetrics and Gynecology 74: 492–495

Board J A, Redwine F O, Moncure C W, Frable W J, Taylor J R 1979 Identification of differing etiologies of clinically diagnosed premature menopause. American Journal of Obstetrics and Gynecology 134: 936–944

Bowden D H, Davis P G, Sommers S C 1963 Ataxia-telangectasia. A case with lesions of ovaries and adenohypophysis. Journal of Neuropathology and Experimental Neurology 22: 549–554

Case Records of the Massachusetts General Hospital 1986 Case No 46-1986. Resistent ovary syndrome with hyalinisation of preantral follicles. New England Journal of Medicine 315: 1336–1344

Case Records of the Massachusetts General Hospital 1987 Case No 46-1987. Autoimmune oophoritis with primary ovarian failure. New England Journal of Medicine 317: 1270–1278

Collen R J, Lippe B M, Kaplan S A 1979 Primary ovarian failure, juvenile rheumatoid arthritis, and vitiligo. American Journal of Diseases of Children 133: 598–600

Coulam C B 1982 Premature gonadal failure. Fertility and Sterility 38: 645–655

Coulam C B 1983 Autoimmune ovarian failure. Seminars in Reproductive Endocrinology 1: 161–167

Coulam C B, Ryan R J 1979 Premature menopause 1. Etiology. American Journal of Obstetrics and Gynecology 133: 639–643

Coulam C B, Kempers R D, Randall R V 1981a Premature ovarian failure: evidence for an autoimmune mechanism. Fertility and Sterility 36: 238–240

Coulam C B, Field C S, Kempers R D 1981b Spontaneous bilateral ovarian hemorrhages as a cause of premature ovarian failure. Mayo Clinic Proceedings 56: 762–764

Coulam C B, Stringfellow S, Hoefnagel D 1983 Evidence for a genetic factor in the etiology of premature ovarian failure. Fertility and Sterility 40: 693–695

Damewood M D, Zacur H A, Hoffman G J, Rock J A 1986 Circulating antibodies in premature ovarian failure. Obstetrics and Gynecology 68: 850–854

De Moraes-Ruehsen M, Blizzard R M, Garcia-Bunuel R, Seegar Jones G 1972 Autoimmunity and ovarian failure. American Journal of Obstetrics and Gynecology 112: 693–703

Dempster A T, de Swiet M, Dewhurst J 1981 Premature ovarian failure associated with the candida endocrinopathy syndrome. British Journal of Obstetrics and Gynaecology 88: 563–565

Devroey P, Wisanto A, Camus M et al 1988 Oocyte donation in patients without ovarian function. Human Reproduction 3: 699–704

Dewhurst C J, de Koos E B, Ferreira H P 1975 The resistant ovary syndrome. British Journal of Obstetrics and Gynaecology 82: 341–345

Edmonds M, Lamki L, Killinger D W, Volpe R 1973 Autoimmune thyroiditis, adrenalitis and oophoritis. The American Journal of Medicine 54: 782–787

Emperaire J C, Audebert A, Greenblatt R B 1970 Premature ovarian failure. Report of seven cases. American Journal of Obstetrics and Gynecology 108: 445–449

Escobar M E, Cigorraga S B, Chiauzzi V A, Charreau E H, Rivarola M A 1982 Development of the gonadotrophic resistant ovary syndrome in myasthenia gravis; suggestion of similar autoimmune mechanisms. Acta Endocrinologica 99: 431–436

Evers J L H, Rolland R 1981 The gonadotrophin resistant ovary syndrome: a curable disease? Clinical Endocrinology 14: 99–103

Fox H 1992 The pathology of premature ovarian failure. Journal of Pathology 167: 357–363

Fraser I S, Russell P, Greco S, Robertson D M 1986 Resistant ovary syndrome and premature ovarian failure in young women with galactosaemia. Clinical Reproduction and Fertility 4: 133–138

Fraser I S, Shearman R P, Smith A, Russell P 1988 An association among blepharophimosis, resistant ovary syndrome, and true premature menopause. Fertility and Sterility 50: 747–751

Friedman C I, Barrows H, Kim M H 1983 Hypergonadotropic hypogonadism. American Journal of Obstetrics and Gynecology 145: 360–372

Friedman C I, Neff J, Kim M H 1984 Immunologic parameters in premature follicular depletion: T and B lymphocytes, T-cell subpopulations, cutaneous reactivity, and serum immunoglobulin concentrations. Diagnostic Immunology 2: 48–52

Friedman C I, Gurgen-Varol F, Lucas J, Neff J 1987 Persistent progesterone production associated with autoimmune oophoritis. Journal of Reproductive Medicine 32: 293–296

Fujii S, Ikeda S, Tachizaki T, Kagiya A, Saito Y 1993 Successful pregnancy in a woman with premature ovarian failure. Asia Oceania Journal of Obstetrics and Gynecology 19: 177–180

Gandar R 1988 Defaillance prematuree des ovaires. Journal de Gynecologie Obstetrique et Biologie de la Reproduction (Paris) 17: 351–361

Gloor E, Hurlimann J 1984 Autoimmune oophoritis. American Journal of Clinical Pathology 81: 105–109

Gloor E, Juillard E, Curchod A, Legeret J C 1982 Ovarian hypoplasia with follicular calcifications. American Journal of Clinical Pathology 78: 857–860

Goldenberg R L, Powell R D, Rosen S W, Marshall J R, Ross G T 1976 Ovarian morphology in women with anosmia and hypogonadotropic hypogonadism. American Journal of Obstetrics and Gynecology 126: 91–94

Hartemann P, Leclère J, Thomas J-L, Genton P, Arbogast J 1983 Syndrome des ovaires résistant aux gonadotrophines et maladie de Wilson; une observation. La Revue de Médicine Interne 4: 353–355

Ho P C, Tang G W, Fu K H, Fan M C, Lawton J W 1988 Immunologic studies in patients with premature ovarian failure. Obstetrics and Gynecology 71: 622–626

Irvine W J 1980 Autoimmunity in endocrine disease. Recent Progress in Hormone Research 36: 509–556

Irvine W J, Barnes E W 1975 Addison's disease, ovarian failure and hypoparathyroidism. Clinics in Endocrinology and Metabolism 4: 379–434

Irvine W J, Chan M M W, Scarth L et al 1968 Immunological aspects of premature ovarian failure associated with idiopathic Addison's disease. Lancet ii: 883–887

Irvine W J, Chan M M W, Scarth L 1969 The further characterization of autoantibodies reactive with extra-adrenal steroid-producing cells in patients with adrenal disorders. Clinical and Experimental Immunology 4: 489–503

Jacquemyn Y, Dumon J, Buytaert P 1989 Ovarian function in the non-mosaic Turner syndrome; a case report. European Journal of Obstetrics Gynecology and Reproductive Biology 30: 187–191

Jones C A, Collin J R O 1984 Blepharophimosis and its association with female infertility. British Journal of Ophthalmology 68: 533–534

Kaufman F, Kogut M D, Donnell G N, Koch R, Goebelsmann U 1979 Ovarian failure in galactosaemia. Lancet ii: 737–738

Kaufman F R, Kogut M D, Donnell G N, Goebelsmann U, March C, Koch R 1981 Hypergonadotropic hypogonadism in female patients with galactosemia. New England Journal of Medicine 304: 994–998

Khastgir G, Abdalla H, Studd J W 1994 The case against ovarian biopsy for the diagnosis of premature menopause. British Journal of Obstetrics and Gynaecology 101: 96–98

Kinch R A H, Plunkett E R, Smout M S, Carr D H 1965 Primary ovarian failure. American Journal of Obstetrics and Gynecology 91: 630–644

Koninckx Ph R, Brosens I A 1977 The 'gonadotropin-resistant ovary' syndrome as a cause of secondary amenorrhea and infertility. Fertility and Sterility 28: 926–931

Kuki S, Morgan R L, Tucci J R 1981 Myasthenia gravis and premature ovarian failure. Archives of Internal Medicine 141: 1230–1232

Levy H L, Driscoll S G, Porensky R S, Wender D F 1984 Ovarian failure in galactosemia. New England Journal of Medicine 310: 50

Lim H T, Meinders A E, de Haan L D, Bronkhorst F B 1984 Anovulation presumably due to the gonadotrophin-resistant ovary syndrome. European Journal of Obstetrics, Gynecology and Reproductive Biology 16: 327–337

Lonsdale R N, Roberts P F, Trowell J E 1991 Autoimmune oophoritis associated with polycystic ovaries. Histopathology 19: 77–81

Loriaux D L 1985 The polyendocrine deficiency syndromes. New England Journal of Medicine 312: 1568–1569

McDonough P G 1980 Diagnosis and therapy of primary amenorrhea. In: Gold J J, Josimovich J B (eds) Gynecological endocrinology. Harper and Row, Hagerstown, MD, p 278

McNatty K P, Short R V, Barnes E W, Irvine W J 1975 The cytotoxic effect of serum from patients with Addison's disease and autoimmune ovarian failure on human granulosa cells in culture. Clinical and Experimental Immunology 22: 378–384

Massai M R, Bergeron C, Martel D et al 1993 Physiological oestradiol and progesterone replacement cycles in women with ovarian failure: a model to study endometrial maturation and sex steroid receptor regulation by exogenous hormones. Human Reproduction 8: 1828–1834

Mattison D R, Evans M I, Schwimmer W B, White B J, Jensen B, Schulman J D 1984 Familial premature ovarian failure. American Journal of Human Genetics 36: 1341–1348

Maxson W S, Wentz A C 1983 The gonadotropin resistant ovary syndrome. Seminars in Reproductive Endocrinology 1: 147–160

Meldrum D R, Frumar A M, Shamonki I M, Benirschke K, Judd H L 1980 Ovarian and adrenal steroidogenesis in a patient with gonadotropin-resistant ovaries and hilus cell hyperplasia. Obstetrics and Gynecology 56: 216–221

Michalak D P, Zacur H A, Rock J A, Woodruff J D 1983 Autoimmunity in a patient with 47,XXX karyotype. Obstetrics and Gynecology 62: 667–669

Miller M E, Chatten J 1967 Ovarian changes in ataxia telangectasia. Acta Paediatrica Scandinavica 56: 559–561

Miyake T, Taguchi O, Ikeda H, Sato Y, Takeuchi S, Nishizuka Y 1988 Acute oocyte loss in experimental oophoritis as a possible model of premature ovarian failure. American Journal of Obstetrics and Gynecology 158: 186–192

Moncayo R, Moncayo H E 1992 Autoimmunity and the ovary. Immunology Today 13: 255–258

Morrison J C, Givens J R, Wiser W L, Fish S A 1975 Mumps oophoritis: a cause of premature menopause. Fertility and Sterility 26: 655–659

Muir A, Maclaren N K 1991 Autoimmune diseases of the adrenal glands, parathyroid glands, gonads, and hypothalamic–pituitary axis. Endocrinology and Metabolism Clinics of North America 20: 619–644

Narahara K, Kamada M, Takahashi Y et al 1992 Case of ovarian dysgenesis and dilated cardiomyopathy supports existence of Malouf syndrome. American Journal of Medical Genetics 44: 369–373

Okuda K, Yoshikawa M, Ushiroyama T, Sugimoto O, Maeda T, Mori H 1989 Two patients with hypergonadotropic ovarian failure due to pituitary hyperplasia. Obstetrics and Gynecology 74: 498–501

Pallister P D, Opitz J M 1979 The Perrault syndrome: autosomal recessive ovarian dysgenesis with facultative, non-sex-limited sensorineural deafness. American Journal of Medical Genetics 4: 239–246

Portuondo J A, Barral A, Melchor J C, Tanago J G, Neyro J L 1984 Chromosomal complements in primary gonadal failure. Obstetrics and Gynecology 64: 757–761

Rabinowe S L, Berger M J, Welch W R, Dluhy R G 1986 Lymphocytic dysfunction in autoimmune oophoritis. Resumption of menses with corticosteroids. American Journal of Medicine 81: 347–350

Rebar R W, Connolly H V 1990 Clinical features of young women with hypergonadotropic amenorrhea. Fertility and Sterility 53: 804–810

Rebar R W, Erickson G F, Yen S S C 1982 Idiopathic premature ovarian failure: clinical and endocrine characteristics. Fertility and Sterility 37: 35–41

Robins D B, Ladda R L, Thieme G A, Boal D K, Emanuel B S, Zackai E H 1989 Prenatal detection of Roberts-SC phocomelia syndrome: report of 2 sibs with characteristic manifestations. American Journal of Medical Genetics 32: 390–394

Robinson A C R, Dockeray C J, Cullen M J, Sweeney E C 1984 Hypergonadotrophic hypogonadism in classical galactosaemia: evidence for defective oogenesis. Case report. British Journal of Obstetrics and Gynaecology 91: 199–200

Russell P, Bannatyne P, Shearman R P, Fraser I S, Corbett P 1982 Premature hypergonadotropic ovarian failure: Clinicopathological study of 19 cases. International Journal of Gynecological Pathology 1: 185–201

Safneck J R, de Sa D J 1986 Structures mimicking sex cord-stromal tumours and gonadoblastomas in the ovaries of normal infants and children. Histopathology 10: 909–920

Santoro N, Schmidt C L 1990 Pregnancy after an unsuccessful oocyte donation cycle. Fertility and Sterility 53: 174–176

Sedmak D D, Hart W R, Tubbs R R 1987 Autoimmune oophoritis: a histopathologic study of involved ovaries with immunologic characterization of the mononuclear cell infiltrate. International Journal of Gynecological Pathology 6: 73–81

Shangold M M, Turksoy R N, Bashford R A, Hammond C B 1977 Pregnancy following the 'insensitive ovary syndrome'. Fertility and Sterility 28: 1179–1181

Shearman R P S 1985 Clinical reproductive endocrinology. Churchill Livingstone, Edinburgh, p 481–507

Smith A, Fraser I S, Noel M 1979 Three siblings with premature gonadal failure. Fertility and Sterility 32: 528–530

Speed R M 1988 The possible role of meiotic pairing anomalies in the atresia of human fetal oocytes. Human Genetics 78: 260–266

Starup J, Sele V 1973 Premature ovarian failure. Acta Obstetricia et Gynecologica Scandinavica 52: 259–268

Talbert L M, Raj M H G, Hammond M G, Greer T 1984 Endocrine and immunologic studies in a patient with resistant ovary syndrome. Fertility and Sterility 45: 741–744

Taparelli F, Squadrini F, de Rienzo B, Lami G, Fornaciari A 1988 Isolation of mumps virus from vaginal secretions in association with oophoritis. Journal of Infection 17: 255–258

Therman E, Susman B 1990 The similarity of phenotypic effects caused by Xp and Xq deletions in the human female: a hypothesis. Human Genetics 85: 175–183

Toth T L, Lanzendorf S E, Sandow B A et al 1994 Cryopreservation of human prophase I oocytes from unstimulated follicles. Fertility and Sterility 61: 1077–1082

Tsuchiya I, Sahashi K, Mitsuma T, Ibi T, Noguchi M 1989 Two cases of myasthenia gravis associated with transient amenorrhea. Rinsho Shinkeigaku 29: 647–650

Tulandi T, Kinch R A H 1981 Premature ovarian failure. Obstetrical and Gynecological Survey 36: 521–527

Van Campenhout J, Vauclair R, Maraghi K 1972 Gonadotropin-resistant ovaries in primary amenorrhea. Obstetrics and Gynecology 40: 6–12

Vasquez A M, Kenny F M 1973 Ovarian failure and antiovarian antibodies in association with hypoparathyroidism, moniliasis, and Addison's and Hashimoto's disease. Obstetrics and Gynecology 41: 414–418

Verhoeven G F M, Wilson J D 1979 The syndromes of

primary hormone resistance. Progress in Endocrinology and Metabolism 28: 253–289

Villanueva A L, Rebar R W 1983 Triple-X syndrome and premature ovarian failure. Obstetrics and Gynecology 62: 70s–73s

Wolfe C D A, Stirling R W 1988 Premature menopause associated with autoimmune oophoritis. Case report. British Journal of Obstetrics and Gynaecology 95: 630–632

9

Intersex

R. Jansen

Intersex, or ambiguous sexual development, usually presents at birth or soon afterwards. The intersex states described in this chapter comprise discrepancies in chromosomal, gonadal, and internal and external genital sexual development. Attention is paid to the gonads that accompany intersex states and the mechanisms by which abnormal genetic and endocrine influences affect formation of the internal and external genitalia.

Normal embryological development of the ovaries is described in Chapter 1. Anomalies of ovarian development and descent unrelated to sexual ambiguity are described in Chapter 6. Gonadal agenesis, or dysgenesis, is described in Chapter 7. The tumors that can develop in the abnormal ovaries of intersex states when Y chromosomal material is present in the genotype, particularly gonadoblastoma, are described in Chapters 40–51.

'Intersex' and 'hermaphroditism' have similar meanings. The term 'true hermaphroditism' is used when an individual has both ovarian and testicular tissue, either in one gonad or separately. 'Pseudohermaphroditism' encompasses all other intersex states. Female intersex implies the absence of a Y chromosome in the genotype and the determining of a gonad with follicular structures. Male intersex implies the presence of Y chromosomal material in the genotype and the determining of a gonad with tubules. More fundamental discrepancies occur in the abnormal gonadal states that are attributable to disorders of chromosomal sex.

CHROMOSOMAL SEX

At least one X chromosome is required for life. Even so, many 45,X conceptuses are aborted spontaneously in the first trimester of pregnancy (Boué et al 1975), often without the embryonic plate having formed. Normal development of the ovaries requires genes that are present on both the short (p) and long (q) arms of the second X chromosome; therefore deletions of either arm of an X chromosome usually produce gonadal agenesis. Normal stature requires genes that are present on the short arm of the X chromosomes. *Turner syndrome* is defined as the association between constitutional short stature and gonadal agenesis or dysgenesis. Chromosomal deletions involving the short arm of the X chromosome (e.g. 46,XXp−) therefore produce Turner syndrome, whereas abnormalities affecting the long arm of the X chromosome (e.g. 46,XXq−) are associated with normal or tall stature, and the condition is known as *pure gonadal dysgenesis* (discussed further, below).

The development of a testis requires the presence of at least one Y chromosome or, more precisely, the terminal short-arm portion of the Y chromosome. This region in the Y-chromosome carries the SRY gene, which encodes *testicular determining factor* (TDF). On the X-chromosome, the corresponding gene is TDFX which, being nonrecombining, is subject to X inactivation. It has been postulated that TDFX functions as a suppresser of the various testis-formation genes (some of which are located on autosomes, perhaps chromosome 9p) (Harley & Goodfellow 1994) and that SRY permits operation of the testis-formation genes by repressing the function of TDFX (Ogata & Matsuo 1994). The combination of SRY and a single active copy of TDFX (as in the 46,XY karyotype) thus leads to normal testis formation. The phenotype of *Klinefelter syndrome* (47,XXY) is male because the normal process of X-inactivation deletes one dose of TDFX. Likewise, 47,XXX and 48,XXXX karyotypes are associated with a normal female phenotype (serial inactivation of excess X chromosomal loci occurs normally), and only occasionally does ovarian dysgenesis occur.

The hypothesis proposes that a genotype of 46,Xp+,Y should be able to cause sex reversal, with a female phenotype, provided X-inactivation of the added X material does not occur (Parkhurst & Meneely 1994). On the other hand, duplication of SRY with a 46,X,Yp+ karyotype has caused gonadal dysgenesis and phenotypic female intersex (Ogata et al 1992). The 47,XYY karyotype, however, is associated with a male phenotype and, usually, normal development. Cause and effect remain cloudy and individual case reports of gender phenotypes and sex determination contrary to expectations are still leading to more refined (or possibly alternative) hypotheses on exactly how normal testicular and ovarian development come about.

Pure gonadal dysgenesis can result from a variety of simpler chromosomal aberrations based on 46,XY (*Swyer syndrome*), such as mutations or deletions of SRY, TDFX, or chromosome 9p. Preservation of SRY but partial loss of TDFX accounts for some cases of pure gonadal dysgenesis with the karyotype 46,XX. Occasionally, 46,XX is associated with normal, even fertile, male development, which is explained by translocation of the SRY gene with unequal interchange between X and Y chromosomes during paternal meiosis, despite an absence of other Y-chromosomal material (López et al 1995). Alternatively, SRY preservation with (a) chromosomal disorder elsewhere, (b) loss of sequences regulatory to SRY, or (c) spread of X inactivation across a nearby X;Y translocation breakpoint (Bogan & Page 1994) can result in frustrated testicular development, as in partial or mixed gonadal dysgenesis. It seems that in cases of absent or faulty gonadal development of whatever cause the presence of Y-chromosomal material close to the centromere predisposes the dysgenetic or streak gonad to the development of gonadoblastoma (e.g. Page 1994) and thus to malignant germ cell tumors.

Historically, estimating chromosomal 'maleness' has involved detecting H-Y antigen, which is governed by a locus close to, but not identical with, SRY. Nowadays, however, the polymerase chain reaction (PCR) can be used for the detection of the SRY sequence itself. Thus true hermaphrodites with 46,XX karyotypes have generally been H-Y positive (Wachtel 1979) and are presumed to have been SRY positive, as have patients with Turner syndrome (45,X) who have gone on to develop germ cell tumors (Kocova et al 1994). By contrast, tests for H-Y antigen have been negative in some patients with 46,XY karyotypes and gonadal agenesis (Wachtel 1979), who can be assumed to have a deletion that involves SRY itself. On present evidence, the best laboratory indicators of predisposition to gonadoblastoma in a dysgenetic gonad are the karyotypic demonstration of either a Y-chromosome remnant or a marker chromosome of unknown origin (Page 1994).

GONADAL SEX

Epithelial sex cord formation takes place in a gonad, irrespective of the presence or absence of germ cells (McCoshen 1982). The direction that gonadal sex differentiation takes is an inherent function of the somatic gonadal elements; the influence of the Y chromosome in somatic cells effects differentiation into testicular tubules (McLaren 1980, McCoshen 1982); in the absence of SRY influence, follicular structures develop to constitute an ovary, irrespective of the karyotype of the primitive germ cells (Sharp et al 1980, McLaren et al 1984).

Thus, when the genotypes of the germ cells and the gonadal somatic cells coincide, there is a concordance of development that produces either ovarian follicles with secondary oocytes held in meiotic arrest or testicular tubules with Sertoli cells and spermatogonia.

The two processes – follicle formation and tubule formation – can coexist in an individual, usually because of chromosomal mosaicism (although this can be difficult to detect on peripheral karyotyping) (Winters et al 1979), accounting for the clinical range of conditions known as *true hermaphroditism* (van Niekerk 1976, Krob et al

1994). The ovarian and testicular tissue in true hermaphrodites can be found in separate gonads or can coexist in one gonad (termed an ovotestis). Other discrepancies occur (McLaren 1980), but atresia of oocytes is likely if follicle formation is imperfect, and spermatogenic failure is probable at or before puberty in testes or ovotestes that have not descended to the scrotum. Reproductive competence is more likely among true hermaphrodites who are phenotypic females than among those who are phenotypic males. A surprising histological diagnosis of ovotestis is occasionally made after an oophorectomy has been performed for unrelated indications in a parous woman (Tiltman & Sweerts 1982). Between these normal extremes true hermaphrodites can show just about any intersex phenotype.

In *ovarian dysgenesis* when the karyotype is 45,X (*Turner syndrome*), follicular oocytes have been present in most fetuses and newborns that have been examined histologically (see Ch. 7), although the numbers of oocytes are considerably reduced in comparison with normal females. In most cases follicular atresia is complete before puberty, accounting for the anatomical outcome of streak gonads. Occasionally (mostly with X chromosome partial deletions, isochromosomes, or mosaic states), follicular oocytes can persist beyond puberty, ovulation can take place, and pregnancies have occurred before secondary amenorrhea and premature menopause (characterized by high serum levels of FSH and LH) have ensued (Nielsen et al 1979).

The gonadal streaks of ovarian dysgenesis are neither morphologically simple nor endocrinologically inert. The fibrous tissue component is that of normal unluteinized ovarian cortical stroma. Mesonephric remnants are found and tubules of the ovarian rete are always present (Jones & Scott 1971). There are hilus cells in the stroma: after puberty, these cells respond to high levels of serum luteinizing hormone by secreting testosterone. Growth of pubic and axillary hair is therefore usual in patients with Turner syndrome by the late teen years, even if they have not been treated with ovarian steroids. In time, hilus cell hyperplasia can occur. Turner syndrome patients who develop clitoromegaly or in whom there is breast development in the absence of estrogen replacement therapy should be suspected of having gonadoblastoma (Jansen 1992) and be reinvestigated.

In men or women with *male intersex*, the testes are usually abdominal or inguinal. As in otherwise normal men with cryptorchid testes, these gonads are characterized by spermatogenic failure, depletion of spermatogonia with time, hyalinization of the seminiferous tubules, and thickening of tubular basement membranes. Spermatogenic failure can occur despite normal testicular descent, as in Klinefelter syndrome. The morphology of the interstitial tissue of testes in intersex states varies according to the abnormality (Table 9.1). In many cases of peripheral androgen resistance, including women with testicular feminization syndrome (see below), there is Leydig cell hyperplasia and circulating levels of testosterone are in the normal male range. In intersex due to androgen synthesis failure, Leydig cell hypoplasia or agenesis may be present. Sertoli cells can persist in the tubules and can aromatize androgens to estrogens accounting, in male intersex, for breast development or gynaecomastia at puberty.

INTERNAL GENITAL SEX

Normal female internal genital differentiation happens by default (Jost 1953). If development of the paramesonephric or mullerian ducts is not specifically inhibited by antimullerian hormone (AMH) secreted by Sertoli cells, these ducts persist and form the fallopian tubes, uterus, and upper vagina. AMH is produced and released from the 6th week of normal male embryonic development (Josso 1986), acting by diffusion to repress development of the ipsilateral duct. During the 7th week, Leydig cell production of testosterone begins to stimulate development of the male internal genitalia, comprising the epididymis, vas deferens, and seminal vesicle, which are derived from the mesonephric (wolffian) duct on each side. Development of these structures therefore fails in normal female fetuses as well as in fetuses that have gonadal dysgenesis. Instead, isolated mesonephric duct remnants unconnected to rete fragments are present in the region of the ovaries or streak gonads.

In *mixed gonadal dysgenesis*, chromosomal

Table 9.1 Anatomical summary of intersex states

Karyotype	Gonadal structure	Internal genitalia	External genitalia and general development
GONADAL DYSGENESIS			
Pure gonadal agenesis (Swyer syndrome if a 46,XY karyotype)			
46,XX; 46,XY	Fibrous streak	Normal female	Normal female: normal or tall stature
Turner syndrome			
45,X; X-deletions	Fibrous streak	Normal female	Normal female: short stature plus other stigmata
Mixed gonadal dysgenesis			
45,X; 46,XY; mosaicism	Fibrous streak; contralateral testis or gonadoblastoma	Uterus invariable; variable ipsilateral epididymis and vas	Labioscrotal fusion, clitoromegaly and short stature
TRUE HERMAPHRODITISM			
46,XX; 46,XY; mosaicism	Ovary and testis or ovotestis	Various	Range from normal male to normal female
FEMALE INTERSEX			
Virilizing congenital adrenal hyperplasia			
46,XX	Normal ovaries	Normal uterus, tubes and upper vagina	**Mild:** labioscrotal fusion, urogenital sinus, clitoromegaly **Severe:** vagina enters urethra above bladder sphincter; phallic urethra; progressive virilisation, especially at puberty
Aromatase deficiency (very rare)			
46,XX	Multicystic ovaries	As above	Labioscrotal fusion, phallic enlargement; further virilization at puberty
Prenatal exposure to exogenous androgens (e.g. danazol, testosterone, some progestins)			
46,XX	Normal ovaries	As above	Labioscrotal fusion, relatively mild phallic enlargement; nonprogressive
Maternal virilizing tumors and tumor-like conditions			
46,XX	Normal ovaries	As above	As above
MALE INTERSEX			
Complete androgen resistance – 'testicular feminization'			
46,XY	Undescended testes	No uterus or tubes; variable rudimentary vas and epididymis; mesonephric cysts	Normal female vulva, blind vagina; sparse sexual hair
Partial androgen resistance			
46,XY	Testes, often incompletely descended; Leydig cell hyperplasia	No uterus or tubes; epididymis and vas often deficient in receptor anomalies, but normal in 5α-hydroxylase deficiency	Varies from male with oligospermia or micropenis, through perineal–scrotal–hypospadias (usual presentation), to female with labioscrotal fusion and clitoromegaly (unusual); virilization at puberty and occasional gynecomastia
Androgen synthesis failure			
46,XY	Undescended testes, Leydig cell hypoplasia	No uterus or tubes; marked deficiency of vas and epididymal development	As above, but more likely to be at female end of spectrum; likely to be virilized at puberty
Prenatal exposure to exogenous androgen-blocking drugs (e.g. cyproterone acetate)			
46,XY	Testes; normal male	As above; virilization at puberty	
*XX-male syndrome**			
46,XX	Testes; normal male	Normal male	Short stature; sterility

*Classified as male intersex as detection of H-Y antigen or SRY gene on PCR implies existence of Y material in karyotype.

mosaicism is associated with the presence of SRY-containing somatic cell lines, and there is a discordance of gonadal development (Table 9.1) that results in the presence of one streak gonad and one testis. The presence or absence of Sertoli cells in a particular gonad correlates with the morphology of the internal genitalia on that side (Bonaventura et al 1979), reflecting the predominantly local, unilateral action of AMH and testosterone in early embryos.

Testicular feminization syndrome (or 'androgen insensitivity syndrome'), in which there is a deficiency of androgen receptors in genetic males, is characterized by a lack of male internal genitalia owing to complete insensitivity to the action of testosterone (Rutgers & Scully 1991). Production of AMH is most often normal or increased (Rey et al 1994), however, and mullerian inhibition is usually complete (Zourlas & Jones 1965), with no uterus and with the female external genitalia ending internally in a short, blind vagina. Children affected are invariably raised as girls. Inheritance is X-linked recessive, so families can include sisters, maternal aunts, and maternal grandmothers with the condition. Breast development takes place at puberty, but pubic hair is, at most, sparse. The clinical diagnosis is confirmed by finding normal male serum levels of testosterone in a phenotypic female.

Partial androgen insensitivity syndromes (including *Reifenstein syndrome*) result in a variety of male intersex disorders in which there is incomplete peripheral failure of androgens to bind to androgen receptors or incomplete failure of post-androgen-receptor translation of androgen action (Lee et al 1980, Kaufman et al 1981, Medina et al 1981, Warne et al 1983). Wolffian development is often deficient (Wilson et al 1974) and external genital development (see below) is ambiguous. Affected infants are usually raised as boys. Gynecomastia can occur at puberty. These instances of virilizing male intersex are described in more detail below.

Male intersex from partial androgen insensitivity due to *5α-reductase deficiency*, also X linked, has little or no effect on development of the epididymis and vas deferens (Imperato-McGinley et al 1979) because, unlike androgen action on the external genitalia (see below), the more local expression of testosterone on the internal genitalia does not require prior enzymatic reduction of testosterone to dihydrotestosterone by 5α-reductase. By contrast, male intersex conditions due to *androgen synthesis failure*, which include Leydig cell hypoplasia from autosomal recessive congenital abnormality of the Leydig cell LH-receptor (Berthezene et al 1976, Kremer et al 1995), are accompanied by marked deficiencies of wolffian development. Prenatal exposure of male fetuses, during the critical time of wolffian development from the 7th to the 14th weeks, to androgen-blocking drugs (e.g. cyproterone acetate and other progestogens) and to non-steroidal estrogens (e.g. diethylstilboestrol), is also accompanied by inhibition in growth of wolffian duct derivatives and ambiguous external genitalia, despite normal and complete mullerian inhibition (Mills & Bongiovanni 1978, Aarskog 1979).

Just as androgen action can fail independently of AMH activity, so mullerian inhibition can fail despite androgenic adequacy. Inguinal or scrotal uteri are occasionally encountered in patients with male phenotypes (Perez-Palacios et al 1978, Josso et al 1983), the so-called *uterine-hernia syndrome*. More commonly, transrectal ultrasound studies of (generally subfertile) men reveal cysts of presumed mullerian origin within the substance of the prostate gland (Jarow 1993). 46,XY women with mixed gonadal dysgenesis sometimes have persistent Sertoli cell function in a unilateral gonad and, instead of the more usual midline uterus with bilateral tubes, there can be a single, contralateral uterine horn and tube (Bonaventura et al 1979), which is then often located in an inguinal hernia (Davidoff & Federman 1973). Cases of testicular feminization syndrome have occasionally been described with inguinal hernias containing a uterus (Oka et al 1984), and a woman with the uterine-hernia syndrome has been reported who presented with primary amenorrhea and a normal 46,XX karyotype (Riggall & Cantor 1980).

EXTERNAL GENITAL SEX

Exposure of the differentiating urogenital sinus to circulating androgens during the 10th to 14th weeks of intrauterine life causes virilization of the external genitalia, with labioscrotal fusion, a penile urethral orifice, and progressive phallic enlargement. These events are normal in male fetuses, in which testosterone secreted by fetal testicular Leydig cells is reduced to dihydrotestosterone (DHT) by the enzyme 5α-reductase in sensitive genital tissues. DHT binds to intracellular DHT receptors, through which androgen action is expressed. These events are frustrated in conditions of virilizing male intersex, mentioned above, in which either androgen production or androgen responsiveness is diminished (Table 9.1), resulting in ambiguous genitalia.

The results of incomplete virilizing events in genetic males can be indistinguishable clinically from *virilizing female intersex*, in which genetically female fetuses have been exposed to abnormally high amounts of androgens (Reschini et al 1985, Conte et al 1994), either endogenous (as in congenital adrenal hyperplasia and in nonadrenal steroid synthesis disorders such as congenital deficiency of aromatase) or exogenous (e.g. maternal danazol ingestion or maternal virilizing tumors during pregnancy) (Table 9.1). The distinction between male and female intersex in cases of ambiguous external genitalia is therefore made on the basis of the karyotype.

DIFFERENTIAL DIAGNOSIS

The discrimination between various causes of ambiguous genitalia at birth is summarized in Table 9.2. In the clinical assessment of ambiguous genitalia no sex assignment should be made until skilled pediatric advice has been obtained. The severity of the developmental deficiency of the phallus generally determines the sex of rearing, perhaps overriding the karyotypic sex or the internal genital sex.

External virilization in females can take place independently of normality or abnormality of internal genital development, both because of the difference in timing of fetal internal and external genital development, and because of the different nature of the inhibitors and evocators. On the one hand, partial or complete labioscrotal fusion can accompany essentially normal uterine and vaginal development in cases of congenital adrenal hyperplasia or maternal hyperandrogenism. On the other hand, in the condition of *mullerian agenesis*, normal female external genitalia are associated with congenital absence of the uterus and vagina.

Table 9.2 Differential diagnosis of ambiguous genitalia at birth

Tests:
1. Karyotype
2. Serum 17-hydroxyprogesterone level
3. Physical examination/ultrasound/urogenital sinography
4. Occasionally, laparotomy

KARYOTYPE 46,XX	
Congenital adrenal hyperplasia	High serum 17-hydroxyprogesterone; hyponatremia can develop
Maternal androgens	Positive history
True hermaphroditism	Laparotomy for diagnosis
Idiopathic embryonic virilisation	Diagnosed by exclusion
KARYOTYPE 46,XY	
Cryptorchid-hypospadic male	Uterus absent
Virilizing male intersex	Internal genitalia defined by laparotomy
True hermaphroditism	Laparotomy for diagnosis
KARYOTYPE 45,X	
Ovarian dysgenesis with clitoromegaly	Laparotomy for diagnosis
Mixed gonadal dysgenesis	Laparotomy for diagnosis
KARYOTYPE 47,XXY	
Klinefelter syndrome with sexual ambiguity	
KARYOTYPE 46,XY/46,XX MOSAICISM	
True (chromosomal) hermaphroditism	

EVENTS AT PUBERTY

The rise of circulating pituitary gonadotrophins that brings about puberty in normal individuals will generally also take place in patients with intersex states. The anatomical and clinical consequences depend on the nature of the responsive tissues in the gonads.

In *gonadal dysgenesis*, high levels of gonadotrophins occur early in childhood; high luteinizing hormone levels eventually stimulate hilus cells in the streak gonads to secrete androgens and to produce pubic and axillary hair growth. Breast development from estrogen secretion in gonadal dysgenesis indicates either persistent follicular activity or the growth of a gonadoblastoma (Saunders et al 1975, Jones 1976); patients in whom breast development cannot be attributed to deliberate estrogen therapy must therefore always be investigated.

Conditions of *virilizing female intersex* due to continuing disorders that involve abnormal adrenal or gonadal androgen secretion progress markedly at puberty. Most female intersex patients with congenital adrenal hyperplasia will have been under treatment with corticosteroids for adrenal suppression by the time of puberty, and corrective surgery for labioscrotal fusion and clitoromegaly will ordinarily have been performed during childhood. But androgen secretion in congenital adrenal hyperplasia continues to be greater than normal, even if these patients are receiving steroid therapy, and puberty occurs early, resulting in relatively short stature and a tendency towards a male body habitus. Exposure of the hypothalamus and higher cerebral centers to androgens in late fetal and early infantile life can compromise female psychosexual orientation and postpubertal cyclical pituitary–ovarian function. Psychosocial studies have indicated a tendency towards masculine, lesbian, or bisexual behavior in a higher than expected proportion of patients with congenital adrenal hyperplasia (Money et al 1984), and persistent oligomenorrhea in adulthood is common.

In *male intersex* due to partial androgen insensitivity, androgen synthesis failure or mixed gonadal dysgenesis, rising luteinizing hormone levels at puberty invariably elicit an increase in gonadal interstitial androgen secretion, producing further virilization. Although not a concern in children raised as boys, virilization must be avoided in children raised as girls. The prospect of masculinization at puberty is one reason for carrying out elective gonadectomy in childhood in such girls.

In male intersex due to 5α-hydroxylase deficiency, puberty produces enlargement of the phallus, further rugosity of the scrotum, and accentuation of male-like behavioral patterns. Clearly an understanding of this condition should encourage male gender assignment in affected individuals at birth. However, even children reared as girls develop such pronounced tendencies towards male identity at puberty that gender reassignment is common. This is presumably so because cerebral androgen effects in late fetal and early neonatal life, as well as at puberty, do not depend on the reduction of testosterone to DHT and have thus taken place as in a normal male. In some communities in which this condition is common, there is cultural recognition of physical and behavioral sex reversal at puberty (Imperato-McGinley et al 1979).

In *testicular feminization syndrome* due to complete androgen insensitivity, the breasts develop normally at puberty; indeed, breast development is substantial in relation to the sparseness of axillary and pubic hair. Body habitus is female and, although the vagina is relatively short and sterility is inevitable, no cerebral androgenization will ever have taken place and psychosexual orientation is thoroughly female.

An approach to differential diagnosis of primary amenorrhea and abnormal pubertal development associated with intersex states is given in Table 9.3.

NEOPLASTIC SEQUELAE IN INTERSEX STATES

During puberty and in adult life, patients with intersex can be at special risk of developing can-

Table 9.3 Differential diagnosis of amenorrhea and virilization at puberty (F = Female; M = Male)

Tests:
1. Karyotype
2. Serum FSH, LH, testosterone

	FSH	LH	Testosterone
KARYOTYPE 46,XX			
Congenital adrenal hyperplasia	Normal	Normal	Normal–high (F)
Prepubertal polycystic ovary syndrome	Low	Normal–high	Normal–high (F)
Virilizing ovarian or adrenal tumor	Low	Low	High (F)
KARYOTYPE 46,XY			
Mixed gonadal dysgenesis	High	High	Low–Normal (M)
Partial androgen insensitivity	Normal	Normal	Normal–high (M)
Androgen synthesis failure	High	High	Low–Normal (M)
True hermaphroditism	Normal–high	Normal–high	Low–Normal (M)

cer. Neoplastic sequelae are noteworthy in three circumstances.

Ovarian failure in phenotypic females requires *estrogen substitution therapy* to avoid genital atrophy, osteoporosis, and other sequelae of estrogen lack. Patients such as those with Turner syndrome have developed endometrial carcinoma due to inadequate additional progestogen therapy (McCarroll et al 1975).

All patients with incomplete sexual differentiation who carry *Y chromosomal material* are at increased risk of developing germ cell tumors, perhaps with serious supervening malignancy, in the abdominal or incompletely descended gonads (Manuel et al 1976, Nagel et al 1984, Page 1994). The risk of gonadoblastoma is highest (20% or more) in patients with mixed gonadal dysgenesis, Swyer syndrome (Villanueva et al 1984), and other gonadal dysgenesis patients who have cytogenetically indeterminate sex chromosomal fragments or who can be demonstrated to carry multiple Y-chromosomal loci with molecular methods (Kocova et al 1994). These patients should have bilateral gonadectomies carried out at diagnosis, preferably prior to puberty. The risk is slightly less for the group of conditions constituting virilizing male intersex. In women with testicular feminization syndrome the risk is still lower, but rises steadily with time, and particularly so after 30 years of age; gonadectomies can be postponed until the third decade to allow spontaneous feminization if a 4% risk of dysgerminoma is accepted (Manuel et al 1976); testicular hamartomas are present in up to 60% of patients (Rutgers & Scully 1991). In Klinefelter syndrome there is no increased risk of testicular tumors, but mediastinal, retroperitoneal, and pineal germ cell tumors are more common, as is carcinoma of the gynecomastic breast (Carlson 1980).

In summary, it is recommended that elective gonadectomy be carried out by the age of 12 years in patients with XY gonadal dysgenesis, and by puberty in patients with male intersex, including testicular feminization. On the other hand, a pathological diagnosis of breast cancer or extragonadal germ cell tumor in a male should lead to a suspicion of Klinefelter syndrome.

Finally, there are rare circumstances in which lower genital tract development is so anomalous that failure of squamous epithelialization of the upper vagina occurs, in a manner similar to the accompanying anomalies of in utero diethylstilbestrol exposure. Cases of *clear cell carcinoma* have been reported in association with such gross pelvic anatomical derangements (Taylor & Weed 1963).

REFERENCES

Aarskog D 1979 Maternal progestins as a possible cause of hypospadias. New England Journal of Medicine 300: 75–78

Berthezene F, Forest M G, Grimaud J A, Claustrat B, Mornex R 1976 Leydig-cell agenesis. A cause of male pseudohermaphroditism. New England Journal of Medicine 295: 969–972

Bogan J S, Page D C 1994 Ovary? Testis? – A mammalian dilemma. Cell 76: 603–607

Bonaventura L M, Roth L M, Cleary R E 1979 The Sertoli cell in mixed gonadal dysgenesis. Obstetrics and Gynecology 53: 324–329

Boué J, Boué A, Lazar P 1975 Retrospective and prospective epidemiological studies of 1500 karyotyped spontaneous human abortions. Teratology 12: 11–26

Carlson H E 1980 Gynecomastia. N Engl J Med 303: 795–799

Conte F A, Grumbach M M, Ito Y, Fisher C R, Simpson E R 1994 A syndrome of female pseudohermaphrodism, hypergonadotropic hypogonadism, and multicystic ovaries associated with missense mutations in the gene encoding aromatase (P450arom). Journal of Clinical Endocrinology and Metabolism 78: 1287–1292

Davidoff F, Federman D D 1973 Mixed gonadal dysgenesis. Pediatrics 52: 725–742

Harley V R, Goodfellow P N 1994 The biochemical role of SRY in sex determination. Molecular Reproduction and Development 39: 184–193

Imperato-McGinley J, Peterson R E, Gautier T, Sturla E 1979 Androgens and the evolution of male-gender identity among male pseudohermaphrodites with 5α-reductase deficiency. New England Journal of Medicine 300: 1233–1237

Jansen R P S 1992 Oncological endocrinology. In Coppleson M (ed), Gynecologic oncology: fundamental principles and clinical practice, 2nd edn. Churchill Livingstone, Edinburgh, p 135–171

Jarow J P 1993 Transrectal ultrasonography of infertile men. Fertility and Sterility 60: 1035–1039

Jones H W Jr 1976 Editorial comment. Obstetrical and Gynecological Survey 31: 217

Jones H W Jr, Scott W W 1971 Hermaphroditism, genital anomalies and related endocrine disorders, 2nd edn. Williams & Wilkins, Baltimore, OH, p 85

Josso N 1986 Antimüllerian hormone: new perspectives for a sexist molecule. Endocrine Reviews 7: 421–433

Josso N, Fekete C, Cachin O, Nezelof C, Rappaport R 1983 Persistence of Müllerian ducts in male pseudohermaphroditism, and its relationship to cryptorchidism. Clinical Endocrinology 19: 247–258

Jost A 1953 Studies on sex differentiation in mammals. Recent Progress in Hormone Research 8: 379–418

Kaufman M, Pinsky L, Feder-Hollander R 1981 Defective up-regulation of the androgen receptor in human androgen insensitivity. Nature 293: 735–737

Kremer H, Kraaij R, Toledo S P A et al 1995 Male pseudohermaphroditism to a homozygous nussense mutation or the luternizing hormonal receptor gene. Nature Genetics 9: 160–164

Kocova M, Siegel S F, Nalesnick M, Trucco M 1994 Detection of Y-chromosomal sequences in gonadal tissue of patients with Turner syndrome (45,X). New England Journal of Medicine 331: 682–683

Krob G, Braun A, Kuhnle U 1994 True hermaphroditism: geographical distribution, clinical findings, chromosomes and gonadal histology. European Journal of Pediatrics 153: 2–10

Lee P A, Danish R K, Mazur T, Migeon C J 1980 Micropenis. III: Primary hypogonadism, partial androgen insensitivity syndrome, and idiopathic disorders. Johns Hopkins Medical Journal 147: 175–181

López M, Torres L, Méndez J P et al 1995 SRY alone can induce normal male sexual differentiation. American Journal of Medical Genetics 55: 356–358

McCarroll A M, Montgomery D A D, Harley J Mc D G, McKeown E F, MacHenry J C 1975 Endometrial carcinoma after cyclical estrogen-progestogen therapy for Turner's syndrome. British Journal of Obstetrics and Gynaecology 82: 421–423

McCoshen J A 1982 In vivo sex differentiation of congeneic germinal cell aplastic gonads. American Journal of Obstetrics and Gynecology 142: 83–88

McLaren A 1980 Oocytes in the testis. Nature 283: 688–689

McLaren A, Simpson E, Tomonari K, Chandler P, Hogg H 1984 Male sexual differentiation in mice lacking H-Y antigen. Nature 312: 552–555

Manuel M, Katayama K P, Jones H W Jr 1976 The age of occurrence of gonadal tumors in intersex patients with a Y chromosome. American journal of Obstetrics and Gynecology 124: 293–300

Medina M, Chavez B, Perez-Palacios G 1981 Defective androgen action at the cellular level in the androgen resistance syndromes. I: Differences between the complete and incomplete testicular feminization syndromes. Journal of Clinical Endocrinology and Metabolism 53: 1243–1246

Mills J L, Bongiovanni A M 1978 Effect of prenatal estrogen exposure on male genitalia. Pediatrics 62: 1160–1165

Money J, Schwartz M, Lewis V G 1984 Adult erotosexual status and fetal hormonal masculinization: 46,XY congenital virilizing adrenal hyperplasia and 46,XY androgen-insensitivity syndrome compared. Psychoneuroendocrinology 9: 405–414

Nagel T, Camrgo M, Tagatz G et al 1984 Gonadal tumors in patients with gonadal dysgenesis and sex chromosomal rings and fragments. American Journal of Obstetrics and Gynecology 150: 76–82

Nielsen J, Sillesen I, Hansen K B 1979 Fertility in Turner's syndrome. Case report and review of literature. British Journal of Obstetrics and Gynaecology 86: 833–835

Ogata T, Matsuo N 1994 Testis determining gene(s) on the X chromosome short arm: chromosomal location and possible role in testis formation. Journal of Medical Genetics 31: 349–350

Ogata T, Hawkins J R, Taylor A, Matsuo N, Hata J, Goodfellow P 1992 Sex reversal in a child with a 46,X,Yp+ karyotype: support for the existence of a gene(s), located in distal Xp, involved in testis formation. Journal of Medical Genetics 29: 226–230

Oka M, Katabuchi H, Munemura M, Mizumoto J, Maeyama M 1984 An unusual case of male pseudohermaphroditism: complete testicular feminization associated with incomplete differentiation of the Müllerian duct. Fertility and Sterility 41: 154–158

Page D C 1994 Y chromosome sequences in Turner's syndrome and risk of gonadoblastoma or virilisation. Lancet 343: 240

Parkhurst S M, Meneely P M 1994 Sex determination and dosage compensation: lessons fom flies and worms. Science 264: 914–932

Perez-Palacios G, Faz R, Benavides S, Manrique J J, Larrea F 1978 Anorchia and persistent Müllerian duct: a variant of the embryonic testicular regression syndrome. Journal of Clinical Endocrinology and Metabolism 47: 812–817

Reschini E, Giustina G, d'Alberton A, Candiani B G 1985 Female pseudohermaphroditism due to maternal androgen administration: 25-year follow-up [letter]. Lancet i: 1226

Rey R, Mebarki F, Forest M G et al 1994 Anti-müllerian hormone in children with androgen insensitivity. Journal of Clinical Endocrinology and Metabolism 79: 960–964

Riggall F C, Cantor B 1980 46,XY hernia uterus inguinale and vaginal agenesis. Obstetrics and Gynecology 56: 265–266

Rutgers J I, Scully R E 1991 The androgen insensitivity syndrome (testicular feminization): a clinicopathologic study of 43 cases. International Journal of Gynecological Pathology 10: 126–145

Saunders D M, Barratt J, Grudzinskas G 1975 Feminization in gonadal dysgenesis associated with ovarian gonadoblastoma. Obstetrics and Gynecology 46: 93–97

Sharp A J, Wachtel S S, Benirschke K 1980 H-Y antigen in a fertile female horse. Journal of Reproduction and Fertility 58: 157–160

Taylor J M, Weed J C 1963 Adenocarcinoma of the cervix associated with multiple congenital anomalies. Obstetrics and Gynecology 21: 446–449

Tiltman A J, Sweerts M 1982 Multiparity in a covert true hermaphrodite. Obstetrics and Gynecology 60: 752–754

van Niekerk W A 1976 True hermaphroditism. An analytic review with a report of 3 new cases. American Journal of Obstetrics and Gynecology 126: 890–907

Villanueva A L, Benirschke K, Campbell J, Wachtel S S, Rebar R W 1984 Complete development of secondary sex characteristics in a case of 46,XY pure gonadal dysgenesis. Obstetrics and Gynecology 64: 68s–72s

Wachtel S S 1979 The genetics of intersexuality: Clinical and theoretic perspectives. Obstetrics and Gynecology 54: 671–685

Warne G L, Gyorki S, Risberger G P, Khalid B A K, Funder J W 1983 Correlations between fibroblast androgen receptor levels and clinical features in abnormal male sexual differentiation and fertility. Australian and New Zealand Journal of Medicine 13: 335–341

Winters S J, Wachtel S S, White B J et al 1979 H-Y antigen mosaicism in the gonad of a 46,XX true hermaphrodite. New England Journal of Medicine 300: 745–749

Zourlas P A, Jones H W Jr 1965 Clinical, histological and cytogenetic findings in male hermaphroditism. II: Male hermaphrodites with feminine external genitalia (testicular feminization). Obstetrics and Gynecology 25: 768–774

10

Ovarian pathology and pregnancy

P. Russell   A. Farnsworth

TUMOR-LIKE LESIONS ASSOCIATED WITH PREGNANCY

There are six currently recognized non-neoplastic ovarian lesions which are encountered exclusively in pregnancy or the puerperium. These are pregnancy luteoma, multiple theca lutein cysts, solitary luteinized follicular cysts of pregnancy and puerperium, intrafollicular granulosa cell proliferations, hilus cell hyperplasia, and deciduosis. These lesions involute spontaneously after termination of the pregnancy (Clement 1993). Other ovarian enlargements not necessarily exclusive to pregnancy are also seen, e.g. corpus luteum cysts, endometriotic cysts, and paraovarian cysts (Buttery et al 1973, Ballard et al 1984).

The six conditions exclusive to pregnancy are grouped together to emphasize the importance of their recognition by pathologists, thus avoiding unnecessarily radical surgery.

Luteomas of pregnancy (nodular theca-lutein hyperplasia)

These are multinodular, often multicentric or bilateral, tumor-like masses of lutein cells which develop during an otherwise normal pregnancy and involute in the puerperium (Heller et al 1990). Most workers favor an origin from the lutein cells found during pregnancy as isolated groups in the stroma or in the walls of atretic follicles (Norris & Taylor 1967, Garcia-Bunuel & Brandes 1976). Some patients have a history suggestive of polycystic ovary syndrome, and luteomas in these patients possibly arise from the hyperplastic, often luteinized, stromal cells existing before the onset of pregnancy (Polansky et al 1974). Human chorionic gonadotrophin (hCG) is necessary for the development of luteomas, but is unlikely to be the only etiological factor since the lesions are not associated with trophoblastic disease or with early pregnancy, when hCG levels are at their highest. There are some morphological and clinical similarities between luteomas and multiple theca-lutein cysts (hyperreactio luteinalis), and some workers regard them as related, cystic, and solid forms of theca-lutein cell hyperplasia (Norris & Taylor 1967, Polansky et al 1974). However, in contrast to luteomas, hyperreactio luteinalis is associated with conditions of pathological hCG elevation, multiple gestations, and abnormal pregnancy states (see below).

Although the typical patient reported in the literature has been multiparous and black, it is thought that neither of these characteristics is a genuine predisposing factor (Scully 1979). Asymptomatic lesions are possibly more common than suspected in all sections of the community. The 'tumors' usually present in the third trimester and are most commonly incidental findings at cesarean section or postpartum tubal ligation. About one-quarter of patients have become hirsute or virilized and masculinization of female fetuses has been reported (Polansky et al 1974, Scully 1979). In these patients urinary excretion of 17 keto-steroids and plasma testosterone levels may be elevated, possibly representing a failure of the placenta to aromatize the excessive circulating androgens.

The lesions are multiple in up to one-half and bilateral in approximately one-third of cases (Scully 1979). Even if a luteoma is macroscopically unilateral, biopsy of the contralateral ovary may show microscopic nodules which are nevertheless morphologically distinct from the physiological aggregates of stromal lutein cells found in normal pregnancies (Krause & Stembridge 1966, Sternberg & Dhurandhar 1977).

Macroscopic features

Luteomas are usually 6–12 cm in diameter, although 20 cm lesions have been recorded. They are well circumscribed nonencapsulated masses which may be multinodular, imparting a bosselated appearance to the external surfaces. The cut surfaces show soft grey-brown or tan tissue, often with a mottled appearance due to focal hemorrhage. Small cystic spaces may be present. A typical corpus luteum of pregnancy can sometimes be detected as an anatomically distinct entity. Luteomas excised in the puerperium may be softer and paler, because of the onset of involutional changes, or may be frankly necrotic. Luteomas which have been biopsied during pregnancy have been shown to have disappeared later without trace or have left only a small scar (Sternberg & Barclay 1966). Luteomas do not require surgical excision but can be safely biopsied for confirmation of diagnosis (preferably by frozen section) and then allowed to regress spontaneously.

Microscopic features

Luteomas are composed of sheets of large eosinophilic cells which are broken up into alveolar groups by numerous delicate blood vessels (Fig. 10.1). A trabecular arrangement is less frequently seen. The cell size is intermediate between that of granulosa and theca lutein cells. The reticulin pattern of fibers around groups of cells rather than individual cells is also intermediate between the abundant pericellular distribution of reticulin fibers in the theca interna and the paucity of fibers in the granulosa layer. Follicular spaces containing colloid-like material may be present (Fig. 10.1B), but the intracellular hyaline droplets ('colloid bodies') typical of corpora lutea of pregnancy are rarely identified (Scully 1979). The cytoplasm is eosinophilic and sometimes finely vacuolated, but there is little stainable lipid. The round central nuclei have a prominent nucleolus and abundant euchromatin. There may be mild nuclear pleiomorphism and mitotic figures can usually be observed but do not often exceed 3/HPF (Fig. 10.1C). The remainder of the ovary shows the physiological changes of pregnancy, but small theca lutein cysts may be evident as well (Norris & Chorlton 1974). Early involutional changes include nuclear pyknosis and increased cytoplasmic vacuolation, but eventually the luteoma is reduced to sheets of necrotic cells (Fig. 10.1d). At this late stage the typical reticulin pattern may still provide a clue to the nature of the lesion.

Differential diagnosis

Nodular stromal hyperthecosis (see Ch. 14) may occur in pregnancy. The ovaries are uniformly enlarged and display multiple microscopic nodules of spindle-shaped luteinized stromal cells, arranged in bundles rather than alveoli. Reticulin fibres invest individual cells which have pale or finely vacuolated cytoplasm containing abundant lipid.

Lipid cell tumors (see Ch. 39) are almost always unilateral (with the exception of stromal luteomas; see Ch. 14) and can sometimes be seen arising in relation to the ovarian hilus. They are solid lobulated tumors composed of eosinophilic or finely vacuolated cells arranged in a diffuse or, less commonly, a trabecular pattern not dissimilar from that of luteomas. Reticulin surrounds single cells or small groups. Mitotic activity is variable but rarely as prominent as in luteomas of pregnancy. The most helpful distinguishing microscopic features are the abundant stainable intracytoplasmic lipid in all lipid cell tumors and

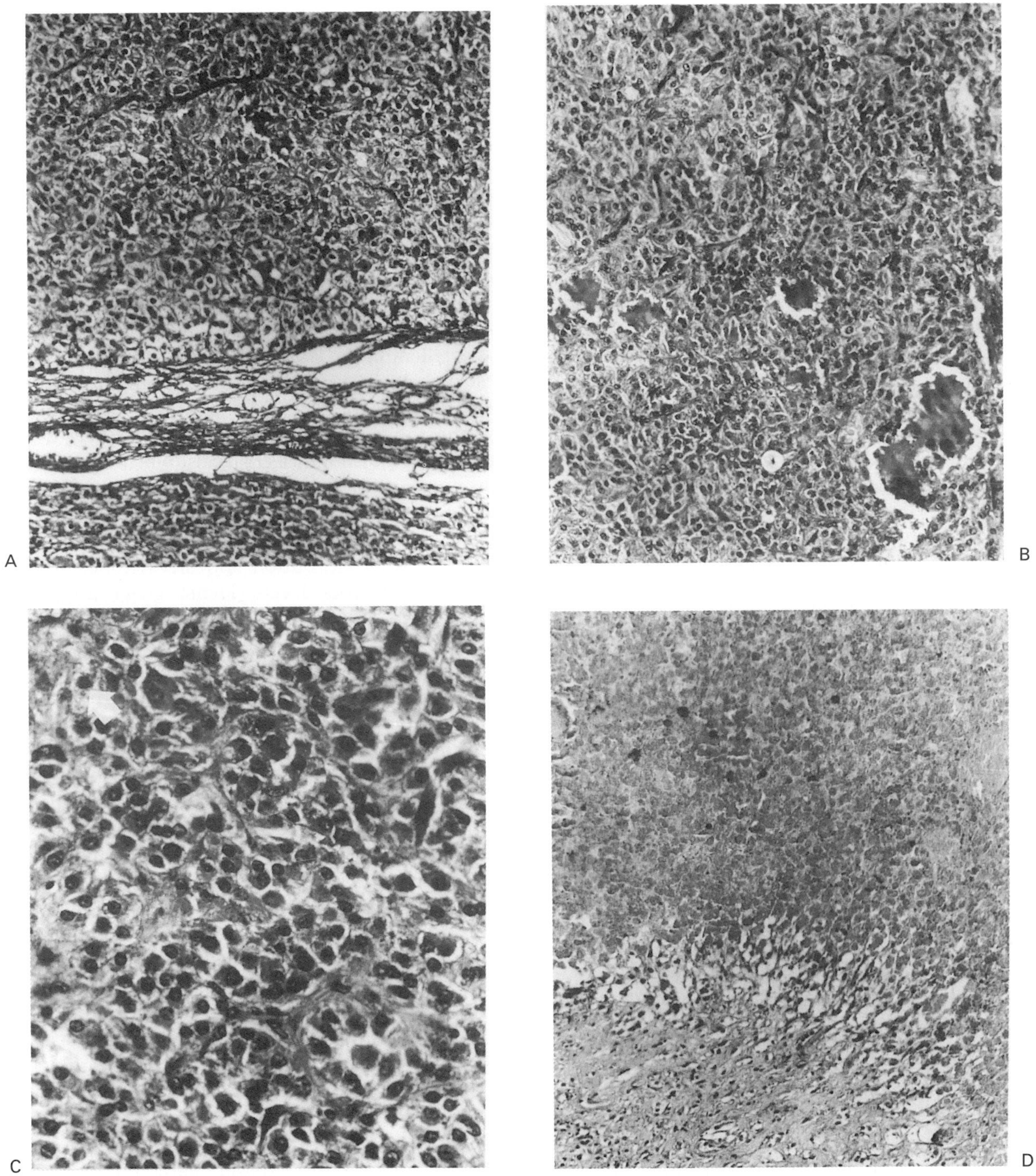

Fig. 10.1 Luteoma of pregnancy, a 4 cm solitary nodule excised at cesarean section. (A) Well-defined 'tumor' margin; stromal luteinization below. H + E ×100. (B) Uniform cells in alveolar groups, and follicular spaces containing colloid-like material. H + E ×100. (C) Luteoma cells with abundant cytoplasm, mildly pleiomorphic nuclei and mitosis (arrow). H + E ×250. (D) Involuted luteoma 5 months postpartum; sheets of ghost cells with some organization (granulation tissue) at margin. H + E ×100

the presence of crystalloids of Reinke in Leydig cell tumors (see Table 39.1).

Thecomas (see Ch. 34) are usually unilateral. They may be focally luteinized in pregnancy and resemble luteomas. However, the basic spindle shape of the cells is still evident. Reticulin stains are helpful in highlighting the abundant fibers around individual cells, and the perivascular hyaline plaques. Mitoses are rare.

Sclerosing stromal tumors (see Ch. 34), closely related to thecomas, display a striking lobulated pattern which is due to bands of edematous immature or mature collagenous stroma (not found in luteomas). Within the lobules there is abundant pericellular reticulin as seen in thecomas. Another helpful distinguishing feature is the mixed population of spindle and polyhedral eosinophilic cells (mostly the latter).

Granulosa cell tumors (see Ch. 33) are rare in pregnancy but, when they occur, are usually of the juvenile type which may closely resemble luteomas (Young et al 1984). However, they display a variegated histological pattern, including macrofollicular and diffuse areas with only focal areas of luteinized thecal cells. There is often patchy but prominent nuclear pleiomorphism and moderate mitotic activity. By contrast, luteomas of pregnancy are fairly uniform in appearance, are composed of only one cell type and do not show nuclear pleiomorphism. Granulosa cell tumors of adult type are less likely to cause confusion unless they are of diffuse pattern with marked luteinization. Reticulin stains show very sparse fibres and no alveolar arrangement. Typical trabecular areas are likely to be present, at least focally.

Multiple theca lutein cysts (hyperreactio luteinalis)

While theca lutein cysts (luteinized follicular cysts) can occur at any age and in many different clinical situations (see Ch. 12), multiple bilateral theca lutein cysts are classically associated with molar pregnancies or choriocarcinoma, in which conditions they are identified in about 25% of cases (Caspi et al 1973, Novak & Woodruff 1979, Scully 1979). They also occur in association with Rh iso-immunization, nonimmune hydrops, or multiple pregnancies (Hatjis 1985) and it has also been reported with a placental chorangioma (King et al 1991). The syndrome has even been described in women with apparently normal pregnancies, although on review half of these had features of toxemia (Caspi et al 1973, Barad et al 1981). A similar clinicopathological picture may result rarely from ovarian hyperstimulation provoked by ovulation-induction agents (see Ch. 11). Although multiple bilateral theca lutein cysts are usually associated with abnormally elevated hCG levels, additional factors are likely to be necessary for their genesis. The cysts may persist into, or appear first in, the puerperium when hCG levels have fallen. In the latter situation it is thought that the cysts initially develop during pregnancy under the influence of hCG but are then maintained by the follicle stimulating hormone (FSH) and luteinizing hormone (LH) levels, which rise soon after parturition if lactation is not established (Clement & Scully 1980, Planner et al 1982). Theca lutein cysts are also reported occurring with maternal virilization and elevated maternal serum testosterone levels (Hensleigh et al 1975, Scully 1979, Ito et al 1987, Okadome et al 1989). The female fetuses in these cases, however, showed no evidence of masculinization.

The hyperreactio luteinalis syndrome presents at any stage of pregnancy and even in the puerperium, and may be associated with considerable morbidity and, rarely, mortality. Marked ovarian edema, gross hemorrhage and torsion may lead to ascites, ovarian rupture, hemoperitoneum, or shock. Ovarian enlargement may be responsible for obstructive symptoms and dystocia. At the other end of the clinical spectrum, the cysts may be incidental findings at caesarean section.

The condition almost always regresses within a few weeks after parturition; for this reason surgery during pregnancy, which is often required for diagnostic purposes or for management of acute abdomen or shock, should be as conservative as the condition of the ovary and surgical techniques allow. Intraoperative frozen section examination of an incisional ovarian biopsy may obviate unnecessarily extensive surgery based on the erroneous presumption of malignant disease. Review of the literature reveals a high percentage of incorrect diagnoses by both gynecological surgeon and pathologist (Scully 1979). Because of the association with gestational trophoblastic disease, this possibility should be investigated if the cysts are identified.

Macroscopic features

Both ovaries are usually involved and measure up to 15 cm in diameter, occasionally larger. The capsular surface is lobulated, smooth and shiny, unless disrupted by hemorrhage. Torsion is frequent and the involved ovary may be dark purple owing to diffuse hemorrhage. Sectioning shows multiple cysts separated by very edematous stroma. Most of the cysts range in size from 1 to 4 cm in diameter. They are filled with yellowish fluid or blood and have a thin smooth lining. A normal corpus luteum of pregnancy may also be recognizable (Fig. 10.2).

Microscopic features

The follicular cysts show hyperplasia and prominent luteinization of the theca interna layer; the granulosa is often luteinized as well (Figs 10.3, 10.4). The edematous stroma may also contain large clusters of luteinized stromal cells.

Differential diagnosis

Solitary luteinized follicular cysts of pregnancy and the puerperium (see below) are very large, unilateral and unilocular. Hemorrhage and edema are usually absent. The lining of luteinized cells shows no distinct separation into granulosa and theca layers and exhibits striking focal nuclear pleiomorphism. Luteomas of pregnancy cause

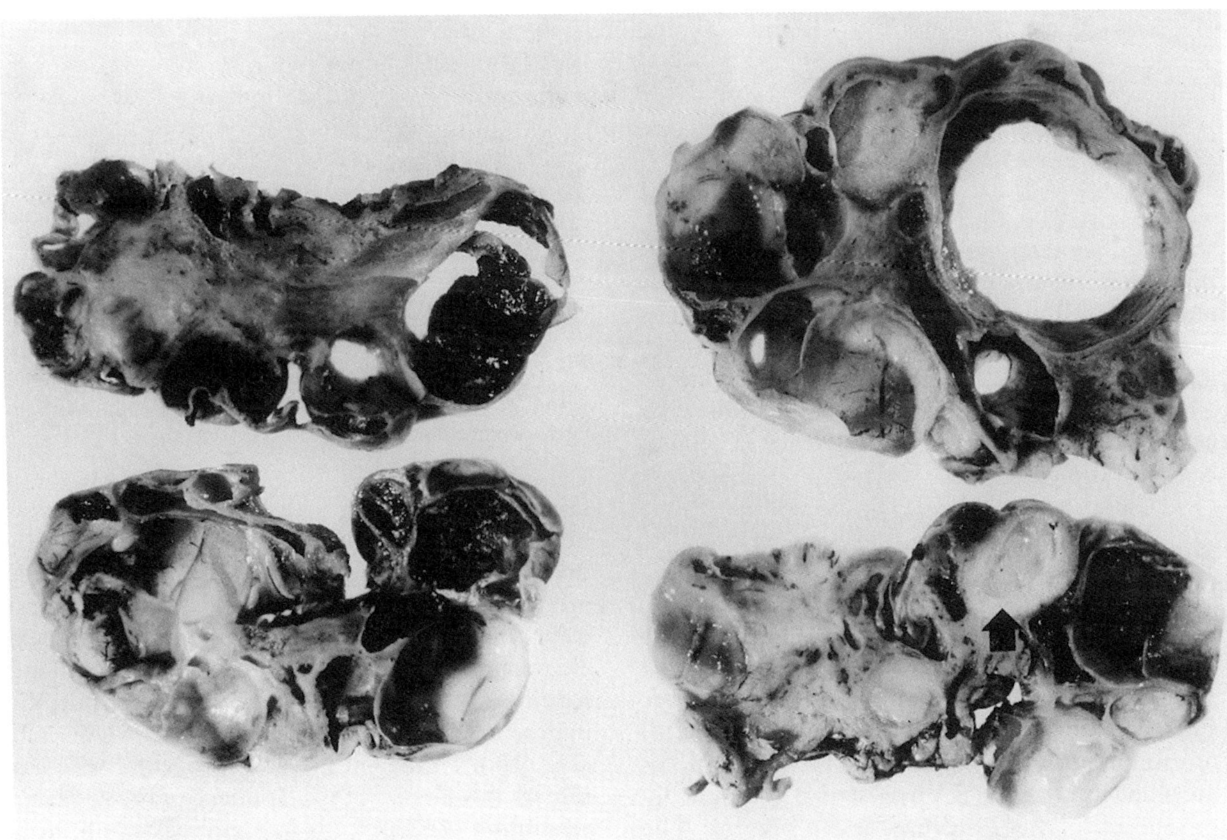

Fig. 10.2 Multiple theca lutein cysts in pregnancy. Both ovaries display multiple cysts and intervening hemorrhagic edematous stroma. The corpus luteum of pregnancy is seen in the slice at the bottom right (arrow). (Tissue courtesy of Dr Warwick Staples, Dubbo, New South Wales)

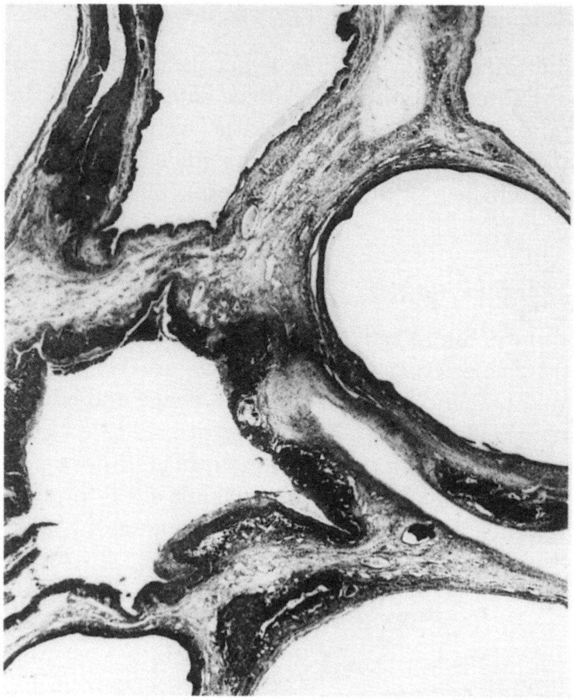

Fig. 10.3 Same case as in Fig. 10.2. Ribbons of luteinized cells line cysts. H + E ×6

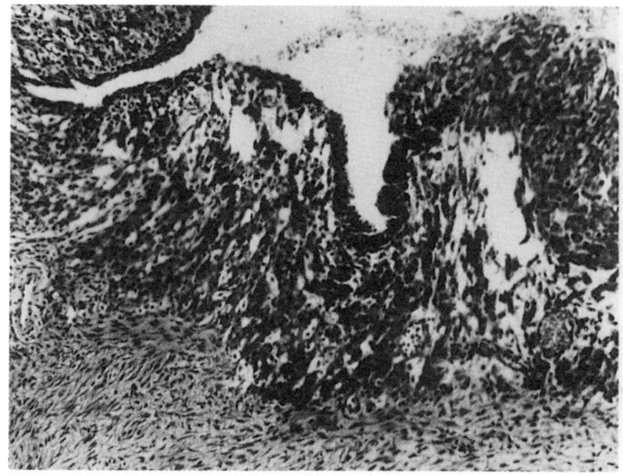

A

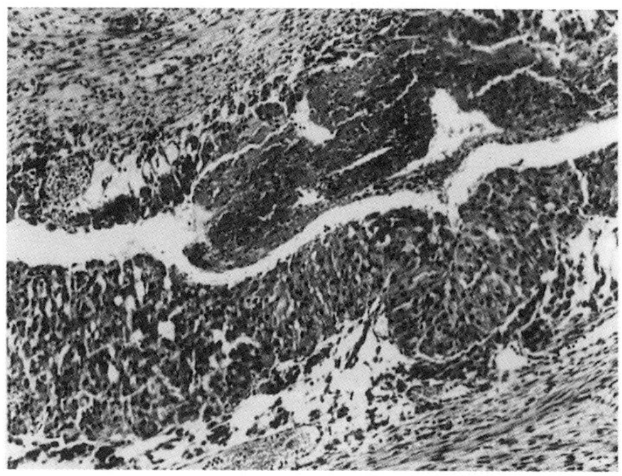

B

Fig. 10.4 Detail of Fig. 10.2. (A) Luteinization of theca predominantly but also of granulosa (right). H + E ×64. (B) Luteinization of both theca and granulosa with some necrosis of the lining (above). H + E ×64

solid, rather than cystic, ovarian enlargement by multinodular masses of luteinized cells. Cystic granulosa cell tumors have not been described in pregnancy but are a potential source of confusion. The tumors may be multicystic and even bilateral. The neoplastic granulosa cells lining the cysts could become luteinized in pregnancy (Clement & Scully 1980).

Solitary luteinized follicular cysts of pregnancy and puerperium

A large distinctive follicular cyst of the ovary occurs during pregnancy (Clement & Scully 1980, Roth et al 1988, Thomas et al 1993). These cysts present as adnexal masses in the third to fourth months of pregnancy or postpartum, or are incidental findings at caesarean section. No clinical endocrine disturbances are present. The involved ovaries exhibit very large (average diameter 25 cm), unilocular, thin-walled cysts which contain clear or mucoid fluid. Microscopically, the cysts are lined by single or multiple layers of large luteinized cells, with only a sparse reticulin network. Similar cells are sometimes also embedded in the fibrous wall of the cysts, but these cells are not obviously thecal in type, i.e. there is no clear definition of the granulosa and thecal elements of the cyst wall (Fig. 10.5). A striking feature is the focal presence of large pleiomorphic hyperchromatic nuclei in the luteinized cells (Fig. 10.6). This latter feature, together with the remarkably large cyst size and lack of recognizable separation of lining cells into granulosa and theca layers, distinguish this entity morphologically from the follicular cysts of nonpregnant women.

Pathogenesis is unknown, but hCG stimulation is probably important. Although the entity has

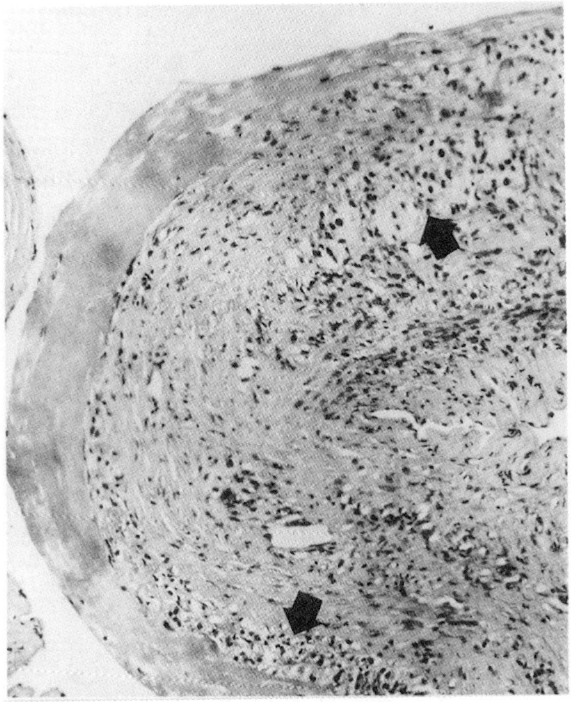

Fig. 10.5 Solitary 23 cm luteinized follicular cyst removed 2 months postpartum following torsion. Groups of pleiomorphic vacuolated luteinized cells (arrows) are present in the fibrous wall. Lumen is lined by fibrin. H + E ×80

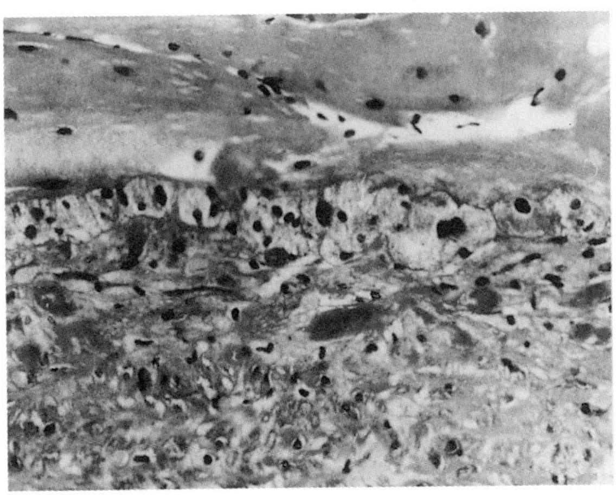

Fig. 10.6 Detail of cyst wall showing luteinized cells with pleiomorphic hyperchromatic nuclei (same case as in Fig. 10.5). H + E ×160

some features in common with hyperreactio luteinalis, the latter is distinguished by multiplicity of cysts, clear distinction between theca and granulosa layers (with luteinization predominantly of the former), widespread stromal edema and hemorrhage, and lack of nuclear pleiomorphism in the cyst lining cells.

Leydig (hilus) cell hyperplasia

This is an uncommonly diagnosed condition which has a close association with pregnancy. It is asymptomatic but may be found incidentally in ovaries biopsied or excised for indications such as tumor (see Ch. 15).

Deciduosis

Deciduosis (extrauterine decidual change), a quasi-physiological process, is not commonly encountered by the surgical pathologist. Decidual change is thought to arise in the subcoelomic mesenchyme as a result of the hormonal stimulus of pregnancy and is thus an expression of mullerianosis (see Ch. 20). It can be identified, if carefully sought, in most ovaries from term or near-term pregnancies (Herr et al 1979); it is found with greater difficulty in the first and second trimesters (Nelson & Greene 1958). Deciduosis also develops on the peritoneal surfaces of other pelvic and abdominal structures. Deciduosis may be exaggerated in patients with trophoblastic disease (see Fig. 53.7). It is also worth noting here that decidual change is regularly observed in the stroma of ovarian endometriotic deposits during pregnancy. Pseudodeciduosis (deciduosis in nonpregnant women) is discussed in Chapter 20.

Macroscopic features

In fresh surgical specimens or as observed at laparotomy, deciduosis appears as a blotchy pink surface change which may assume a gyriform or geographical pattern. The individual foci are flat, verrucous, or nodular and red or pink, consequent upon their vascularity, but blanch after fixation.

Microscopic features

Decidual foci consist of superficial discrete collections of cells cytologically similar to the decidual

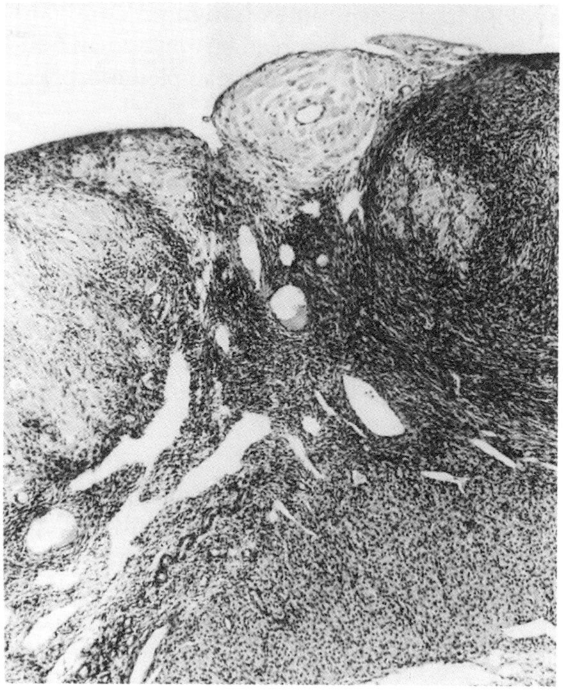

Fig. 10.7 Ovarian deciduosis. Subserosal plaque, with central capillary, plus clustered decidual cells in adjacent cortex. Note stromal luteinization below. H + E ×80

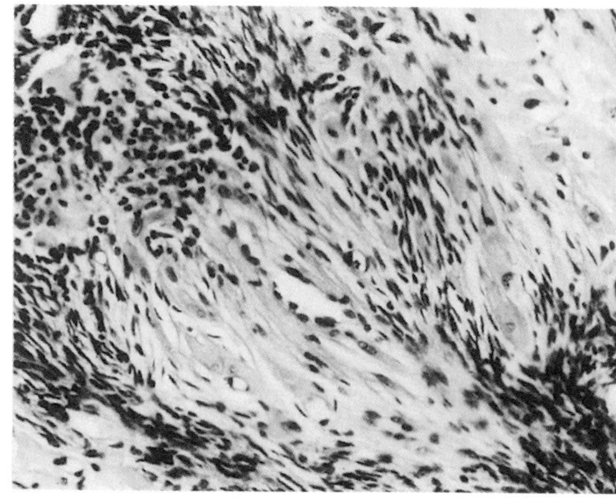

A

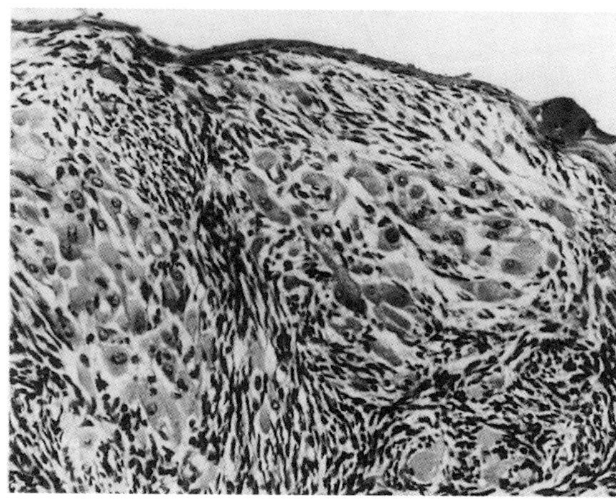

B

Fig. 10.8 Detail of deciduosis. (A) Same case as in Fig. 10.7. Group of decidual cells around capillary and adjacent cluster of lymphocytes. H + E ×160. (B) Decidual cells showing abundant cytoplasm, round to oval nuclei with prominent nucleoli. H + E ×160

cells of gestational endometrium, i.e. distinct cell margins, abundant slightly eosinophilic finely granular cytoplasm, and round pale nuclei with conspicuous nucleoli. Capillaries are prominent and the decidual cells sometimes appear to unsheathe them. There is often a sprinkling of lymphocytes (Figs 10.7, 10.8). Most commonly the foci are nodular or plaque like, but some lie just beneath the serosal surface and are surrounded by edematous stroma. Decidual foci may become confluent. Individual decidual cells may be seen as well, usually adjacent to the larger foci described above (Israel et al 1954).

Ovarian granulosa cell proliferations of pregnancy

Proliferations of granulosa cells that stimulate small neoplasms have been reported as incidental findings in pregnant women (Clement et al 1988). The lesions are usually multiple and are present within atretic follicles. The arrangement of the granulosa cells mimic similar patterns in granulosa cell tumors i.e. solid, microfollicular trabecular, or insular. In all but two of nine cases described, the granulosa cells contained scanty cytoplasm and grooved nuclei resembling the cells of the adult-type granulosa cell tumor. In one of the cases the cells were luteinized with ungrooved nuclei of variable size; in the other case there was a sertoliform pattern and the cytoplasm of the cells was vacuolated, suggesting the presence of lipid.

It is thought that these lesions are a non-neoplastic response to the normal status of pregnancy. The differential diagnosis, however, is that of a small granulosa or Sertoli cell tumor or, where there are luteinized cells, a pregnancy luteoma. The microscopic size, multifocality, and confinement to atretic follicles support the lesions being present.

OTHER OVARIAN LESIONS ASSOCIATED WITH PREGNANCY

Torsion

Torsion of both tumorous and nontumorous ovaries is more common in pregnant than in nonpregnant patients. This is thought to be due to physiological dislocation of the ovaries in pregnancy and to the softening and edema of the pelvic tissues, especially ligaments (see Ch. 17).

Leiomyomatosis peritonealis disseminata

This condition is characterized by the presence of innumerable nodules, 2–3 mm in diameter, scattered throughout the peritoneal cavity but particularly conspicuous in the pelvis and omentum. Ovarian involvement is present in 25% of cases. The nodules are superficial, discrete, and well circumscribed. They are composed of whorled smooth muscle, similar to the familiar uterine leiomyomas, but may also contain some fibroblasts and decidual cells. The condition usually presents in association with pregnancy or use of the oral contraceptive pill. Resolution may be spontaneous postpartum, but can also be accelerated by progesterone. Leiomyomatosis peritonealis disseminata is discussed fully in Chapter 26.

Neoplasms in pregnancy

The true incidence of ovarian neoplasms in pregnancy is difficult to assess from the literature and to a great extent depends on the method of diagnosis (clinical or surgical) and whether nonneoplastic lesions have been included. Most series have excluded all benign lesions less than 5 cm in diameter, although tumors smaller than this have caused clinical problems in pregnancy (Buttery et al 1973). Large series from referral centers probably do not reflect the incidence and distribution of ovarian tumors in pregnancy in the general population (Novak et al 1975). A reasonable figure based on multiple series seems to be of the order of one tumor diagnosed or removed in each 1000 pregnancies, of which 2–5% can be expected to be malignant (contrasted with 20% of ovarian tumors in general). This is in accord with our experience (Table 10.1).

Table 10.1 Primary ovarian tumors diagnosed or removed during pregnancy (119 157 pregnancies, KGV Hospital, 1950–1975)

Surface epithelial–stromal tumors	
Serous:	
Benign	13
Atypically proliferating	1
Mucinous:	
Benign	24
Atypically proliferating	1
Malignant	1
Sex cord–stromal tumors	
Thecoma	1
Sclerosing stromal tumor	1
Fibroma	1
Germ cell tumors	
Teratomas:	
Immature	1
Mature	67
Monodermal (struma)	2
TOTAL	113

The majority of tumors are detected in the first trimester, most commonly following presentation with abdominal pain (due to torsion in half the cases). Discovery by clinical examination at routine antenatal examination or incidental finding at caesarean section are also frequently reported (Buttery et al 1973). Virilization is a rare presentation, even in tumors of stromal origin, presumably because the placenta is capable of aromatizing to estrogens the excessive androgens produced (Verhoeven et al 1973, Hensleigh et al 1975, Young et al 1984). However metastatic tumors with stromal luteinisation, especially those of Krukenberg type, are more commonly associated with virilisation in pregnant, contrasted with nonpregnant, hosts and may also be responsible for masculinisation of a female fetus (see Ch. 55). This complication is less commonly associated with primary epithelial tumors (Verhoeven et al 1973). Torsion and rupture of tumors occur more commonly in pregnant than nonpregnant patients.

It is generally considered that cystic lesions less

than 10 cm in diameter identified in the first trimester should be followed clinically until about the 16th week; by this time the cyst, if dysfunctional in type, may already be undergoing involution (Barber 1981, Young et al 1984, Struyk & Treffers 1984). This expectant management obviates surgery in early pregnancy with its high risk of precipitating an abortion. Solid lesions, as determined by ultrasound, require immediate surgery, with frozen section control, because of the greater possibility of malignancy. Intraoperative diagnosis of benign or non-neoplastic lesions, e.g. luteomas, will then allow partial ovarian conservation. Pregnancy does not exert an adverse effect on the prognosis of ovarian cancers. On the contrary, tumors first detected in pregnancy have a better outcome statistically, probably because the regular antenatal examinations result in tumors being discovered at an earlier stage than might otherwise have occurred (Creasman et al 1971). Also, malignant tumors identified in pregnant women tend to be of low histological grade (Novak et al 1975).

The most common benign tumors associated with pregnancy are mature cystic teratomas (dermoid cysts), which constitute very close to 50% of tumors in most series. The next most frequent lesions are the cystadenomas; varying ratios of mucinous to serous subtypes have been recorded, but in the larger series mucinous tumors have been more frequent, reflecting their incidence in women overall (Buttery et al 1973, Russell 1979, Struyk & Treffers 1984).

Malignant tumors are too infrequent for any center to have collected sufficient cases for meaningful analysis of their histological distribution. Surface epithelial–stromal tumors appear to outnumber germ cell tumors, despite the relative youth of the population under study. Most other types of primary ovarian tumors have also been reported in pregnancy. Metastatic tumors, especially those of Krukenberg type, are not infrequently reported.

The histological appearance of tumors in pregnancy is generally the same as that seen in the non-pregnant patients. Notable exceptions are the sex cord–stromal tumors which may show prominent edema and also a degree of luteinization, which sometimes results in difficulty in classification (Young et al 1984). Metastatic carcinomas, and, to a lesser extent, primary epithelial–stromal tumors, may show stromal luteinization.

Ovarian pregnancy

Ovarian nidation occurs about once in every 10 000 pregnancies and accounts for approximately 1% of ectopic gestations (Hallatt 1982, Grimes et al 1983). The ratio of ovarian to tubal pregnancies is increased in users of intrauterine contraceptive devices (IUDs), which confer some protection against the latter (Berger & Blechner 1978, Rivera et al 1988). There is no definite evidence that use of an IUD predisposes to ovarian pregnancy (Lehfeldt et al 1970). In marked contrast to patients with tubal ectopics, most series have shown that patients with ovarian pregnancies are highly fertile and have a lower than average incidence of pelvic inflammatory disease and endometriosis (Boronow et al 1965, Hallatt 1982).

The clinical presentation in most cases is similar to that of tubal ectopic gestation. Hemoperitoneum is frequent, but blood loss is often greater than with the tubal equivalent. The greater vascularity of the ovary probably accounts for the higher percentage of ovarian pregnancies, compared with tubal, which proceed beyond the first trimester. The review by Boronow et al (1965) revealed that 91% of ovarian pregnancies terminated in the first trimester, 5.3% in the second, and 3.7% in the third. An exceptional case presented at term with obstructed labor. Such cases have a high risk of perinatal mortality, but livebirths have been reported (Mofid et al 1976, Williams et al 1982). Ovarian pregnancy, like its tubal equivalent, may also be subclinical, with spontaneous death and resorption of the conceptus (Hallatt 1982).

The pathogenesis is best explained by chance fertilization of an unexpectedly mature ovum within the fimbriae, or on the ovarian surface, and subsequent implantation in the ovarian parenchyma. Intrafollicular implantation and development of the conceptus within the corpus luteum itself is considered highly unlikely. This is not only because the ovum would not have completed its first meiotic division and matured to the point of being able to accept fertilization, but also because of the inhospitable environment in the hemorrhagic corpus luteum. Ovarian endometriosis is thought to play no role in local nidation.

Definitive diagnosis of ovarian pregnancy requires proof of ovarian nidation and exclusion of tubal nidation with secondary ovarian involvement, and the following criteria are applicable:

- The tube must be intact and clearly separate from the ovary
- The fetal sac should occupy the normal position of the ovary and be connected to the uterus by the utero-ovarian ligament
- Definite ovarian tissue must be present in the sac wall

These criteria obviously become more difficult to establish in more advanced gestations, and in these cases it has been suggested that confirmation of ovarian pregnancy requires the demonstration of ovarian tissue at several places in the fetal sac wall, including at a point between the sac and any adherent structures (Boronow et al 1965).

Macroscopic features

The typical first trimester ovarian pregnancy is seen as a hemorrhagic cyst, which is often ruptured. Distinction from a corpus luteum may be difficult for both surgeon and pathologist, particu-

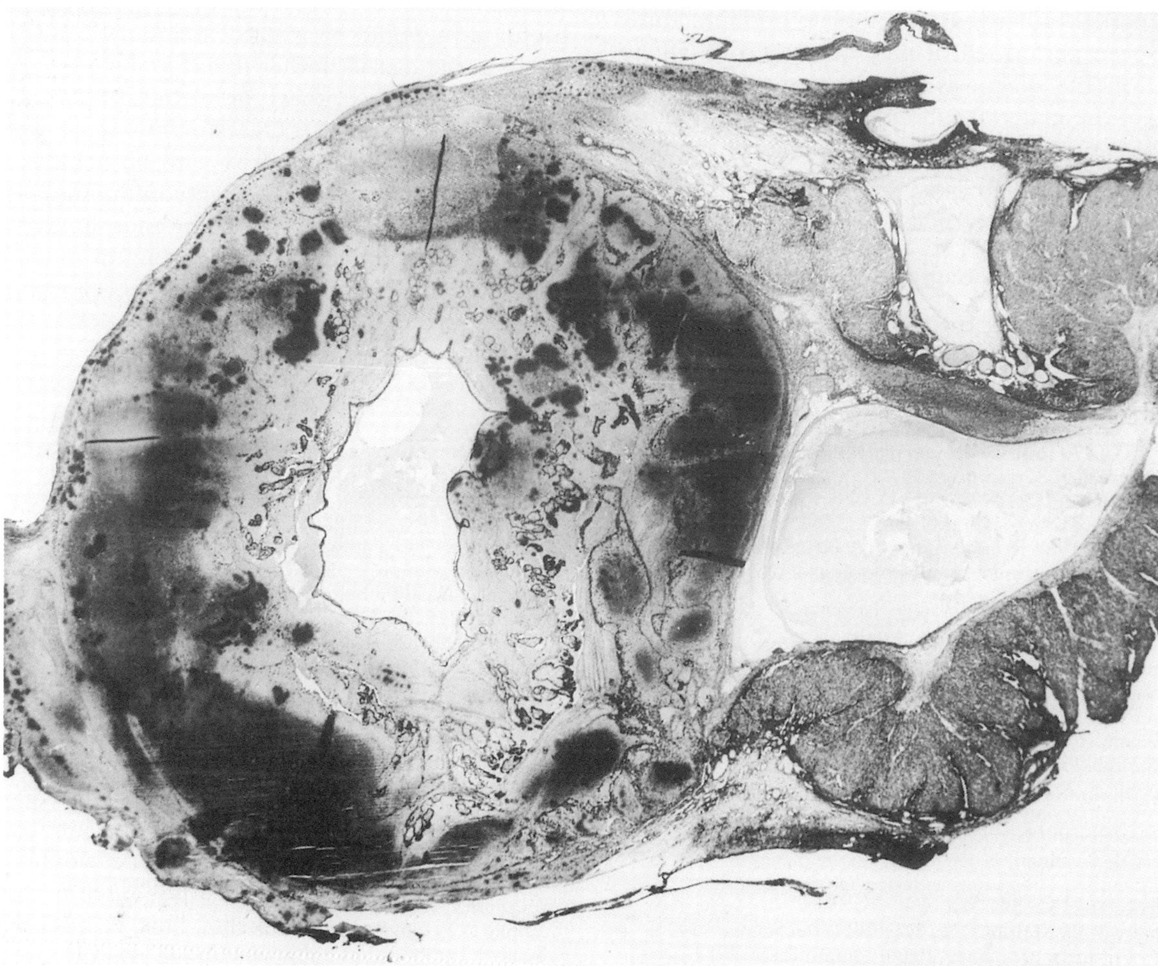

Fig. 10.9 Ectopic ovarian pregnancy. Chorionic vesicle and immature villi surrounded by blood clot. Corpus luteum at right. H + E ×8

larly since a corpus luteum is always also present, often in contiguity, with an ovarian pregnancy. In less than half the reported cases a sac containing an embryo can be identified. The fallopian tube, if submitted, is distinctly separate from the ovary and is usually free of disease.

Microscopic features

Histological examination is necessary to confirm that trophoblastic tissue is present in juxtaposition to unequivocal ovarian structures. A corpus luteum of pregnancy can often be identified close to the hemorrhagic implantation site (Fig. 10.9). Deciduosis and other pregnancy-associated alterations may be noted in the adjacent parenchyma. If a partial rather than a complete oophorectomy has been performed, it may be more difficult to confirm the diagnosis by pathological examination of the material submitted, and consideration of the surgeon's operative findings may be required to arrive at the correct diagnosis.

Primary ovarian trophoblastic disease

Ovarian hydatidiform mole is an extremely rare lesion which is considered to develop subsequent to ovarian pregnancy. The ovary is grossly enlarged and replaced by an encapsulated hemorrhagic mass of vesicles. Confirmation of primary ovarian origin requires exclusion of extension of molar disease from the uterus or fallopian tube, as well as demonstration that the molar tissue is intraovarian (Adli 1978, Jock et al 1981, d'Aguillo et al 1982).

Gestational choriocarcinoma in the ovary may be either metastatic from the uterus or a primary tumor developing subsequent to ovarian pregnancy. Exclusion of the former beyond reasonable doubt is implicit in confirming the latter possibility, something which is extraordinarily difficult to do (Fox & Langley 1976, Benjamin & Rorat 1978, Axe et al 1985). It has been suggested that a useful term would be 'choriocarcinoma occurring solely in the ovary', rather than forcing a particular case into the primary or metastatic category (Veridiano et al 1980). Ovarian choriocarcinoma has been reported to coexist with an apparently normal uterogestation, further confounding the issue (Cunanan et al 1980). The morphology of choriocarcinoma and the problems in diagnosis of nongestational choriocarcinoma (germ cell tumor) are discussed in Chapter 45.

REFERENCES

Adli A G 1978 Primary ovarian hydatidiform mole. International Surgery 63: 103

Axe S R, Klein V R, Woodruff J D 1985 Choriocarcinoma of the ovary. Obstetrics and Gynecology 66: 111–114

Ballard C A 1984 Ovarian tumors associated with pregnancy termination patients. American Journal of Obstetrics and Gynecology 149: 384–387

Barad D H, Gimovsky M L, Petrie R H, Bowe E T 1981 Diagnosis and management of bilateral theca lutein cysts in a normal term pregnancy. Diagnostic Gynecology and Obstetrics 3: 27–30

Barber H R K 1981 Malignant disease in the pregnant woman. In: Coppleson M (ed) Gynecologic oncology. Churchill Livingstone, Edinburgh, p 795–806

Benjamin F, Rorat E 1978 Primary gestational choriocarcinoma of the ovary. American Journal of Obstetrics and Gynecology 131: 343–345

Berger B, Blechner J N 1978 Ovarian pregnancy associated with copper-7 intrauterine device. Obstetrics and Gynecology 52: 597–600

Boronow R C, McElin T W, West R H, Buckingham J C 1965 Ovarian pregnancy. Report of four cases and a thirteen-year survey of the English literature. American Journal of Obstetrics and Gynecology 91: 1095–1106

Buttery B W, Beischer N A, Fortune D W, Macafee C A J 1973 Ovarian tumors in pregnancy. Medical Journal of Australia 1: 345–349

Caspi E, Schreyer P, Bukovsky J 1973 Ovarian lutein cysts in pregnancy. Obstetrics and Gynecology 42: 388–398

Clement P B 1993 Tumour-like lesions of the ovary associated with pregnancy. International Journal of Gynaecological Pathology 12: 108–115

Clement P B, Scully R E 1980 Large solitary luteinised follicle cyst of pregnancy and puerperium. A clinicopathological analysis of eight cases. American Journal of Surgical Pathology 4: 431–438

Clement P B, Young R H, Scully R E 1988 Ovarian granulosa cell proliferations of pregnancy: a report of nine cases. Human Pathology 19: 657–662

Creasman W T, Rutledge F, Smith J P 1971 Carcinoma of the ovary associated with pregnancy. Obstetrics and Gynecology 38: 111–116

Cunanan R G, Lippes J, Tancinco P A 1980 Choriocarcinoma of the ovary with coexisting normal pregnancy. Obstetrics and Gynecology 55: 669–672

d'Aguillo A F, Goldberg M I, Kamalamma M, Yuliano S E, Scully J T 1982 Primary ovarian hydatidiform mole. Human Pathology 13: 279–281

Fox H, Langley F A 1976 Tumours of the ovary. Heinemann, London, p 196–209

Garcia-Bunuel R, Brandes D 1976 Luteoma of pregnancy: ultrastructural features. Human Pathology 7: 205–214
Grimes H G, Nosal R A, Gallagher J C 1983 Ovarian pregnancy: a series of 24 cases. Obstetrics and Gynecology 61: 174–180
Hallatt J G 1982 Primary ovarian pregnancy: A report of 25 cases. American Journal of Obstetrics and Gynecology 143: 55–60
Hatjis C G 1985 Nonimmunologic fetal hydrops associated with hyperreactio luteinalis. Obstetrics and Gynecology 65: 11s–13s
Heller D S, Frydman C P, Klein M J 1990 Luteoma of pregnancy. Mount Sinai Journal of Medicine 57: 40–42
Hensleigh P A, Carter R P, Grotjan H E 1975 Fetal protection against masculinization with hyperreactio luteinalis and virilization. Journal of Clinical Endocrinology and Metabolism 40: 816–823
Herr J C, Platz C E, Heidger P M, Curet L B 1979 Smooth muscle within ovarian decidual nodules: a link to leiomyomatosis peritonealis disseminata? Obstetrics and Gynecology 53: 451–456
Israel S L, Rubenstone A, Meranze D R 1954 The ovary at term. 1. Decidua-like reaction and surface cell proliferation. Obstetrics and Gynecology 3: 399–407
Ito M, Tohya T, Yoshimura T, Matsui K, Fujisaki S, Okamura H 1987 Theca lutein cysts with maternal virilization and elevated serum testosterone in pregnancy. Acta Obstetricia et Gynaecologica Scandinavica 66: 565–566
Jock D E, Schwartz P E, Portnoy L 1981 Primary ovarian hydatidiform mole: addition of a sixth case to the literature. Obstetrics and Gynecology 58: 657–659
King P A, Lopes A, Tang M H, Lam S K, Ma H K 1991 Theca-lutein cysts associated with placental chorangioma. Case report. British Journal of Obstetrics and Gynaecology 98: 322–323
Krause D E, Stembridge V A 1966 Luteomas of pregnancy. American Journal of Obstetrics and Gynecology 95: 192–206
Lehfeldt H, Tietze C, Gorstein F 1970 Ovarian pregnancy and the intrauterine device. American Journal of Obstetrics and Gynecology 108: 1005–1009
Mofid M, Rhee M W, Lankerani M 1976 Ovarian pregnancy with delivery of a live baby. Obstetrics and Gynecology 47: 5s–8s
Nelson W W, Greene R R 1958 Some observations on the histology of the human ovary during pregnancy. American Journal of Obstetrics and Gynecology 76: 66–90
Norris H J, Taylor H B 1967 Nodular theca-lutein hyperplasia of pregnancy (so-called 'pregnancy luteoma'). A clinical and pathological study of 15 cases. American Journal of Clinical Pathology 47: 557–566
Norris H J, Chorlton I 1974 Functioning tumors of the ovary. Clinical Obstetrics and Gynecology 17: 189–228
Novak E R, Lambrou C D, Woodruff J D 1975 Ovarian tumors in pregnancy. An Ovarian Tumor Registry review. Obstetrics and Gynecology 46: 401–406
Novak E R, Woodruff J D 1979 Novak's Gynecologic and obstetric pathology with clinical and endocrine relations, 8th edn. W B Saunders, Philadelphia, p 651–688
Okadome M, Kaku T, Tsukamoto M et al 1989 Hyperreactio luteinalis in normal singleton pregnancy. International Journal of Gynaecology and Obstetrics 29: 365–371
Planner R S, Abell D A, Barbaro C A, Beischer N A 1982 Australian and New Zealand Journal of Obstetrics and Gynaecology 22: 96–100
Polansky S, DePapp E W, Ogden E B 1974 Virilisation associated with bilateral luteomas of pregnancy. Obstetrics and Gynecology 45: 516–522
Rivera F H, Torres F J, Rodriguez A F 1988 Ovarian pregnancy; a clinicopathological study of eight cases. European Journal of Obstetrics and Gynaecology 29: 339–345
Roth L M, Ehrlich C E, Ellis G H 1988 Large luteinized follicular cyst of pregnancy and puerperium Southern Medical Journal 81: 805–806
Russell P 1979 The pathological assessment of ovarian neoplasms. 1: Introduction to the common 'epithelial' tumors and analysis of benign 'epithelial' tumors. Pathology 11: 5–26
Scully R E 1979 Tumors of the ovary and maldeveloped gonads. In: Atlas of tumor pathology, fascicle 16, second series. Armed Forces Institute of Pathology, Washington, p 364–399
Sternberg W H, Barclay D L 1966 Luteoma of pregnancy. American Journal of Obstetrics and Gynecology 95: 165–181
Sternberg W H, Dhurandhar H N 1977 Functional ovarian tumors of stromal and sex cord origin. Human Pathology 8: 565–582
Struyk A P H B, Treffers P E 1984 Ovarian tumors in pregnancy. Acta Obstetricia et Gynecologica Scandinavica 63: 421–442
Thomas S, Krishnasawami H, Seshadri L 1993 Large solitary luteinized follicle cyst of pregnancy and puerperium. Acta Obstetricia et Gynecologica Scandinavica 72: 678–679
Verhoeven A T M, Mastboom J L, Van Leusden H A I M, Van Der Velden W H M 1973 Virilization in pregnancy coexisting with an (ovarian) mucinous cystadenoma: a case report and review of virilizing ovarian tumors in pregnancy. Obstetrical and Gynecological Survey 28: 597–622
Veridiano N P, Gal D, Delke I, Rosen Y, Tancer M L 1980 Gestational choriocarcinoma of the ovary. Gynecologic Oncology 10: 235–240
Williams P C, Malvar T C, Kraft J R 1982 Term ovarian pregnancy with delivery of a live female infant. American Journal of Obstetrics and Gynecology 142: 589–591
Young R H, Dudley A G, Scully R E 1984 Granulosa cell, Sertoli–Leydig cell and unclassified sex cord-stromal tumors associated with pregnancy: a clinicopathological analysis of thirty-six cases. Gynecologic Oncology 18: 181–205

11

Iatrogenic, traumatic, and hemorrhagic lesions

P. Russell A. Farnsworth

A classification of iatrogenic, traumatic, and hemorrhagic lesions is given in Table 11.1.

SEQUELAE OF SURGERY OR TRAUMA

Ovarian remnant syndrome

This condition is said to exist if a patient, who is thought to have had a total bilateral oophorectomy, later develops a palpable mass or experiences pelvic pain or other symptoms referable to ovarian tissue that has been left behind (Symmonds & Pettit 1979, Muram & Drouin 1982, Pettit & Lee 1988). The incomplete oophorectomy is usually the consequence of difficult surgical dissection secondary to adhesions caused by endometriosis or pelvic inflammatory disease, which is often complicated further by previous surgery. In a premenopausal patient, climacteric symptoms fail to develop and, if the uterus has been left behind, continuing cyclic vaginal bleeding may occur. In these patients clinical suspicions of the syndrome will be confirmed if the serum follicle stimulating hormone (FSH) and leuteinizing hormone (LH) are found to be still within the premenopausal range.

At re-exploration, ovarian remnants may be found attached by usually dense adhesions to any of the residual pelvic structures, including the uterus (Fig. 11.1), or the pelvic wall. Remnants may be grossly enlarged by the presence of endometriotic or dysfunctional cysts, but some consist simply of normal functional ovarian parenchyma (Symmonds & Pettit 1979). Obstruction or compression of the ureter, the colon, or bladder may occur. Clinical and surgical management of the syndrome is discussed by Price et al (1990). Ectopic ovarian remnants should not be confused with accessory or supernumerary ovaries (see Ch. 6).

Table 11.1 Iatrogenic, traumatic, and hemorragic ovarian lesions

Sequelae of surgery or trauma
Ovarian remnant syndrome
Splenosis (autotransplantation of splenic tissue)
Ovarian failure (Ch. 8)
Hypogonadotrophic hypogonadism (Ch. 8)
Foreign body granulomas and adhesions (Ch. 19)
Effects of radiotherapy
Effects of drugs and other exogenous substances
Chemotherapeutic and immunosuppressive drugs
Anticoagulants
Hormones and related drugs:
oral contraceptives
progesterone
danazol
gonadotrophin-releasing hormone analogs
ovulation-induction agents
Alcohol
Cigarette smoke
Carotene
Haemorrhage and rupture (hemoperitoneum)

Splenosis (autotransplantation of splenic tissue)

This most often follows trauma, usually a motor vehicle accident, which has resulted in splenic rupture necessitating splenectomy (Widman & Laubscher 1971, Brewster 1973, Fleming et al 1976). Symmers (1978) reports that the condition can also occur following rupture of a diseased spleen. Nodules of splenic tissue, usually less than 1 cm in diameter, are randomly distributed in the peritoneal cavity and may be found on the ovaries (Fig. 11.2). There is clinical and experimental

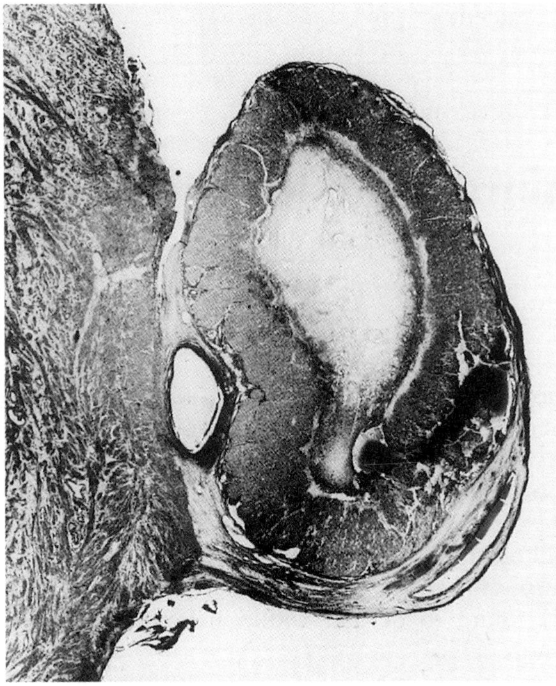

Fig. 11.1 Ovarian remnant, consisting chiefly of a fresh corpus luteum, adherent to the uterine wall in a 46-year-old woman with abnormal uterine bleeding following 'total' bilateral salpingo-oophorectomy. H + E ×5

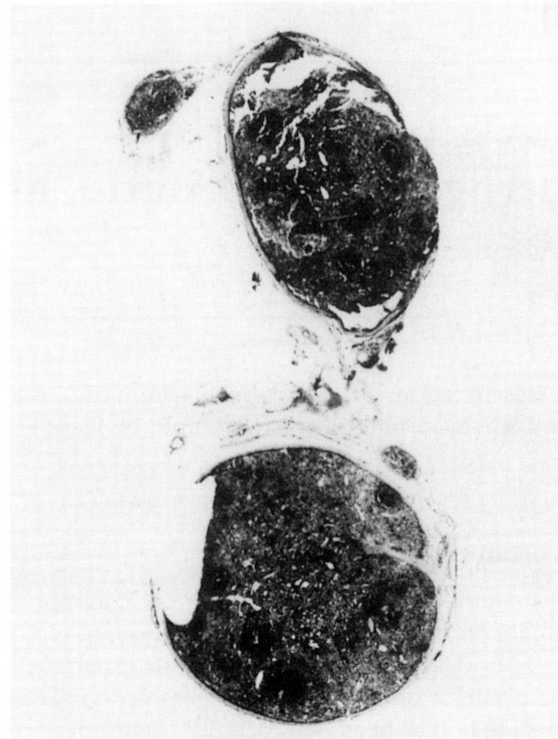

Fig. 11.2 Peritoneal splenotic nodules, thought to represent endometriosis at laparotomy, in a 28-year-old woman with infertility. History of motor vehicle accident followed by splenectomy 17 years previously. H + E ×7

evidence that the implants perform normal splenic function (Fleming et al 1976). Splenosis is generally asymptomatic, but may cause abdominal or pelvic pain simulating endometriosis (Overton 1982, Auerbach et al 1985), or produce intestinal obstruction due to the development of adhesions. The gynecological surgeon may encounter splenosis as an incidental finding, or mistakenly interpret the widespread fleshy reddish-brown or purplish peritoneal nodules as deposits of endometriosis. Clinical confusion is increased if the two conditions coexist (Sinder et al 1965). The implants are encased by fibrous tissue which simulates a splenic capsule, but lacks smooth muscle and elastic fibres. In the larger nodules, all the histological components of normally sited splenic parenchyma are apparent (Fig. 11.3) but, in smaller lesions, red pulp only may be evident. Splenunculi can be distinguished from splenotic foci by their restricted distribution, limited numbers, regular shapes, presence of a capsule and miniature hilus, and lack of associated adhesions.

EFFECTS OF RADIOTHERAPY

The ovaries may be exposed to external high-dose ionising radiation for a variety of reasons – most commonly for the treatment of malignant disease, both in children and adults. In the past, radiotherapy has been used to induce an artificial menopause and to treat some nonmalignant conditions such as endometriosis.

Apart from achieving the desired radiotherapeutic effect on tumor growth, the most important issue at stake for young patients undergoing treatment for malignant disease is that of subsequent fertility. In cases of accidental exposure or inadvertent irradiation of a pregnant woman, the effect on the fetus also has to be considered.

In contrast to gametogenesis in males, proliferation of oogonia ceases in utero and the number of oocytes is then fixed and cannot be replenished. Destruction of these germ cells in utero may lead to ovarian dysgenesis and, postnatally, to prema-

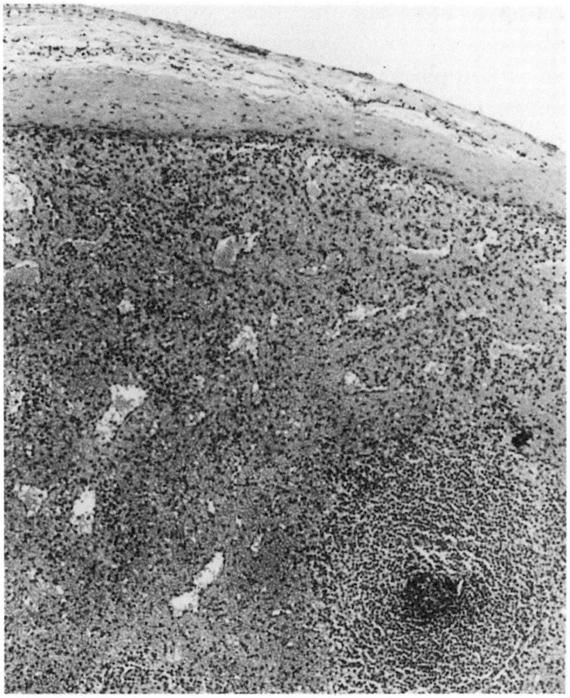

Fig. 11.3 Ovarian splenotic nodule showing fibrous 'capsule', red and white pulp. H + E ×64

ture ovarian failure (Verp 1983, 1985; see Ch. 8). The mitotically active oogonia are much more sensitive to radiation than oocytes which are in a resting phase (prophase of their first meiotic division) until just before ovulation (Baker 1971, Casarett 1980). Ovarian follicles also vary in their sensitivity; actively growing follicles appear to be most vulnerable, possibly because their rapidly proliferating granulosa cells are radiosensitive, and their destruction may lead to death of the oocyte which they invest (Casarett 1980).

The effect of radiation on any particular organ or tissue depends not only on the type of radiation, its dose, and rate of delivery, but also on environmental and host factors (Baker 1971). Doses of less than 150 rad are not harmful to the ovaries of young women, but may be catastrophic for the fetal germ cells and somatic tissues. A dose of 400 rad will render most women over 40 years permanently amenorrheic; 800 rad (acute or fractionated) will sterilize virtually all women. Intermediate doses will cause a variable number of younger women to have temporary or permanent amenorrhea. Children display a greater resistance to radiation-induced ovarian failure. However, high doses (2000–3000 rad), as used in the treatment of abdominal malignancies, will produce permanent ovarian failure (Shalet et al 1976, Stillman et al 1981). Oophoropexy and lead shielding are only partially successful in preserving fertility (le Floch et al 1976, Thomas et al 1976). As is also the case with chemotherapy, return of regular menses or even pregnancy after treatment does not necessarily mean that the ovaries have not been damaged. It may be years before the reduction in the oocyte pool becomes evident as premature ovarian failure (Chapman 1982, Verp 1983, 1985).

Microscopic features

The first observable light microscopic change in irradiated oocytes is nuclear pyknosis. Condensation of chromatin and damage to the nuclear envelope are evident ultrastructurally. The cytoplasmic damage which follows is manifest as eosinophilia. Granulosa cells exhibit pyknosis and karyolysis very soon after a radiation insult and, if a sufficient number of these cells are destroyed and regeneration is inadequate, the oocyte will die and the follicle will undergo atresia (Baker 1971, Casarett 1980). Granulosa lutein cells show cytoplasmic vacuolation. The chronic effect on the follicular apparatus is a decrease in follicular activity, demonstrated by a progressive reduction in the numbers of growing and involuting follicles and corpora lutea, culminating in primordial follicle depletion (Himelstein-Braw et al 1977, Casarett 1980). This irreversible stage is reached more readily in older patients because the pre-irradiation reserve of oocytes is smaller (Verp 1983, 1985).

The acute and chronic irradiation effects in the nonspecialized ovarian structures are similar to those documented more often in other organs (Fajardo & Berthrong 1978). Stromal edema and fibrin exudation progress to stromal hyalinization, fibrosis, and capsular adhesions. Vascular changes are most conspicuous in arteries, which show fibrinoid necrosis, thrombosis, hyalinization of the media, foam cell accumulation, and myointimal proliferation. However, damage to the microvasculature is considered to be the prime mediator of delayed radiation injury, particularly ischemic necrosis and fibrosis (Fajardo & Berthrong 1978).

EFFECTS OF DRUGS AND OTHER EXOGENOUS SUBSTANCES

Chemotherapeutic and immunosuppressive drugs

From limited morphological studies, it would appear that antineoplastic drugs have a similar general effect on the ovary as ionizing radiation – namely death of selected cells, especially those which are proliferating at the time of the insult. Individual drugs have a variable ovarian toxicity, and the factors that influence the response of patients to radiotherapy also operate with respect to chemotherapy. The most important variable is patient age, older women being more likely to develop temporary or permanent amenorrhea due to oocyte destruction (Verp 1983, 1985). By contrast, prepubertal children treated for cancer with cytotoxics alone have good prospects of subsequent fertility (Verp 1983, 1985). This favorable situation has been attributed to the low level of ovarian follicular activity before puberty (Chapman 1982). An attempt to simulate this quiescent state, and thus mitigate the damaging effect of chemotherapy in adults, has been made by giving oral contraceptives during therapy for Hodgkin's disease, with some encouraging clinical results supported by ovarian biopsies, assessed semiquantitatively pre- and posttherapy (Chapman & Sutcliffe 1981, Familiari et al 1993).

Busulphan, one of the earlier cytotoxic drugs, used in the treatment of leukemia, has been noted to render approximately 40% of exposed women amenorrheic; the risk of ovarian failure appears to be age related (Verp 1983, 1985).

Cyclophosphamide is used as an immunosuppressant in various nonmalignant conditions such as rheumatoid arthritis, systemic lupus erythematosus, and glomerulonephritis, and also as a component of combined chemotherapy regimes for malignant disease. When used alone, it causes ovarian failure in about half of treated adult women, the response being related to patient age and dose (Verp 1983, 1985). The demonstration of oocyte depletion in a child treated with cyclophosphamide suggested the mode of ovarian toxicity (Miller et al 1971). Warne et al (1973) examined ovarian biopsies in six treated adults and showed a lack of follicular maturation and (in four cases) oocyte depletion. Their observations suggested a progressive loss of ovarian function with continued drug exposure.

Chlorambucil and nitrogen mustards have caused ovarian failure, but the degree of risk is not well established. The vinca alkaloids appear to have a relatively low potential for ovarian toxicity, while actinomycin D and methotrexate, as used in the treatment of trophoblastic disease, are associated with a negligible risk of subsequent ovarian failure (Verp 1983, 1985).

Combination chemotherapy is likely to cause permanent amenorrhea in about half of treated patients, and the ovarian damage may be progressive (Chapman 1982, Verp 1983, 1985). Biopsies in such patients have shown capsular thickening, perioophoritis, stromal fibrohyalinization, necrotizing vasculitis, hemorrhage, and 'general disintegration of the follicular apparatus' (Morgenfeld et al 1972).

Chemotherapy and radiotherapy

This combination is potentially more damaging to the ovary than either therapeutic modality given alone, and permanent amenorrhea occurs in at least half of adults so treated (Horning et al 1981, Verp 1985). Children also react adversely to these regimes (Himelstein-Braw et al 1977, Stillman et al 1981). In a study of children who survived acute lymphoblastic leukemia treated with combination of chemotherapy and cranial irradiation (Quigley et al 1989), normal or relatively early puberty was observed. Autopsy studies of ovaries of children dying from cancer after such treatment have shown a reduction in the number of follicles and their activity (Himelstein-Braw et al 1978, Nicosia et al 1985).

Hormones and related drugs

Oral contraceptives

Combined estrogen–progestogen contraceptive pills inhibit ovulation by suppressing the release of pituitary gonadotrophins. Morphological effects on the ovaries depend on the type of preparation administered (Sanchez-Rivera et al 1968). High-dose formulas suppress all functional activity, and the ovaries shrink to postmenopausal size. Follicular growth is inhibited, no corpora lutea are formed, and the ovarian stroma becomes dense and fibrous. The basement membrane around primordial follicles is thickened (Mestwerdt & Kranzfelder 1980), but oocytes are unaffected. After several months of therapy, corpora albicantes may be the only evidence of previous follicular activity. With low-dose preparations, there may be continuing folliculogenesis, including the development of mature (Graafian) follicles in which, however, there are subtle morphological aberrations, such as vacuolation of granulosa and thecal cells (more readily observable by electron microscopy (Mestwerdt & Kranzfelder 1980)). Ovulation is still inhibited, the follicles undergo atresia and corpora lutea do not form.

Although practical problems in differential diagnosis are unlikely to arise, it is worth noting here that similar morphological ovarian changes, correlating with functional arrest, are also seen in women with hypogonadotrophic hypogonadism, resistant ovary syndrome (see Ch. 8) and prolonged hyperprolactinemia.

Progesterone

Short-term high-dose progesterone therapy is used in the management of various gynecological disorders, including endometriosis and abnormal uterine bleeding, especially that due to anovulation. Follicular activity is suppressed and ovulation can be inhibited. Foci of pseudodeciduosis (see Ch. 20) may be noted in the ovarian cortex and elsewhere beneath the pelvic peritoneum (Fig. 11.4). Ovarian (and extraovarian) endometriotic lesions may exhibit a progestogenic effect similar to that more commonly encountered in the endometrium. The endometriotic glands are small, poorly developed and relatively inactive, while the stroma shows a pseudodecidual reaction (see Fig. 21.12A).

Low-dose progestogens, as used in the contraceptive 'mini-pill', do not cause the conspicuous morphological alterations noted above. Follicular activity usually continues and ovulation, with the

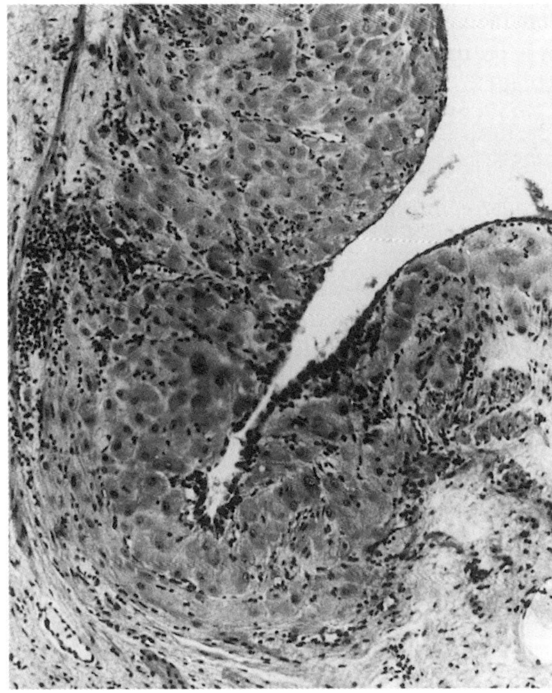

Fig. 11.4 Pseudodeciduosis in the lining of a pelvic mesothelial cyst in a women recently treated with progesterone. A band of large eosinophilic cells is present beneath the mesothelium. H + E ×80

formation of a normal corpus luteum, occurs in about 40% of cases. There is defective ovulation in a further 30% (Landgren & Diczfalusy 1980). Follicular (estrogenic) cysts have been noted in some patients (Tayob et al 1985).

Danazol

This steroid hormone, used in the treatment of endometriosis, dysfunctional uterine bleeding, benign breast disease and angioneurotic edema, causes profound ovarian suppression and inhibits ovulation. It has a complex action, interfering with cyclical FSH and LH production, directly inhibiting follicular development and steroidogenesis, and also having a weak impeded androgenic effect. The ovaries become small and follicular activity is arrested. Endometriotic lesions shrink and may be difficult to identify, even microscopically. The endometriotic glands become very small and are lined by atrophic cuboidal cells which display characteristic ultrastructural changes

(Pedersen & Rank 1984). The endometriotic stroma is compact and similarly inactive, and may be difficult to differentiate from cortical stroma (see Fig. 21.12B).

Gonadotrophin-releasing hormone (GnRH) analogs

These are powerful suppressers of ovarian function (by inhibition of pituitary gonadotrophin secretion) and are used to treat endometriosis and other conditions in which inhibition of estrogen secretion is desired. The ovaries become small and follicular activity ceases.

Ovulation-induction agents

Ovulation-induction agents, especially clomiphene citrate, pulsatile gonadotrophin releasing hormone (GnRH) therapy and human menopausal gonadotrophins, may produce an iatrogenic form of hyperreactio luteinalis (see Ch. 10) known as ovarian hyperstimulation syndrome. This complication develops only after human chorionic gonadotrophin (hCG) is given at the time of ovulation, and is particularly prone to occur in women with the polycystic ovary syndrome (Navot et al 1988, Tulandi et al 1984). A mild form of this syndrome, detectable by ultrasound, is said to occur in as many as 65% of women undergoing ovulation induction (McArdle et al 1983).

In severe cases the ovaries become massively enlarged (Magnus et al 1988) and, although surgical intervention is usually not required, pathological examination shows changes identical to multiple theca lutein cysts as well as one or more corpora lutea. The syndrome may be life threatening, with the development of ascites, hydrothorax (Kingsland et al 1989), or coagulation disturbances resulting in thromboembolic phenomena (Mills et al 1992). The pathophysiology of the condition is discussed by Schenker & Polishuk (1975) and Haning et al (1985).

Tamoxifen

Tamoxifen is being increasingly used as adjuvent therapy in premenopausal women with breast cancer. The hormonal effects of tamoxifen in premenopausal women are associated with increased levels of estradiol and progesterone, whereas FSH and LH remain normal or increase slightly (Spicer et al 1991). Tamoxifen is structurally similar to clomiphene, and is equivalent for induction of ovulation. It is suggested that the elevated serum levels of estrogen and progesterone are due to multiple maturation of ovarian follicles.

There have been recent reports of the development of multiple and single ovarian follicular cysts in premenopausal women treated with tamoxifen (Cohen et al 1994, Terada et al 1993). Both necrosis (Jolles et al 1990) and torsion (Barbieri et al 1993) have also been reported as complications of the development of these cysts.

Alcohol

The ovaries, in contrast to the testes, appear to be resistant to germ cell injury induced by alcohol. Ethanol causes ovarian suppression in rats but its effect on human ovaries has not been adequately studied (Verp 1983, 1985). Inhibition of follicular maturation has been suggested (Galvaõ-Teles et al 1986).

Cigarette smoke

An inverse relationship between number of cigarettes smoked per day and age of menopause has been claimed, based on epidemiological studies. Derivatives of cigarette smoke have been found to be ovotoxic in animal systems, but their effect on human ovaries has not been established (Verp 1983, 1985).

Carotene

Women with excessive intake of carotene-containing foodstuffs and consequent hypercarotenemia have been shown to have 'golden ovaries' which are uniformly bright yellow and display widespread fine lipid granules which stain positively for carotenoid pigments. Two of the six reported cases were young undernourished women with oligomenorrhea/amenorrhea (anorexia nervosa), while the others were older well-nourished women with irregular uterine bleeding (Page 1971).

OVARIAN HEMORRHAGE AND RUPTURE (HEMOPERITONEUM)

Small hemorrhages are common in normally functioning ovaries. The well-vascularized theca interna of developing follicles is prone to hemorrhage, but usually only a small intrafollicular or perifollicular hematoma is formed. Slight bleeding occurs with follicular rupture at ovulation. Bleeding also occurs regularly in the vascularization stage of the corpus luteum; this is usually slight, but if excessive may lead to the formation of a corpus luteum cyst (see Ch. 12).

On occasions, profuse hemorrhage from the above sources may cause ovarian rupture and hemoperitoneum (Fig. 11.5). Most cases have been associated with corpora lutea, especially if

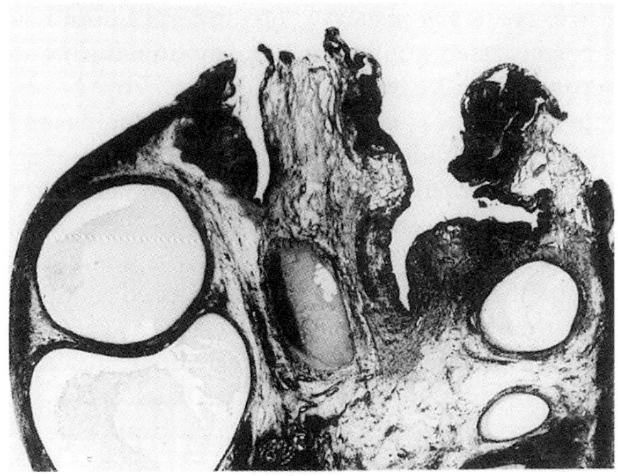

Fig. 11.5 Ruptured hemorrhagic ovulatory follicle from young woman with an acute abdomen. H + E ×5

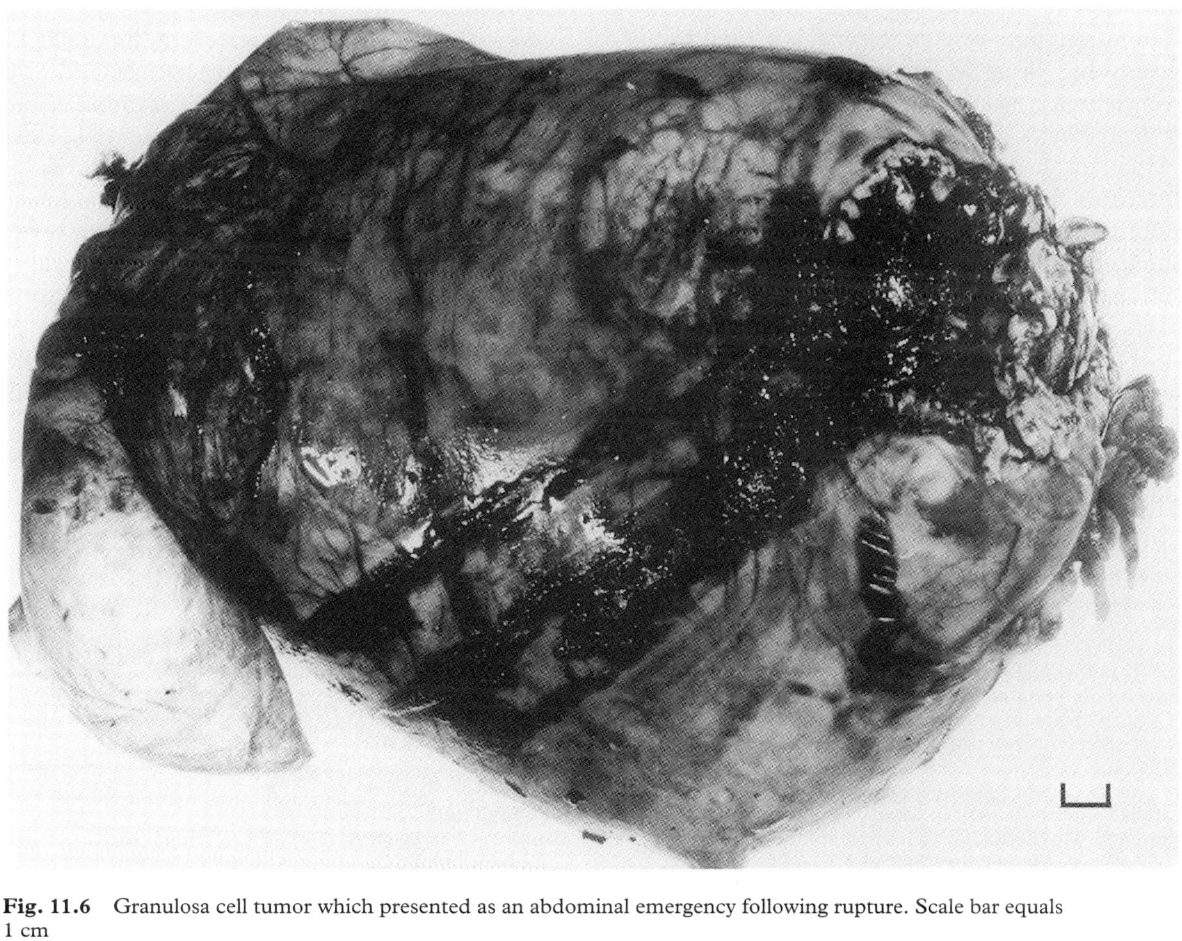

Fig. 11.6 Granulosa cell tumor which presented as an abdominal emergency following rupture. Scale bar equals 1 cm

cystic (Peters et al 1979). Hemoperitoneum from a corpus luteum may occur at any time during the reproductive years, but especially during pregnancy (Hallatt et al 1984). The risk is increased in patients receiving anticoagulants of any type, and may occur even if the coagulation indices are in the therapeutic range (Peters et al 1979, Itskovitz et al 1982, Hill & Kassam 1984). In this clinical group, hemoperitoneum has exceeded 2000 ml and there is an appreciable risk of a recurrent episode (Peters et al 1979). Rupture occurs most often on day 20–26 of the menstrual cycle, and two-thirds of cases involve the right ovary; the relative sparing of the left ovary is considered to be due to its cushioning by the rectosigmoid colon. The clinical features and surgical management are discussed fully by Hallatt et al (1984). Massive ovarian hemorrhage has also been reported in von Willebrand's disease (Weinstein et al 1983). Inhibition of ovulation by oral contraception or bilateral salpingo-oophorectomy and total hysterectomy has been recommended as prophylactic treatment for women at high risk (Peters et al 1979, Itskovitz et al 1982, Weinstein et al 1983).

Ovarian hemorrhage from nonphysiological structures is associated most commonly with endometriosis. Intracystic or large intraovarian hematomas may progress to ovarian rupture and hemoperitoneum. Torsion can lead to hemorrhagic infarction, but rarely to rupture (see Ch. 17). A less common cause is neoplasia; choriocarcinomas, granulosa cell and endodermal sinus tumors are particularly prone to hemorrhage or rupture and may present initially as abdominal emergencies (Fig. 11.6). Rare causes are ectopic (ovarian) pregnancies, hyperreactio luteinalis (see Ch. 10), and the ovarian hyperstimulation syndrome (see above). Pathological examination of the excised tissues (oophorectomy, wedge excision, or cystectomy) will readily identify the source of the bleeding, except when extensive interstitial hemorrhage has obscured morphological detail. In these cases, the operative findings and clinical features should provide a presumptive diagnosis. Sometimes examination of blood clot evacuated from the peritoneal cavity may yield diagnostic material such as groups of lutein cells, chorionic villi, or tumor fragments (Fig. 11.7).

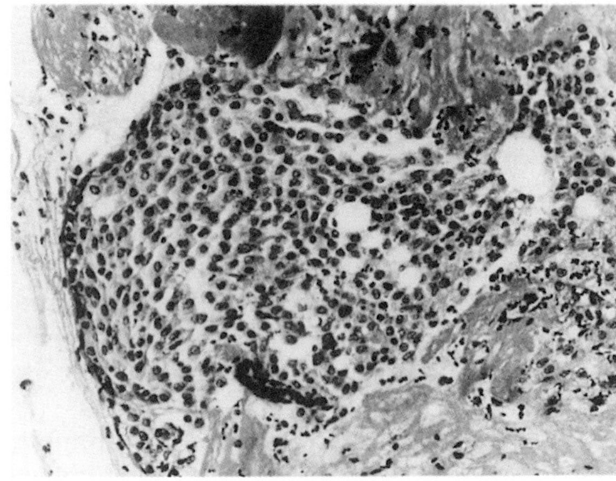

Fig. 11.7 Peritoneal blood clot, containing granulosa cells, retrieved at laparotomy from young woman with ruptured follicular cyst. H + E ×160

REFERENCES

Auerbach R D, Kohorn E I, Cornelius E A, Chambers J T 1985 Splenosis: a complicating factor in total abdominal hysterectomy. Obstetrics and Gynecology 65: 65s–68s

Baker T G 1971 Radiosensitivity of mammalian oocytes with particular reference to the human female. American Journal of Obstetrics and Gynecology 110: 746–761

Barbieri R L, Ferracci A L, Droesch J N, Rochelson B L 1993 Ovarian torsion in a premenopausal woman treated with tamoxifen for breast cancer. Fertility and Sterility 59: 459–460

Brewster D C 1973 Splenosis. Report of two cases and review of the literature. American Journal of Surgery 126: 14–19

Casarett G W 1980 Radiation histopathology. CRC Press, Boca Raton, FL, vol 2, p 75–94

Chapman R M 1982 Effect of cytotoxic therapy on sexuality and gonadal function. Seminars in Oncology 9: 84–94

Chapman R M, Sutcliffe S B 1981 Protection of ovarian function by oral contraceptives in women receiving chemotherapy for Hodgkin's disease. Blood 58: 849–851

Cohen I, Rosen D J, Attaras M, Beyth Y, Shapira J, Yigael D 1994 Tamoxifen treatment in premenopausal breast cancer patients may be associated with ovarian overstimulation, cyst formation and fibroid overgrowth. British Journal of Cancer 69: 620–621

Fajardo L F, Berthrong M 1978 Radiation injury in surgical pathology. Part I. American Journal of Surgical Pathology 2: 159–199

Familiari G, Caggiati A, Nottola S A, Ermini M, Di Benedetto M R, Motta P M 1993 Ultrastructure of human ovarian primordial follicles after combination chemotherapy for Hodgkin's disease. Human Reproduction 8: 2080–2087

Fleming C R, Dickson E R, Harrison E G 1976 Splenosis: autotransplantation of splenic tissue. American Journal of Medicine 61: 414–419

Galvaõ-Teles A, Monteiro E, Gavaler J S, Van Thiel D H 1986 Gonadal consequences of alcohol abuse: lessons learned from the liver. Hepatology 6: 135–140

Hallatt J G, Steele C H, Snyder M 1984 Ruptured corpus luteum with hemoperitoneum: a study of 173 surgical cases. American Journal of Obstetrics and Gynecology 149: 5–8

Haning R V, Strawn E Y, Nolten W E 1985 Pathophysiology of the ovarian hyperstimulation syndrome. Obstetrics and Gynecology 66: 220–224

Hill J A, Kassam S H 1984 Ovarian haemorrhage in ovulating women receiving anticoagulant therapy. A report of two cases. Journal of Reproductive Medicine 29: 205–208

Himelstein-Braw R, Peters H, Faber M 1977 Influence of irradiation and chemotherapy on the ovaries of children with abdominal tumors. British Journal of Cancer 36: 269–275

Himelstein-Braw R, Peters H, Faber M 1978 Morphological study of the ovaries of leukaemic children. British Journal of Cancer 38: 82–87

Horning S J, Hoppe R T, Kaplan H S, Rosenberg S A 1981 Female reproductive potential after treatment for Hodgkin's disease. New England Journal of Medicine 304: 1377–1382

Itskovitz J, Brandes J M, Urbach J, Fisher M 1982 Ovarian hematoma and hemoperitoneum complicating anticoagulant therapy. International Surgery 67: 533–534

Jolles C J, Smotkin D, Ford K L, Jones K P 1990 Cystic ovarian necrosis complicating tamoxifen therapy for breast cancer in a premenopausal woman. A case report. Journal of Reproductive Medicine 35: 229–300

Kingsland C R, Collins J V, Rizk B, Mason B A 1989 Ovarian hyperstimulation presenting as acute hydrothorax after in vitro fertilization. American Journal of Obstetrics and Gynecology 161: 381–382

Landgren B-M, Diczfalusy E 1980 Hormonal effects of the 300 mg norethisterone (NET) minipill. Contraception 21: 87–113

le Floch O, Donaldson S S, Kaplan H S 1976 Pregnancy following oophoropexy and total nodal irradiation in women with Hodgkin's disease. Cancer 38: 2263–2268

McArdle C, Sdibel M, Hann L E et al 1983 The diagnosis of ovarian hyperstimulation OHS: the impact of ultrasound. Fertility and Sterility 39: 464–467

Magnus O, Tanbo T, Henriksen T, Abyholm T 1988 Severe ovarian hyperstimulation syndrome. Case reports. Acta Europaea Fertilitatis 19: 89–92

Mestwerdt W, Kranzfelder D 1980 Morphologic findings in the human ovary under physiologic conditions and after contraceptive use. In: Dallenbach-Hellweg G (ed) Functional morphologic changes in female sex organs induced by exogenous hormones. Springer-Verlag, Berlin, p 168–179

Miller J J, Williams G F, Leissring J C 1971 Multiple late complications of therapy with cyclophosphamide, including ovarian destruction. American Journal of Medicine 50: 530–535

Mills M S, Eddowes H A, Fox R, Wardle P G 1992 Subclavian vein thrombosis: a late complication of ovarian hyperstimulation syndrome. Human Reproduction 7: 370–371

Morgenfeld M C, Goldberg V, Parisier H, Bugnard S C, Bur G E 1972 Ovarian lesions due to cytostatic agents during the treatment of Hodgkin's disease. Surgery, Gynecology and Obstetrics 134: 826–828

Muram D, Drouin P1982 Ovarian remnant syndrome. Canadian Medical Association Journal 127: 399–400

Navot D, Relov A, Birkenfeld A, Rabinowitz R, Brezinski A, Margalioth E J 1988 Risk factors and prognostic variables in the ovarian hyperstimulation syndrome. American Journal of Obstetrics and Gynecology 159: 210–215

Nicosia S V, Matus-Ridley M, Meadows A T 1985 Gonadal effects of cancer therapy in girls. Cancer 55: 2364–2372

Overton T H 1982 Splenosis: a cause of pelvic pain. American Journal of Obstetrics and Gynecology 143: 969–970

Page S W 1971 Golden ovaries. Australian and New Zealand Journal of Obstetrics and Gynaecology 11: 32–36

Pedersen H, Rank F 1984 Morphology of endometriosis before and during treatment with danazol. Acta Obstetricia et Gynecologica Scandinavica 123 (suppl): 13–14

Peters W A, Thiagarajah S, Thornton W N 1979 Ovarian hemorrhage in patients receiving anticoagulant therapy. Journal of Reproductive Medicine 22: 82–86

Pettit P D, Lee R A 1988 Ovarian remnant syndrome: diagnostic dilemma and surgical challenge. Obstetrics and Gynecology 71: 580–583

Price F V, Edwards R, Buchsbaum H J 1990 Ovarian remnant syndrome: difficulties in diagnosis and management. Obstetrical and Gynecological Survey 45: 151–156

Quigley C, Cowell C, Jimenez M et al 1989 Normal or early development of puberty despite gonadal damage in children treated for acute lymphoblastic leukaemia. New England Journal of Medicine 321: 143–151

Sanchez-Rivera G, Merlo J G, Escudero M, Botella-Llusia J 1968 Action of several synthetic steroids of the human ovary. American Journal of Obstetrics and Gynecology 101: 665–671

Schenker J G, Polishuk W Z 1975 Ovarian hyperstimulation syndrome. Obstetrics and Gynecology 46: 23–28

Shalet S M, Beardwell C G, Morris Jones P H, Pearson D, Orrell DH 1976 Ovarian failure following abdominal irradiation in childhood. British Journal of Cancer 33: 655–658

Sinder C, Dochat G R, Wentsler N E 1965 Splenoendometriosis. American Journal of Obstetrics and Gynecology 92: 883–884

Spicer D V, Pike M C, Henderson B E 1991 Ovarian cancer and long-term tamoxifen in premenopausal women. Lancet 337: 1414

Stillman R J, Schinfeld J S, Schiff I et al 1981 Ovarian failure in long-term survivors of childhood malignancy. American Journal of Obstetrics and Gynecology 139: 62–66

Symmers W St C 1978 The lymphoreticular system. In: Systemic pathology, 2nd edn. Churchill Livingstone, Edinburgh, vol 2, p 728

Symmonds R E, Pettit P D M 1979 Ovarian remnant syndrome. Obstetrics and Gynecology 54: 174–177

Tayob Y, Adams J, Jacobs H S, Guillebaud J 1985 Ultrasound demonstration of increased frequency of functional ovarian cysts in women using progestogen-only oral contraception. British Journal of Obstetrics and Gynecology 92: 1003–1009

Terada S, Uchide K, Suzuki N, Akosofu K 1993 A follicular cyst during tamoxifen therapy in a premenopausal breast cancer woman. Gynecological and Obstetric Investigation 35: 62–64

Thomas P R M, Winstanly D, Peckham M J, Austin D E, Murray M A F, Jacobs H S 1976 Reproductive and endocrine function in patients with Hodgkin's disease: effects of oophoropexy and irradiation. British Journal of Cancer 33: 226–231

Tulandi T, McInnes R A, Arronet G H 1984 Ovarian hyperstimulation following ovulation induction with human menopausal gonadotropin. International Journal of Fertility 29: 113–117

Verp M S 1983 Environmental causes of ovarian failure. Seminars in Reproductive Endocrinolgy 1: 101–111

Verp M S 1985 Environmental factors causing ovarian failure in humans. In: Sciarra J W (ed) Gynecology and obstetrics. Harper & Row, Philadelphia, vol 5, p 1–11

Warne G L, Fairley K F, Hobbs J B, Martin F I R 1973 Cyclophosphamide-induced ovarian failure. New England Journal of Medicine 289:1159–1162

Weinstein D, Rabinowitz R, Malach D, Mor-Yosef S, Eldor A, Schenker J G 1983 Ovarian hemorrhage in women with Von Willebrand's disease. A report of two cases. Journal of Reproductive Medicine 28: 500–502

Widman W D, Laubscher F A 1971 Splenosis. A disease or beneficial condition? Archives of Surgery 102: 152–158

12

Dysfunctional cysts

P. Russell   A. Farnsworth

The term 'dysfunctional' refers to ovarian cysts derived from the follicular apparatus either before or after ovulation. They can be classified as outlined in Table 12.1. Dysfunctional cysts can be either the result or the cause of disordered hypothalamic–pituitary–ovarian function. Although the cysts are not always functional in the sense of producing steroid hormones, they all have or have had the potential to do so at some stage in their development. It should be noted that functional activity is not exclusive to ovarian cysts of follicular origin, since hormonal activity may be associated with some neoplastic cysts as a result of the steroidogenic activity of contiguous stromal cells.

The incidence of dysfunctional cysts is unknown, but they are generally considered to be common. Many are undoubtedly subclinical. Ultrasound examination is now used widely in the diagnosis and surveillance of dysfunctional cysts, which achieve clinical importance if they are larger than 3 cm in diameter and do not disappear on repeat scanning 2–3 weeks later. Although dysfunctional cysts usually resolve spontaneously after a few weeks or months, their resolution can be accelerated by transvaginal ultrasound-guided needle drainage. This procedure can be both diagnostic and therapeutic. Such management may prevent unnecessary ovarian surgery (Turetz et al 1980). A further discussion of this procedure and the cytology of the aspirated fluid is given below.

Table 12.1 Classification of dysfunctional ovarian cysts

Cysts derived from preovulatory follicles
Follicular cyst – unluteinized
Follicular cyst – luteinized:
granulosa lutein cyst
theca lutein cyst
Follicular cyst – atretic
Cysts derived from corpus luteum
Cystic corpus luteum
Corpus luteum cyst
Corpus albicans cyst
Simple cysts

We have avoided using the terms 'luteal' or 'lutein cyst' which have been used by others to describe any luteinized dysfunctional ovarian cyst. These nonspecific terms do not indicate the pathogenesis of the lesions and are not useful without further qualification. 'Luteinization' is a morphological term which indicates a resemblance of the cells to those of the corpus luteum. This means an increase in eosinophilic or finely vesicular cytoplasm due to accumulation of lipid. Luteinization correlates with increased steroidogenic activity, often progestogenic.

'Polycystic' is a term which should be reserved for the abnormal ovaries found in association with the Stein–Leventhal and related clinical syndromes (see Ch. 13). The ovaries commonly have thick white capsules, and display multiple cystic follicles and small luteinized follicular cysts of atretic type, and occur with a characteristic disturbance of hypothalamic–pituitary function. Ovaries displaying several cysts, but otherwise not fitting into this category, should be called 'multicystic' in order to avoid confusion.

CYSTS DERIVED FROM THE PRE-OVULATORY FOLLICLES

Follicular cysts

The antral, or Graafian, follicle which develops

under the influence of follicle stimulating hormone (FSH) reaches a maximum diameter of 2.5–3.0 cm as determined by sequential ultrasound examinations during normal menstrual cycles (Robertson et al 1979, Lentz 1985). Experience of ovum pick-up procedures from the stimulated ovaries of women undertaking assisted reproduction indicates that follicles of this size or greater do not contain viable oocytes. This gives validity to an erstwhile arbitrary separation between physiological (smaller) and pathological (larger) cysts derived from preovulatory follicles.

The etiology of follicular cysts is not always obvious, but in most cases reflects disordered function of the pituitary–ovarian axis. Pathological cystic change may develop either in the follicular growth phase or during atresia. The biochemical nature of aspirated cyst fluid and the histological appearance of the lining provide some clues to pathogenesis. Unluteinized follicular cysts, which produce predominantly estradiol, result from excessive ovarian stimulation (either by endogenous FSH or by ovulation-induction agents) or an abnormal response to normal stimulation.

Granulosa lutein cysts are follicular cysts with luteinization predominantly of the granulosa cells (which are internal to the basal lamina) (Fig. 12.1); like corpora lutea, they secrete progesterone. An unknown proportion of granulosa lutein cysts are the result of failure of follicular rupture at the expected time of ovulation. This circumstance is the basis of the luteinized unruptured follicle (LUF) syndrome, which describes infertile women with regular menses and presumptive evidence of ovulation (raised basal body temperature, raised serum progesterone levels, and a secretory endometrial histology), but without release of an ovum (Koninckx et al 1980, Holtz et al 1985, Schenken et al 1986). The syndrome can be diagnosed by direct observation of the ovarian surface at laparoscopy (lack of an ovulation stigma), serial ultrasonographic evaluations of the ovary (continuing follicle growth rather than collapse), or steroid assays of peritoneal fluid (peritoneal fluid/plasma ratios of less than 5.0 for estradiol or progesterone). Although this syndrome has been most clearly studied in infertile women with endometriosis, there is no reason to suppose that follicular luteinization associated with failure of ovulation does not occur in other clinical groups (Dmowski et al 1980).

Theca lutein cysts are follicular cysts with luteinization predominantly of the theca interna (which is external to the basal lamina) (Fig. 12.1); androstenedione is the characteristic steroid product. These cysts develop when there is prolonged exposure to LH or human chorionic gonadotrophin (hCG), either endogenous, such as in polycystic ovary syndrome (see Ch. 13) or hyperreactio luteinalis syndrome of pregnancy (multiple theca lutein cysts; see Ch. 10), or exogenous, as in the ovarian hyperstimulation syndrome (see Ch. 11). Atretic follicular cysts are also capable of elaborating androstenedione.

Clinical features

Follicular cysts may thus secrete estradiol, progesterone, or androstenedione as their major products, but not necessarily in sufficient quantities to produce endocrine symptoms. Piver et al (1970) found that two-thirds of patients with surgically excised follicular cysts had menstrual irregularities, although a causal relationship could not be established. The mere physical presence of the cyst, or complications such as rupture or torsion, may precipitate clinical presentation. Follicular cysts occur at any age and the clinical manifestations vary accordingly.

Use of high resolution antenatal ultrasound has led to an increased detection of ovarian cysts in the fetus. They are very uncommon, with an estimated incidence of one in 2625 fetuses (Kirkinen & Jouppila 1985). The diagnosis is usually made in the third trimester. Their exact etiology is unclear, but the development of these cysts may be related to the active folliculogenesis that occurs in utero as an abnormal response to maternal hCG, and fetal gonadotrophins which normally stimulate follicular development from the fourth gestational month (O'Hagen et al 1985). They rarely occur with other congenital abnormalities (Rizzo et al 1989). The cysts are usually unilateral and range in size from 2 to 11 cm (Sakala et al 1991). Complications such as torsion, rupture, intestinal obstruction, and dystocia have been reported (Montag et al 1983, Sakala et al 1991). Other organ compression may occur, especially

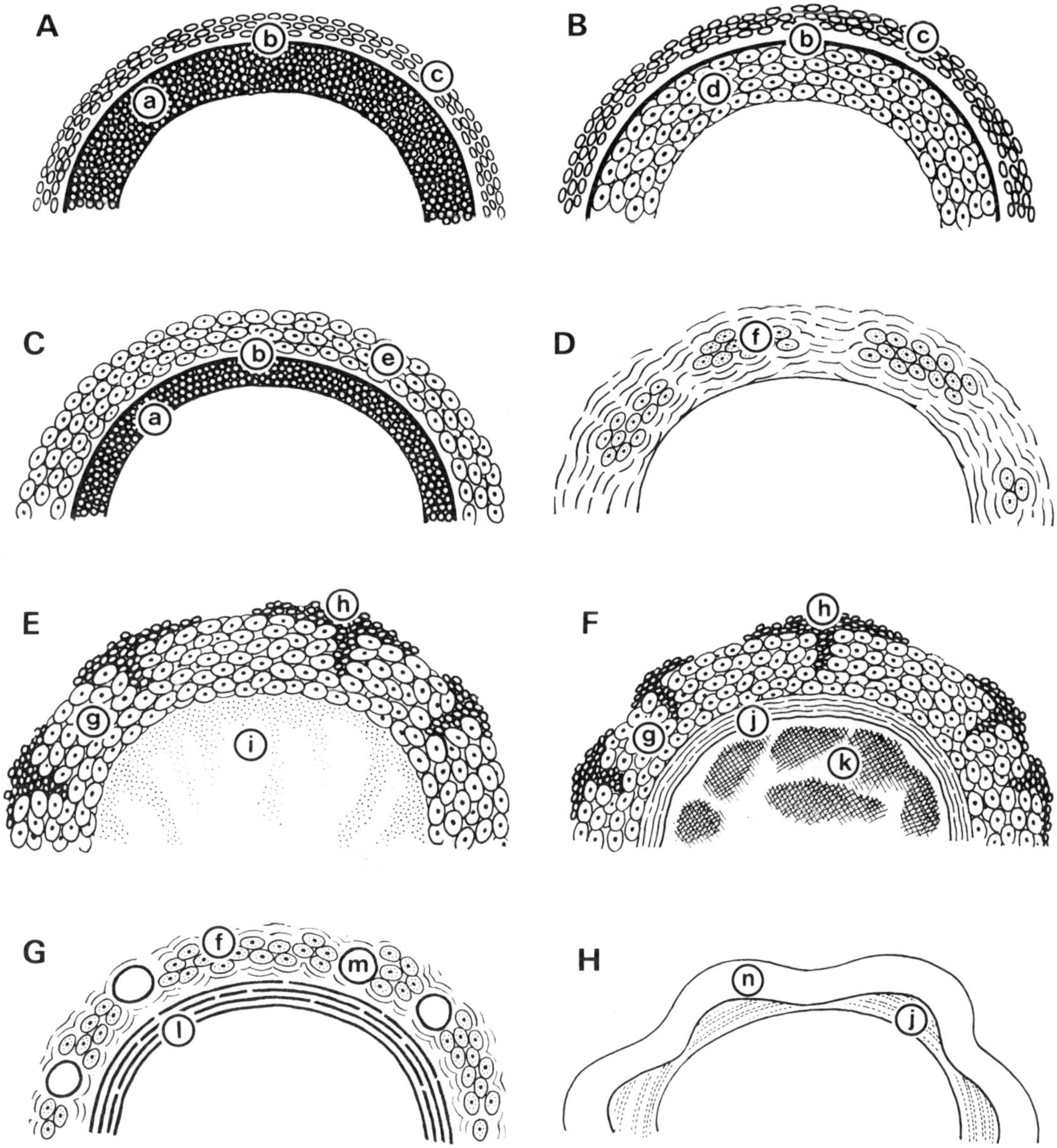

Fig. 12.1 Comparative morphology of dysfunctional cysts. (A) Unluteinized follicular cyst. (B) Granulosa lutein cyst. (C) Theca lutein cyst. (D) Involuting follicular cyst. (E) Cystic corpus luteum (F) Corpus luteum cyst (early). (G) Corpus luteum cyst (late). (H) Corpus albicans cyst. (a) Unluteinized granulosa, (b) basal lamina, (c) unluteinized theca interna, (d) luteinized granulosa, (e) luteinized theca, (f) involuting luteinized cells, (g) granulosa lutein layer, (h) theca (para) lutein layer, (i) fibrin, (j) loose fibrous tissue, (k) blood, (l) dense fibrous tissue, (m) prominent blood vessels, (n) acellular hyalinized fibrous tissue

with the larger ovarian cysts, and this has been associated with polyhydramnios (Rizzo et al 1989). Management, especially of the asymptomatic lesion, is still controversial (Suita et al 1991). Aspiration in utero has been attempted (Montag et al 1983, Kirkinen & Jouppila 1985, Landrum et al 1986, Meagher et al 1993). Surgical removal with preservation of as much ovarian tissue as possible has been recommended by Zachariou et al (1989) and a more conservative approach by Suita et al (1991). In a recent review of 230 cases in the literature, Brandt et al (1991) suggested that simple cysts tend to resolve spontaneously and should be treated conservatively. If the cyst is larger than 4 cm, aspiration or removal may be indicated. Complex cystic masses, symptomatic ovarian cysts, or cysts that do not resolve should be removed.

In prepubertal girls, follicular cysts form a significant proportion of ovarian lesions that come to surgical intervention (Adelman et al 1975, Bower & Adkins 1981). The most common clinical presentations are pain, vomiting, diarrhea, and constipation. More than half the cysts are palpable (Adelman et al 1975). Appendicitis is often the preoperative diagnosis. Clinical presentation may be precipitated by ovarian torsion. A less common, but well recognized, association is with isosexual pseudoprecocity, either idiopathic or associated with hypothyroidism or the McCune–Albright syndrome (Danon et al 1975, Lindsay et al 1983, Lightner & Kelch 1984). It is generally considered that the cysts develop as a consequence of precocious puberty, although there are instances of clinical regression following surgical excision of the ovarian lesions (Wieland et al 1976).

During the reproductive years, follicular cysts may be responsible for minor nonspecific pelvic symptoms, menstrual irregularities, virilization, ovarian torsion, hemorrhage, or rupture. The latter complications are usually spontaneous, but may be precipitated by anticoagulant therapy (Peters et al 1979; see Ch. 11). Unluteinized follicular cysts may produce sufficient estradiol to cause irregular or prolonged (dysfunctional) uterine bleeding. The endometrium in such cases may show disordered proliferative phase changes or hyperplasia. Granulosa lutein cysts secrete progesterone, but rarely in sufficient amounts to disturb the menstrual cycle. However, an inappropriate progestogenic effect may be noted in the endometrium. They are also associated with the LUF syndrome (see above) in which progesterone production is sufficiently close to normal for there to be difficulty in distinguishing the abnormality from normal corpus luteum development. Atretic cysts, if numerous (as in the polycystic ovary syndrome), may synthesize sufficient androstenedione to produce hirsutism or virilization.

During pregnancy, pre-existing follicular cysts may become luteinized. New cysts rarely develop but a notable exception is the hyperreactio luteinalis syndrome (multiple theca lutein cysts; see Ch 10). Clement & Scully (1980) have described large solitary luteinized follicular cysts which presented as adnexal masses in the third to fourth months of pregnancy or postpartum, or were incidental findings at caesarean section. There were no clinical endocrine disturbances beyond those that characterize normal pregnancy (see Ch. 10).

Patients with chronic renal failure, undergoing regular hemodialysis, have a high incidence of follicular cysts. There is a risk of hemorrhage and rupture because of concurrent anticoagulant therapy (Thaysen et al 1975). The endocrinological features of these patients suggest that uremia may produce a polycystic ovary-like syndrome (Handelsman et al 1984). Cystic fibrosis patients, if menstruating, have a high incidence of ovarian cysts, presumed follicular, as determined by ultrasound examinations (Shawker et al 1983). Multiple cystic follicles and follicular cysts have been noted in women with anorexia nervosa during the phase of weight gain; the changes observed by sequential ultrasound in these patients appear to parallel those of normal prepubertal development (Treasure et al 1985).

Symptomatic follicular cysts are rare after the menopause, although some sporadic follicular activity (generally without ovulation) continues in the early years. Estrogenic cysts (associated with breast enlargement and tenderness and mucoid vaginal discharge) have been reported up to 6 years after endocrinologically proven menopause. On uterine curettage, the endometrial glands may show the effect of estrogenic stimulation, ranging from weak proliferative activity to complex hyperplasia (Stevens & Plotka 1977, Strickler et al 1984).

Macroscopic features

Follicular cysts are usually single, but multiple cysts are characteristic of the polycystic ovary syndrome, ovarian hyperstimulation from exogenous gonadotrophin therapy, and the hyperreactio luteinalis syndrome of pregnancy. The diameter of unluteinized follicular cysts is greater than 3 cm (which distinguishes them from physiological cystic follicles), but rarely exceeds 10 cm. The excep-

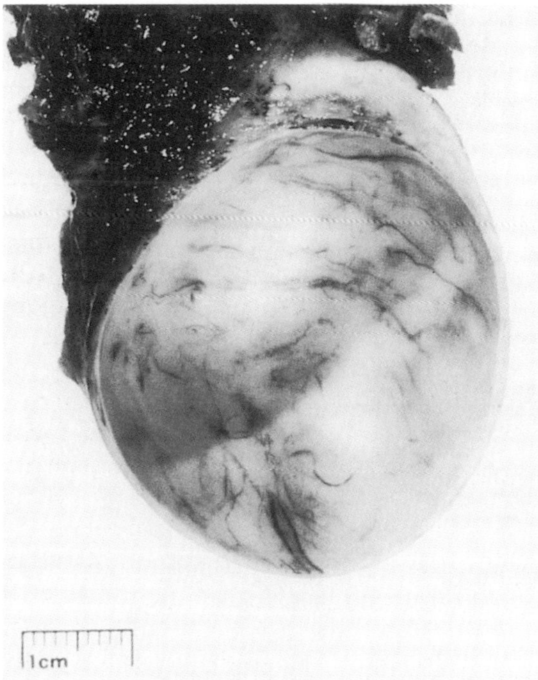

Fig. 12.2 Follicular cyst. Cut surface showing typical smooth shiny lining with prominent underlying blood vessels. Residual attenuated ovarian tissue is present in the cyst wall, above and at right

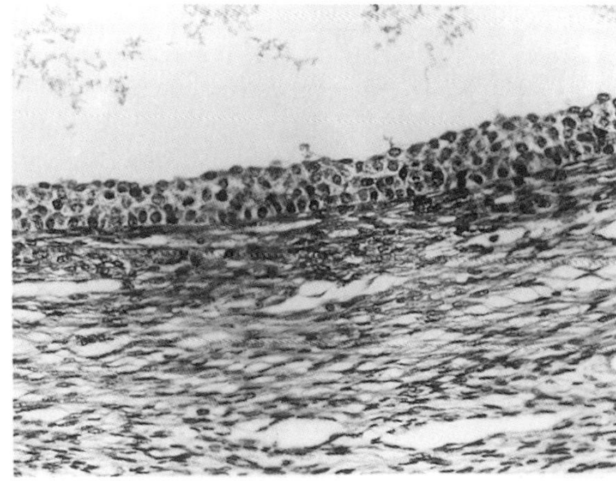

Fig. 12.3 Unluteinized follicular cyst. About four layers of uniform small granulosa cells are present above the basal lamina. H + E ×80

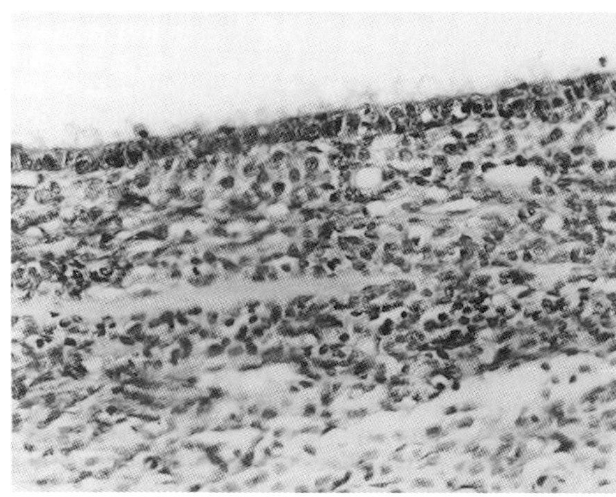

Fig. 12.4 Unluteinized follicular cyst. The attenuated lining of granulosa cells is only one to two cells thick, simulating a benign epithelial cyst. H + E ×80

tion is the large solitary luteinized follicle cyst of pregnancy and puerperium (median reported diameter 25 cm) (see Ch. 10). Luteinized follicular cysts are very variable in size; atretic cysts are generally about 1 cm in diameter. Follicular cysts cause symmetrical or asymmetrical ovarian enlargement. The cysts are round or ovoid with smooth shiny linings. They contain clear fluid (which coagulates to a curd-like material after FAA fixation), or fresh or altered blood. The surrounding ovarian tissue may be very attenuated and distorted (Fig. 12.2).

Microscopic features

Unluteinized follicular cysts show the microscopic features of physiological growing cystic follicles, with well-preserved granulosa and theca layers separated by a basal lamina (Fig. 12.3). However, the cumulus oophorus and oocyte are no longer present. The lining may be somewhat attenuated secondary to dilatation (Fig. 12.4). There is no trace of the festooned pattern of a corpus luteum. In the stage of involution the lining is often incomplete and later is represented only by small clusters of lutein cells in the compressed ovarian stroma, which becomes progressively fibrotic (Fig. 12.5). As involution continues, it becomes increasingly difficult to identify any distinguishing features, and definitive diagnosis may not be possible; in this situation the cyst is better designated 'simple' (see below).

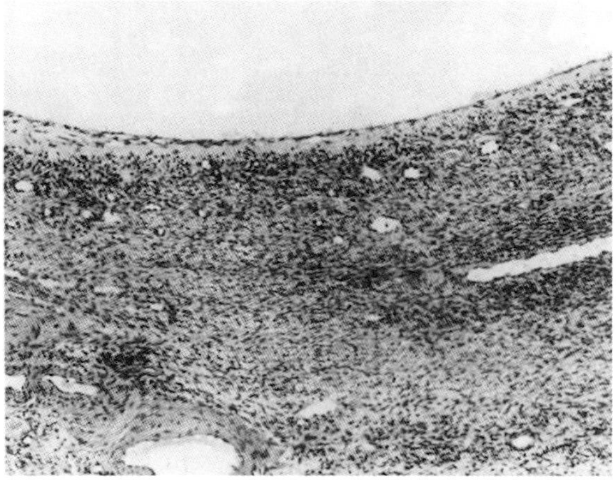

Fig. 12.5 Involuting follicular cyst with smooth internal contour and fibrous wall in which there are clusters of small follicular cells. H + E ×64

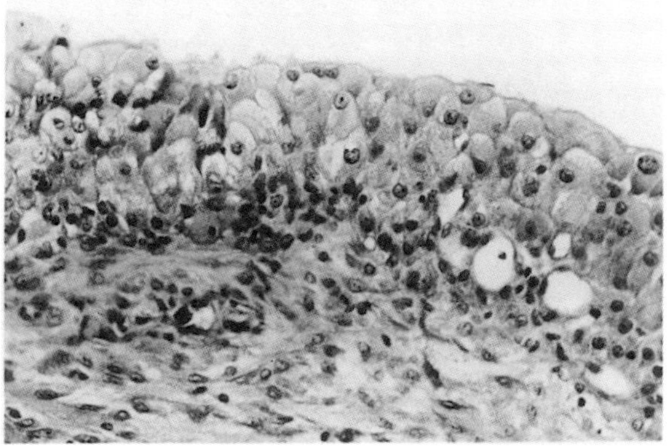

Fig. 12.6 Granulosa lutein cyst lined by large eosinophilic cells. The thecal layer is inconspicuous. H + E ×160

Luteinized follicular cysts show the general features of unluteinized follicular cysts as described above, but in addition there is luteinization of some of the cellular components of the cyst wall – either the granulosa (granulosa lutein cyst; Fig. 12.6) or theca layer (theca lutein cyst; see Figs 10.3, 10.4, 12.7–12.9), or occasionally both, although the cyst is classified according to the layer predominantly affected. Luteinization is recognized by cellular enlargement caused by an increase in eosinophilic or finely vacuolated cytoplasm; the changes are analogous to those seen in the development of a corpus luteum.

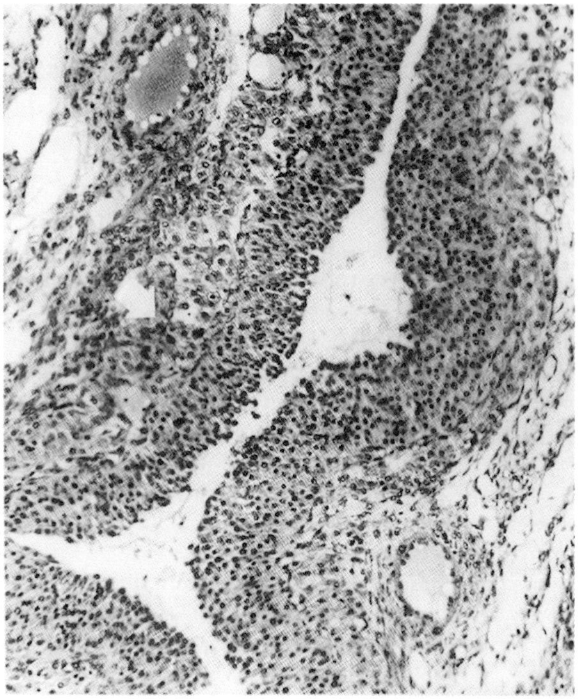

Fig. 12.7 Theca lutein cyst. Thick lining of small granulosa cells with large luteinized theca cells beneath basal lamina (most conspicuous at left; arrow). H + E ×80

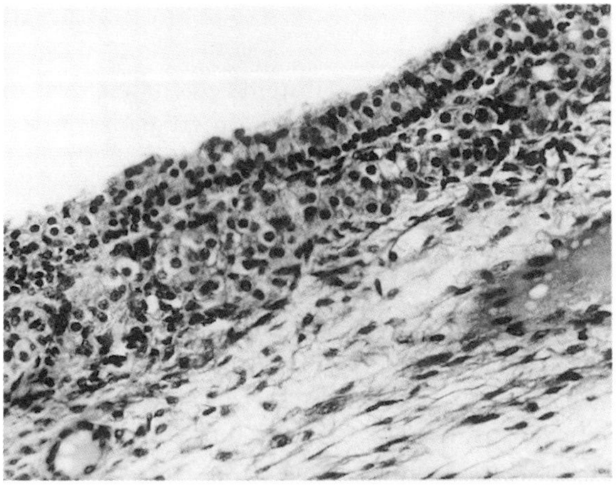

Fig. 12.8 Theca lutein cyst. Detail of large luteinized theca cells beneath basal lamina. H + E ×160

Atretic follicular cysts are lined by ovarian stroma in which there are small clusters of luteinized thecal cells. They may be indistinguishable from involuting follicular cysts of other types (Figs. 12.10, 12.11).

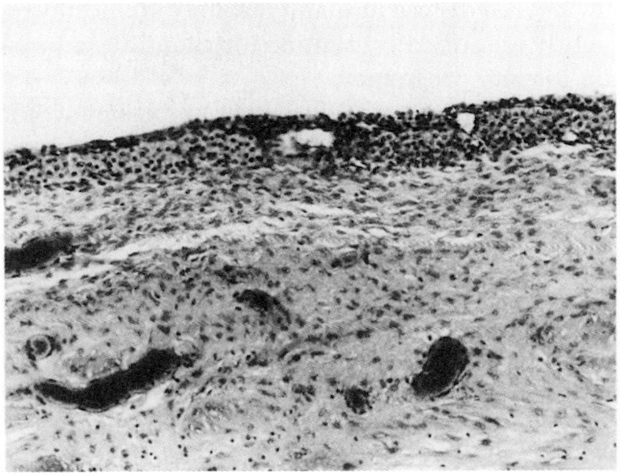

Fig. 12.9 Theca lutein cyst. Well preserved theca layer but most of granulosa is lost. Note distinct basal lamina. H + E ×80

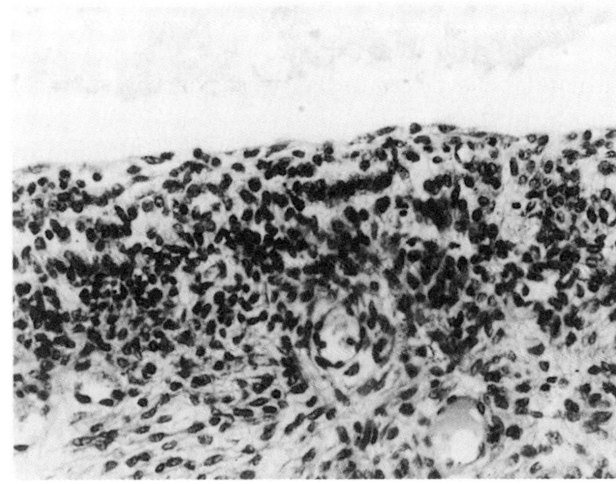

Fig. 12.11 Detail of Fig. 12.10. Clusters of follicular cells of uncertain type close to cyst lumen. H + E ×160

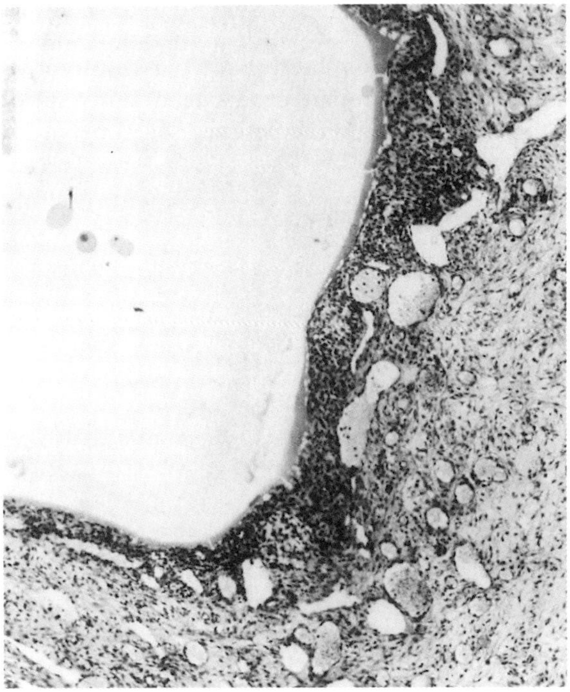

Fig. 12.10 Atretic cyst from patient with polycystic ovary syndrome. Note smooth internal contour and fibrous wall. H + E ×64

Other histological alterations may be seen in the ovary if follicular cysts are associated with some specific clinicopathological syndromes. For example, polycystic ovaries also show subcapsular fibrosis and focal stromal luteinisation (see Ch. 13), and the ovaries in hyperreactio luteinalis and the hyperstimulation syndrome exhibit marked stromal edema and hemorrhage (see Ch. 10).

The distinguishing features of the various types of follicular cysts are illustrated diagrammatically in Fig. 12.1.

Differential diagnosis

Cysts derived from a corpus luteum can be distinguished from luteinized follicular cysts by their retention, partially or focally, of their convoluted lining with invaginations of paralutein cells, and by their innermost lining of fibrous tissue (the result of organization of the central hematoma). In addition, a well-defined vascular zone may be evident.

Benign epithelial cysts may be indistinguishable from follicular cysts macroscopically, but microscopy will reveal the diagnostic lining of mullerian epithelium, most commonly serous (tubal) in type. Care should be taken not to misinterpret an attenuated layer of granulosa cells as an epithelial lining (see Figs 3.22, 12.4)

Simple parovarian cysts are sometimes submitted as ovarian lesions. If the complete adnexa are received, this type of cyst can be readily recognized to be extraovarian; if not, microscopy will demonstrate that the cyst lies in the loose fibrous tissues of the mesovarium, often in close proximity to other (noncystic) paramesonephric tubules. They are lined by a single layer of tubal-type epithelial cells surrounded by a narrow cuff of smooth muscle.

Cystic granulosa cell tumors may be difficult to distinguish from follicular cysts. They are often considerably larger and are always unilateral. The neoplastic cells lining the cysts usually show prominent luteinization and may display mitotic activity. Although most granulosa cell tumors are estrogenic, one-sixth to one-third of the cystic variant are clinically androgenic, a feature not associated with follicular cysts except in the specific clinical situations mentioned above (Norris & Chorlton 1974, Nakashima et al 1984).

CYSTS DERIVED FROM THE CORPUS LUTEUM

These cysts are derived from the follicular apparatus but show evidence of prior ovulation, which distinguishes them from the follicular cysts already described. Ovulation is indicated by convolution of the cyst lining (which results from collapse of the follicle) with the characteristic invaginations of theca lutein (paralutein) cells into the inner zone of granulosa lutein cells (see Ch. 3). A layer of fibrous tissue lining the inner surface of the cyst, resulting from organization of the corpus luteum hematoma, is also a good indicator that ovulation has occurred. The distinguishing features of the various types of cysts derived from the corpus luteum are illustrated diagrammatically in Fig. 12.1.

Cystic corpora lutea

Corpora lutea of menstruation do not usually exceed 3 cm in diameter (average size 2 cm), but may do so if there is an unusually large fluid-filled central cavity. Such cystic corpora lutea usually function and involute normally and are unassociated with any clinical endocrine disturbance. Their clinical significance is that they are more prone to spontaneous rupture than their noncystic counterparts (Hallatt et al 1984). The risk of this complication is increased in patients on anticoagulant therapy (Peters et al 1979). Cystic corpora lutea of pregnancy can often exceed 5 cm and may exceed 10 cm in diameter; they are not infrequently identified on routine ultrasound examination in early pregnancy.

Cystic corpora lutea display all the macroscopic and microscopic features of their noncystic counterparts (see Ch. 3). The distension leads to some attenuation of the convolutions, but without loss of distinction of cell layers (Fig. 12.12).

Corpus luteum cysts

This is a cyst derived from a corpus luteum of menstruation or pregnancy which results from excessive central hemorrhage (Piver et al 1970). Small physiological hemorrhages occur 2–4 days after ovulation during the stage of vascularization of the corpus luteum (see Ch. 3) and usually organize rapidly. However, if hemorrhage is excessive and the corpus luteum becomes overdistended with blood, there is likely to be delayed involution. Although most are probably asymptomatic, in the nonpregnant patient this delayed involution of the corpus luteum (sometimes called persistent

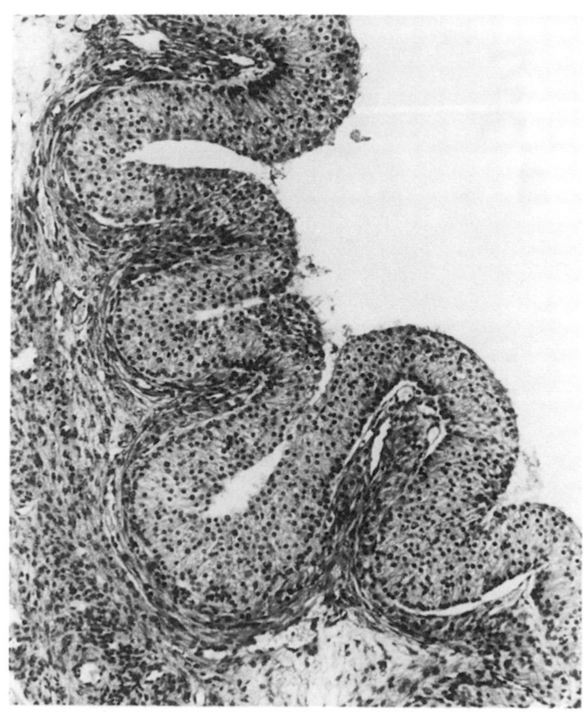

Fig. 12.12 Wall of ruptured cystic corpus luteum with early luteinization of granulosa and theca. H + E ×80

corpus luteum) and its continuing production of progesterone may result in minor menstrual disturbances. Clinical observations suggest that in some patients the cysts are the result of an underlying endocrine disturbance rather than an accident of vascularization. Piver et al (1970) reviewed the clinical findings in 66 cases of corpus luteum cysts and found that, of 42 patients without other pathological lesions that may have influenced menstrual function, 25 had abnormal menstrual histories, most commonly menorrhagia or metrorrhagia. The endometrium in such patients may show an inappropriate progestogenic effect, Arias–Stella change, or the picture of irregular shedding. As with a cystic corpus luteum, there is also a risk of spontaneous rupture and hemoperitoneum.

Macroscopic features

Corpus luteum cysts are solitary and have an average diameter of 5.5 cm (Piver et al 1970). They are unilocular and contain clear yellowish fluid or altered blood. Rupture may be evident. They have a smooth internal lining of grey fibrous tissue and, if excised early in their natural history, there is an incomplete band of bright yellow tissue in the wall of the cyst which represents the luteinized tissues. The convoluted pattern of a normal corpus luteum is not evident grossly.

Microscopic features

The corpus luteum cyst shows evidence of ovulation as indicated above. The lining of fibrous tissue contains mature collagen which can be demonstrated by use of a trichrome connective tissue stain. Although hemorrhage in the cyst wall and surrounding stroma may partially obscure morphological features, vestiges of the convoluted lining can be seen microscopically if carefully sought. Peripheral clusters of small paralutein (theca lutein) cells may still be seen between larger groups of granulosa lutein cells (see Figs 3.15, 12.13). The granulosa and theca lutein cells are smaller than those seen in a fresh corpus luteum. The nuclei are small, hyperchromatic, and lack mitotic activity, while the cytoplasm is usually finely vesicular. With progressive involution, fewer and smaller islands of lutein cells are found within the increasingly fibrotic wall, but a well-defined zone of small blood vessels remains as a marker of the phase of vascularization (Figs 12.14–12.16).

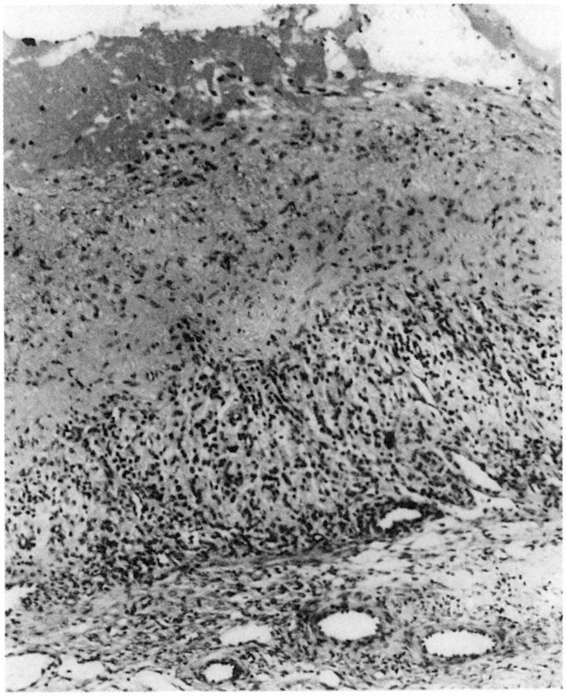

Fig. 12.13 Early corpus luteum cyst with organising hematoma at top and thin zone of involuting vacuolated luteinized cells below. H + E ×80

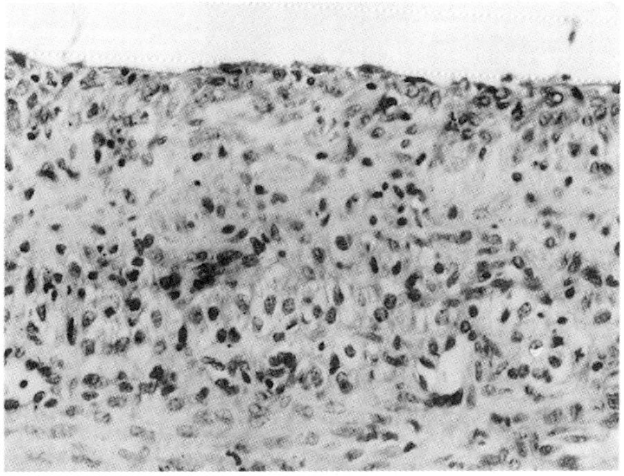

Fig. 12.14 Late corpus luteum cyst. Inner zone of fibrous tissue with involuting vacuolated luteinized cells beneath. H + E ×200

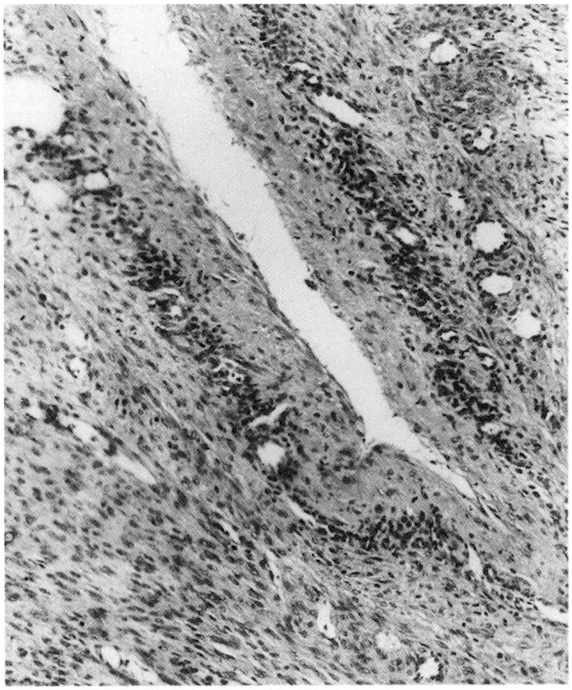

Fig. 12.15 Late corpus luteum cyst. Inner ragged layer of fibrous tissue with clusters of involuting luteinized cells in well-vascularized zone beneath. H + E ×100

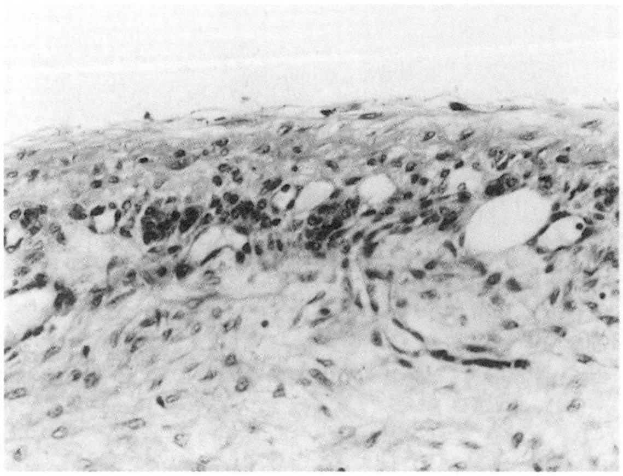

Fig. 12.16 Detail of Fig 12.15. Involuting luteinized cells in vascular zone. H + E ×200

Differential diagnosis

Cystic corpora lutea are likely to contain a fresh coagulum rather than profuse altered blood. Luteinized tissue can still be readily recognized and the convoluted lining is usually still apparent. Microscopy will show distinct theca and granulosa lutein layers with only early involutional changes. The innermost lining consists of organizing fibrin and blood rather than mature collagenous fibrous tissue.

Luteinized follicular cysts may have similar macroscopic features to corpus luteum cysts, but are less likely to be hemorrhagic. The microscopic distinction hinges around evidence of ovulation as indicated above. Follicular cysts generally lack the zone of vascularization. Some long-standing cysts may be very difficult to classify and are then best designated 'simple' cysts (see below).

Endometriotic cysts may be impossible to distinguish macroscopically from corpus luteum cysts, but may be suspected if there is evidence of endometriosis elsewhere in the submitted specimens or if the diagnosis is indicated clinically. The microscopic identification of endometrial glands and stroma quickly excludes this lesion from the differential diagnosis.

Corpus albicans cysts

The corpus albicans is typically a small solid hyalinized fibrous scar, but occasionally it has a central cavity containing clear fluid. The cysts are rarely more than 1 cm in diameter. They may follow involution of a corpus luteum or corpus luteum cyst. The mechanism of fluid retention or accumulation is not known. Microscopically the cyst wall is composed of a convoluted ribbon-like band of hyalinized acellular fibrous tissue, usually with an innermost lining of looser fibrous connective tissue with a smoother outline (Fig. 12.17). The cysts are nonfunctional and are too small to produce symptomatic adnexal masses.

SIMPLE CYSTS

These are ovarian cysts or cyst-like structures which lack identifiable linings. Some produce symptomatic adnexal masses, but most are incidental findings by the surgeon or pathologist; they are unlikely to be associated with any disturbance of menstrual function.

The cysts are usually less than 10 cm in diameter, solitary, and have a smooth internal surface

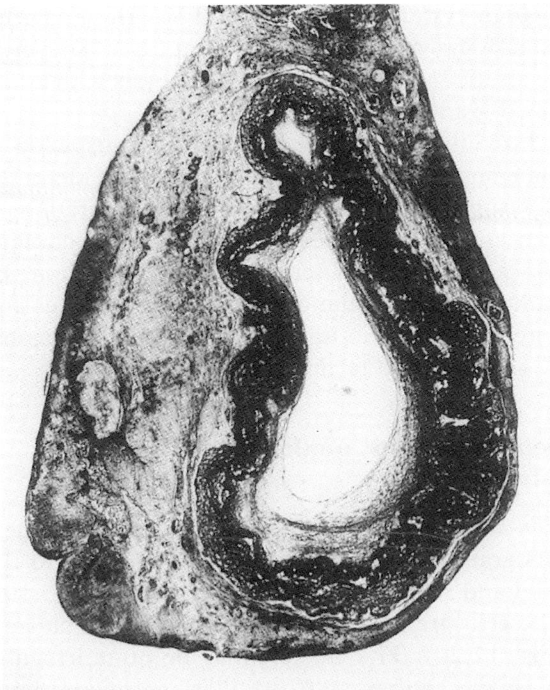

Fig. 12.17 Corpus albicans cyst. Outer ribbon of hyalinised fibrous tissue and inner zone of loose fibrous tissue. Masson's trichrome ×7

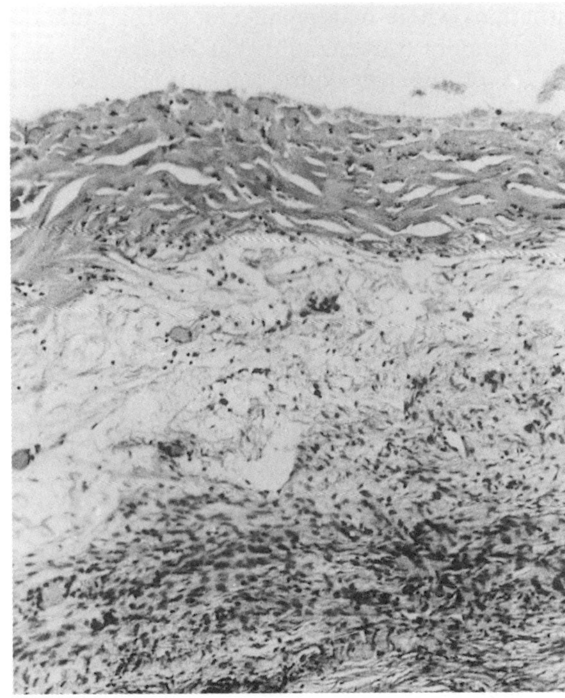

Fig. 12.18 Simple cyst lined by dense fibrous tissue; no distinguishing features present. H + E ×80

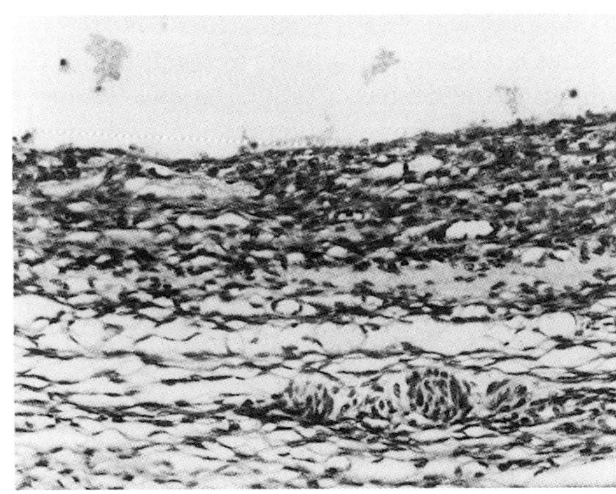

Fig. 12.19 Simple cyst lined by ovarian stroma; epithelial or follicular lining has been lost. H + E ×160

and a variable content of clear fluid or altered blood. The lining usually consists only of a narrow band of dense fibrous tissue or compressed ovarian stroma (Figs 12.18, 12.19). There may be occasional small clusters of involuting lutein cells in the cyst wall, suggesting an origin from the follicular apparatus. Sometimes there is a complete or partial lining of apparent epithelial cells which are too attenuated for their origin to be identified; these cysts may represent epithelial cystomas. Some are lined by granulation tissue or organizing hematoma; such lesions may be endometriotic in origin, but all the necessary diagnostic features are not present (see Ch. 21). There is probably no benefit in precisely categorising 'simple' cysts. All are benign and most are non-neoplastic.

CYTOLOGY OF DYSFUNCTIONAL OVARIAN CYSTS

Cystic lesions of the ovary may be diagnosed by aspiration with cytological examination of the cyst fluid, made possible by recent technical advances in laparoscopy and ultrasound (de Crespigny et al 1989). Aspiration of ovarian cysts is an increasingly common procedure in association with assisted reproductive technology or other clinical situations where maintenance of ovarian function is paramount (Greenbaum et al 1992).

Use of the procedure remains controversial, and technical limitations need to be understood. The main problems are:

- If the lesion is malignant there is a consequent risk of spilling malignant cells into the peritoneal cavity
- Inaccuracy of cytological examination may lead to unacceptable rates of false-negative and false-positive cytology predictions, in inexperienced hands.

Aspiration is not usually recommended if there is *any* clinical suspicion of malignancy (Roden et al 1989). It is therefore important to be able to predict, using high resolution ultrasonography, those cysts likely to be malignant (Herrman et al 1987, see Ch. 58), and base a decision to aspirate accordingly. In cases of suspected malignancy, complete removal of the cyst with subsequent histopathological examination is the treatment of choice.

Cytological interpretation also has its limitations. Although the exact rates are unknown, false-positive and false-negative results (as with all cytology) will always occur (Koss 1980). False-positive results are most likely to result from overestimating the degree of cellular atypia (Nunez & Diaz 1992) or from contamination with tissues included during aspiration (Nadji et al 1974).

One of the major criticisms of this technique relates to false-negative results in the presence of malignant cysts. In one series of cystic and solid lesions, 6% of malignant tumors were incorrectly identified (Kjellgren & Ångström 1982). In another study, cytological examination failed to identify five of seven malignant cysts (Diernaes et al 1987). False-negative results are more commonly associated with attempted aspiration of solid tumors or semisolid lesions when the correct area is not sampled. Other fluid samples, usually cyst fluid, may not be diagnostic, and in these cases no interpretation should be given. Fluid which contains only lymphocytes or macrophages, large amounts of blood, or only very scanty cellular material may be inadequate for assessment. Under these circumstances, a diagnosis of malignancy must not be excluded. Such findings may present in fluid aspirated from many types of ovarian cyst, e.g. follicular, endometriotic, corpus luteum cysts, or surface inclusion cysts. They may be atretic follicles or old follicular cysts with attenuated granulosa cell lining.

Providing that there is no clinical suspicion of malignancy and that ultrasound has not identified any solid or multiloculated cysts, aspiration of ovarian cysts may then be a worthwhile technique (Buckley 1989). Increasing familiarization by pathologists with the cytological appearances and potential pitfalls in this area will improve diagnostic accuracy and facilitate utilization.

Follicular cysts: nonluteinized and luteinized

Non-luteinized follicular cysts will contain numerous granulosa cells that have been shed into the fluid and reflect the normal lining (see Fig. 3.10). The cells are arranged singly and in tight clusters (Fig. 12.20). The clusters may be quite irregular in shape, some with papillary configurations. Granulosa cells contain round to oval nuclei and a small rim of distinct cytoplasm. The chromatin is coarsely granular and nuclear grooves may be present, but are usually absent. Mitoses may be identified. The cells are uniform with negligible variation from cell to cell. Degenerative changes may be present.

Luteinized follicular cysts contain single and/or clusters of granulosa cells, some or all of which are luteinized. The clusters may form papillary or spherical groups. Luteinized granulosa cells have round to oval nuclei with coarse chromatin and may have small prominent nucleoli (Fig. 12.21). Cell cytoplasm is ample and foamy. Mitotic figures are not unusual in the cell clusters. The cells are predictable and show no pleiomorphism. Degenerative changes may be present in single cells with obvious nuclear pyknosis (Fig. 12.22).

Differential diagnosis

The cytological appearances of follicular cyst fluids may present an alarming appearance to the unwary, due to the abundant cellularity, immature appearance of the cells, granularity of the chromatin, and presence of mitotic figures (Nunez & Diaz 1992).

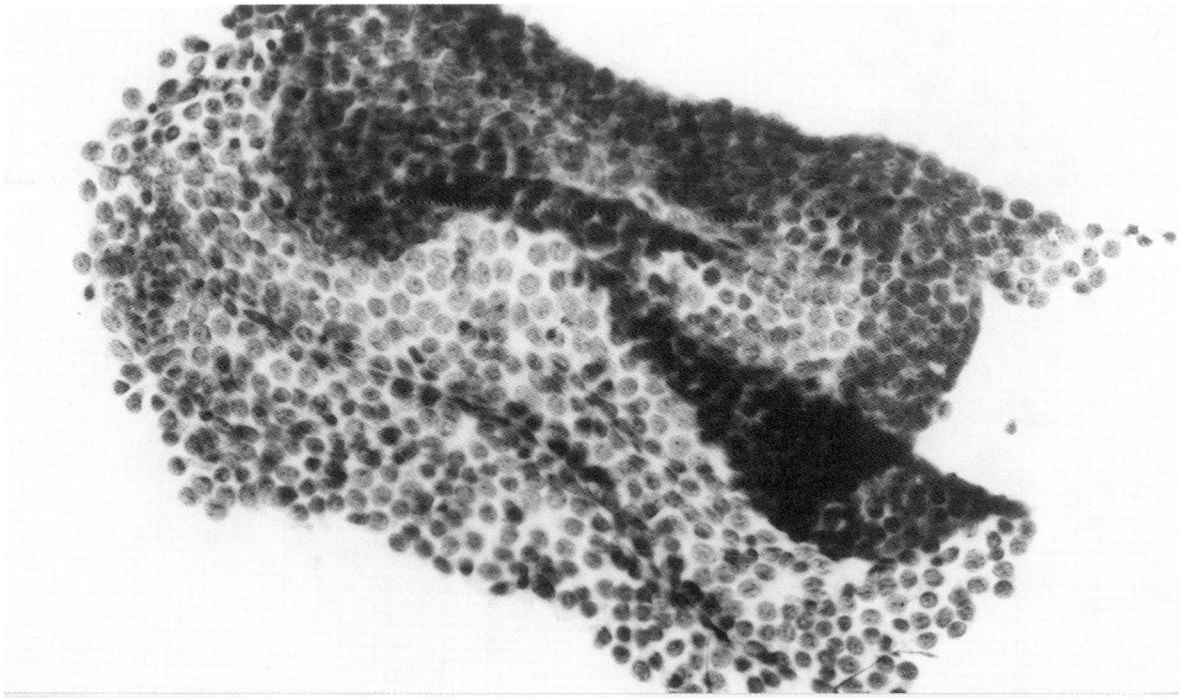

Fig. 12.20 Nonluteinized follicular cyst fluid. Folded sheet of well-preserved, uniform, nonluteinized granulosa cells. Note high Nuclear Cytoplasmic ratio and relatively coarse chromatin, and occasional nuclear grooves. Pap stain ×350

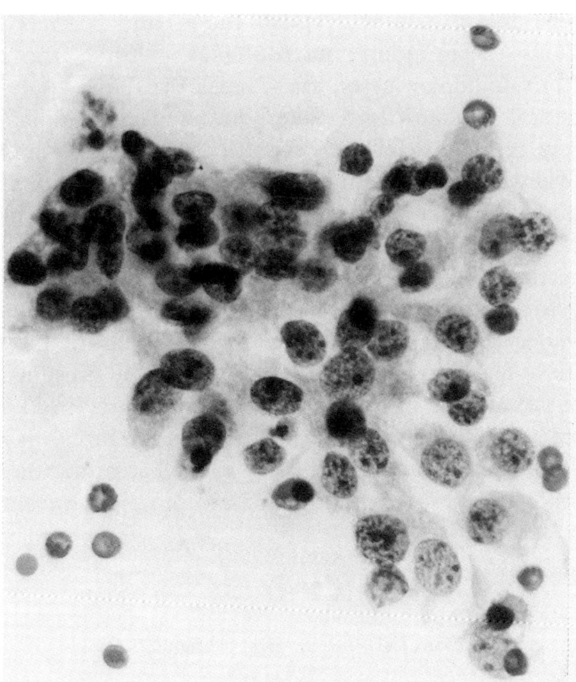

Fig. 12.21 Luteinized follicular cells. Groups of large cells with granular chromatin and lacy cytoplasm. Some degenerative changes are also present at top left. Note red blood cells at lower left for comparison. Pap stain ×462

Follicular cysts have to be distinguished from granulosa cell tumors, particularly the cystic juvenile type. Helpful features are the presence of Call–Exner bodies in tumors and pronounced indented irregular nuclei corresponding to the longitudinally grooved nuclei seen in tissue sections. The nuclear chromatin in tumor cases is also usually finer and small nucleoli are often noted.

In cases where epithelial malignancies are unexpectedly encountered, pathologists should avail themselves of the clinical findings, i.e. ultrasound and laparoscopic appearances. Most neoplastic cysts are large, multilocular, and may have excrescences, capsular irregularities, or may be solid. Frankly malignant cytological criteria and coarse irregular nuclear chromatin, irregular nuclear margins, and true cellular pleiomorphism are harbingers of such a diagnosis. Carcinoid tumors and

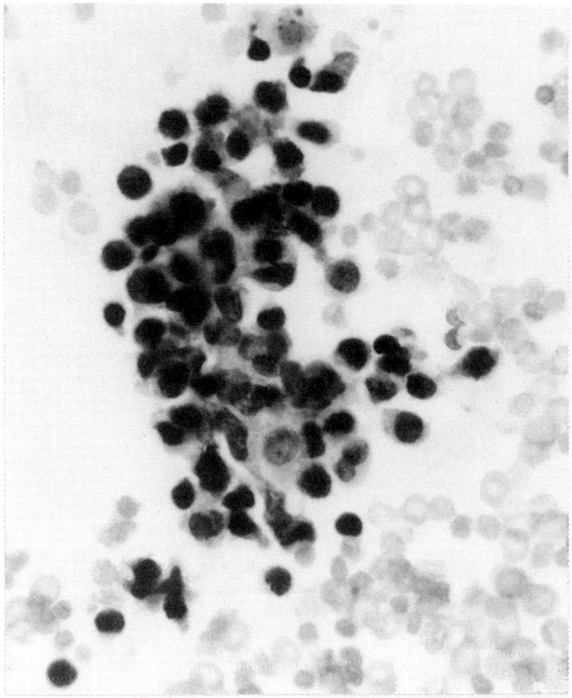

Fig. 12.22 Degenerate nonluteinized follicular cells. These may be abundant, with dense small pyknotic nuclei. Pap stain ×462

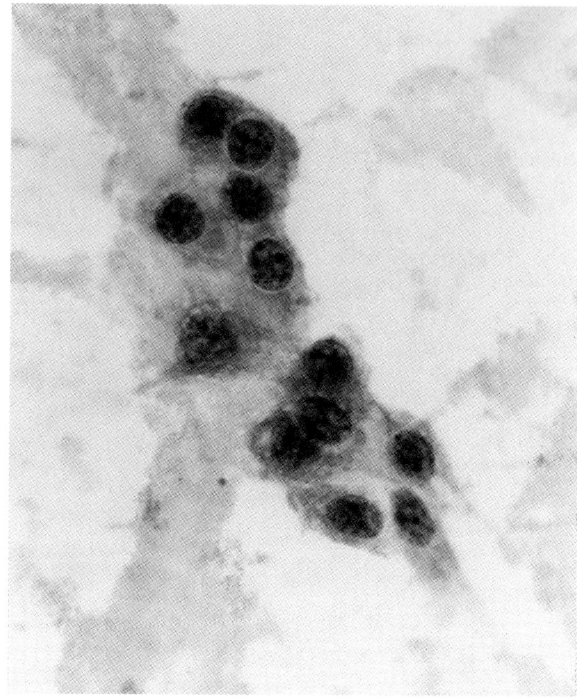

Fig. 12.23 Luteinized follicular cells may form sheets, single cells, clusters (as here), and papillary fragments. Hemosiderin-laden macrophages may also be present (not in this field). Pap stain ×462

serous neoplasms may also need to be specifically excluded.

Carcinoid tumors contain cells which, cytologically, may resemble granulosa cells with rounded nuclei and coarse chromatin. Clinical correlation may be necessary, and confirmation supplied by demonstrating the argyrophilia of carcinoids and immunoreactivity for NSE, serotonin, chromogranin, and neuronal peptides (see Ch. 49). *Serous neoplasms* will have abundant papillary clusters of epithelial cells with atypical nuclei, containing obvious nucleoli. Psammoma bodies may be present.

Cysts derived from corpus luteum

Hemorrhagic corpus luteum contains numerous fully luteinized granulosa cells singly and in clusters and mixed with fresh blood and scattered hemosiderin-laden macrophages. Unlike those from follicular cysts, these cells are large, polyhedral in shape, and have a low nuclear cytoplasmic ratio. Nuclei are eccentric, round to slightly oval with finely granular chromatin and prominent nucleoli. Nuclear grooves are not present and binucleation may be present. Cytoplasm is ample, finely granular, and contains tiny vacuoles. Yellowish cytochrome pigment may also be present. *Hemorrhagic corpus luteum* cysts may be identified by these features (Fig. 12.23) as well as the presence of abundant fibrin and some fibroblasts in the smear background. Regressing corpora lutea may contain large luteinized cells, as well as numerous macrophages with yellow hematoidin pigment.

REFERENCES

Adelman S, Benson C D, Hertzler J H 1975 Surgical lesions of the ovary in infancy and childhood. Surgery, Gynecology and Obstetrics 141: 219–222

Bower R J, Adkins J C 1981 Surgical ovarian lesions in children. American Surgeon 47: 474–478

Brandt M L, Luks F I, Filiatrault D, Garel L, Desjardins J G,

Youssef S 1991 Surgical indications in acute natally diagnosed ovarian cysts. Journal of Paediatric Surgery 26: 276–281
Buckley C M 1989 Is needle aspiration of ovarian cysts adequate for diagnosis? British Journal of Obstetrics and Gynaecology 96: 1021–1023
Clement P B, Scully R E 1980 Large solitary luteinized follicle cyst of pregnancy and puerperium. A clinicopathological analysis of eight cases. American Journal of Surgical Pathology 4: 431–438
Danon M, Robboy S J, Kim S, Scully R, Crawford J D 1975 Cushing syndrome, sexual precocity, and polyostotic fibrous dysplasia (Albright syndrome) in infancy. Journal of Pediatrics 87: 917–921
de Crespigny L C, Robinson H P, Davoren R A M, Fortune D 1989 The simple ovarian cyst: aspirate or operate? British Journal of Obstetrics and Gynaecology 96: 1035–1039
Diernaes E, Rasmussen J, Sorensen T, Hasch E 1987 Ovarian cysts: management by puncture. Lancet ii: 1084
Dmowski W P, Rao R, Scommegna A 1980 The luteinized unruptured follicle syndrome and endometriosis. Fertility and Sterility 33: 30–34
Greenbaum E, Mayer J R, Stangel J J, Hughes P 1992 Aspiration cytology of ovarian cysts in in-vitro fertilization patients. Acta Cytologica 36: 3601–3611
Hallatt J G, Steele C H, Snyder M 1984 Ruptured corpus luteum with hemoperitoneum: a study of 173 surgical cases. American Journal of Obstetrics and Gynecology 149: 5–8
Handelsman D J, McDowell I F W, Caterson I D, Tiller D J, Hall B M, Turtle J R 1984 Ovarian function after renal transplantation: comparison of cyclosporin A with azathioprine and prednisone combination regimens. British Journal of Obstetrics and Gynaecology 91: 802–807
Herrman U J, Locher G W, Goldhirsch A 1987 Sonographic patterns of ovarian tumors: prediction of malignancy. Obstetrics and Gynecology 69: 777–781
Holtz G, Williamson H O, Mathur R S, Landgrebe S C, Moore E E 1985 Luteinized unruptured follicle syndrome in mild endometriosis. Journal of Reproductive Medicine 30: 643–645
Kirkinen P, Jouppila P 1985 Perinatal aspects of pregnancy complicated by fetal ovarian cyst. Journal of Perinatal Medicine 13: 245–251
Kjellgren O, Ångström T 1982 Aspiration biopsy cytology of ovarian tumors. In: Blaustein A (ed) Pathology of the female genital tract, 2nd edn. Springer-Verlag, New York, p 741–751
Koninckx P R, De Moor P, Brosens I A 1980 Diagnosis of luteinized unruptured follicle syndrome by steroid hormone assays on peritoneal fluid. British Journal of Obstetrics and Gynaecology 87: 929–934
Koss L G 1980 Thin needle aspiration biopsy [editorial]. Acta Cytologica 24: 1–3
Landrum B, Ogburn P L, Feinberg S et al 1986 Intrauterine aspiration of a large fetal ovarian cyst. Obstetrics and Gynecology 68: 11s–14s
Lentz S 1985 Ultrasonic study of follicular maturation, ovulation and development of corpus luteum during normal menstrual cycles. Acta Obstetricia et Gynecologica Scandinavica 64: 15–19
Lightner E S, Kelch R P 1984 Treatment of precocious pseudopuberty associated with ovarian cysts. American Journal of Diseases of Children 138: 126–128
Lindsay A N, Voorhess M L, MacGillivray M H 1983 Multicystic ovaries in primary hypothyroidism. Obstetrics and Gynecology 61: 433–437
Meagher S E, Fisk N M, Boogert A, Russell P 1993 Foetal ovarian cysts: diagnostic and therapeutic role for intrauterine aspiration. Foetal Diagnosis and Therapy 8: 195–199
Montag T W, Auletta F J, Gibson M 1983 Neonatal ovarian cyst: prenatal diagnosis and analysis of the cyst fluid. Obstetrics and Gynecology 61: 38s–41s
Nadji M, Greening S E, Seuai B U, Averette H E, Nordqvsit S R B, Ng A B P 1979 Fine needle aspiration cytology in gynecologic oncology. II. Morphologic aspects. Acta Cytologica 23: 380–388
Nakashima N, Young R H, Scully R E 1984 Androgenic granulosa cell tumors of the ovary; a clinicopathologic analysis of 17 cases and review of the literature. Archives of Pathology and Laboratory Medicine 108: 786–791
Norris H J, Chorlton I 1974 Functioning tumors of the ovary. Clinical Obstetrics and Gynecology 17: 189–228
Nunez C, Diaz J I 1992 Ovarian follicular cysts: a potential source of false positive diagnoses in ovarian cytology. Diagnostic Cytopathology 8: 532–536
O'Hagen D B, Pudifin J, Mickel R E 1985 Antenatal detection of foetal ovarian cyst by real time ultrasound. A case report. South African Medical Journal 67: 471
Peters W A, Thiagarajah S, Thornton W N 1979 Ovarian hemorrhage in patients receiving anticoagulant therapy. Journal of Reproductive Medicine 22: 82–86
Piver M S, Williams L J, Marcuse P M 1970 Influence of luteal cysts on menstrual function. Obstetrics and Gynecology 35: 740–751
Rizzo N, Gabrielli S, Perolo A 1989 Prenatal diagnosis and management of foetal ovarian cysts. Prenatal Diagnosis 9: 97
Robertson R D, Picker R H, Wilson PC, Saunders D M 1979 Assessment of ovulation by ultrasound and plasma estradiol determinations. Obstetrics and Gynecology 54: 686–691
Roden A, Coltart J M, Chapman M G 1989 Needle aspiration of simple ovarian cysts in pregnancy. British Journal of Obstetrics and Gynaecology 96: 994–996
Sakala E P, Leon Z A, Rouse G A 1991 Management of antenatally diagnosed foetal ovarian cyst. Obstetrical and Gynaecological Survey 46: 407–414
Schenken R S, Werlin L B, Williams R F, Prihoda T J, Hodgen G D 1986 Histologic and hormonal documentation of the luteinized unruptured follicle syndrome. American Journal of Obstetrics and Gynecology 154: 839–847
Shawker T H, Hubbard V S, Reichert C M, Guerreiro de Matos O M 1983 Cystic ovaries in cystic fibrosis: an ultrasound and autopsy study. Journal of Ultrasound in Medicine 2: 439–444
Stevens M L, Plotka E D 1977 Functional lutein cyst in a postmenopausal woman. Obstetrics and Gynecology 50: 27s–29s
Strickler R C, Kelly R W, Askin F B 1984 Postmenopausal ovarian follicle cyst: an unusual cause of estrogen excess. International Journal of Gynecological Pathology 3: 318–322
Suita S, Sakaguchi T, Ikeda K, Nakama H 1991 Therapeutic dilemmas associated with antenatally detected ovarian cysts. Surgery Gynaecology and Obstetrics 171: 502–508
Thaysen J H, Ølgaard K, Jensen H G 1975 Ovarian cysts in women on chronic intermittent haemodialysis. Acta Medica Scandinavica 197: 433–437

Treasure J L, Gordon P A L, King E A, Wheeler M, Russell G F M 1985 Cystic ovaries: a phase of anorexia nervosa. Lancet ii: 1379–1382

Turetz F, Smulewicz J, Wallach R C 1980 Evolution of functional ovarian cysts: sonographic appearance and management. International Journal of Gynaecology and Obstetrics 17: 312–322

Wieland R G, Bendezu R, Hallberg M C, Tang P, Webster K 1976 Hormonal evaluation of premature menarche produced by a follicular cyst. American Journal of Obstetrics and Gynecology 126: 731–733

Zachariou Z, Roth H, Boos R, Troger J, Daum R 1989 Three years experience with large ovarian cysts diagnosed in utero. Journal of Paediatric Surgery 24 (5): 478–82

13

Polycystic ovary syndrome

J. Eden

The current paradigm of polycystic ovary syndrome has come a long way from the clinical syndrome described by Stein and Leventhal in 1935. Whereas previous reports had emphasized irregular heavy menstrual loss in association with polycystic ovaries, these investigators were first to describe the syndrome of amenorrhea, hirsutism, and enlarged polycystic ovaries. It is now clear that women who exhibit these symptoms represent the severe end of a spectrum of disease. Studies using high resolution ultrasound have suggested that more than 20% of normal women have ultrasound evidence of polycystic ovaries (Polsen et al 1988, Clayton et al 1992). Glucose intolerance and acanthosis nigricans are rare presentations. Endometrial carcinoma is an underestimated complication of anovulation associated with polycystic ovary syndrome and may rarely be the presenting illness (Goldzieher 1981).

Many authors use the term 'polycystic ovaries' to describe asymptomatic women with typical ultrasound features and reserve the term 'polycystic ovary syndrome' for those women who have morphological features of polycystic ovaries associated with clinical symptoms such as hirsutism, scalp hair loss, oily skin or acne, or oligomenorrhea (Adams et al 1986, Eden 1989). Some women will present with dysfunctional uterine bleeding. In many cases, the ovarian cycle lengthens as these women put on weight, and weight loss in obese women with polycystic ovary syndrome is often associated with a resumption of regular menses (Stein & Leventhal 1935, Eden 1989, Conway & Jacobs 1993). It has been postulated that polycystic ovaries may simply represent that subset of women who seem to ovulate best when thin, unlike their (normal) counterparts who need a certain amount of fat to ovulate regularly and thus become amenorrheic when pathologically thin. Skin symptoms such as acne or hirsutism are not determined only by serum androgen levels but also by the activity of the skin's hormone receptors and the activity of enzymes such as 5α-reductase.

Etiology of polycystic ovaries

It is likely that polycystic ovaries result from many divergent causes and probably do not represent a single disease entity. Thus women with clearly defined androgen excess problems such as congenital adrenal hyperplasia often have coexistent polycystic ovaries. Some proposed pathogeneses include androgen excess by the adrenal glands or ovaries (McKenna 1988), abnormal secretion of luteinizing hormone mediated by a hypothalamic pituitary lesion (Yen 1980), enzymatically abnormal ovarian follicular steroid synthesis (Kirschner & Jacobs 1971), hyperinsulinemia (Conway & Jacobs 1993), a genetic lesion (Franks 1991), or a derangement of intraovarian growth factors (Conway & Jacobs 1993).

Ultrasound features of polycystic ovaries

The most commonly used criteria are those of Adams et al (1986). The most consistent ultrasound feature is the presence of more than 10 peripherally placed symmetrical small follicles (2–6 mm in diameter) in association with increased stroma and often an ovarian volume greater than 12 cm^3 (see Ch. 58). This appearance should not be confused with that of 'multicystic ovaries' commonly found in association with hypothalamic amenorrhea. The multicystic ovary usually has 3–6 asymmetrical follicles with normal stroma. In our experience, transvaginal ultrasound is usually necessary to accurately identify the ovarian morphology.

Biochemical features of polycystic ovary syndrome

The biochemical profiles of these patients are characterized by the following:

1. Many have sustained high luteinizing hormone levels due to an increase in luteinizing hormone pulse size and frequency. These high levels of luteinizing hormone appear to play a part in the excessive theca cell growth and consequent androgen production. There is some evidence that, amongst women with polycystic ovary syndrome, it is this subgroup with high serum luteinizing hormone levels that is at increased risk of infertility and miscarriage (Jacobs et al 1990, Franks 1991, Piper & Poretsky 1994).
2. Most authors have found normal or slightly lower levels of follicle stimulating hormone (Eden 1989, Franks 1991).
3. Most patients have demonstrable androgen excess with raised levels of total testosterone or androstenedione or dehydroepiandrostene sulfate. About 40% of women with polycystic ovary syndrome will have at least one of these androgens elevated (Yen 1980, McKenna 1988, Eden 1989).
4. Obese and anovulatory women with polycystic ovary syndrome usually have low levels of sex hormone binding globulin, resulting in high free testosterone levels (Eden 1989, Conway & Jacobs 1993).
5. Recently, many authors have stressed the importance of hyperinsulinemia or abnormalities of the insulin-like growth factor axis. Certainly many obese anovulatory women with polycystic ovary syndrome appear to have hyperinsulinemia. Insulin inhibits sex hormone binding globulin production and stimulates ovarian androgen production (Blackard et al 1991, Conway & Jacobs 1993).

Macroscopic features

Both ovaries are generally symmetrically enlarged two to threefold, but may be of normal size, and rarely only one ovary is enlarged (Delahunt et al 1975). Unlike the slightly flattened ovaries of normal women, the enlarged ovaries of polycystic ovary syndrome are ovoid or globular. Dilated vessels are frequently visible on the thickened capsular surface, which is often not only thickened but also pearly white with bluish areas overlying multiple cortical follicles. The cut surfaces typically show a linear subcapsular aggregation of these multiple small follicles up to about 8 mm in diameter and contain a clear protein-rich follicular fluid.

Microscopic features

The tunica albuginea is usually, but not always, increased in thickness, often threefold but occasionally up to tenfold, with an accentuation of the layered interlacing bundles of acellular fibrocollagenous connective tissue (Fig. 13.1). This finding is not specific for polycystic ovary syndrome and is found in many anovulatory states.

Follicular development deviates markedly from normal in many ways. Primordial follicles are present in appropriate or slightly reduced numbers and there are many cystic follicles at about the 4–10 mm stage of development (Fig. 13.2). The relative uniformity of size of the cystic follicles is a

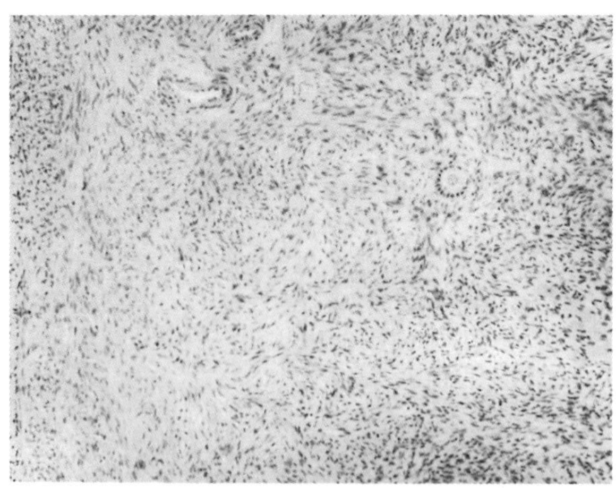

Fig. 13.1 Low power of thickened and somewhat fibrotic tunica delimited by the serosa (left) and a solitary primordial follicle. H + E ×60

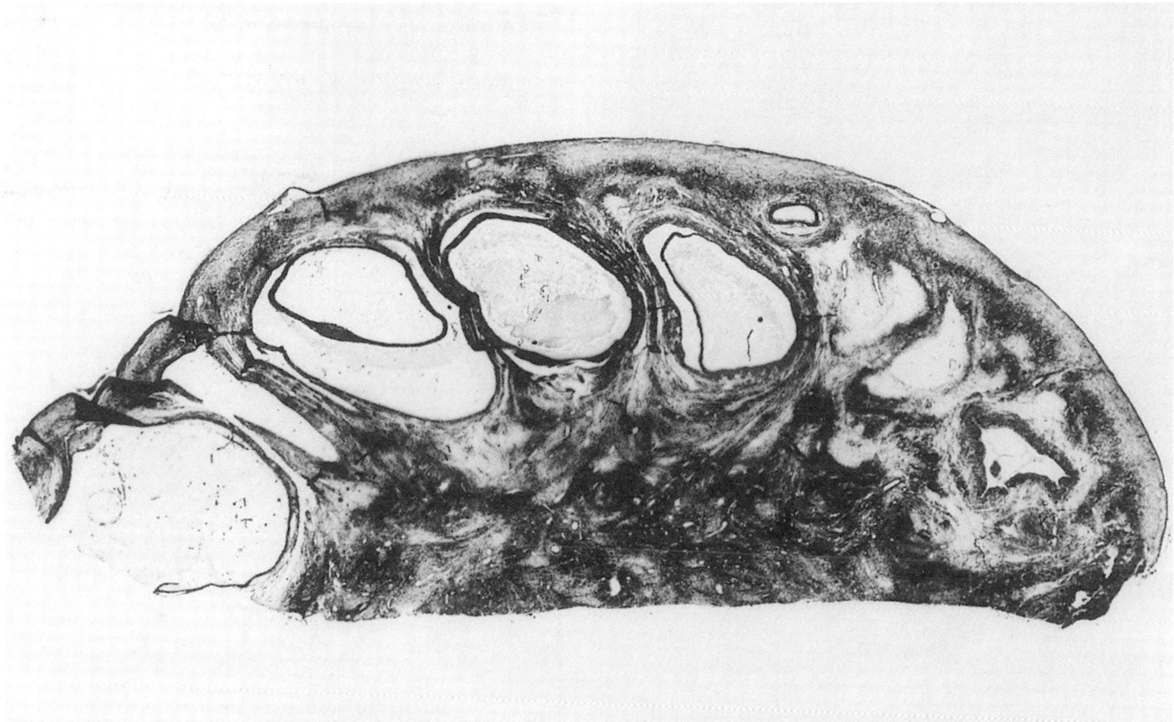

Fig. 13.2 Polycystic ovary. Note the relative uniformity of size of the developing and regressing cystic follicles and absence of stigmata of ovulation. H + E ×5

typical feature of polycystic ovary syndrome. Anovulatory women will have a conspicuous absence of residua of ovulation. Follicular atresia is prominent. Apart from aberrant follicular development theca cell hyperplasia is seen in all cases (Greenblatt & Mahesh 1976). The theca interna layer is often two to three times thicker than normal. The theca cells may be larger than normal with more obvious eosinophilic cytoplasm or appear frankly luteinized. The granulosa of these follicles is either indistinguishable from normal or exhibits early regressive changes with disaggregation and lack of mitotic activity (Fig. 13.3). Atretic follicles may also show persistence of the prominent theca cell layer (Fig. 13.4). The persistence of these theca cells, often to the point where other components of the atretic follicles have completely disappeared (Futterweit 1984), offers a possible explanation for the infrequent, isolated aggregates or clusters of such cells in the deep cortical and medullary stroma (Fig. 13.5). These

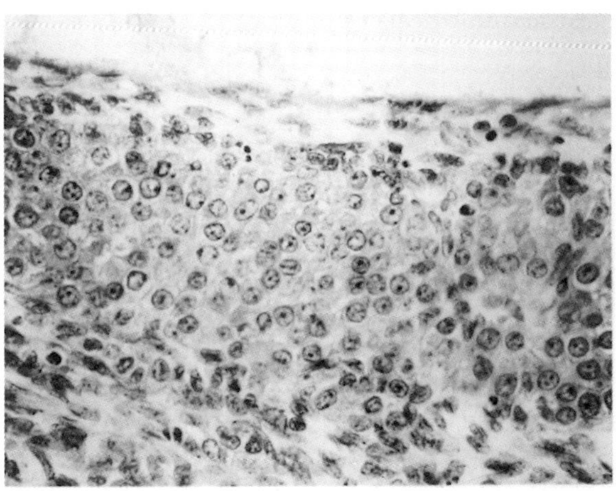

Fig. 13.3 Hyperplastic and partly luteinized theca interna and an attenuated, effete granulosa (top) are typical changes in many of the cystic follicles. H + E ×250

clusters are occasionally seen in normal ovaries, but are much more prominent in, and are typical of, hyperthecosis. This latter entity and polycystic

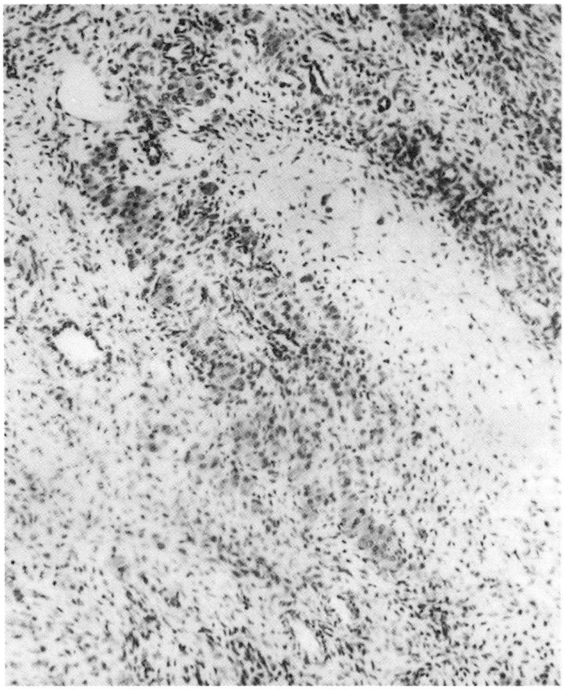

Fig. 13.4 Old atretic follicular remnant with residual and luteinized theca cells around its perimeter. H + E ×75

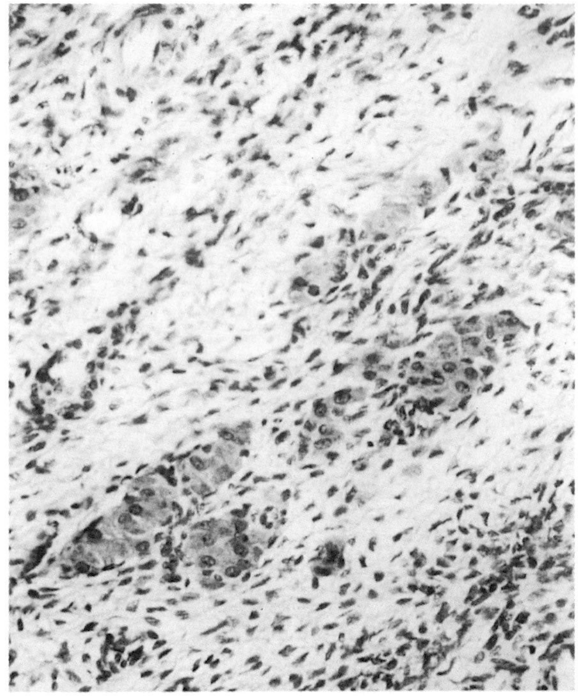

Fig. 13.5 Clusters of prominent stromal lutein cells with rounded nuclei and eosinophilic slightly granular cytoplasm. The prominence of these cells is enhanced through staining by an immunoperoxidase technique for estradiol. ×150

ovary syndrome are thought by some (Givens 1977, Scully 1979) to be elements in a single clinicopathological continuum.

Differential diagnosis

Using pelvic ultrasound, polycystic ovaries and multicystic ovaries may be difficult to distinguish, although the main characteristic feature of polycystic ovaries is the presence of more than 10 peripheral small follicles in association with increased stroma. Clinically, late onset congenital adrenal hyperplasia and other virilizing disorders may mimic polycystic ovaries. For the pathologist, other conditions which may resemble polycystic ovary syndrome include the ovarian hyperstimulation syndrome, the swollen ovary syndrome and hyperreactio luteinalis with multiple theca lutein cysts, and prominence of luteinized stromal cells in enlarged ovaries. The clinical context of this latter condition associated with a pregnancy episode or trophoblastic disease hardly lends itself to ready confusion.

REFERENCES

Adams J, Franks S, Polson D W 1986 Prevalence of polycystic ovaries in women with anovulation and idiopathic hirsutism. British Medical Journal 293: 355–359

Blackard W G, Clore J N, Matt D W et al 1991 A direct effect of hyperinsulinaemia on serum sex hormone binding globulin levels in obese women with the polycystic ovary syndrome. Journal of Clinical Endocrinology and Metabolism 72: 83–89

Clayton R N, Hodgkinson J, Dyer S et al 1992 How common are polycystic ovaries in normal women and what is their significance for the fertility of the population? Clinical Endocrinology 37: 127–134

Conway G S, Jacobs H S 1993 Clinical implications of hyperinsulinaemia in women. Clinical Endocrinology 39: 623–632

Delahunt J W, Clements R V, Ramsay I D, Newton J, Collins W P, Landon J 1975 The polycystic ovary syndrome. British Medical Journal 4: 621

Eden J A 1989 The polycystic ovary syndrome. Australian

and New Zealand Journal of Obstetrics and Gynaecology 29: 403–416
Franks S 1991 The ubiquitous polycystic ovary. Journal of Endocrinology 129: 317–319
Futterweit W 1984 Polycystic ovarian disease. Springer-Verlag, New York, p 41–46
Givens J R 1977 Polycystic ovarian disease. In: Givens J R (ed) Gynecologic endocrinology. Year Book, Chicago, IL, p 127–142
Goldzieher J W 1981 Polycystic ovarian disease. Fertility and Sterility 35: 371–394
Greenblatt R B, Mahesh V B 1976 The androgenic polycystic ovary. American Journal of Obstetrics and Gynecology 125: 712–726
Jacobs H S, Owen E J, Regan L 1990 Hypersecretion of luteinizing hormone, infertility and miscarriage. Lancet 336: 1141–1144
Kirschner M A, Jacobs J B 1971 Combined ovarian and adrenal vein catheterization to determine the sites of androgen over-production in hirsute women. Journal of Clinical Endocrinology and Metabolism 33: 199–209
McKenna T J 1988 Pathogenesis and treatment of the polycystic ovary syndrome. New England Journal of Medicine 318: 558–562
Piper B, Poretsky L 1994 Insulin resistance, hypersecretion of luteinizing hormone: a dual-defect hypothesis for the pathogenesis of polycystic ovary syndrome. Obstetrics and Gynecology 84: 613–621
Polsen D W, Adams J, Franks S, Wadsworth J 1988 Polycystic ovaries – a common finding in normal women. Lancet 870–872
Scully R E 1979 Tumors of the ovary and maldeveloped gonads, AFIP Fascicle 16, 2nd series. Armed Forces Institute of Pathology, Washington, DC
Stein I F, Leventhal M L 1935 Amenorrhea associated with bilateral polycystic ovaries. American Journal of Obstetrics and Gynecology 29: 181–191
Yen S S C 1980 The polycystic ovary syndrome. Clinical Endocrinology 12: 177–208

14

Stromal hyperplasia and hyperthecosis

P. Russell   A. Farnsworth

Hyperplasia of the cortical and medullary stroma of mild degree is a sufficiently common finding in the ovaries of perimenopausal and postmenopausal women to warrant some degree of caution in attaching clinicopathological significance to such changes. Stromal hyperplasia is essentially always diffusely bilateral. Thus, while sampling is not an important factor in assessment, the apparent severity of the changes does not correlate well with clinical symptomatology. It is our practice, consonant with that of other authors (Scully 1979), to reserve the term for definite and florid cases, and our minimum criteria are obliteration of the normal distinction between cortex and medulla or at least some nodularity to the proliferating stroma. The majority of women with stromal hyperplasia, as defined above, are in the older age group and many are postmenopausal. Indeed, it may be found in up to a third of such women (Snowden et al 1989). Clinical symptoms are due to excess androgen (androstenedione) production by the hyperplastic stroma, with or without dominant peripheral aromatization to estrone. Diabetes, hypertension, and particularly obesity are associated with the latter.

Hyperthecosis is defined as the presence of luteinized stromal cells (of thecal origin; see Ch. 3) at a distance from the follicles and either clustered or scattered diffusely in the stroma. It regularly occurs in association with ovarian stromal hyperplasia on the one hand, and merges imperceptibly with the polycystic ovary syndrome on the other. Some reports, however, have tended to stress the validity of separating hyperthecosis as a distinct clinical, hormonal and pathological entity (Aiman et al 1978, Karam & Hajj 1979) not responding to the usual means of induction of ovulation. Like stromal hyperplasia, it may on occasion be asymptomatic, but is more usually accompanied by marked defeminization and virilization (due to elaboration of dihydrotestosterone, testosterone, and androstenedione), and only occasionally estrogenic (Nagamani et al 1988, Sasano et al 1989, Snowden et al 1989). A single case has been associated with progesterone production (Ravinsky 1984). Although isolated luteinized stromal cells are common in postmenopausal ovaries, clinical hyperthecosis occurs mostly in women of reproductive age (Leedman et al 1989, Nuovo 1989) and may rarely present as virilization in pregnancy, ameliorating spontaneously after delivery (Erkkola et al 1985). Two examples of virilizing hyperthecosis have been reported in association with placental site trophoblastic tumor (Nagelberg & Rosen 1985, Nagamani et al 1990). There have been reported familial occurrences (Judd et al 1973, Wilroy et al 1975). It is almost always bilateral. An apparently genuine unilateral case has been recorded (Farber et al 1981), while others have been complicated by massive edema, which cannot be ruled out as an antecedent cause of the hyperthecosis (see Ch. 16). Virilizing hyperthecosis, unlike polycystic ovary syndrome, tends not to respond to clomiphene treatment, but a measure of success has been achieved with the use of gonadotrophin-releasing hormone agonists (Steingold et al 1986).

Macroscopic features

In stromal hyperplasia, with or without hyperthecosis, both ovaries are enlarged up to twice their normal size and assume a more rounded shape.

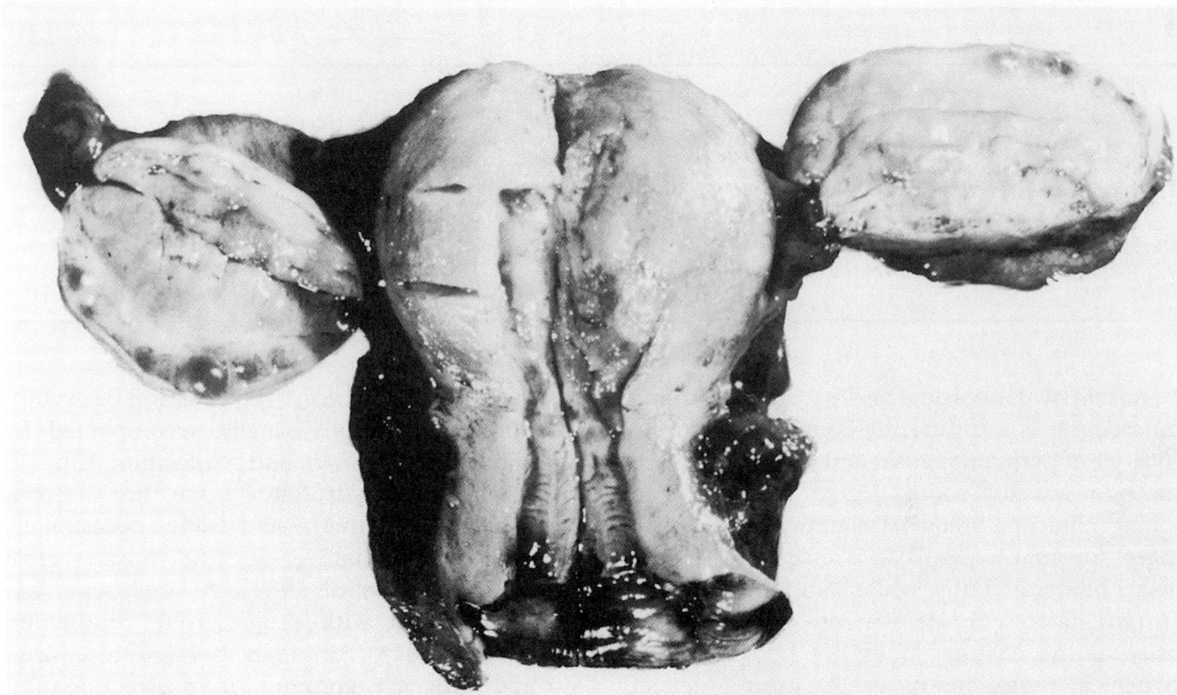

Fig. 14.1 Radical hysterectomy for endometrial adenocarcinoma. Uterus is opened posteriorly revealing an ill-defined tumor mass in the fundus (right side). Both ovaries are uniformly enlarged with blurring of the usual distinction between cortex and medulla – stromal hyperplasia. A few small cystic follicles are present in the left ovary.

The tunica albuginea is thickened, and cystic follicles (smaller and less numerous than those typical of the polycystic ovary syndrome) will be present in those of young women (Fig. 14.1). The cut surface of each ovary is uniformly pale yellow to fawn and, in severe cases, there is absence of the usual division into cortex and medulla. In rare cases a nodular appearance is obvious macroscopically, and this should alert one to the possibility of nodular stromal hyperthecosis and stromal luteoma.

Microscopic features

Stromal hyperplasia is characterized by a variable but marked proliferation of plump but otherwise undistinguished spindled stromal cells, each invested by reticulin fibrils, recapitulating the swathes and whorls of normal ovarian stroma (Fig. 14.2). The medulla is most altered by this proliferation and the usually obvious corticomedullary interface

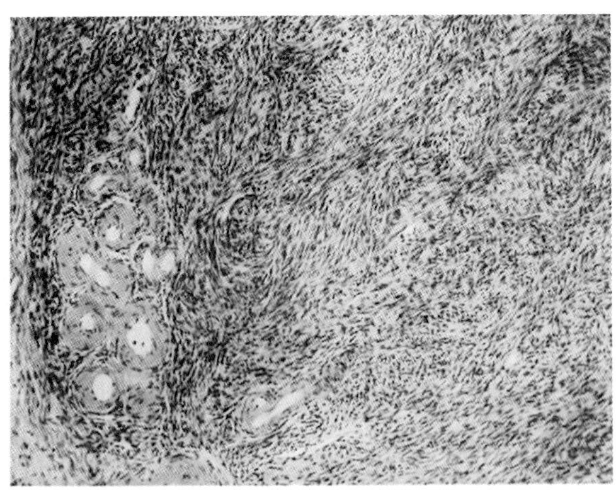

Fig. 14.2 Cortical stromal hyperplasia characterized by swirls and bands of small spindle cells, more cellular but otherwise indistinguishable from normal ovarian cortex. H + E ×60

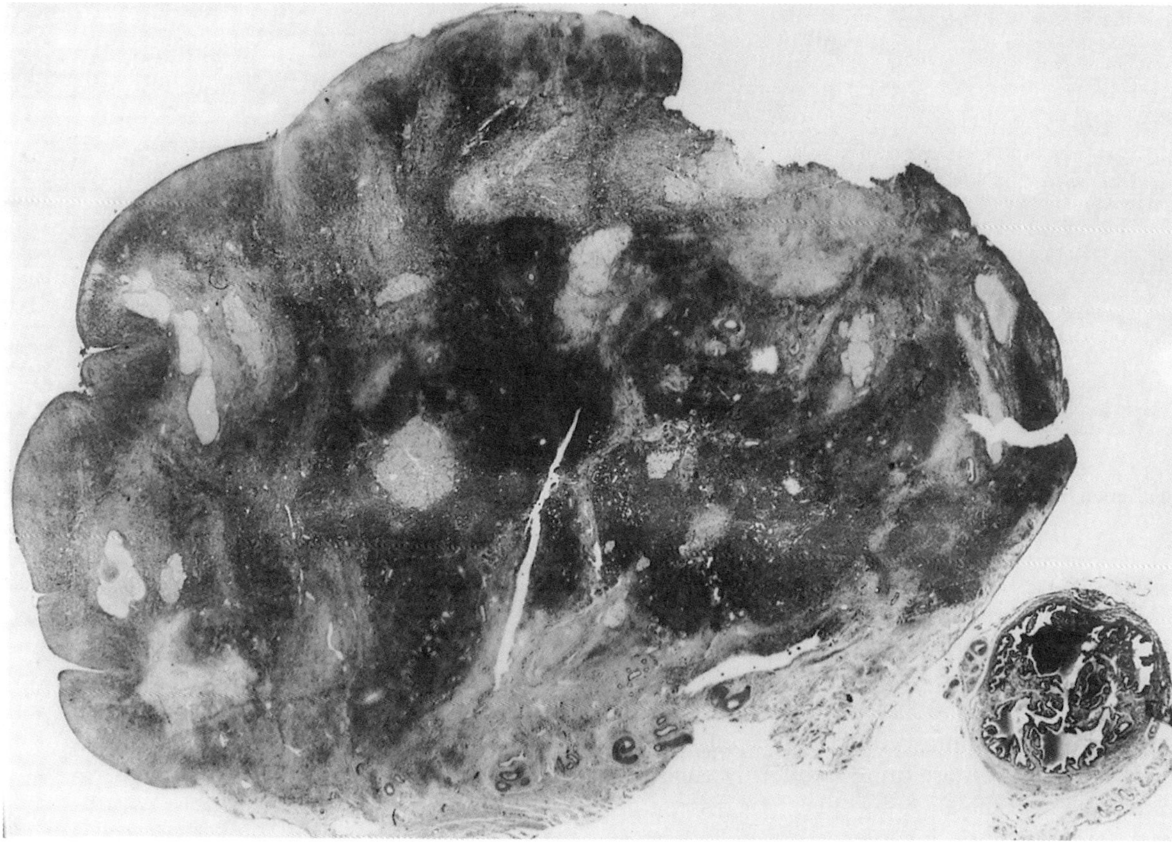

A

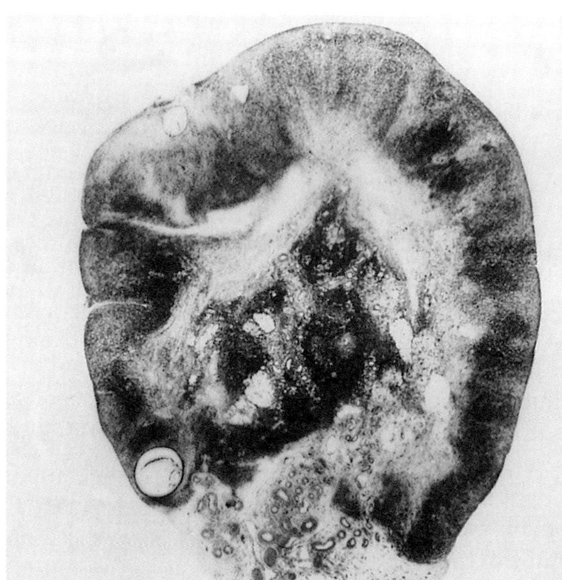

B

Fig. 14.3 (A) Section of diffusely hyperplastic postmenopausal ovary. Note obliteration of normal corticomedullary junction. (B) Normal postmenopausal ovary for comparison. H + E ×6

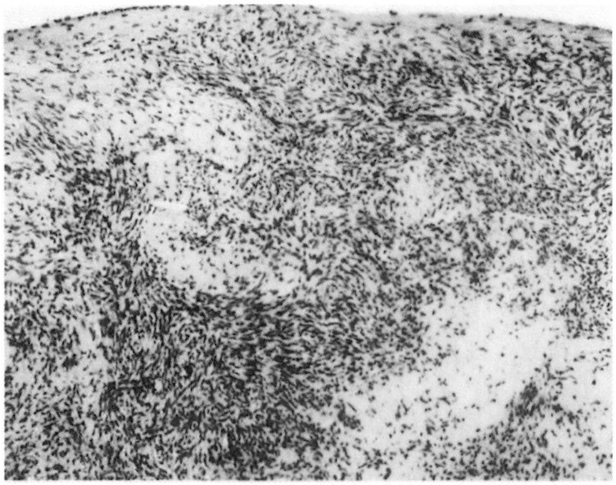

Fig. 14.4 Cortical stromal hyperplasia with focal hyalinization but no 'granulomas'. H + E ×60

may be obliterated. Stromal hyperplasia may be entirely diffuse (Fig. 14.3), but rather more commonly a focal or widespread nodular pattern is generated, particularly in the cortex. Despite the absence of luteinized cells (by definition), fat stains performed on frozen sections will usually reveal widespread intracytoplasmic lipid. Small foci of hyalinization are quite frequently encountered in the superficial cortex (Fig. 14.4); some of these lesions include histiocytes which impart a 'granulomatous' character to the lesions which are generally considered to be the end result of regression in small cortical aggregates of luteinized stromal cells (see Fig. 14.6).

Stromal hyperthecosis is typified by isolated or aggregated lutein-like cells throughout each ovary. These cells tend to be more numerous in the medulla than the cortex, and they are large and polyhedral with abundant eosinophilic granular or finely vacuolated cytoplasm and rounded central nuclei, each with a single small nucleolus (Fig. 14.5). Focal regression is sometimes seen with hyalinization and a mild lymphohistiocytic infiltrate (Fig. 14.6). A continuum exists between such diffuse cases and those in which the lutein cells form multiple discrete small nodules (Fig. 14.7; nodular stromal hyperthecosis). The cortex frequently contains small cystic follicles, each with a prominent luteinized theca interna layer. Stigmata of recent ovulation are absent, but follicular atresia is sometimes increased (Nuovo 1989).

In occasional cases, one or more of these

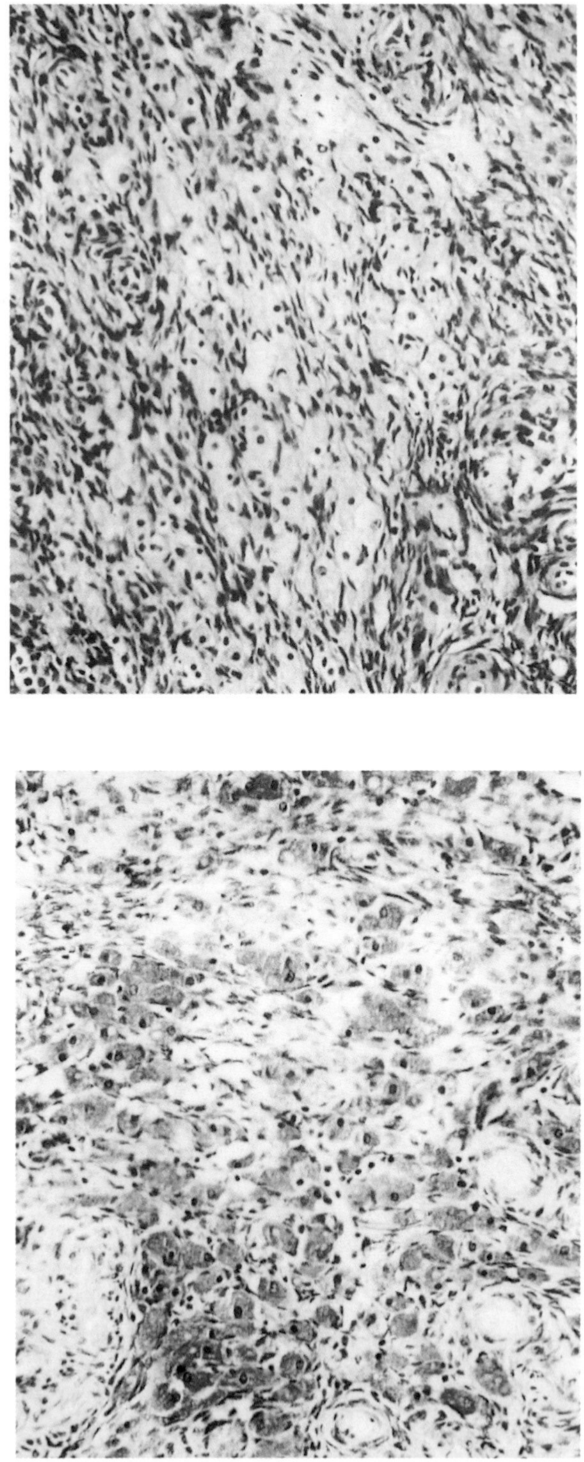

A

B

Fig. 14.5 Stromal hyperthecosis. Clusters of luteinized stromal cells. (A) H + E ×150. (B) Immunoperoxidase for estradiol. ×150

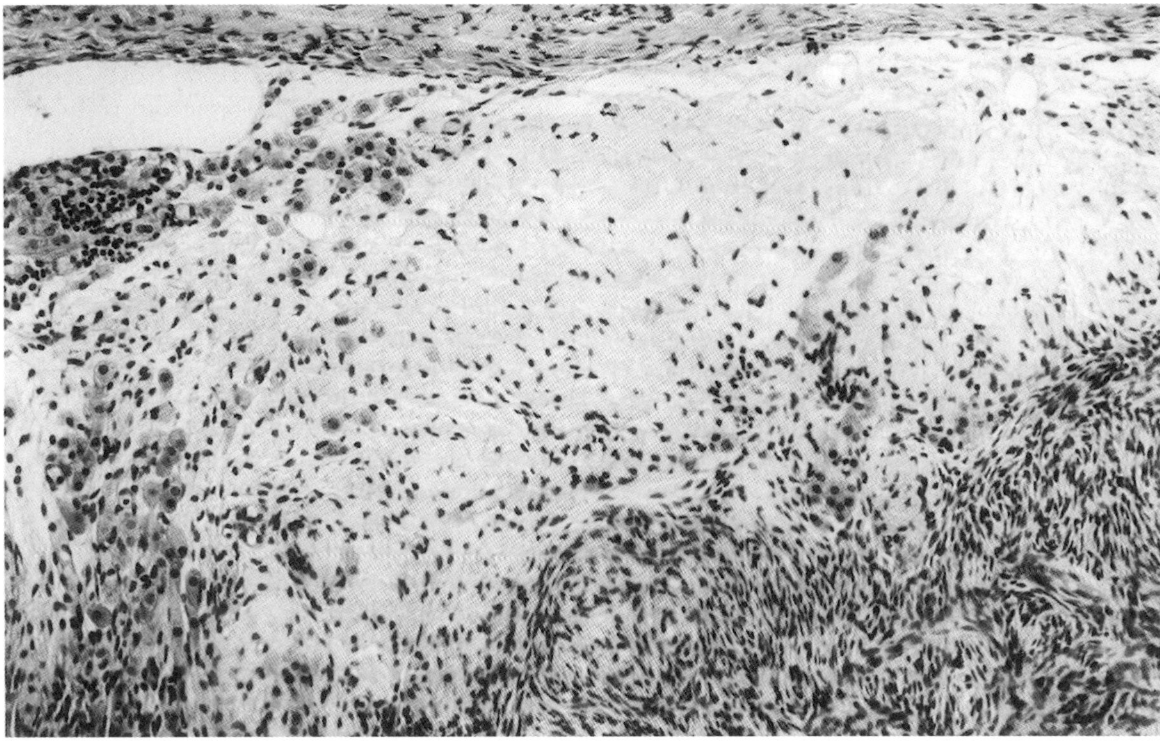

Fig. 14.6 Hyperthecosis with a small collection of residual luteinized stromal cells immediately beneath the tunica (top). A mild chronic inflammatory infiltrate is noted at the top left while the remainder of the focus has undergone hyalinization. H + E ×125

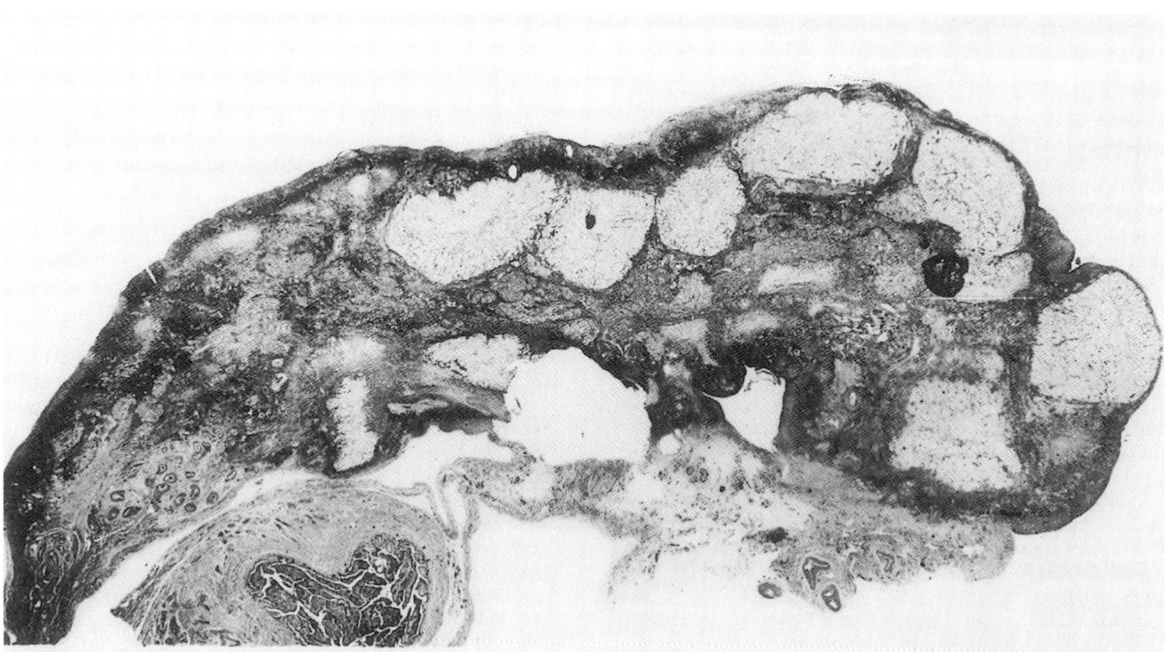

Fig. 14.7 Nodular stromal hyperthecosis from a virilized woman. Multiple discrete nodules of large pale lutein cells against a background of stromal hyperplasia. H + E ×5

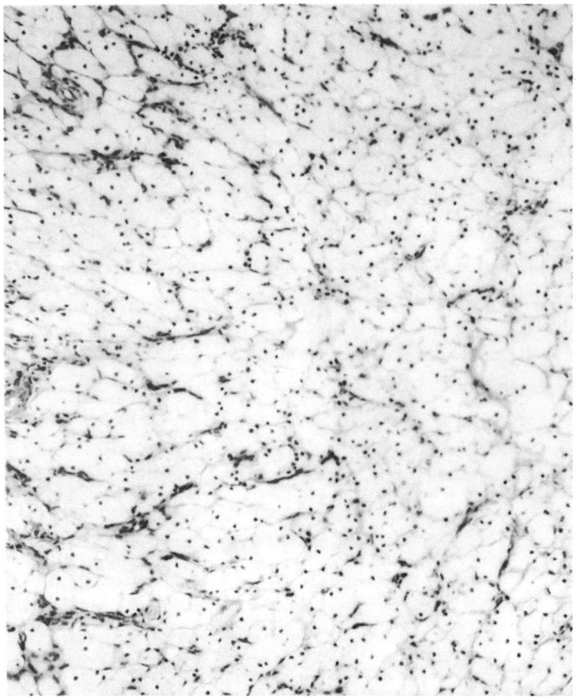

Fig. 14.8 Stromal luteoma. Large vacuolated lutein cells from a solitary 9 mm nodule. H + E ×75

nodules becomes dominant, suggesting to some authors a specific neoplasm – stromal luteoma (Sternberg & Dhurandhar 1977, Hayes & Scully 1987). It is our view that, in accord with similar pathological processes in other endocrine glands (e.g. thyroid and parathyroid), the diagnosis of stromal luteoma should be made with caution in the presence of multiple hyperplastic nodules of theca-like cells, and the term is best reserved for those lipid cell tumors of stromal origin which arise in the absence of such diffuse or nodular ovarian stromal hyperplasia or hyperthecosis. These tumor-like nodules are composed entirely of large rounded lutein cells (Fig. 14.8), and average about 1 cm in diameter (Hayes & Scully 1987). Reinke's crystals are absent, distinguishing them from Leydig cell tumors of stromal (or non-hilar) origin. Paradoxically, Leydig cell hyperplasia and Leydig cell tumors (Sternberg & Roth 1973) may also occur in association with hyperthecosis. The spindled nonluteinized theca-like cells of partly luteinized thecomas (see Ch. 34) are also absent, as are the perivascular hyaline plaques typical of thecomas.

REFERENCES

Aiman J, Edman C D, Worley R J, Vellios F, MacDonald P C 1978 Androgen and estrogen formation in women with ovarian hyperthecosis. Obstetrics and Gynecology 51: 1–9

Erkkola R, Seppala P, Klemi P J 1985 Virilization during pregnancy due to bilateral hyperthecosis. Hormone Research 21: 83–87

Farber M, Madanes A, O'Brian D S, Millan V G, Turksoy R N, Rule A H 1981 Asymmetric hyperthecosis ovarii. Obstetrics and Gynecology 57: 521–525

Hayes M C, Scully R E 1987 Stromal luteoma of the ovary: a clinicopathological analysis of 25 cases. International Journal of Gynecological Pathology 6: 313–321

Judd H L, Scully R E, Herbst A L, Yen S S C, Ingersol F M, Kliman B 1973 Familial hyperthecosis; comparison of endocrinologic and histologic findings with polycystic ovarian disease. American Journal of Obstetrics and Gynecology 117: 976–982

Karam K, Hajj S 1979 Hyperthecosis syndrome. Clinical, endocrinologic and histologic findings. Acta Obstetricia et Gynecologica Scandinavica 58: 73–79

Leedman P J, Bierre A R, Martin F I R 1989 Virilizing nodular ovarian stromal hyperthecosis, diabetes mellitus and insulin resistance in a postmenopausal woman. Case report. British Journal of Obstetrics and Gynaecology 96: 1095–1098

Nagamani M, Hannigan E V, van Dinh T, Stuart CA 1988 Hyperinsulinemia and stromal luteinization of the ovaries in postmenopausal women with endometrial cancer. Journal of Clinical Endocrinology and Metabolism 67: 144–148

Nagamani M, Kaspar H G, Hannigan E V, Smith E 1990 Hyperthecosis of the ovaries in a woman with a placental site trophoblastic tumor. Obstetrics and Gynecology 76: 931–935

Nagelberg S B, Rosen S W 1985 Clinical and laboratory investigation of a virilized woman with placental-site trophoblastic tumor. Obstetrics and Gynecology 65: 527–534

Nuovo G J 1989 Virilizing stromal thecosis of the ovary associated with multiple corpora atretica. American Journal of Clinical Pathology 92: 505–508

Ravinsky E 1984 Ovarian hyperthecosis associated with pseudosarcomatous changes in the endometrial stroma. American Journal of Surgical Pathology 8: 939–943

Sasano H, Fukunaga M, Rojas M, Silverberg S G 1989 Hyperthecosis of the ovary. Clinicopathologic study of 19 cases with immunohistochemical analysis of steroidogenic enzymes. International Journal of Gynecological Pathology 8: 311–320

Scully R E 1979 Tumors of the ovary and maldeveloped gonads, AFIP Fascicle 16, 2nd series. Armed Forces Institute of Pathology, Washington, DC, p 369–371

Snowden J A, Harkin P J R, Thornton J G, Wells M 1989 Morphometric assessment of ovarian stromal proliferation – a clinicopathological study. Histopathology 14: 369–379

Steingold K A, Judd H L, Nieberg R K, Lu J K H, Chang R J 1986 Treatment of severe androgen excess due to ovarian hyperthecosis with a long-acting gonadotrophin-releasing hormone agonist. American Journal of Obstetrics and Gynecology 154: 1241–1248

Sternberg W H, Dhurandhar H M 1977 Functional ovarian tumors of stromal and sex cord origin. Human Pathology 8: 565–582

Sternberg W H, Roth L M 1973 Ovarian stromal tumors containing Leydig cells. I: Stromal–Leydig cell tumor and non-neoplastic transformation of ovarian stroma to Leydig cells. Cancer 32: 940–951

Wilroy R S, Givens J R, Wiser W L, Coleman S A, Anderson R N, Summitt R L 1975 Hyperthecosis: an inheritable form of polycystic ovarian disease. Birth Defects 11: 81–86

15

Leydig cell hyperplasia

P. Russell   A. Farnsworth

Hilus or Leydig cells are infrequently observed in routine sections of the ovary unless specifically sought, despite their documented presence in at least 80% of ovaries (see Ch. 3). It is this inconspicuousness in the average ovarian biopsy which draws immediate attention to prominence or proliferation of these cells. Such a proliferation or hyperplasia is rare, but is most regularly seen in response to raised gonadotrophin levels during pregnancy or at the menopause. It is generally of mild degree and unassociated with clinical endocrine disturbance. Occasionally the pregnancy-associated hilus or Leydig cell hyperplasia is more severe, sufficient to produce visible mitotic activity in these cells (an otherwise extremely rare occurrence in our experience). In nonpregnant women, hilus cell hyperplasia most frequently occurs against a background of stromal hyperplasia and hyperthecosis. Although there is no consistent endocrine profile associated with, or regarded as specific for, hilus cell hyperplasia, it may be a cause of increased serum testosterone levels (McLellan et al 1990).

Macroscopic features

The ovaries are not necessarily enlarged and do not reveal specific identifiable gross features.

Microscopic features

The hyperplasia is characterized by clusters and nodules of typical rounded or polygonal Leydig cells with moderately sized, vesicular, central nuclei and eosinophilic, granular to finely vacuolated cytoplasm (Fig. 15.1). Yellow-brown intracytoplasmic lipochrome (lipofuscin) pigment is often focally observed, and Reinke's crystals (see Ch. 3) are usually found in some cells, although they may be very sparse indeed and their prominence does not correlate with the severity of the hyperplasia. Nuclear pleiomorphism is not a regular feature, although, as recorded by Scully (1979), bizarre hyperchromatic nuclei may be encountered in the hyperplastic Leydig cells of postmenopausal women.

The nodules or clusters of Leydig cells vary greatly from area to area and, although most prominent in the ovarian hilus, may extend into the mesovarium and, in an apparently unique case, into the adjacent fallopian tubes (Lewis 1964). Small capillary vessels are identifiable amongst the Leydig cells, and nonmyelinated nerves can be disclosed in apposition to many of the cell clusters by immunohistochemical techniques.

In pregnant women, the remainder of the ovary shows a variety of physiological changes, as outlined in Chapters 3 and 10. In the nonpregnant patient with Leydig cells hyperplasia, there is likely to be an accompanying cortical and medullary stromal hyperplasia, with histological features ranging from polycystic ovary syndrome to nodular stromal hyperthecosis and, rarely, other related stromal 'tumors' such as stromal luteoma (Scully 1964) or stromal–Leydig cell tumor (Sternberg & Roth 1973).

Leydig cells (with typical Reinke's crystals) may also be found in a limited range of hyperplastic and neoplastic conditions, derived from the ovarian stroma and distinct from the ovarian hilus cells. These non-neoplastic stromal Leydig cells may be seen in simple stromal hyperplasias (Scully 1953), stromal proliferations reactive to

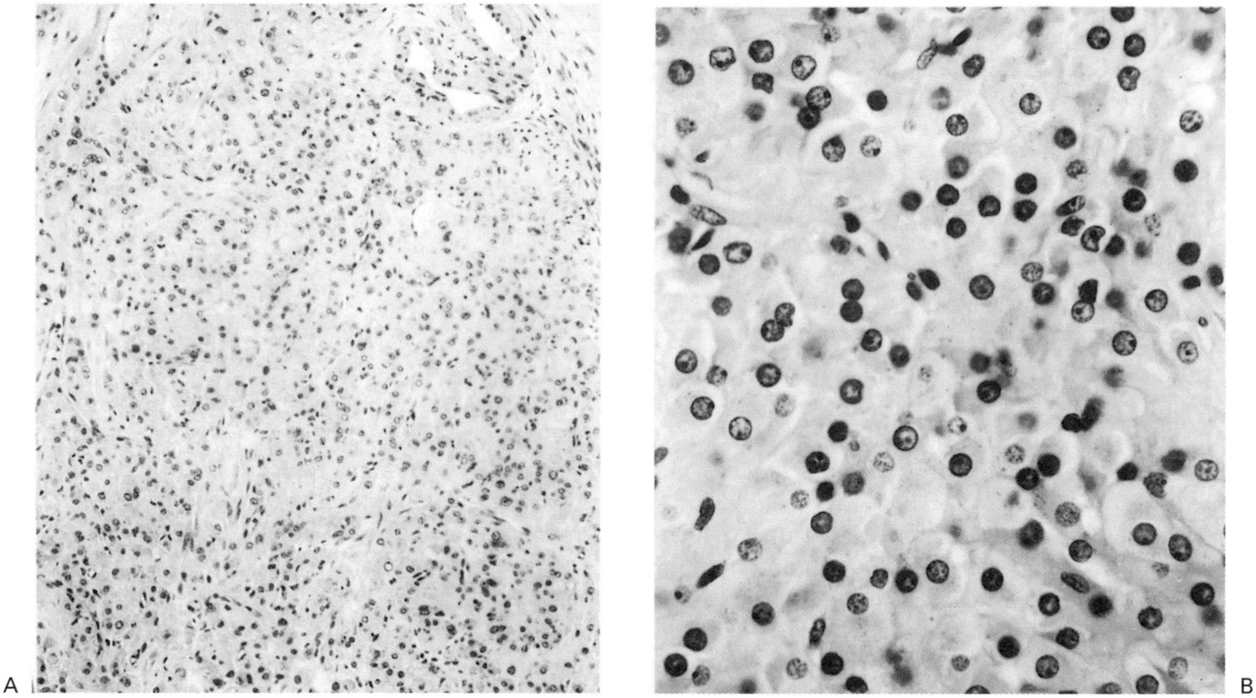

Fig. 15.1 Leydig cell hyperplasia. (A) Large nodule of typical polygonal Leydig cells associated with a number of small vessels. H + E ×75. (B) Leydig cells with uniform, rounded, central, vesicular nuclei and eosinophilic, slightly granular cytoplasm. H + E ×300

metastatic carcinomas (Sternberg & Roth 1973; see Ch. 53), or primary epithelial ovarian neoplasms (see Fig. 24.16; Novak et al 1970, Hameed 1972). Rarely, typical Leydig cells are noted in benign ovarian stromal tumors – the so-called stromal–Leydig cell tumors and pure Leydig cell tumors of non-hilar type (Roth & Sternberg 1973, Sternberg & Roth 1973). Unlike Leydig cell tumors of hilus cell origin, these lesions are characteristically multinodular, bilateral, and found in ovaries with stromal hyperplasia and hyperthecosis. It is a moot point, therefore, whether these lesions (particularly the stromal–Leydig cell tumors of Sternberg & Roth (1973)) are true neoplasms or multinodular hyperplasias, a faint echo of the analogous argument relating to thecomas (see Ch. 34).

REFERENCES

Hameed K 1972 Brenner tumor of the ovary with Leydig cell hyperplasia. A histologic and ultrastructure study. Cancer 30: 945–952

Lewis J D 1964 Hilus-cell hyperplasia of ovaries and tubes. Obstetrics and Gynecology 24: 728–731

McLellan A R, Mowat A, Cordiner J et al 1990 Hilus cell pathology and hirsutism. Clinical Endocrinology 32: 203–212

Novak D J, Lauchlan S C, McCawley J C, Fairman C 1970 Virilization during pregnancy. Case report and review of literature. American Journal of Medicine 49: 281–290

Roth L M, Sternberg W H 1973 Ovarian stromal tumors containing Leydig cells. II: Pure Leydig cell tumor, non-hilar type. Cancer 32: 952–960

Scully R E 1953 Hyperestrinism in old women. Report of a case with cortical and medullary hyperplasia of the ovaries and possible adrenal hyperactivity. American Journal of Obstetrics and Gynecology 65: 1248–1256

Scully R E 1964 Stromal luteoma of the ovary. A distinctive type of lipoid-cell tumor. Cancer 17: 769–778

Scully R E 1979 Tumors of the ovary and maldeveloped gonads, AFIP fascicle 16, 2nd series. Armed Forces Institute of Pathology, Washington, DC, p 388–390

Sternberg W H, Roth L M 1973 Ovarian stromal tumors containing Leydig cells. I: Stromal–Leydig cell tumor and non-neoplastic transformation of ovarian stroma. Cancer 32: 940–951

16

Massive edema and fibromatosis

P. Russell A. Farnsworth

This rare tumor-like entity is typified by 'marked enlargement of one or both ovaries by an accumulation of edema fluid in the stroma, separating normal follicular structures' (Serov et al 1973). Of the 60 or so reported cases, 80% have occurred in women in their second and third decades (rarely in prepubertal girls). Most have presented with acute abdominal pain and/or a palpable adnexal mass, and less commonly with menstrual disturbances. Masculinization of varying degrees is sometimes present (Vasquez et al 1982), clinically suggestive of the polycystic ovary syndrome in some cases – a pathological condition which may coexist with massive ovarian edema (Sageshima et al 1990, Eden 1994), and a single instance of isosexual pseudoprecocity in a 6-year-old girl has been reported (Sternberg & Dhurandhar 1977). It is possible that both the edema and the abnormal hormone production are the result of a local paraendocrine factor (Eden 1994). Meigs syndrome occasionally accompanies massive ovarian edema (Slotky et al 1982, Fukuda et al 1984, Lacson et al 1989), as does fibromatosis (see below).

Massive ovarian edema was first described by Kalstone et al (1969) and is thought to result from partial or intermittent torsion of an otherwise normal ovary (observed at operation in one-half of cases), compromising venous and lymphatic drainage but not causing ischemic necrosis. Although some reported cases include a specific denial that torsion was present at laparotomy, the presence of complete torsion of the contralateral ovary in some cases (Chervenak et al 1980), a quite striking right-sided predominance (two-thirds of cases) which accords with a similar pattern of torsion of otherwise normal fallopian tube and ovary (see Ch. 17), a low frequency (10%) of bilaterality, and examples of massive ovarian edema caused by lymphatic obstruction due to lymphangiitis carcinomatosa (Young & Scully 1984, Wong 1989), all argue for a mechanical pathogenesis.

Unilateral salpingo-oophorectomy has been the traditional surgical procedure for massive ovarian edema. It is almost universally unilateral; furthermore, it is argued, exclusion of an underlying neoplastic process which may have predisposed to the partial torsion in an individual case cannot be achieved without microscopic examination of the enlarged ovary (Mainguene et al 1993). The young age of the patients and the consequent importance of retention of reproductive capacity, however, suggest a more conservative approach – namely intraoperative frozen section examination of a large wedge biopsy of the affected ovary to exclude underlying neoplasia and to confirm viability of the edematous ovary, followed by surgical tethering of the ovary to the uterus or side wall of the pelvis. This course of action has been employed with an acceptable measure of clinical success (Elkins & Stock 1982, Young & Scully 1984, Hill et al 1993). An alternative conservative approach has involved use of oral contraceptive agents (Hubbell et al 1993).

Macroscopic features

The enlarged ovary may measure up to 35 cm in diameter (Nassar et al 1976) with an average size of 11 cm. It presents a soft pearly external surface, often with follicles visible under the capsule. The cut surface has an almost featureless but nevertheless characteristic myxoid appearance (Fig. 16.1),

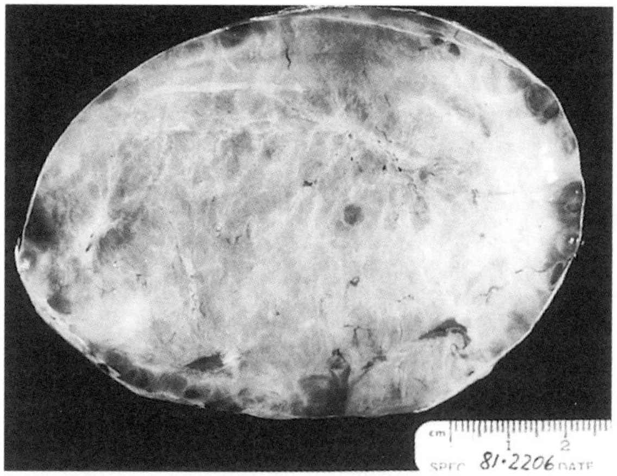

Fig. 16.1 Featureless cut surface of an ovary with massive edema from which protein-rich fluid readily exudes. Follicles are apparent beneath the capsule

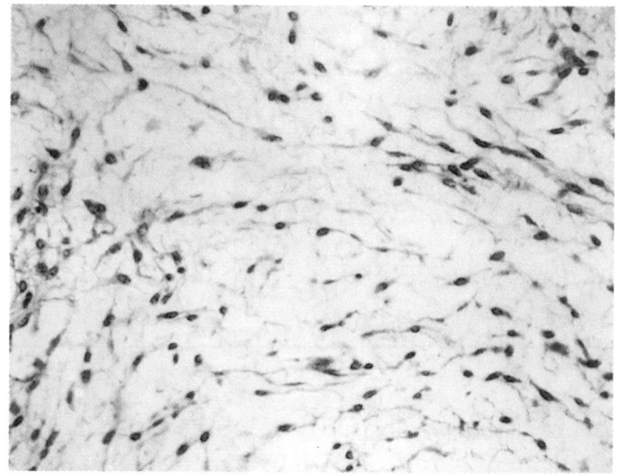

Fig. 16.3 Stellate stromal cells widely separated by gross interstitial edema. H + E ×125

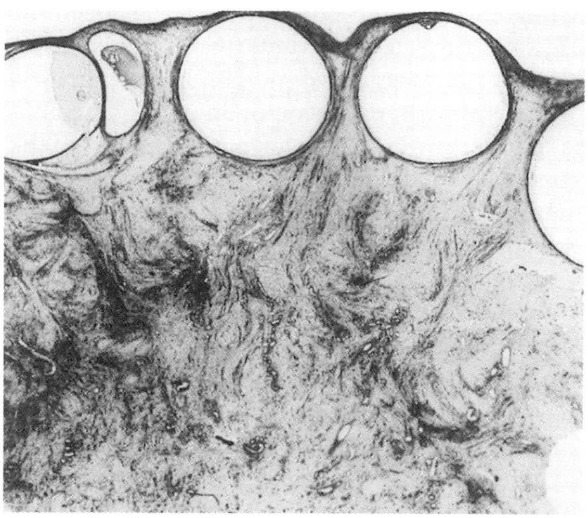

Fig. 16.2 Massive ovarian edema, maximal in the deeper cortex and medulla, with relative sparing of the superficial cortex. H + E ×4

from which colorless, protein-rich edema fluid readily exudes.

Microscopic features

The typical features are diffuse edema of the medulla and inner cortex with relative sparing of the superficial cortex and tunica albuginea, which are often thick and fibrotic. Cystic follicles beneath the tunica (Fig. 16.2) and other normal cortical and medullary structures such as corpora albicantes may also be noted, separated by loose myxoid tissue. Small fields of normal-appearing ovarian stroma may be present in less edematous areas. The marked edema widely separates stellate stromal cells and scanty intervening collagen (Fig. 16.3), making vascular and lymphatic channels abnormally prominent. There may be some congestion and foci of red cell extravasation and, rarely, small numbers of lymphocytes, mast cells and macrophages may be observed (Roth et al 1979). Focal necrosis is rarely observed (Young & Scully 1984). Over 40% of examples show isolated or clustered luteinized stromal cells (Tiltman & Nel 1984, Young & Scully 1984), thought to be the source of excess steroid hormone production in those patients presenting with virilization. The luteinization is confined to edematous areas, but may be seen in the contralateral edematous or nonedematous ovary. It appears to be related directly to the duration of symptoms.

Differential diagnosis

Massive ovarian edema is to be distinguished from other ovarian lesions that may show marked focal or generalized edema. These would include ovarian fibromas or thecafibromas (see Ch. 34), in which ovarian architecture is distorted or replaced by circumscribed masses of predominantly fibrous tissue. The relationship between massive ovarian edema and the so-called fibromatosis of Young & Scully (1984) is yet to be settled and, in our view, is more likely to represent disparate responses to the same pathological stimulus rather than one (fibromatosis) being a precursor of the other (massive ovarian edema). Various forms of hyperthecosis such as polycystic ovaries are always bilateral and show obvious stromal hyperplasia, while sclerosing stromal tumors (see Ch. 34) tend to compress the surrounding normal ovarian tissue and have a pseudolobular pattern with focal hyalinization. Metastatic carcinomas and malignant lymphomas may be sufficiently edematous that they grossly resemble massive ovarian edema. This applies particularly to Krukenberg tumors, in which the diagnostic signet ring cells may be quite sparse indeed.

FIBROMATOSIS

The protean manifestations of non-neoplastic proliferations of the 'undifferentiated' ovarian stroma collectively may be described as 'fibromatosis'. The term was first applied to a tumor-like condition of unknown cause, characterized by florid overgrowth of collagen-producing spindle cells which envelop normal follicular structures and lead to thickening of the superficial cortex (Young & Scully 1984). Their cases morphologically showed relatively acellular fascicles of fibroblastic cells with rare foci of stromal edema and/or luteinized stromal cells. The strong clinical overlap with massive edema (young age, clinical manifestations of menstrual irregularities, abdominal pain and, less commonly, virilization, and identification of torsion in some cases at operation) all suggested to these authors that pathogenetically massive ovarian edema was simply fibromatosis followed by torsion and the accumulation of fluid.

It is our view that the relationship is much stronger than this, and perhaps an inverse one to that proposed above. Quite apart from acellular collagen-rich 'fibromatosis' being a rarer entity than massive ovarian edema to which it is said to predispose, massive ovarian edema is not regularly described with significant areas of residual acellular fibrocollagenosis, a process which is illogical to accept as reversible. Rather than fibromatosis being merely one of a number of otherwise loosely related precursors to massive edema, we believe that the examples initially reported by Young & Scully (1984) represent the 'burnt-out' or 'mature' result of a florid reactive proliferative process which has, at the 'acellular' end of the morphological spectrum, typical massive ovarian edema and, at the other end of this spectrum, a rare collection of 'immature' highly cellular fibroblastic tumor-like lesions which have been variously reported in the literature as 'thecomas' (Faber 1962, Schweisguth et al 1971), 'secondary massive edema' (Lacson et al 1989), 'sarcoma-like ovarian nodules' (Khan & Pandey 1994), 'malignant luteinized thecoma' (Dudzinski et al 1989), 'fibromatosis' (Byrne et al 1989, Roche & du Boulay 1989), and 'luteinized thecoma with sclerosing peritonitis' (Clement et al 1994). The characteristics of this combined group are: firstly, their young age (mean age 23.5 years, range 4–76 years), abdominal pain and swelling associated with pelvic masses, and ascites/pleural effusions in many cases; secondly, a frequent association between abdominal fibromatosis/sclerosing peritonitis and ovarian fibromatosis/massive ovarian edema (Lacson et al 1989, Roche & du Boulay 1989, Antoniuk et al 1993, Regan et al 1993, Khan & Pandey 1994, Clement et al 1994); thirdly, occasional exposure to antiepileptic drugs or to β-adrenergic blocking agents (particularly in patients under 10 years of age); and, fourthly, a personally observed case of massive edema in one ovary and florid 'immature' fibromatosis in the other. One patient from this group has suffered a fatal outcome, but only as a result of progressive peritoneal disease (Roche & du Boulay 1989); in the majority of patients, the associated peritoneal disease has been self-limited or has responded to conservative management (Antoniuk et al 1993). All patients have had their ovarian masses removed, and the potential resolution of the ovarian pathology, as has been observed with massive ovarian edema, has not been tested.

Although the underlying mechanism for ovarian fibromatosis is at the moment unknown, it is speculated that local tissue injury (e.g. surgery, or incomplete or intermittent ovarian torsion) stimulates platelets and macrophages to secrete locally acting growth factors, which in turn induce massive fibroblastic proliferation and/or edema

(Roche & du Boulay 1989). It may be that patients who present in the acute phase of this process exhibit either massive ovarian edema or florid mitotically active 'immature' fibromatosis with or without associated peritoneal pathology, and those who present in a subacute or resolving phase exhibit the better documented 'mature' form of acellular sclerotic fibromatosis.

Macroscopic features

The ovaries are always at least somewhat enlarged. Those cases showing only slight enlargement are described as firm and either smooth surfaced or showing some exaggeration of the surface nodularity. The mature, fibrous, or acellular variants can range up to 12 cm in diameter, these being firm, pale, smooth-surfaced masses with the cut surfaces showing persistence of obvious follicular structures in about one-third of cases.

The immature or cellular variants are usually large solid masses averaging 15 cm in diameter (range 5–30 cm) and may weigh up to 3000 g. Unlike cases of massive ovarian edema, they are frequently bilateral. The external surface is tan-white and smooth, but may be hemorrhagic with fibrinous adhesions. The cut surfaces are solid but may show occasional fluid-filled cysts and vary in consistency from firm and pink-grey or sarcoma like to extremely edematous. Focal hemorrhage is often described.

Microscopic features

The mature variant of fibromatosis is characterized by collagen-producing spindle cells which proliferate around and between normal follicles (Fig. 16.4) and produce a thickened fibrotic cortex. The proliferative process varies from densely acellular bands of collagen to intersecting bundles of spindle cells with a storiform pattern resembling ovarian cortex. Minor foci of uninvolved cortex and edema may be present (Fig. 16.5), as may rare luteinized cells in the fibromatous zones or adjacent normal cortex (Young & Scully 1984). Microscopic foci of sex cord differentiation have been recorded (Young & Scully 1984, Byrne et al 1989). These may be isolated epithelial-like structures (Fig. 16.6), or may be aggregated around areas of hypercellularity suggesting development from old follicular remnants.

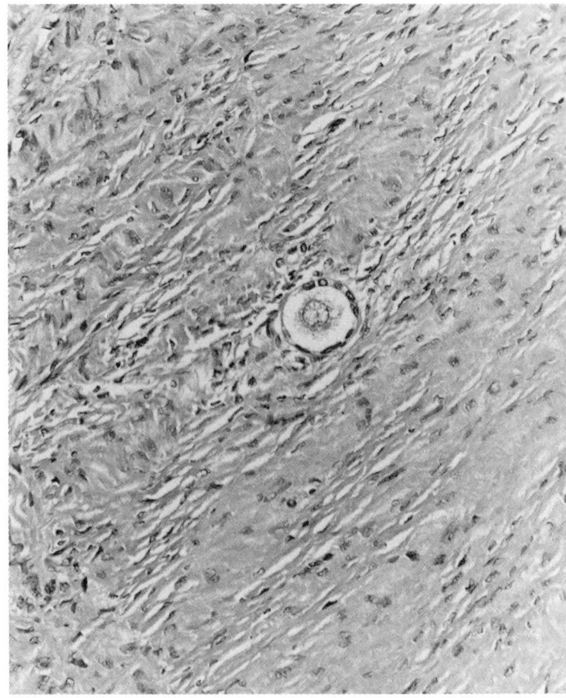

Fig. 16.4 Ovarian fibromatosis characterized by uniform, dense fibrocollagenous connective tissue. An entrapped primordial follicle is present. H + E ×116

'Immature' ovarian fibromatosis is characterized by densely cellular swathes and intersecting bundles of spindle-shaped fibroblasts or myofibroblasts (Fig. 16.7). Areas of apparent maturation of the myofibroblastic stroma (Fig. 16.8) suggest a transition from 'immature' fibromatosis towards more typical or familiar examples of fibromatosis (see Figs 16.4, 16.5). In most instances, this process totally obliterates the normal architecture of the ovary, but in ovaries which are only slightly enlarged it may be confined to the cortex (Clement et al 1994, Khan & Pandey 1994). The proliferating myofibroblastic cells, which are immunoreactive for vimentin and smooth-muscle actin, have scanty cytoplasm and round to oval, vesicular, but remarkably bland nuclei. Nucleoli are small or inapparent. Mitoses are very numerous, regularly exceeding 20/10 HPF; atypical mitoses are not seen (Fig. 16.9). Reticulin stains show a fine pericellular meshwork of fibrils. Hemorrhage is seen focally, but no necrosis.

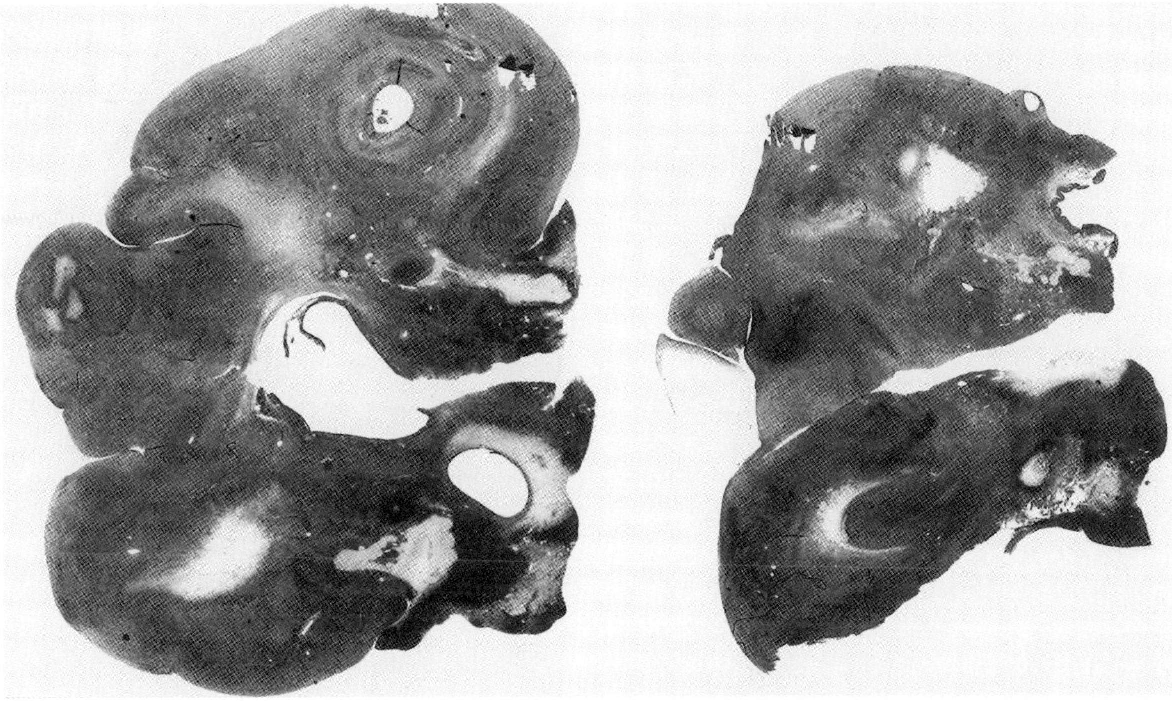

Fig. 16.5 Low power survey of ovarian fibromatosis. Irregular replacement by dense sclerotic fibrous tissue is seen with focal edema, entrapped follicular remnants and small areas of uninvolved cortex. H + E ×3.3

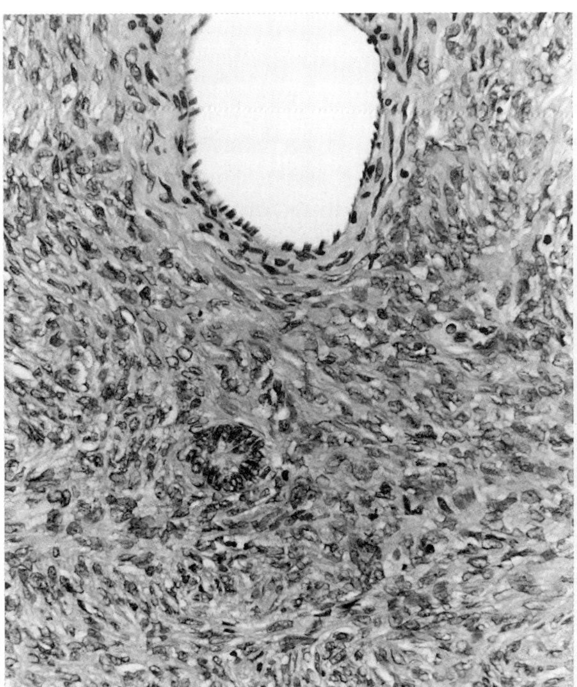

Fig. 16.6 Ovarian fibromatosis showing rare sex cord-like structure, deep within the fibroblastic nodule. H + E ×116

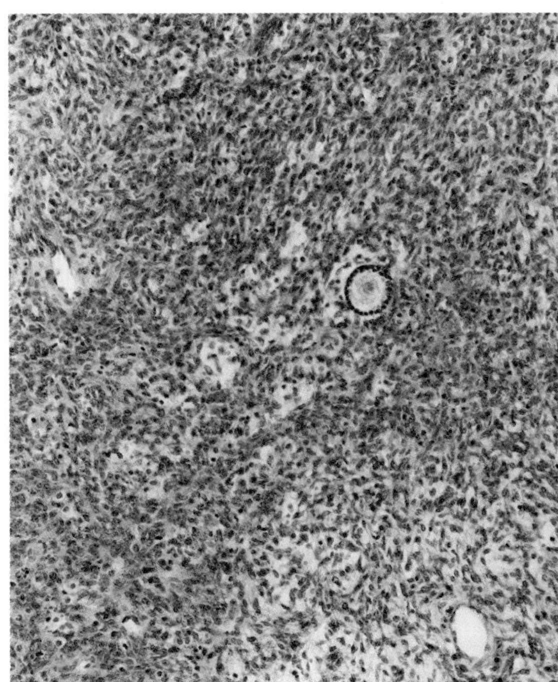

Fig. 16.7 'Immature fibromatosis' with plump spindle shaped myofibroblastic cells enveloping residual primordial follicle. H + E ×60

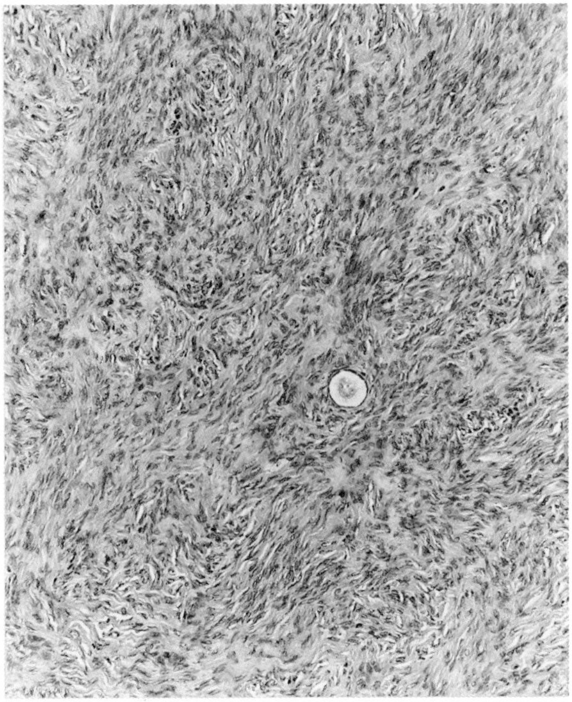

Fig. 16.8 Ovarian fibromatosis exhibiting stromal cellularity intermediate between that shown in Fig. 16.7 and that of 'end-stage' disease shown in Fig. 16.4. H + E ×60

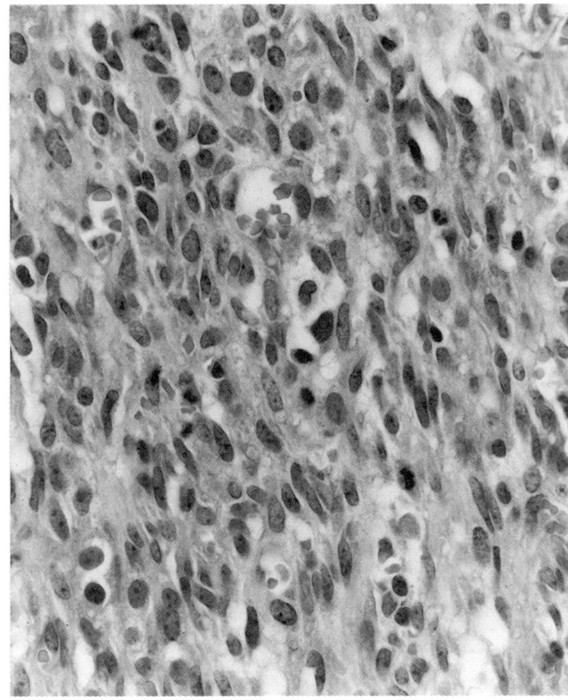

Fig. 16.9 'Immature fibromatosis'. Higher power of proliferating myofibroblastic cells shown in Fig. 16.7. Note bland oval nuclei, but numerous mitoses. H + E ×231

This architectural pattern merges into areas more typical of massive ovarian edema with conspicuous intercellular edema fluid, microcyst formation, dilated lymphatics and sinusoidal blood vessels, and interstitial hemorrhages. At the interfaces, the proliferating fibroblasts assume a 'tissue-culture' appearance (Fig. 16.10).

Scattered in both the cellular fibroblastic and edematous areas are single or nested lutein-like cells. These cells exhibit small to moderate amounts of eosinophilic cytoplasm and rounded central nuclei, often with an obvious central nucleolus (Fig. 16.11). Cells intermediate between the lutein-like cells and fibroblasts are seen.

Another important morphological feature, which has been reported in some cases, is the identification of entrapped follicular structures; this is crucial, because (as with massive ovarian edema) it represents strong evidence that the process is not neoplastic. These are usually unremarkable primordial follicles (Roche & du Boulay 1989, Clement et al 1994; see Figs 16.4, 16.7, 16.8), but may be 'dysplastic' (Byrne et al 1989).

Differential diagnosis

The expansion of the entity of fibromatosis presented here is based on what appears to be an emerging pattern of association between massive ovarian edema, various forms of reactive intra-abdominal fibromatoses, exposure to drugs known to cause sclerosing peritonitis/retroperitoneal fibromatosis, and morphological appearances which do not favor a benign expansile or malignant infiltrative neoplastic process.

Stromal hyperthecosis (see Ch. 14), like many cases of 'immature' fibromatosis, is commonly bilateral and occurs in young women. However, it is not associated with ascites or an acute presentation, does not cause gross enlargement of the ovaries, does not obliterate ovarian architecture, and is not associated with either collagen production or proliferating mitotically active fibroblastic cells.

Luteinized thecomas, the neoplasms which most closely resemble 'immature' fibromatosis, may occur in young women (Zhang et al 1982), but

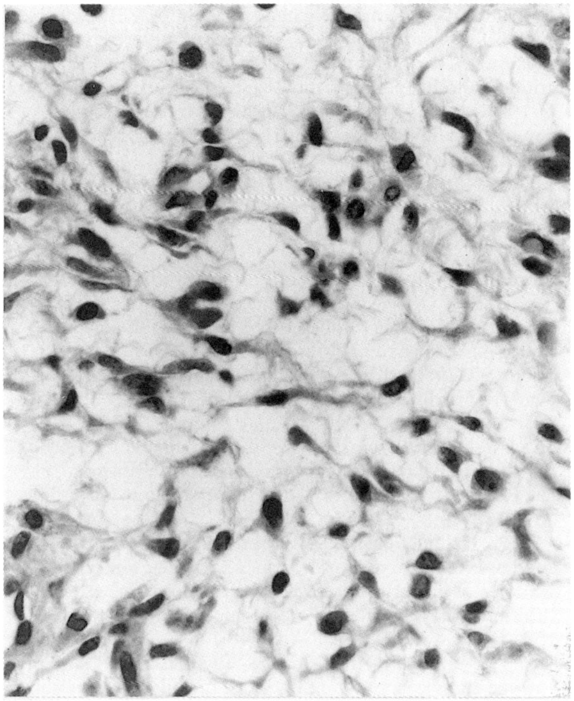

Fig. 16.10 'Immature fibromatosis'. Intercellular edema imparts a 'tissue culture' appearance to proliferating mesenchymal cells, and a morphological pattern which overlaps that of massive ovarian edema. H + E ×231

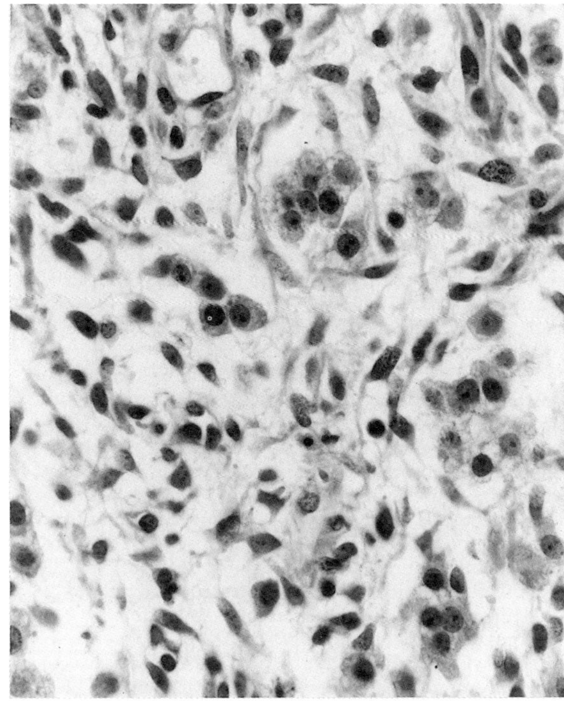

Fig. 16.11 Nests of small to medium sized lutein cells with eosinophilic granular cytoplasm, rounded nuclei each with a central nucleolus. H + E ×231

with only vanishing rarity under the age of 20 years, while almost one-half of patients with fibromatosis showing florid proliferative features are younger than 20 years of age, and some are under 10 years. Most luteinized thecomas are estrogenic (>50%), unilateral (>90%), and unassociated with ascites or peritoneal pathology, while fibromatosis is endocrinologically inactive or occasionally androgenic, commonly bilateral, and may present in association with similar fibroblastic peritoneal lesions. Histologically, luteinized thecomas are not edematous (Zhang et al 1982) and do not incorporate native ovarian follicles.

REFERENCES

Antoniuk P, Tjandra J J, Lavery I C 1993 Diffuse intra-abdominal fibromatosis in association with bilateral ovarian fibromatosis and edema. Australian and New Zealand Journal of Surgery 63: 315–318

Byrne P, Vella E J, Rollason T, Frampton J 1989 Ovarian fibromatosis with minor sex cord elements. Case report. British Journal of Obstetrics and Gynaecology 96: 245–248

Chervenak F A, Castadot M-J, Wiederman J, Sedlis A 1980 Massive ovarian edema: review of the world literature and report of two cases. Obstetrical and Gynecological Survey 35: 677–684

Clement P B, Young R H, Hanna W, Scully R E 1994 Sclerosing peritonitis associated with luteinized thecomas of the ovary. A clinicopathological analysis of six cases. American Journal of Surgical Pathology 18: 1–13

Dudzinski M, Cohen M, Ducatman B 1989 Ovarian malignant thecoma – an unusual tumor in an adolescent. Gynecologic Oncology 35: 104–109

Eden J A 1994 Massive ovarian edema. British Journal of Obstetrics and Gynaecology 101: 456–458

Elkins T E, Stock R J 1982 Recurrent massive edema of the ovary. Southern Medical Journal 75: 478–480

Faber H K 1962 Meigs' syndrome with thecomas of both ovaries in a 4-year-old girl. Journal of Pediatrics 61: 769–773

Fukuda O, Munemura M, Tohya T, Maeyama M, Iwamasa T 1984 Massive edema of the ovary associated with hydrothorax and ascites. Gynecologic Oncology 17: 231–237

Hill L M, Pelekanos M, Kanbour A 1993 Massive edema of an ovary previously fixed to the pelvic side wall. Journal of Ultrasound in Medicine 12: 629–632

Hubbell G P, Punch M R, Elkins T E, Abrams G D 1993

Conservative management of bilateral massive edema of the ovary. A case report. Journal of Reproductive Medicine 38: 61–64
Kalstone C E, Jaffe R B, Abell M R 1969 Massive edema of the ovary simulating fibroma. Obstetrics and Gynecology 38: 564–571
Khan E M, Pandey R 1994 Sarcoma-like ovarian nodules associated with retractile mesenteritis and retroperitoneal fibrosis. Histopathology 24: 276–278
Lacson A G, Alrabeeah A, Gillis D A, Salisbury S, Grantmyre E B 1989 Secondary massive ovarian edema with Meig's syndrome. American Journal of Clinical Pathology 91: 597–603
Mainguene C, Laporte J L, Zakhama A, Kambouchner M, Mulard C, Amouroux J 1993 Une pseudo-tumeur ovarienne rare: l'oedeme massif de l'ovaire. Journal de Gynecologie Obstetrique et Biologie de la Reproduction (Paris) 22: 39–42
Nassar T R, Virgilio L A, Abdul-Karim R W 1976 Massive edema of the ovary. A case report and review of the literature. Obstetrics and Gynecology 47: 77s–80s
Regan F, Tran T, Crofton M E 1993 Case report: idiopathic retroperitoneal fibrosis: an unusual cause of an ovarian mass. British Journal of Radiology 66: 558–560
Roche W R, du Boulay C E H 1989 A case of ovarian fibromatosis with disseminated intra-abdominal fibromatosis. Histopathology 14: 101–107
Roth L M, Deaton R L, Sternberg W H 1979 Massive ovarian edema. American Journal of Surgical Pathology 3: 11–21
Sageshima M, Masuda H, Kawamura K, Shozawa T 1990 Massive ovarian edema associated with polycystic ovary. Acta Pathologica Japonica 40: 73–78
Schweisguth O, Gerard-Marchant R, Plainfosse B, Lemerle J, Watchi J M, Seringe P 1971 Bilateral nonfunctioning thecoma of the ovary in epileptic children under anticonvulsant therapy. Acta Paediatrica Scandinavica 60: 6–10
Serov S F, Scully R E, Sobin L H 1973 Histological typing of ovarian tumors. International histological classification of tumors No. 9. World Health Organization, Geneva
Slotky B, Shrivastav R, Lee B M 1982 Massive edema of the ovary. Obstetrics and Gynecology 59: 92s–94s
Sternberg W H, Dhurandhar H M 1977 Functional ovarian tumors of stromal and sex cord origin. Human Pathology 8: 565–582
Tiltman A J, Nel C P 1984 Massive edema of the ovary. South African Medical Journal 66: 924–926
Vasquez S B, Sotos J F, Kim M H 1982 Massive edema of the ovary and virilization. Obstetrics and Gynecology 59: 95s–99s
Wong S Y 1989 Bilateral massive ovarian edema – report of a case due to lymphangiitis carcinomatosa. Virchows Archiv [A] Pathological Anatomy and Histopathology 414: 355–358
Young R H, Scully R E 1984 Fibromatosis and massive edema of the ovary, possibly related entities: a report of 14 cases of fibromatosis and 11 cases of massive edema. International Journal of Gynecological Pathology 3: 153–178
Zhang J, Young R H, Arseneau J, Scully R E 1982 Ovarian stromal tumors containing lutein or Leydig cells (luteinized thecomas and stromal Leydig cell tumors). A clinicopathological analysis of 50 cases. International Journal of Gynecological Pathology 1: 270–285

17

Adnexal torsion

Torsion of the fallopian tube and ovary is an uncommon but not rare gynecological occurrence. It presents most frequently during the reproductive years, but about one-quarter of reported cases have involved children (Lee & Welch 1967, James et al 1970). Occurrence in neonates and infants has been previously considered very rare (Grosfeld 1969), but more recent reviews of pediatric surgical ovarian lesions revealed 11 of 22 cases of adnexal torsion to have occurred in infants less than 8 months of age (Bower & Adkins 1981). Otherwise unexplained absence of an ovary has been attributed to subclinical torsion and consequent autoamputation occurring in childhood or perhaps even in utero (Nissen et al 1977, Kennedy et al 1981, Beyth & Bar-On 1984). Some cases of ovarian dystopia (see Ch. 6) are due to the same mechanism, the amputated organ attaching itself to an abdominal structure, most commonly the omentum. Massive ovarian edema may be a variation on the theme of torsion, the clinicopathological differences being dictated by the degree and speed of torsion and the stage at which the condition is diagnosed (see Ch. 16).

The clinical presentation always includes lower abdominal pain, and there is often a history of previous similar but less severe episodes (Lee & Welch 1967, James et al 1970). Nausea and vomiting are common. Fever and leucocytosis are variably present. Clinical examination reveals a palpable tender tense pelvic mass in most adult patients. In children, rectal examination identifies a mass (at the pelvic brim) in a smaller percentage of cases (James et al 1970). Ovarian rupture and hemoperitoneum may provide additional signs of peritonism and shock. The provisional diagnosis preoperatively is commonly acute appendicitis. By the time the patient comes to surgery, ovarian infarction has often already occurred, and oophorectomy or salpingo-oophorectomy is indicated. Torsion may rarely be subclinical, leading to spontaneous recovery or autoamputation as alluded to above. Such patients can sometimes provide a remote history of unexplained abdominal pain, usually in childhood (Case Records of the Massachusetts General Hospital 1971, Azoury et al 1980).

The tube and ovary usually undergo torsion as a single unit, rotating around the broad ligament as an axis. Less commonly, the ovary twists alone, around the mesovarium. Very rarely, the tube alone undergoes torsion (Lee & Welch 1967, Provost 1972, Bernardus et al 1984). The right side is more commonly affected, the left ovary being less freely mobile because of the presence of the sigmoid colon (James et al 1970). In accordance with Küstner's rule, the right ovary twists in a clockwise manner and the left counterclockwise (Guileyardo 1982). Bilateral torsion occurs very rarely (Azoury et al 1980, Bower & Adkins 1981, Guileyardo 1982).

In adults, most cases of adnexal torsion are secondary to pathological ovarian enlargements (Lee & Welch 1967, Bider et al 1991). Once adult ovaries exceed a diameter of 6 cm, they are lifted out of the confines of the pelvis and become more freely mobile. A wide range of cystic and neoplastic diseases have been identified in twisted ovaries, the most common lesions being cystic teratomas or cystadenomas. Dysfunctional ovarian cysts are also frequent predisposing factors, while malignant tumors account for less than 5% of instances. Ovarian enlargements associated with adhesions resulting in anatomical fixation are, however, unlikely to be implicated, e.g. inflammatory conditions and endometriosis, or malignant disease with

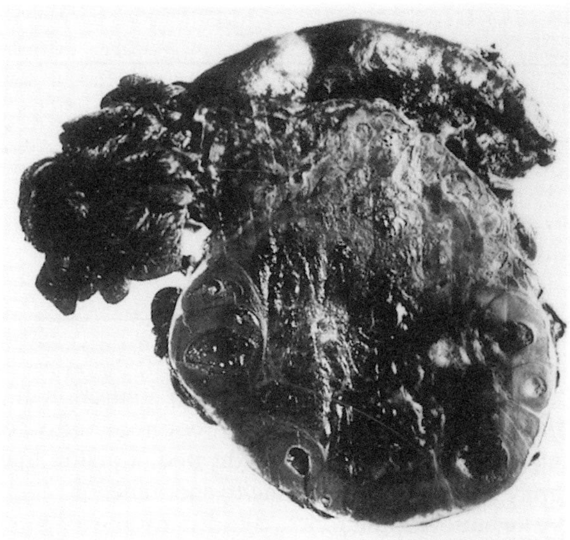

Fig. 17.1 Idiopathic adnexal torsion in a young woman. Several cystic follicles are evident in the hemorrhagic infarcted ovary, but no cyst or neoplasm could be identified

infiltration into adjacent structures. In a smaller number of cases, tubal disease, e.g. hydrosalpinx, appears to be responsible for adnexal torsion (Lee & Welch 1967). Bernardus et al (1984) have since demonstrated that isolated tubal torsion may be a complication of some methods of tubal sterilization, especially if the venous drainage of the fimbrial segment has been compromised. There is an increased risk of torsion of normal fallopian tube and ovary in pregnancy because of increased ovarian mobility within the abdomen during this period (McGowan 1983). Torsion has also been described as occurring in association with ovarian hyperstimulation syndrome. Intraoperative unwinding of the adnexa was successfully performed in these

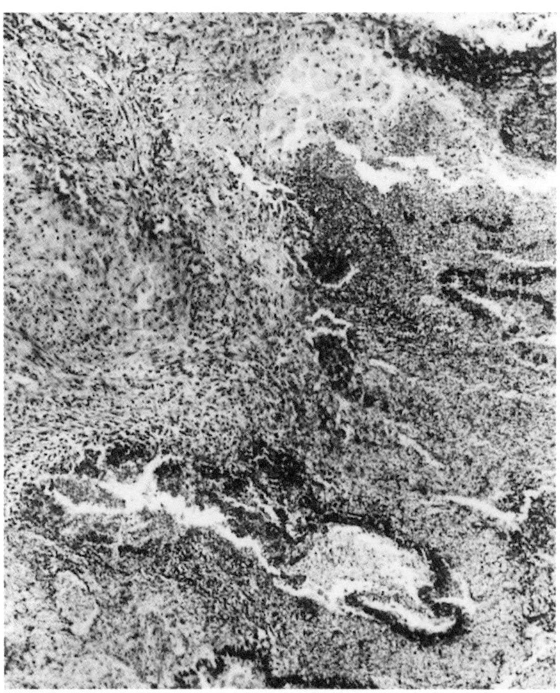

Fig. 17.2 Torsion of endometrioid tumor. Glands are still recognizable within the necrotic zone below and right. Granulation tissue and foamy macrophages are present above and left. H + E ×50

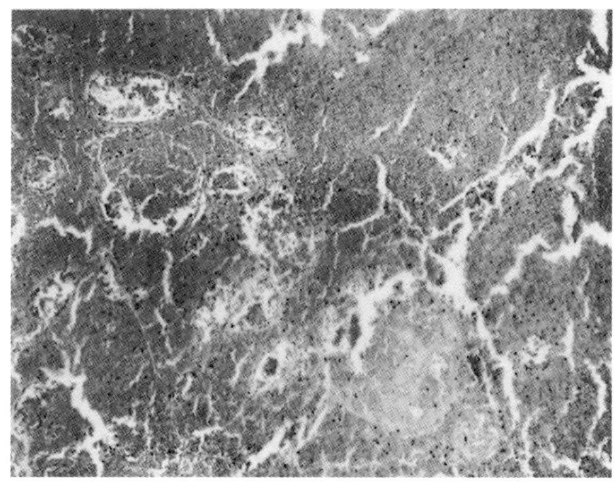

A

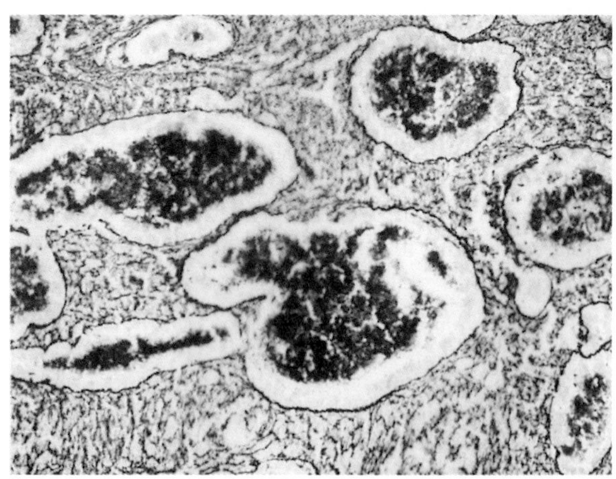

B

Fig. 17.3 Torsion of benign mucinous tumor.
(A) Featureless hemorrhagic necrotic area. H + E ×60
(B) Similar area with glandular morphology highlighted by reticulin stain. ×60

patients where salvage of their ovaries was crucial (Mashiach et al 1990).

In children, torsion of apparently normal ovaries accounts for approximately one-third of cases (Lee & Welch 1967, Case Records of the Massachusetts General Hospital 1971, Ward & Frazier 1978). The relatively large size of prepubertal ovaries, with respect to the uterus, and their intra-abdominal location, encourages torsion. Minor anatomical variations may be additional contributing factors. Isolated torsion of the fallopian tube has been reported very rarely in premenarcheal girls (Barnes et al 1977). The range of pathological ovarian enlargements associated with adnexal torsion in children is similar to that in adults.

Macroscopic features

The affected ovary is always enlarged, ranging from 6 cm (4 cm in children) to 15 cm in diameter. Rupture is sometimes evident. The cut surface is edematous and hemorrhagic, and possibly necrotic, so that both normal and abnormal structures may be obscured (Fig. 17.1). The presence of a teratoma can be assumed if sebaceous material, hair, or cartilage are found, but other varieties of cyst and tumor may be less readily recognizable. Examination of the ovarian pedicle may reveal thrombosis of the hilar blood vessels. In the rare case of autoamputation, the ovary is reduced to a degenerate cystic or partially calcified mass which lies free in the peritoneal cavity or is attached to abdominal structures, most commonly the omentum.

Microscopic features

Microscopy confirms edema, hemorrhage, ischemic change, and often frank necrosis (Fig. 17.2). Normal structures may be difficult to identify. Multiple blocks of more solid or apparently viable areas, especially cyst walls, should be examined to determine the nature of any underlying pathological condition and to exclude the possibility of a malignant neoplasm. We have found that reticulin stains are particularly helpful in clarifying the architecture of degenerate tissue and determining the broad category of cyst or tumor to which individual cases belong (Fig. 17.3). The special features of massive ovarian edema are discussed in Chapter 16. The accompanying fallopian tube, if torted, may show similar ischaemic changes and, less frequently, the apparent cause of adnexal torsion, such as a hydrosalpinx (Lee & Welch 1967, Azoury et al 1980).

REFERENCES

Azoury R S, Chehab R M, Mufarrij I K 1980 The twisted adnexa. A clinical pathological review. Diagnostic Gynecology and Obstetrics 2: 185–191

Barnes W S, Schantz J C, Shochat S J 1977 Torsion of the fallopian tube in a premenarcheal female patient. American Journal of Diseases of Children 131: 1297–1298

Bernardus R E, van der Slikke J W, Roex A J M, Dijkhuizen G H, Stolk J G 1984 Torsion of the fallopian tube: Some considerations on its etiology. Obstetrics and Gynecology 64: 675–678

Beyth Y, Bar-On E 1984 Tuboovarian autoamputation and infertility. Fertility and Sterility 42: 932–934

Bider D, Mashiach S, Dulitzky M, Kokia E, Lipitz S, Ben Rafael Z 1991 Clinical surgical and pathological findings of adnexal torsion in pregnant and non pregnant women. Surgery Gynecology and Obstetrics 173: 363–366

Bower R J, Adkins J C 1981 Surgical ovarian lesions in children. American Surgeon 47: 474–478

Case Records of the Massachusetts General Hospital 1971 Case No 9–1971. New England Journal of Medicine 284: 491–496

Grosfeld J L 1969 Torsion of normal ovary in the first two years of life. American Journal of Surgery 117: 726–727

Guileyardo J M 1982 Neonatal ovarian torsion. American Journal of Diseases of Children 136: 945–946

James D F, Barber H R K, Graber E A 1970 Torsion of normal uterine adnexa in children. Report of three cases. Obstetrics and Gynecology 35: 226–230

Kennedy L A, Pinckney L E, Currarino G, Votteler T P 1981 Amputated calcified ovaries in children. Pediatric Radiology 141: 83–86

Lee R A, Welch J S 1967 Torsion of the uterine adnexa. American Journal of Obstetrics and Gynecology 97: 974–977

McGowan L 1983 Surgical diseases of the ovary in pregnancy. Clinical Obstetrics and Gynecology 26: 843–852

Mashiach S, Bider D, Moran O, Goldenberg M, Ben Rafael Z 1990 Adnexal torsion of hyperstimulated ovaries in pregnancies after gonadotropin therapy. Fertility and Sterility 53: 76–80

Nissen E D, Kent D R, Nissen S E, Feldman B M 1977 Unilateral tuboovarian autoamputation. Journal of Reproductive Medicine 19: 151–153

Provost R W 1972 Torsion of the normal fallopian tube. Obstetrics and Gynecology 39: 80–82

Ward M J A, Frazier T G 1978 Torsion of normal uterine adnexa in childhood: Case report. Pediatrics 61: 573–574

SECTION 3

Inflammatory lesions

18

Infectious lesions

P. Russell A. Farnsworth

Bacterial oophoritis
Pelvic inflammatory disease
Isolated ovarian abscess
Xanthogranulomatous oophoritis (inflammatory pseudotumor)
Malacoplakia
Actinomycosis
Tuberculosis
Viral oophoritis
Mumps
Cytomegalovirus
Parasitic oophoritis
Schistosomiasis (Bilharziasis)
Enterobiasis
Echinococcosis
Fungal oophoritis
Coccidioidomycosis
Blastomycosis

Microorganisms may reach the ovaries in a number of ways. The most common is ascending spread (either mucosally or interstitially) from a focus of infection in the lower genital tract – pelvic inflammatory disease (PID). Most such infections are sexually transmitted, but others are postpartum or postabortal complications, or are associated with use of an intrauterine contraceptive device (IUD). Direct spread from an adherent infected pelvic or abdominal structure, e.g. colonic diverticulum or appendix, may occur. Hematogenous seeding of organisms into the ovary is the predominant mechanism of involvement in tuberculosis, coccidioidomycosis, echinococcosis, and viral oophoritis. Schistosomal worms and ova reach the ovarian parenchyma via the venous route. Transcoelomic spread of scolices (following rupture of hepatic hydatid cysts) accounts for some cases of ovarian echinococcosis. Enterobius worms gain access to the ovaries by ascending the genital tract following their excretion from the anus. It has been suggested that microbial entry to the ovary is facilitated by breaches in the ovarian capsule such as ovulation stigmas or cyst perforations (Willson & Black 1964, Niebyl et al 1978, Wetchler & Dunn 1985). The bloody content of corpora lutea or hemorrhagic endometriotic cysts provides an excellent culture medium (Niebyl et al 1978, Egger & Weigmann 1982).

To facilitate differential diagnosis, it is helpful to divide oophoritis into groups showing common histological reactions, e.g. suppurative, eosinophilic, lymphoplasmacytic, or granulomatous (Table 18.1). In this book, 'granulomatous' inflammation refers to reactions which include discrete granulomas as defined by Robbins et al (1984): 'small 0.5–2.0 mm collections of modified macrophages called epithelioid cells usually surrounded by a rim of lymphocytes'.

BACTERIAL OOPHORITIS

Pelvic inflammatory disease

Most acute and chronic suppurative oophoritis is associated with PID. This is the syndrome of ascending, often recurrent, infection of the female genital tract which tends to localize in the fallopian tubes, but may also involve adjacent structures such as peritoneum and ovaries. Gonococci and chlamydiae are the bacteria most commonly isolated. The pattern of spread of ascending pelvic infection varies somewhat with different inciting microorganisms – gonococci tend to adhere to mucosal surfaces of the genital tract, while streptococci spread via both mucosal and interstitial routes and thus are more likely to be responsible for pelvic abscesses. Once tissue damage has occurred, secondary bacterial invaders, chiefly anaerobic,

Table 18.1 Oophoritis: differential diagnosis by tissue reaction (note that an etiological agent may be associated with more than one type of reaction)

Acute or chronic suppuration
Acute diffuse oophoritis associated with PID
Ovarian abscess associated with PID
Isolated ovarian abscess
Actinomycosis
Foreign body
Coccidioidomycosis, blastomycosis
Schistosomiasis (R)
Acute serositis (without parenchymal inflammation)
Ruptured tubal ectopic gestation
Generalized peritonitis
Peritoneal carcinomatosis
Eosinophilic infiltration
Foreign body reactions, especially starch (S)
Enterobiasis (S)
Schistosomiasis (S)
Autoimmune oophoritis (R)
Isolated noninfectious granulomatous oophoritis (R)
Lymphoplasmacytic infiltration
Autoimmume oophoritis
Resolving phase of suppurative oophoritis
Cytomegalovirus oophoritis
Foreign body granulomas
Exogenous substances, e.g. sutures, talc, starch, radiographic media, parasites, intestinal contents
Endogenous substances, e.g. contents of mature cystic teratomas, keratin from uterine adenoacanthomas, cauterized tissue
Sarcoidal granulomas
Sarcoidosis
Crohn's disease
Foreign body reactions, especially starch (S)
'Cortical granulomas'
Autoimmune oophoritis (R)
Necrotizing granulomas
Tuberculosis (S)
Foreign body reactions, especially starch (R)(S), radiographic media (R)(S)
Enterobiasis (S)
Coccidioidomycosis, blastomycosis
Isolated noninfectious granulomatous oophoritis
Schistosomiasis (R)

(R) Rare feature of the condition. (S) Predominantly serosal lesions.

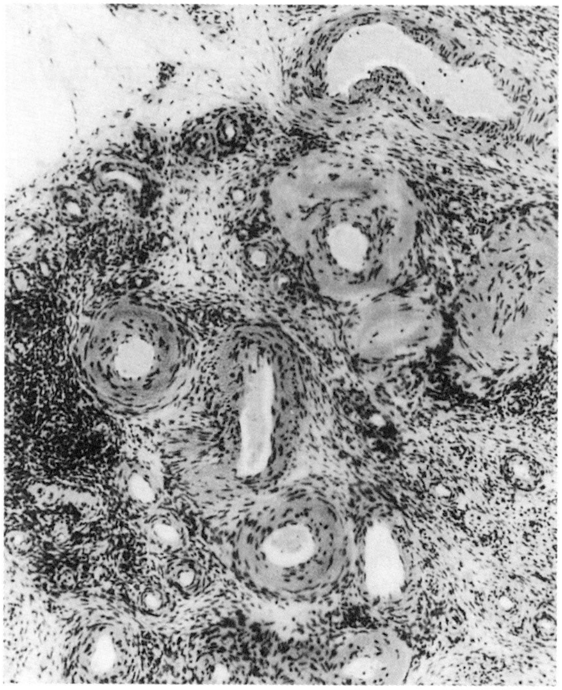

Fig. 18.1 Ovarian amyloidosis in patient with gross bilateral pyosalpinges. Walls of arterioles are asymmetrically thickened by hyaline material (which showed apple green birefringence after staining with Congo red). Ovarian stroma is not inflamed. H + E ×80

may replace the initial organisms. Acute salpingitis results in the production of inflammatory exudate, including fibrin, from the tubal serosa and ostia, leading to adhesions to adjacent pelvic, and sometimes abdominal organs.

The ovaries appear to be able to resist the invasion of pathogenic bacteria, and their involvement in PID is often limited to a perioophoritis, even in the presence of tubo-ovarian inflammatory masses. We have seen a case of gross chronic pyosalpinges, producing amyloidosis (demonstrated in both liver and ovaries; Fig. 18.1), in which the ovaries were essentially uninflamed. However, recurrent or severe PID may result in ovarian parenchymal involvement – initially an acute diffuse oophoritis. Abscess formation, usually in continuity with a pyosalpinx (tubo-ovarian abscess), sometimes follows and this may result in permanent loss of ovarian parenchyma. In chronic PID there may be an increase in cystic follicles and follicular or corpus luteum cysts, but chronic PID did not influence growth of follicles or ability to ovulate (Byckov 1990).

Some studies have shown the presence of an IUD gives a 1.6–9.3 times risk of developing PID compared with nonusers (Burkman 1980), and such patients are also likely to be host to a wider range of microorganisms, especially nongonococcal, including actinomycetes (see below) and anaerobes (Holmes et al 1980). Polymicrobial infections are also more common in this group of women (Mårdh 1980). But other studies have shown that when the number of sexual partners is controlled for, there is no increased risk of PID (Eschenbach et al 1977, Kaufman et al 1980).

Oophoritis may complicate other pelvic and abdominal infections such as diverticulitis and appendicitis. The latter is a particular problem in prepubertal girls, in whom the ovaries lie within the abdominal cavity and hence are in closer proximity to the appendix than in adults (Mueller et al 1986).

Isolated ovarian abscesses

Isolated ovarian abscesses, unassociated with salpingitis, are unusual lesions. In almost all cases there is a predisposing factor such as a recent gynecological operation, childbirth, or IUD use. They may also be secondary to direct or lymphatic spread from nongynecological pelvic inflammatory process such as diverticulitis or inflammatory bowel disease. *Escherichia coli* and bacteroides species are the most common organisms isolated (Willson & Black 1964, Niebyl et al 1978, Wetchler & Dunn 1985). As opposed to the insidious development of ovarian abscesses in association with PID, isolated abscesses have an acute presentation, usually with abdominal pain. Physical examination usually reveals abdominal tenderness and a pelvic mass. Rupture is likely if surgical treatment is not prompt; acute peritonitis and pelvic abscess are likely sequelae.

Secondary infection of pre-existing cysts is a recognized clinical risk. One per cent of mature cystic teratomas (dermoid cysts) are said to become infected, usually by coliforms. *Salmonella typhi* has been responsible for infecting ovarian mucinous cystadenomas (Evans-Jones & French 1983) and mature cystic teratomas (Hingorani et al 1963), as well as causing abscesses ab initio (Soloff & Hermann 1935). Endometriotic cysts are also prone to secondary suppurative inflammation (Egger & Weigmann 1982), but the frequency of this complication is not uniformly reported.

Macroscopic features

Infected ovaries are slightly or moderately enlarged, with adhesions on the serosal surfaces. Although they may be bound to inflamed fallopian tubes and incorporated into tubo-ovarian masses, careful dissection of such specimens usually enables the ovaries to be separated. In acute infections the ovaries are tense, with superficial fibrinous exudate. Sectioning reveals edematous hyperemic parenchyma. Abscesses may be confined to the ovary, but are more commonly in continuity with a pyosalpinx – forming a tubo-ovarian abscess. Abscesses have a central soft necrotic zone or cavity surrounded by shaggy grey tissue. Focal hemorrhages may be present. If chronic, an outer layer of dense fibrous tissue is usually present.

Microscopic features

In acute diffuse oophoritis there is polymorph infiltration, edema, vascular dilatation, and focal hemorhage. Follicular structures may be involved (Fig. 18.2). Abscesses display central accumula-

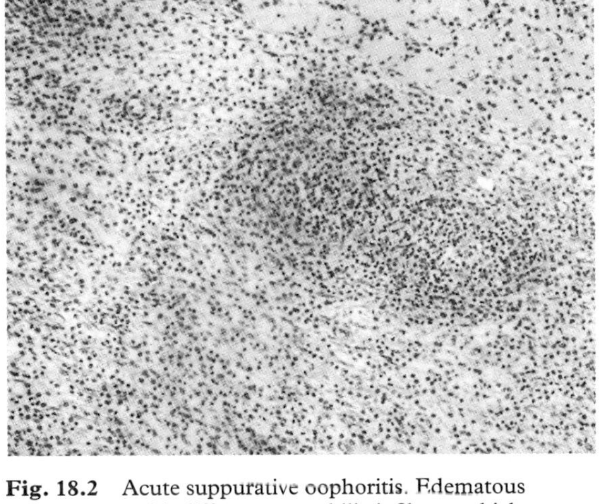

Fig. 18.2 Acute suppurative oophoritis. Edematous parenchyma with diffuse neutrophilic infiltrate which even involves a corpus fibrosum. H + E ×90

tions of necrotic debris or cavities lined by granulation tissue admixed with inflammatory cells, including polymorphs, lymphocytes, plasma cells, and macrophages (Figs 18.3, 18.4). Large foamy lipid-laden macrophages (xanthoma cells) may be conspicuous if there has been a lot of hemorrhage and necrosis. Hemosiderin and lipofuscin (ceroid) pigment may also be demonstrable.

Acute perioophoritis is characterized by polymorph infiltration and fibrin exudation. Groups of peritoneal macrophages adhere to the serosal surfaces. The exudate becomes organized by the ingrowth of proliferating fibroblasts and capillaries – granulation tissue. Concurrent with this reparative process there is a proliferation of mesothelial cells, which may be quite exuberant (see Ch. 20). Perioophoritis resolves, but leaves behind adhesions, scattered lymphocytes, and sometimes psammoma bodies as residua of the inflammatory process.

Chronic diffuse oophoritis is rarely observed in patients with PID (Fig. 18.5). Focal lympho-

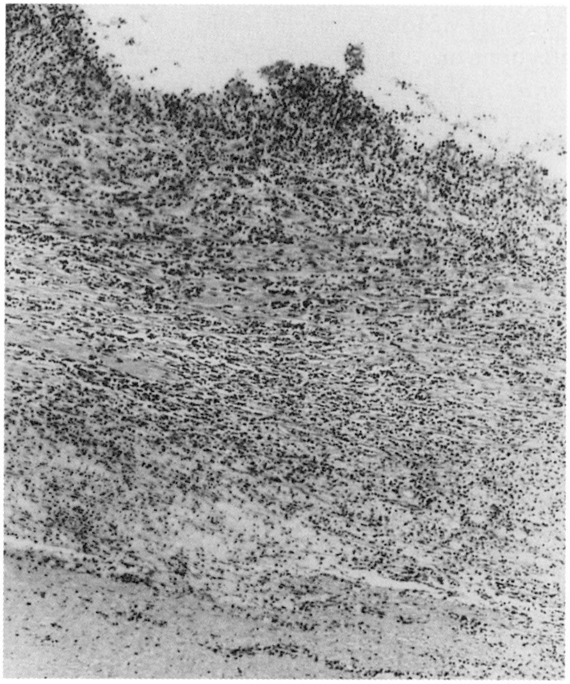

A

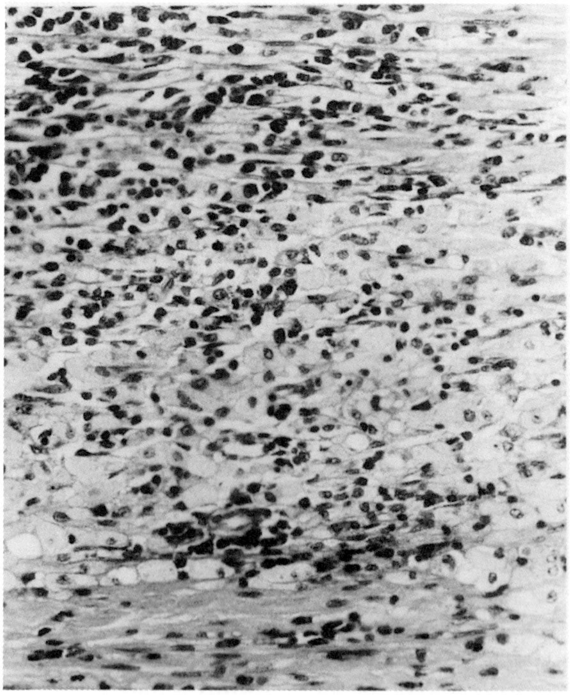

B

Fig. 18.4 Ovarian abscess (chronic phase). (A) Thick fibrous wall with shaggy lining. Heavy infiltrate of chronic inflammatory cells. H + E ×50. (B) Detail of cellular infiltrate – plasma cells, lymphocytes and foamy macrophages. H + E ×200

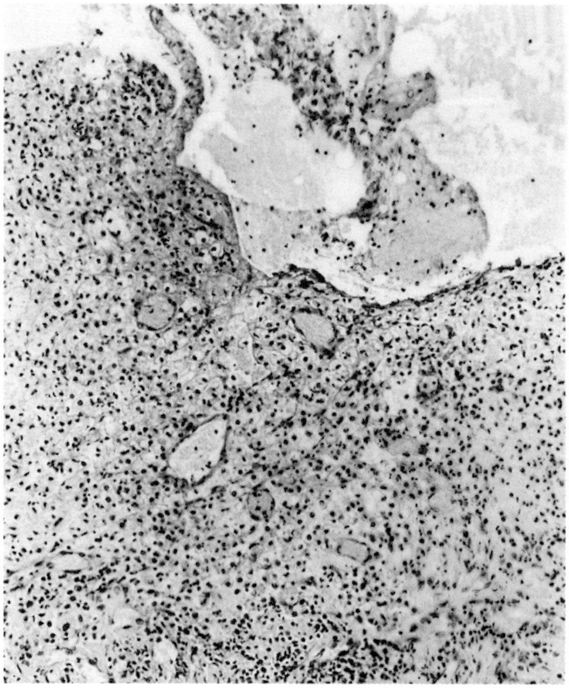

Fig. 18.3 Ovarian abscess (acute phase). Wall of edematous granulation tissue infiltrated by acute inflammatory cells. Exudate and debris in cavity. H + E ×80

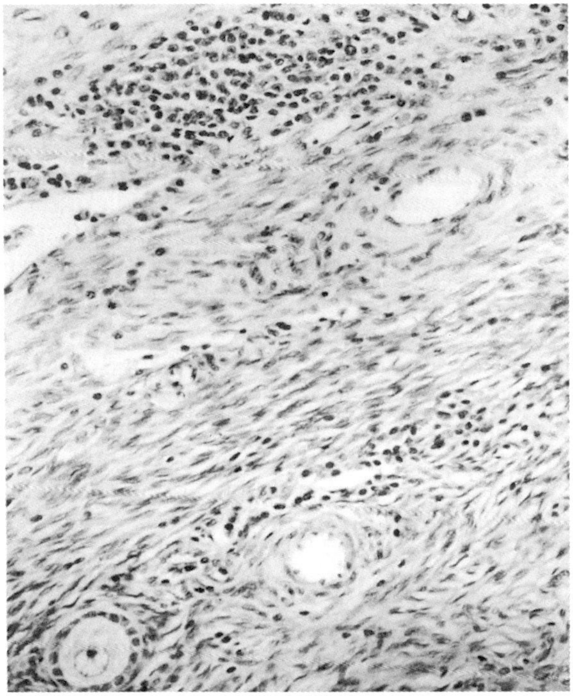

Fig. 18.5 Chronic lymphoplasmacytic oophoritis. Patchy infiltrate adjacent to a resolving abscess. H + E ×175

cytic infiltrates are associated with autoimmune oophoritis (see below).

In most cases of suppurative oophoritis, the fallopian tubes are also inflamed. However, in cases of isolated ovarian abscess, endosalpingitis is absent, by definition, although there may be tubal edema and perisalpingitis.

Xanthogranulomatous oophoritis (inflammatory pseudotumor)

This is a rare variant of chronic oophoritis and only two cases have been reported, both in young women with a history of PID (Minkowitz et al 1965, Pace et al 1984). Two further cases of anatomically less well defined adnexal inflammatory pseudotumors have also been described (Kunakemakorn et al 1976, Shalev et al 1982). Bacteroides species have been isolated from two of the cases (Shalev et al 1982, Pace et al 1984). Inflammatory pseudotumors probably result from exaggerated prolonged repair reactions in cases of oophoritis which have involved an unusual degree of necrosis or hemorrhage, with consequent abundance of lipid breakdown products. The pathological features are similar to those of the more commonly encountered xanthogranulomatous pyelonephritis.

Macroscopically, pseudotumors are firm, yellow, well-circumscribed masses (4–8 cm in diameter), with foci of hemorrhage and necrosis. Stigmata of PID are generally present elsewhere.

Microscopically, the picture is dominated by sheets of foamy macrophages interpersed with nonvacuolated, sometimes multinucleated histiocytes, plasma cells, lymphocytes, and neutrophils. The foamy cells contain lipid as well as PAS-positive cytoplasmic granules (which have the ultrastructural characteristics of lysosomes). Hemosiderin deposition and fibroblastic proliferation are usually present.

Malacoplakia

This chronic inflammatory process rarely involves the female genital tract, being more often identified in the renal pelvis and bladder. The lower genital tract (especially the vagina) is more commonly affected than the ovaries; most patients are postmenopausal (Chalvardjian et al 1980). The components of the inflammatory infiltrate are very similar to those of xanthogranulomatous oophoritis (as described above), with the additional presence of the pathognomonic Michaelis–Gutmann bodies within histiocytes (von Hansemann cells) and extracellularly. These basophilic structures are nuclear sized, sometimes with a bull's-eye appearance, and contain stainable iron and calcium. Ultrastructurally they are electron dense with a variable core of lysosome-like material. The macrophages also exhibit numerous secondary lysosomes which contain partially digested bacteria and neutrophils. There is good evidence that malacoplakia results from an acquired inability to destroy ingested bacteria (Abdou et al 1977).

Actinomycosis

Actinomycetes are bacteria, most closely related to the corynebacteria and mycobacteria, but superficially resembling fungi. *Actinomyces israelii* is a common commensal in the pharynx, and passes through the gastrointestinal tract if swallowed. It may gain access to the vagina following inoculation via orogenital or rectovaginal transfer. Although it is not generally considered to be a normal vaginal inhabitant, it can be identified, using meticulous techniques, from the lower genital tract of many sexually active women, irrespective of type of contraception (Persson & Holmberg 1984). Pelvic actinomycosis is rare, and in older reports was almost always secondary to ileocaecal disease (MacCarthy 1955). Although actinomycotic PID, associated with IUD use, has been recognized since the 1920s, the popularization of the new generation IUDs in the 1960s was followed by a spate of reports (Schiffer et al 1975) and reports continue to occur (Sandin et al 1993). There appears to be a correlation with prolonged IUD usage (Burkman et al 1982, Hsu et al 1990). Cervicovaginal smears may provide an easy and useful means of identifying IUD users who are at risk of developing actinomycotic PID (Luff et al 1978, Burkman et al 1982). The organism is readily identified in cervicovaginal smears of 8–30% of IUD users, but only rarely, and in small numbers, in nonusers (Jones et al 1979, Burkman et al 1982). Up to 25% of those with positive smears develop clinical PID (not necessarily due to actinomycosis), which is likely to be more severe clinically and with a higher probability of developing a tubo-ovarian abscess than PID not associated with the identification of actinomycetes in the smear (Bhagavan & Gupta 1978).

Culture of the organisms is successful in less than one-third of the histologically confirmed cases, but other anaerobic bacteria are isolated from the abscesses in most cases (Lomax et al 1976). Almost all patients with actinomycotic

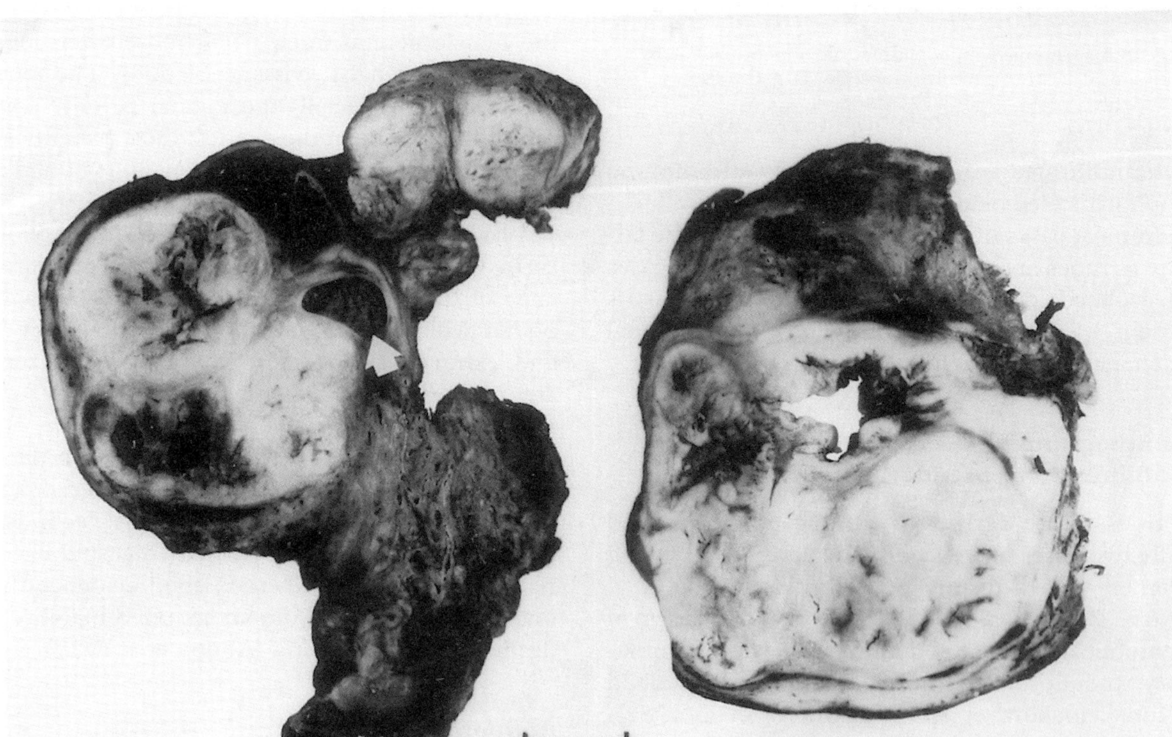

Fig. 18.6 Ovarian actinomycosis. Slices of right adnexal mass from a 43-year-old woman who had been using an IUD for 10 years. Thick-walled necrotic cavities in ovary and thickened fallopian tube (above). A residual cystic follicle is recognizable at left (arrow). Scale bar equals 1 cm

PID have an actinomycotic endometritis; uterine curettings and tissue adherent to a removed IUD can also be used for histological examination and culture.

Macroscopic features

Adnexal involvement is frequently unilateral (Schmidt et al 1980), and usually involves both fallopian tube and ovary to form a tubo-ovarian mass. Fistula formation is rare. The fallopian tube is thickened and distorted and bound by adhesions to the ovary. Ovarian involvement causes moderate enlargement, up to 10 cm in diameter, and sectioning shows multiple abscesses separated by dense fibrous tissue (Fig. 18.6). The abscesses have a shaggy grey lining and contain purulent, sometimes bloodstained, material. Sulfur granules may be evident macroscopically; multiple blocks may be necessary to identify them microscopically.

Microscopic features

The actinomycotic colonies are located in the center of abscesses and are surrounded by polymorphs and necrotic debris (Fig. 18.7A,B). Occasional multinucleated histiocytes may be seen in close proximity to the colonies (Fig. 18.7B). Foamy histiocytes are often conspicuous in the adjacent granulation tissue. Plasma cells and lymphocytes are more obvious in the peripheral zone of fibrous tissue. The colonies consist of branching filaments (Fig. 18.7C); the central denser portion is hematoxylinophilic, but the peripheral radiating clubs are eosinophilic. The organisms are Gram positive and usually non-acid-fast. Away from the colony the filaments may be found broken up into coccal or bacillary forms.

Tuberculosis

Genital tuberculosis is still common in some parts

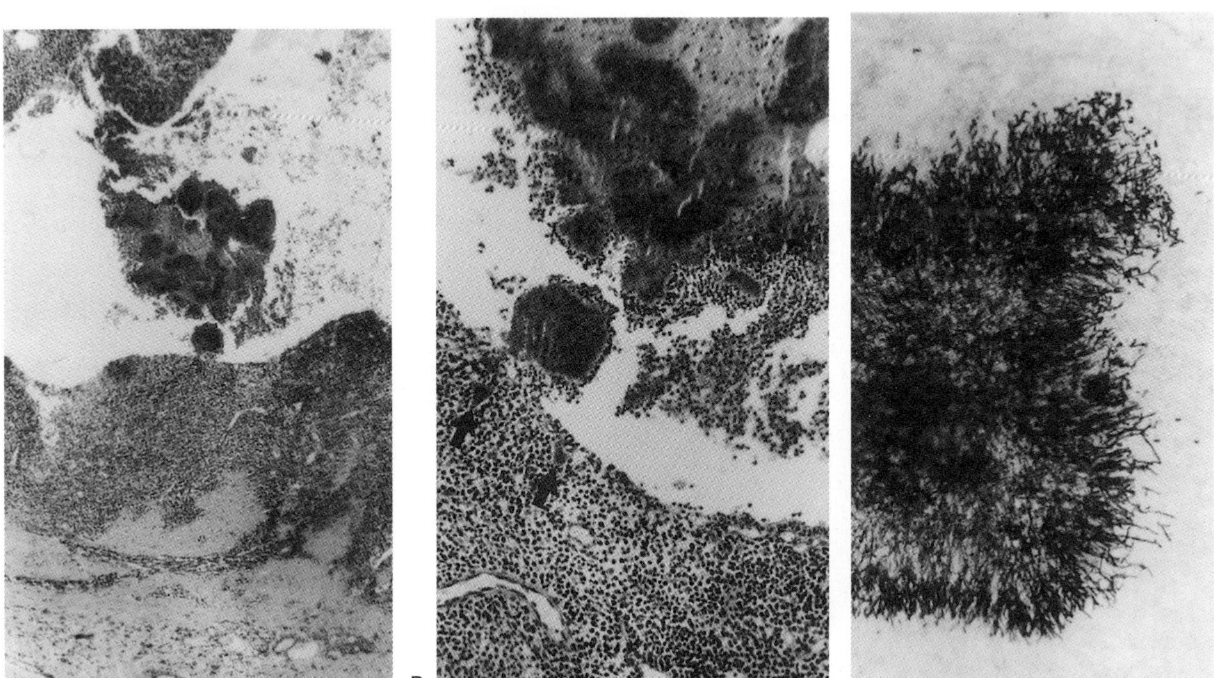

A B C

Fig. 18.7 Actinomycosis (same case as in Fig. 18.6). (A) Bacterial colony in cavity, surrounded by granulation tissue, and peripheral zone of fibrotic ovarian stroma. H + E ×32. (B) Detail of cellular infiltrate composed of lymphocytes, plasma cells, neutrophils (in lumen adjacent to colony) and a few multinucleated histiocytes (arrows). H + E ×80. (C) Filamentous structure of actinomycetes highlighted by methenamine silver stain. H + E ×320 of the world (India, Eastern Europe, South America, the Middle and Far East), where it is an important cause of infertility. Although most genital tuberculosis is thought to be bloodborne from a pulmonary focus, less than half the patients have a history of tuberculosis or an abnormal chest X-ray. Within the pelvis, tubercle bacilli have a predilection to lodge in the fallopian tubes, from which direct spread to the ovaries may occur. Less commonly, the infection spreads via lymphatics from a tuberculous focus in the urinary or gastrointestinal tracts. Overall, the ovaries are involved in 20–63% of patients with genital tuberculosis (Sutherland 1985, Agarwal & Gupta 1993). They may also be involved incidentally in tuberculous peritonitis (Fig. 18.8). Elevation of serum calcium-125 may be noted mimicking ovarian cancer (Hoffman 1989).

Macroscopically, tuberculous oophoritis is most commonly manifest as small white capsular tubercles associated with serosal adhesions. Granulomas may extend into the ovarian cortex and, infrequently, frank caseous necrosis with cavitation occurs (Fig. 18.9). Tuberculous fallopian tubes typically show nodular thickening with relative sparing of the ostia (Wheeler 1994). The microscopic appearance of the granulomas is typical of tuberculosis elsewhere. The diagnosis should be confirmed by demonstrating tubercle bacilli by the Ziehl–Neelsen or auramine–rhodamine (fluorescent) stains, or by culture of fresh ovarian tissue. Differential diagnoses include sarcoidosis and other inflammatory processes which may exhibit tuberculoid granulomas (Table 18.1). If a definitive diagnosis cannot be reached on ovarian histology (including special stains) or culture, uterine curettage may provide diagnostically useful material. The endometrium is involved in up to 90% of patients with genital tuberculosis, and curettage can provide material for microbiological culture as well as histological examination.

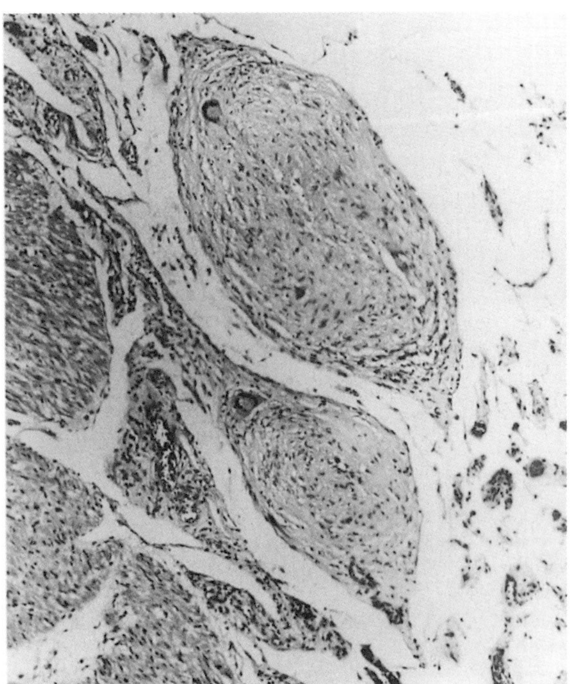

Fig. 18.8 Tuberculous peritonitis. Multiple discrete tubercles are present, some with central necrosis. Langhans giant cells are conspicuous. H + E ×64

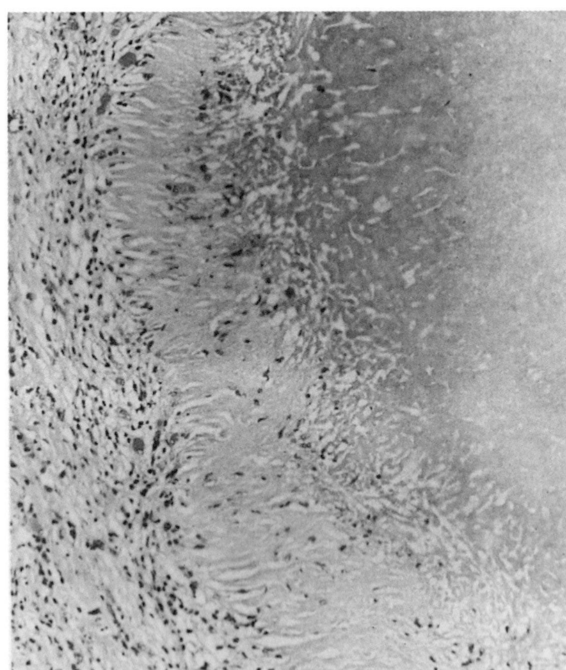

Fig. 18.9 Ovarian tuberculosis. From 10 cm necrotic ovarian mass in a 78-year-old woman. Cellular reaction in this case is limited to palisading histiocytes and sparse lymphocytes. Rare acid-fast bacilli were identified. Compare with Fig. 19.8 (isolated noninfectious granuloma). H + E ×100 (material courtesy of Dr H Y Yeung, Hong Kong)

VIRAL OOPHORITIS

Mumps

Transient acute oophoritis may occur during the course of mumps and the exanthems (Blaustein 1982). While orchitis is a well-known manifestation of mumps infection in males, said to occur in 20% of patients, the occurrence of oophoritis in infected females is less well recognized and is said to be less frequent (of the order of 5%) (Morrison et al 1975). There are no reports in the literature of the histological features of mumps oophoritis. As in the testis, infection may result in irreversible tissue damage; mumps oophoritis has been put forward as a possible cause of premature menopause in a small proportion of patients (Morrison et al 1975, Cramer et al 1983).

Cytomegalovirus

Cytomegalovirus (CMV) infection of the female genital organs is probably secondary to viremia, but venereal transmission is also a possibility (McCracken et al 1974). CMV oophoritis is rare, and has been reported only in immunosuppressed patients (Iwasaki et al 1988, Sharma et al 1994). In most cases, the ovaries show focal hemorrhagic cortical necrosis, associated with polymorph and lymphoplasmacytic infiltration (Fig. 18.10). Within and bordering this area, infected stromal and endothelial cells are readily identified by their enlargement and pleiomorphism; the characteristic basophilic intranuclear inclusions are easily found and intracytoplasmic inclusions may also be present (Fig. 18.11). A chronic inflammatory cell infiltrate is present in the surrounding viable parenchyma.

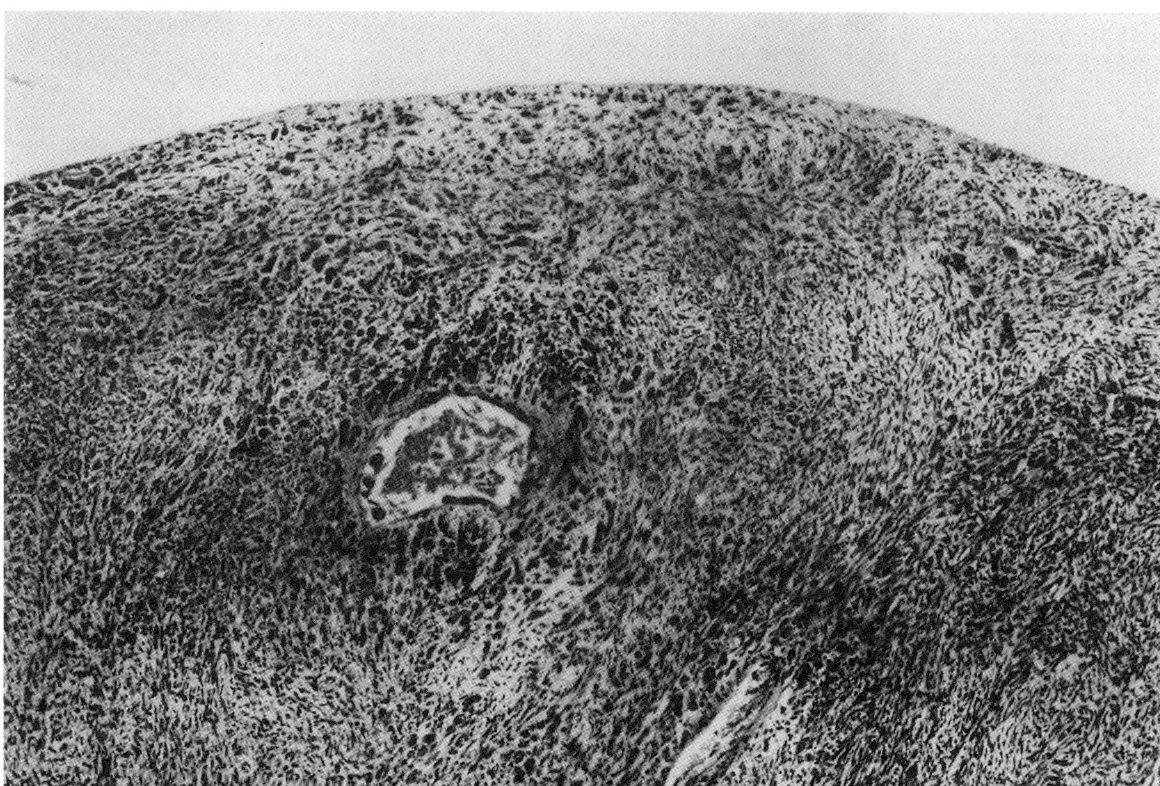

Fig. 18.10 Cytomegalovirus oophoritis from an immunosuppressed 37-year-old woman. Wedge-shaped cortical infarct. H + E ×80

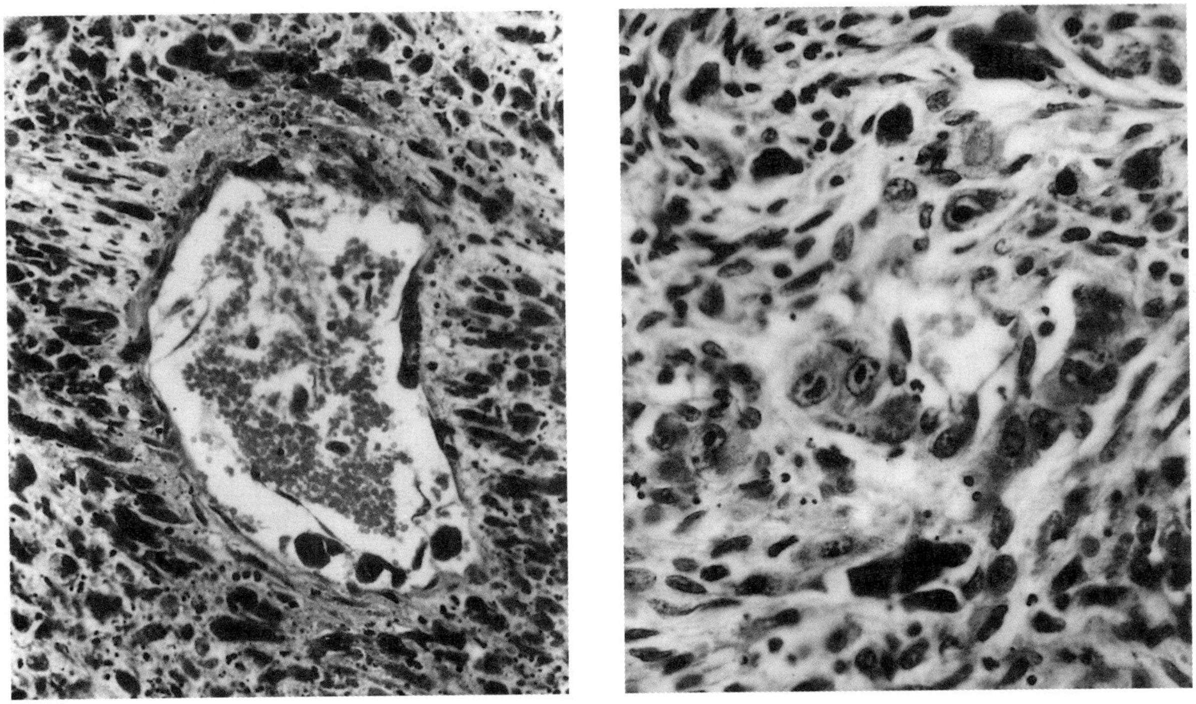

A B

Fig. 18.11 Detail of Fig. 18.10. (A) Vessel at base of infarct showing infected endothelial cells. H + E ×200. (B) Infected stromal cells with intranuclear and intracytoplasmic inclusions. H + E ×350

PARASITIC OOPHORITIS

Schistosomiasis (bilharziasis)

The three principal pathogenic schistosomes are *Schistosoma mansoni*, *S. haematobium*, and *S. japonicum*. The most widely distributed geographically is *S. mansoni* and this is found in Central and South America, Africa and the Middle East. *S. haematobium* is found throughout Africa and the Middle East, while *S. japonicum* is restricted to South East Asia and Japan. However, modern migration and travel patterns mean that infestations may be found in patients remote from endemic areas (Mahmood 1975).

Genital schistosomiasis is rare and represents so-called ectopic disease, i.e. not related directly to the life cycle of the organism. Worms preferentially lodge in the mesenteric and portal (*S. mansoni* and *S. japonicum*) or vesical veins (*S. haematobium*), but may gain access to the genital tract via venous anastomoses such as those between the hemorrhoidal and hypogastric veins, and between mesenteric and ovarian veins. It is usually an incidental finding, although some patients with upper genital tract infections have symptoms suggestive of PID (Areán 1956). Involvement of the female genital tract occurs more frequently in *S. haematobium* than in *S. mansoni* infection; however, whereas *S. haematobium* predominantly involves the lower genital tract, *S. mansoni* has a predilection for tubes and ovaries (Areán 1956, Berry 1966, Mahmood 1975). Involvement of genital organs by *S. japonicum* is usually an incidental finding.

If the schistosomal infection is merely an incidental finding, the ovaries are likely to be of normal size. Small white nodules are present on their surfaces, and often elsewhere on the pelvic peritoneum as well; this appearance may simulate metastatic carcinoma. In patients with clinical disease, the ovaries may be enlarged up to three times normal size and display necrosis, abscesses, and hemorrhages (Areán 1956, Bahary et al 1967); tubo-ovarian adhesions are always present and adhesions to other pelvic structures are present in the majority.

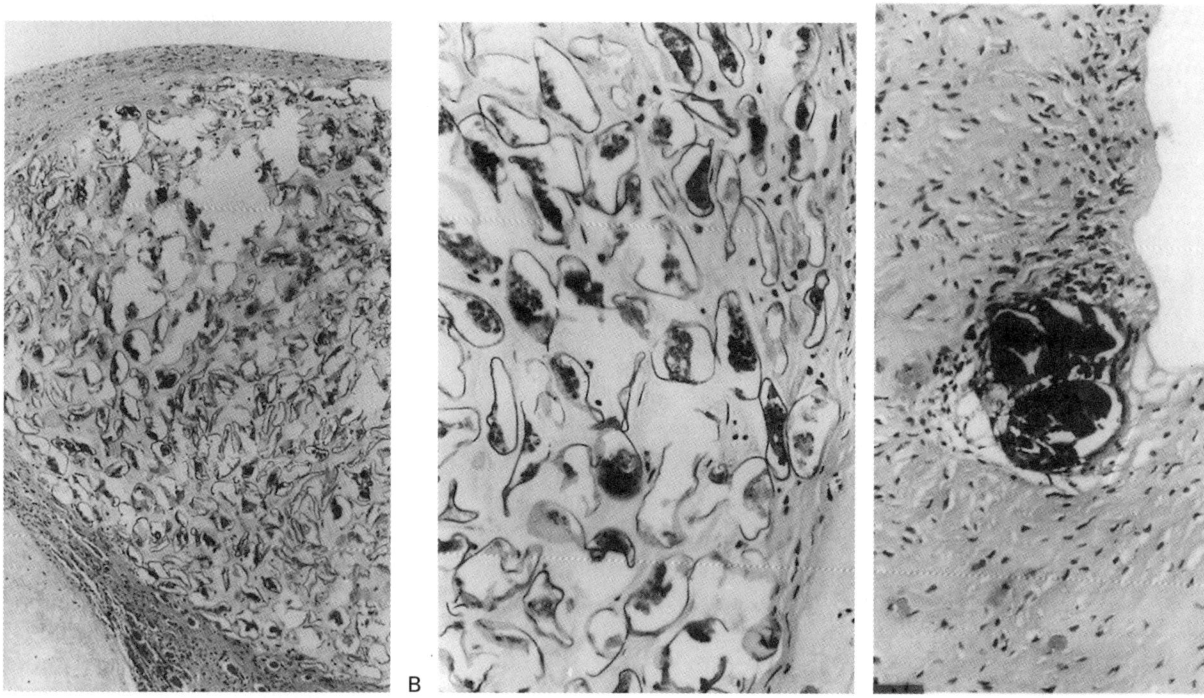

A B C

Fig. 18.12 Ovarian schistosomiasis. (A) Large group of *S. japonicum* ova in ovarian cortex. H + E ×64 (B) Detail of rather distorted ova. No tissue reaction. H + E ×200. (C) Calcified ova beneath ovarian capsule, probably in a lymphatic channel. H + E ×200. (Courtesy of Dr L Ma & Dr H Y Yeung, Hong Kong)

Living worms and dead ova appear to provoke little tissue reaction, but dead worms and living ova, when they enter the tissues, provoke a granulomatous reaction (Berry 1966). Ova are more commonly identified than worms (Fig. 18.12). The cellular infiltrate consists of epithelioid cells, foreign body giant cells, lymphocytes, plasma cells, and eosinophils. Some granulomas appear tuberculoid. Sometimes the cellular reaction to freshly laid ova is predominantly eosinophilic, with formation of abscesses. The Splendore–Hoeppli phenomenon (radiating eosinophilic deposits around ova) may also be observed. The peripheral zone of the granulomas is composed of fibrous tissue, which gradually increases in amount and may replace entire lesions. Dead ova frequently calcify and these are not uncommonly found, not only within the ovarian parenchyma (Fig. 18.12c), but (more often) within veins of the outer uterine wall or broad ligament.

Schistosomal ova can be readily differentiated from each other in histological preparations if spines are visible in the plane of section. The ova of each of the species are in the size range 80–160 μm in length and 30–90 μm in width. *S. haematobium* and *S. mansoni* are elongate; *S. haematobium* have a terminal spine while *S. mansoni* has a lateral one. *S. japonicum* is round to ovoid and has a lateral spine which is less prominent than that of *S. mansoni* (Fig. 18.13).

Enterobiasis

Pelvic peritoneal granulomas due to *Enterobius* (*Oxyuris*) *vermicularis* (pin worm, threadworm) are rare complications of gastrointestinal infestation and have been reported in females only. Parasites are thought to gain entry to the peritoneal cavity by ascending the genital tract after migrating to the introitus from the anus. The identification of enterobius-related granulomas in the cervix, endometrium, and fallopian tubes supports this mechanism (FitzGerald et al 1974, Beckman & Holland 1981). On reaching the peri-

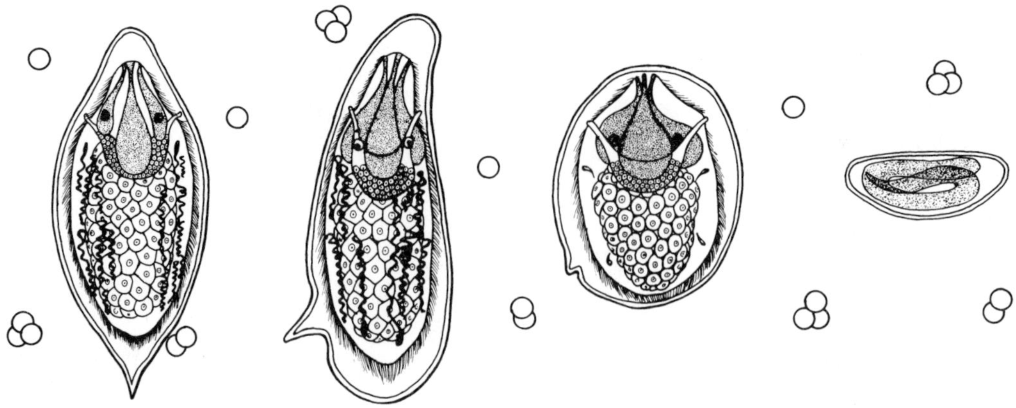

Fig. 18.13 Parasitic ova. From left to right: *S. haematobium*, *S. mansoni*, *S. japonicum*, *E. vermicularis*. Circles represent the size of red blood cells.

toneal cavity the worms die and their ova are released, inciting the inflammatory reaction. The granulomas are usually located in the pelvis and may involve the serosal surfaces of the ovaries. If numerous, they may simulate peritoneal carcinomatosis (Sinniah et al 1991).

Macroscopically, ovarian granulomas are small soft yellow-brown serosal nodules, up to 1 cm in diameter, sometimes associated with adhesions. Larger lesions may show central softening. They are generally superficial, but an exception to this was the case of a ruptured tubo-ovarian abscess (with generalized purulent peritonitis) in the wall of which granulomas containing enterobius ova were identified (Kahn et al 1981). Microscopically, the granulomatous inflammation is centered around the ova which are oval (up to 60 μm long and 30 μm wide) with double-contoured smooth shells, flattened on one side, in which embryonic structures may be identified (Fig. 18.13). Degenerate worms are rarely identified (Neafie et al 1976, Viñuela et al 1979, Beckman & Holland 1981). Ova (and worms) are surrounded by necrotic debris containing numerous eosinophils and, beyond this, there is a zone of granulation tissue which includes epithelioid histiocytes and lymphocytes. The granulomas show peripheral fibrosis. The ova and, indeed, entire granulomas may undergo calcification.

The finding of large necrotizing pelvic granulomas, particularly if associated with an eosinophilic infiltrate, should prompt a search for a possible causative parasite by processing additional tissue and cutting step-sections if appropriate. Enterobius ova can be distinguished from those of schistosoma by their smaller size and lack of spines (Fig. 18.13). Peripheral blood eosinophilia is usually not observed, and examination of the feces for ova is usually negative (FitzGerald et al 1974, McMahon et al 1984).

Echinococcosis

Echinococcosis is an infestation by the cestode *Echinoccocus granulosus* which is prevalent in sheep and cattle raising areas of Australia, New Zealand, and South America, and also in the Middle East, Iceland, and some European countries. Genital involvement is rare, occurring in only 0.1–0.3% of infected females; the uterus is more commonly affected than the ovary (Georgakopoulos et al 1979, 1980, Fabre et al 1983). Ovarian involvement may represent primary infection (if embryos emerging from the gut pass through both liver and lungs before establishing themselves in the tissues) or secondary infection (if it follows rupture of a primary hepatic cyst, either into the vascular system or peritoneal cavity).

Pelvic hydatid cysts measure up to 16 cm in diameter (Georgakopoulos et al 1980) and show the characteristic triple-layered wall consisting of innermost germinal epithelium (with its brood capsules and scolices), hyaline laminated membrane, and outermost adventitial fibrous tissue (of

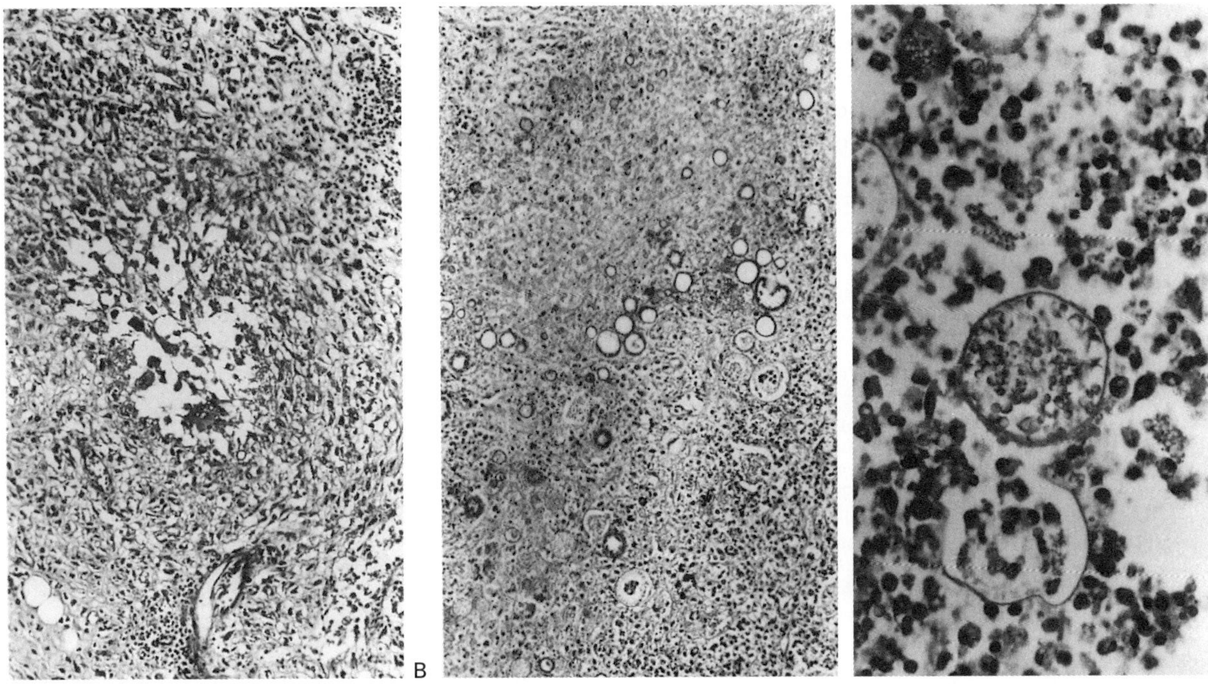

Fig. 18.14 Coccidioidomycosis (nonovarian). Typical tissue reactions. (A) Necrotizing granulomas. H + E ×80. (B) Necrotic suppurative lesion with numerous spherules of variable size. H + E ×80. (C) Detail of spherules with refractile walls and content of endospores. Numerous free endospores are also present in the adjacent inflammatory infiltrate. H + E ×320

host origin). Calcification of the cyst wall (a very useful radiological sign), is usually associated with regression of the cyst following death of the parasite.

FUNGAL OOPHORITIS

Coccidioidomycosis

This fungal disease is endemic in certain semi-arid areas of North, Central, and South America. Genital infection is rare, even in cases of disseminated fatal coccidioidomycosis (which generally occurs in immunosuppressed patients). As in tuberculosis, genital involvement results from bloodborne spread of organisms from a pulmonary lesion which is generally radiologically inactive or apparently healed. Pelvic coccidioidomycosis is usually associated with peritonitis (Saw et al 1975, Bylund et al 1986).

In cases of uterine adnexal involvement, the tubes and ovaries show dense serosal adhesions and multiple small white nodules are apparent on the serosal surfaces (Bylund et al 1986). In addition, the ovaries may contain abscess cavities (Saw et al 1975). The inflammatory reaction to *Coccidioides immitis* is either tuberculoid granulomatous, which may progress to caseation and cavitation, or suppurative with microabscess formation (Fig. 18.14A,B). The fungal elements are seen in tissues as spherules (sporangia) measuring 20–200 μm in diameter, which have thin doubly refractile walls. The enclosed endospores (2–3 μm diameter) are released into the tissues upon rupture of the spherules (Fig. 18.14C). A rapid diagnosis of pelvic coccidioidomycosis may be made by identifying the spherules in wet preparations of peritoneal fluid or purulent exudates. Similar material or fresh tissue from the ovary, endometrial curettings, or vaginal discharge can be used for culture. Serology and coccidioidin skin tests are also helpful.

Blastomycosis

Genital tract involvement in North American

blastomycosis is rare and results from venereal transmission, or hematogenous spread from a pulmonary lesion. Murray et al (1984) described a patient with a blastomycotic tubo-ovarian abscess, considered to be a complication of reactivated pulmonary infection, in whom the diagnosis of pelvic blastomycosis was initially made on a cervical smear. *Blastomyces dermatitidis* was cultured from the fallopian tube and uterus. The tissue reaction to the fungus is similar to that seen in coccidioidomycosis, i.e. either suppurative or tuberculoid granulomatous inflammation. The budding thick-walled yeast bodies (8–20 μm diameter) are readily found in sections.

REFERENCES

Abdou N I, NaPombejara C, Sagawa A et al 1977 Malacoplakia: evidence for monocyte lysosomal abnormality correctable by cholinergic agonist in vitro and in vivo. New England Journal of Medicine 297: 1413–1419

Agarwal J, Gupta J K 1993 Female genital tuberculosis – a retrospective clinico-pathological study of 501 cases. Indian Journal of Pathological Microbiology 36: 389–397

Areán V M 1956 Manson's schistosomiasis of the female genital tract. American Journal of Obstetrics and Gynecology 72: 1038–1053

Bahary C M, Ovadia Y, Neri A 1967 *Schistosoma mansoni* of the ovary. American Journal of Obstetrics and Gynecology 98: 290–292

Beckman E N, Holland J B 1981 Ovarian enterobiasis – a proposed pathogenesis. American Journal of Tropical Medicine and Hygiene 30: 74–76

Berry A 1966 A cytopathological and histopathological study of bilharziasis of the female genital tract. Journal of Pathology and Bacteriology 91: 325–338

Bhagavan B S, Gupta P K 1978 Genital actinomycosis and intrauterine contraceptive devices. Cytopathologic diagnosis and clinical significance. Human Pathology 9: 567–578

Blaustein A 1982 Pathology of the female genital tract, 2nd edn. Springer-Verlag, New York, p 442–448

Burkman R T 1980 Intrauterine device use and the risk of pelvic inflammatory disease. American Journal of Obstetrics and Gynecology 138: 861–863

Burkman R, Schlesselman S, McCaffrey L, Gupta P K, Spence M 1982 The relationship of genital tract actinomycetes and the development of pelvic inflammatory disease. American Journal of Obstetrics and Gynecology 143: 585–589

Bychkov V 1990 Ovarian pathology in chronic pelvic inflammatory disease. Gynecological and Obstetrical Investigation 30: 31–33

Bylund D J, Nanfro J J, Marsh W L 1986 Coccidioidomycosis of the female genital tract. Archives of Pathology and Laboratory Medicine 110: 232–235

Chalvardjian A, Picard L, Shaw R, Davey R, Cairns J D 1980 Malacoplakia of the female genital tract. American Journal of Obstetrics and Gynecology 138: 391–394

Cramer D W, Welch W R, Cassells S, Scully R E 1983 Mumps, menarche, menopause and ovarian cancer. American Journal of Obstetrics and Gynecology 147: 1–6

Egger H, Weigmann P 1982 Clinical and surgical aspects of ovarian endometriotic cysts. Archives of Gynecology 233: 37–45

Eschenbach D A, Harrish J P, Holmes K K 1977 Pathogenesis of acute pelvic inflammatory disease: role of contraception and other risk factors. American Journal of Obstetrics and Gynecology 128: 838–850

Evans D J, Lampert I A 1978 Ovarian involvement by cytomegalovirus (letter). Human Pathology 9: 122

Evans-Jones J C, French G L 1983 An ovarian cyst infected with *Salmonella typhi*. Case report. British Journal of Obstetrics and Gynaecology 90: 680–682

Fabre M, Paillas J, Quillard J 1983 Le kyste hydatique tubo-ovarien. A propos d'une observation. Semaine des Hôpitaux de Paris 59: 1842–1844

FitzGerald T B, Mainwaring A R, Ahmed A 1974 Pelvic peritoneal oxyuriasis simulating metastatic carcinoma. A case report. Journal of Obstetrics and Gynaecology of the British Commonwealth 81: 248–250

Georgakopoulos P A, Hadgidakis E, Belios B, Bersis A 1979 Primäre ovariale Echinokokkiasis. Zentralblatt für Gynäkologie 104: 1288–1291

Georgakopoulos P A, Gogas C G, Sariyannis H G 1980 Hydatid disease of the female genitalia. Obstetrics and Gynecology 55: 555–559

Hingorani V, Narula R K, Bhalla S 1963 *Salmonella typhi* infection in an ovarian dermoid. Obstetrics and Gynecology 22: 118–120

Hoffman M S 1989 Peritoneal tuberculosis, large ovarian thecoma and an elevated serum Ca 125 level mimicking ovarian cancer. Journal of Florida Medical Association 76: 388–389

Holmes K K, Eschenbach D A, Knapp J S 1980 Salpingitis: Overview of etiology and epidemiology. American Journal of Obstetrics and Gynecology 138: 893–900

Hsu S P, Wang K G, Yang Y C, Lan C C 1990 Pelvic actinomycosis associated with intrauterine contraceptive devices. A review of 6 cases. Chung Hua I Hsueh Tsa Chin Taipei 46: 289–292

Iwasaki T, Sakuma T, Satodate R, Takano N, Sata T, Kurata T 1988 Cytomegalovirus oophoritis with cortical necrosis during remission of acute lymphocytic leukaemia. Acta Pathologica Japonica 38: 1069–1076

Jones M C, Buschmann B O, Dowling E A, Pollock H M 1979 The prevalence of actinomycetes-like organisms found in cervicovaginal smears of 300 IUD wearers. Acta Cytologica 23: 282–286

Kahn J S, Steele R J C, Stewart D 1981 *Enterobius vermicularis* infestation of the female genital tract causing generalised peritonitis. British Journal of Obstetrics and Gynaecology 88: 681–683

Kaufman D W, Shapiro S, Rosenberg L et al 1980 Intrauterine contraceptive device use and pelvic inflammatory disease. American Journal of Obstetrics and Gynecology 136: 159–162

Kunakemakorn P, Ontai G, Balin H 1976 Pelvic inflammatory pseudotumor: a case report. American Journal of Obstetrics and Gynecology 126: 286–287

Lomax C W, Harbert G M, Thornton W M 1976 Actinomycosis of the female genital tract. Obstetrics and Gynecology 48: 341–346

Luff R D, Gupta P K, Spence M R, Frost J K 1978 Pelvic actinomycosis and the intrauterine contraceptive device. A cyto-histomorphologic study. American Journal of Clinical Pathology 69: 581–586

MacCarthy J 1955 Actinomycosis of the female pelvic organs with involvement of the endometrium. Journal of Pathology and Bacteriology 69: 175–178

McCracken A W, D'Agostino A N, Brucks A B, Kingsley W B 1974 Acquired cytomegalovirus infection presenting as viral endometritis. American Journal of Clinical Pathology 61: 556–560

McMahon J N, Connolly C E, Long S V, Meehan F P 1984 Enterobius granulomas of the uterus, ovary and pelvic peritoneum. Two case reports. British Journal of Obstetrics and Gynaecology 91: 289–290

Mahmood K 1975 Granulomatous oophoritis due to *Schistosoma mansoni*. American Journal of Obstetrics and Gynecology 123: 919–920

Mårdh P-A 1980 An overview of infectious agents of salpingitis, their biology, and recent advances in methods of detection. American Journal of Obstetrics and Gynecology 138: 933–951

Minkowitz S, Friedman F, Henniger G 1965 Xanthogranuloma of the ovary. Archives of Pathology 80: 209–213

Morrison J C, Givens J R, Wiser W L, Fish S A 1975 Mumps oophoritis: A cause of premature menopause. Fertility and Sterility 26: 655–659

Mueller B A, Daling J R, Moore D E et al 1986 Appendectomy and the risk of tubal infertility. New England Journal of Medicine 315: 1506–1508

Murray J J, Clark C A, Lands R H, Heim C R, Burnett L S 1984 Reactivation blastomycosis presenting as a tuboovarian abscess. Obstetrics and Gynecology 64: 828–830

Neafie R C, Connor D H, Meyers W M 1976 Enterobiasis. In: Binford C H, Connor D H (eds) Pathology of tropical and extraordinary diseases. Armed Forces Institute of Pathology, Washington, DC, p 455–459

Niebyl J R, Parmley T H, Spence M R, Woodruff J D 1978 Unilateral ovarian abscess associated with the intrauterine device. Obstetrics and Gynecology 52: 165–168

Pace E H, Voet R L, Melancon J T 1984 Xanthogranulomatous oophoritis: an inflammatory pseudotumor of the ovary. International Journal of Gynecological Pathology 3: 398–402

Persson E, Holmberg K 1984 A longitudinal study of *Actinomyces israelii* in the female genital tract. Acta Obstetricia et Gynecologica Scandinavica 63: 207–216

Robbins S L, Cotran R S, Kumar V 1984 Pathologic basis of disease, 3rd edn. W B Saunders, Philadelphia, p 64

Sandin R L, Green J N, Sarzier J S et al 1993 Pelvicabdominal actinomycosis associated with an intrauterine contraceptive device. A case of liver dissemination mimicking metastic ovarian cancer. Annals of Clinical Laboratory Science 23: 448–455

Saw E C, Smale L E, Einstein H, Huntington R W 1975 Female genital coccidioidomycosis. Obstetrics and Gynecology 45: 199–202

Schaefer G 1976 Female genital tuberculosis. Clinical Obstetrics and Gynecology 19: 223–239

Schiffer M A, Elguezabal A, Sultana M, Allen A C 1975 Actinomycosis infections associated with intrauterine contraceptive devices. Obstetrics and Gynecology 45: 67–72

Schmidt W A, Bedrossian C W M, Ali V, Webb J A, Bastian F O 1980 Actinomycosis and intrauterine contraceptive devices. The clinicopathologic entity. Diagnostic Gynecology and Obstetrics 2: 165–177

Shalev E, Zuckerman H, Rizescu I 1982 Pelvic inflammatory pseudotumor (xanthogranuloma). Acta Obstetricia et Gynecologica Scandinavica 61: 285–286

Sharma T M, Nadasdy T, Leech R W, Kingma D W, Johnson L D, Hanson Painton O 1994 In-situ DNA hybridization study of 'primary' cytomegalovirus (CMV) oophoritis. Acta Obstetricia et Gynecologica Scandinavica 73: 429–431

Sinniah B, Leopairut J, Neafie R C, Connor D H, Voge M 1991 Enterobiasis: a histopathological study of 259 patients. Annals of Tropical Medicine and Parasitology 85: 625–635

Soloff L A, Hermann C S 1935 Chronic typhoid abscess of the ovary. American Journal of Obstetrics and Gynecology 30: 290–292

Subietas A, Depppisch L M, Astarloa J 1977 Cytomegalovirus oophoritis: ovarian cortical necrosis. Human Pathology 8: 285–292

Sutherland A M 1985 Genital tuberculosis: analysis of a personal series of 710 cases. Australian and New Zealand Journal of Obstetrics and Gynaecology 25: 203–207

Viñuela A, Fernandez-Rojo F, Martinez-Merino A 1979 Oxyuris granulomas of pelvic peritoneum and appendicular wall. Histopathology 3: 69–77

Wetchler S J, Dunn L J 1985 Ovarian abscess. Report of a case and a review of the literature. Obstetrical and Gynecological Survey 40: 476–485

Wheeler J E 1994 Diseases of the fallopian tube. In: Kurman R J (ed) Blaustein's pathology of the female genital tract, 4th edn. Springer-Verlag, New York, p 529–561

Willson J R, Black J R 1964 Ovarian abscess. American Journal of Obstetrics and Gynecology 90: 34–43

19

Noninfectious inflammatory lesions

P. Russell A. Farnsworth

SARCOIDOSIS

Sarcoidosis rarely involves the female genital tract, even in the active stage of the disease when granulomas may be widely disseminated throughout the body. It is not known what gynecological symptoms, if any, are directly attributable to pelvic sarcoidosis or whether it is detrimental to reproductive function (Ho 1979). The uterus is more often affected than the adnexa. Most reported cases have been in patients with current or recent evidence of pulmonary sarcoidosis. Elevated serum calcium-125 may be present (Trimble et al 1991).

Ovarian granulomas are distributed at random through the cortex, medulla, and hilus (Winslow & Funkhouser 1968, Chalvardjian 1978); one case with apparent selective localization at the margins of corpora lutea and albicantes has been described (Sommers 1983). As in extragenital sites, the discrete noncaseating granulomas are composed of epithelioid histiocytes with small numbers of giant cells of Langhans or foreign body type, sometimes containing crystalloid inclusions. A diagnosis of ovarian sarcoidosis in the absence of systemic disease should be made with great caution, since the histological changes alone are not pathognomonic (see Table 18.1, Fig. 19.1). Tuberculosis and mycoses, especially if endemic in the patient's locality, should be excluded by the appropriate special stains, and preferably culture as well. The sections should be screened, with the aid of polarizing filters, for foreign bodies, particularly starch granules (see below) and parasitic elements (see Ch. 18).

CROHN'S DISEASE

Crohn's disease (regional enteritis) characteristically involves the terminal ileum and, because of the tendency to perforation and abscess formation, right iliac fossa or pelvic masses may develop. These may masquerade as ovarian tumors or tubo-ovarian abscesses, a situation which sometimes leads to laparotomies and intestinal resections which might be considered inappropriate for the long-term management of Crohn's disease (Donaldson 1978). The ovary is very rarely and only 'accidentally' involved in Crohn's disease and, in two of four reported cases, was a surprise finding at laparotomy for presumed gynecological disease. Ovarian involvement is the result of direct extension of the inflammatory process from the adherent segment of intestine. The right ovary, by virtue of its proximity to the terminal ileum, is more commonly affected, but left adnexal involvement has also been reported – in a patient with a 5-year history of rectosigmoid disease (Brooks & Wheeler 1977).

Ovarian granulomas may be restricted to the serosa and superficial cortex, or widely distributed in the parenchyma (Wlodarski & Trainer 1975,

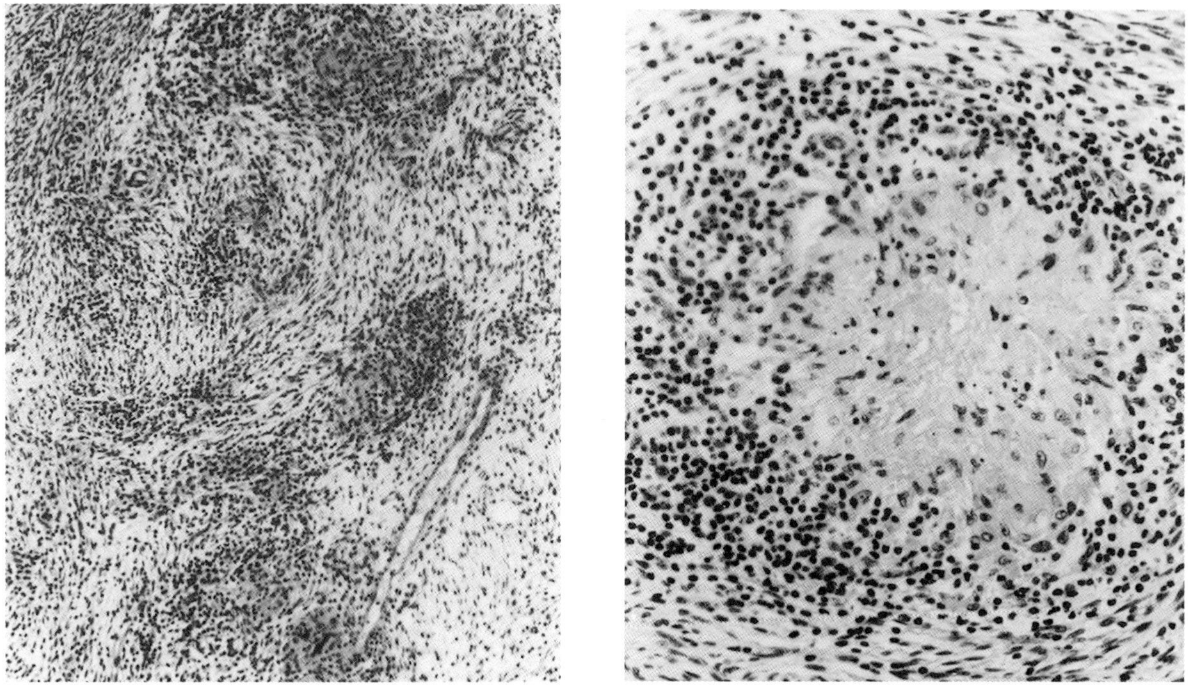

A B

Fig. 19.1 Sarcoidal granulomas which were incidental findings in a postmenopausal woman with no clinical features of sarcoidosis. No microorganisms or foreign bodies could be identified and the cause of the granulomas remains obscure. (A) Multiple medullary granulomas. H + E ×80. (B) Detail of cortical granuloma with a suggestion of central necrosis. H + E ×200

Frost et al 1981). They are sarcoidal in type and set in a background of lymphocytic infiltration. A more destructive combined suppurative and granulomatous reaction has also been described, in association with an ileal–ovarian 'fistula' (Honoré 1981). The ipsilateral fallopian tube is generally involved as well. There should be no problem in differential diagnosis once the clinical and surgical details are available. However, it is prudent to exclude infective causes of granulomatous oophoritis, such as actinomycosis or tuberculosis (see Table 18.1), which may also be associated with ileocaecal disease.

FOREIGN BODY GRANULOMAS

These are usually related to the presence of exogenous foreign material, but similar reactions to endogenous tissue components may also be encountered. The nature of the foreign material may be difficult to determine in tissue sections (Fig. 19.2).

Suture material

Foreign body granulomas in the ovary are most commonly associated with suture material retained following previous surgery. The sutures may consist of dense hyaline material, in varying degrees of disintegration (Figs 19.3A,B), or translucent threads (Fig. 19.3C). The foreign body component of the granulomas can be highlighted with the use of polarizing filters. The cellular reaction consists of macrophages, some multinucleated (Touton giant cells), and lymphocytes. There is local fibrosis and serosal adhesions.

Talc and starch

Surgical glove powders, both talc and starch-based, are a common cause of peritoneal granulomas. The widespread peritoneal granulomas may simulate carcinomatosis or tuberculosis at subsequent laparotomy. Case reports suggest that starch granulomas resolve within a few months, leaving

A 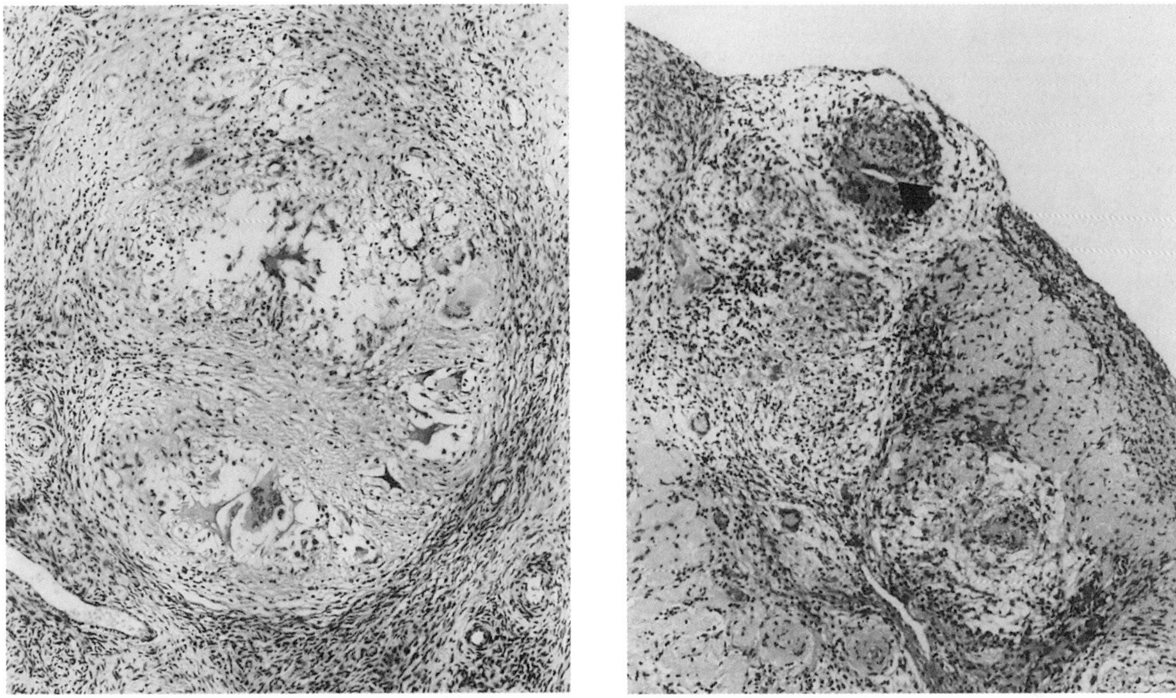 B

Fig. 19.2 Foreign body granulomas. (A) Granuloma from patient with history of previous ovarian surgery. Giant cells and fibrous tissue are conspicuous. H + E ×80. (B) Granulomas in ovarian cortex with an unusually prominent eosinophilic infiltrate. A spicule of foreign material of unknown origin is present in the serosal granuloma (arrow). H + E ×50

no residua or only adhesions (Cox 1970). Although usually of no clinical significance, some patients develop a chronic fibrosing peritonitis, while others suffer an acute illness (abdominal pain and fever) 2–4 weeks postoperatively (Nissim et al 1981). Starch is less irritant than talc but, although carefully modified for surgical use, is apparently poorly absorbed by some patients. A hypersensitivity reaction may be involved. As well as being surgically introduced, talc and starch may enter the peritoneal cavity by ascending the genital tract; the source in these cases is powder from contraceptives, deodorants, and gloves used for vaginal examination. Mostafa et al (1985) found small cortical granulomas, containing foreign material consistent with talc, in 9% of oophorectomy specimens; a history of previous abdominal surgery was present in only 44% of these cases.

Talc granulomas are of typical foreign-body type. Multinucleated giant cells are usually numerous and contain pleiomorphic spiculate crystals; they are readily demonstrated by polarized light.

Starch granulomas show a variety of histological patterns. The most common is a typical foreign body reaction. Some lesions include prominent polymorphonuclear leucocytes, especially eosinophils, to the extent of forming microabscesses. An uncommon pattern is sarcoidal or tuberculoid granulomas, which may include foci of necrosis (Fig. 19.4A). The latter appearance may lead to an erroneous diagnosis of tuberculosis (Nissim et al 1981). This mistake can be avoided by being aware of the possibility of starch granulomas and searching for the granules when appropriate. Their presence can usually be suspected in H + E sections if, with careful focusing, polyhedral translucent blue-green bodies 10 μm in diameter are found (Fig. 19.4B). Their nature can be confirmed by examining the section with polarized light, which reveals the pathognomonic Maltese crosses (Fig. 19.4C). They can also be stained with PAS, Ziehl–Neelsen, methenamine silver, or Lugol's iodine (Nissim et al 1981). Freshly introduced starch can be excluded by its

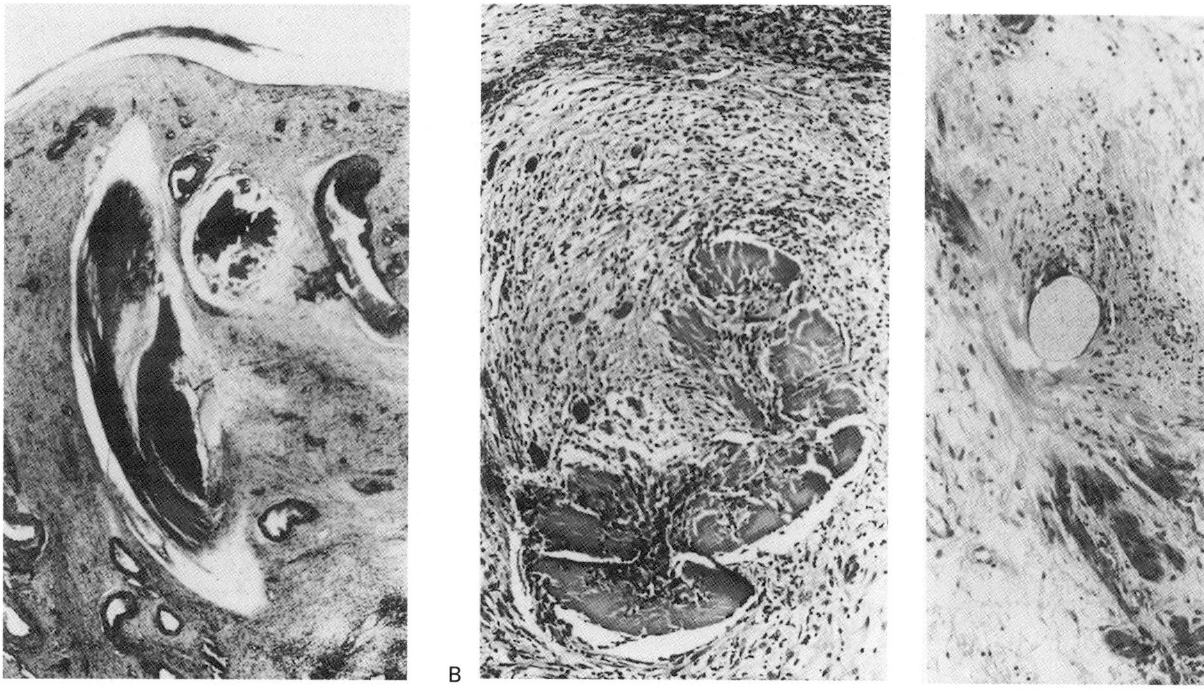

A B C

Fig. 19.3 Reactions to suture material. (A) Amorphous suture material surrounded by dense fibrous tissue, but negligible inflammation. H + E ×25. (B) Partially disintegrated suture material surrounded by fibrous tissue and a mixed inflammatory infiltrate. H + E ×100. (C) Vicryl™ suture (used in microsurgical procedures), distinguished by its translucent blue appearance in H + E sections. Histiocytes are closely applied to the foreign material, but other inflammatory cells are sparse. Fibrosis is typically minimal. (Section from mesovarium.) H + E ×80

microanatomical location. Rarely, fat necrosis and rheumatoid-type necrotizing foci are identified as reactions to starch (Davies & Neely 1972).

Hysterosalpingographic contrast media

Peritoneal granulomas may develop following hysterosalpingography. Oil-based contrast media are only slowly absorbed from the peritoneal cavity, and lipogranulomas sometimes form. There is a foreign body giant cell reaction orientated around clear vacuoles from which lipid has been removed during processing (similar to the pattern seen in lymph nodes following lymphangiograms or cholecystograms). The granulomas sometimes become confluent, and focal necrosis may occur (Fig. 19.5). If uterine or tubal tissue is available for examination, lipogranulomas and foamy macrophages may be evident in the endometrial stroma and tubal submucosa. Peritoneal granulomas have also been reported, but less frequently, after the use of water-based contrast media (Soules & Spadoni 1982).

Parasites

Reactions to parasites and their ova include a foreign body granulomatous component (see Ch. 18).

Intestinal contents

Ovarian foreign body granulomas may be seen following intestinal perforation (such as in Crohn's disease or diverticulitis). The granulomas are generally confined to the serosa, but plant material and barium (from a perforated colon) have been identified in the parenchyma (Benirschke et al 1984).

Contents of mature cystic teratomas

A foreign body reaction is commonly seen in rela-

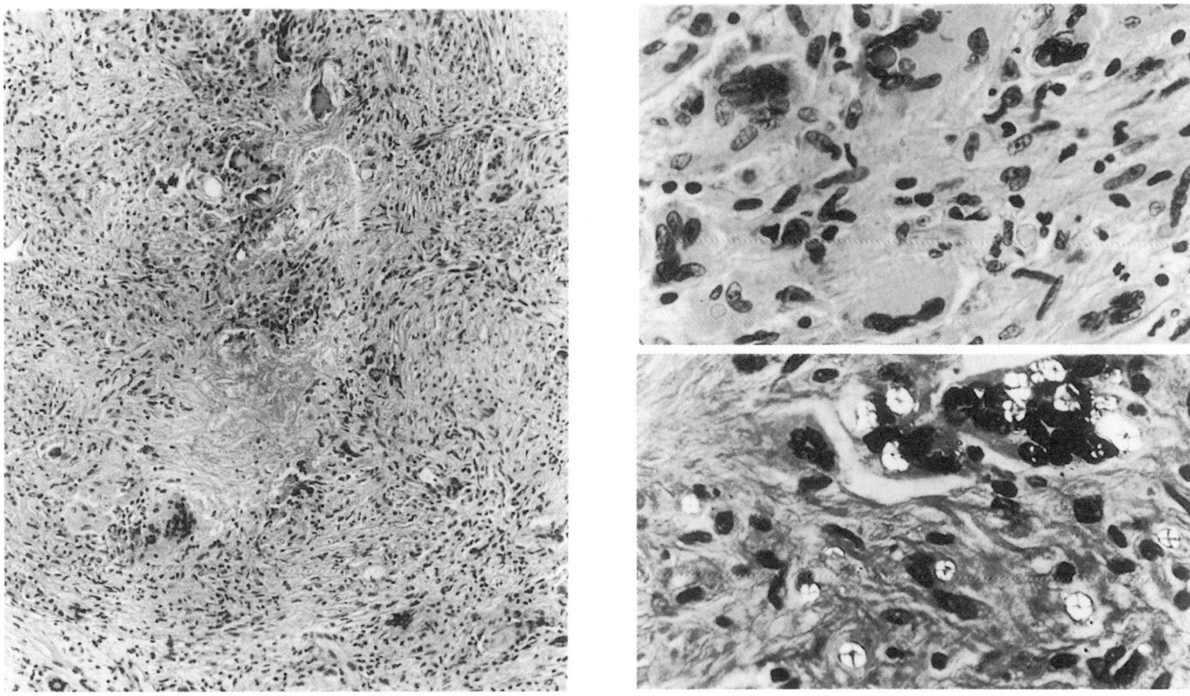

A B C

Fig. 19.4 Starch granulomas 6 weeks after laparotomy. (A) Thickened fibrotic peritoneum with necrotising granulomas. H + E ×80. (B) Detail of granuloma; refractile round foreign bodies in giant cells. H + E ×256. (C) Similar area viewed with polarised light; foreign bodies display typical Maltese cross appearance of starch granules. H + E ×256

tion to mature cystic teratomas (dermoid cysts). Squames, hairs, and sebum may be extruded into the surrounding ovarian tissue, where they incite an inflammatory response. Widespread peritoneal granulomas and adhesions may develop if the cyst ruptures (see Ch. 46).

Keratin from genital tract adenoacanthomas

Peritoneal foreign body granulomas may be found in association with endometrial or ovarian adeno-acanthomas, and uterine examples are considered to result from reflux of acellular keratinous debris through the fallopian tubes (Chen et al 1978, Kim & Scully 1990). The lesions have been seen on the serosal surfaces of the adnexa, uterus, colon, and appendix. Care must be taken not to misinterpret

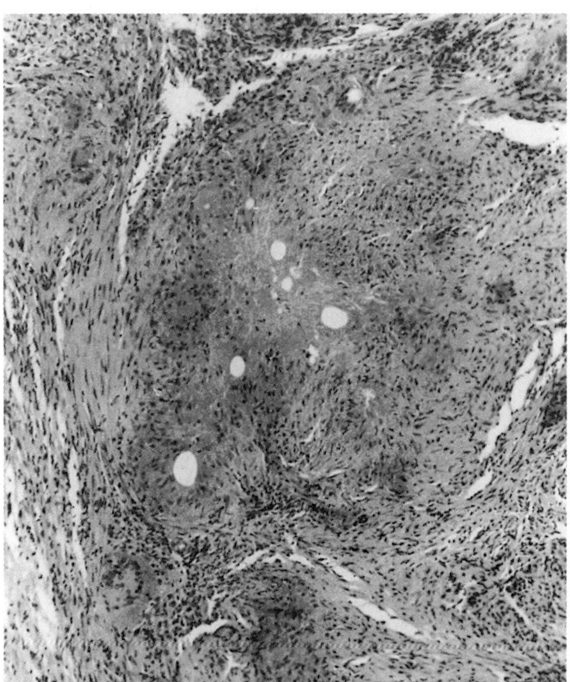

Fig. 19.5 Lipiodol™ granuloma. Necrotizing peritoneal granulomas were identified after recent hysterosalpingogram; similar granulomas were present in synchronously sampled endometrium. The clear spaces in the center of the granuloma indicate where foreign lipid has been dissolved out during processing. H + E ×80

these granulomas as deposits of metastatic carcinoma, as this has serious implications for staging.

Postcautery granulomas

Florid foreign body granulomatous reactions in pelvic peritoneal and ovarian biopsies are occasionally encountered in patients who have had endometriotic or other lesions cauterized in the weeks or months prior to biopsy. The lesions show central eosinophilic, focally refractile, amorphous material (representing the coagulated tissue and carbonaceous debris), surrounded by large numbers of multinucleated foreign body giant cells and a peripheral lymphocytic infiltrate (Fig. 19.6).

OTHER GRANULOMAS

Cortical granulomas

'Cortical granulomas' in postmenopausal ovaries were first described by Hertig (1944), who considered that they represented regressing hyperplastic stromal nodules. Boss et al (1965), in their analysis of ovarian changes at autopsy in 90 adult women, found cortical granulomas in 16% and noted an association with stromal 'proliferation'. We have observed similar lesions which could be interpreted morphologically as representing transitional stages in the involution of hyperthecosis (Fig. 19.7). Hughesdon (1976) regards the lesions as manifestations of endometriosis – 'stromatosis' (see Ch. 20). Others have related them to germinal inclusion cysts (Roddick & Green 1958, Mostafa et al 1985). The granulomas are well circumscribed, 100–500 μm in diameter and consist of loose ovarian stroma containing small numbers of lymphocytes and epithelioid cells (which may represent either luteinized stromal cells or macrophages), multinucleated giant cells, and occasional anisotropic fat crystals. The lesions are well vascularized, but eventually become fibrotic and hyalinized.

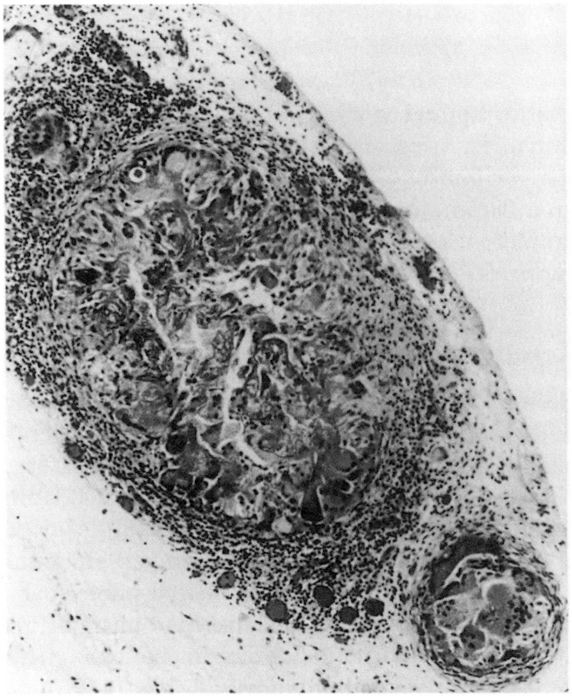

Fig. 19.6 Postcautery peritoneal granulomas. Central amorphous coagulated tissue surrounded by innumerable multinucleated giant cells and peripheral zone of lymphocytes. History of cautery to peritoneal endometriosis 6 weeks previously. H + E ×80

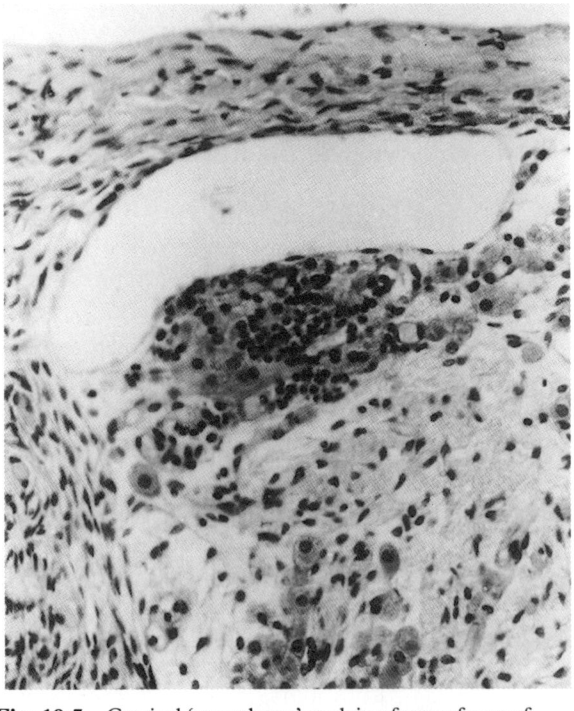

Fig. 19.7 Cortical 'granuloma' evolving from a focus of stromal luteinization. Aggregate of lymphocytes and epithelioid cells adjacent to blood vessel. H + E ×200

Isolated noninfectious granulomas

Isolated noninfectious granulomas were described by Herbold et al (1984). Typically, they occur in premenopausal women with no evidence of systemic granulomatous disease or of genital tract infection of potentially granulomatous type. In the majority of patients the granulomas are incidental findings and there is a history of previous surgery (6 months to 12 years) involving the now affected ovary. The granulomas are multiple and may be bilateral. The granulomas are small, with an acellular hyaline core bordered by palisading histiocytes and peripheral fibrosis. A history of prior surgery suggests the possibility that the granulomas may be a reaction to traumatized or devitalized tissues (Al Dawoud et al 1991, Kernohan et al 1991). The lesions resemble the necrobiotic rheumatoid-like granulomas which may be found in the cervix following cone biopsy (Evans et al 1984; Fig. 19.8). In one case where there was no history of prior surgery, but subacute torsion and subsequent ischemia may be a possible cause of the necrotizing process as well.

AUTOIMMUNE OOPHORITIS

Some patients with premature ovarian failure have a chronic oophoritis which is considered to be autoimmune in origin, by virtue of the nature and specificity of the inflammatory infiltrate for follicular structures (Bannatyne et al 1990), the association with other autoimmune conditions, as well as the presence of antiovarian antibodies in a small proportion of cases. The clinical features and relationship to other types of premature ovarian failure are discussed in Chapter 8.

Macroscopic features

The ovaries may be of normal size but many are markedly enlarged (up to five times normal). They are often multicystic (Biscotti et al 1989,

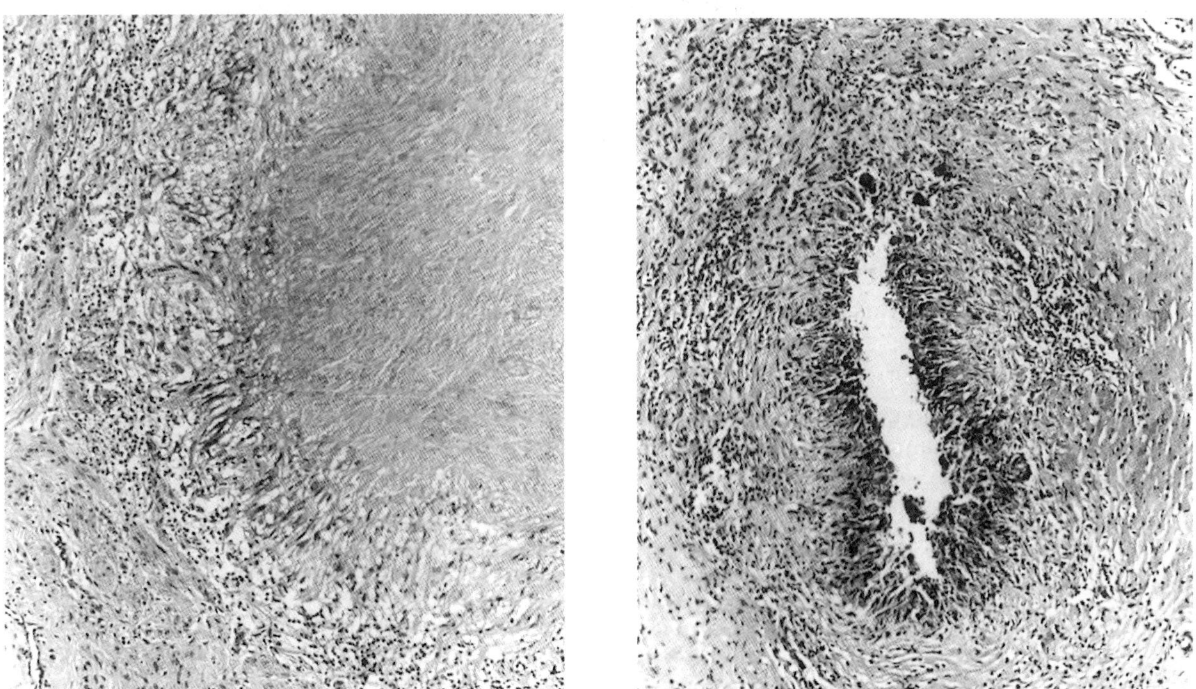

A B

Fig. 19.8 Isolated non-infectious granulomas (from cervix after cone biopsy). (A) Large amorphous necrotic area bordered by palisading histiocytes and lymphocytes. Compare with Fig. 18. 9 – ovarian tuberculosis. H + E ×80. (B) Smaller necrotising granuloma with more intense inflammatory infiltrate which includes a few multinucleated giant cells (best seen above). H + E ×80

Lonsdale et al 1991). The patients may present with an adnexal mass.

Microscopic features

All cases have shown inflammatory infiltrates very specifically directed at follicular cells. The infiltrates consist of lymphocytes and plasma cells, or more rarely show a granulomatous and eosinophilic reaction (Lewis 1993), directed at follicular cells as well (Figs 19.9, 19.10).

The usual histological pattern is that of a lymphoplasmacytic infiltrate in close apposition to the theca interna of developing follicles – the more advanced the follicles, the denser the inflammatory infiltrate and the greater the preponderance of plasma cells. The granulosa of affected follicles is only focally and sparsely infiltrated by inflammatory cells, but secondary degenerative features, such as hydropic change and apoptosis, may be observed. The follicular fluid contains few, if any, inflammatory cells (Figs 19.11–19.14). Primordial follicles are apparently entirely spared this process. With atresia of developing follicles, the inflammatory infiltrate subsides to some extent, though rarely completely (Fig. 19.15). Dysplastic follicles may also be seen (Fig. 19.16), similar to those described in the resistant ovary syndrome (see Ch. 8). If ovulation occurs, corpora lutea, both granulosa and theca lutein layers, are heavily infiltrated by lymphocytes and plasma cells; focal necrosis may be present (Figs 19.17, 19.18); the infiltrate is occasionally predominantly eosinophilic (Fig. 19.19). Immunohistochemical characteriza-

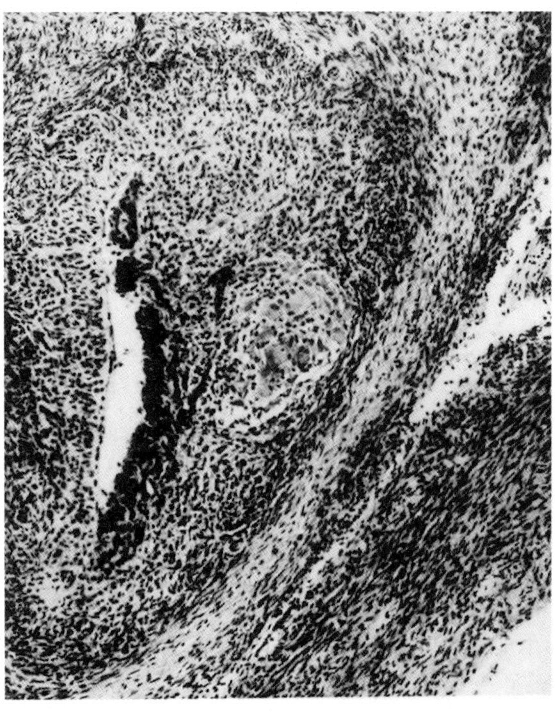

Fig. 19.9 Chronic oophoritis in an 18-year-old girl with premature ovarian failure. Perifolliculitis which includes a well-formed, sarcoid-like granuloma. H + E ×90. (Reproduced, with permission, from Russell et al 1982)

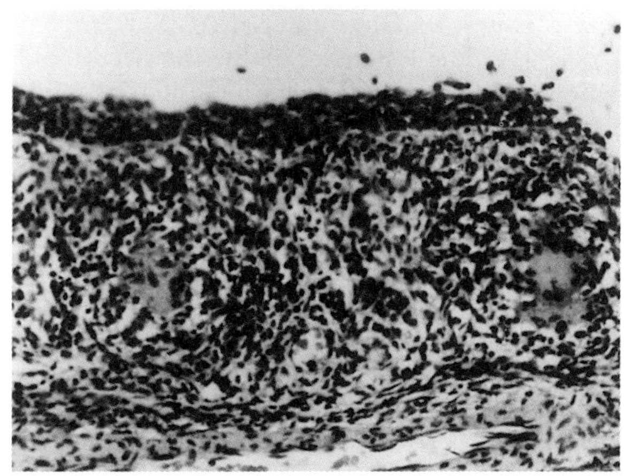

A

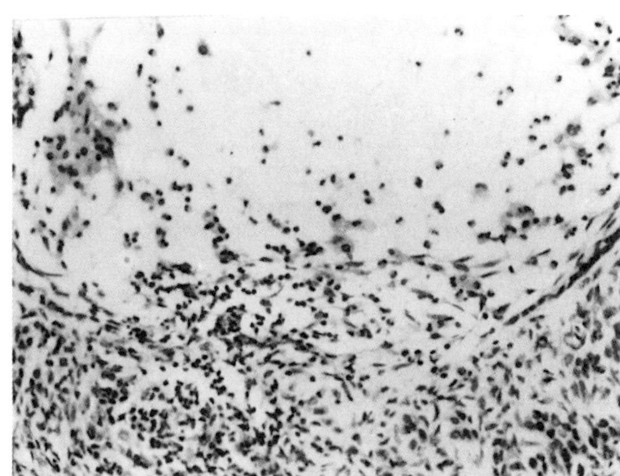

B

Fig. 19.10 Same case as in Fig 19.9. (A) Follicle with infiltrate consisting of lymphocytes and histiocytes, some multinucleated, in theca. Granulosa is relatively unaffected. H + E ×160. (B) Follicle with disruption of theca and granulosa by infiltrate which includes numerous eosinophils. Multinucleated histiocyte at left. H + E ×160

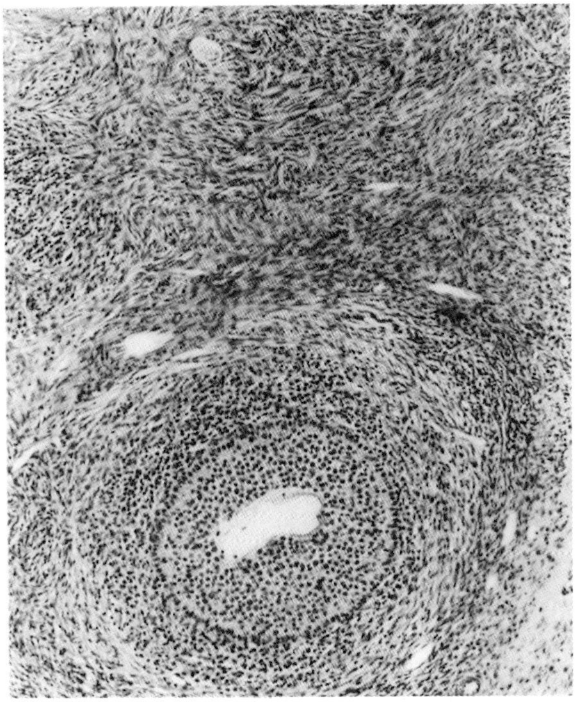

Fig. 19.11 Chronic autoimmune oophoritis. Primary follicle (with disrupted zona pellucida) cuffed by an inflammatory infiltrate in the theca interna. Normal primordial follicle above. A few lymphocytes are present close to an atretic follicle (below right) and another follicular structure (out of picture) at left. Stroma elsewhere is not infiltrated. H + E ×80

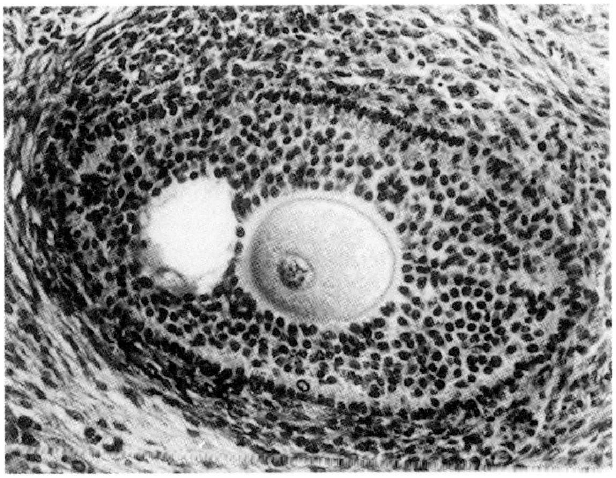

Fig. 19.12 Lymphoplasmacytic infiltrate surrounding otherwise normal early antral follicle. H + E ×200

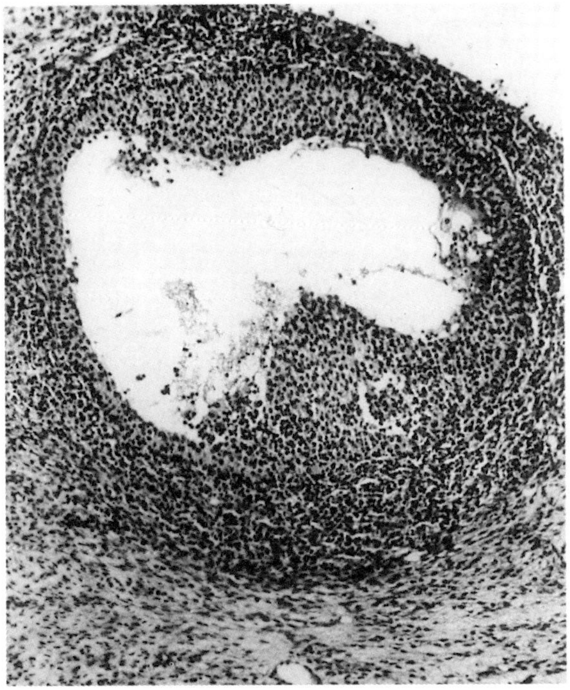

Fig. 19.13 Antral follicle with heavy chronic inflammatory infiltrate in theca and lighter infiltrate in granulosa which appears degenerate especially in region of cumulus oophorus. Follicular fluid contains fibrin and a few inflammatory cells. H + E ×80

tion of the infiltrate in one case has revealed a mixture of B cells (including plasma cells), T cells (both T4+ and T8+), macrophages, and a few natural killer cells (Sedmak et al 1987). The cystic structures seen macroscopically are generally developing follicles or involuting corpora lutea. They are most likely due to elevated levels of pituitary gonadotrophins (Biscotti et al 1989). The intervening stroma is unremarkable.

ARTERITIS

Arteritis is rarely encountered in ovarian specimens. In most cases, it is an incidental finding, but in some it has called attention to previously undiagnosed systemic disease. Pathological varieties which have been reported are necrotising arteritis, giant cell arteritis and polyarteritis nodosa. Classification depends on the size of vessels involved, the presence or absence of fibrinoid necrosis, and the nature of the inflammatory

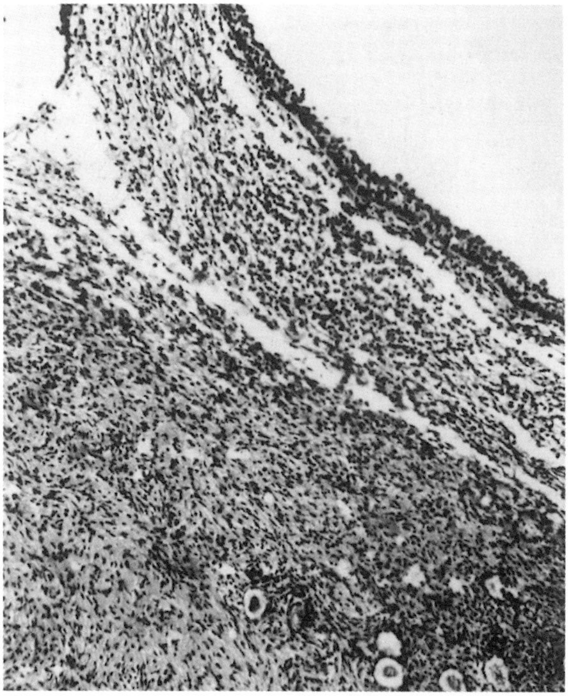

Fig. 19.14 Cystic follicle with moderate chronic inflammatory cell infiltrate in theca. Numerous primordial follicles (without associated inflammation) in cortical stroma below. H + E ×90 (Reproduced, with permission, from International Journal of Gynaecological Pathology)

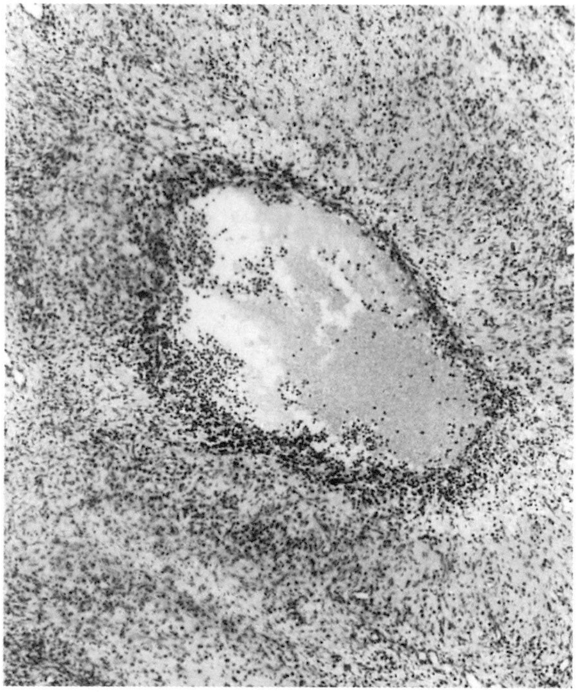

Fig. 19.15 Atretic follicle with diffuse lymphoplasmacytic infiltrate. H + E ×64

infiltrate, especially with respect to giant cells and eosinophils.

Necrotizing arteritis

A small proportion of patients with necrotizing arteritis suffer from a systemic connective tissue disorder such as lupus erythematosus, while others give a history of drug therapy, especially penicillin, suggesting an allergic basis to the lesion (Wilansky et al 1980). A solitary case of a necrotizing vasculitis following in vitro fertilization (Ilbery et al 1991) has been reported which was associated with a major intra-abdominal hemorrhage. In the majority, however, no underlying cause can be identified, and these appear to be cases of idiopathic isolated visceral necrotizing vasculitis, similar to that first described in the appendix by Plaut (1932). Further investigation and follow-up of asymptomatic patients with uterine and adnexal involvement has been unrewarding in uncovering systemic disease (Ansell et al 1974, Wilansky et al 1980).

Medium-sized arteries and arterioles are affected (Fig. 19.20). The most striking feature is fibrinoid necrosis of the media with some associated disruption of the internal elastic lamina. Fibrin is often seen in the lumen, but thrombosis and tissue infarction do not occur. An inflammatory infiltrate, chiefly lymphocytic, is present throughout the vessel wall and adventitia. Neutrophils and eosinophils, but not giant cells, may be present in small numbers. If eosinophils are prominent, the possibility of polyarteritis nodosa should be considered (see below).

Giant cell arteritis

Classical giant cell arteritis affects large and medium-sized arteries, especially the temporal and intracranial vessels. Less commonly, giant cell arteritis affects smaller arteries and arterioles, and this variant may be either disseminated or anatomically restricted (Lie 1978). In the latter

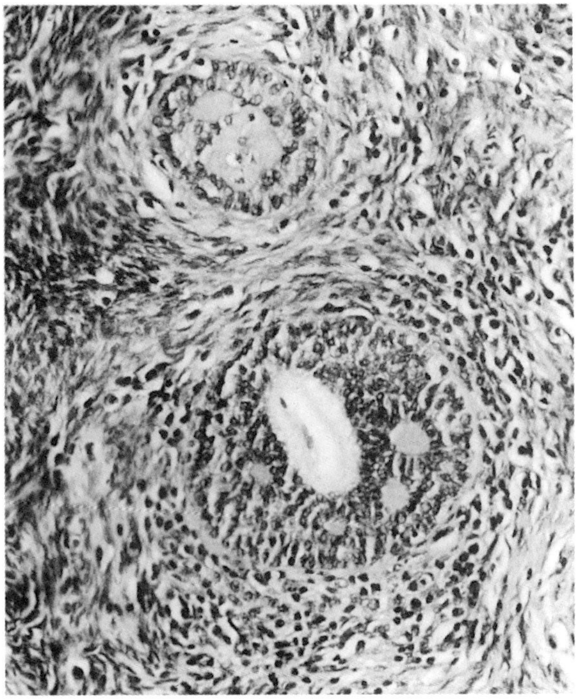

Fig. 19.16 Dysplastic primary follicles in auto-immune oophoritis. Nodules of hyaline material becoming confluent in upper follicle. Lower follicle resembles structures seen in sex cord tumors with annular tubules. H + E ×200

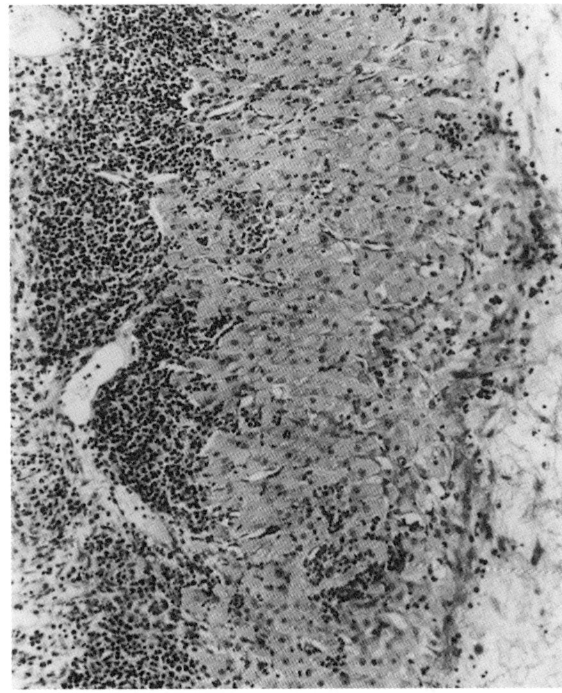

Fig. 19.17 Autoimmune oophoritis from a 48-year-old woman with menorrhagia; past history of Addison's and Hashimoto's disease. Fresh corpus luteum with inflammatory infiltrate involving chiefly theca lutein layer. Only sparse inflammatory cells in central coagulum at right. H + E ×50

group, the female genital organs are commonly involved, including the ovaries in about half of these (Pirozynski 1976, Petrides et al 1979, Bell et al 1986, Lhote et al 1992). All the reported cases have been in postmenopausal women, of whom about one-half suffered from polymyalgia rheumatica. In asymptomatic women, in whom the diagnosis is an incidental finding, treatment appears to be unnecessary (Bell et al 1986, Summers et al 1991).

Small arteries and arterioles show random segmental involvement. There is intimal edema and fibrosis which results in luminal narrowing. The media is expanded by a granulomatous inflammatory infiltrate consisting of lymphocytes and histiocytes, some epithelioid, and multinucleated giant cells. There is destruction of elastic fibers, especially in the internal elastic lamina. Inflammatory cells, mainly lymphocytes, extend into the intima and adventitia. Eosinophils are conspicuous by their absence. Fibrinoid necrosis and thromboses are rarely seen.

Polyarteritis nodosa

The female genital tract, including the ovaries, may be involved in polyarteritis nodosa (Patalano & Sommers 1961) and, rarely, is the source of tissue in which the diagnosis is first made (Lombard et al 1986). Radiographic demonstration of microaneurysms, which have a predilection for arterial bifurcations, is important in confirming the diagnosis. Medium and small sized arteries are affected; they show fibrinoid necrosis and an acute, predominantly eosinophilic, inflammatory infiltrate. In older lesions, lymphocytes and plasma cells are also present. Thromboses may develop, and these may result in infarction of distal tissues.

PUERPERAL OVARIAN VEIN THROMBOPHLEBITIS

Puerperal ovarian vein thrombophlebitis and

A 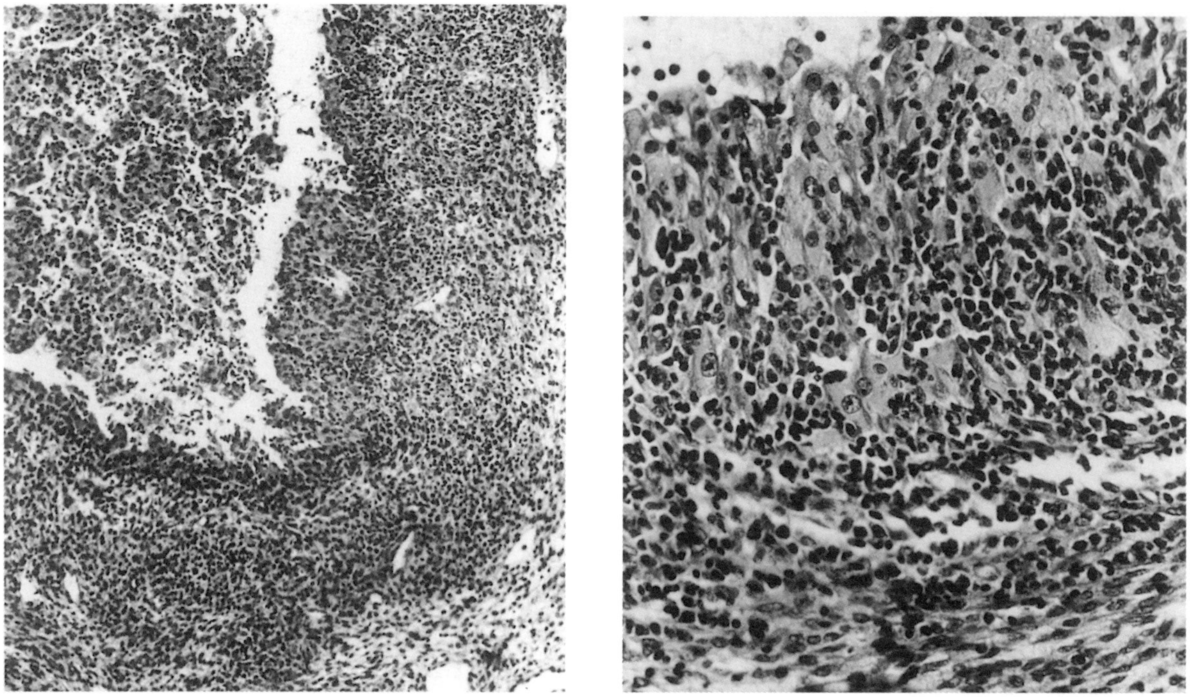 B

Fig. 19.18 Autoimmune oophoritis in 26-year-old woman with secondary infertility. (A) Heavy inflammatory infiltrate in wall of fresh corpus luteum with disruption and sloughing of granulosa cells. H + E ×80. (B) Detail of lymphoplasmacytic infiltrate involving both granulosa and theca lutein layers. H + E ×200

thrombosis is rarely encountered by the pathologist because standard management does not include oophorectomy. The condition has been reported to complicate one in 600 deliveries (Brown & Munsick 1971) and, less frequently, abortions (Gardstein et al 1973, Allan et al 1976, Adachi et al 1984). It is part of the spectrum of pelvic thrombophlebitis, but selective involvement of the ovarian veins makes the condition clinically distinct from nonpuerperal cases, in which the uterine and iliac veins are predominantly affected. The condition is considered by some to be infective, with the primary source being the placental bed; positive bacterial cultures from the ovarian veins have been obtained in a few cases (Munsick & Gillanders 1981). Postpartum hypercoagulability, together with dilatation and stasis,

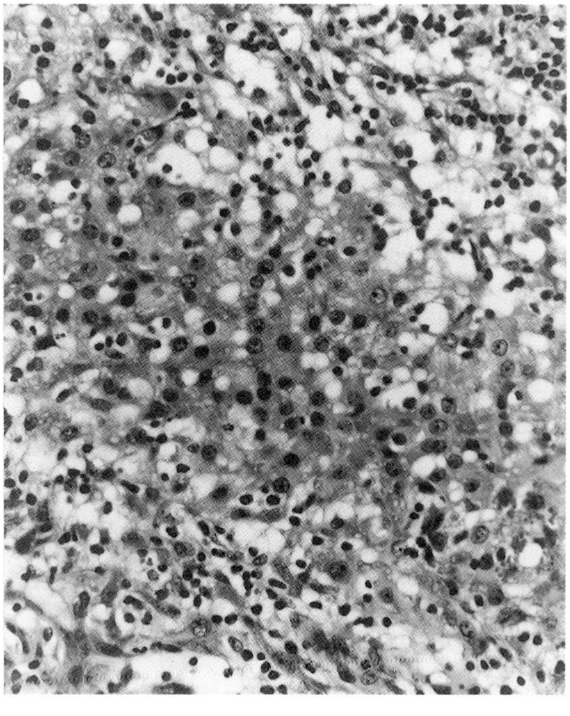

Fig. 19.19 Autoimmune oophoritis in which the inflammatory infiltrate concentrated at the margins of the granulosa lutein layer contains mostly eosinophils rather than plasma cells. H + E ×116. (Material courtesy of Dr J Lewis, Perth)

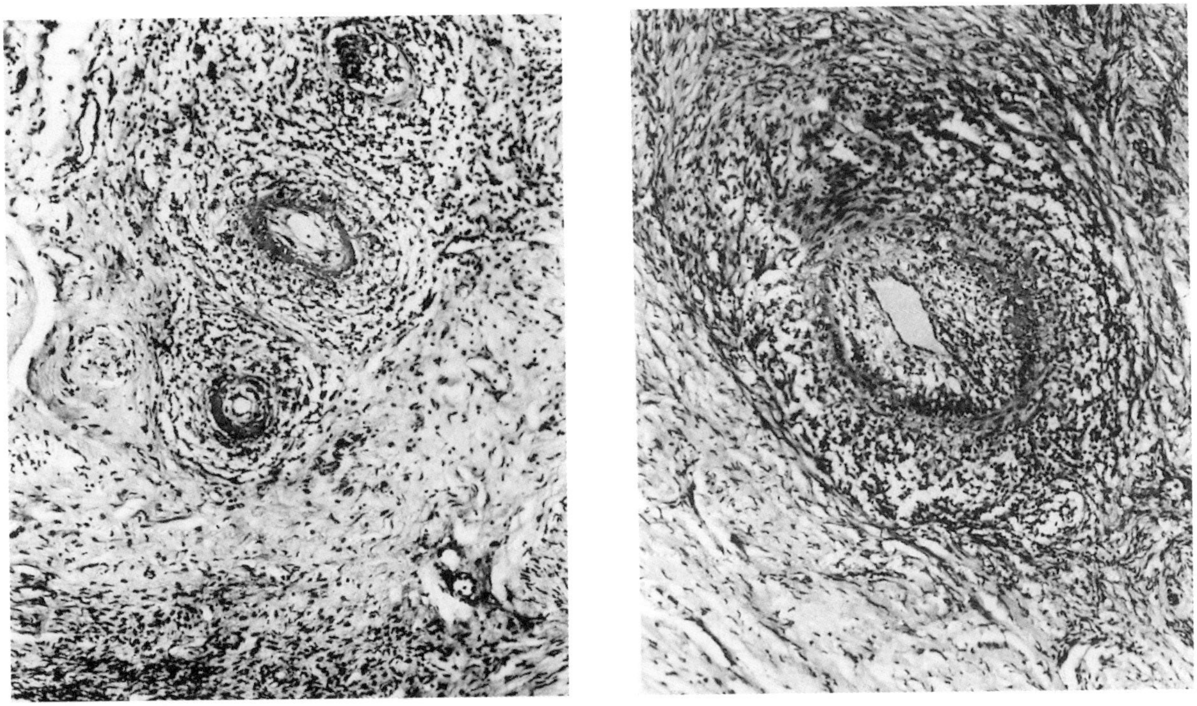

A B

Fig. 19.20 Isolated necrotising arteritis. Incidental finding in an ovary which also contained a small Brenner tumor. No evidence of systemic vasculitis. (A) Small artery showing conspicuous fibrinoid necrosis and transmural infiltrate of lymphocytes and polymorphs. H + E ×80. (B) Larger vessel showing less conspicuous fibrinoid necrosis, but prominent intimal fibrosis. H + E ×80

potentiate thrombosis in the inflamed veins. Peculiarities in ovarian venous blood flow postpartum (antegrade on the right, but retrograde on the left) result in preferential spread of infection to the right side (Munsick & Gillanders 1981). Amniotic fluid embolism has also been described in one case (Kern & Duff 1981).

The usual presentation is with severe lower abdominal pain and fever 2 or 3 days postpartum. Physical examination reveals a tender rope-like mass extending laterally and cephalad from the uterine cornu, but the physical findings may be insignificant. The right side is involved in 90% of unilateral cases, and 14% of all cases are bilateral (Munsick & Gillanders 1981). Venography, ultrasonography, and computer-assisted tomographic scanning (see Ch. 58) have been used to facilitate noninvasive diagnosis (Khurana et al 1988, Baka et al 1989). The preferred treatment is heparinization and antibiotic therapy but, if this is unsuccessful after 3–5 days, operative intervention (ovarian vein ligation) is indicated (Hughey et al 1979, Munsick & Gillanders 1981, Tang et al 1985). Pulmonary embolism is a rare complication, but has proved fatal in four reported cases (Munsick & Gillanders 1981).

At laparotomy, the thrombosed ovarian veins are markedly enlarged (up to 10 cm in diameter), tortuous, tense, and firm; thrombus sometimes extends into the ovaries. The inferior vena cava, left renal vein or both may be involved in continuity. The ovaries and fallopian tubes are dark and congested, but their viability is not usually compromised and reports of infarction are rare (Gardstein et al 1973, Munsick & Gillanders 1981). The ovarian veins, if available for histological examination, show thrombophlebitis (Munsick & Gillanders 1981).

REFERENCES

Adachi A, Segan J, Li J K H 1984 Ovarian vein thrombosis mimicking ectopic pregnancy. New York State Journal of Medicine 84: 567–568

Al Dawoud, Yates R, Foulis A K 1991 Post-operative necrotizing granulomas in the ovary. Journal of Clinical Pathology 44: 524–525

Allan T R, Miller G C II, Wabrek A J, Burchell R C 1976 Postpartum and postabortal ovarian vein thrombophlebitis. Obstetrics and Gynecology 47: 525–528

Ansell I D, Evans D J, Wight D G D 1974 Asymptomatic arteritis of the uterine cervix. Journal of Clinical Pathology 27: 664–668

Baka J J, Leu-Toaff A S, Friedman A C et al 1989 Ovarian vein thrombosis with atypical presentation. Role of sonography and duplex doppler. Obstetrics and Gynecology 73: 887–889

Bannatyne P, Russell P, Shearman R P 1990 Auto-immune oophoritis: a clinicopathologic assessment of 12 cases. International Journal of Gynecological Pathology 9: 191–207

Bell D A, Mondschein M, Scully R E 1986 Giant cell arteritis of the female genital tract. A report of three cases. American Journal of Surgical Pathology 10: 696–701

Benirschke K, Bonin M L, Rost T 1984 Plant material in ovary following barium enema. Archives of Pathology and Laboratory Medicine 108: 359–360

Biscotti C V, Hart W R, Lucas J G 1989 Cystic ovarian enlargement resulting from auto-immune oophoritis. Obstetrics and Gynecology 74: 492–495

Boss J H, Scully R E, Wegner K H, Cohen R B 1965 Structural alterations in the adult ovary – clinical significance. Obstetrics and Gynecology 25: 747–764

Brooks J J, Wheeler J E 1977 Granulomatous salpingitis secondary to Crohn's disease. Obstetrics and Gynecology 49: 31s–33s

Brown T K, Munsick R A 1971 Puerperal ovarian vein thrombophlebitis: A syndrome. American Journal of Obstetrics and Gynecology 109: 263–273

Chalvardjian A 1978 Sarcoidosis of the female genital tract. American Journal of Obstetrics and Gynecology 132: 78–80

Chen K T K, Kostich N D, Rosai J 1978 Peritoneal foreign body granulomas to keratin in uterine adenoacanthoma. Archives of Pathology and Laboratory Medicine 102: 174–177

Cox K R 1970 Starch granuloma (pseudo-malignant seedlings). British Journal of Surgery 57: 650–653

Davies J D, Neely J 1972 The histopathology of peritoneal starch granulomas. Journal of Pathology 107: 265–278

Donaldson L B 1978 Crohn's disease: 'its gynecologic aspect'. American Journal of Obstetrics and Gynecology 131: 196–202

Evans C S, Goldman R L, Klein H Z, Kohout N D 1984 Necrobiotic granulomas of the uterine cervix. A probable postoperative reaction. American Journal of Surgical Pathology 8: 841–844

Frost S S, Elstein M P, Latour F, Roth J L A 1981 Crohn's disease of the mouth and ovary. Digestive Diseases and Sciences 26: 568–571

Gardstein H F, Ferenczy A, Richart R M 1973 Asymptomatic bilateral ovarian infarction and venous thrombosis. American Journal of Obstetrics and Gynecology 11: 1164–1166

Gloor E, Hurlimann J 1984 Autoimmune oophoritis. American Journal of Clinical Pathology 81: 105–109

Herbold D R, Frable W J, Kraus F T 1984 Isolated non-infectious granulomas of the ovary. International Journal of Gynecological Pathology 2: 380–391

Hertig A T1944 The aging ovary – a preliminary note. Journal of Clinical Endocrinology 4: 581–582

Ho K L 1979 Sarcoidosis of the uterus. Human Pathology 10: 219–222

Honoré L H 1981 Combined suppurative and noncaseating granulomatous oophoritis associated with distal ileitis (Crohn's disease). European Journal of Obstetrics, Gynecology and Reproductive Biology 12: 91–94

Hughesdon P E 1976 The endometrial identity of benign stromatosis of the ovary and its relation to other forms of endometriosis. Journal of Pathology 119: 201–209

Hughey M, McElin T W, Caprini J A 1979 Nonsurgical diagnosis and management of puerperal ovarian vein thrombophlebitis. American Journal of Obstetrics and Gynecology 133: 461–463

Ilbery M, Lyons B, Sundaresan V 1991 Ovarian necrotizing vasculitis causing major intra-abdominal haemorrhage after IVF. British Journal of Obstetrics and Gynaecology 98: 596–569

Kern S B, Duff P 1981 Localized amniotic fluid embolism presenting as ovarian vein thrombosis and refactory post-operative fever. American Journal of Clinical Pathology 76: 476–480

Kernohan N M, Best P V, Janial V, Kitchener H C 1991 Palisading granuloma of the ovary. Histopathology 19: 279–280

Khurana B K, Rao J, Friedman S A, Cho K C 1988 Computed tomographic features of puerperal ovarian vein thrombosis. American Journal of Obstetrics and Gynecology 159: 905–908

Kim K R, Scully R E 1990 Peritoneal keratin granulomas with carcinomas of endometrium and ovary and atypical polypoid adenomyoma of endometrium. A clinicopathologic analysis of 22 cases. American Journal of Surgical Pathology 14: 925–932

Lewis J 1993 Eosinophilic perifolliculitis: a variant of autoimmune oophoritis? International Journal of Gynecological Pathology 12: 360–364

Lhote F, Mainguere C, Grische-Wiseler V, Fior R, Feintuch M J, Royer I 1992 Giant cell arteritis of the female genital tract with temporal arteritis. Annals of Rheumatoid Disease 51: 900–903

Lie J T 1978 Disseminated visceral giant cell arteritis. Histopathologic description and differentiation from other granulomatous vasculitides. American Journal of Clinical Pathology 69: 299–305

Lombard C M, Moore M H, Seifer D B 1986 Diagnosis of systemic polyarteritis nodosa following total abdominal hysterectomy and bilateral salpingo-oohorectomy: A case report. International Journal of Gynecological Pathology 5: 63–68

Lonsdale R N, Roberts P F, Trowell J E 1991 Auto-immune oophoritis associated with polycystic ovaries. Histopathology 19: 77–81

Mostafa S A M, Bargeron C B, Flower R W, Rosenshein N B, Parmley T H, Woodruff J D 1985 Foreign body granulomas in normal ovaries. Obstetrics and Gynecology 66: 701–702

Munsick R A, Gillanders L A 1981 A review of the syndrome of puerperal ovarian vein thrombophlebitis. Obstetrical and Gynecological Survey 36: 57–66

Nissim F, Ashkenazy M, Borenstein R, Czernobilsky B 1981 Tuberculoid cornstarch granulomas with caseous necrosis. A diagnostic challenge. Archives of Pathology and Laboratory Medicine 105: 86–88

Patalano V J, Sommers S C 1961 Biopsy diagnosis of polyarteritis nodosa. Archives of Pathology 72: 1–7

Petrides M, Robertson I G, Fox H 1979 Giant cell arteritis of the female genital tract. British Journal of Obstetrics and Gynaecology 86: 148–151

Pirozynski W J 1976 Giant cell arteritis of the uterus. Report of two cases. American Journal of Clinical Pathology 65: 308–313

Plaut A 1932 Focal arteriolitis. American Journal of Pathology 8: 620–621

Roddick J W, Greene R R 1958 The relation of nonmalignant postmenopausal endometrial changes to ovarian morphology. American Journal of Obstetrics and Gynecology 75: 235–239

Russell P, Bannatyne P, Shearman R P, Fraser I S, Corbett P 1982 Premature hypergonadotropic ovarian failure: clinicopathological study of 19 cases. International Journal of Gynecological Pathology 1: 185–201

Sedmak D D, Hart W R, Tubbs R R 1987 Autoimmune oophoritis: a histopathologic study of involved ovaries with immunologic characterization of the mononuclear cell infiltrate. International Journal of Gynecological Pathology 6: 73–81

Sommers S C 1983 Female genital tract granulomas. In: Ioachim H L (ed) Pathology of granulomas. Raven Press, New York, p 395–409

Soules M R, Spadoni L R 1982 Oil versus aqueous media for hysterosalpingography; a continuing debate based on many opinions and few facts. Fertility and Sterility 38: 1–11

Summers P R, Biswas M K, Boulware D W, Green L, Herrera E H, O'Quinn A G 1991 A case report of giant cell arteritis of the uterus and adnexa. American Journal of Obstetrics and Gynecology 164: 540–542

Tang L C H, Woo J S K, Choo Y C 1985 Puerperal ovarian vein thrombophlebitis. Postgraduate Medical Journal 61: 179–180

Trimble E L, Saigo P E, Frieberg G W, Rubin S C, Hoskins W J 1991 Peritoneal sarcoidosis and elevated Ca 125. Obstetrics and Gynecology 78: 976–977

Wilansky R, MacLean J N, Miro R et al 1980 Necrotising vasculitis in gynecological surgery. European Journal of Obstetrics, Gynecology and Reproductive Biology 10: 401–406

Winslow R C, Funkhouser J W 1968 Sarcoidosis of the female reproductive organs. Report of a case. Obstetrics and Gynecology 32: 285–289

Wlordarski F M, Trainer T D 1975 Granulomatous oophoritis and salpingitis associated with Crohn's disease of the appendix. American Journal of Obstetrics and Gynecology 122: 527–528

SECTION 4

Mullerianosis and surface proliferative lesions

20

Mullerianosis and reactive mesothelial lesions

MULLERIANOSIS

There is no widely accepted generic term for the various manifestations of mullerian-directed metaplasias and non-neoplastic proliferations (both epithelial and mesenchymal) which can be identified on, and immediately beneath, the ovarian surface, the pelvic peritoneum, and omentum, and in retroperitoneal lymph nodes. 'Endometriosis' is the established term for the lesions in this group which exhibit endometrial epithelium and stroma. 'Endosalpingiosis' describes lesions composed of tubal epithelium and, similarly, 'endocervicosis' indicates the rare but analogous mucinous epithelial lesions. 'Mullerian or paramesonephric metaplasia', 'benign glandular inclusions', 'inclusion cysts', 'benign tubular lesions', and 'implants' (if associated with ovarian carcinoma) are some other terms in current usage. Lauchlan (1972, 1994) has used the term 'secondary mullerian system' to refer to all mullerian-type epithelium (including endometriotic lesions) located outside the cavities of the original mullerian ducts. 'Mullerianosis' (Bassis 1960) is a simple term, sufficiently descriptive of the spectrum of differentiation seen in these lesions to justify wider use, and will be adopted in this text.

The pathogenesis of these lesions is unclear. Metaplasia is an appropriate term only if it is accepted that, in the development of these lesions, one adult tissue, i.e. ovarian surface epithelium (or pelvic mesothelium), is replaced by another type, e.g. mucinous epithelium. Acknowledging that this transformation may proceed via intermediate undifferentiated or stem cells (Lugo & Putong 1984), 'metaplasia' is probably the best term available. The undifferentiated cells involved in the genesis of mullerianosis are those of the subcoelomic mesenchyme, which contributes substantially to the embryogenesis of the mullerian ducts but is inapparent in postnatal life. Thus, the pelvic and abdominal peritoneum retain a potential for mullerian differentiation conditioned by their embryonic origin. This potential is greatest in the ovaries and decreases with increasing distance from them (Lauchlan 1972, 1994).

A dysontogenetic origin cannot be excluded. It is possible that embryonic cell rests are present in the observed anatomical distribution of mullerianosis and are stimulated after puberty in a manner akin to that of acquired common skin naevi – an analogy we find entirely appropriate given their natural history and premalignant potential.

Mullerianosis is generally considered to be acquired; the lesions have not been described in premenarcheal girls (Blaustein et al 1982). It is likely that the lesions are induced by changes in the hormonal milieu which follow puberty. The additional factors which cause a small proportion of women to develop florid mullerianosis (endometriosis and/or endosalpingiosis) are unknown. As well as being hormonally induced, the lesions show variable hormone dependence and sensitivity. The most obvious example of hormone sensitivity is endometriosis, and is responsible for its spectacular pathology and clinical manifestations. Mullerianotic lesions (including endometriosis) atrophy after the menopause and may eventually degenerate and be resorbed (Tutscha & Lauchlan 1980, Zinsser & Wheeler 1982). There is anecdotal evidence of regression of extraovarian endosalpingiotic lesions after oophorectomy, but whether this effect is coincidental, due to alteration of the hormonal environment or removal of the 'influence of the parent tumor', is unclear (Burmeister et al 1969).

Our experience is that mullerianosis, especially endosalpingiosis, is a very common incidental finding in gynecological specimens and that, if specifically sought by careful macroscopic examination and multiple blocks, it could be identified in most, if not all, women at one or more sites in the parietal or visceral pelvic peritoneum, especially on the ovarian surfaces. An attempt to assess the incidence of endosalpingiosis was made by Zinsser & Wheeler (1982), who prospectively studied omenta from surgical and autopsy material in both women and men; lesions were found only in surgically removed omenta from females (in 25.7% of cases) and were never identified in men.

Despite its frequency, mullerianosis cannot be considered physiological. The adverse clinical complications of endometriosis are well known. In addition, and perhaps more importantly, all mullerianotic lesions have the potential to develop neoplasia if they are the target of carcinogenic influences (Czernobilsky & Lancet 1972, Parmley & Woodruff 1974, Scully 1979). The surface epithelial–stromal tumors are generally considered to arise ultimately from the surface epithelium of the ovary; Scully (1979) states that their origin is specifically from the metaplastic epithelium of inclusion cysts.

Ovarian mullerianosis involves not only simple metaplastic transformation of surface epithelium, but also the formation of papillae, cysts, and tubules (Burmeister et al 1969, Tutscha & Lauchlan 1980). The latter may result from passive invaginations caused by traction, similar to the mechanism described below for the formation of cortical inclusion cysts. Alternatively, the metaplastic epithelium may grow spontaneously in these tubular forms in a manner observed experimentally in rabbit surface epithelial cell cultures (Nicosia et al 1985). In addition to occurring *de novo* on the ovarian surface, mullerian metaplasia may also develop in ovarian cortical inclusion cysts and mesothelial cysts (discussed below), and these occurrences can be considered to be within the spectrum of 'mullerianosis'.

The most common type of epithelial differentiation is tubal, perhaps reflecting the fact that this is the prototypic mullerian epithelium. Endometrial epithelial differentiation, without the appearance of stroma, is also frequent. Mucinous and clear cell forms are very uncommon, and have been reported only on the ovaries. Transitional cell or urothelial metaplasia (Walthard's rests) cannot strictly be considered to be a form of mullerian differentiation, but is discussed here for convenience because it is known to occur within the fallopian tubes and cervix (Egan & Russell 1996A,B), and, like the various forms of mullerianosis, is the probable precursor of one type of surface epithelial–stromal neoplasm – the transitional cell or Brenner tumor.

The spectrum of mullerianosis which involves the ovary includes not only epithelial metaplasias but also mesenchymal and mixed forms. Endometriosis, an example of the latter, is discussed fully in Chapter 21. A schema indicating the potential paths of mullerian differentiation (both metaplastic and neoplastic) is given in Table 20.1.

Epithelial metaplasias

The simplest histological form of ovarian mullerianosis is focal metaplasia of the single-layered surface epithelium without any architectural reorganization. However, mullerianosis more often presents as superficial cortical tubules or cysts, sometimes clustered, surrounded by prominent basement membranes (Figs 20.1, 20.2). Similar lesions may result from epithelial metaplasia in cortical inclusion cysts (see below). The most common epithelial type is serous or tubal; endometrial and endocervical types are less frequently observed, while clear cell, transitional cell

Table 20.1 Classification of mullerianosis with corresponding mullerian neoplasms

Mullerianosis (metaplasia)	Mullerian tumors (neoplasia)
Epithelial	
Tubal (endosalpingiosis)	Serous
Endometrial	Endometrioid
Endocervical (endocervicosis)	Mucinous
Clear cell	Clear cell
Squamous	Squamous
Mesothelial	Mesothelial
Transitional cells (Walthard's rests)	Brenner, transitional cell
Mesenchymal	
Endometrial stromal (deciduosis)	Endometrial stromal
Smooth muscle (Leiomymatosis peritoneales dissemineta)	Smooth muscle
Epithelial/mesenchymal	
Endometrial/stromal (endometriosis)	Mixed mullerian

(Walthard's rests) and squamous metaplasia are rare. The lining epithelium, especially if tubal, may show papillary infoldings covered by a single, sometimes pseudostratified, layer of epithelial cells (Fig. 20.3).

Endosalpingiotic foci may exhibit epithelial proliferation considered to be in excess of that expected in benign lesions, and the criteria used for their assessment are the same as those used for serous tumors in general (see Ch. 23). Psammoma bodies (calcospherites) are commonly present, and may be in continuity with the epithelium or lie apparently free in the lumen or in the adjacent ovarian stroma (Figs 20.2, 20.3). The lesions are not associated with mesothelial reactions, adhesions or inflammation, apart from occasional lymphocytes.

Papillations are exophytic mullerianotic lesions

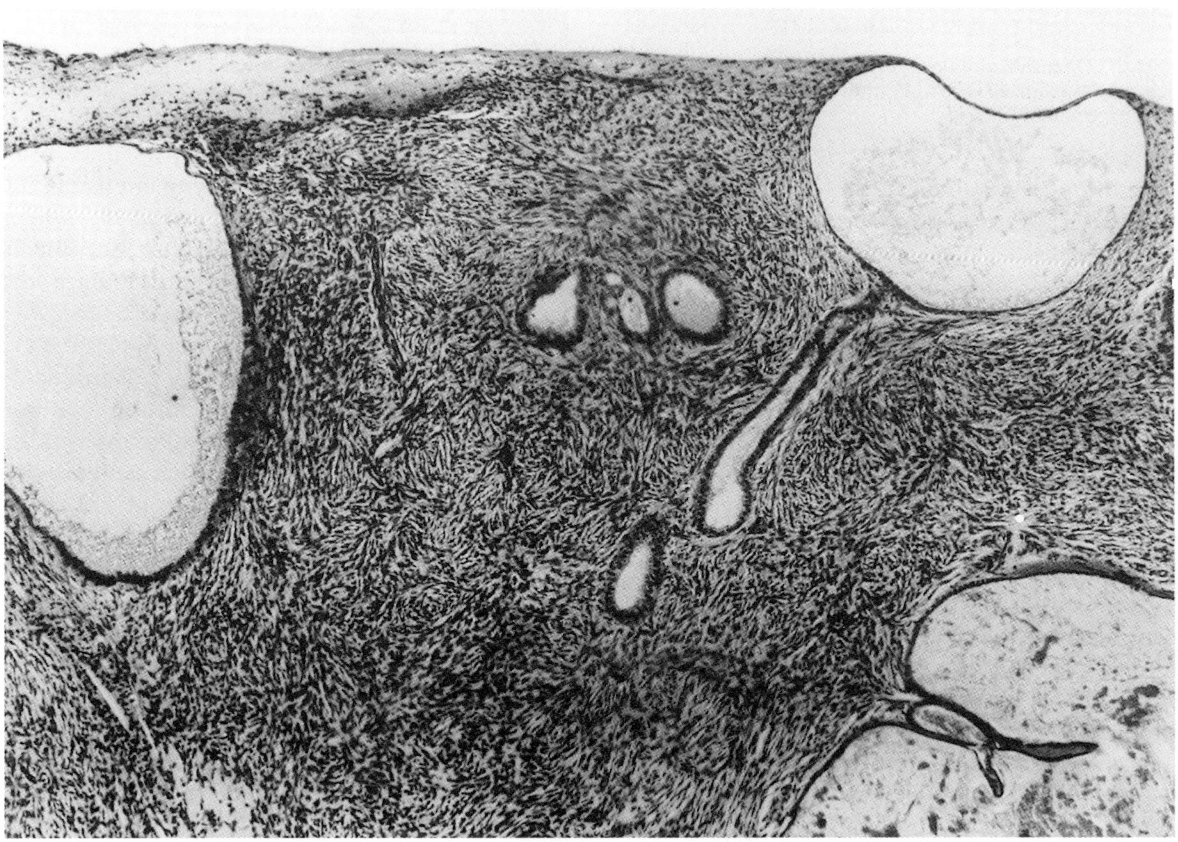

Fig. 20.1 Ovarian mullerianosis in a postmenopausal woman. The tubular structures are lined by tubal epithelium but the lining of the cysts is too attenuated for identification. H + E ×80

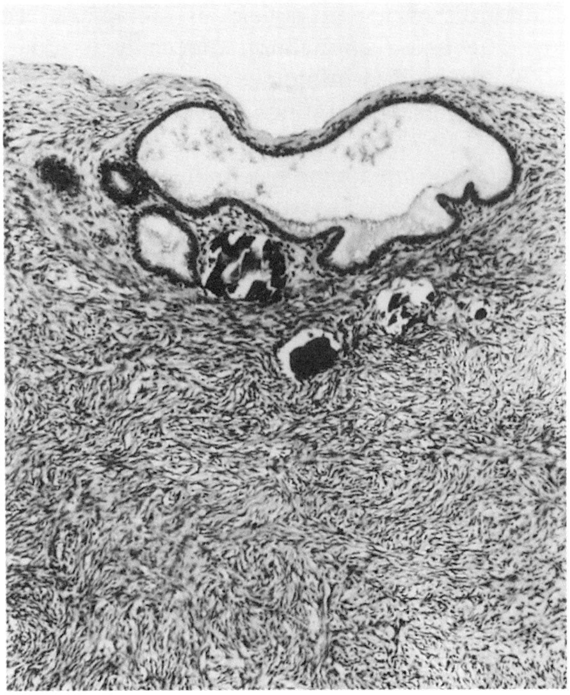

Fig. 20.2 Ovarian endosalpingiosis. Cluster of epithelial structures in superficial cortex. Psammoma bodies in adjacent stroma. H + E ×80

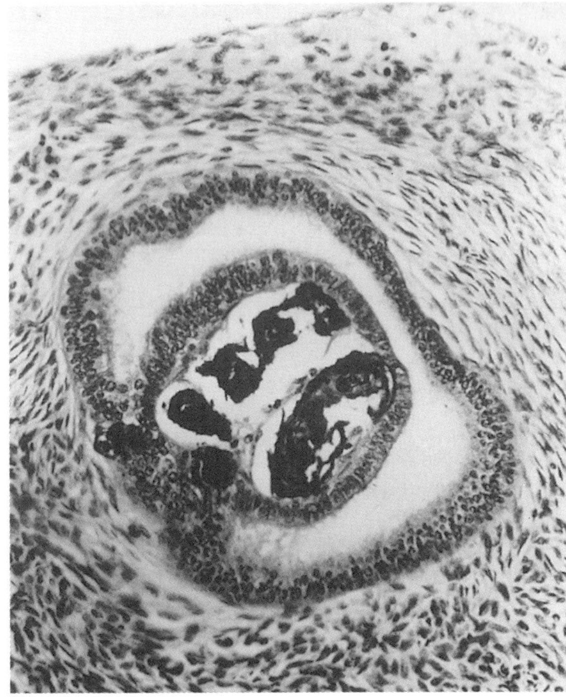

Fig. 20.3 Ovarian endosalpingiosis. This lesion displays an epithelial infolding with subjacent psammoma bodies. The epithelium is ciliated. H + E ×200

most often encountered in peri- or post-menopausal ovaries. They are, by convention only, smaller than 1 cm in maximum dimension; most larger lesions qualify as serous adenofibromas, serous papillomas, or papillary mesotheliomas (see Chs 23, 31). They are wart-like excrescences with similar color and texture to ovarian cortical tissue, but sometimes firmer. They have a papillary structure with a broad base (Fig. 20.4). The relatively thick papillae are composed of dense fibrous tissue covered by a single layer of cytologically benign small cuboidal cells resembling those of ovarian surface epithelium, mesothelium, or tubal mucosa (Fig. 20.5).

An important differential diagnosis is between endosalpingiosis and metastatic serous carcinoma (Coffin et al 1985). Deposits of metastatic carcinoma have infiltrative margins, lack peripheral basement membranes, and are associated with mesothelial proliferations or desmoplastic stromal reactions. Carcinoma, although sometimes forming glandular or tubular structures, lacks the orderly cellular arrangements of endosalpingiosis. Nuclear atypia and mitotic activity are usual, and focal necrosis may be observed. Cilia are unlikely to be encountered in serous carcinoma, but are common in endosalpingiosis; psammoma bodies can be expected in both entities.

Walthard's rests are very commonly observed on or beneath the tubal serosa but are less frequently found on the ovaries. They can be observed macroscopically, usually near the hilus, as 1–2 mm translucent nodules or blebs which contain clear fluid. Histologically, they consist of subserosal groups of epithelial cells with distinct cell margins, clear cytoplasm, and ovoid nuclei which often have longitudinal grooves ('coffee bean' nuclei). The cellular groups often have eccentrically located lumens, and these are sometimes lined by mucinous epithelial cells (Fig. 20.6). *Squamous metaplasia* may be observed (Fig. 20.6B). No local reactive features are present. Ultrastructural studies show close similarities between the cells comprising Walthard's rests and native transitional cells, and there is also a histogenetic relationship with transitional cell tumors (see Ch. 28).

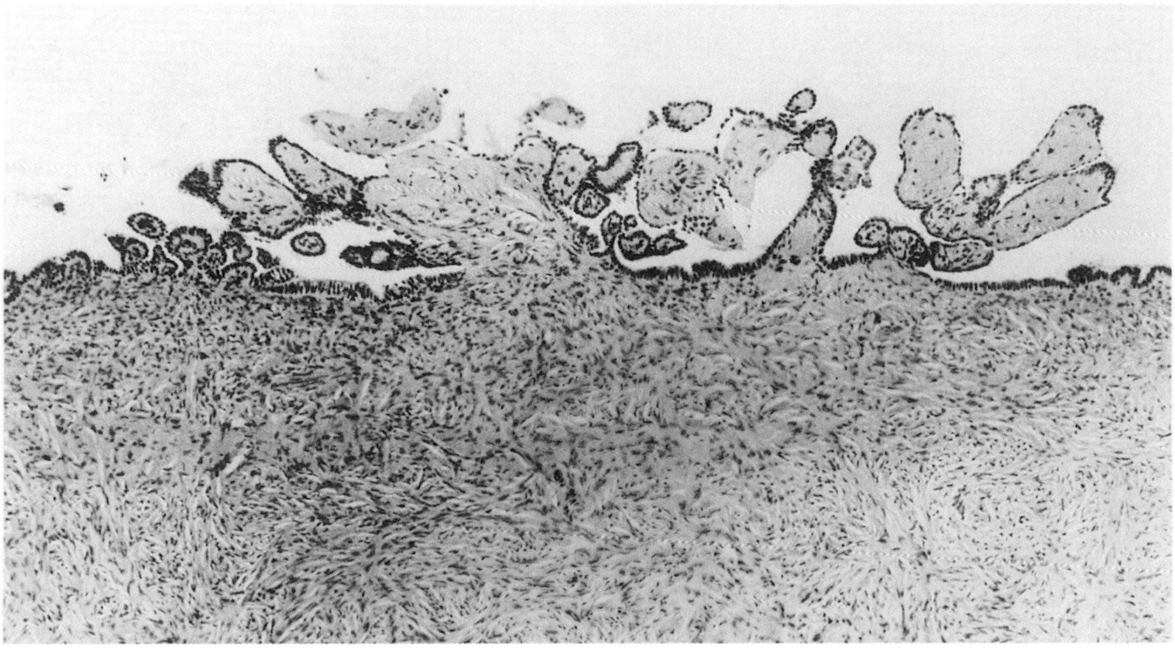

Fig. 20.4 Papillation. Broad-based superficial papillary lesion. Underlying cortical stroma is sclerotic. H + E ×80

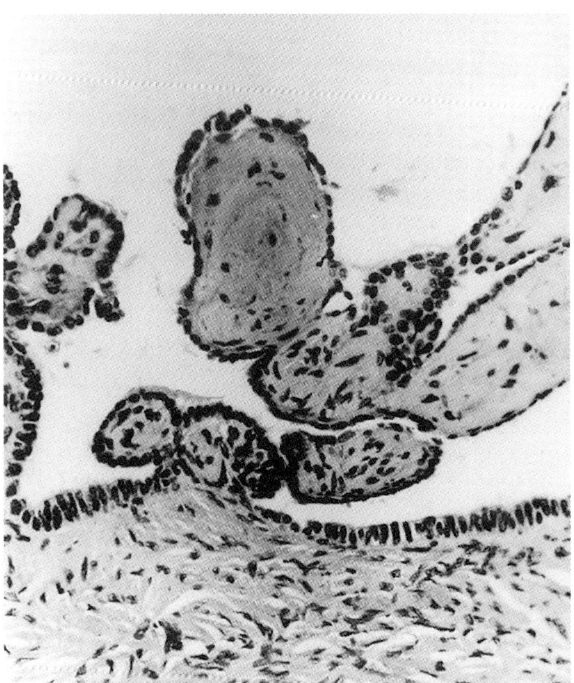

Fig. 20.5 Detail of Fig. 20.4. Papillae are composed of dense fibrous tissue covered by cuboidal and columnar epithelium. H + E ×200

Mesenchymal metaplasias

Recognized paths of mesenchymal differentiation are towards endometrial stroma and smooth muscle. The former is involved in the development of deciduosis and, together with endometrial epithelial metaplasia, of endometriosis. The latter is involved in leiomyomatosis peritonealis disseminata (see Ch. 26) and as a minor component of some endometriotic and endosalpingiotic lesions.

Deciduosis is observed classically in pregnancy (see Ch. 10); groups of decidual cells, indistinguishable from those found in gestational endometrium, appear beneath the ovarian surface epithelium (and elsewhere in the pelvic and lower abdominal peritoneum and lymph nodes). Patients with trophoblastic disease also regularly exhibit deciduosis (see Fig. 53.7), mediated, as in a normal pregnancy, by high plasma levels of chorionic gonadotrophins. Ectopic decidual reactions in the absence of pregnancy or gestational trophoblastic disease (pseudodeciduosis) are most commonly associated with exogenous progesterone administration (see Ch. 11). They occur rarely in the absence of such histories and have mostly been identified in premenopausal women.

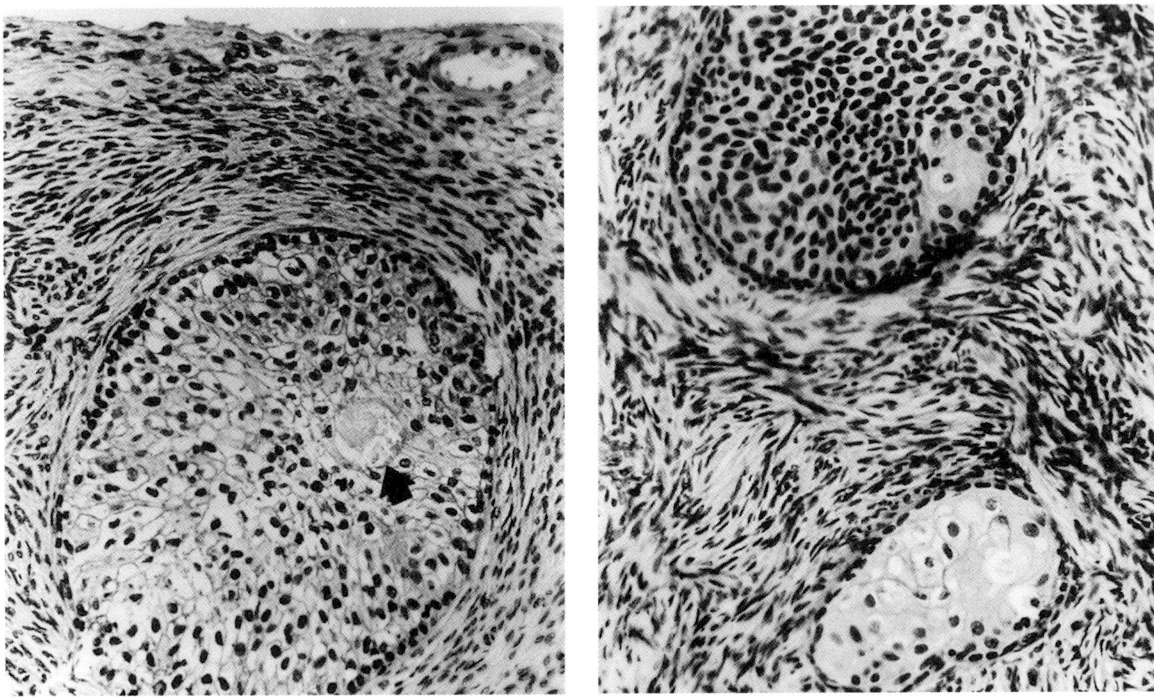

A B

Fig. 20.6 Ovarian Walthard's rests – superficial cortical lesions. (A) Nest of transitional cells with small eccentric lumen (arrow). Note distinct cell margins, abundant cytoplasm and elongate nuclei. H + E ×200. (B) Squamous metaplasia, more obvious in the small lesion below. H + E ×200

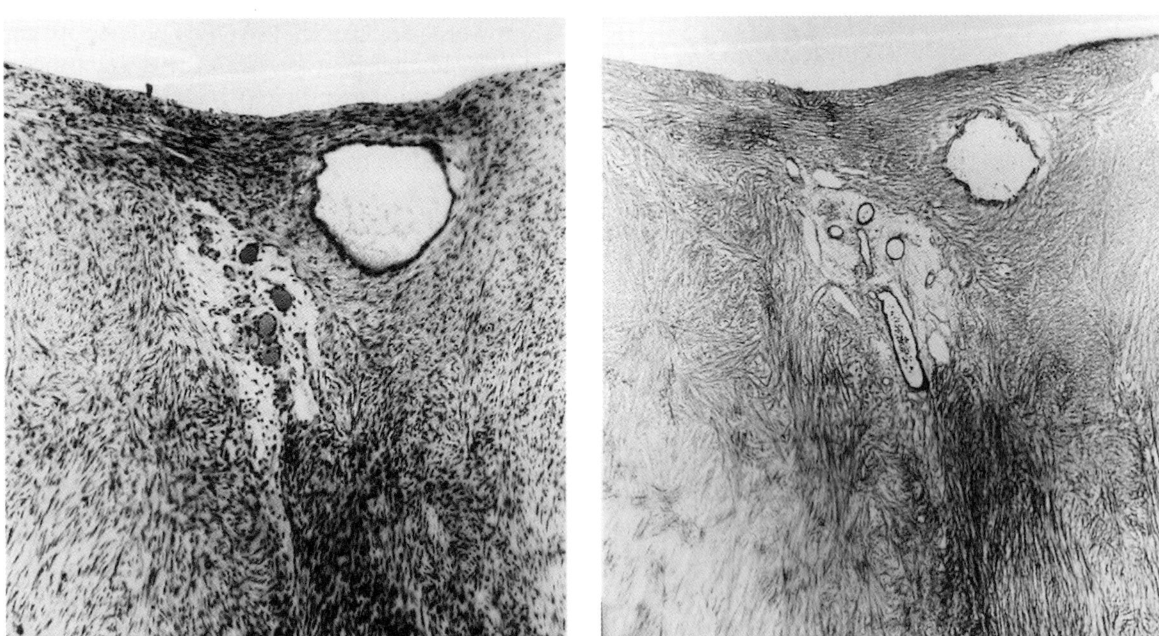

A B

Fig. 20.7 'Benign stromatosis'. Isolated focus of loose vascular connective tissue consistent with endometrial stroma and distinguished from adjacent ovarian stroma by its paucity of reticulin fibres. Small endosalpingiotic lesion at right. (A) H + E ×80. (B) Reticulin stain ×80

The decidua-like cells in most cases are located close to corpora lutea, suggesting that high local levels of progesterone may have etiological significance. Decidual change is usually not seen in synchronously sampled endometrium (Bassis 1956, Ober et al 1957). Bassis (1956) reported a high percentage of associated ovarian stromal hyperplasia, but also, like Ober et al (1957), observed examples in postmenopausal women (with atrophic ovaries) in whom an adrenal source of progesterone was postulated. Care must be taken not to mistake foci of pseudodeciduosis for deposits of metastatic carcinoma, e.g. breast, especially in the postmenopausal ovary in which the large eosinophilic decidua-like cells make such a striking contrast with the surrounding atrophic ovarian parenchyma.

Hughesdon (1972, 1976) has used the term *benign stromatosis* to refer to all lesions consisting of isolated endometrial stroma in the ovarian cortex, whether showing decidualization or not. The endometrial stroma which constitutes the nodules is distinguished from ovarian stroma by its finer reticulin framework (Fig. 20.7). The lesions do not exhibit hemorrhagic manifestations, but eventually become acellular and hyaline. Only a small proportion of cases show concurrent endometriosis. Hughesdon (1972, 1976) found stromatosis to be very common in women over the age of 45 years, but other workers have not had outstanding success in identifying these lesions. The granulomatous variant resembles the cortical 'granulomas' seen, not infrequently, in patients with cortical stromal hyperplasia (see Chs 14, 19).

Differentiation of the subcoelomic mesenchyme in the direction of smooth muscle, with the formation of multiple tumor-like nodules in the peritoneum, including the ovarian surface, is the purported pathogenesis of leiomyomatosis peritonealis disseminata (see Ch. 26). Some degree of smooth muscle differentiation can sometimes be seen around inclusion cysts and endometriotic lesions.

Mixed epithelial and mesenchymal differentiation

Metaplasia and differentiation towards both endometrial epithelium and stroma is the pathogenic basis of many, and probably most, cases of endometriosis (see Ch. 21).

CORTICAL INCLUSION CYSTS

These lesions are included as a separate category in the World Health Organization classification of ovarian tumors (Appendix B). They are small epithelial lined cysts and are frequently found within the cortex of ovaries. They occur so regularly that it would not be inappropriate to include them in the section on normal ovarian histology. They are thought to arise when cortical clefts and invaginations become pinched off from the capsular surface (Lauchlan 1972, Radisavljecvic 1977, Blaustein 1981) (Fig 20.8). These invaginations are seen in fetal and premenarcheal ovaries, as well as in women of reproductive age when the ovarian surface is disrupted as a result of ovulation. It has been proposed that scarring results in traction of the surface epithelium and its subsequent invagination. The microscopic cysts are often multiple, and have a round or stellate outline. They are initially lined by the same cuboidal epithelium which covers the ovarian surface, but mullerian epithelial metaplasia usually ensues. At this stage they are indistinguishable from cystic and tubular forms of mullerianosis. Although tubal metaplasia most frequently occurs, endometrial, endocervical, clear cells, and mixed epithelial cellular differentiation have all been observed (Scully 1979). Although it is argued that some degree of epithelial proliferation and papillary projections are necessary before the term 'mullerianosis' is used (Bell & Scully 1989), to try to distinguish these two lesions (i.e. mullerianosis versus mullerian metaplasia) in a cortical inclusion cyst is of little practical importance.

Of more importance is to distinguish these cysts or tubular lesions from small benign cyst adenomas. This is done, according to convention, by size. A lesion is designated a cystadenoma if it is more than 1 cm in diameter (see Ch 23).

REACTIVE MESOTHELIAL PROLIFERATIONS AND CYSTS ASSOCIATED WITH THE OVARY

Proliferative changes on the surface of the ovaries

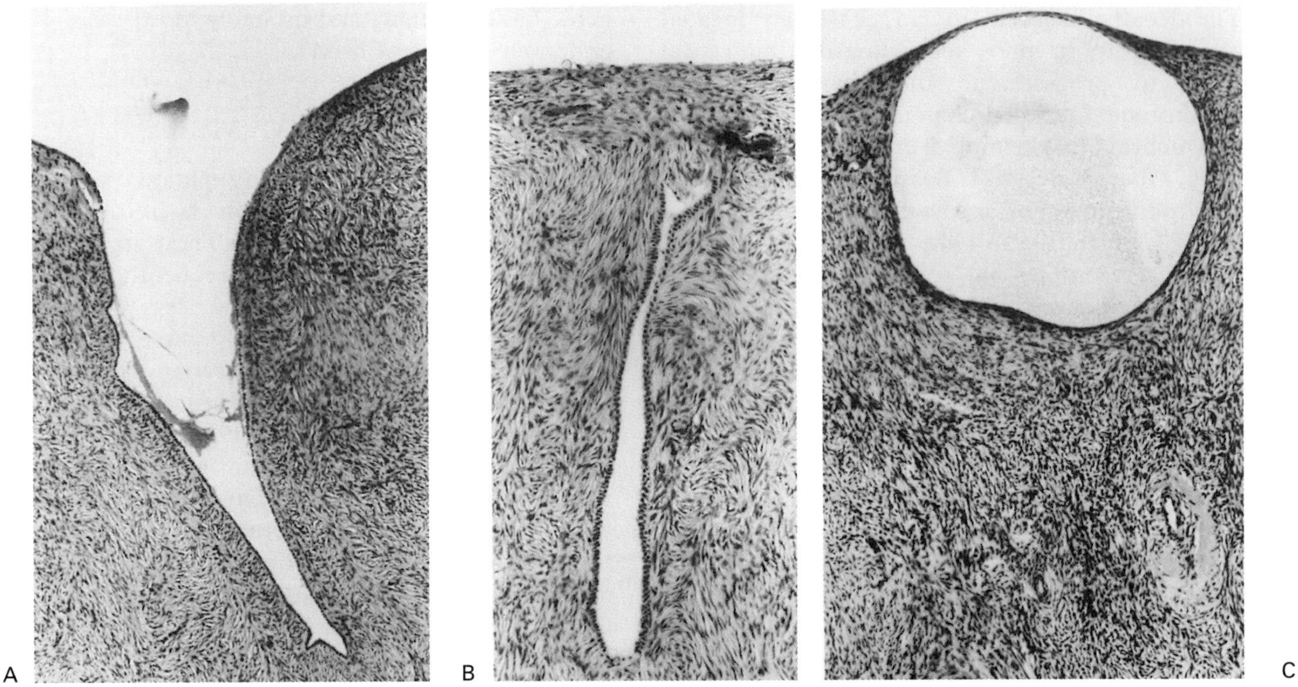

Fig. 20.8 Pathogenesis of cortical inclusion cyst. (A) Deep cortical cleft. H + E ×64. (B) Similar cleft pinched off by fibrous tissue. H + E ×80. (C) Distension of epithelial inclusion to form a cyst. H + E ×64

are most commonly associated with pelvic inflammatory disease or ruptured ectopic tubal pregnancies. More remote inflammatory foci such as appendicitis or diverticulitis may also be inciting factors. Some unusual ovarian mesothelial inclusions with a pseudo-infiltrative patterns have been noted in patients with endometriosis (Kerner et al 1981).

The development of granulation tissue and adhesions in perioophoritis is discussed in Chapter 18. Mesothelial cells take an active part in these surface proliferations and appear in ribbons, sheets, clusters, tubules, and papillary formations, not only in the position of the original serosal surface, but also extending into the overlying organizing exudate (Figs 20.9–20.11). Mesothelial cells are uniform in appearance, with small regular round or oval nuclei (with central nucleoli) and eosinophilic, sometimes vacuolated, cytoplasm. They may be bi- or multinucleated. Despite their benign cytological appearance, their exuberant and sometimes pseudo-infiltrative growth, together with frequently observed (albeit modest) mitotic activity, may lead to a false impression of primary or metastatic carcinoma (Farhi & Silverberg 1982). Carcinoma cells are distinguished by their relatively sparse cytoplasm, nuclear pleiomorphism, and conspicuous mitotic activity. Exuberant surface proliferations, sometimes forming sessile or polypoid nodules, can also raise the suspicion of mesothelioma, a problem also encountered in the walls of hernial sacs (Rosai & Dehner 1975). The degree of cellular proliferation and atypia is important in making the distinction (McCaughey et al 1985).

The source of these proliferating mesothelial cells on the ovaries is worthy of discussion. Although the ovarian surface epithelial cells have many morphologic features in common with mesothelial cells (Blaustein 1984), there are also noteworthy differences and they patently differ, even at light microscopic level, from the mesothelial cells of the adjacent pelvic peritoneum. Both are, however, of coelomic epithelial origin and it is plausible that ovarian surface epithelial cells may differentiate (i.e. revert) to typical meso-

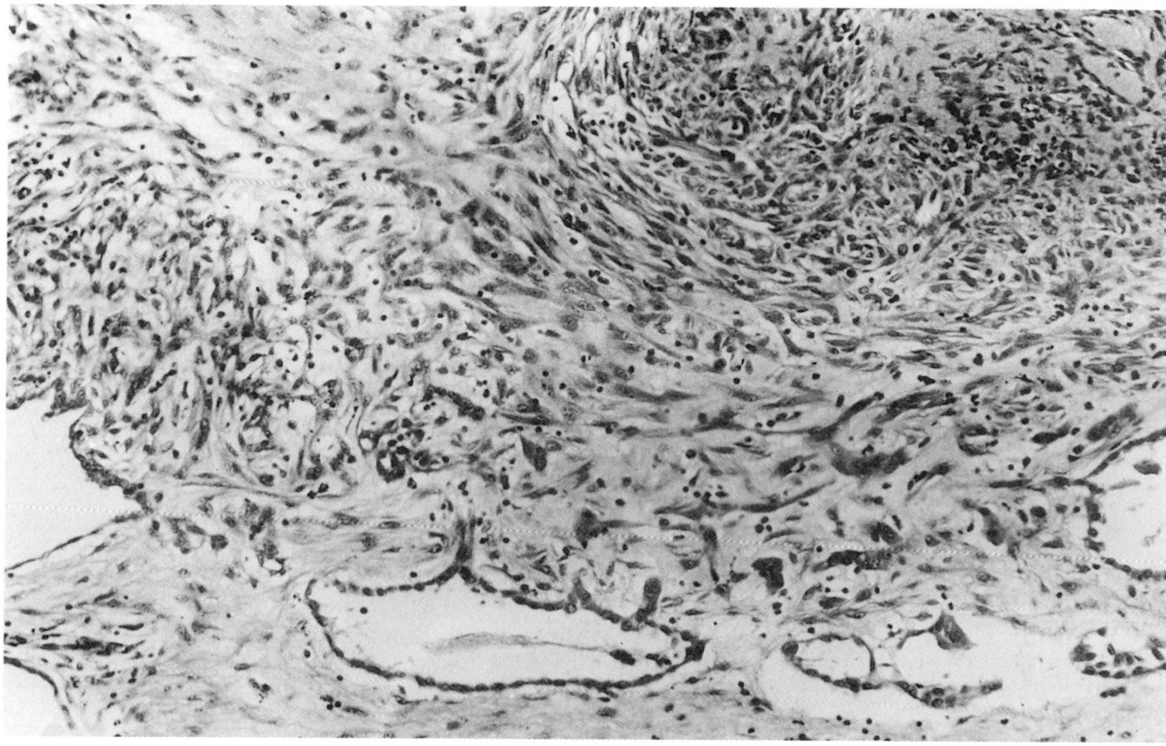

Fig. 20.9 Perioophoritis; exuberant ovarian surface proliferative lesion in response to ruptured ectopic tubal pregnancy. Granulation tissue and streams of elongate mesothelial cells are seen above the original serosal surface which is indicated by elongate horizontal cystic spaces lined by smaller cuboidal mesothelial cells. There is a sparse inflammatory infiltrate, chiefly lymphocytic. H + E ×128

thelial cells. Origin from subperitoneal connective tissue fibroblasts has also been suggested (Raftery 1973).

Resolution of surface proliferative lesions and inflammatory exudates may leave adhesions of variable density, ranging from delicate strands of loose connective tissue to broad bands of dense well-vascularized collagenous fibrous tissue. Entrapment of inflammatory exudate within granulation tissue and proliferating sheets of mesothelial cells may lead to mesothelial (peritoneal) cyst formation. These may not become clinically apparent until months or years after the precipitating events. Pain is the most common symptom. Some lesions are incidental findings at laparotomy for unrelated problems.

Extraovarian mesothelial cysts are usually less than 1 cm in diameter and are often multiple. Occasionally large cysts up to 20 cm in diameter are present and may form multilocular masses simulating ovarian cystadenomas (Gussman et al 1986). The cysts are thin walled and contain clear proteinaceous fluid (Fig. 20.12). The walls consist of fibrous tissue lined by attenuated mesothelial cells (Fig. 20.13). Metaplasia of the epithelial lining of mesothelial cysts is common; it is usually tubal in type and this development represents one origin of endosalpingiosis (see above). Inflammatory reactions, if present at all, are limited to sparse lymphocytic infiltrations. Some cysts show more marked inflammation as well as mural proliferations of mesothelial cells with (pseudo-infiltrative patterns) similar to those seen in perioophoritis as described above (McFadden & Clement 1986) (Fig. 20.14). The differential diagnosis of reactive mesothelial proliferations and cysts from benign cystic mesotheliomas may be extremely difficult, and in part relies on the macroscopic appearance and clinical history of the lesions (see Ch. 31).

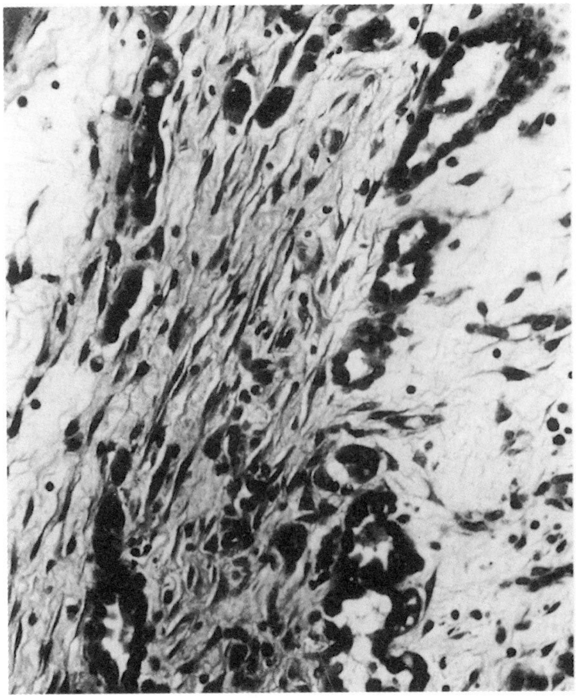

Fig. 20.10 Proliferating mesothelial cells forming ribbons and tubules. Note regular ovoid nuclei with central nucleoli. H + E ×200

Psammoma bodies are commonly encountered in reactive surface proliferative and endosalpingiotic lesions. They are found just beneath the surface epithelium or in adhesions (see Figs 20.2, 20.3, 20.10). Papillary mesothelial clusters and psammoma bodies shed from the peritoneum may also find their way into the lumens of the fallopian tubes, and their presence there does not necessarily imply tubal disease. Psammoma bodies begin to develop intracellularly as dystrophic calcium salt deposits on intermediate cytoplasmic filaments, probably as a result of cellular hypoxia. Extruded calcium salts and cellular debris in the stroma become the nidus for further calcification.

PERITONEAL PIGMENTATIONS

Melanosis peritonei

Melanosis peritonei may involve the ovarian surface as well as the general peritoneum. The condition most commonly follows rupture of mature

A

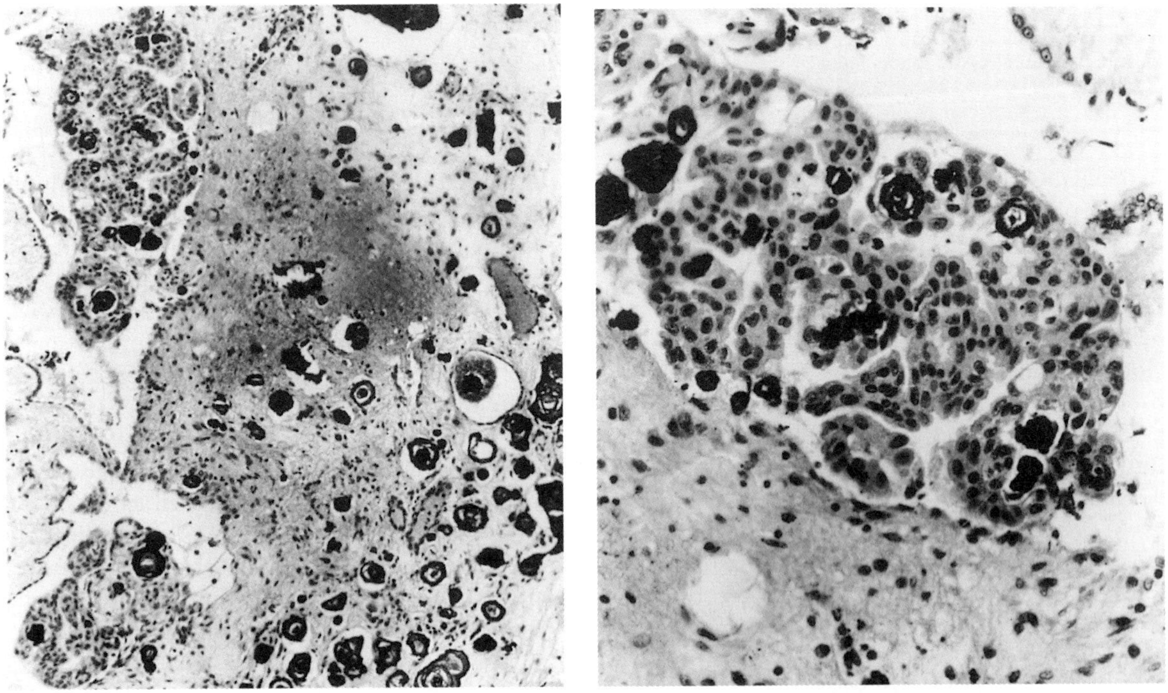

B

Fig. 20.11 Chronic perioophoritis. (A) Fibrous serosal adhesion which includes numerous psammoma bodies. Marked mesothelial proliferation between adhesion and serosal surface at left. H + E ×80. (B) Detail of papillary mesothelial cluster. Cells have slightly irregular ovoid nuclei and abundant cytoplasm. The differential diagnosis of such a process includes an extraovarian proliferating serous neoplasm. H + E ×200

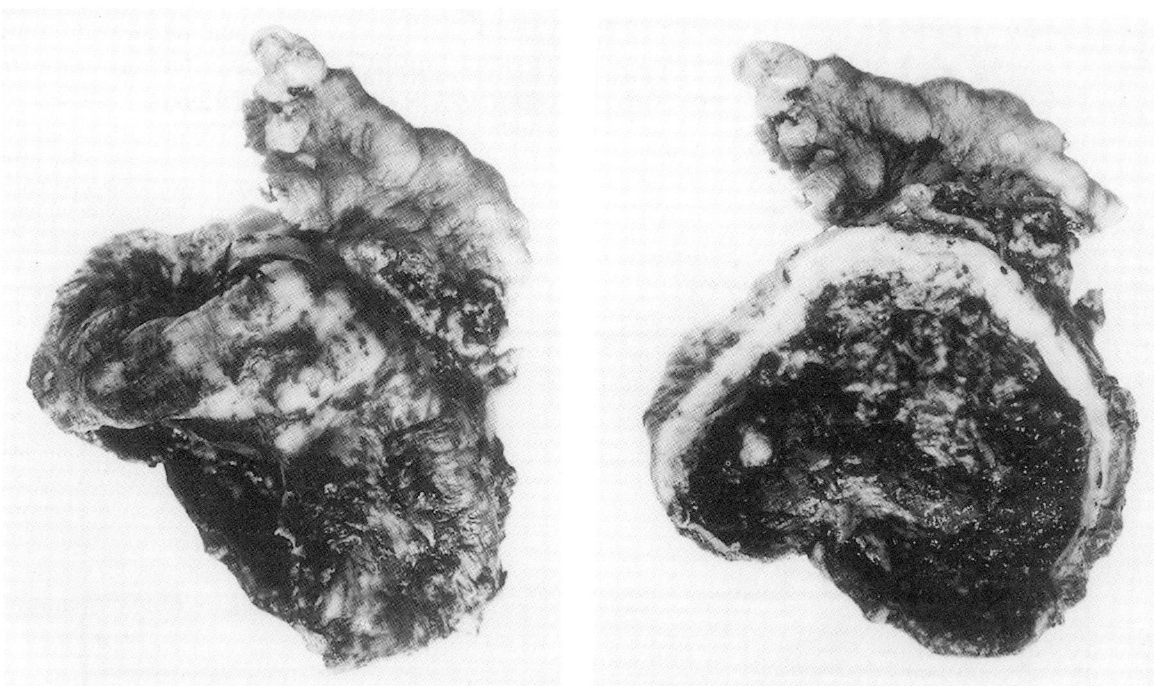

A B

Fig. 21.2 Chronic endometriotic ovarian cyst which ruptured during excision. (A) External surface shows dense hemorrhagic adhesions. (B) Cut surface shows thick fibrous wall and rough hemorrhagic lining with adherent altered blood

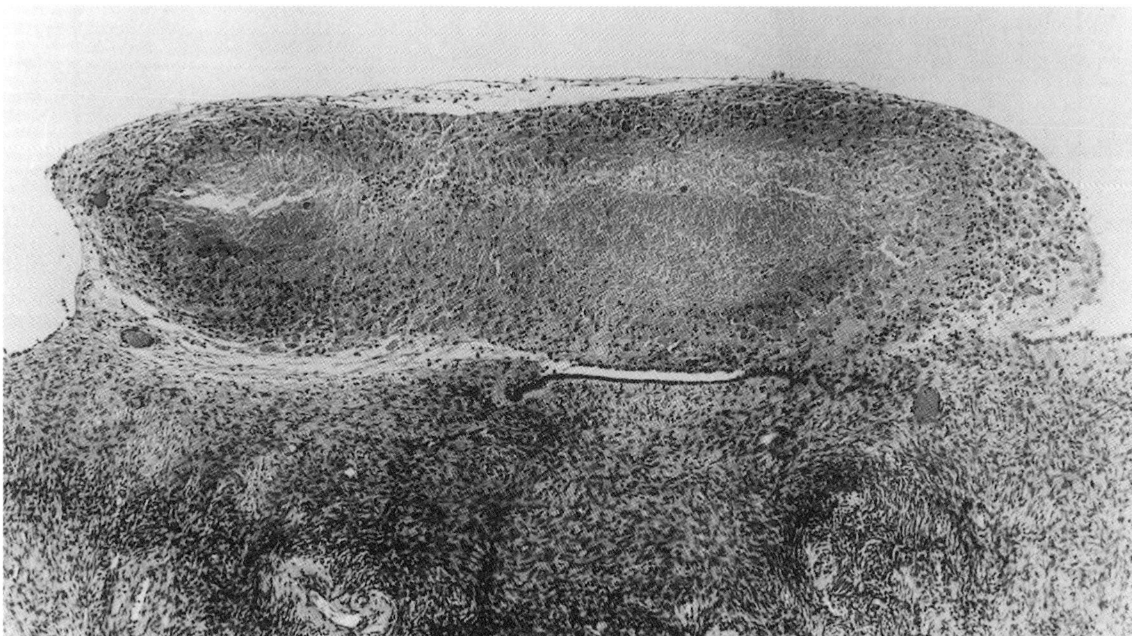

Fig. 21.3 Cellular debris adherent to ovarian surface from patient with freshly ruptured endometriotic cyst. Similar peritoneal nodules were widespread in the pelvis. The lesion includes macrophages and other inflammatory cells; central necrotic area imparts a granulomatous appearance. H + E ×80

THE AMERICAN FERTILITY SOCIETY
REVISED CLASSIFICATION OF ENDOMETRIOSIS

Patient's Name ______________________ Date ______________

Stage I (Minimal) - 1-5
Stage II (Mild) - 6-15
Stage III (Moderate) - 16-40
Stage IV (Severe) - >40
Total ______________

Laparoscopy ________ Laparotomy ________ Photography ________
Recommended Treatment ______________________

Prognosis ______________

PERITONEUM	**ENDOMETRIOSIS**	<1cm	1-3cm	>3cm
	Superficial	1	2	4
	Deep	2	4	6
OVARY	R Superficial	1	2	4
	Deep	4	16	20
	L Superficial	1	2	4
	Deep	4	16	20
	POSTERIOR CULDESAC OBLITERATION	Partial		Complete
		4		40
OVARY	**ADHESIONS**	<1/3 Enclosure	1/3-2/3 Enclosure	>2/3 Enclosure
	R Filmy	1	2	4
	Dense	4	8	16
	L Filmy	1	2	4
	Dense	4	8	16
TUBE	R Filmy	1	2	4
	Dense	4*	8*	16
	L Filmy	1	2	4
	Dense	4*	8*	16

*If the fimbriated end of the fallopian tube is completely enclosed, change the point assignment to 16.

Additional Endometriosis: ______________________

Associated Pathology: ______________________

To Be Used with Normal Tubes and Ovaries

L R

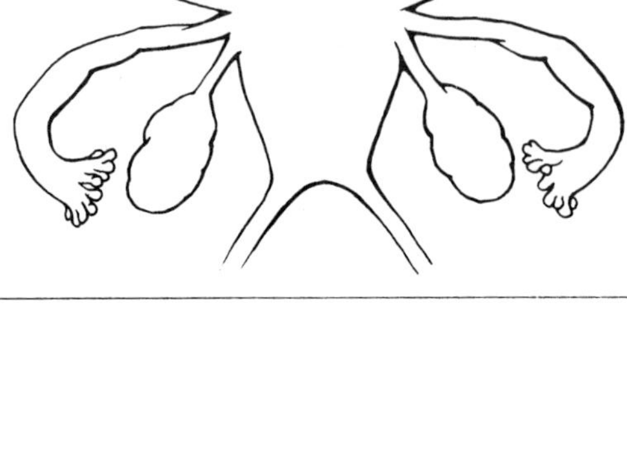

To Be Used with Abnormal Tubes and/or Ovaries

L R

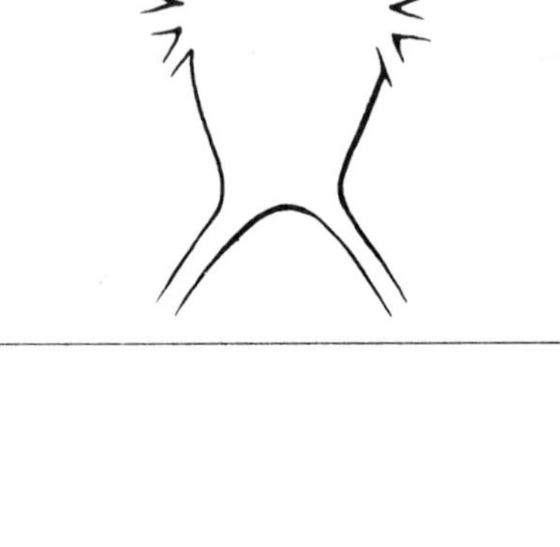

EXAMPLES & GUIDELINES

STAGE I (MINIMAL)

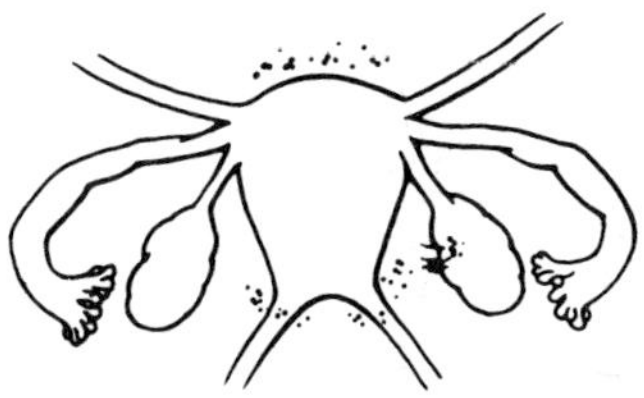

PERITONEUM
Superficial Endo – 1-3cm - 2
R. OVARY
Superficial Endo – < 1cm - 1
Filmy Adhesions – < 1/3 - 1
TOTAL POINTS 4

STAGE II (MILD)

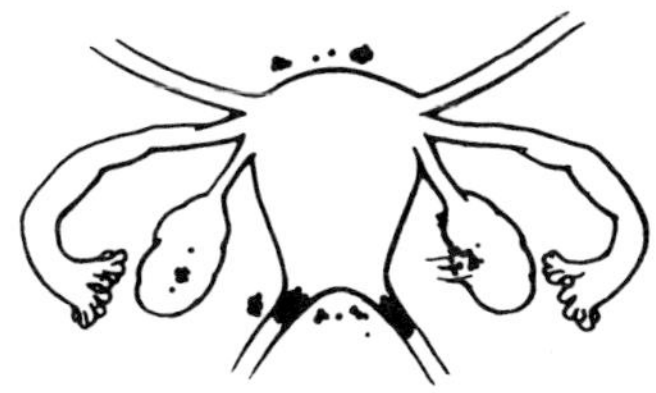

PERITONEUM
Deep Endo – > 3cm - 6
R. OVARY
Superficial Endo – < 1cm - 1
Filmy Adhesions – < 1/3 - 1
L. OVARY
Superficial Endo – < 1cm - 1
TOTAL POINTS 9

STAGE III (MODERATE)

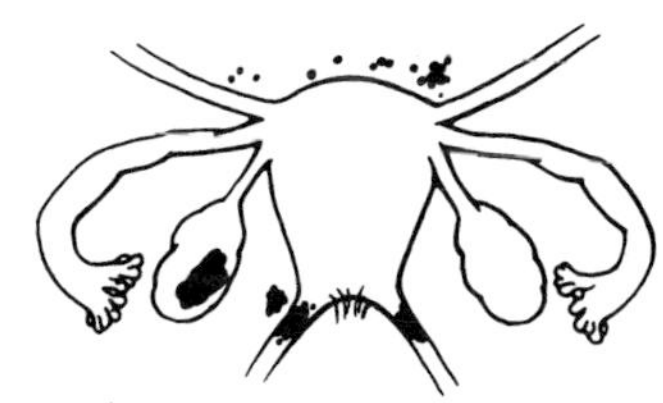

PERITONEUM
Deep Endo – > 3cm - 6
CULDESAC
Partial Obliteration - 4
L. OVARY
Deep Endo – 1-3cm - 16
TOTAL POINTS 26

STAGE III (MODERATE)

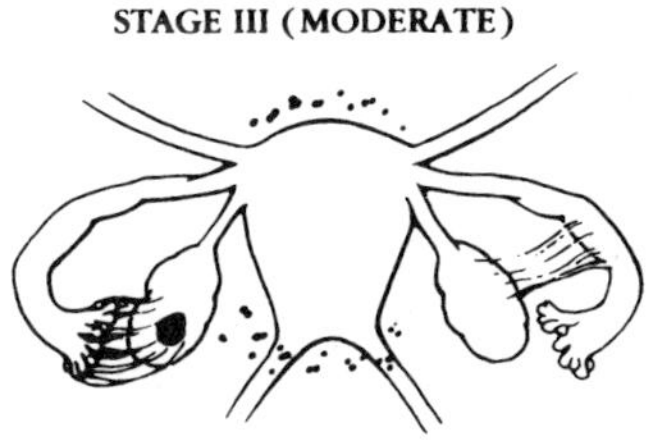

PERITONEUM
Superficial Endo – > 3cm - 3
R. TUBE
Filmy Adhesions – < 1/3 - 1
R. OVARY
Filmy Adhesions – < 1/3 - 1
L. TUBE
Dense Adhesions – < 1/3 - 16*
L. OVARY
Deep Endo – < 1 cm -4
Dense Adhesions – < 1/3 -4
TOTAL POINTS 29

STAGE IV (SEVERE)

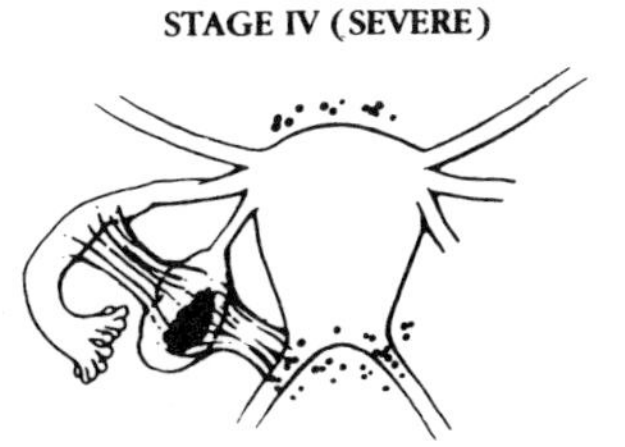

PERITONEUM
Superficial Endo – > 3cm - 3
L. OVARY
Deep Endo – 1-3cm - 32**
Dense Adhesions – < 1/3 - 8**
L. TUBE
Dense Adhesions – < 1/3 -8**
TOTAL POINTS 51

*Point assignment changed to 16
**Point assignment doubled

STAGE IV (SEVERE)

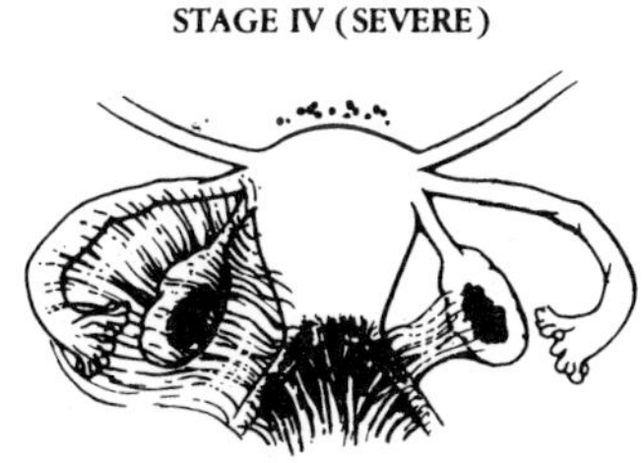

PERITONEUM
Deep Endo – > 3cm - 6
CULDESAC
Complete Obliteration - 40
R. OVARY
Deep Endo – 1-3cm - 16
Dense Adhesions – < 1/3 - 4
L. TUBE
Dense Adhesions – > 2/3 - 16
L. OVARY
Deep Endo – 1-3cm - 16
Dense Adhesions – > 2/3 - 16
TOTAL POINTS 114

Determination of the stage or degree of endometrial involvement is based on a weighted point system. Distribution of points has been arbitrarily determined and may require further revision or refinement as knowledge of the disease increases.

To ensure complete evaluation, inspection of the pelvis in a clockwise or counterclockwise fashion is encouraged. Number, size and location of endometrial implants, plaques, endometriomas and/or adhesions are noted. For example, five separate 0.5cm superficial implants on the peritoneum (2.5 cm total) would be assigned 2 points. (The surface of the uterus should be considered peritoneum.) The severity of the endometriosis or adhesions should be assigned the highest score only for peritoneum, ovary, tube or culdesac. For example, a 4cm superficial and a 2cm deep implant of the peritoneum should be given a score of 6 (not 7). A 4cm deep endometrioma of the ovary associated with more than 3cm of superficial disease should be scored 20 (not 24).

In those patients with only one adenexa, points applied to disease of the remaining tube and ovary should be multipled by two. **Points assigned may be circled and totaled. Aggregation of points indicates stage of disease (minimal, mild, moderate, or severe).

The presence of endometriosis of the bowel, urinary tract, fallopian tube, vagina, cervix, skin etc., should be documented under "additional endometriosis." Other pathology such as tubal occlusion, leiomyomata, uterine anomaly, etc., should be documented under "associated pathology." All pathology should be depicted as specifically as possible on the sketch of pelvic organs, and means of observation (laparoscopy or laparotomy) should be noted.

Fig. 21.4 Revised American Fertility Society classification of endometriosis: 1985. (Reproduced with permission of The American Fertility Society from Fertility and Sterility 43: 351–352)

The relationship between mild endometriosis and infertility has received much attention in the literature, but remains enigmatic. In these patients there is minimal anatomical distortion of the adnexa so that mechanical impairment of tubal motility and inadequate ovum pick-up are unlikely. There are many proposed mechanisms of infertility in this clinical group, none of which are universally accepted; they are not necessarily mutually exclusive and multiple factors may operate in individual patients (Muse & Wilson 1982). Those which have received most attention include: altered prostaglandin secretion (Weed 1980, Moon et al 1981); anovulation associated with the luteinized unruptured follicle syndrome (see above); alterations in the volume, cellular, or biochemical characteristics of peritoneal fluid (Drake et al 1980, Haney et al 1981, Halme & Hall 1982, Muscato et al 1982); and autoimmune phenomena (Weed & Arquembourg 1980, Dmowski & Radwanska 1984).

Macroscopic features

Early superficial endometriotic lesions may be impossible to identify macroscopically in excised ovaries, but their presence may be marked by adhesions which are often hemorrhagic. The gynecologist can more readily recognize these tiny lesions at laparoscopy or laparotomy, where they appear as white, red, purple, or flesh-colored blebs, dimples, plaques, or papules, sometimes associated with adhesions.

Ovarian endometriosis progresses by growth and coalescence of endometriotic foci which now involve the ovarian parenchyma, as well as the addition of superficial lesions. The ovarian architecture is disrupted by the expanding lesions, and normal follicular structures become progressively more difficult to identify. Dense capsular adhesions are usually present at this stage, as well as intraovarian fibrosis (Fig. 21.1). Individual lesions are soft and hemorrhagic, and frequently become cystic. Excised chronic endometriotic cysts are generally 5–10 cm in maximum diameter; cysts larger than 20 cm are rare. The lumens usually contain fresh or altered blood which give them their common name of 'chocolate' cysts. They are lined by rough granular tissue which is orange or brown or frankly hemorrhagic; smooth velvety areas are occasionally seen. The outer portion of the cyst wall is composed of tough pale fibrous tissue. There is often evidence of cyst rupture; endometriotic cysts may be very friable and rupture spontaneously or during removal (Fig. 21.2). Fragments of extruded degenerate endometriotic tissue may be found adherent to the ovarian capsule, forming granuloma-like lesions (Fig. 21.3).

The fallopian tubes may be inextricably adherent to the ovaries and may themselves exhibit serosal endometriotic lesions (see Fig. 21.1). The uterus may also be involved, especially the serosal surface of the posterior wall (Pouch of Douglas) and the uterosacral ligaments.

The progression of pelvic endometriosis is reflected in the clinical classification of endometriosis as presented by the American Fertility Society (1985) and reproduced in Figure 21.4.

Microscopic features

The diagnosis of endometriosis rests on the identification of ectopic endometrial tissue, including both glandular and stromal elements. The presence of either one without the other does not permit the exclusion of several lesions discussed in the differential diagnosis below.

Endometrial epithelium is characterized by tall columnar cells with elongate cigar-shaped nuclei showing regular vertical orientation. Occasional ciliated cells may be present. The glands usually appear relatively inactive, with only sparse mitoses, but florid proliferative and secretory activity may at times be observed (Fig. 21.5).

Endometrial stroma consists of small spindle-shaped cells with inconspicuous cytoplasm. The cells are supported by a delicate reticulin network which is much finer than that of native ovarian stroma, as can be demonstrated by silver impregnation staining. All degrees of decidualization of the stromal cells may be seen if the endometriotic focus is cyclically functional (Fig. 21.5). Smooth muscle fibers may be associated with the stromal component of endometriotic foci, most commonly as randomly arranged small groups, but sometimes forming an incomplete sheath around chronic cysts (Fig. 21.6).

The earliest detectable endometriotic lesions

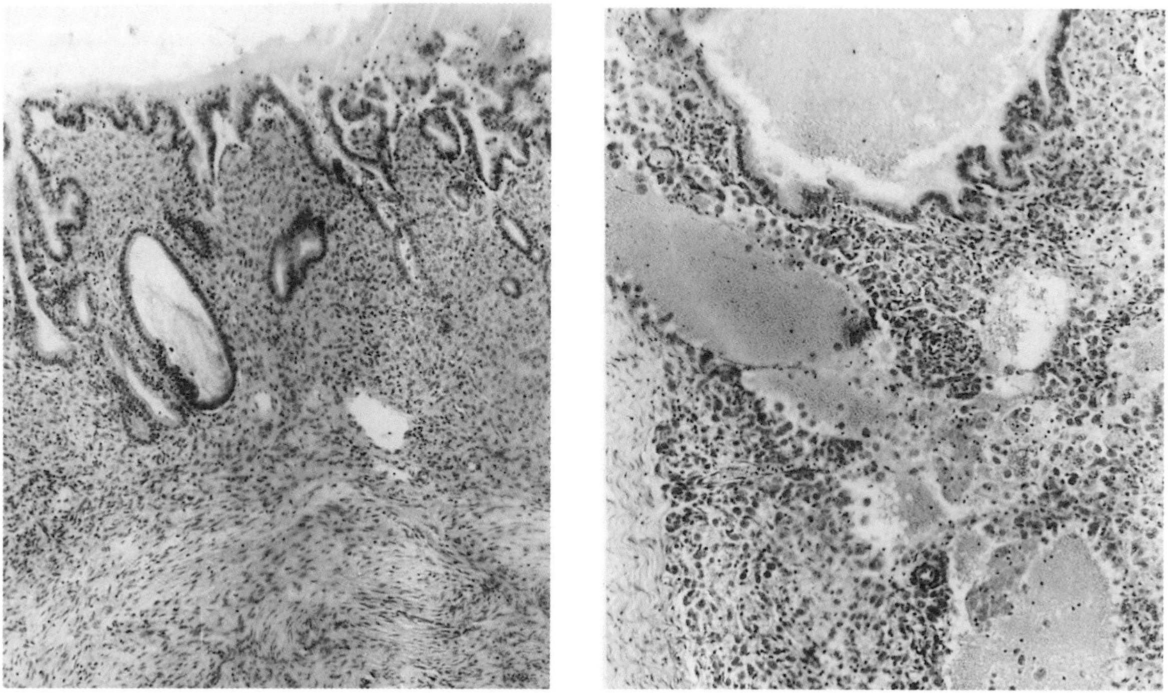

A B

Fig. 21.5 Cyclical activity in endometriosis. (A) Well-developed secretory activity with abundant stromal predecidualization. H + E ×64. (B) 'Menstrual' disintegration in endometriotic focus. Dissociated predecidualized cells are seen best at top right. Epithelium is secretory. H + E ×80

consist of small pieces of endometrial tissue which form plaques on the ovarian capsular surface or appear to be only loosely attached to the serosa (Fig. 21.7A). Initially, there may be only a little attached fibrin or blood, but the endometriotic tissue soon becomes encased by adhesions (Fig. 21.7B). These superficial endometriotic lesions are separated from the underlying cortex by fibrous tissue in which the original peritoneal surface may still be marked by a discontinuous line of mesothelial cells forming cleft-like or tubular spaces (Figs 21.7C,D).

Small parenchymal lesions (less than 1 cm in diameter) consist of islands of endometrial stroma in which glands are usually randomly distributed but sometimes show orientation towards a central lumen, simulating a diminutive uterine cavity (Fig. 21.8A). The stroma may include deposits of hemosiderin, but the glands are well preserved

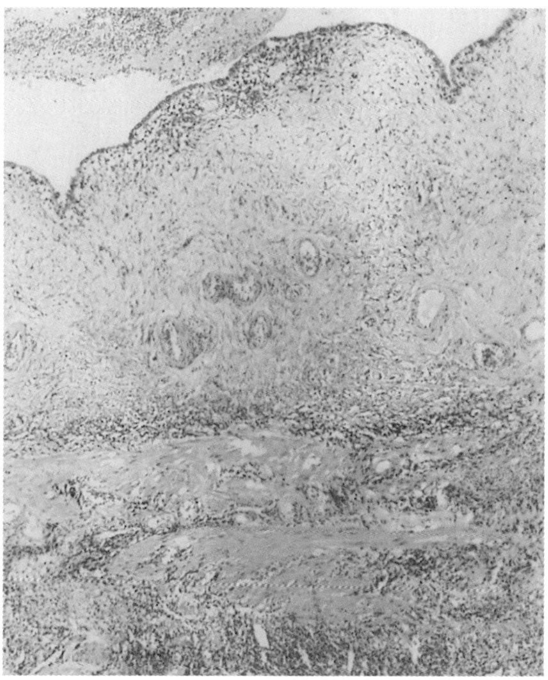

Fig. 21.6 Chronic endometriotic ovarian cyst; bands of smooth muscle are seen beneath zone of fibrous tissue. H + E ×50

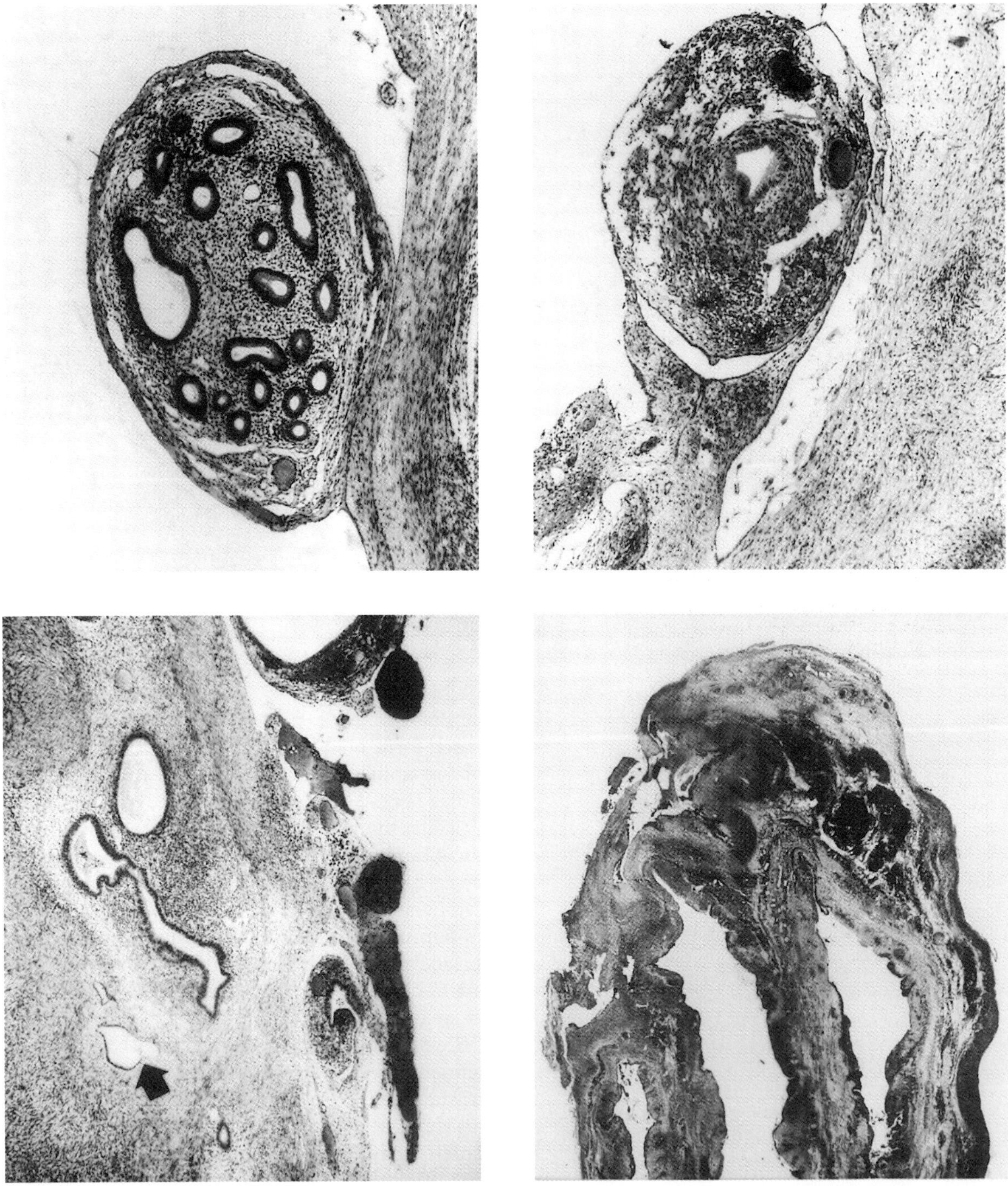

A B C D

Fig. 21.7 Progression of ovarian endometriosis.(A) Microscopic focus of endometrial tissue with tenuous connection to capsule. H + E ×50. (B) Similar tiny endometriotic lesion, in this case associated with adhesions. H + E ×64. (C) Capsular endometriotic lesions bound by dense fibrous adhesions. Original serosal surface is marked by slit-like spaces lined by mesothelial cells (arrow). H + E ×35. (D) Parenchymal endometriosis with cysts separated by fibrotic ovarian stroma. Serosal endometriosis is seen at left associated with hemorrhage and dense fibrous adhesions. H + E ×4

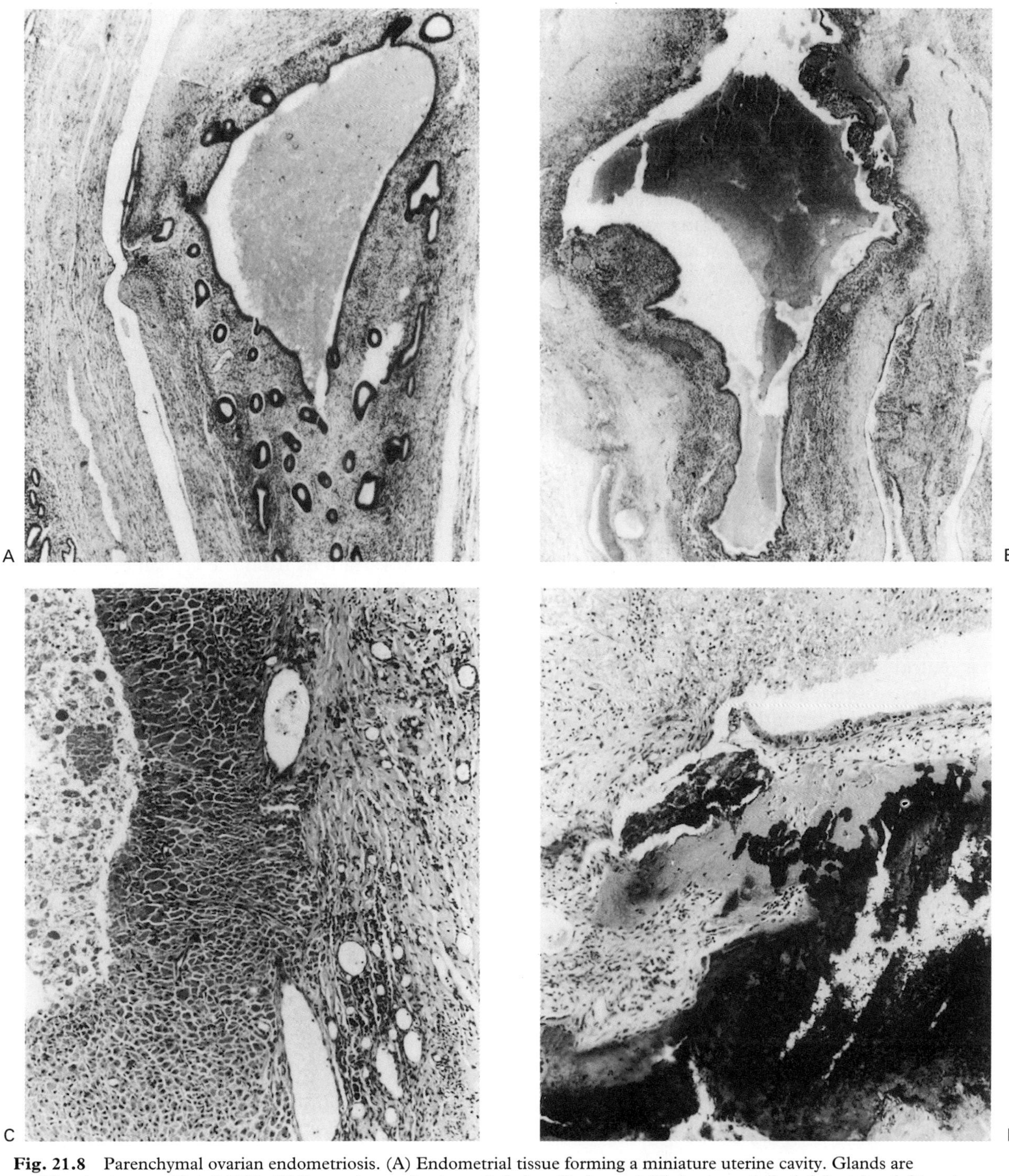

Fig. 21.8 Parenchymal ovarian endometriosis. (A) Endometrial tissue forming a miniature uterine cavity. Glands are proliferative in type. H + E ×25. (B) Larger hemorrhagic cystic lesion. Endometrial lining is partially deficient (top left) and replaced by granulation tissue. Serosal endometriosis and adhesions at right. H + E ×20. (C) Part of cyst lining composed only of densely packed hemosiderin-laden macrophages. Hemosiderin is also present in underlying fibrous tissue. H + E ×50. (D) Dystrophic ossification in wall of chronic endometriotic cyst. H + E ×80

morphologically at this stage. Larger parenchymal lesions are generally cystic; they are lined by endometrium which is frequently focally deficient and replaced by granulation tissue (Fig. 21.8B). Within the endometrial stroma or granulation tissue it is common to find sheets of foamy or hemosiderin-laden macrophages (Figs 21.8C, 21.9A). Lipofuscin (ceroid) pigment is sometimes present. The whole lesion is surrounded by a zone of fibrous tissue, itself containing coarse hemosiderin granules (Fig. 21.8C). Calcification in the cyst wall is encountered uncommonly, and ossification very rarely (Fig. 21.8D). A chronic non-specific inflammatory infiltrate, including plasma cells, is frequently seen as a reactive or repair process in the cyst lining (Czernobilsky & Morris 1979) (Figs 21.9, 21.10). In an apparently unique case, amyloid deposits have been identified in the wall of a chronically inflamed cyst (Salomonowitz 1980).

A number of cases have been reported of the development of necrotic pseudoxanthomatous nodules in association with endometriosis (Clement et al 1988, Carey & Kirk 1993). The lesions are found in both ovary and peritoneum, and consist of granulomatous nodules composed of a central focus of necrotic tissue surrounded by histiocytes (pseudoxanthoma cells), hyalinized connective tissue, or both. Endometriotic glands and stroma were typically absent in the nodules and their immediate vicinity. Foci of recognizable endometriosis were found in the ovaries in all cases. The most important lesion to distinguish these nodules from is metastatic tumor.

It is at this stage of florid clinical endometriosis that the microscopic diagnosis may be the most difficult. The endometrial tissue may have undergone 'self-destruction' and, despite the examination of multiple blocks, all that can be found in the cyst walls are dense fibrous tissue, sheets of macrophages, and granulation tissue. Although the diagnosis of endometriosis requires the demonstration of both endometrial glands and stroma, there would seem to be no merit in diagnostic criteria that are so rigid they exclude many clinically obvious cases of endometriosis. We feel that circumstantial evidence is admissible and that it is reasonable to conclude that the findings are 'compatible with endometriosis' if lesions are typical apart from the lack of endometrial glands, and definite endometriosis is present in other parts of the submitted specimens.

Several variations from the typical endometriotic morphology described above may be encountered, reflecting the fact that, on occasion, ectopic endometriotic tissue may exhibit any of the physiological and pathological changes of its uterine counterpart. Functional changes (in addition to the cyclical changes mentioned above) may be observed, such as hypersecretory change and

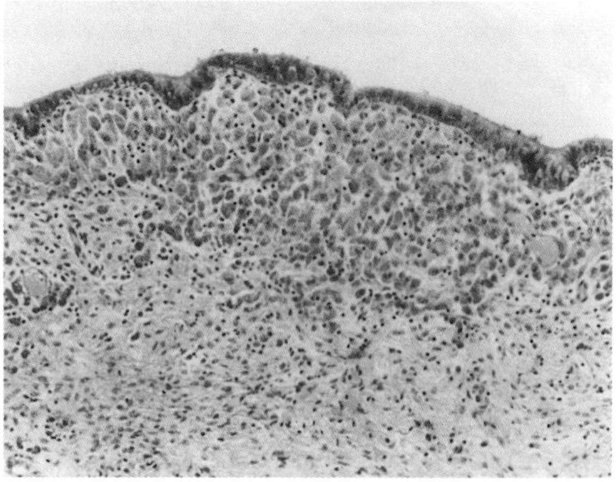

A

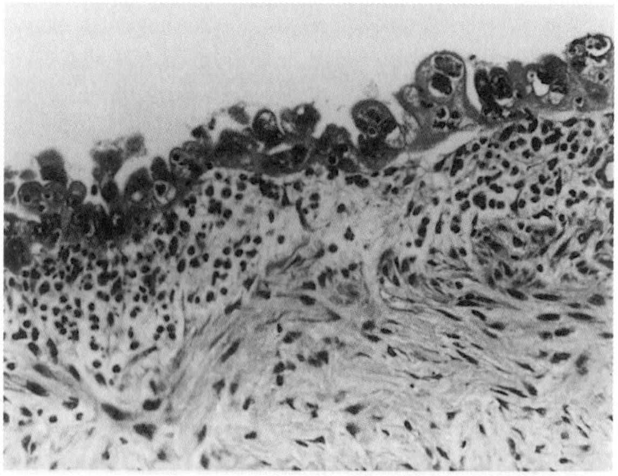

B

Fig. 21.9 Inflammation in chronic endometriotic cysts. (A) Endometrial stroma beneath epithelium contains numerous plasma cells and lymphocytes as well as hemosiderin-laden macrophages. H +E ×80. (B) Cyst lining is infiltrated by inflammatory cells, chiefly neutrophils. Epithelial cells show degenerative changes including nuclear atypia. H + E ×160

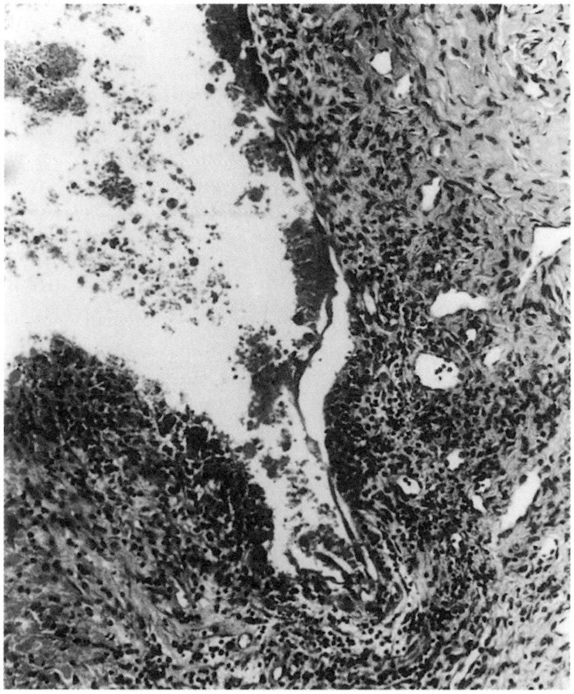

Fig. 21.10 Regenerative epithelial atypia in wall of chronic endometriotic cyst. Heavy chronic inflammatory infiltrate beneath the denuded epithelial lining. H + E ×100

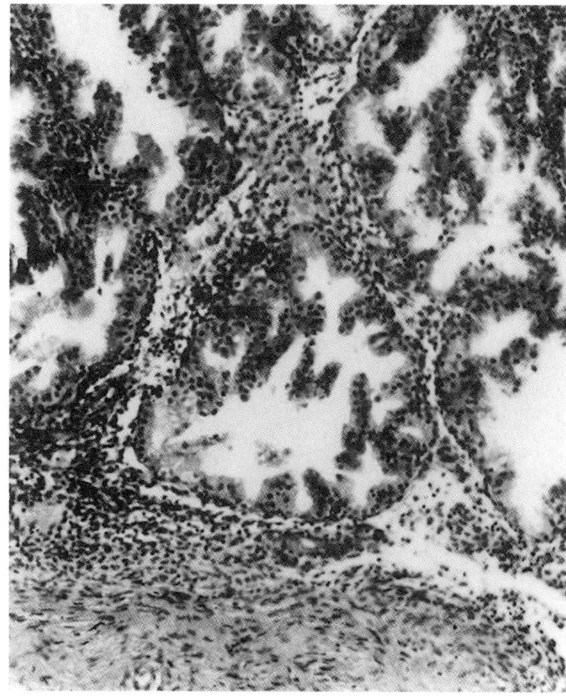

Fig. 21.11 Hypersecretory change in lining of endometriotic cyst excised in pregnancy. H + E ×100

stromal decidualization in pregnancy (Fig. 21.11), or atrophy induced by danazol therapy (see Ch. 11; Fig. 21.12). Rarely, hypersecretory glandular activity may be observed in close proximity to a corpus luteum, suggesting a response to high local levels of progesterone.

Epithelial 'metaplasias' are commonly encountered. Tubal metaplasia (alternating groups of ciliated and secretory cells) is the most frequent (found in about 25% of cases), and may be either focal or widespread (Lauchlan 1966, Czernobilsky & Morris 1979) (Fig. 21.13A). Endometriotic lesions showing prominent tubal metaplasia have been called 'endosalpingiosis', but we prefer to reserve this term for serosal inclusion cysts lined by metaplastic tubal epithelium (see Ch. 20). Mucinous metaplasia is much less frequently observed and is usually focal (Lauchlan 1966) (Fig. 21.13B). Squamous metaplasia has been reported to occur in long-standing endometriotic cysts (Blaustein 1982). Clear cell metaplasia has also been described, but this can be difficult to distinguish from secretory changes, particularly the Arias–Stella reaction (Czernobilsky & Morris 1979).

Atypical and preneoplastic changes

In endometriotic epithelium, these have received scant attention in the literature. Czernobilsky & Morris (1979) found mild atypia considered to be of a regenerative or reactive nature in 43 of 194 cases of ovarian endometriosis. The typical finding was of large polygonal or flattened cells with abundant eosinophilic cytoplasm and enlarged hyperchromatic nuclei (Figs 21.9, 21.10, 21.14). Four further cases showed foci of adenomatous hyperplasia analogous to that more commonly encountered in uterine endometrium. These hyperplastic changes have been interpreted as probable precursors of endometrioid malignancy (Hyman 1977, Czernobilsky & Morris 1979), a notion which is supported by the identification of such changes adjacent to carcinomas arising in endometriotic cysts. A further six cases have been

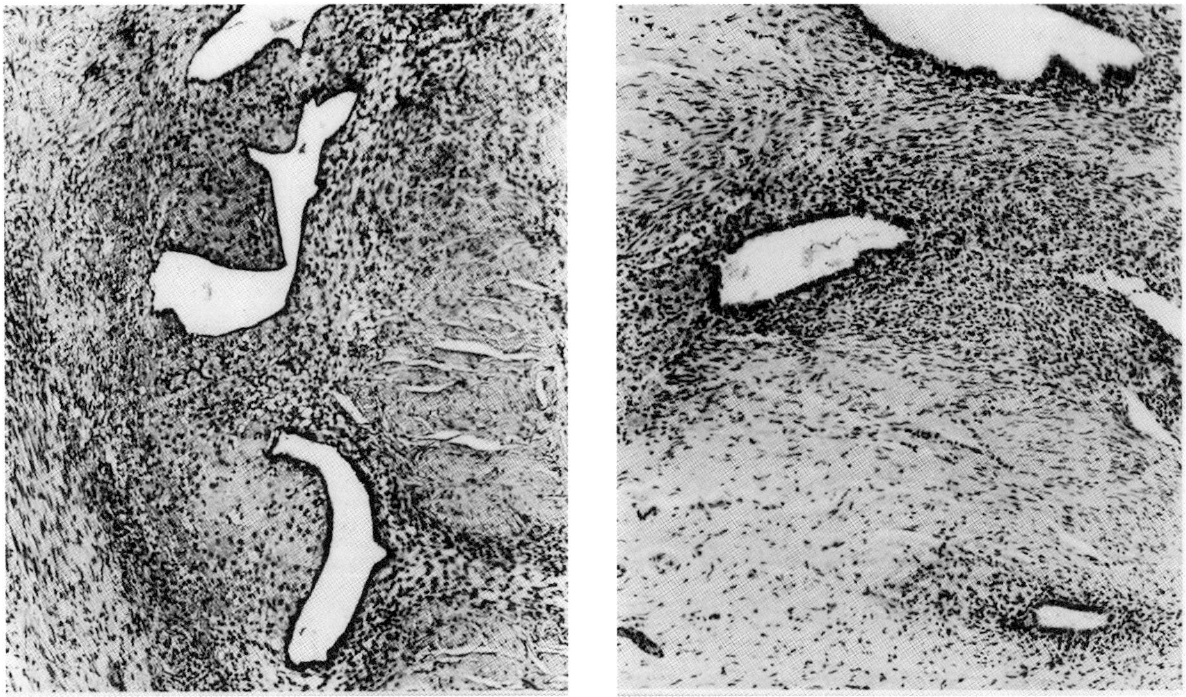

A B

Fig. 21.12 Iatrogenic changes in endometriosis. (A) Pseudodecidual stromal reaction and glandular atrophy induced by high-dose progesterone therapy. H + E ×80. (B) Atrophy of glands and stroma induced by danazol. H + E ×100

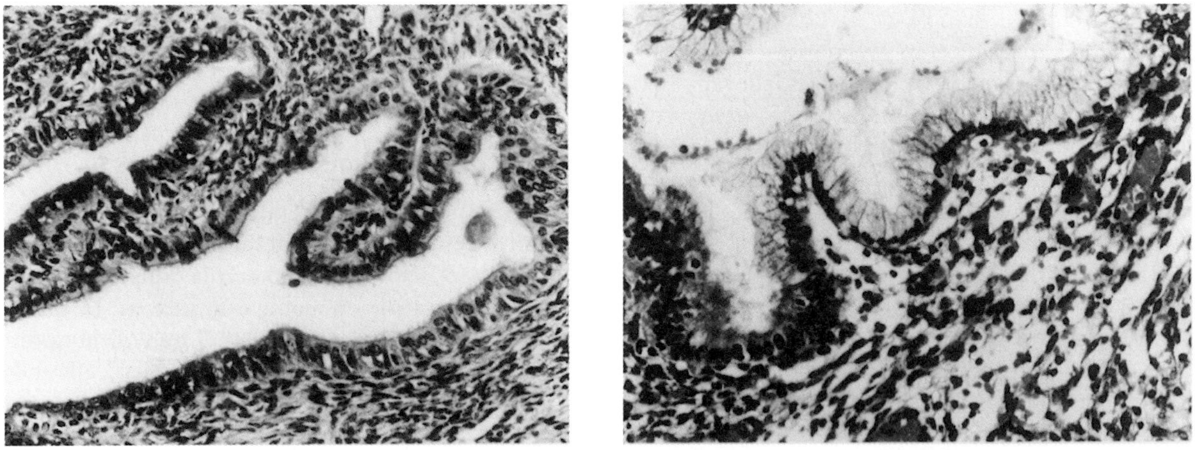

A B

Fig. 21.13 Epithelial metaplasia in endometriosis. (A) Tubal; alternating groups of ciliated and secretory cells. H + E ×200. (B) Mucinous, resembling endocervical epithelium; small basal nuclei and abundant mucin-filled cytoplasm. H + E ×160

reported of atypical glandular epithelial changes in endometriosis associated with the development of ovarian carcinoma (La Grenade & Silverberg 1988, Moll et al 1990).

Smooth muscle is not uncommon within and surrounding endometriotic lesions, but is rarely conspicuous (Scully 1981) (see Fig. 21.6). An adenomyoma, a tumor-like mass of endometrium and smooth muscle analogous to the familiar uterine lesion, has been reported in the wall of an

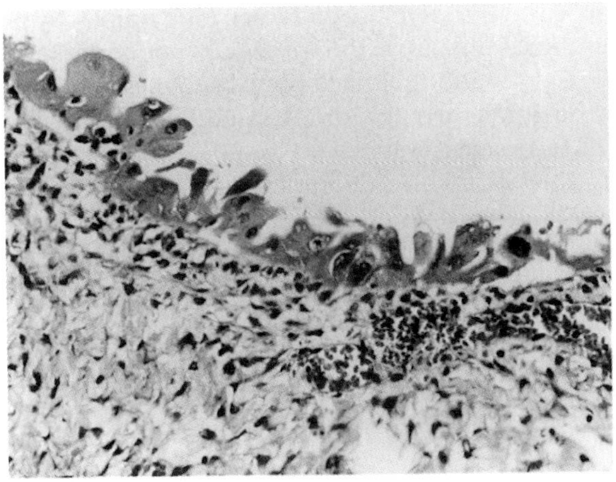

Fig. 21.14 Epithelial atypia in chronic endometriotic cyst. Pleiomorphic cells with abundant eosinophilic cytoplasm and nuclear atypia. Inflammation and epithelial ulceration were present nearby. H + E ×160

endometriotic cyst (McDougal & Roth 1986). Bizarre ovarian lesions, consisting of endometrial tissue surrounded by a thick layer of smooth muscle, resembling a uterus, have been reported (Cozzutto 1981, Pueblitz-Peredo et al 1985); it is as yet unclear whether they represent variants of endometriosis (endomyometriosis) or sequestered horns of congenitally malformed uteri. Leiomyomatosis peritonealis disseminata is another lesion in which endometrium and smooth muscle coexist, although the latter is the dominant component (see Ch. 26).

Endometriosis may be associated with the development of Liesegang rings (Clement et al 1989, Schwartz & Bellin 1991). These eosinophilic acellular laminated structures are usually found in the kidneys or synovium within cysts or areas of inflammation. They can be associated with an

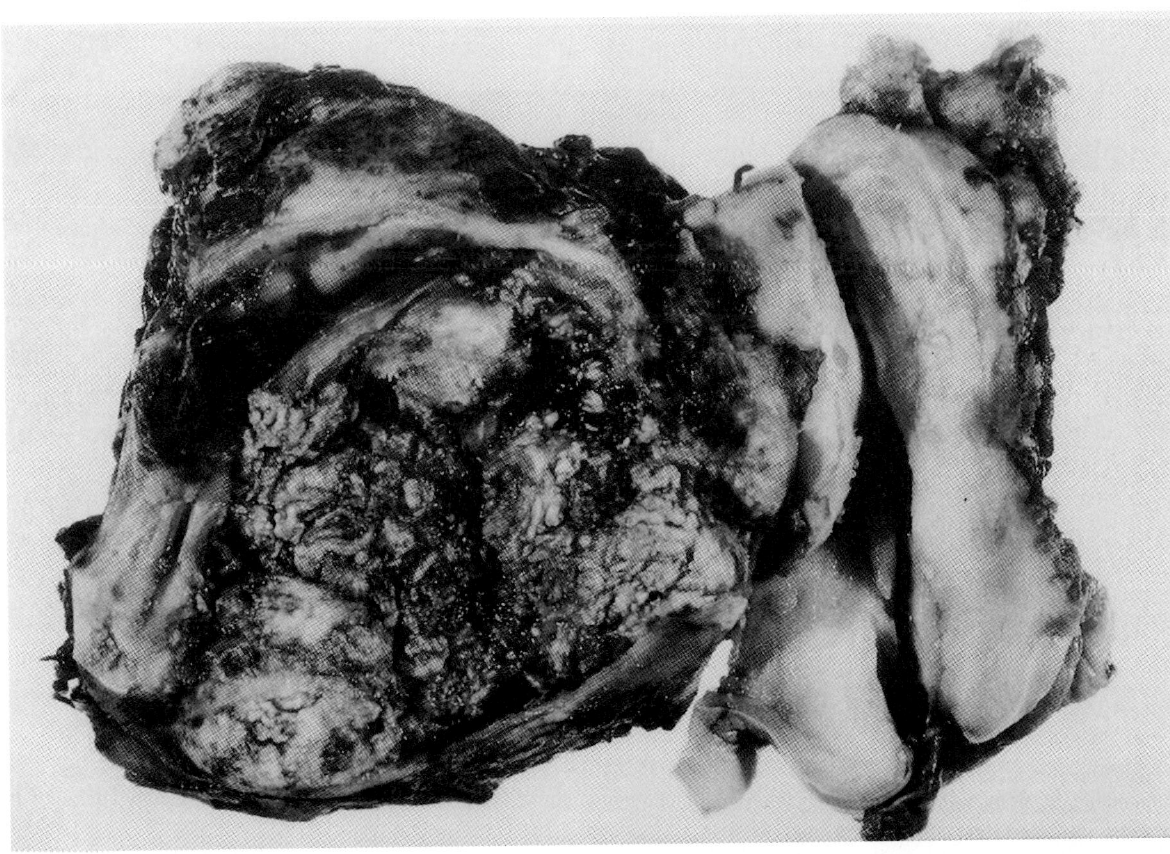

Fig. 21.15 Adenosquamous carcinoma arising in endometriosis. Tumor tissue almost fills large cyst and directly infiltrates the uterine wall. Smaller chronic endometriotic cyst with smooth lining, surrounded by white fibrotic ovarian tissue, is seen above

endometriotic cyst. It is important to distinguish them from parasites or foreign material.

Differential diagnosis

Corpus luteum cysts (see Ch. 12) are the lesions most likely to be confused macroscopically with chronic endometriotic cysts, since both have a ragged hemorrhagic internal surface. Microscopically, both are lined, at least focally, by fibrous tissue and granulation tissue in which are clusters of pale vacuolated cells. Hemosiderin is not as conspicuous as in endometriotic cysts. Endometrial glands and stroma are, of course, absent.

Serosal inclusion cysts (see Ch. 20) are very common superficial cortical lesions, lined by cuboidal cells of surface epithelial type or by metaplastic epithelium, usually tubal (endosalpingiosis). They are commonly associated with psammoma bodies. The lesions are distinguished from small superficial endometriotic lesions by an epithelial lining which is generally not endometrial in type, and their lack of cytogenic endometrial stroma, hemorrhage, or associated adhesions.

Mesothelial cysts (see Ch. 20) are very superficial lesions which do not impinge on the ovarian cortex. They are lined by cuboidal cells with small round nuclei which are readily distinguished from columnar endometrial cells with their cigar-shaped nuclei. Endometrial stroma is absent. They are usually the end result of inflammatory processes involving the ovarian capsular surface, so that adhesions and chronic inflammatory cells are often present.

Rete ovarii and parovarian vestigial remnants may superficially resemble endometriotic foci. The rete has a characteristic ramifying pattern (see Fig. 3.24) and is surrounded by condensed ovarian, rather than endometriotic, stroma without evidence of hemorrhage. It is lined by cuboidal or

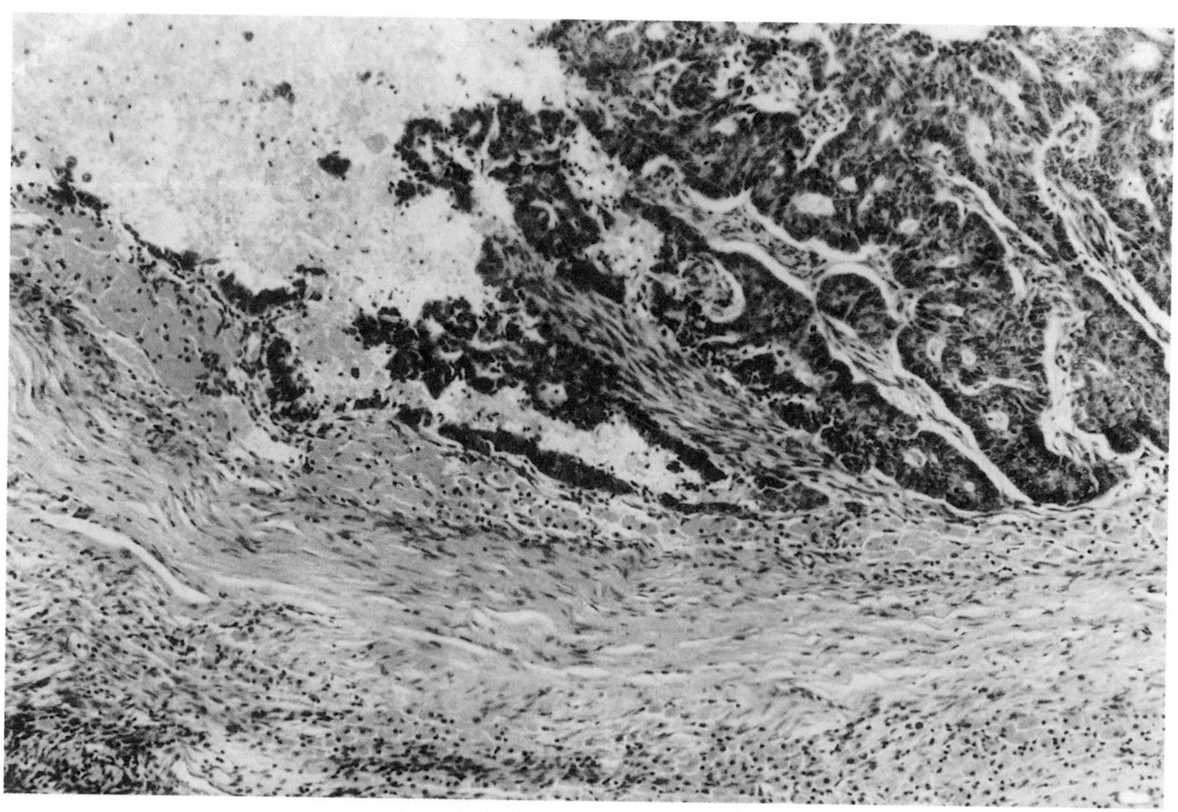

Fig. 21.16 Endometrioid carcinoma arising from the lining of a chronic endometriotic cyst. A single layer of atypical endometrial epithelium, subtended by hemosiderin-laden macrophages, lines the cyst at left. H +E ×100

columnar cells. Paramesonephric and mesonephric remnants are lined by tubal and cuboidal epithelium respectively, with cuffs of smooth muscle.

Mature adult cystic teratomas (see Ch. 46) should not cause confusion if there is an opportunity to examine the surgical specimen macroscopically, or if multiple blocks have been sectioned. However, individual slides may show a cyst lining composed of macrophages, granulation tissue, and fibrous tissue – a picture also seen in endometriotic (and corpus luteum) cysts. Close scrutiny of the macrophage zone should reveal the pathognomonic hair fragments or squames.

Deciduosis and pseudodeciduosis are manifestations of mullerianosis occurring in the pregnant (see Ch. 10) and the nonpregnant state (see Ch. 20), respectively. The subperitoneal decidual foci resemble the endometriotic lesions of pregnant women or patients receiving progesterone therapy. The absence of endometrial glands excludes endometriosis.

Endometrioid cystadenomas (see Ch. 25), benign tumors analogous to mucinous, and serous cystadenomas, are uncommonly reported but possibly underdiagnosed. They are lined by typical endometrial epithelium subtended by ovarian stroma without intervening endometrial stroma. There are usually no signs of hemorrhage and no associated adhesions. Endometrioid cystadenofibromas display a complex architectural pattern with irregular gland-like spaces separated by abundant dense fibrous tissue; endometrial stroma is absent.

Low grade endometrial stromal sarcomas (endolymphatic stromal myosis) occur as primary or secondary tumors in the ovary (see Ch. 26). Secondary tumors are readily recognized macroscopically by their worm-like extensions within the broad ligament extending from the primary tumor in the uterine wall. Both are distinguished microscopically from endometriosis by their mitotic activity and lack of endometrial glands.

Development of malignancy

A relationship between ovarian endometriosis and carcinoma was first noted by Sampson (1925). For many years afterwards, the diagnosis of endometrioid ovarian carcinoma demanded the demonstration of its origin in a focus of endometriosis. More recently, it has become clear that the majority of endometrioid carcinomas, like others of the surface epithelial–stromal group, are of coelomic epithelial origin and arise in ovaries unblemished by endometriosis (see Ch. 25). It is also now apparent that histological types of ovarian carcinoma, other than endometrioid, can develop in endometriotic lesions.

Of endometrioid carcinomas, 5–10% can be demonstrated to arise in endometriotic foci, and in an additional 5–10% endometriosis is present elsewhere in the same ovary (Scully 1979, Mostoufizadeh & Scully 1980, Fox & Buckley 1984). Overall, pelvic endometriosis (not necessarily ovarian) is evident in up to 28% of patients (Hyman 1977, Russell 1979, Mostoufizadeh & Scully 1980). These figures may be underestimates, since rapidly growing carcinomas may destroy evidence of their endometriotic origins.

Endometrioid carcinomas (usually well differentiated) are the most common tumors to develop

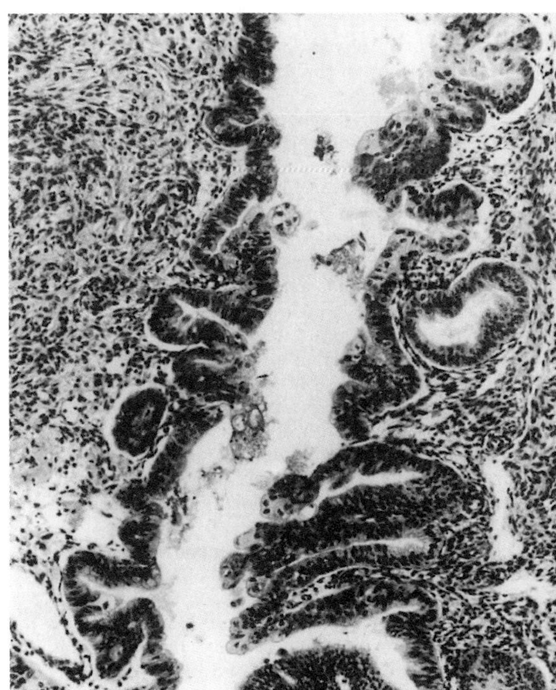

Fig. 21.17 Preneoplastic change in endometriosis. Hyperplastic endometrial epithelium in small endometriotic cyst found in mesovarium adjacent to tumor illustrated in Fig. 21.15. H + E ×80

in association with endometriosis, followed by clear-cell carcinomas and mixed mullerian tumors. Serous, mucinous, and squamous carcinomas are rarely implicated (Mostoufizadeh & Scully 1980). The relationship between endometriosis and carcinoma may in fact be closer in clear-cell rather than endometrioid types, based on a significantly higher frequency of concurrent ovarian endometriosis (Russell 1979).

The risk of development of carcinoma in patients with ovarian endometriosis, although difficult to assess, would seem to be less than 1% (Mostoufizadeh & Scully 1980). Malignancy may also complicate endometriosis in extraovarian sites, notably the rectovaginal septum (Brooks & Wheeler 1977, Hyman 1977). It is worth noting that, in postmenopausal women, ovarian and extraovarian endometriotic deposits, like uterine endometrium, can be stimulated by estrogen replacement therapy, and possible neoplastic transformation should be considered in patients with a history of endometriosis if a pelvic mass develops (Brooks & Wheeler 1977, Case Records of the Massachusetts General Hospital 1980).

Macroscopically, carcinomas arising in endometriotic cysts tend to be papillary or polypoid masses protruding into the lumen (Figs 21.15, 21.16). An intimate anatomical association between the tumor and the endometriotic lesion should be demonstrated in order to establish a causal relationship. Atypical proliferation may be noted in the endometriotic epithelium adjacent to the tumor (Fig. 21.17). A number of cases have now been reported of atypical endometrial proliferation in endometriosis associated with the development of malignancy such as clear-cell and endometrioid carcinoma (La Grenade & Silverberg 1988). One case of clear-cell carcinoma developed 3 years after observation of an atypical focus (Moll et al 1990). It is recommended that patients with foci of atypical epithelium in endometriosis be followed carefully.

REFERENCES

American Fertility Society 1985 Revised American Fertility Society classification of endometriosis: 1985. Fertility and Sterility 43: 351–352

Baiocchi G, Kavanagh J J, Whaton J T 1990 Endometrioid stromal sarcomas arising from ovarian and extraovarian endometriosis: report of two cases and review of the literature. Gynecologic Oncology 36: 147–151

Bergqvist A, Ljungberg O, Myhre E 1984 Human endometrium and endometriotic tissue obtained simultaneously: a comparative histological study. International Journal of Gynecological Pathology 3: 135–145

Blaustein A 1982 Pathology of the female genital tract, 2nd edn. Springer-Verlag, New York, p 464–478

Brooks J J, Wheeler J E 1977 Malignancy arising in extragonadal endometriosis. A case report and summary of the world literature. Cancer 40: 3065–3073

Carey M, Kirk M E 1993 Necrotic pseudoxanthomatous nodules of the omentum and peritoneum: a peculiar reaction to endometriotic cyst contents. Obstetrics and Gynecology 82: 650–652

Case Records of the Massachusetts General Hospital 1980 Case 23–1980. New England Journal of Medicine 302: 1354–1358

Clement P B, Young R G, Scully R E 1988 Necrotic pseudoxanthomatous nodules of ovary and peritoneum in endometriosis. American Journal of Surgical Pathology 12: 390–397

Clement P B, Young R H, Scully R E 1989 Liesegang rings in the female genital tract. A report of three cases. International Journal of Gynecological Pathology 8: 271–276

Cozzutto C 1981 Uterus-like mass replacing ovary. Report of a new entity. Archives of Pathology and Laboratory Medicine 105: 508–511

Czernobilsky B, Morris W J 1979 A histologic study of ovarian endometriosis with emphasis on hyperplastic and atypical changes. Obstetrics and Gynecology 53: 318–323

Dmowski W P, Radwanska E 1984 Current concepts on pathology, histogenesis and etiology of endometriosis. Acta Obstetricia et Gynecologica Scandinavica 123: 29–33

Drake T S, Metz S A, Grunert G M, O'Brien W F 1980 Peritoneal fluid volume in endometriosis. Fertility and Sterility 34: 280–281

Egger H, Weigmann P 1982 Clinical and surgical aspects of ovarian endometriotic cysts. Archives of Gynecology 233: 37–45

El-Mahgoub S, Yaseen S 1980 A positive proof for the theory of coelomic metaplasia. American Journal of Obstetrics and Gynecology 137: 137–140

Fox H 1985 XIIIth World Congress of Anatomic and Clinical Pathology, Brighton, 3 October [gynaecological slide seminar]

Fox H, Buckley C H 1984 Current concepts of endometriosis. Clinics in Obstetrics and Gynaecology 11: 279–287

Halme J, Hall J L 1982 Effect of pelvic fluid from endometriosis patients on human sperm penetration of zona-free hamster ova. Fertility and Sterility 37: 573–576

Haney A F, Muscato J J, Weinberg J B 1981 Peritoneal fluid cell populations in infertility patients. Fertility and Sterility 35: 696–698

Hyman M P 1977 Extraovarian endometrioid carcinoma. Review of the literature and report of two cases with unusual features. American Journal of Clinical Pathology 68: 522–527

Jansen R P S, Russell P 1986 Nonnpigmented endometriosis. Clinical, laparoscopic and pathologic definition. American Journal of Obstetrics and Gynecology 155: 1154–1159

Kistner R W 1971 Gynecology: principles and practice, Year Book, Chicago, IL, p 441

Koninckx P R, Ide P, Vandenbroucke W, Brosens I A 1980 New aspects of the pathophysiology of endometriosis and associated infertility. Journal of Reproductive Medicine 24: 257–260

Lauchlan S C 1966 The cytology of endometriosis. American Journal of Obstetrics and Gynecology 94: 533–535

La Grenade A, Silverberg S G 1988 Ovarian tumors associated with atypical endometriosis. Human Pathology 19: 1080–1084

Liu D T Y, Hitchcock A 1986 Endometriosis: its association with retrograde menstruation, dysmenorrhoea and tubal pathology. British Journal of Obstetrics and Gynaecology 93: 859–862

McDougal R A, Roth L M 1986 Ovarian adenomyoma associated with an endometriotic cyst. Southern Medical Journal 79: 640–642

Merrill J A 1966 Endometrial induction of endometriosis across Millipore filters. American Journal of Obstetrics and Gynecology 94: 780–790

Moll U M, Chumas J C, Chalas E, Mann W J 1990 Ovarian carcinoma arising in atypical endometriosis. Obstetrics and Gynecology 75: 537–539

Moon Y S, Leung P C S, Yuen B A, Gomel V 1981 Prostaglandin F in human endometriotic tissue. American Journal of Obstetrics and Gynecology 141: 344–345

Mostoufizadeh M, Scully R E 1980 Malignant tumors arising in endometriosis. Clinical Obstetrics and Gynecology 23: 951–963

Muscato J J, Haney A F, Weinberg J B 1982 Sperm phagocytosis by human peritoneal macrophages. A possible cause of infertility in endometriosis. American Journal of Obstetrics and Gynecology 144: 503–510

Muse K N, Wilson E A 1982 How does mild endometriosis cause infertility? Fertility and Sterility 38: 145–152

Pellicano M, Magri G, Lacchi L 1994 A case of ovarian endometriosis in late menopause. Clinics in Obstetrics and Gynecology 21: 57–58

Pueblitz-Peredo S, Luévano-Flores E, Rincón-Taracena R, Ochoa-Carrillo F J 1985 Uteruslike mass of the ovary: endomyometriosis or congenital malformation? A case with a discussion of histogenesis. Archives of Pathology and Laboratory Medicine 109: 361–364

Ranney B 1971 Endometriosis IV. Hereditary tendency. Obstetrics and Gynecology 37: 734–737

Ranney B 1980 Etiology, prevention and inhibition of endometriosis. Clinical Obstetrics and Gynecology 23: 875–883

Ridley J H 1968 The histogenesis of endometriosis. A review of facts and fancies. Obstetrical and Gynecological Survey 23: 1–35

Rosenfeld D L, Lecher B D 1981 Endometriosis in a patient with Rokitansky–Kuster–Hauser syndrome. American Journal of Obstetrics and Gynecology 139: 105

Russell P 1979 The pathological assessment of ovarian epithelial neoplasms. III. The malignant 'epithelial tumors'. Pathology 11: 493–532

Salomonowitz E 1980 Tumorförmige amyloidose des ovars. Geburtshilfe und Frauenheilkunde 40: 644–647

Sampson J A 1921 Perforating hemorrhagic (chocolate) cysts of the ovary. Their importance and especially their relation to pelvic adenomas of the endometrial type ('adenomyoma' of the uterus, rectovaginal septum, sigmoid etc.). Archives of Surgery 3: 245–323

Sampson J A 1925 Endometrial carcinoma of the ovary, arising in endometrial tissue of that organ. Archives of Surgery 10: 1–72

Sanfilippo J S, Wakim N G, Schikler K N, Yussman M A 1986 Endometriosis in association with uterine anomaly. American Journal of Obstetrics and Gynecology 154: 39–43

Schwartz D A, Bellin H J 1991 Liesegang rings developing with intraperitoneal endometriotic implants. A case report. Journal of Reproductive Medicine 36: 403–406

Schweppe K-W, Wynn R M 1981 Ultrastructural changes in endometriotic implants during the menstrual cycle. Obstetrics and Gynecology 58: 465–473

Schweppe K-W, Wynn R M 1984 Endocrine dependency of endometriosis: an ultrastructural study. European Journal of Obstetrics, Gynecology and Reproductive Biology 17: 193–208

Scully R E 1979 Tumors of the ovary and maldeveloped gonads. Atlas of tumor pathology, fascicle 16, 2nd series. Armed Forces Institute of Pathology, Washington, DC, p 92–110

Scully R E 1981 Smooth-muscle differentiation in genital tract disorders. Archives of Pathology and Laboratory Medicine 105: 505–507

Simpson J L, Elias S, Malinak L R, Buttram V C 1980 Heritable aspects of endometriosis I. Genetic studies. American Journal of Obstetrics and Gynecology 137: 327–337

Weed J C 1980 Prostaglandins as related to endometriosis. Clinical Obstetrics and Gynecology 23: 890–895

Weed J C, Holland J B 1977 Endometriosis and infertility: an enigma. Fertility and Sterility 28: 135–140

Weed J C, Arquembourg P C 1980 Endometriosis: can it produce an autoimmune response resulting in infertility? Clinical Obstetrics and Gynecology 23: 885–893

Williams T J, Pratt J H 1977 Endometriosis in 1000 consecutive celiotomies: Incidence and management. American Journal of Obstetrics and Gynecology 129: 245–250

SECTION 5

Mullerian epithelial and mesenchymal tumors

22

Introduction, clinical perspective, and principles of management

A. Ferrier

Definition

From a purely practical point of view, a common histogenesis ultimately from the surface epithelium (modified mesothelium) of the ovary is a very convenient and readily understood concept by which the so-called surface epithelial/stromal tumors may be grouped and differentiated from germ cell, gonadal stromal, or other ovarian tumors. However, evidence supporting this genesis varies, in individual tumors taken in isolation, from fairly conclusive to flimsy. The common thread is said to be the embryological development of the mullerian ducts and their derivatives (fallopian tubes, uterine body and cervix, and upper vagina) from this same coelomic epithelium (see Ch. 1). The ovarian and nearby pelvic and abdominal mesothelial surface is thus thought to express a retained potential for mullerian differentiation in neoplasms derived from it. This is, however, a classification of best fit, and theoretical anomalies based on this premise include probable 'non-surface-epithelial' origins of some mucinous, transitional cell, squamous and wolffian tumors, as well as possible coelomic epithelial origin of the primitive sex cords (see Ch. 1) and thus their neoplastic derivatives. This group of tumors is diverse, many with homologs within the mullerian duct derivatives, but some without. Homologous tumors have been reported elsewhere in the female pelvis, quite commonly in the broad ligaments (Rojansky et al 1985), widespread throughout the peritoneal cavity (see Ch. 23), and in testicular and paratesticular tissues in men (Young & Scully 1986). Considering them as a single neoplastic spectrum has led to blurring in the literature of well-defined and distinct patterns of genesis, metastasis, pathological correlates, therapeutic responses, and clinical outcomes. For example, virtually all primary mucinous ovarian carcinomas are of 'intestinal' rather than endocervical type, and their response to chemotherapy (or lack of it) should be more akin to that of colorectal adenocarcinomas than to 'mullerian' tumors. Yet this has not been tested, and there remains a dogged persistence amongst our clinical colleagues, in dealing with such carcinomas, to regard them as part of a mullerian spectrum. One of the implicit aims of this text, and particularly the next nine chapters, is to facilitate histological differentiation between the various neoplastic entities and to stress differences rather than similarities. Important differences between these tumor types are the parameters used for grading. Whilst these are generally architectural and cytological (Bichel & Jakobsen 1989), they are employed with variable reliability (Stalsberg et al 1988, Haapasalo et al 1990, Lund et al 1991, Tyler et al 1991, Sakamoto et al 1994) and different emphases are placed in the various tumor types.

Precursor lesions

Of some importance is whether or not such lesions as serosal inclusions, surface proliferations, metaplasias, or endometriosis (see Chs 20, 21), in the ovary (or elsewhere), represent possible precursor lesions in the genesis of the surface epithelial/stromal tumors. The nature and distribution of the inclusions are central to understanding such tumors, for it may well be they which demonstrate the mullerian potential of the surface 'epithelium' of the ovary and, in turn, dictate the relative frequency and histological range of the tumors seen (Pickartz 1993). An emerging concept is the link between the ovarian mullerian epithelial and mesenchymal tumors and those histologically indistinguishable extraovarian neoplasms based on a similar origin from such focal peritoneal lesions in the female pelvis and abdomen, the most important of these being serous in type (see Ch. 23). There appears merit in considering the female genital tract, ovaries, and peritoneal cavity as a single organ system, as envisaged by Lauchlan (1994). This approach would remove many of the staging anomalies occasioned by our current obeisance to organ pathology and the dogma of a single notional primary for all neoplastic processes (Russell et al 1985).

Proliferative spectrum

Of equal significance is the subdivision of these tumors according to degree of proliferation/malignancy. Recommendations of both International Federation of Gynecology and Obstetrics (FIGO) and the World Health Organization (WHO) (Serov et al 1973) are to subgroup the surface epithelial/stromal ovarian tumors into benign, 'borderline' ('proliferating', 'tumor of low malignant potential' – defined as neoplasms exhibiting an unusual degree of cellular proliferation, greater than that encountered in a benign form of the same type of tumor, but showing no destructive invasion of the stromal component) (Scully 1979), and malignant categories.

There is good circumstantial evidence that ovarian epithelial/stromal malignancies arise, by progressive transformation, from the epithelium of benign epithelial precursors (inclusion cysts or tumors) (Steinback 1981, Plaxe et al 1990). Transitions from 'benign' through 'proliferating' to 'malignant' are commonly observed in ovarian epithelial tumors of serous, mucinous, endometrioid, clear cell, and transitional cell types (Russell 1979a,b, Powell et al 1992), representing an adenoma–carcinoma sequence in such lesions. Powell et al (1992) have speculated that the series of molecular genetic events necessary for this transformation, may occur rapidly or more slowly. In the former event the transition from inclusion cyst to carcinoma might occur in the absence of a benign tumor phase (or, alternatively, it might not be appreciated pathologically). In the latter event, or if only the initial phases of this molecular cascade were to take place, then a benign or proliferating tumor might result, followed by a carcinoma only after further steps. Our understanding of these molecular genetic events is starting to emerge but, in the meantime, there appears logic in grading the neoplastic process according to the most advanced changes observed in the tissues at the time of clinical presentation. Earlier or 'pre-existing' changes should be commented upon. The criteria currently advocated to distinguish the atypically proliferating tumors (our preferred term) from their benign counterparts or precursors include the significant presence (i.e. >10% of the tissue available for review; lesser foci can be dismissed) in the same tumor of any *two* of the following:

- Epithelial budding – epithelial cell proliferation, usually in the form of small papillae without connective tissue cores, with a tendency for single cells or cell clusters to detach into the cyst lumen
- Multilayering of epithelium – stratification of epithelial cells covering papillae or lining glandular spaces, or production of solid morules of cells where a single layered epithelium is usual in the corresponding benign tumor
- Mitotic activity – an increase over the very low mitotic activity of most benign tumors or, in the case of mucinous tumors, an alteration in distribution of mitoses
- Nuclear atypia – an increase in nuclear/cytoplasmic ratio, alterations in nuclear chromatin pattern, abnormalities of size, shape, and number of nucleoli

The original reason for creating the proliferating group of ovarian tumors was to explain the remarkably good prognosis in a small number of women with serous ovarian tumors showing pathological features suggesting malignancy (Taylor 1929) and evidence, at laparotomy, of apparent widespread metastases (these latter now termed 'implants'). It is our contention that the vast majority of the extraovarian manifestations of serous tumors with atypical proliferation are a result of widespread multifocal in situ neoplasia arising from peritoneal serous inclusions (endosalpingiosis) and correspond to part of the same neoplastic spectrum which has been delineated in the ovaries (Russell 1984). As a consequence of this, in our view, the general term 'proliferating surface epithelial/stromal tumor' carries more the connotations of 'atypical hyperplasia', 'premalignant atypia', 'ovarian intraepithelial neoplasia' (Yoonessi et al 1988), or 'adenocarcinoma in situ' superimposed upon a previous benign epithelial tumor, rather than 'tumor of low malignant potential' as advocated by Scully (1982) and Zaloudek & Kurman (1983). Pathological discussion of individual tumors in the following chapters reflects this approach, grouping tumors which histologically show atypical proliferation into a noninvasive (pre-invasive?) category with benign tumors (as one would do for tumors of the other major organ systems of the body).

A more critical point of discrimination in the range of tumor proliferation is, therefore, between atypically proliferating tumors and frank carcinomas, the latter defined by the presence of destructive stromal invasion (epithelial tumor cells invading the surrounding supportive stroma and inducing a desmoplastic response in this stroma). Such appearances are to be distinguished from the plethora of patterns generated by pseudo-invasion or benign intrusion of the stromal component in cystic tumors and the increasingly complex proliferative pattern of glands in solid tumors. The problem is least difficult in serous tumors and greatest in mucinous and endometrioid lesions, although destructive invasion, an ill-defined concept, is not even constant in cases of serous carcinoma. We feel this is a perceptual rather than conceptual problem. Our practice is to pay particular attention to the following histological markers in identifying areas of invasion:

- In mostly cystic tumors, a change in architectural contour at the epithelial/stromal interface of the tumor from broad front to focal irregularities and polymorphic epithelial structures projecting into the stroma. In mainly solid tumors, a haphazard arrangement of irregular sized and shaped glandular structures. Such changes represent a true qualitative change in the orientation of epithelial elements to each other, whereas within tumors showing atypical proliferation there is merely a quantitative increase of epithelium with an architectural configuration in keeping with that seen in the benign equivalent.
- Alteration in the character of the tumor stroma from hypercellular, fibrous ovarian, or hyalinized stroma to edematous immature stroma with dilated thin-walled sinusoidal vessels, resembling reparative granulation tissue.
- Presence of chronic inflammatory cells. Lymphocytes or plasma cells, while sometimes absent in invasive tumors, are only occasionally prominent in noninvasive or borderline tumors, and their presence may be a marker of stromal invasion, particularly if focal and if closely applied to areas of irregular epithelial growth.

It is our intention, in the following chapters, to critically apply these principles to the appraisal of the surface epithelial–stromal tumors of the ovary, which account for about 60% of all ovarian neoplasms and 80–90% of primary ovarian malignancies (Katsube et al 1982). Their approximate relative frequencies according to a modified WHO classification (Appendix B) are shown in Table 22.1.

Burden of disease

In most Western countries epithelial ovarian

Table 22.1 Percentage histological distribution of 1000 consecutive surface epithelial–stromal tumors encountered at King George V Hospital

	Non-invasive		Invasive carcinomas	Total
	Benign	Proliferating		
Serous	23	7	16	46
Mucinous	29.5	5	2	36.5
Endometrioid	–†	1.5	6	7.5
Mullerian mesenchymal	–†	–†	0.7	0.7
Clear cell	–†	–†	3	3
Transitional cell	2	–†	–†	2
Squamous*	–†	–	–†	–†
Mixed epithelial	1.5	0.5	0.5	2.5
Undifferentiated carcinomas	–	–	1.5	1.5
Unclassified epithelial	–†	–†	0.3	0.3
Total	56	14	30	100

*Squamous cell neoplasms of nonteratomatous origin.
†Rarely encountered tumors.

malignancy is the fifth commonest cancer affecting women and ranks fourth in cancer mortality (Cannistra 1993). In the USA, it is currently estimated that there will be 24 000 new cases of epithelial ovarian cancer and 13 600 deaths from the disease each year (Boring et al 1994). Rarely diagnosed in women under age 40 years, ovarian cancer has a peak incidence in the seventh decade of 55/100 000 population (American Cancer Society 1991). Median age at diagnosis is 61 years. The lifetime risk of ovarian cancer is approximately 1% among most Caucasian populations, and varies from 0.45% in Japan to 1.7% in Sweden (Muir et al 1987). There appears to be no clear trend in the incidence of ovarian neoplasia during the last 20 years, although some reports refer to a decreasing incidence in younger women, attributed to the oral contraceptive pill (Villard-Mackintosh et al 1989). In the USA, there has been a 3.6% increase in the age-adjusted incidence of ovarian cancer amongst black women in the period 1975–1984, and a small decrease of 1.9% in white women (National Cancer Institute 1986).

Survival has changed little over the last 20 years. The 5-year survival statistics demonstrate an overall survival probability of approximately 40%. Three-quarters of cases present with widespread metastatic disease. Survival at 5 years in this group is 10–20%. Patients diagnosed with early stage disease confined to the ovary or pelvis demonstrate a 5-year survival rate of 80%.

Risk factors

Hereditary ovarian cancer is responsible for about 5% of all diagnosed cases. Three familial cancer syndromes have been described involving epithelial ovarian cancer: breast–ovarian cancer, site-specific ovarian cancer, and the Lynch II syndrome characterized by inherited ovarian, endometrial, and nonpolyposis colorectal cancer (Lynch et al 1990a). The pattern of inheritance appears to be autosomal dominant with incomplete penetrance. The risk of inheritance in some affected families is estimated to be 40% (Lynch et al 1990b). Familial ovarian cancer is characterized by an early age of diagnosis. The median age is 49 years (Lynch et al 1993). The genetic pattern demonstrates loss of heterozygosity on chromosome 17q. Linkage studies in families with early onset breast–ovarian cancer have indicated a gene (BrCA1) mapping to 17q12–21, which accords an inherited susceptibility to both breast and ovarian cancer (Hall et al 1990). It is estimated that the first-degree relatives of women diagnosed with breast cancer, who are perimenopausal, have a comparable risk (two-fold) of developing ovarian cancer as they do breast cancer (Thompson & Schildkraut 1990). These ovarian neoplasms are frequently high-grade serous carcinomas which manifest a clinically aggressive course. There is also evidence from retrospective studies of women who have undergone prophylactic oophorectomy that there is also a high risk of primary peritoneal serous carcinoma (Tobacman et al 1982).

There is an increasing body of evidence that reproductive factors and some forms of infertility treatment are risk factors in the pathogenesis of epithelial ovarian cancer (Purdie et al 1995). Many of these data are consistent with the incessant ovulation theory (Fathalla 1971). Fathalla proposed that repeated involvement of the surface (germinal) epithelium during the process of ovulation without adequate physiological rest was associated with development of ovarian neoplasia. Malignant transformation results from repetitive trauma to the surface epithelium followed by cellular proliferation, infolding, and the formation of inclusion cysts. This concept may explain why factors increasing the risk of ovarian cancer include low parity, prolonged unprotected sexual intercourse, and the administration of ovulation-induction agents, particularly where conception was not achieved. Protective factors include high parity, combined hormonal contraception and lactation (Table 22.2).

Ovarian cancer prevention

Ovarian cancer is associated with more deaths than all other gynecological malignancies combined. Several screening strategies have been proposed. A successful screening program needs three prerequisites: a disease which is prevalent enough to justify screening; a well-defined natural history where early detection will allow treatment to improve outcome; and a cost-effective

Table 22.2 Risk factors for surface epithelial–stromal ovarian cancer

Reference	Factor	Cases/controls	Source of controls	Crude odds ratio (95% CI)	Adjusted odds ratio (95% CI)
Kerlikowske et al 1992	Family history*				
	Nil			1.0	NA
	1 relative or first-degree relative			3.1 (2.2–4.4)	NA
	2 or 3 relatives			4.6 (1.1–18.4)	NA
	Hereditary ovarian cancer	(50% lifetime risk)		NA	NA
Harlow et al 1992	Perineal talc exposure			1.3 (1.1–1.6)	
Mettlin & Piver 1990	Whole-milk consumption (>1 glass/day)	36/27	Hospital	3.1 (1.8–5.5)	NA
Whittemore et al 1992	*Reproductive factors*				
	Fertility drugs	20/11	Community		2.8 (1.3–6.1)
	Duration of unprotected intercourse (>15 years)	133/171	Community		1.6 (1.2–2.2)
	Parity (any term pregnancy)	1041/4644	Community		0.47 (0.4–0.56)
	Lactation	392/2472	Community		0.81 (0.68–0.95)
	OCP (>6 years)	351/2472	Community		0.30 (0.23–0.41)
	Hysterectomy (<40 years)	65/445	Community		0.76 (0.57–1.0)
	Tubal ligation	29/193	Community		0.59 (0.38–0.93)

*estimated odds ratios.

screening test. Clinical (pelvic) examination lacks sufficient sensitivity or specificity as a screening test. Considerable attention has been directed to serum tumor markers and pelvic ultrasound. The most extensively evaluated serum tumor marker, calCA-125, is of limited value as a screening test. In early stage, potentially curable disease, calCA-125 determinations are positive in only 50% of cases (Olt et al 1990). Transabdominal and transvaginal ultrasound have demonstrated improved sensitivity and specificity. In a prospective study of 5479 self-referred asymptomatic women, five women with early ovarian cancer were detected and another four with metastatic disease. Despite an apparent sensitivity of 100%, 2.3% of the scan results were false-positives resulting in 317 women being recommended to have unnecessary surgery (Campbell et al 1989). The cost of ultrasonography, in addition to the risks and costs associated with subsequent evaluation of false-positive tests, prevents its implementation for routine population based screening. Screening for high-risk populations, in particular early-onset ovarian cancer families, poses additional problems, with no evidence of improved life expectancy (Schapira et al 1993). The current recommendations of the Committee on Gynecologic Practice of the American College of Obstetricians and Gynecologists (ACOG) where there is a strong family history of ovarian cancer are: where preservation of fertility is important, 6 monthly transvaginal ultrasonography to be undertaken and prophylactic oophorectomy to be considered when the family has been completed or not planned. The oral contraceptive should also be prescribed to young women who are not planning a family (ACOG Committee 1993). The efficacy of the oral contraceptive has not been proven in high-risk groups.

Surface epithelial–stromal ovarian tumors do not produce specific symptoms. As they grow, local symptoms referable to size and weight, such as urinary frequency, constipation and a sense of heaviness within the pelvis, may be experienced.

Larger or more rapidly growing tumors consistently present with pelvic or lower abdominal pain or discomfort (in 50% of cases), abdominal swelling (50%), abnormal uterine bleeding in one-third, gastrointestinal symptoms (such as dyspepsia, nausea, cramps, and diarrhea) in about 20% of patients, and weight loss and urinary symptoms only slightly less frequently. Acute abdominal symptoms, due to rupture, torsion, or hemorrhage, are uncommon (less rare in benign than malignant tumors), and a plethora of unusual paraneoplastic syndromes may occasionally draw the clinician's attention to the ovarian lesion (see Appendix D).

The diagnosis of ovarian tumors ultimately depends upon histological examination of biopsy material following exploratory laparotomy. A recent trend of ultrasound-guided aspiration of ovarian cysts and cytological examination of the cyst fluid has been widely criticised, as 50% of histologically malignant cysts do not demonstrate malignant cells on examination of the cyst aspirate (Trimbos & Hacker 1993). FIGO staging of the proliferating and invasive malignant tumors (Appendix C) is based on laparotomy findings, and includes the final histological typing and grading as well as cytology of peritoneal fluid (including washings taken in the absence of clinical ascites). Cytological examination of pleural fluid and fine needle aspirates of liver metastases and supraclavicular nodes are required to confirm FIGO stage 4 disease. Parallel assessments of tumor tissue removed at laparotomy for cellular DNA content (Friedlander et al 1984, Rodenburg et al 1987), estrogen and progesterone receptor levels (Schwartz et al 1985), and tumor markers (Kabawat et al 1983, Casper et al 1984), offer additional prognostic data, and it is important that the pathologist be aware of the requirements of these techniques (see Ch. 4). It has been standard practice for some time to remove the omentum as part of both staging and primary therapy of ovarian cancer, as well as to excise peritoneal lesions and biopsy subdiaphragmatic tissue, pelvic peritoneum, and retroperitoneal lymph nodes (Chen & Lee 1984).

The importance of adequate surgical staging has been clearly demonstrated. When 100 patients thought to have early stage disease on initial surgical assessment were re-explored, 30% were upstaged, of whom 77% actually had stage 3 disease (Young et al 1983). A subsequent study of 291 patients with ovarian cancer found that 46% of those cases had been incorrectly staged. Of patients explored by gynaecological oncologists, 97% were correctly staged, while staging was correct in only 52% by specialist gynecologists and 35% by general surgeons (McGowan 1985).

Primary therapy of these tumors is surgical removal. This is adequate for benign tumors and the majority of proliferating tumors. Intraoperative frozen section or cytological examination (see Ch. 57) plays a role in our institution in the typing of these tumors and the exclusion of frank malignancy when the preservation of fertility is desirable and conservative surgery is planned. The paradox of a limited surgical approach for the preservation of fertility is that extensive surgical staging of the peritoneal cavity is required to confirm the absence of occult microscopic disease. As part of this procedure, an ipsilateral pelvic and para-aortic lymph node dissection is frequently carried out in addition to omentectomy and multiple peritoneal biopsies.

There is considerable evidence that early stage proliferating ovarian tumors have been overtreated. In a review of four randomized trials including 253 patients with proliferating tumors, the corrected survival was 99%. Although 83% of the patients underwent total abdominal hysterectomy, bilateral salpingo-oophorectomy, and omentectomy, none of the patients with less extensive surgery recurred. Adjuvant treatment does not appear to improve corrected survival and is associated with significant toxicity (Trope et al 1993).

The management of early stage invasive ovarian neoplasia has been the subject of five randomized trials. Adjuvant treatment included melphalan, phosphorus-32, cisplatin, and pelvic radiotherapy (Dembo et al 1979a, Young et al 1990, Bolis et al 1989). FIGO stage Ia grade I and II lesions do not appear to have an improved survival advantage following adjuvant treatment. Observation is therefore the current recommended management strategy. Relapse rates of 20%, associated with high-grade lesions, positive peritoneal cytology, cyst capsule rupture, and all stage 2 lesions, warrant adjuvant treatment with as yet undetermined optimal therapy.

The role of radiotherapy in the treatment of ovarian cancer remains unclear. There are few randomized trials assessing the efficacy of radiotherapy and those that have been attempted have been flawed by inadequate surgical staging or poor patient accrual. Current data would suggest that the role of radiotherapy is restricted to whole abdominal and pelvic prescription, with a pelvic boost for a subset of patients with early stage disease, demonstrating no macroscopic residuum, well or moderately differentiated morphology, and non-clear-cell histology (Dembo et al 1979b).

In the majority of cases the surgeon is confronted with advanced, large volume disease widely disseminated throughout the peritoneal cavity. Occasionally, the histological diagnosis confirms a noninvasive or proliferating lesion. Thorough surgical debulking of these lesions is recommended, as there is no proven adjuvant therapy. Furthermore, a complete cytoreductive procedure is needed to exclude invasive foci (invasive 'implants'), which appear to confer a poorer prognosis and may warrant adjuvant therapy (Bell et al 1988). A number of reports have documented favorable 5-year survival rates for patients with proliferating lesions, but a steady decline after 5 years. In a recent report of long-term follow-up of patients with proliferating lesions, patients with stage 3 disease demonstrated a recurrence rate of 54%, but a long-term disease-specific mortality rate of only 26% (Leake et al 1992).

Radical cytoreductive surgery is considered the current standard for the management of large volume invasive disease. The theoretical justification for such an approach is that removal of large volume disease improves subsequent response to chemotherapy, reduces the discomfort of bulky disease, allows the patient to enhance her nutritional status, and reduces harmful metabolic effects of the tumor (Griffiths 1986). The mathematical model, proposed by Goldie & Coldman (1979), would also support this view, stating that the spontaneous tumor cell mutation rate is related to the number of tumor cells and their rate of growth. There are no randomized trials which address the efficacy of maximum cytoreductive surgery, and the current support for this approach comes from indirect evidence. Pooled analysis from 12 studies shows a median survival of 39 months for optimally debulked patients and 17 months for suboptimally cytoreduced patients (Ozols et al 1992). The Gynecologic Oncology Group attempted to test the hypothesis that cytoreductive surgery improved survival by comparing patients with low volume disease who had been optimally debulked with patients who initially had large volume disease who were optimally cytoreduced surgically. Both groups received the same cisplatin containing combination chemotherapy. Those patients diagnosed with large volume disease demonstrated a poorer outcome than the small volume group, suggesting that tumor biology rather than the radical nature of the surgical procedure determines treatment outcome (Hoskins et al 1992). Furthermore, in a metanalysis of 58 studies, maximum cytoreductive surgery appeared to have a small effect on treatment outcome (Hunter et al 1992).

Since the late 1970s, cisplatin combination chemotherapy has been the standard for adjuvant therapy. Clinical response rates of 60% are consistently reported, with a pathologically confirmed complete response rate of 30%. Median survival is reported to be approximately 24 months (Omura et al 1989). Despite the improvement in progression-free interval and median survival, the proportion of patients who present with advanced disease alive 5 years after initial treatment remains a dismal 10–20%.

Taxol, a new chemotherapy agent, has recently been shown to be active against ovarian carcinoma. Initial studies suggested that in patients resistant to cisplatin-based chemotherapy, 30% would respond to Taxol (McGuire et al 1989), while a subsequent clinical trial comparing Taxol plus cisplatin with the current standard, cyclophosphamide and cisplatin, demonstrated a statistically significant recurrence-free and median survival advantage with the Taxol group (McGuire et al 1996). Taxol or Taxol-like chemotherapy may become the standard first-line therapy in the future.

Second-look laparotomy continues to be advocated in many centers as a standard component of the management regimen. There is no evidence that this procedure prolongs survival. Moreover, 50% of patients with negative second-look operations following cisplatin chemotherapy subsequently recur, in one-half of cases at sites not assessable by laparotomy (Rubin et al 1988). If second-look procedures are considered a diagnostic test, this is equivalent to a sensitivity of 0.5, similar to a toss of a coin predicting 'heads'. Second-look laparotomies should remain part of investigational protocols exclusively. Secondary cytoreductive surgery, commonly confused with second-look laparotomy, is done where there is clear evidence of recurrent disease. The intent is to further reduce tumor volume resistant to initial chemotherapy. There have been no prospective randomized trials assessing the survival impact of secondary debulking surgery. Survival following surgical re-exploration appears to be related to progression-free interval following initial therapy. Although 25% of patients undergoing secondary cytoreductive surgery will have the tumor volume reduced to a microscopic residuum (Hoskins et al 1989) and demonstrate a survival benefit, other groups have demonstrated no survival advantage for patients who are successfully cytoreduced compared to those with macroscopic residual disease (Luesley et al 1984).

Finally, autopsy examination is all too frequently the final exposure of the pathologist to the patient with ovarian carcinoma, and adherence to a full standard autopsy protocol can still yield useful information (Dvoretsky et al 1988, Rose et al 1989).

REFERENCES

American Cancer Society 1991 Cancer Facts and Figures 1991. American Cancer Society, Atlanta, GA

Bell D A, Weinstock M A, Scully R E 1988 Peritoneal implants of ovarian serous borderline tumors: histologic features and prognosis.Cancer 62: 2212–2222

Bichel P, Jakobsen A 1989 A new histologic grading index in ovarian carcinoma. International Journal of Gynecological Pathology 8: 147–155

Bolis G, Beni S, Favalli G et al 1989 Multicenter controlled trial in patients with epithelial ovarian cancer stage I. Proceedings of the International Gynecologic Cancer Society 157

Boring C C, Squires T S, Tong T, Montgomery S 1994 Cancer statistics 1994 Ca. A Cancer Journal for Clinicians 44: 7–26

Campbell S, Bhan V, Royston P, Whitehead M I, Collins W P 1989 Transabdominal ultrasound screening for early ovarian cancer. British Medical Journal 299: 1363–1367

Cannistra S A 1993 Cancer of the ovary. New England Journal of Medicine 329: 1550–1559

Casper S, van Nagell J R, Powell D F et al 1984 Immunohistochemical localization of tumor markers in epithelial ovarian cancer. American Journal of Obstetrics and Gynecology 149: 154–158

Chen S S, Lee L 1984 Prognostic significance of morphology of tumor and retroperitoneal lymph nodes in epithelial carcinoma of the ovary. Gynecologic Oncology 18: 87–93

Dembo A J, Bush R S, Beale F A, Bean H A, Pringle J F, Sturgeon J F 1979a The Princess Margaret Hospital study of ovarian cancer: Stage I, II and asymptomatic III presentations. Cancer Treatment Report 63: 249–254

Dembo A J, Bush R S, Beale F A et al 1979b Improved survival following abdominopelvic irradiation in patients with a completed pelvic operation. American Journal of Obstetrics and Gynecology 134: 793–800

Dvoretsky P, Richards K, Angel C et al 1988 Distribution of disease at autopsy in 100 women with ovarian cancer. Human Pathology 19: 57–63

Fathalla M F 1971 Incessant ovulation – a factor in ovarian neoplasia. Lancet Jul 17; 2(716): 163

Friedlander M L, Hedley D W, Taylor I W, Russell P, Coates AS, Tattersall M H N 1984 Influence of cellular DNA content on survival in advanced ovarian cancer. Cancer Research 44: 397–400

Goldie J H, Coldman A J 1979 A mathematical model for relating the drug sensitivity of tumors to their spontaneous mutation rate. Cancer Treatment Report 63: 1727–1733

Griffiths C 1986 Surgery at the time of diagnosis in ovarian cancer. In: Blackledge G, Chan K K (eds) Management of ovarian cancer. Butterworth, London, p 60

Haapasalo H, Collan Y, Seppa Gidlund A L, Atkin N B, Pesonen E 1990 Prognostic value of ovarian carcinoma grading methods – a method comparison study. Histopathology 16: 1–7

Hall J M, Lee M K, Newman B et al 1990 Linkage of early-onset familial breast cancer to chromosome 17q21. Science 250: 1684–1689

Harlow B L, Cramer D W, Bell D A, Welch D R 1992 Perineal exposure to talc and ovarian cancer risk. Obstetrics and Gynecology 80: 19–26

Hoskins W J, Rubin SC, Dulaney E et al 1989 Influence of secondary cytoreduction at the time of second-look laparotomy on the survival of patients with epithelial ovarian cancer. Gynecolic Oncology 34: 365–371

Hoskins W J, Bundy B N, Thigpen J T, Omura G A 1992 The influence of cytoreductive surgery on recurrence-free interval and survival in small-volume stage III epithelial ovarian cancer: A Gynecologic Oncology Group Study. Gynecologic Oncology 47: 159–166

Hunter R W, Alexander N D E, Soutter W P 1992 Meta-analysis of surgery in advanced ovarian carcinoma; is maximum cytoreductive surgery an independent determinant of prognosis? American Journal of Obstetrics and Gynecology 166: 504–511

Kabawat S E, Bast R C, Welch W R, Knapp R C, Colvin R B 1983 Immunopathologic characterization of a monoclonal antibody that recognizes common surface antigens of human ovarian tumors of serous, endometrioid and clear cell types. American Journal of Clinical Pathology 79: 98–104

Katsube Y, Berg J W, Silverberg S G 1982 Epidemiologic

pathology of ovarian tumors. International Journal of Gynecological Pathology 1: 3–16

Kerlikowske K, Brown J S, Grady D G 1992 Should women with familial ovarian cancer undergo prophylactic oophorectomy? Obstetrics and Gynecology 80: 700–707

Lauchlan S C 1994 The secondary mullerian system revisited. International Journal of Gynecological Pathology 13: 73–79

Leake J F, Currie J L, Rosenshein N E, Woodruff J D 1992 Long-term follow-up of serous ovarian tumors of low malignant potential. Gynecologic Oncology 47: 150–158

Luesley D M, Chan K K, Fielding J W, Hurlow R, Blackledge G R, Jordon J A 1984 Second-look laparotomy in the management of epithelial ovarian carcinoma: an evaluation of fifty cases. Obstetrics and Gynecology 64: 421–426

Lund B, Thomsen H K, Olsen J 1991 Reproducibility of histopathological evaluation in epithelial ovarian carcinoma. Clinical implications. Acta Pathologica Microbiologica et Immunologica Scandinavica 99: 353–358

Lynch H T, Fitzsimmons M L, Conway T A, Bewtra C, Lynch J 1990a Hereditary carcinoma of the ovary and associated cancers: a study of two families. Gynecologic Oncology 36: 48–55

Lynch H T, Conway T, Lynch J 1990b Hereditary ovarian cancer. In: Sharp F, Mason W P, Leake R E (eds) Ovarian cancer: biological and therapeutic challenges. Chapman & Hall Medical, Cambridge, p 719

Lynch H T, Watson P, Lynch J F, Conway T A, Fili M 1993 Heterogeneity in age at onset. Cancer 71: 573–581

McGowan L, Lesher L P, Norris H J, Barnett M 1985 Misstaging of ovarian cancer. Obstetrics and Gynecology 65: 568–572

McGuire W P, Rowinski E K, Rosenheim N E et al 1989 Taxol: a unique antineoplastic agent with significant activity in advanced ovarian epithelial neoplasms. Annals of Internal Medicine 111: 273–279

McGuire W P, Hoskins W J, Brady M F et al 1996 Cyclophosphamide and cisplatin compared with paclitaxel and cisplatin in patients with stage III and stage IV ovarian cancer. New England Journal of Medicine 334: 1–6

Mettlin C, Piver M S 1990 A case-control study of milk-drinking and ovarian cancer. American Journal of Epidemiology 132: 871–876

Muir C, Waterhouse J, Mack T, Powell J, Whelan S 1987 Cancer in five continents, vol V. IARC Scientific Publications No. 88. IARC, Lyon

National Cancer Institute 1986 Division of Cancer Prevention and Control: Annual Cancer Statistics Review. NIH Publication No. 87–2789. NIH, Bethseda, MD

Olt G J, Berchuck A, Bast R C 1990 Gynecologic tumor markers. Seminars in Surgical Oncology 6: 305–313

Omura G A, Bundy B N, Berek J S, Curry S, Delgado G, Mortel R 1989 Randomised trial of cyclophosphamide and cisplatin with or without doxorubicin in ovarian carcinoma: a Gynecologic Oncology Group Study. Journal of Clinical Oncology 7: 457–465

Ozols R F, Rubin S C, Dembo A J, Robboy S 1992 Epithelial Ovarian Cancer. In: Hoskins W J, Perez C A, Young R C (eds) Principles and practice of gynecologic oncology. J D Lippincott, Philadelphia, PA, p 754

Pickartz H 1993 Differential diagnosis of peritoneal lesions of müllerian type and similar epithelial tumors of the peritoneum. International Journal of Gynecological Pathology 12: 116–119

Plaxe S C, Deligdisch L, Dottino P R et al 1990 Ovarian intraepithelial neoplasia demonstrated in patients with stage 1 ovarian carcinoma. Gynecologic Oncology 38: 367–372

Powell D E, Puls L, van Nagell J Jr 1992 Current concepts in epithelial ovarian tumors: does benign to malignant transformation occur? Human Pathology 23: 846–847

Purdie D, Green A, Bain C et al 1995 Reproductive and other factors and risk of epithelial ovarian cancer: an Australian case-control study. International Journal of Cancer 62: 678–684

Rodenburg C J, Cornelisse C J, Heintz P A M, Hermans J, Fleuren G J 1987 Tumor ploidy as a prognostic factor in advanced ovarian cancer. Cancer 59: 317–323

Rojansky N, Ophir E, Sharony A, Spira H, Suprun H 1985 Broad ligament adenocarcinoma – its origin and clinical behavior. A literature review and report of a case. Obstetrical and Gynecological Survey 40: 665–671

Rose P G, Piver M S, Tsukada Y, Lau T S 1989 Metastatic patterns in histologic variants of ovarian cancer. An autopsy study. Cancer 64: 1508–1513

Routine Cancer screening. ACOG Committee Opinion: Committee on Gynecologic Practice number 128. October 1993. Int J Gynaecol Obstet 43: 344–8

Rubin S C, Hoskins W J, Hakes T B, Markman M, Cain J M, Lewis J L Jr 1988 Recurrence after negative second-look laparotomy in advanced ovarian cancer. Analysis of risk factors. American Journal of Obstetrics and Gynecology 159: 1094–1098

Russell P 1979a The pathological assessment of ovarian neoplasms. II: The proliferating 'epithelial' tumours. Pathology 11: 251–282

Russell P 1979b The pathological assessment of ovarian neoplasms. III: The malignant 'epithelial' tumors. Pathology 11: 493–532

Russell P 1984 Borderline epithelial tumors of the ovary: a conceptual dilemma. Clinics in Obstetrics and Gynaecology 11: 259–277

Russell P, Bannatyne P M, Solomon H J, Stoddard L D, Tattersall M H N 1985 Multifocal tumorigenesis in the upper female genital tract – implications for staging and management. International Journal of Gynecological Pathology 4: 192–210

Sakamoto A, Sasaki H, Furusato M et al 1994 Observer disagreement in histological classification of ovarian tumors in Japan. Gynecologic Oncology 54: 54–58

Schapira M M, Matchar D B, Young M J 1993 The effectiveness of ovarian cancer screening: a decision analysis model. Annals of Internal Medicine 118: 838–843

Schwartz P E, Merino M J, LiVolsi V A, Lawrence R, MacLusky N, Eisenfeld A 1985 Histopathologic correlations of estrogen and progestin receptor protein in epithelial ovarian carcinomas. Obstetrics and Gynecology 66: 428–433

Scully R E 1979 Tumors of the ovary and maldeveloped gonads, AFIP Fascicle 16, 2nd series. Armed Forces Institute of Pathology, Washington, DC, p 53–151

Scully R E 1982 Common epithelial tumors of borderline malignancy (carcinomas of low malignant potential). Bulletin de Cancer (Paris) 69: 228–238

Serov S F, Scully R E, Sobin L H 1973 Histological typing of ovarian tumors. International histological classification of tumors No. 9. World Health Organization, Geneva

Stalsberg H, Abeler V, Blom G P, Bostad L, Skarland E, Westgaard G 1988 Observer variation in histologic classification of malignant and borderline ovarian tumors. Human Pathology 19: 1030–1035

Steinback F 1981 Benign, borderline and malignant serous cystadenomas of the ovary. Pathology Research and Practice 172: 58–72

Tobacman J K, Greene M H, Tucker M A, Costa J, Kase R, Fraumeni J F Jr 1982 Intra-abdominal carcinomatosis after prophylactic oophorectomy in ovarian cancer-prone families. Lancet ii: 795–797

Taylor H C Jr 1929 Malignant and semimalignant tumours of the ovary. Surgery Gynecology and Obstetrics 48: 204–230

Thompson W D, Schildkraut J M 1990 Family history of gynaecological cancers: relationship to the incidence of breast cancer prior to ade 55. International Journal of Epidemiology 20: 595–602

Trimbos J B, Hacker N F 1993 The case against aspirating ovarian cysts. Cancer 71: 1551–1558

Trope C, Kaern J, Vergote I B, Kristensen G, Abeler V 1993 Are borderline tumors of the ovary overtreated both surgically and systemically? A review of four prospective randomised trials including 253 patients with borderline tumors. Gynecologic Oncology 51: 236–243

Villard-Mackintosh L, Vessey M P, Jones L 1989 The effects of oral contraceptives and parity on ovarian cancer trends in women under 55 years of age. British Journal of Obstetrics and Gynaecology 96: 783–788

Whittemore A S, Harris R, Itnyre J and the Collaborative Ovarian Cancer Group 1992 Characteristics relating to ovarian cancer risk: collaborative analysis of 12 US case-control studies. American Journal of Epidemiology 136: 1175–1184

Yoonessi M, Crickard K, Celik C, Yoonessi S 1988 Borderline epithelial tumors of the ovary: ovarian intraepithelial neoplasia. Obstetrical and Gynecological Survey 43: 435–444

Young R H, Scully R E 1986 Testicular and paratesticular tumors and tumor-like lesions of ovarian common epithelial and Mullerian types. A report of four cases and review of the literature. American Journal of Clinical Pathology 86: 146–152

Young R C, Decker D G, Wharton J T et al 1983 Staging laparotomy in early ovarian cancer. Journal of the American Medical Association 250: 3072–3076

Young R C, Walton L A, Ellenberg S S et al 1990 Adjuvant therapy in stage I and II epithelial ovarian cancer. Results of two prospective randomised trials. New England Journal of Medicine 322: 1021–1027

Zaloudek C, Kurman R J 1983 Recent advances in the pathology of ovarian cancer. Clinics in Obstetrics and Gynaecology 10: 155–185

23

Serous tumors

P. Russell A. Farnsworth

The principal architectural and cytological features of these tumors are based on the proclivity of the epithelium to produce, to a greater or lesser extent, fine papillary structures, and for the epithelial cells to resemble those of the native fallopian tube mucosa (secretory, ciliated, intercalary, and intraepithelial vacuolated cells being present) (Fig. 23.1) or, less commonly, the surface epithelium of the ovary. Similar tumors may be found in all anatomical divisions of the mature female genital tract (Bannatyne & Russell 1981, Russell et al 1985, Sherman et al 1992, Zheng et al 1996). Additionally, they are well documented in parovarian cysts (Chandraratnam & Leong 1983, Rojansky et al 1985, Seltzer et al 1988, Aslani et al 1988, Jensen & Nielsen 1989, Aslani & Scully 1989, Kaur et al 1990), retroperitoneum (Ulbright et al 1983) or pelvic lymph nodes (Farhi & Silverberg 1982), umbilicus (Hernandez et al 1993), pelvic and abdominal peritoneum and omentum (Genadry et al 1981, Lindeque et al 1985, Chen & Flam 1986, McCaughey et al 1986, Austin et al 1987, Bell et al 1988, Dalrymple et al 1989, Wick et al 1989, Fromm et al 1990, Ransom et al 1990, Truong et al 1990, Rosen et al 1992, Maasen & Debus-Theide 1993), with or without a coexisting serous ovarian neoplasm (Feuer et al 1989), and sometimes years after removal of normal ovaries (Tobacman et al 1982, Chen et al 1985, Kemp et al 1992, Piver et al 1993). Rare examples have been described in the testes of male patients (Axiotis 1988, Kosmehl et al 1989, Remmele et al 1992, Jones et al 1995).

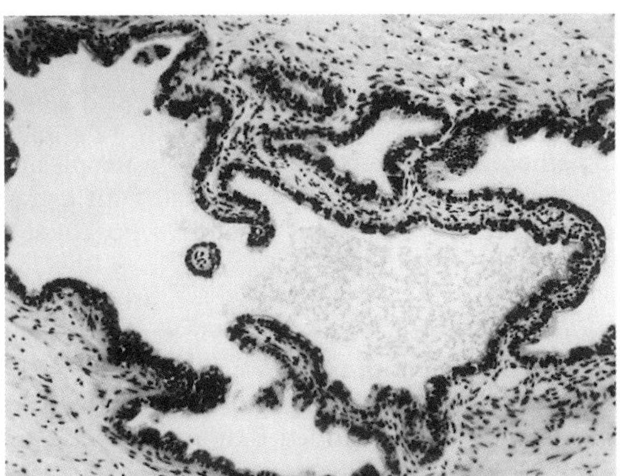

Fig. 23.1 A focus from a benign serous ovarian tumor showing the quite remarkable similarity between the epithelial component and the normal endosalpinx. H + E ×60

Rounded, laminated, microscopic calcifications, psammoma bodies, are present in varying numbers (e.g. about 15% of benign tumors) in the stroma, but they are not specific diagnostic features (being occasionally found in non-neoplastic fallopian tube mucosa as well as in other mullerian and nonmullerian tumors). Some cells produce mucin, which is mostly extracellular in histological sections – the luminal borders of the cells exhibiting diastase-resistant PAS-positive and mucicarmine-positive glycocalyx. Obvious intracellular mucin should suggest a diagnosis other than pure serous tumor. A plethora of immunohistochemical tumor markers such as amylases (van Kley et al 1981, Bruns et al 1982), CA1, CA-125 antigen, EMA, S100 protein, Leu-M1, B72.3 antigen, and CEA (Kabawat et al 1983, Fleuren & Nap 1988, Wick et al 1989) are all used in characterizing the cell type (Table 23.1), but in our cxpcrience are only infrequently of assistance with the difficult diagnostic problem. Cytoplasmic argyrophilia may be seen in up to

Table 23.1 Immunophenotype of serous carcinomas

Antibody against	Expression (%)
Cytokeratins (AE1/AE3, CAM 5.2)	100
Epithelial membrane antigen (EMA)	100
HMFG-IIIC12	100
CA-125 antigen	85
OV-TL3	85
B72.3 antigen	85
Ber-EP4	85
S100 protein	80
Mov18	80
OV632	75
GFAP	60
Leu M1	45
Vimentin	40
Carcinoembryonic antigen (CEA)	10

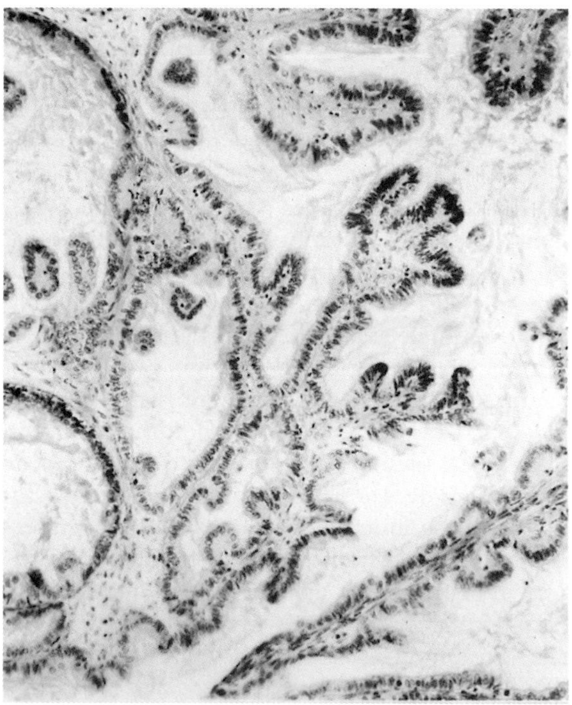

Fig. 23.2 Benign serous tumor with marked prominence of the ciliated cells, producing small fan-like projections. This should not be misinterpreted as true 'proliferation.' H + E ×90

30% of serous tumors (and 40% of serous carcinomas), but this is not associated with neurosecretory granules on ultrastructural examination (Lin et al 1991). Ciliated cells are characteristically found in benign serous tumors (Fig. 23.2), less frequently in proliferating serous tumors, and rarely in other than well-differentiated carcinomas. The cells of moderately and poorly differentiated serous carcinomas (Fig. 23.3) are usually small with round to slightly oval nuclei and prominent nucleoli. Cytoplasm is generally scant and basophilic or amphophilic with indistinct cell borders (Fig. 23.3A). The cells may be somewhat spindled in areas of poorly differentiated carcinoma (Fig. 23.4). Occasional cellular variants include those in which abundant eosinophilic cytoplasm (Fig. 23.3B) gives rise to large polyhedral cells (but the nuclei remain small), others with evidence of secretion in tall columnar cells (Fig. 23.5) with subnuclear or supranuclear vacuoles (but quite different from the large pavement-like cells of clear cell carcinoma), and rare tumors with a focal cribriform or mesothelioma-like pattern in which the cells are greatly attenuated and distorted (Fig. 23.6). While a distinctive feature of serous carcinomas is the relative uniformity of cell size and staining characteristics from one field to another, an equally typical feature is the presence of randomly distributed single mononuclear tumor giant cells, sometimes clustered in areas of ischemic degeneration (see Figs 23.3C, 23.35).

Although encountered at any age, benign lesions show a peak incidence in the fourth and fifth decades. Bilaterality rates of 12–20% overall have been reported (Russell 1979a, Scully 1979), but this rate is significantly higher in elderly patients. Apparently unilateral tumors may be associated with very small or microscopic cortical adenofibromas in the contralateral ovary, and bilaterality rates are thus influenced by a particular pathologist's minimal criteria for a neoplasm. Rarely, benign tumors are associated with extraovarian epithelial inclusions of serous type (Russell 1979a, Bell & Scully 1990a).

The mean age of incidence for proliferating serous tumors is similar to that for benign serous tumors. They are more commonly bilateral (35%) than totally benign serous tumors, although again some of these are included only on the basis of microscopic lesions in the contralateral ovary showing atypical epithelial proliferation (Fig. 23.7). In about 35% of cases, they are associated with serous epithelial lesions in extraovarian sites

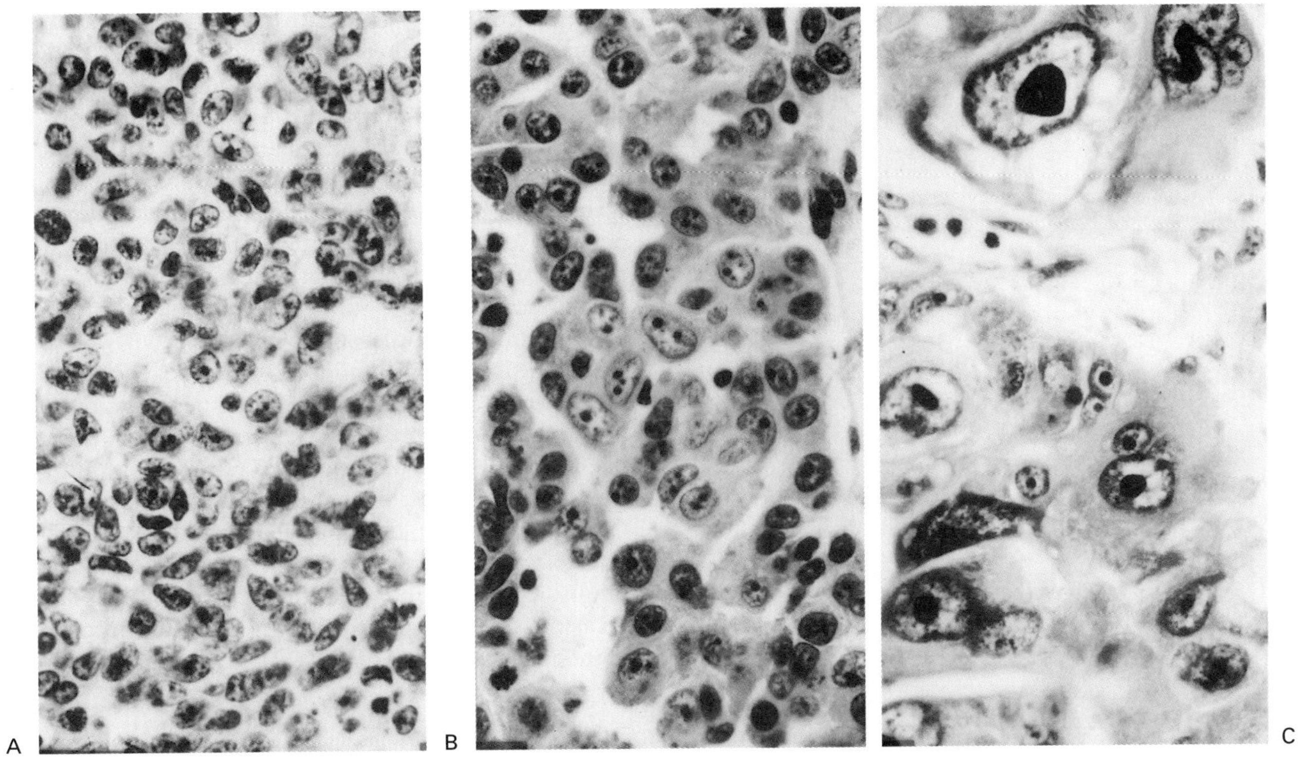

Fig. 23.3 Poorly differentiated serous carcinoma. (A) High power of the commonly encountered cellular variants including those with eosinophilic cytoplasm (B), and bizarre mononuclear giant cells (C). H + E ×350

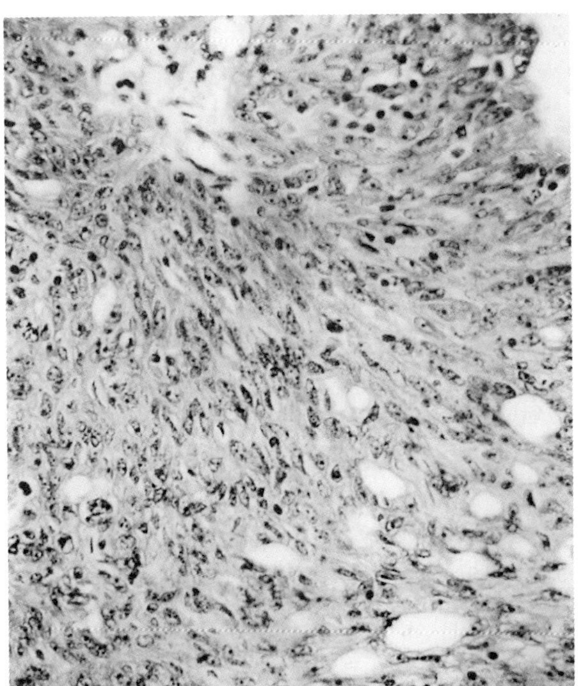

Fig. 23.4 Poorly differentiated serous carcinoma. Focus in which the tumor cells are distinctly spindle-shaped. H + E ×175

(Fig. 23.8). The presence of these often widely distributed peritoneal lesions is, in turn, associated, in approximately 20–25% of patients only, with a progressive but not necessarily fatal clinical course, patients sometimes exhibiting extremely prolonged survival with known residual bulky disease (Nagata et al 1990). This invites an alternative interpretation of their significance other than straightforward metastases or 'implants'. Clinical life table analysis for *all* patients with atypically proliferating serous tumors indicates 5-, 10-, 15-, and 20-year survival rates of 97, 95, 92, and 89%, respectively (Massad et al 1991, Leake et al 1992). All patients with tumor confined to the ovaries and without 'positive' peritoneal washings can be expected to survive without recurrence (Yoonessi et al 1988, Manchul et al 1992, Kurman & Trimble 1993), with the very rare late

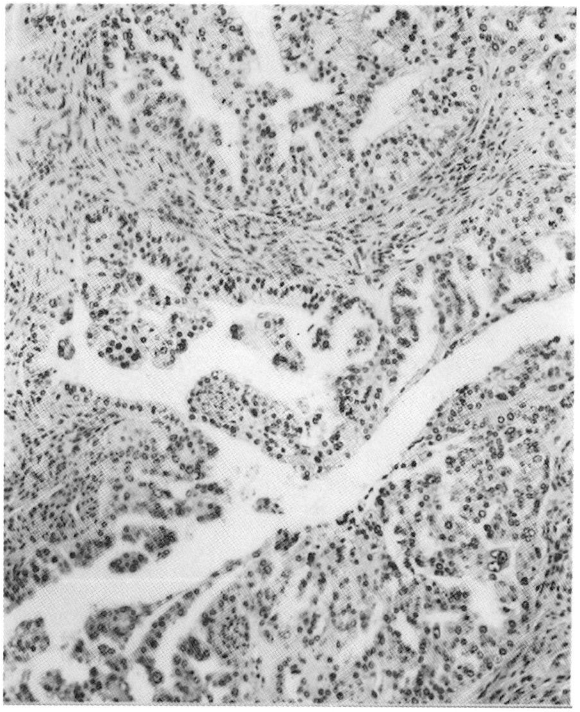

Fig. 23.5 oderately differentiated serous carcinoma with secretory change prominent in the upper half. The cells, however, remain tall columnar and do not resemble the polyhedral cells of clear cell carcinomas (see Ch. 27). H + E ×90

'recurrences' being accounted for by serous carcinomas arising in the peritoneal cavity (i.e. new disease). The probability of tumor-associated death for those patients with extraovarian lesions is estimated as 4% at 5 years and 13% at 10 years (Bell et al 1988). Adjuvant therapy does not seem to improve the overall corrected survival of those patients with high stage disease (Trope et al 1993) and, in our view and that of others, may be counterproductive in these patients (Kurman & Trimble 1993). Rare examples of atypically proliferating serous lesions in the fallopian tube (Zheng et al 1996) or the pelvic and abdominal peritoneum in the absence of a coexisting ovarian tumor have been recorded in young women (Raju et al 1989, Bell & Scully 1989, 1990a, Biscotti & Hart 1992). One such patient developed low grade invasive serous carcinoma of the peritoneum (Bell & Scully 1990a) but, in the absence of local invasion, conservative therapy is generally recommended (Biscotti & Hart 1992).

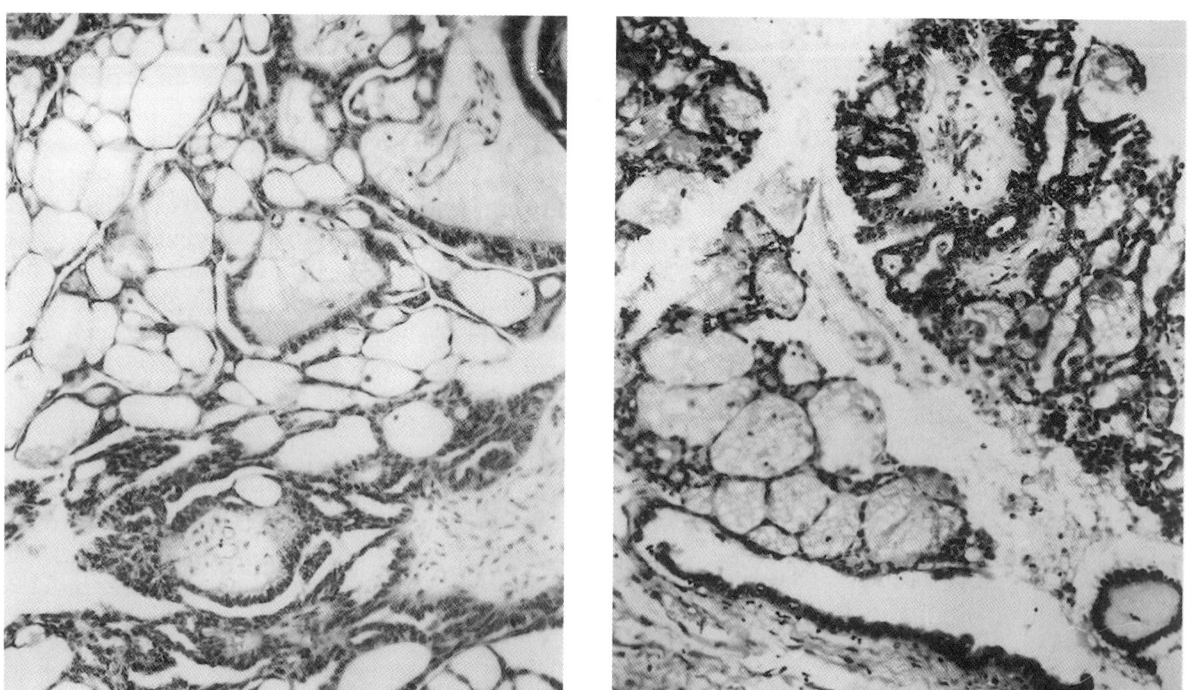

Fig. 23.6 Focal cribriform patterns with mesothelial-like attenuation of the epithelial cells may be seen in both proliferating (as here) and invasive malignant serous tumors. H + E ×90

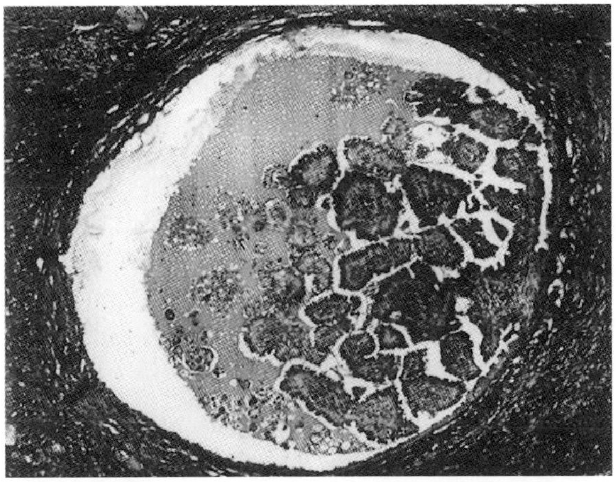

Fig. 23.7 Microscopic ovarian serous lesion showing the architectural features of mild epithelial proliferation. H + E ×90

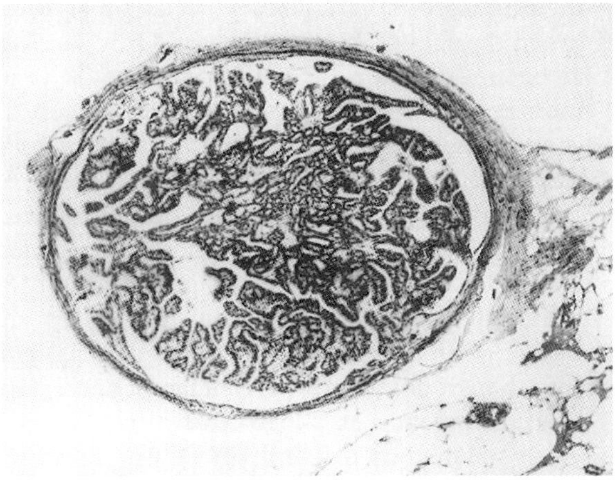

Fig. 23.8 A circumscribed serous papillary lesion or 'implant' of so-called 'noninvasive epithelial type' (Bell et al 1988) in the greater omentum of a woman with bilateral proliferating serous ovarian tumors. H + E ×35

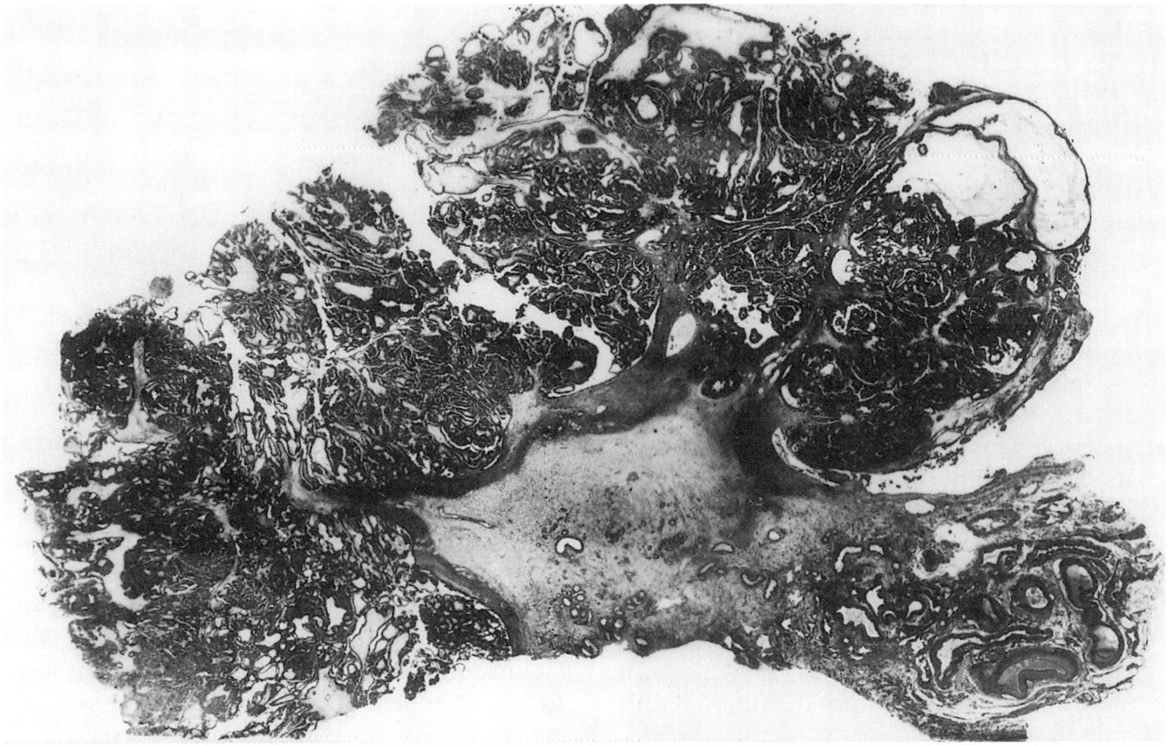

Fig. 23.9 The typical exophytic growth pattern of so-called serous surface papillary carcinoma of the ovary. Invasion of the underlying ovarian stroma is rarely a prominent feature in such cases. H + E ×5

Invasive serous carcinomas occur most often between the ages of 45 and 65 years. Only 30 cases have been reported in women under age 20 years (Moen et al 1994), of which only three were in advanced stage. They are bilateral in about two-thirds of all cases (one-third of stage 1 cases). As well as being by far the most commonly bilateral ovarian neoplasms, they are the most often widely disseminated at the time of diagnosis (80–85% exhibit widespread intraperitoneal tumor deposits at laparotomy). It is our contention that a significant (though unknown) percentage of such stage 3 cases commence as widespread intraperitoneal disease – analogous to the atypically proliferating serous tumors with 'implants' referred to above (Russell et al 1985, Bell et al 1988). A considerable proportion of stage 3 serous carcinomas (up to 10%) (Gooneratne et al 1982, White et al 1985) show only a minor superficial or surface ovarian serous papillary carcinoma (Fig. 23.9), and perhaps a further 10% are entirely extraovarian abdominal serous carcinomas (Russell 1979c, Foyle et al 1981, Tobacman et al 1982, Ulbright et al 1983, Russell et al 1985, Austin et al 1987, Lele et al 1988, Mills et al 1988, Dalrymple et al 1989, Raju et al 1989, Wick et al 1989, Fromm et al 1990, Ransom et al 1990, Truong et al 1990, Altaras et al 1991, Tsujimura et al 1991, Killackey & Davis 1993, Maasen & Debus-Theide 1993, Mulhollan et al 1994, Rothacker & Möbius 1995) in which the notional primary site (ovary) is excluded as the source of the neoplastic process. In the very early stages of tumor development in such patients, microscopic foci of carcinoma can be seen on the surface of the ovaries, within clefts or cortical inclusions or in the superficial cortex (Bell & Scully 1994). The following descriptions of the microscopic features of ovarian serous tumors are intended to apply equally to their extraovarian homologs.

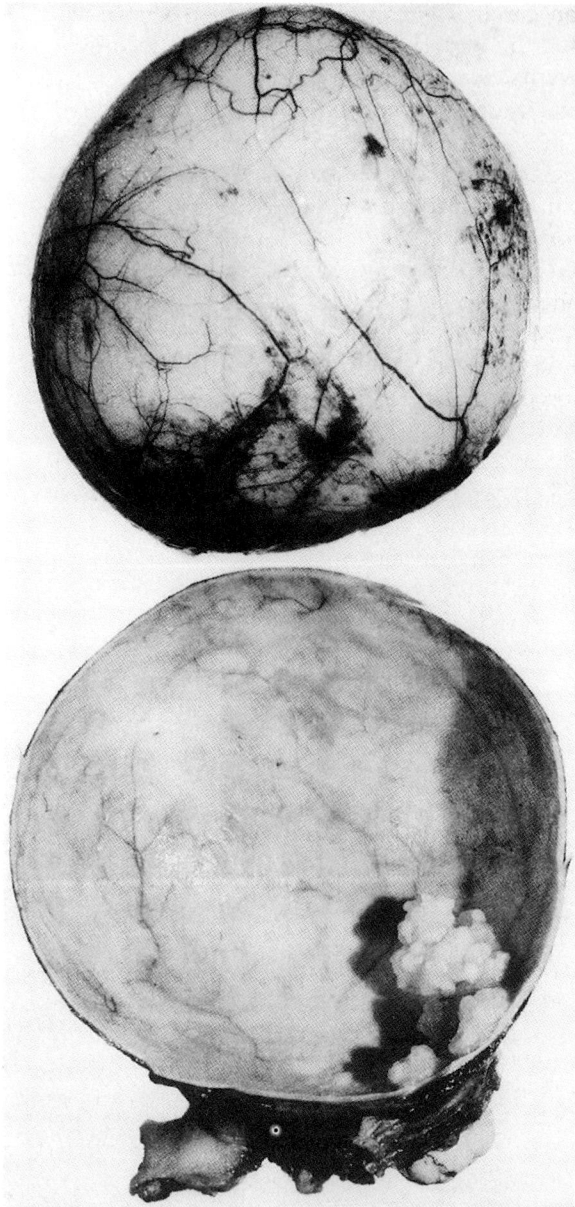

Fig. 23.10 Benign serous cystadenoma with occasional small luminal papillary excrescences

Cytogenetic and molecular genetic studies

DNA ploidy and cell cycle studies suggest that, on average, 5–10% of benign serous tumors, about one-quarter of atypically proliferating serous tumors, and about two-thirds of serous carcinomas are aneuploid (Klemi et al 1988, de Nictolis et al 1992, Griffiths et al 1993).

Clonal karyotypic abnormalities are occasionally seen in benign serous tumors, including monosomy X and trisomy 12 (Pejovic et al 1990). Cytogenetic studies suggest that loss of heterozygosity on chromosomes 6 and 17, and amplification of the HER-2/neu protooncogene may be involved in the early stages of serous ovarian carcinogenesis, while losses on chromosomes 3, 13q, 11p, and 15q are suggested as critical late events, seen in poorly differentiated or progressive carcinomas (Zheng et al 1991, Dodson et al 1993, Kiechle-Schwartz et al 1993). However, allelic losses on 11p, typical of poorly differentiated carcinomas, also may be seen in adjacent low-grade carcinomatous or benign areas, indicative of at least a predisposition to the high-grade carcinoma phenotype (Zheng et al 1993).

Molecular genetic techniques have been used to study the patterns of allelic deletion on chromosome 17 (Tavassoli et al 1993, Tsao et al 1993) and loss of heterozygosity at other polymorphic chromosomal loci (Jacobs et al 1992, Li et al 1993) with a view to establishing the clonality of widespread serous carcinoma (see below). Each of these studies suggest a unifocal origin of high grade, high stage serous carcinomas. Studies on low grade or early stage tumors, which would be more likely to reveal evidence of multifocal tumorigenesis, have not been performed. Studies into the mutational pattern of the p53 gene in patients with widespread ovarian cancer have reached similar conclusions (Mok et al 1992).

Macroscopic features

Benign serous tumors present three basic patterns: cystic, surface papillary and adenofibromatous. Cystic tumors are filled with clear watery (serous) fluid, occasionally thin mucoid material, and rarely the thick tenacious mucus more typical of the mucinous tumors. The external surface of the thin-walled cysts is smooth and glistening, often with a marked vascular pattern. Most are unilocular, but locularity varies greatly, as does the size (averaging 10 cm in diameter, but occasionally measuring greater than 30 cm across) (Hori et al 1991). Because small papillary projections arising from the ovarian surface and serosal inclusion cysts are common (see Ch. 20), a diam-

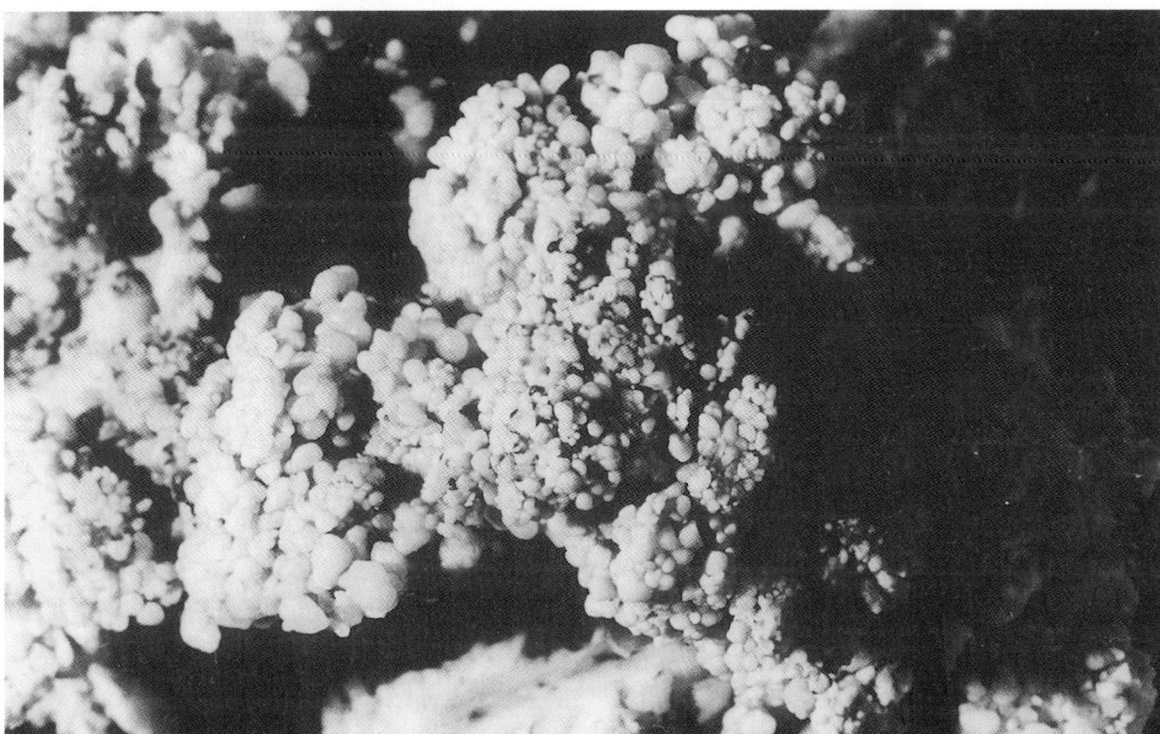

Fig. 23.11 Benign serous surface papilloma showing coarse gelatinous papillae. This patient had similar lesions widespread in the pelvis, but pursued a benign clinical course following their removal

eter of 1 cm or greater is set as an arbitrary dividing line between such lesions and benign neoplasms. The cyst linings are entirely flat or may exhibit grossly visible coarse papillary projections (Fig. 23.10). While, in totally benign tumors such papillary excrescences rarely cover the entire inner surface of the cysts, increasing epithelial proliferation parallels a more diffuse distribution of finer, more friable, and less gelatinous or fibrous papillary structures. Papillae may be present on the external surface of the cysts (Fig. 23.11), and again continua occur both with respect to a decreasing prominence of the cystic component and the fineness and friability of the papillary excrescences themselves. Serous tumors showing more marked epithelial proliferation (Fig. 23.12)

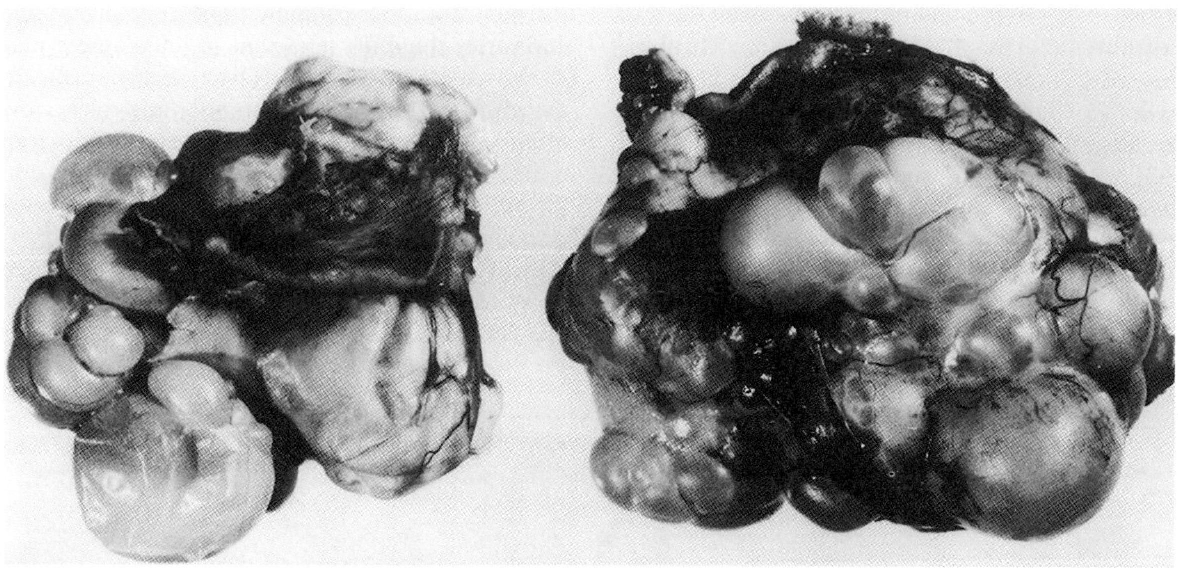

A

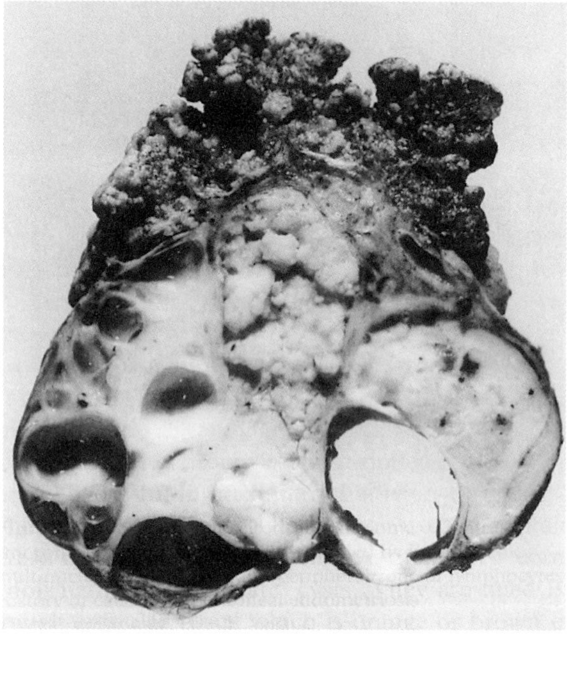

B

Fig. 23.12 Serous tumors with atypical epithelial proliferation. Variability in the prominence of the surface papillary component and the locularity is noted between examples (A) and (B) are more prone than their totally benign counterparts to be bilateral (see above) and to have a surface papillary component (up to 70% of cases in some series) (McCaughey et al 1984). We regard this latter feature as a minor factor only in explaining the extraovarian lesions or 'implants', although the contrary view is supported by a statistical association (Segal & Hart 1992). The third (adenofibromatous) variant comprises solid neoplasms (Fig. 23.13) composed of tough, rubbery fibrous tissue interspersed with glandular spaces of various sizes. The latter may grow and become variably prominent. Clinical and pathological differences between these various gross appearances, such as greater frequency of bilaterality and older mean age of adenofibromatous types, greater frequency of ascites, and peritoneal 'implants' with exophytic or surface papillary types, are more apparent than real and of little consequence.

The gross appearance of invasive serous carcinomas varies according to the differentiation or grade of the lesion. Size ranges from virtually microscopic to 20 cm or so in diameter. Well-differentiated carcinomas are predominantly cystic, multilocular tumors with soft friable papillae partly or mostly filling the cavities. Fluid, if present, is usually turbid or bloody. The external surfaces may be smooth or bosselated and sometimes exhibit a surface papillary component. Tumor adhesions to surrounding organs are common and care should be taken to ensure sampling of these areas as part of tumor assessment in early (stages 1 and 2) cases. Less well-differentiated serous carcinomas (Fig. 23.14) contain solid areas of crumbly pink to grey tissue with less obvious papillary foci. Such areas, however, particularly in bilateral ovarian tumors, are typical enough to allow a presumptive diagnosis of serous differentiation from the gross appearances alone. Nonspecific features such as necrosis and hemorrhage are, of course, often present.

Microscopic features

In benign tumors, the architecture parallels the gross appearance, producing relatively thin-walled cysts (Fig. 23.15), papillary structures (Fig. 23.16),

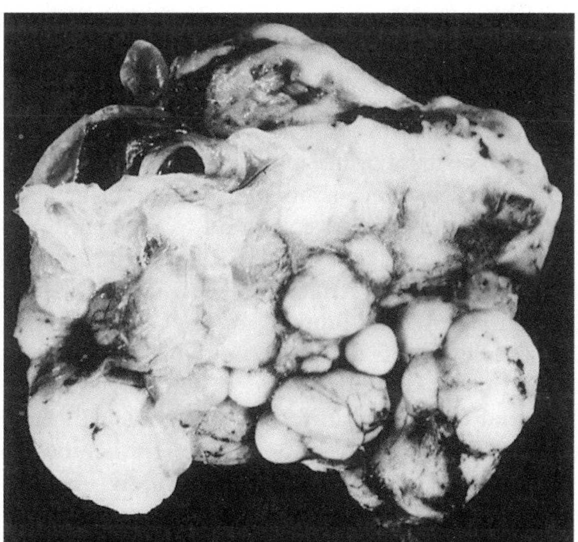

Fig. 23.13 Benign serous adenofibroma. Such tumors are commonly bilateral and, when multinodular as here, are likely to be mistaken for metastases by the surgeon

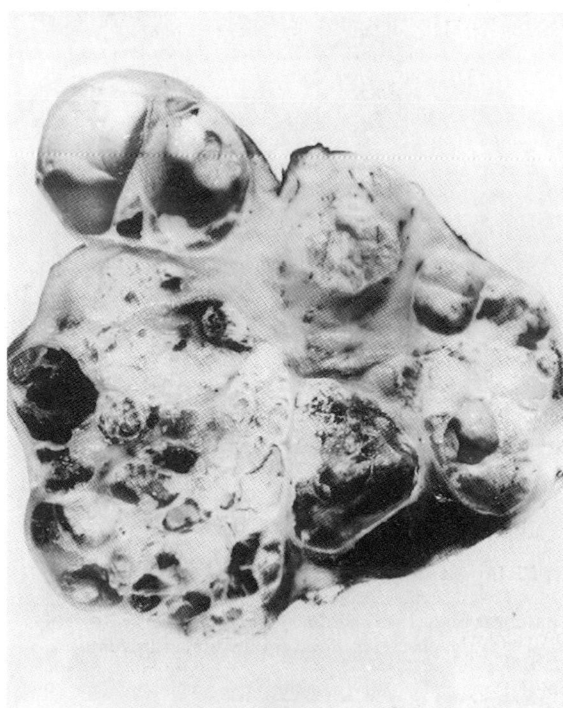

Fig. 23.14 Poorly differentiated multilocular serous carcinoma with a bosselated external surface and solid nodules of friable and partly necrotic carcinoma on the cut surface

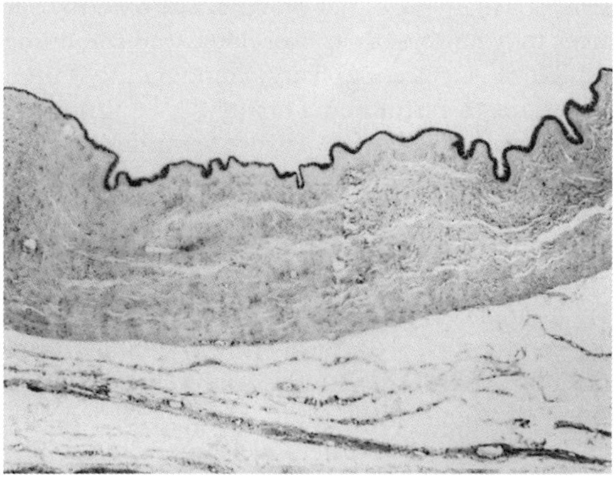

Fig. 23.15 Benign serous cyst. A single-layered epithelium is separated by a thin acellular zone from the underlying dense fibrous stroma of the cyst wall. H + E ×25

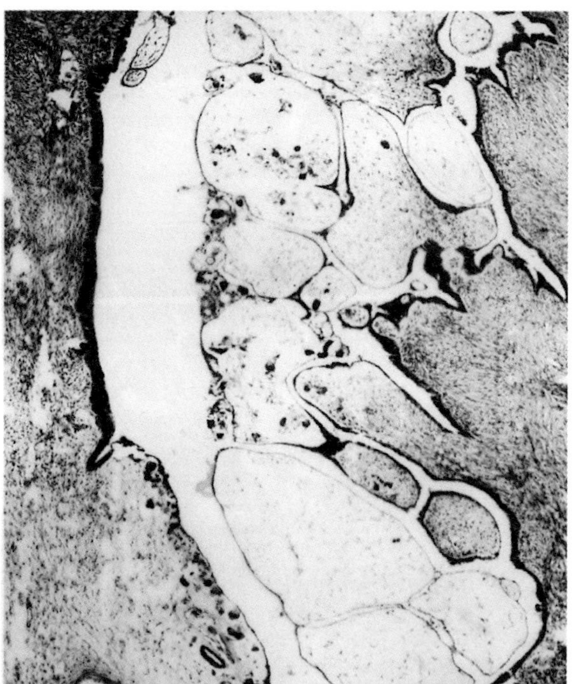

Fig. 23.16 Benign papillary serous cystadenoma. Coarse papillary excrescences project into variably sized cystic spaces. Psammoma bodies are prominent. There is marked regional variation in the character of the epithelium and stroma. H + E ×35

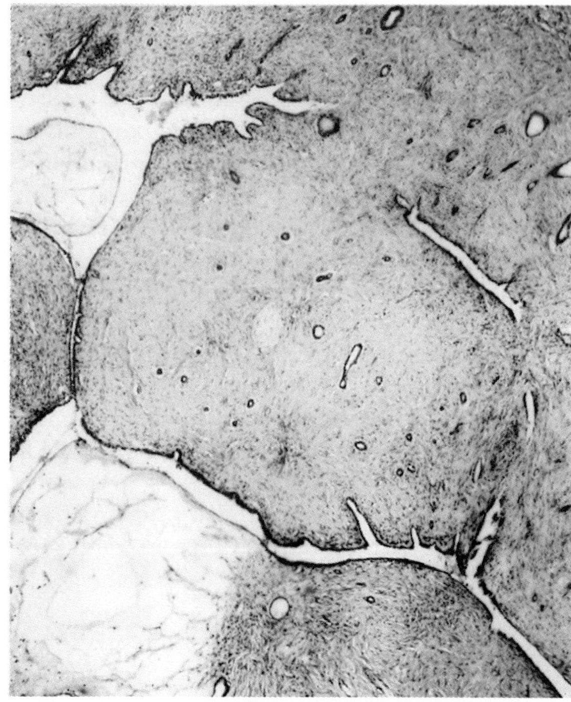

Fig. 23.17 Benign serous adenofibroma. Small epithelial clefts and glandular spaces in dense ovarian stroma. H + E ×35

or glandular spaces embedded in fibrous stroma (adenofibromas) (Fig. 23.17), or more commonly a mixture of these patterns. The epithelium of both smooth and papillary areas is often pseudostratified and tubal in type (see Figs 23.1, 23.2), with the characteristic elongate (secretory cell) or rounded (ciliated cell) nuclei; this epithelium may show histological changes analogous to those of the endosalpingeal mucosa during different phases of the menstrual cycle, including secretory change with tall columnar vacuolated or even clear cells. Secretory and ciliated cells tend to occur in clusters. The difference in height between the two cell types may be quite marked (see Fig. 23.2) and, particularly with 'fanning' of the ciliated cells, causes unevenness of the free epithelial border. Less commonly, it is a single layer of regular flattened to cuboidal cells with uniform basal nuclei. In large cysts, pressure may induce the epithelium to become attenuated. Mitoses are rarely encountered. There is no nuclear atypia. A complex papillary pattern should not be confused with epithelial proliferation (Fig. 23.18). The stroma of the cyst walls and papillary structures ranges from highly cellular and fibrous to almost acellular hyalinized

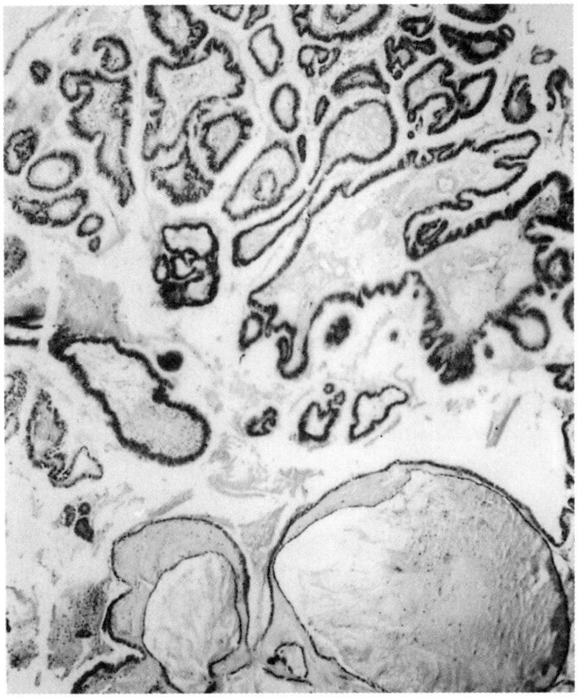

Fig. 23.18 Benign papillary serous cystadenoma with a complex papillary pattern but no epithelial 'proliferation' as defined in Chapter 22. H + E ×90

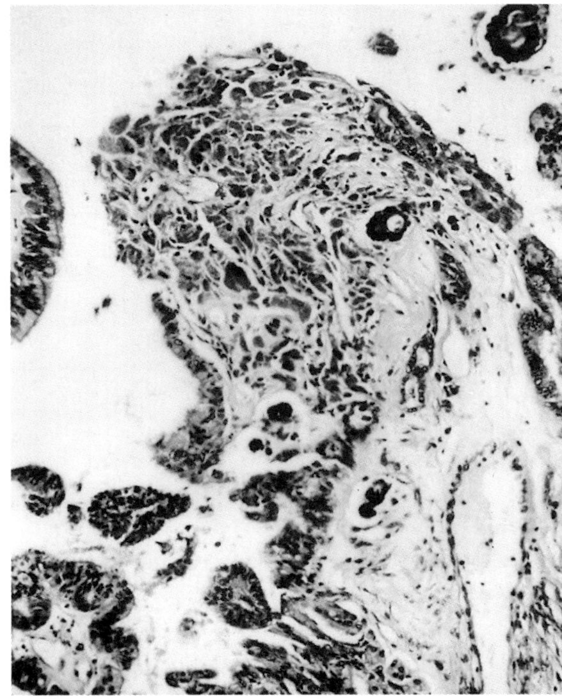

Fig. 23.19 Focal old subepithelial hemorrhage with pigment-laden macrophages and chronic inflammation. H + E ×90

tissue, with marked stromal edema also a common finding (see Figs 23.16, 23.17). There is typically a narrow, acellular zone between the epithelial cells and fibrous stroma of the papillae or cyst wall (see Fig. 23.15), which is thought to correspond to a similar zone in the cortex of normal ovary.

Sometimes there are small foci of old or recent hemorrhage in the stroma, and this may be associated with hemosiderin-laden macrophages (Fig. 23.19). Eosinophilic pseudoxanthoma cells beneath the epithelium are a much more common finding (Fig. 23.20), and when prominent may produce 'ceroid granulomas' (Amazon & Rywlin 1980). The light brown pigment such cells contain is ceroid (lipofuscin), not hemosiderin, and care should be taken not to misinterpret either of these appearances as associated endometriosis. Stromal fatty degeneration has been noted in cyst walls. Rare cases have been reported of pronounced stromal luteinization causing virilization in postmenopausal women (Okolo et al 1990) or associated with pregnancy (Fayez et al 1974).

In proliferating serous tumors, there is a graded prominence and complexity of the papillae lining most cystic spaces. Covering these papillary excrescences, the epithelium also shows a variable distribution and/or severity of the proliferative features noted in Chapter 22. These proliferative changes tend to run pari passu, but the two most easily quantifiable for serous epithelial lesions are stratification of the epithelial lining of papillae and epithelial budding or tufting (Fig. 23.21). Examples with high grade proliferation (Fig. 23.21B) have recently been interpreted as noninvasive 'micropapillary serous carcinomas'; they are more likely than low grade proliferating tumors to have associated extraovarian lesions and these are, in turn, more likely to be invasive (Burks et al 1996). Given the relative uniformity of serous neoplasms from area to area, this is not an unexpected observation. At the low end of the proliferative spectrum, there is no easy answer to the question of how much epithelial proliferation is required to separate such tumors

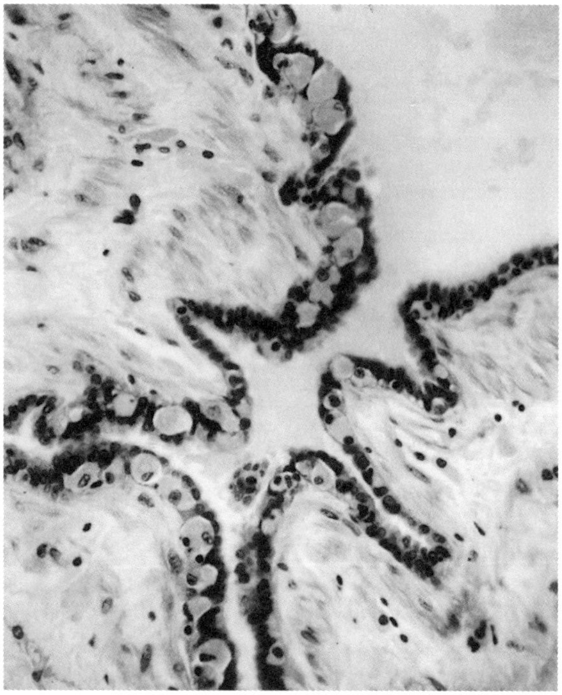

A

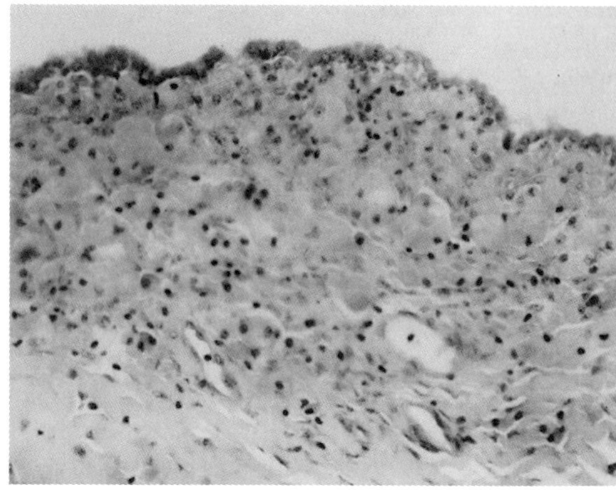

B

Fig. 23.20 Benign serous tumors with lipofuscin-containing 'pseudoxanthoma' cells. (A) Single cells, apparently intraepithelial. H + E ×125. (B) Massed cells beneath the epithelium forming so-called ceroid granulomas. H + E ×125

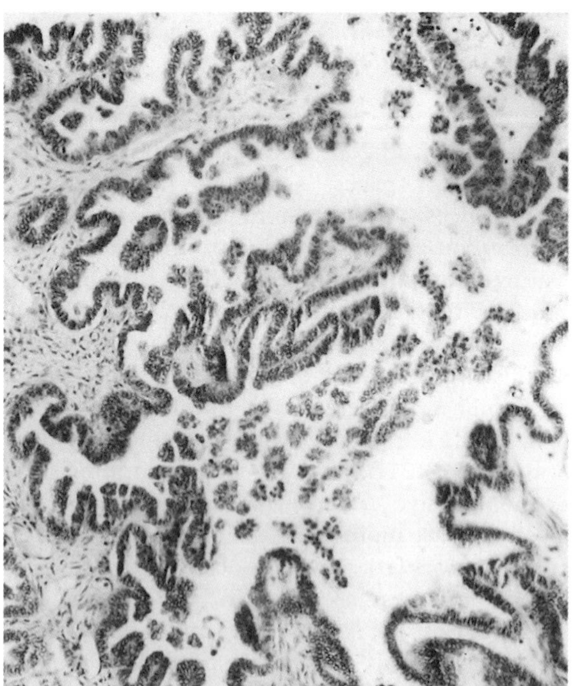

A

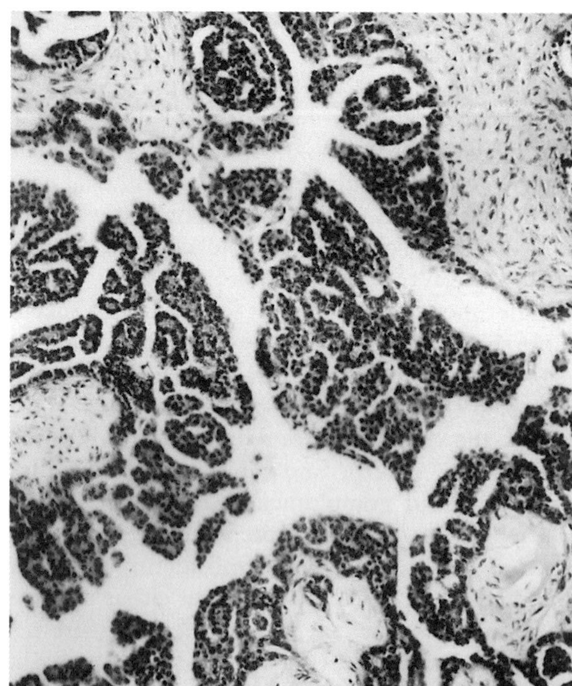

B

Fig. 23.21 Serous tumors showing atypical epithelial proliferation but no stromal invasion. (A) Low grade proliferative activity with budding and tufting. (B) High grade tumor showing more severe epithelial growth with multilayering and hyperchromatic rounded nuclei – the so-called 'micropapillary' pattern (Burks et al 1996). H + E ×90 from their nominally benign counterparts (see Ch. 22), and mixtures of benign and atypically proliferating areas are commonly encountered in the same tumors (Puls et al 1992). Nuclei vary from those seen in benign tumors by being more hyperchromatic and rounded, with obvious, though not prominent, nucleoli and less clear distinction into secretory and ciliated cell populations. Mitoses uncommonly exceed 4/10HPF (Katzenstein et al 1978, Russell 1979b), and bizarre nuclei and tumor giant cells are not seen. As in 'benign' tumors, focal secretory changes are observable as well as extracellular mucin and rare squamoid morules. Attenuation of epithelial cells so as to resemble mesothelium may also be noted (see Fig. 23.6); such patterns have also been described as 'cribriform'. Psammoma bodies and stromal inflammatory infiltrates are seen in up to half of these tumors, but these latter are mild, lymphocytic, and not directed to focal irregularities of architecture such as to suggest invasive carcinoma. Epithelial proliferation in adenofibromatous serous tumors is a rare variation which is difficult to assess (Fig. 23.22). Although more completely documented in mucinous tumors (see Ch. 24), rare proliferating serous tumors may exhibit mural 'sarcoma-like' nodules with osteoclast-like giant cells admixed with pleiomorphic carcinoma cells (de Rosa et al 1991), or true sarcomatous nodules of smooth muscle or rhabdomyosarcomatous differentiation (Allen et al 1992). An apparently unique conjunction of a proliferating serous tumor and a primary diffuse large B-cell lymphoma has been reported (Skodras et al 1994).

Separation of atypically proliferating but noninvasive tumors from frankly invasive cancers according to orthodox criteria clearly implies a transition signaled by microinvasion, and this is occasionally observed. Such microfoci are characterized by single cells or small papillary groups of tumor cells, with increased amounts of eosinophilic cytoplasm, within the stroma (Fig. 23.23); occasionally

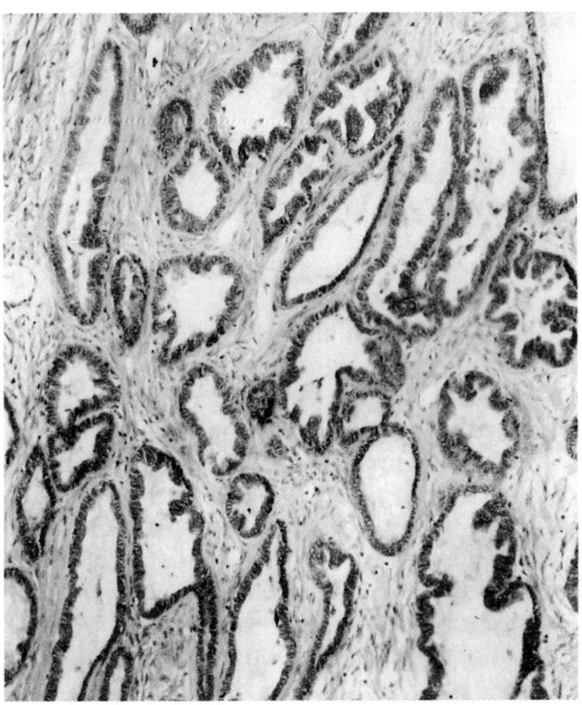

Fig. 23.22 Proliferating serous adenofibroma. Crowded atypical glandular structures with some epithelial tufting and nuclear atypia. H + E ×90

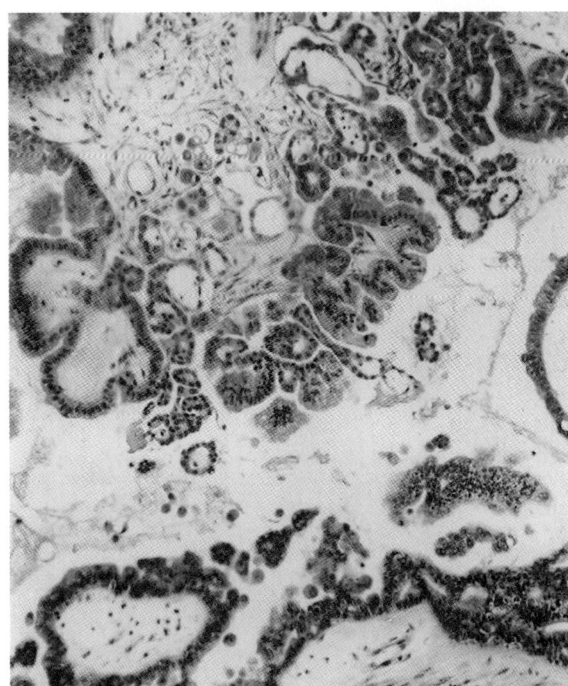

Fig. 23.23 Proliferating serous tumor showing a focus of stromal microinvasion (top centre). Note the plump single and clustered epithelial cells apparently invading, but no recognizable stromal response. H + E ×90

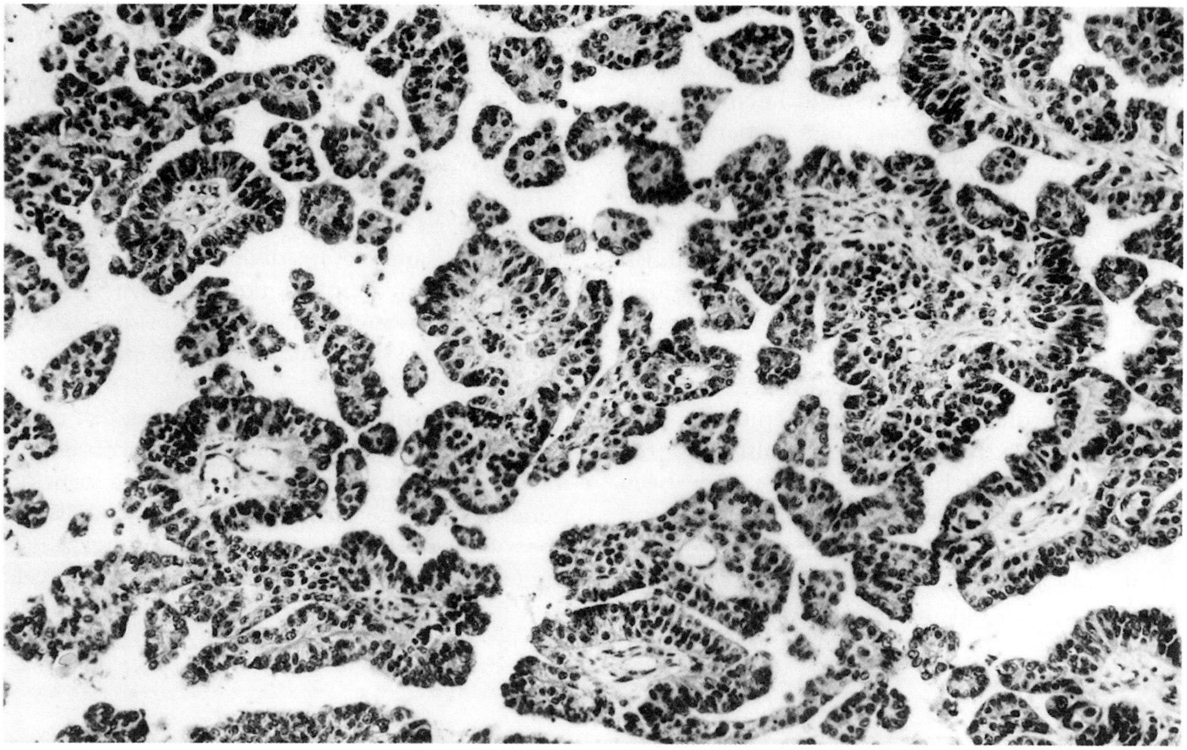

Fig. 23.24 Well-differentiated serous carcinoma with the typical papillary architecture. H + E ×125

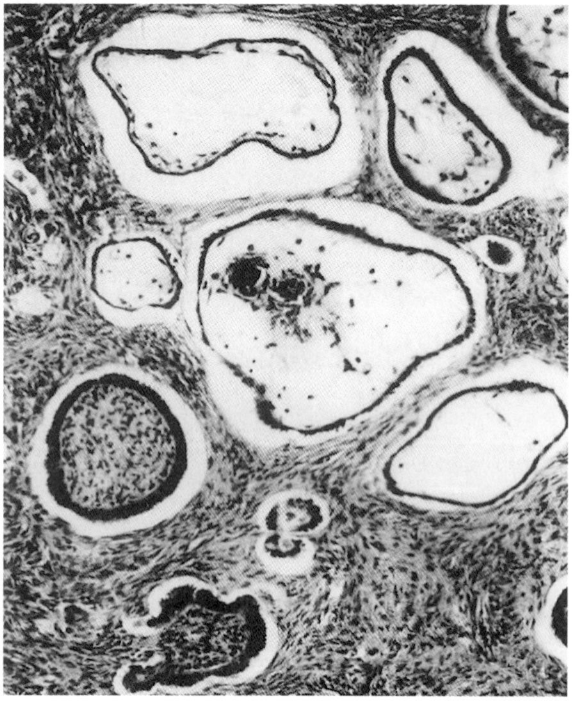

appearing to be in lymphatic spaces. Interpretation of such findings is still controversial, especially as the stroma in the immediate vicinity of the 'infiltrating' cells does not usually show the typical desmoplastic changes of destructive invasion. Although too few cases have been reported to establish their prognostic significance reliably, early indications suggest no material alterations to prognosis or management for such patients (Tavassoli 1988, Bell & Scully 1990b); our anecdotal evidence is supportive. Identification of microinvasion is aided by use of immunohistochemical techniques (Hanselaar et al 1993). It is relevant to note that 'microinvasion' in these circumstances has been shown to be associated with type IV collagenase, capable of degrading basement membrane components (Campo et al 1992), legitimizing this interpretation of the changes reported.

Fig. 23.25 Well-differentiated serous carcinoma in which papillae appear to be growing within dilated lymphatic spaces. H + E ×90

In well-differentiated serous carcinomas, the papillary structures are clearly formed (Fig. 23.24), but with an immature connective tissue core differing from that seen in noninvasive and benign tumors. These exophytic papillae grow into cystic spaces or on the tumor surface. They are also prominent in the cellular, immature stroma of fibrous, or solid portions of tumor. These papillae may occasionally be somewhat larger and appear to be in lymphatic spaces (Fig. 23.25). Psammoma bodies are common in well-differentiated serous carcinomas (60–70%). Their prominence has been correlated positively with clinical outcome (Kuhn et al 1988), but this is probably not an independent prognostic variable. Occasionally, they are very prominent, producing 'psammomatous carcinomas' (Fig. 23.26) or 'psammocarcinoma' (Gilks et al 1990). Care should be taken clearly to identify cytological features of malignancy in the tumor cells which are obscured by the massive overburden of calcispherules. An extreme example of this phenomenon may be the explanation for the unique 'complete psammomatous degeneration' of a 23 cm ovarian mass described by Schneider et al (1985). Spicules of new bone of dystrophic origin have been reported rarely in the stroma of well-differentiated serous carcinomas (Barua & Cox 1982, Bosscher et al 1990). Less common, but nevertheless characteristic, tumor patterns include those in which glandular spaces are more rounded (Fig. 23.27; see also lower portion of Fig. 23.30); such tumors may be difficult to differentiate from endometrioid carcinomas, or may represent intermediate differentiation between these entities. Rarely encountered histological variants are the malignant adenofibromas (Fig. 23.28) in which the epithelial but not the fibrous element is malignant; this pattern may be seen focally in otherwise typical serous carcinomas. Occasionally, acute inflammatory cell infiltrates, unassociated with foci of necrosis, are seen in relation to the epithelium (Fig. 23.29), although not as frequently as in 'mullerian-type' mucinous tumors

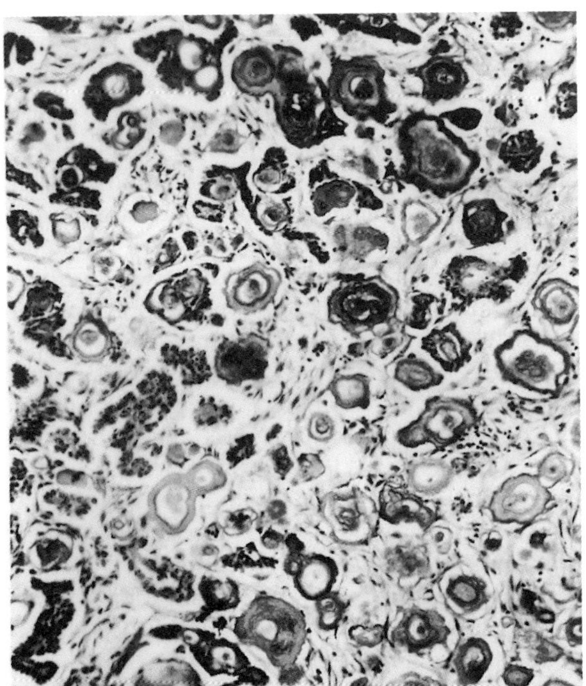

Fig. 23.26 Well-differentiated so-called 'psammomatous' serous carcinoma. H + E ×90

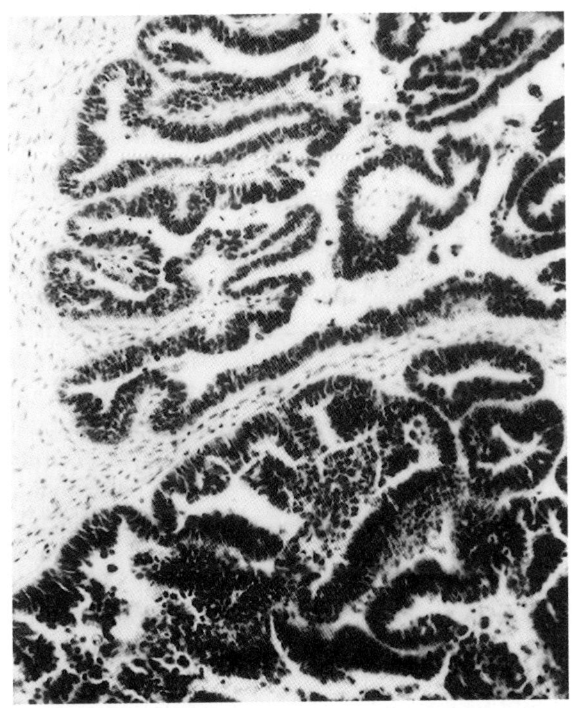

Fig. 23.27 Well-differentiated serous carcinoma in which the epithelial clefts and glandular spaces are broader and blunter than usual – a not uncommon pattern which is to be distinguished from endometrioid carcinoma. H + E ×90

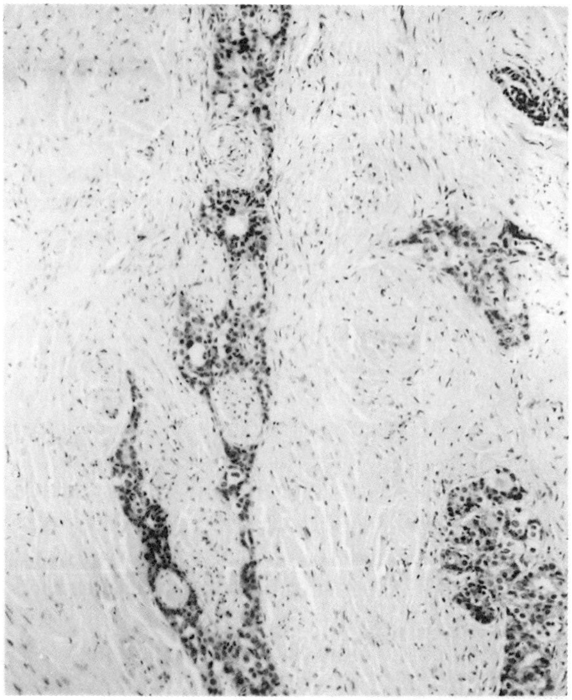

Fig. 23.28 Rare malignant serous adenofibroma with solid nests and cords of malignant cells in benign, relatively acellular fibrous stroma. H + E ×90

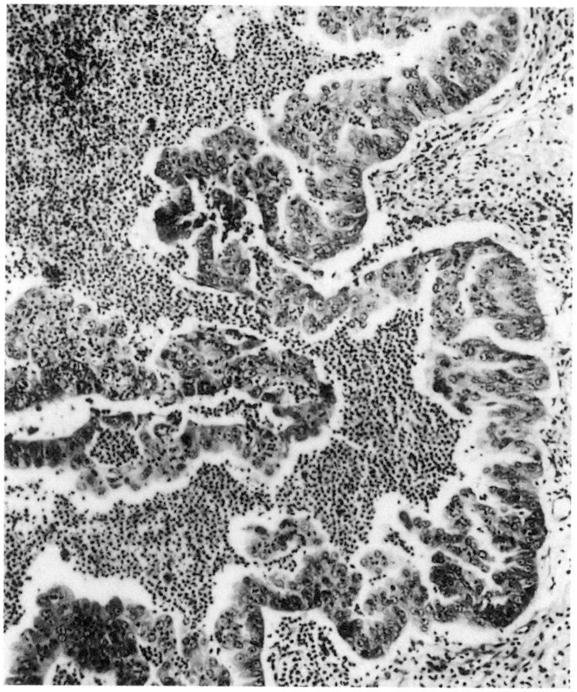

Fig. 23.29 Well-differentiated serous carcinoma with a florid acute inflammatory infiltrate in the cyst lumen, unassociated with obvious tissue necrosis. The patient was afebrile and organisms could not be identified in the exudate. H + E ×90

(see Fig. 24.14). In our experience, these changes are almost always incidental findings in carcinomas from patients who do not exhibit systemic symptoms of infection.

In moderately differentiated serous carcinomas (Fig. 23.30), the papillae are finer and more crowded. An important, and quite characteristic, pattern to recognize in the spectrum of serous carcinoma is the lace-like appearance (Fig. 23.31), which may only be focal but often predominates, and is due to a very fine micropapillary arrangement of the cells which grow centripetally (Fig. 23.31A) and subsequent bridge or partially coalesce (Fig. 23.31B). The slit-like spaces created between these micropapillae tend to be uniform in size and oriented radially. The cells are small and uniform. Other less commonly observed variants are noted in Figures 23.32 and 23.33. It should be remembered that glandular patterns do not exclude serous carcinoma, and the discrimination between poorly differentiated endometrioid carcinoma and serous carcinoma with a predominantly microglandular pattern is usually difficult and sometimes impossible. The rare finding of focal squamous differentiation in otherwise typical serous carcinomas (Ulbright et al 1990) should also be borne in mind in differentiating between these two entities. Psammoma bodies are seen less commonly (approximately 20–30%). Secretory activity may also be present (see Fig. 23.5).

In poorly differentiated serous carcinomas, micropapillary patterns as described above are largely obliterated (Fig. 23.34) and the tumors appear to be made up of solid sheets of small uniform cells (often somewhat spindled) (see Fig. 23.4). The cells at the margins of these small cell masses are not palisaded (unlike granulosa cell tumors), and only rarely produce microglandular aggregates (unlike endometrioid carcinomas). A coarsely papillary configuration with multilayering of the epithelium is not rare and should not be misinterpreted as evidence of transi-

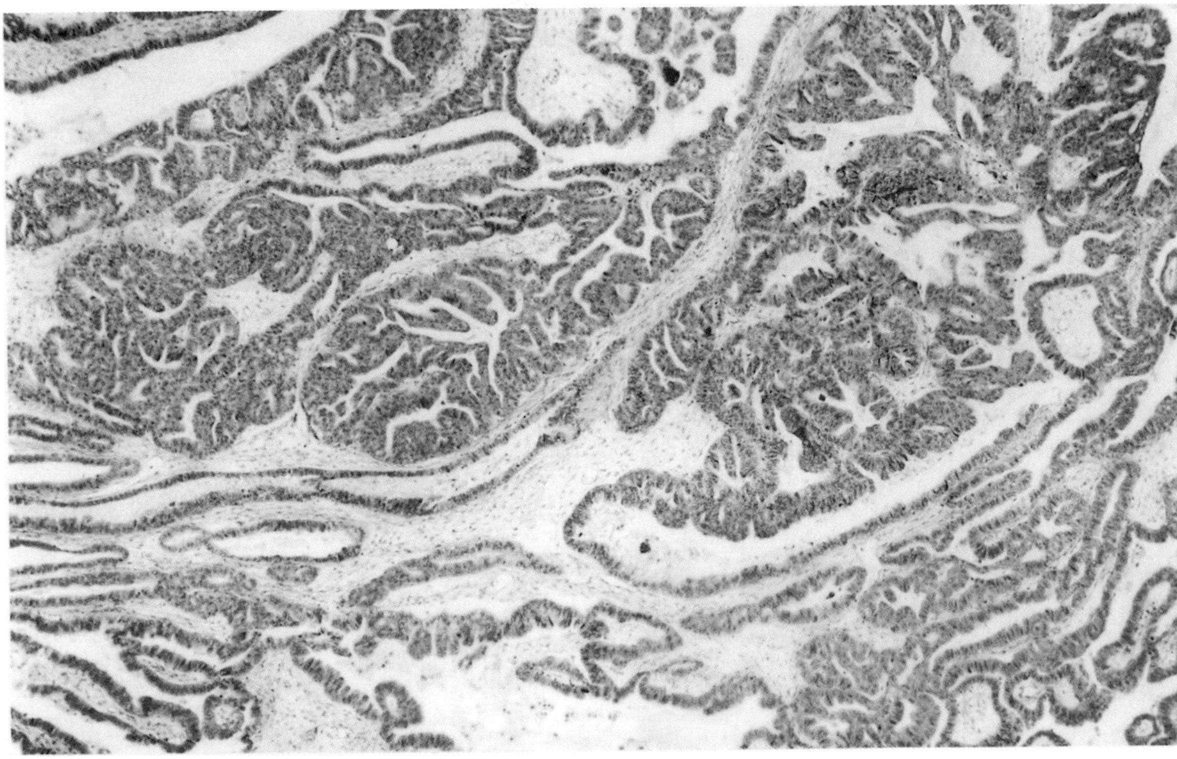

Fig. 23.30 Moderately differentiated serous carcinoma with a fine, complex micropapillary pattern. More broadly contoured glandular spaces are present in the lower portion of the figure. H + E ×125

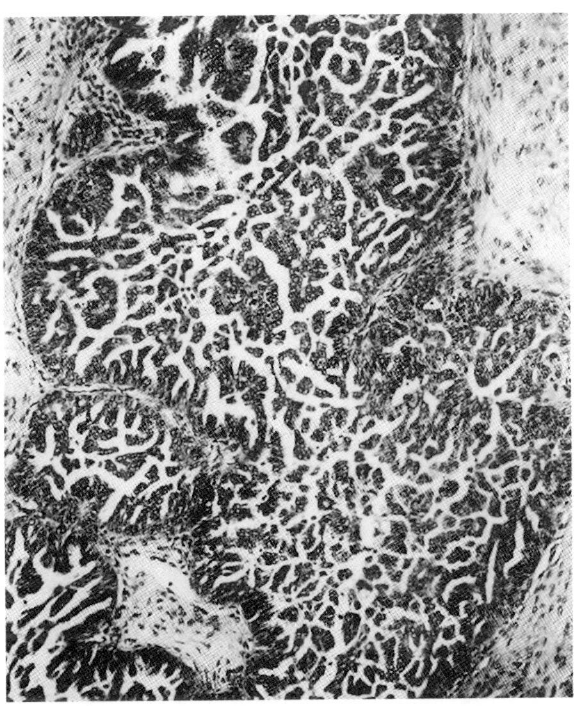

A

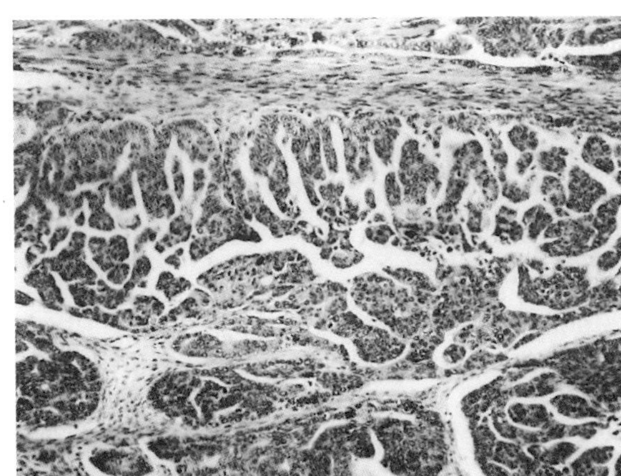

B

Fig. 23.31 Moderately differentiated serous carcinoma with the characteristic lacy appearance, due to a fine micropapillary epithelial growth, either with (A) or without (B) coalescence of the tips of the papillae. H + E ×90

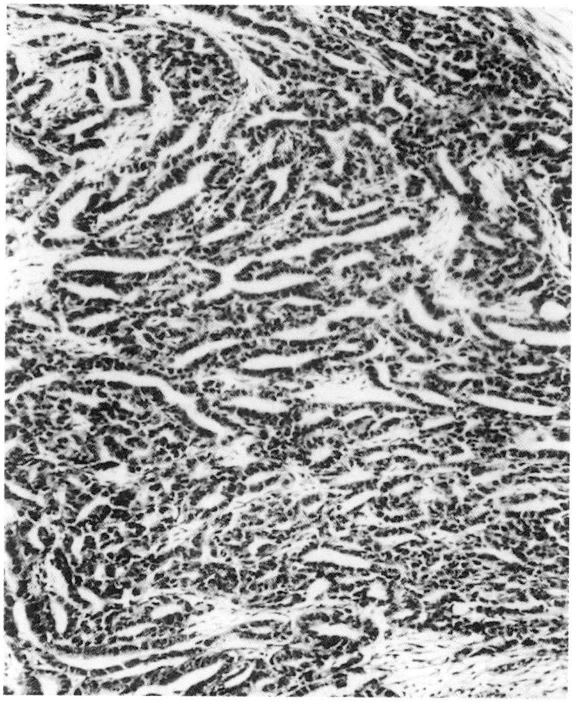

Fig. 23.32 Moderately differentiated serous carcinoma with a complex adenocarcinomatous pattern. The glandular spaces are still elongate and slit-like, differentiating them from those typical of endometrioid adenocarcinomas. H + E ×90

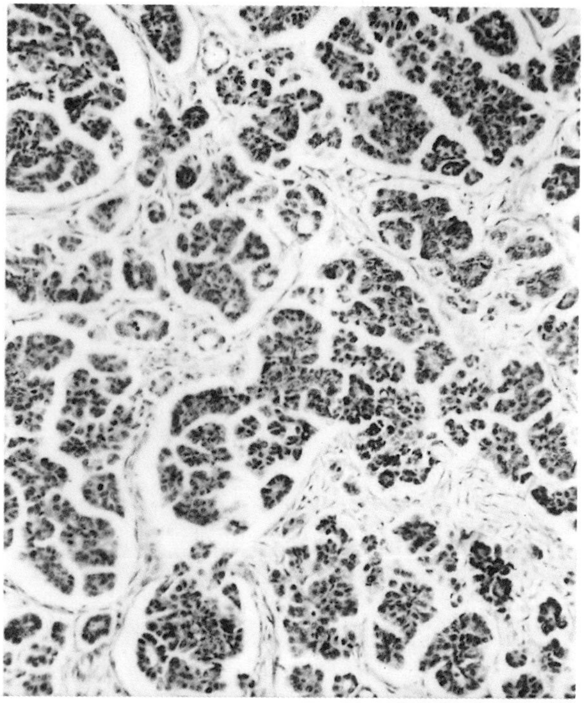

Fig. 23.33 Moderately differentiated serous carcinoma with small morules and papillary clusters of tumor cells in immature stroma. H + E ×90

tional differentiation. A further useful histological marker, seen often in somewhat better differentiated serous carcinomas, is the presence, amongst such sheets of small uniform cells, of occasional bizarre mononuclear giant cells (see Fig. 23.3C) or syncytial-like aggregates (Fig. 23.35). These may be the only features suggestive of serous neoplasia in otherwise undifferentiated carcinomas. An immunophenotype of CA-125 antigen, B72.3 antigen, and S100 protein positivity is strongly suggestive of mullerian serous differentiation (see Table 23.1). Mitoses are usually very numerous and tumor necrosis is often pronounced. Serous carcinomas tend to be uniform throughout, and it is quite uncommon to find a conjunction of poorly differentiated and well-differentiated serous carcinoma (Fig. 23.36).

Unlike many epithelial neoplasms, but certainly like immature ovarian teratomas (see Ch. 47), the histological assessment of the extraovarian lesions is an integral and critical part of pathologically grading as well as staging of serous ovarian neoplasms, and the surgeon should be encouraged to biopsy as many of these as practicable at the time of definitive surgery. They are frequently found on or beneath the surface of pelvic viscera or the omentum in association with serous ovarian tumors, uncommonly in the retroperitoneal lymph nodes and rarely outside the peritoneal cavity (Dugan et al 1991), and in general exhibit the same epithelial characteristics as the dominant ovarian mass, including papilla formation and psammoma bodies, but generally lack much of a stromal component. However, apparent discrepancies occur, particularly when extraovarian epithelial lesions are found in association with the atypically proliferating serous tumors, and both doubt and controversy still accompany the interpretation of the various patterns encountered.

On the one hand, such lesions are accepted as having arisen in situ when histologically benign (Clausen 1991, Maasen & Hiller 1994) and when accompanying benign tumors (Fig. 23.37), but

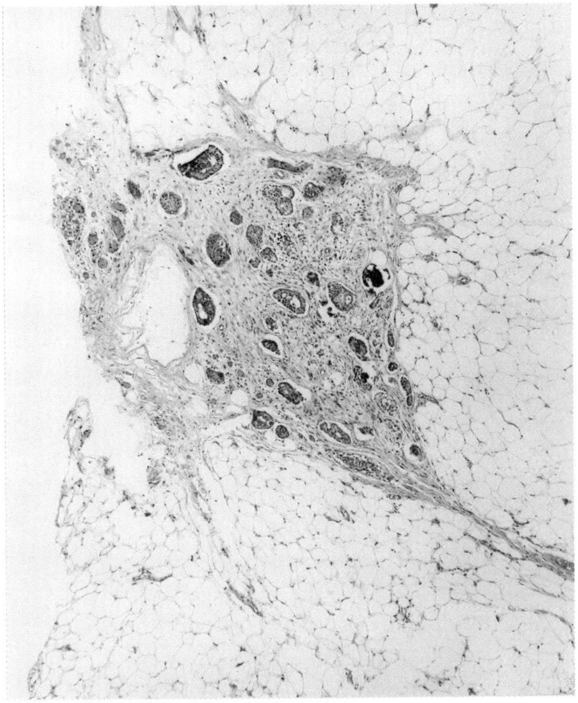

A

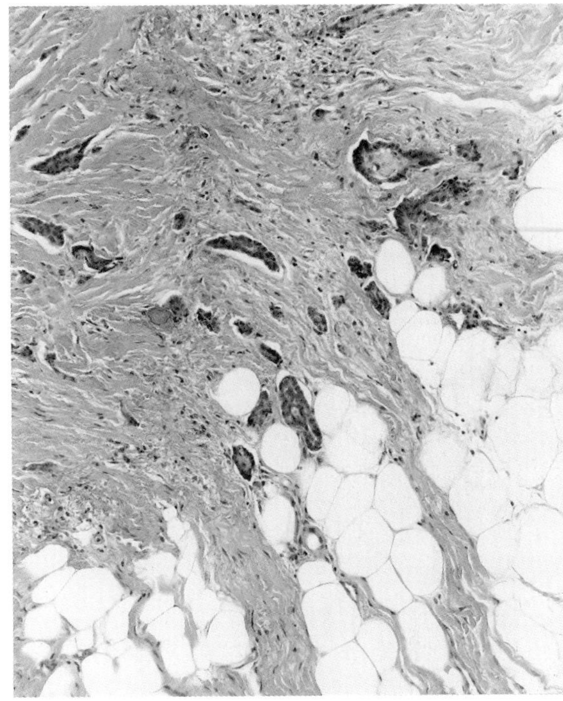

B

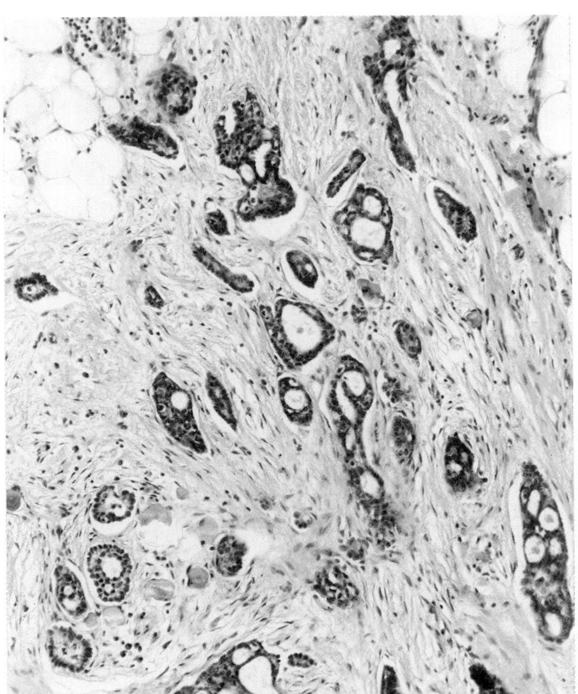

C

Fig. 23.41 Focal lesions of well-differentiated serous carcinoma at various sites in the peritoneal cavity, associated with proliferating (i.e. noninvasive) serous ovarian tumors. These correspond to so-called invasive 'implants'. (A) Low power of an omental lesion showing the radiating glandular pattern tentacular margin and the infiltration into the underlying fatty tissue. H + E ×23. (B) Higher power of infiltrative margin with adipose cells incorporated into the destructive process and the radial orientation of the infiltrating glandular elements. Stroma is densely sclerotic tumor stroma. H + E ×59. (C) Cribriform, micropapillary and microcystic structures, and some semblance of order due to the radial growth of these foci are characteristic of well-differentiated serous carcinoma which are easily differentiated from the complete disorganization of so-called 'noninvasive desmoplastic implants' (see Fig. 23.43). Stroma is desmoplastic and contains a patchy, but usually sparse lymphocytic inflammatory infiltrate. H + E ×59.

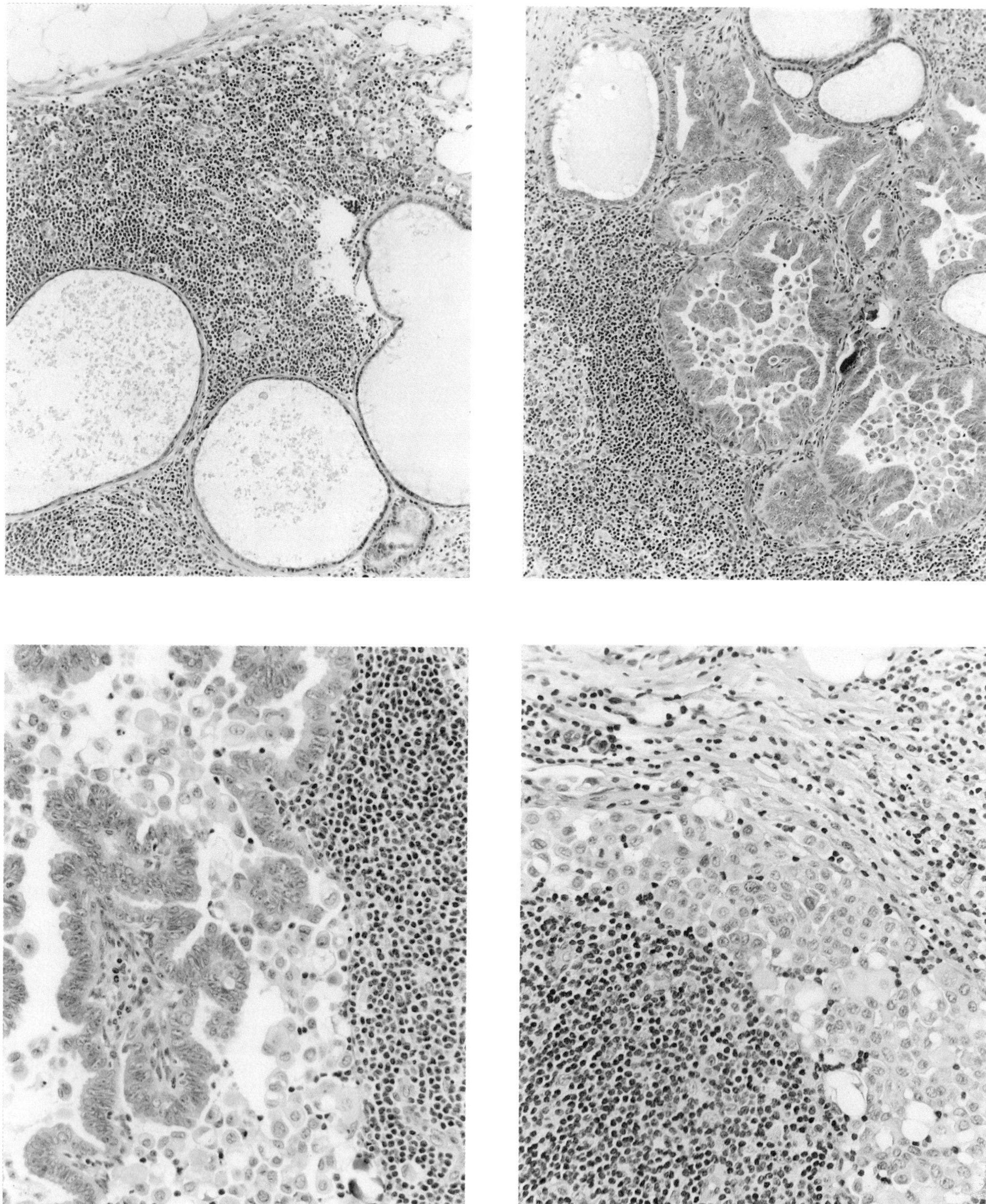

A B C D

should not, in our view, be interpreted as metastatic carcinoma mandating aggressive therapy. Some of these cells derive from the intranodal serous neoplastic process (Fig. 23.42), some are reactive mesothelial cells and some are presumably deported serous epithelial cells from the associated ovarian or peritoneal lesions. Epithelial hyperplasia of the fallopian tube mucosa accompanying proliferating serous ovarian tumors is regarded as evidence of a field effect in mullerian carcinogenesis (Robey & Silva 1989), in the same way that precursor lesions in the contralateral ovaries of women with serous ovarian carcinoma are regarded as evidence of a diffuse field effect (Resta et al 1993).

As outlined in Chapter 22, our philosophy is that these lesions described above arise in situ by a process of mullerian metaplasia, and their histological features must be taken into account when assessing the disease process as a whole. In our experience (Russell & Merkur 1979, Russell 1984), and that of other investigators (McCaughey et al 1984, Bell et al 1988, de Nictolis et al 1992), those occasionally encountered 'implants' showing patterns of locally invasive carcinoma (Fig. 23.41), marked cellular atypia, or mitotic activity (and found in about 10–15% of patients with peritoneal lesions), appear most likely to reflect unfavorably upon the biological aggressiveness of the neoplastic process and the clinical outcome for the patient. Our practice, and that of others (Kurman & Trimble 1993), has been to upgrade such cases to the status of stage 3 low grade serous carcinoma and to recommend that patients be managed accordingly. Those extraovarian lesions which are benign ('endosalpingiosis') or proliferating but noninvasive (of both 'epithelial' and 'desmoplastic' types as defined by Bell et al (1988)) and illustrated in Figures 23.8, 23.37, 23.38, 23.40, 23.42, and 23.43, are noted, and just careful clinical follow-up of the patient is recommended. The same principles apply to the very rare cases of extraovarian serous lesions which, in the absence of a dominant ovarian mass, show similar atypical proliferation (Bell & Scully 1990a). The precise nature of purely extraovarian ('primary peritoneal') psammocarcinoma, characterized by mild cytological atypia, absent mitoses, and florid diffuse microcalcification (Gilks et al 1990) is not clear, but may well be another closely related entity.

The most difficult lesions to assess are those showing marked inflammation, sometimes with reactive mesothelial proliferation and scattered psammoma bodies (Fig 23.43), all of which obscure the possible underlying presence of atypical epithelial cells. Rare instances of degenerate papillary fragments associated with a local inflammatory response are encountered. These are all interpreted as true implants, corresponding to the subgroup of 'desmoplastic noninvasive implants' of Bell et al (1988) and, we believe, add further weight to the argument for in situ genesis of the other very different lesions described above. It may be this subset of peritoneal lesions which specifically account for the increased likelihood of extraovarian 'implants' in association with proliferating tumors with a surface papillary component (Segal & Hart 1992). Useful features in discriminating between desmoplastic noninvasive (i.e. 'true') implants and locally invasive well-differentiated carcinomatous lesions include:

- The superficial location of the 'implant' on the surface of the peritoneum or between lobules of omental fat (as opposed to penetrating invasion of the carcinomatous deposit)
- The circumscription of the lesions (as opposed to an infiltrative, tentacular margin of carcinoma)

Fig. 23.42 Serous epithelial lesions in lymph nodes of patients with proliferating serous ovarian tumors. (A) Totally benign serous inclusions lined by a single layer of inactive tubal-type epithelium. H + E ×59. (B) Proliferating serous inclusions in para-aortic lymph nodes with budding and tufting. A mixture of proliferating and benign serous lesions are seen in the same node. H + E ×59. (C) Proliferating serous nodal inclusions in which there is focal disruption of the integrity of the peripheral epithelium and 'spillage' of enlarged, dishesive, eosinophilic tumor cells into the surrounding nodal sinuses. These plump cells are similar to those described in microinvasive serous carcinoma (see Fig. 23.23) and do not connote, in our view, infiltrative carcinoma. H + E ×116. (D) Sheets of large eosinophilic cells in the subcapsular sinus of a retroperitoneal node. Some of these may have arisen as a result of the process seen in (c), some may be reactive mesothelial cells, and some may have been transported from similar lesions in the peritoneal cavity. Again we do not think, in the absence of a stromal response, that these cells represent metastatic carcinoma. H + E ×116

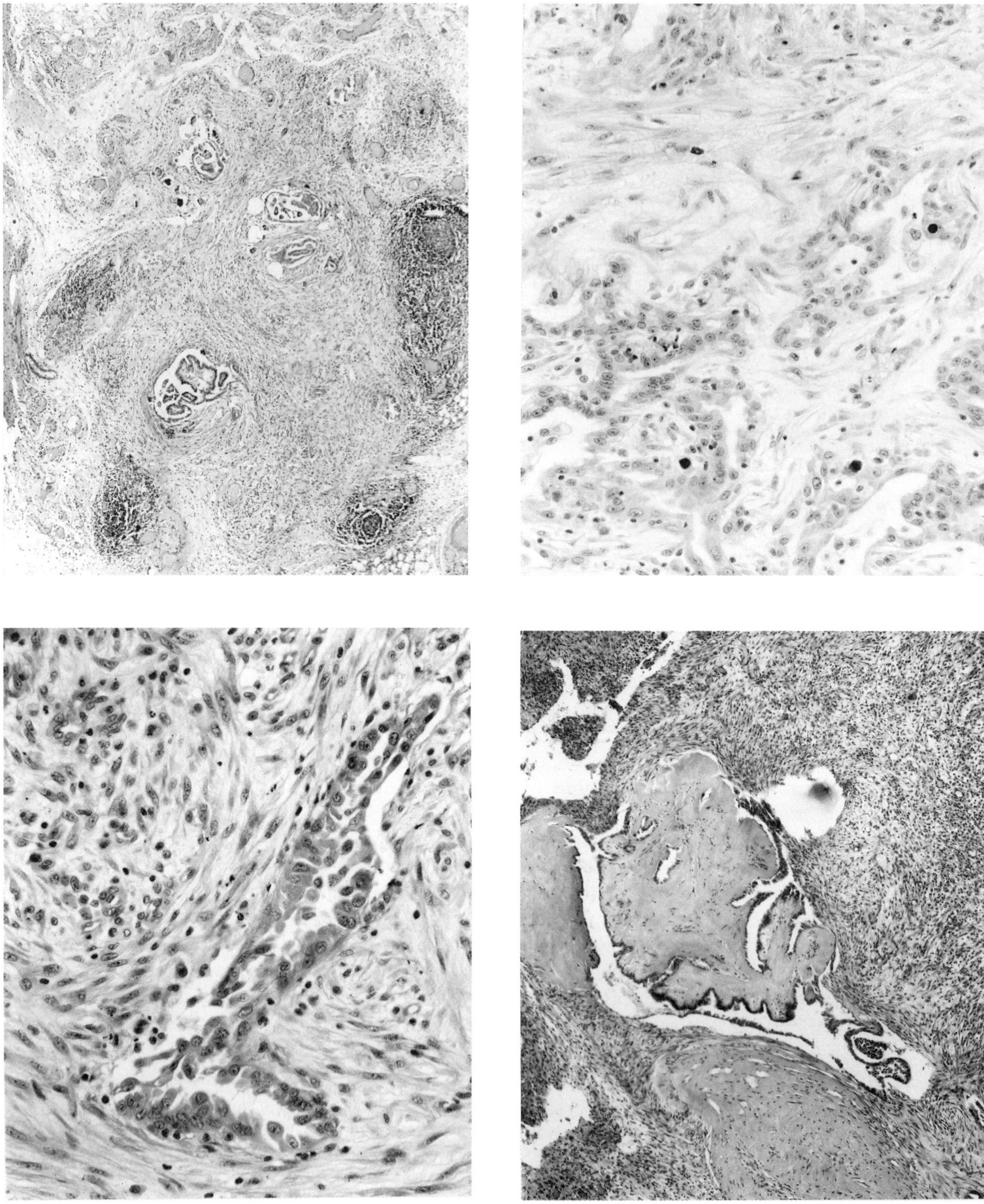

A B C D

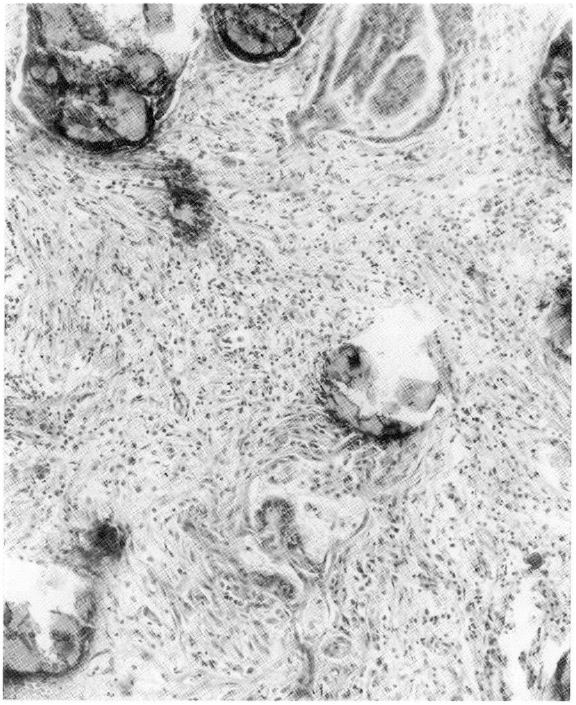

E

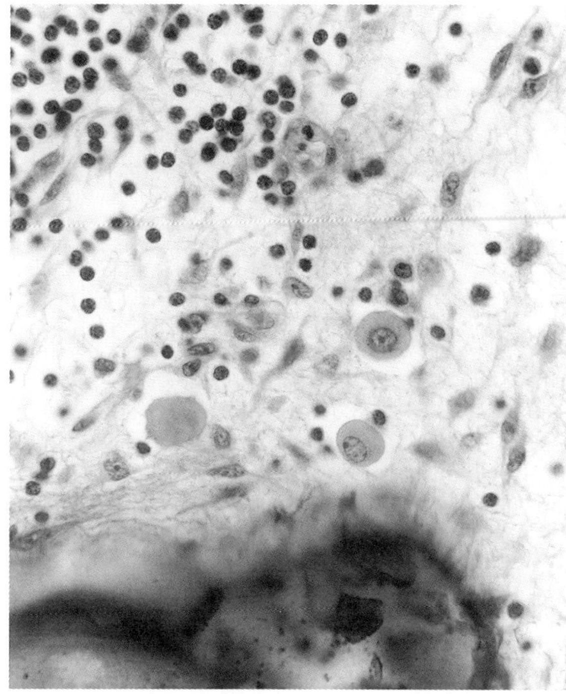

F

Fig. 23.43 So-called 'noninvasive desmoplastic' implants as defined by Bell et al (1988), which are, in our view, probably true implants derived from surface papillary fragments either from the ovarian tumors or even from peritoneal lesions. (A) Totally disorganized and haphazard arrangement of epithelial structures, psammoma bodies, and inflammatory aggregates set in maturing granulation tissue. H + E ×23. (B) Epithelial elements are bland, disorganized, and merge with epithelial-like and spindled elements of mesothelial origin. Stroma is immature granulation tissue with 'tissue-culture' type fibroblasts or spindled mesothelial cells. H + E ×116. (C) Reactive mesothelial cells with eosinophilic cytoplasm and active but bland nuclei may produce small gland-like structures which also must be distinguished from invasive carcinoma. H + E ×116. (D) True implantation of dislodged surface papillary fragments from proliferating serous ovarian tumors, seen here in the pelvis, gives an appearance markedly different from the much more common peritoneal or omental lesions described above. H + E ×23. (E) Haphazard distribution of relatively bland papillary fragments and psammoma bodies in immature granulation tissue. Because such lesions probably derive from surface fragments of ovarian or peritoneal neoplastic processes, their presence does not carry implications of grade or biological aggressiveness (as might, for example, the high grade noninvasive implants shown in Figs 23.40C, D). The inflammatory infiltrate is frequently of mixed cellularity. H + E ×59. (F) Higher power image of Figure 23.43e showing three large eosinophilic epithelial cells of the type described in microinvasive serous carcinoma. As before, these do not represent significant malignant potential. H + E ×231

- The resemblance of the stromal response to organizing granulation tissue with a mixed inflammatory cell infiltrate (as opposed to laminated, fibroblastic tumor-type stroma)
- The totally haphazard and disorganized arrangement of the epithelial elements, psammoma bodies, and mesothelial cells and inclusions, some of which may appear degenerate (as opposed to a somewhat more ordered radiating growth of relatively uniform cribriform or papillary aggregates of serous tumor cells in carcinoma).

Cytological assessment of peritoneal washings in association with atypically proliferating (Johnson et al 1988) and invasive serous ovarian tumors is also an integral part of staging (see Appendix C) and examples of positive washings are given in Figure 23.44. Immunocytochemical identification of CA-125 antigen, B72.3 antigen, Ber-EP4, Leu M1, BMA-120, and CEA, and negative staining for vimentin are useful discriminators between serous tumor cells and other cells in peritoneal washings and ascitic fluids (Guzman et al 1988, Khoury et al 1990, Tickman et al 1990, Skov & Bichel 1991, van Niekerk et al 1991).

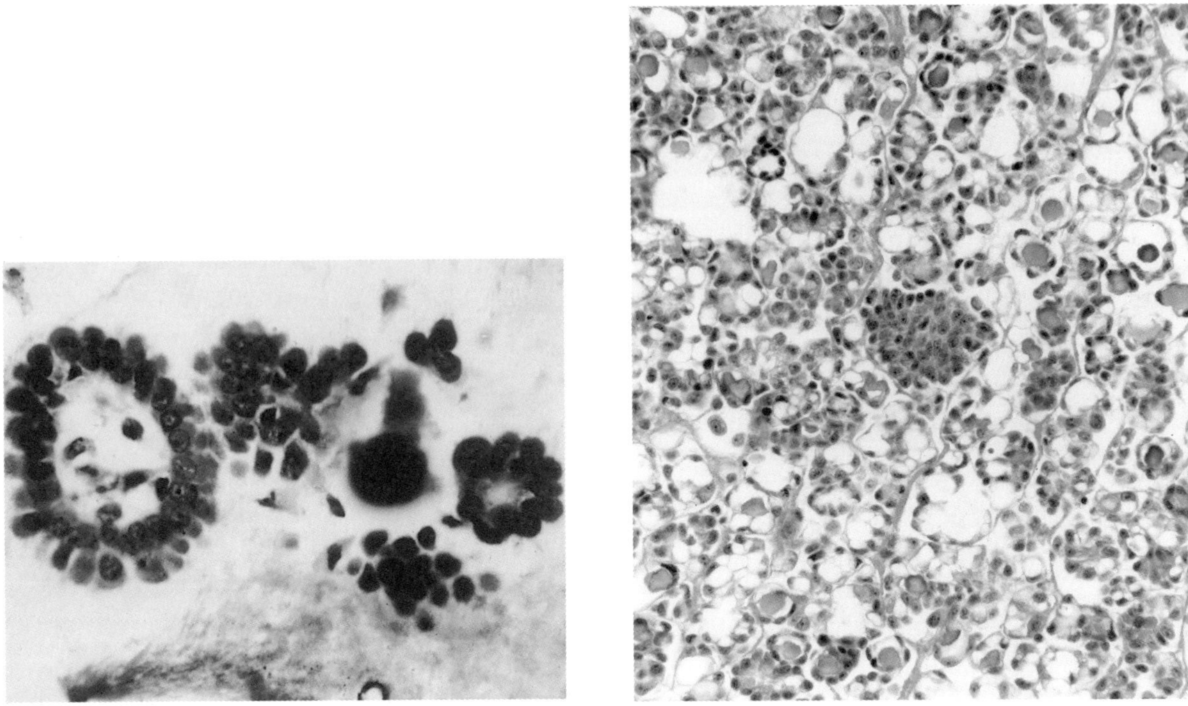

A B

Fig. 23.44 Positive cytological material. (a) Peritoneal washings from a patient with stage 3 well-differentiated serous ovarian carcinoma showing papillary clusters of cytologically malignant epithelial cells. H + E ×231. (b) Densely cellular cell-button prepared from peritoneal washing of recurrent disease in a chemotherapy-treated patient with a proliferating serous ovarian tumor and well-differentiated 'invasive implants' shown in Figure 23.41A. H + E ×116

Differential diagnosis

Discriminating between moderate to poorly differentiated serous and endometrioid ovarian carcinomas is difficult due to their being closely related mullerian tumors and, as a consequence, showing a good deal of overlap in their histological and clinical features. Endometrioid carcinomas are less likely to be bilateral (28% versus 70% overall, and 13% versus 35% of stage 1 cases) or to be widely disseminated in the abdominal cavity at the time of diagnosis (25% versus 85%). Endometrioid carcinomas are more likely to be associated with coexistent adenocarcinoma of the uterine endometrium (in 25–30% of cases) and with non-neoplastic endometriosis in the ovaries or elsewhere in the pelvis (about 30%) than their serous counterparts (Russell 1979a), although synchronous or metachronous serous ovarian carcinomas and uterine endometrioid carcinomas have been reported (Piura & Glezerman 1989, Rose & Reale 1991). Histologically, endometrioid carcinomas vary more from area to area than do serous carcinomas (Table 23.2), and tend to have a microglandular rather than micropapillary pattern, and will show evidence of squamous differentiation in up to one-third of cases.

Poorly differentiated mucinous carcinomas (see Fig. 24.28) may focally resemble serous carcinomas, although such tumors are usually sufficiently variable that further sampling will reveal typical areas of mucin-secreting adenocarcinoma. Mucicarmine and PAS stains should demonstrate intracellular mucins in mucinous carcinomas. Immunohistochemical stains for intestinal epithelial mucins and CEA will usually be positive in mucinous carcinomas, while CA-125 antigen is nearly always negative. In serous carcinomas, CA-125 antigen is focally positive in 85% of tumors, while CEA is positive in only 10% or less of cases in our experience.

Metastatic breast carcinoma has presented diagnostic problems from time to time, particularly in the clinical context of a patient with wide-

Table 23.2 Differential diagnosis: serous versus endometrioid carcinoma of ovary

Serous carcinoma	Endometrioid carcinoma
Clinical	
Disseminated in 85%	Confined to pelvis in 80%
Bilateral in 70–80% of cases (35% in stage 1)	Bilateral in 28% of cases (13% in stage 1)
No association with endometrial carcinoma	Coexistent endometrial tumor in 25–30%
No specific association with pelvic endometriosis	Pelvic endometriosis in 30% (including ovaries)
Histological	
Micropapillary, lacy or solid patterns	Microglandular or trabecular patterns
Slit-like glandular spaces	Tubules or round acinar spaces
Relatively uniform appearance	Variable from area to area
Small round nuclei, prominent nucleoli	Elongate nuclei, coarse granular chromatin
Scanty basophilic cytoplasm	Usually eosinophilic cytoplasm
Very rare squamoid foci	Squamous elements in 30%
Occasional bizarre mononuclear giant cells	Endometriotic origin in some

spread abdominal carcinomatosis and biopsy material being limited to omental or peritoneal tumor tissue, or with apparently normal ovaries.

Cell and nuclear size are similar to that observed in poorly differentiated serous carcinomas. However, nucleoli tend not to be as prominent, and chromatin not as coarse, in breast carcinoma (Mallonee et al 1987) while the dishesive and 'single-file' infiltrative patterns typical of breast carcinomas are rarely seen serous carcinomas. The demonstration of intracellular mucin or immunohistochemical positivity for HMFG-1 and α-lactalbumin are useful and may obviate the need for electron microscopy. Conversely, a newly described entity, invasive micropapillary carcinoma of the breast (Siriaunkgul & Tavassoli 1993), requires differentiation from ovarian serous papillary carcinoma metastatic to the breast (Loredo et al 1990).

Small cell undifferentiated carcinomas may be histologically mistaken for serous carcinomas. These tumors occur in young women (almost never over the age of 40 years), are frequently (60%) associated with paraneoplastic hypercalcemia, and are almost always unilateral (see Ch. 31). Differentiation between serous carcinomas and malignant mesotheliomas is also discussed in Chapter 31.

REFERENCES

Allen C, Stephens M, Williams J 1992 Combined high grade sarcoma and serous ovarian neoplasm. Journal of Clinical Pathology 45: 263–264

Altaras M M, Aviram R, Cohen I, Cordoba M, Weiss E, Beyth Y 1991 Primary peritoneal papillary serous adenocarcinoma: clinical and management aspects. Gynecologic Oncology 40: 230–236

Amazon K, Rywlin A M 1980 Ceroid granulomas in a tubo-ovarian cyst. Southern Medical Journal 73: 1067–1070

Aslani M, Scully R E 1989 Primary carcinoma of the broad ligament. Report of four cases and review of the literature. Cancer 64: 1540–1545

Aslani M, Ahn G-W, Scully R E 1988 Serous papillary cystadenoma of borderline malignancy of broad ligament. A report of 25 cases. International Journal of Gynecological Pathology 7: 131–138

Austin M B, Mills S E, Fechner R E, Anderson W A 1987 Serous surface carcinoma (SCC) of the peritoneum [Abstract]. Laboratory Investigation 56: 3a

Axiotis C A 1988 Intratesticular serous papillary cystadenoma of low malignant potential: an ultrastructural and immunohistochemical study suggesting mullerian differentiation. American Journal of Surgical Pathology 12: 56–63

Bannatyne P M, Russell P 1981 Early adenocarcinoma of the fallopian tubes. A case for multifocal tumorigenesis. Diagnostic Gynecology and Obstetrics 3: 49–60

Barua R, Cox L W 1982 Occurrence of bone in serous cystadenocarcinoma of the ovary. Australian and New Zealand Journal of Obstetrics and Gynaecology 22: 183–186

Bell D A, Scully R E 1989 Benign and borderline serous lesions of the peritoneum in women. Pathology Annual 24 (2): 1–21

Bell D A, Scully R E 1990a Serous borderline tumors of the peritoneum. American Journal of Surgical Pathology 14: 230–239

Bell D A, Scully R E 1990b Ovarian serous borderline tumors with stromal microinvasion: a report of 21 cases. Human Pathology 21: 397–403

Bell D A, Scully R E 1994 Early de novo ovarian carcinoma. A study of fourteen cases. Cancer 73: 1859–1864

Bell D A, Weinstock M A, Scully R E 1988 Peritoneal implants of ovarian serous borderline tumors: histologic features and prognosis. Cancer 62: 2212–2222

Biscotti C V, Hart W R 1992 Peritoneal serous micropapillomatosis of low malignant potential (serous borderline tumors of the peritoneum). A clinicopathologic study of 17 cases. American Journal of Surgical Pathology 16: 467–475

Bosscher J, Barnhill D, O'Connor D, Doering D, Nash J, Park R 1990 Osseous metaplasia in ovarian papillary cystadenocarcinoma. Gynecologic Oncology 39: 228–231

Burks R T, Sherman M E, Kurman R J 1996 Micropapillary serous carcinoma of the ovary and peritoneum: a distinctive low-grade carcinoma related to serous borderline tumors. (Submitted for publication)

Bruns D E, Mills S E, Savory J 1982 Amylase in fallopian tube and serous ovarian neoplasms. Immunohistochemical localization. Archives of Pathology and Laboratory Medicine 106: 17–20

Campo E, Merino M J, Tavassoli F A, Charonis A S, Stetler-Stevenson W G, Liotta L A 1992 Evaluation of basement membrane components and the 72 kDa type collagenase in serous tumors of the ovary. American Journal of Surgical Pathology 16: 500–507

Chandraratnam E, Leong A S-Y 1983 Papillary serous cystadenoma of borderline malignancy arising in a parovarian paramesonephric cyst. Light microscopic and ultrastructural observations. Histopathology 7: 601–611

Chen K T K, Flam MS 1986 Peritoneal papillary serous carcinoma with long-term survival. Cancer 58: 1371–1373

Chen K T K, Schooley J L, Flam MS 1985 Peritoneal carcinomatosis after prophylactic oophorectomy in familial ovarian cancer syndrome. Obstetrics and Gynecology 66: 93s–94s

Clausen I 1991 Peritoneal endosalpingiosis. Zentralblatt für Gynäkologie 113: 329–332

Dalrymple J C, Bannatyne P, Russell P et al 1989 Extraovarian peritoneal serous papillary carcinoma. A clinicopathologic study of 31 cases. Cancer 64: 110–115

de Nictolis M, Montironi R, Tommasoni S et al 1992 Serous borderline tumors of the ovary. A clinicopathologic, immunohistochemical, and quantitative study of 44 cases. Cancer 70: 152–160

de Rosa G, Donofrio V, de Rosa N, Fulciniti F, Zeppa P 1991 Ovarian serous tumor with mural nodules of carcinomatous derivation (sarcomatoid carcinoma): report of a case. International Journal of Gynecological Pathology 10: 311–318

Dodson M K, Hartmann L C, Cliby W A et al 1993 Comparison of loss of heterozygosity patterns in invasive low-grade and high-grade epithelial ovarian carcinomas. Cancer Research 53: 4456–4460

Dugan T, Balsara G, Dunton C J, Hernandez E 1991 Cutaneous involvement by an ovarian serous tumor of low malignant potential. Acta Obstetricia et Gynecologica Scandinavica 70: 625–628

Farhi D C, Silverberg S G 1982 Pseudometastases in female genital cancer. Pathology Annual 17: 47–76

Fayez J A, Bunch T R, Miller G L 1974 Virilization in pregnancy associated with an ovarian serous cystadenoma. American Journal of Obstetrics and Gynecology 120: 341–346

Feuer G A, Shevchuk M, Calanog A 1989 Normal-sized ovary carcinoma syndrome. Obstetrics and Gynecology 73: 786–792

Fleuren G J, Nap M 1988 Carcinoembryonic antigen in primary and metastatic ovarian tumors. Gynecologic Oncology 30: 407–415

Foyle A, Al-Jabi M, McCaughey W T E 1981 Papillary peritoneal tumors in women. American Journal of Surgical Pathology 5: 241–249

Fromm G L, Gershenson D M, Silva E G 1990 Papillary serous carcinoma of the peritoneum. Obstetrics and Gynecology 75: 89–95

Genadry R, Poliakoff S, Rotmensch J, Rosenhein N B, Parmley T H, Woodruff J D 1981 Primary papillary peritoneal neoplasia. Obstetrics and Gynecology 58: 730–734

Gershenson D M, Silva E G 1990 Serous ovarian tumors of low malignant potential with peritoneal implants. Cancer 65: 578–585

Gilks C B, Bell D A, Scully R E 1990 Serous psammocarcinoma of the ovary and peritoneum. International Journal of Gynecological Oncology 9: 110–121

Gooneratne S, Sassone M, Blaustein A, Talerman A 1982 Serous surface papillary carcinoma. A clinicopathologic study of 16 cases. International Journal of Gynecological Pathology 1: 258–269

Griffiths A P, Cross D, Kingston R E, Harkin P, Wells M, Quirke P 1993 Flow cytometry and AgNORs in benign, borderline, and malignant mucinous and serous tumors of the ovary. International Journal of Gynecological Pathology 12: 307–314

Guzman J, Hilgarth M, Bross K J et al 1988 Malignant ascites of serous papillary ovarian adenocarcinoma. An immunocytochemical study of the tumor cells. Acta Cytologica 32: 519–522

Hanselaar A G, Vooijs G P, Mayall B, Ras-Zeijlmans G J, Chadha-Ajwani S 1993 Epithelial markers to detect occult microinvasion in serous tumors. International Journal of Gynecological Pathology 12: 20–27

Hernandez N, Medina V, Alvarez-Arguelles H, Guitierrez R, Perez-Palma J, Diaz-Flores L 1993 Primary papillary psammomatous adenocarcinoma of the umbilicus. Histology and Histopathology 8: 593–598

Hori M, Imai A, Sugiyama T, Yamagiwa S, Miyashita T, Tamaya T 1991 Massive ovarian serous cystadenoma with uneventful postoperative recovery. Gynecological and Obstetrical Investigation 32: 245–246

Jacobs I J, Kohler M F, Wiseman R W et al 1992 Clonal origin of epithelial ovarian carcinoma: analysis by loss of heterozygosity, p53 mutation, and X-chromosome inactivation. Journal of the National Cancer Institute 84: 1793–1798

Jensen M L, Nielsen M N 1989 Broad ligament mucinous and serous cystadenomas of borderline malignancy. Acta Obstetricia et Gynecologica Scandinavica 68: 663-667

Johnson T L, Kumar N B, Hopkins M, Hughes J D (1988) Cytological features of ovarian tumors of low malignant potential. Acta Cytologica 32: 513–518

Jones M A, Young R H, Srigley J R, Scully R E 1995 Paratesticular serous papillary carcinoma. Report of six cases. American Journal of Surgical Pathology 19: 1359–1365

Kabawat S E, Bast R C, Welch W R, Knapp R C, Colvin R B 1983 Immunopathologic characterization of a monoclonal antibody that recognizes common surface antigens of human ovarian tumors of serous, endometrioid and clear cell types. American Journal of Clinical Pathology 79: 98–104

Katzenstein A-L A, Mazur M T, Morgan T E, Kao M-S 1978 Proliferative serous tumors of the ovary. Histologic features and prognosis. American Journal of Surgical Pathology 2: 339–355

Kaur K, Gopalan S, Gupta S K, Dhaliwal L K 1990 Parovarian cystadenocarcinoma: a case report. Asia Oceania Journal of Obstetrics and Gynaecology 16: 131–135

Kemp G M, Hsui J G, Andrews M C 1992 Papillary peritnoeal carcinomatosis after prophylactic oophorectomy. Gynecologic Oncology 47: 395–397

Khoury N, Raju U, Crissman J D, Zarbo R J, Greenawald K A 1990 A comparative immunohistochemical study of peritoneal and ovarian serous tumors, and mesotheliomas. Human Pathology 21: 811–819

Kiechle-Schwartz M, Bauknecht T, Weinker T, Walz L, Pfleiderer A 1993 Loss of heterozygosity on chromosome 11p in human ovarian cancer. Positive correlation with grade of differentiation. Cancer 72: 2423–2432

Killackey M A, Davis A R 1993 Papillary serous carcinoma of the peritoneal surface: matched-case comparison with papillary serous ovarian carcinoma. Gynecologic Oncology 51: 171–174

Klemi P J, Joensuu H, Kiilholma P, Maenpaa J 1988 Clinical significance of abnormal nuclear DNA content in serous ovarian tumors. Cancer 62: 2005–2010

Kosmehl H, Langbein L, Kiss F 1989 Papillary serous carcinoma of the testis. International Urology and Nephrology 21: 169–174

Kuhn W, Kaufman M, Feichter G E, Schmid H, Hanke J, Rummel H H 1988 Psammomabody content and DNA-flow cytometric results as prognostic factors in advanced ovarian carcinoma. European Journal of Gynaecological Oncology 9: 234–241

Kurman R J, Trimble C L 1993 The behaviour of serous tumors of low malignant potential: are they ever malignant? International Journal of Gynecological Pathology 12: 120–127

Leake J F, Rader J S, Woodruff J D, Rosenshein N B 1991 Retroperitoneal lymphatic involvement with epithelial ovarian tumors of low malignant potential. Gynecologic Oncology 42: 124–130

Leake J F, Currie J L, Rosenhein N B, Woodruff J D 1992 Long-term follow-up of serous ovarian tumors of low malignant potential. Gynecologic Oncology 47: 150–158

Lele S B, Piver M S, Matharu J, Tsukada Y 1988 Peritoneal papillary carcinoma. Gynecologic Oncology 31: 315–320

Li S, Han H, Resnik E, Carcangiu M L, Schwartz P E, Yang Feng T L 1993 Advanced ovarian carcinoma: molecular evidence of unifocal origin. Gynecologic Oncology 51: 21–25

Lin M, Hanai J, Wada A et al 1991 Argyrophilia in ovarian serous tumors. A comparative study in 127 epithelial ovarian tumors. Histology and Histopathology 6: 477–484

Lindeque B G, Cronje H S, Deale C J C 1985 Prevalence of primary papillary peritoneal neoplasia in patients with ovarian carcinoma. South African Medical Journal 67: 1005–1007

Loredo D S, Powell J L, Reed W P, Rosenbaum J M 1990 Ovarian carcinoma metastatic to the breast: a case report and review of the literature. Gynecologic Oncology 37: 432–436

Maasen V, Hiller K 1994 Glandular inclusions in lymph nodes: pattern of distribution and metaplastic transformation. Archives of Gynecology and Obstetrics 255: 1–8

Maasen V, Debus-Theide G 1993 Das seros-papillare Karzinom des Peritoneums; eine multizentrische Primarerkrankung. Zentralblatt für Gynäkologie 115: 347–354

McCaughey W T E, Kirk M E, Lester W, Dardick I 1984 Peritoneal epithelial lesions associated with proliferative serous tumors of ovary. Histopathology 8: 195–208

McCaughey W T E, Schryer M J P, Lin X-S, Al-Jabi M 1986 Extraovarian pelvic serous tumor with marked calcification. Archives of Pathology and Laboratory Medicine 110: 78–80

Mallonee M M, Lin F, Hassanien R 1987 A morphologic analysis of the cells of ductal carcinoma of the breast and of adenocarcinoma of the ovary in pleural and abdominal effusions. Acta Cytologica 31: 441–447

Manchul L A, Simm J, Levin W et al 1992 Borderline epithelial ovarian tumors: a review of 81 cases with an assessment of the impact of treatment. International Journal of Radiation Oncology and Biological Physics 22: 867–874

Massad L S Jr, Hunter V J, Szpak C A, Clarke-Pearson D L, Creasman W T 1991 Epithelial ovarian tumors of low malignant potential. Obstetrics and Gynecology 78: 1027–1032

Mills S E, Andersen W A, Fechner R E, Austin M B 1988 Serous surface papillary carcinoma. A clinicopathologic study of 10 cases and comparison with stage III–IV ovarian serous carcinoma. American Journal of Surgical Pathology 12: 827–834

Moen M D, Cliby W A, Wilson T O 1994 Stage III papillary serous cystadenocarcinoma of the ovary in a 15-year-old female. Gynecologic Oncology 53: 274–276

Mok C H, Tsao S W, Knapp R C, Fishbaugh P M, Lau C C 1992 Unifocal origin of advanced human epithelial ovarian cancers. Cancer Research 52: 5119–5122

Mulhollan T J, Silva E G, Tornos C, Guerreiri C, Fromm G L, Gershenson D 1994 Ovarian involvement by serous surface papillary carcinoma. International Journal of Gynecological Pathology 13: 120–126

Nagata O, Aramaki S, Iino H et al 1990 A serous cystadenoma of the ovary of borderline malignancy with a fifteen-year history. A case report. Gan No Rinsho 36: 669–673

Okolo S O, Darley C, Melville H A, Kirkham N 1990 Virilizing ovarian serous cystadenoma. Case report. British Journal of Obsterics and Gynaecology 97: 269–271

Pejovic T, Heim S, Mandahl N et al 1990 Trisomy 12 is a consistent chromosomal aberration in benign ovarian tumors. Genes Chromosomes and Cancer 2: 48–52

Piura B, Glezerman M 1989 Synchronous carcinomas of endometrium and ovary. Gynecologic Oncology 33: 261–264

Piver M S, Jishi M F, Tsukada Y, Nava G 1993 Primary peritoneal carcinoma after prophylactic oophorectomy in women with a family history of ovarian cancer. A report of the Gilda Radner Familial Ovarian Cancer Registry. Cancer 71: 2751–2755

Puls L E, Powell D E, de Priest P D et al 1992 Transition from benign to malignant epithelium in mucinous and serous ovarian cystadenocarcinoma. Gynecologic Oncology 47: 530–57

Prade M, Spatz A, Duvillard P et al 1993 Les inclusions glandulaires benignes dans les ganglions lymphatiques inguinaux et abdominopelviens en pathologie gynecologique. Annals de Pathologie 13: 317–323

Raju U, Fine G, Greenawald K A, Ohorodnik J M 1989 Primary papillary serous neoplasia of the peritoneum: a clinicopathologic and ultrastructural study of eight cases. Human Pathology 20: 426–436

Ransom D T, Patel S R, Keeney G L, Malkasian G D, Edmondson J H 1990 Papillary serous carcinoma of the peritoneum. A review of 33 cases treated with platin-based chemotherapy. Cancer 66: 1091–1094

Remmele W, Kaiserling E, Zerban U et al 1992 Serous papillary cystic tumor of borderline malignancy with focal carcinoma arising in testis: case report with immunohistochemical and ultrastructural observations. Human Pathology 23: 75–79

Resta L, Russo S, Colucci G A, Prat J 1993 Morphologic precursors of ovarian epithelial tumors. Obstetrics and Gynecology 82: 181–186

Robey S S, Silva E G 1989 Epithelial hyperplasia of the fallopian tube. Its association with serous borderline tumors of the ovary. International Journal of Gynecological Pathology 8: 214–220

Rojansky N, Ophir E, Sharony A, Spira H, Suprun H 1985 Broad ligament adenocarcinoma – its origin and clinical behavior. A literature review and report of a case. Obstetrical and Gynecological Survey 40: 665–671

Rose P G, Reale F R 1991 Papillary serous carcinoma of the peritoneum following endometrial cancer. Obstetrics and Gynecology 78: 980–983

Rosen H R, Rosen A C, Preiser J, Stierer M, Klein M Hanak H 1992 Non-ovarian peritoneal papillary serous carcinoma with high Ca125 levels. Archives of Gynecology and Obstetrics 251: 199–202

Rothacker D, Möbius G 1995 Varieties of serous surface papillary carcinoma of the peritoneum in northern Germany: a thirty-year autopsy study. International Journal of Gynecological Pathology 14: 310–318

Russell P 1979a The pathological assessment of ovarian neoplasms. I: Introduction to the common 'epithelial' tumors and analysis of benign 'epithelial' tumors. Pathology 11: 5–26

Russell P 1979b The pathological assessment of ovarian neoplasms. II: The proliferating 'epithelial' tumors. Pathology 11: 251–282

Russell P 1979c The pathological assessment of ovarian neoplasms. III: The malignant 'epithelial' tumors. Pathology 11: 493–532

Russell P 1984 Borderline epithelial tumors of the ovary: a conceptual dilemma. Clinics in Obstetrics and Gynaecology 11: 259–277

Russell P, Merkur H 1979 Proliferating ovarian 'epithelial' tumors: a clinicopathological analysis of 144 cases. Australian and New Zealand Journal of Obstetrics and Gynaecology 19: 45–51

Russell P, Bannatyne P M, Solomon H J, Stoddard L D, Tattersall M H N 1985 Multifocal tumorigenesis in the upper female genital tract – implications for staging and management. International Journal of Gynecolgical Pathology 4: 192–210

Schneider J, Gonzalez-Rodilla I, Eizaguirre M J, Garcia-Satue E 1985 Complete psammomatous degeneration of the ovary. Case report. British Journal of Obstetrics and Gynaecology 92: 419–422

Scully R E 1979 Tumors of the ovary and maldeveloped gonads, AFIP fascicle 16, 2nd series. Armed Forces Institute of Pathology, Washington, DC, p 53–151

Segal G H, Hart W R 1992 Ovarian serous tumors of low malignant potential (serous borderline tumors). The relationship of exophytic surface tumor to peritoneal 'implants'. American Journal of Surgical Pathology 16: 577–583

Seltzer V L, Molho L, Fougner A, Hong P, Kereszti B, Gero M, Spitzer M 1988 Parovarian cystadenocarcinoma of low malignant potential. Gynecologic Oncology 30: 216–221

Sherman M E, Bitterman P, Rosenshein N B, Delgado G, Kurman R J 1992 Uterine serous carcinoma. A morphologically diverse neoplasm with unifying clinicopathologic features. American Journal of Surgical Pathology 16: 600–610

Siriaunkgul S, Tavassoli F A 1993 Invasive micropapillary carcinoma of the breast. Modern Pathology 6: 660–662

Skodras G, Fields V, Kragel P J 1994 Ovarian lymphoma and serous carcinoma of low malignant potential arising in the same ovary. Archives of Pathology and Laboratory Medicine 118: 647–650

Skov R V, Bichel P 1991 OC-125 as a diagnostic aid in the cytological evaluation of ascitic cells in patients with ovarian carcinoma. Virchows Archiv [A] Pathologic Anatomy and Histopathology 419: 59–62

Tan L K, Flynn S D, Carcangiu M L 1994 Ovarian serous borderline tumors with lymph node involvement. Clinicopathologic and DNA content study of seven cases and review of the literature. American Journal of Surgical Pathology 18: 904–912

Tavassoli F A 1988 Serous tumor of low malignant potential with early stromal invasion (serous LMP with microinvasion). Modern Pathology 1: 407–414

Tavassoli M, Ruhrburg C, Beaumont V et al 1993 Whole chromosome 17 loss in ovarian cancer. Genes, Chromosomes and Cancer 8: 195–198

Tickman R J, Cohen C, Varna V A, Fekete P S, de Rose P B 1990 Acta Cytologica Distinction between carcinoma cells and mesothelial cells in serous effusions. Usefulness of immunohistochemistry. Acta Cytologica 34: 491–496

Tobacman J K, Greene M H, Tucker M A, Costa J, Kase R, Fraumeni J F Jr 1982 Intra-abdominal carcinomatosis after prophylactic oophorectomy in ovarian cancer-prone families. Lancet ii: 795–797

Trope C, Kaern J, Vergote I B, Kristensen G, Abeler V 1993 Are borderline tumors of the ovary overtreated both surgically and systemically? A review of four prospective randomized trials including patients with borderline tumors. Gynecologic Oncology 51: 236–243

Truong L D, Maccato M L, Awalt H, Cagle P T, Schwartz M R, Kaplan A L 1990 Serous surface carcinoma of the peritoneum: a clinicopathologic study of 22 cases. Human Pathology 21: 99–110

Tsao S W, Mok C H, Knapp R C et al 1993 Molecular genetic evidence of a unifocal origin for human serous ovarian carcinomas. Gynecologic Oncology 48: 5–10

Tsujimura T, Takeda M, Terada N, Uramoto H 1991 Two cases of peritoneal papillary adenocarcinoma. Acta Pathologica Japonica 41: 642–646

Ulbright T M, Mosley D J, Roth L M, Berkow R L 1983 Papillary serous serous carcinoma of the retroperitoneum. American Journal of Clinical Pathology 79: 633–637

Ulbright T M, Roth L M, Sutton G P 1990 Papillary serous carcinoma of the ovary with squamous differentiation. International Journal of Gynecological Pathology 9: 86–94

van Kley H, Cramer S, Bruns D E 1981 Serous ovarian neoplastic amylase (SONA): a potentially useful marker for serous ovarian tumors. Cancer 48: 1444–1449

van Niekerk C C, Boerman O C, Ramaekers F C, Poels L G 1991 Marker profile in different phases in the transition of normal human ovarian epithelium to ovarian carcinomas. American Journal of Pathology 138: 455–463

White P F, Merino M J, Barwick K W 1985 Serous surface papillary carcinoma of the ovary: a clinical, pathologic, ultrastructural, and immunohistochemical study of 11 cases. Pathology Annual 20: 403–418

Wick M R, Mills S E, Dehner L P, Bollinger D J, Fechner R E 1989 Serous papillary carcinomas arising from the peritoneum and ovaries. A clinicopathologic and immunohistochemical comparison. International Journal of Gynecological Pathology 8: 179–188

Yoonessi M, Crickard K, Celik C, Yoonessi S 1988 Borderline epithelial tumors of the ovary. Ovarian intraepithelial neoplasia. Obstetrical and Gynecological Survey 43: 435–444

Zheng J P, Robinson W R, Ehlen T, Yu M C, Dubeau L 1991 Distinction of low grade from high grade human ovarian carcinomas on the basis of losses of heterozygosity on chromosomes 3, 6, and 11 and HER-2/neu gene amplification. Cancer Research 51: 4045–4051

Zheng J, Wan M, Zweizig S, Velicescu M, Yu M C, Dubeau L 1993 Histologically benign or low-grade malignant tumors adjacent to high-grade ovarian carcinomas contain molecular characteristics of high-grade carcinomas. Cancer Research 53: 4138–4142

Zheng W, Wolf S, Kramer E E, Cox K A, Hoda S A 1996 Borderline papillary serous tumor of the fallopian tube. American Journal of Surgical Pathology 20: 30–35

24

Mucinous tumors

P. Russell A. Farnsworth

The characteristic epithelium of benign mucinous cystadenomas is a uniform single layer of tall columnar cells with clear, homogeneous cytoplasm and small basal nuclei. At both the light and electron microscopic levels, two types of mucin-filled cells have been identified, resembling those of the endocervix and gastrointestinal mucosa (Langley et al 1972, Fenoglio et al 1975, 1976a,b, Ball et al 1990, Shiozawa et al 1992, Tenti et al 1992), a cardinal feature which is reflected in the new World Health Organization (WHO) classification (see Appendix B). In tumors with a mixed or predominantly intestinal character to the epithelium, goblet cells are common; argentaffin or argyrophil neuroendocrine cells are frequently observed (Klemi 1978, Klemi & Nevalainen 1978, Louwerens et al 1983, Aguirre et al 1984, Sasaki et al 1989) and even Paneth cells are very rarely seen. The bulk of tumor cells contain abundant diastase-resistant PAS-positive and mucicarmine-positive glycoproteins, some of which is like intestinal mucin in many of its staining (de Boer et al 1981) and immunohistochemical characteristics (Pant et al 1986). Benign ovarian mucinous tumors are predominantly mullerian ('endocervical like') and lesser proportions are mixed or show exclusively intestinal differentiation (Fulcheri et al 1990). Once proliferative changes are present, however, this ratio changes markedly. About 85% of proliferating tumors are intestinal in pattern (Szymanska et al 1983, Rutgers & Scully 1988) and essentially all invasive mucinous carcinomas are of this genre. Why the malignant end of the endocervical (mullerian) neoplastic spectrum is so rarely represented in the ovary (as contrasted with the endometrial and serous–tubal equivalents) is not known. Invasive cervical adenocarcinomas only very infrequently resemble intestinal carcinomas (Azzopardi & Hou 1965) or produce pseudomyxomatous (colloid carcinoma) patterns. Paradoxically, mucinous ovarian tumors of intestinal type are associated with mullerian-type adenocarcinomas of the cervix (Young & Scully 1988). Occasional reports of morphologically equivalent mucinous tumors occurring in retroperitoneal tissues (Fujii et al 1986, Banerjee & Gough 1988, Cohen et al 1988, Nelson et al 1988, Pennell & Gusdon 1989, Park et al 1991, Sondergaard & Kapersen 1991, Gotoh et al 1992, Rothacker et al 1993, Motoyama et al 1994), uterine broad ligaments (Jensen & Nielsen 1989, Aslani & Scully 1989), spleen (Morinaga et al 1992), and even lung (Graeme-Cook & Mark 1991, Pelletier et al 1993) further confuse the issue of pathogenesis.

Table 24.1 Immunophenotype of mucinous carcinomas

Antibody against	Expression (%)
Cytokeratins (AE1/AE3, CAM 5.2)	100
Cytokeratin 7	100
Cytokeratin 20	75
Epithelial membrane antigen (EMA)	100
HMFG-IIIC12	100
CA 19–9	90
Carcinoembryonic antigen (CEA)	85
HAM-56	75
α-Amylase	75
Vimentin	0
S100 protein	0
CA-125 antigen	0

Benign mucinous cystadenomas occur most frequently during the third to fifth decades, although they may be encountered in quite young women. This age distribution accounts for their being one of the most commonly encountered ovarian neoplasms in pregnancy. They are bilateral in only about 2–3% of cases. The uncommonly large size of some tumors as well as their relative frequency in pregnancy both contribute to their being disproportionately represented amongst ovarian masses presenting with acute torsion.

Proliferating tumors (10–15% of all mucinous tumors) have a peak incidence in the middle of the fourth decade (mean age of intestinal subtype is about 40 years, and of the mullerian subtype about 30 years), but may rarely occur in young girls (Deprest et al 1992). Furthermore, the intestinal subtypes are bilateral in 6–8%, while the mullerian or 'endocervical-like' examples are bilateral in 40% of instances (Rutgers & Scully 1988). It is interesting to note that, in our experience, the age distribution of those patients with ovarian intestinal type mucinous tumors associated with pseudomyxoma ovarii (with or without associated pseudomyxoma peritonei) is significantly older than those without (Russell 1987).

Invasive mucinous carcinomas occur mostly in women in their fourth to seventh decades, are bilateral in about 15–20% of instances and are mostly (95%) confined to the ovaries at laparotomy.

Pseudomyxoma peritonei. It is relevant to mention here pseudomyxoma peritonei (Fig. 24.1), or disseminated peritoneal adenomucinosis as it has also recently been called (Ronnett et al 1995b). This poorly understood condition is due to spread of the contents of mucinous ovarian cysts or gastrointestinal neoplasms (with or without some cellular component) into the general peritoneal

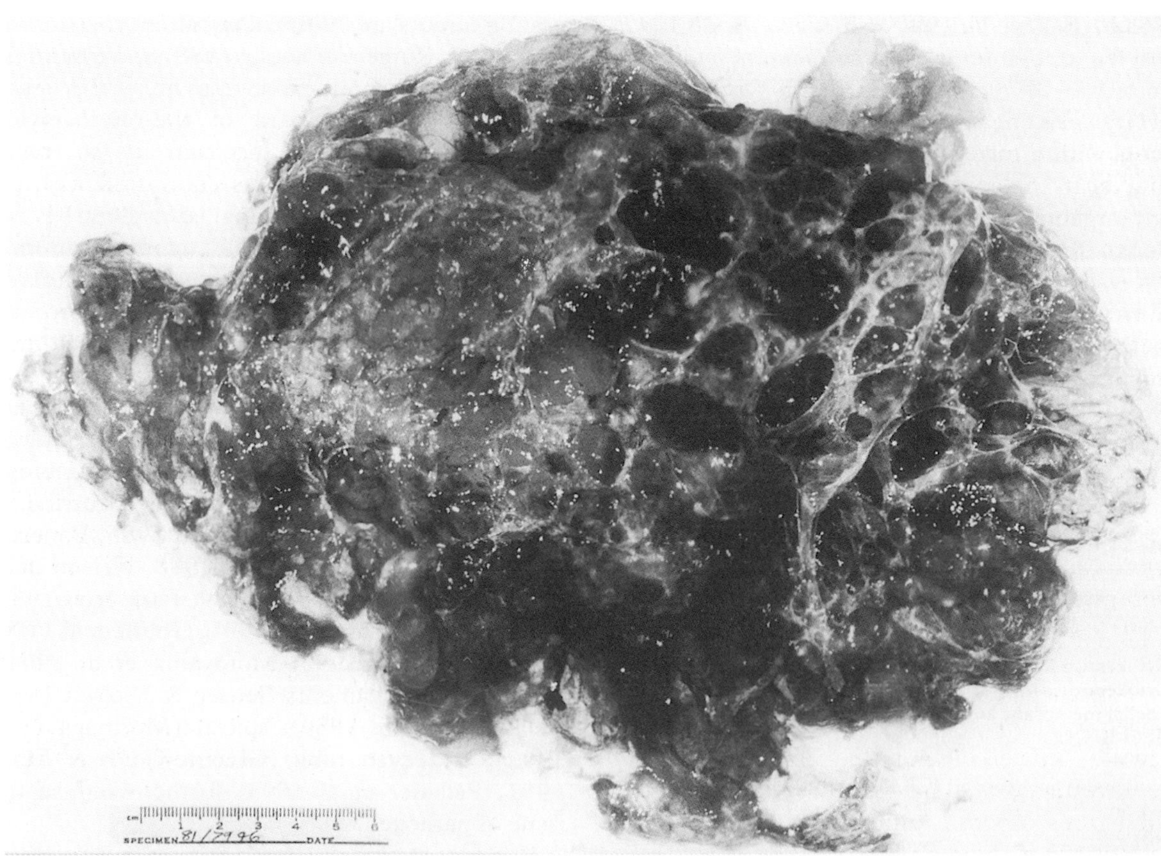

Fig. 24.1 Pseudomyxoma peritonei. Masses of soft jelly-like material removed from the peritoneal cavity of a woman with bilateral ovarian cysts (see Fig. 24.2A,B)

cavity. Theories of genesis include gross rupture of the ovarian cysts, but pseudomyxoma is almost invariably present at the time of initial surgery (whether or not an obvious rupture can be demonstrated) and does not follow accidental rupture during surgical removal. The associated ovarian neoplasm is often bilateral (two-thirds of cases) (Campbell et al 1973, Young et al 1991), and always seems to show an insidious penetration of its stroma by pools and tracts of mucin, giving a pattern referred to as 'pseudomyxoma ovarii' (Figs 24.2, 24.23, 24.27). This appearance may be associated with mucinous ovarian neoplasms at any point in the proliferative spectrum, but most usually at the lower end. On the one hand, pseudomyxoma peritonei is, in our experience, the sole neoplastic extraovarian manifestation of those 15% or so of atypically proliferating mucinous tumors of intestinal type which present with associated disease beyond the ovaries. On the other hand, Rutgers & Scully (1988) have described extraovarian 'implants' analogous to those seen with serous tumors (see Ch. 23) in association with 15% of atypically proliferating mucinous tumors of 'endocervical-like' differentiation. These are two entirely separate and distinct processes, the former progressive, the latter not. Pseudomyxoma ovarii, in turn, appears to be due to break down in the integrity of the epithelium of cysts or smaller acini in the tumor with little or no stromal reaction to the mucins released. This points to the probable pathogenesis of generalized disease; it is unclear whether this process is prima facie evidence of biological malignancy (Michael et al 1987) or a special form of nonmalignant dissemination (Hart & Norris 1973). Precisely the same histological spectrum can be observed in appendiceal mucocoeles, which may or may not also progress to generalized pseudomyxoma (Higa et al 1973, Ronnett et al 1995a,b).

The frequent, but far from universal, synchronous (Wertheim et al 1994) or metachronous (Nogales et al 1991) presence of cytologically similar tumors in the appendix and ovaries has led some investigators to propose that the appendiceal lesions are the notional primary sites of neoplastic transformation and the ovarian masses, along with the peritoneal disease, are manifestations of a metastatic process (Young et al 1991, Prayson et al 1994, Ronnett et al 1995a,b). The concept of independent primary neoplasms is favored by ourselves and others (Kahn & Demopoulos 1992, Sumithran & Susil 1992, Seidman et al 1993). This is an issue of no small moment, as establishment of a 'metastatic' nature of the ovarian tumors in such patients casts genuine doubt upon the very existence of ovarian mucinous tumors 'of low malignant potential', in the same way as an understanding of the multifocal nature of serous type neoplasms casts doubt on the 'low malignant potential' of proliferating ovarian serous tumors. Relevant observations in women with this condition include pseudomyxoma ovarii being more common than pseudomyxoma peritonei (Fig. 24.2C,D), and the coexistence of ovarian mucinous cysts with appendiceal mucinous cystomas without the additional 'linking' presence of pseudomyxoma peritonei (Russell 1979a,b). These would be difficult to explain if pseudomyxoma peritonei is supposed to give rise to pseudomyxoma ovarii. But these are balanced by the almost 100% long-term survival of women with stage I proliferating mucinous tumors, suggesting a negligible propensity to insensible spread by the time of diagnosis (i.e. no malignant potential). Pseudomyxoma peritonei can rarely be due to mucinous lesions of the fallopian tubes (Minguillon et al 1992) and even extra-abdominal neoplasms (Kurita et al 1994). Notwithstanding these controversies, the evidence suggests that a small, but specific, subgroup of gastrointestinal and/or ovarian mucinous tumors (included amongst those showing intestinal epithelial differentiation) is responsible for development of pseudomyxoma peritonei (Russell 1979a), a disorder for which the standard protocols of cytoreductive surgery at initial presentation and repeated palliative debulking, mucolytic agents, chemotherapy, and/or radiotherapy have done relatively little to modify the natural history (Wertheim et al 1994, Look et al 1995). The 1-, 5-, and 10-year survival rates are 98%, 53–65%, and 32–50%, respectively (Carter et al 1991, Gough et al 1994).

Cytogenetic and molecular genetic studies

DNA aneuploidy is reported in 11% of mucinous carcinomas (Griffiths et al 1993). Clonal kary-

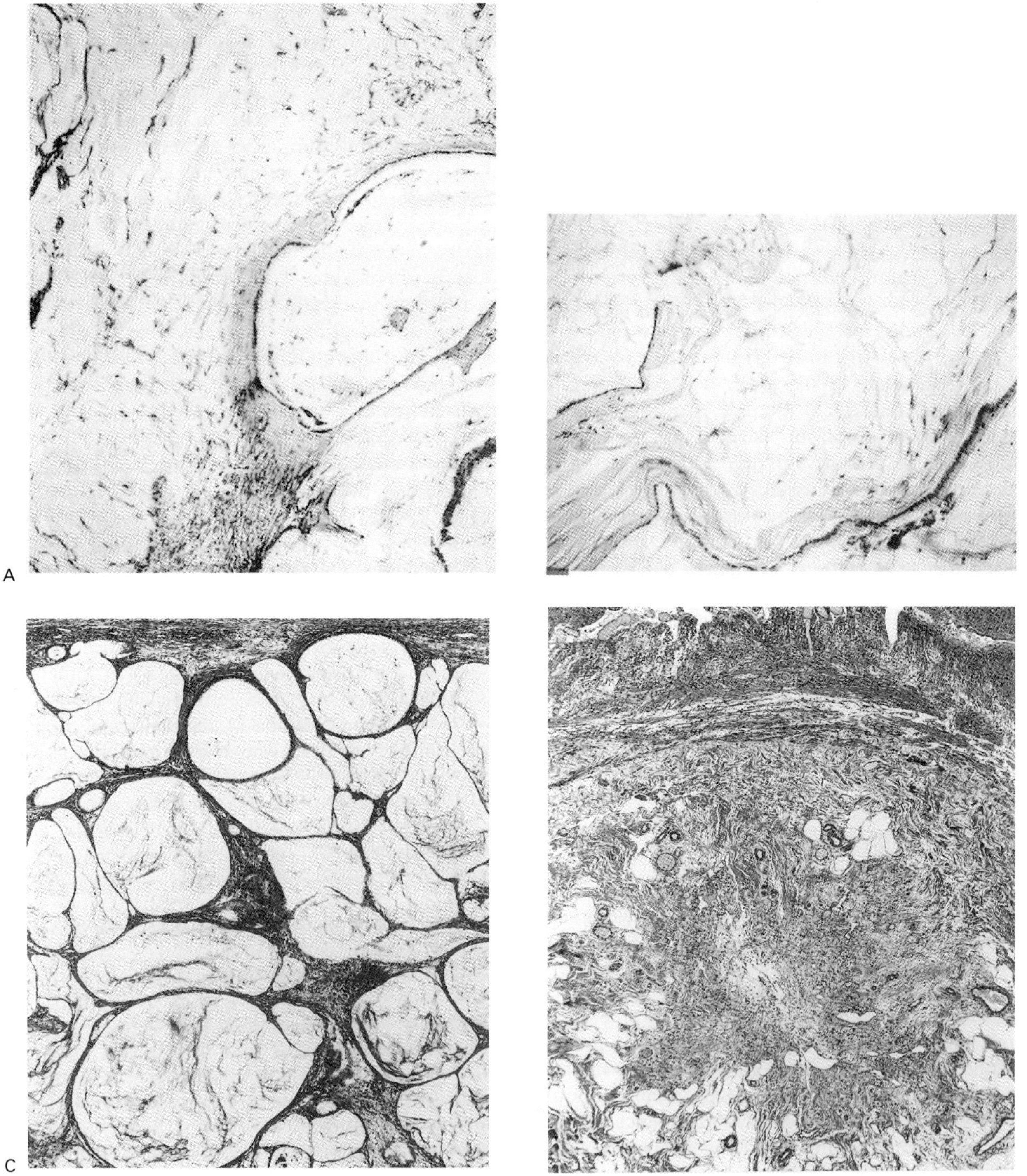

Fig. 24.2 (A) Pseudomyxoma pattern within a cytologically benign mucinous ovarian tumor ('pseudomyxoma ovarii'). Residual ovarian stroma is present in the lower center portion of the figure. H + E ×35. (B) An identical pattern was seen throughout the peritoneal cavity of this patient (see Fig. 24.1). H + E ×60. (C) Pseudomyxoma ovarii in a very low grade proliferating mucinous tumor, in a patient without peritoneal disease. H + E ×23. (D) The associated appendix in this patient was attenuated and fibrotic, without any residual mucosa. H + E ×23

otypic abnormalities such as trisomy 12 have been reported in benign mucinous tumors (Pejovic et al 1990).

Macroscopic features

Benign mucinous tumors are nearly always cystic and multilocular and range in size up to 50 cm in diameter (rare gigantic lesions weighing over 100 kg have been documented) (O'Hanlan 1994). The usually thick-walled opaque capsules have a smooth surface. The cysts contain a thick, tenacious mucinous material – occasionally somewhat more watery in consistency. Typically the locules are multiple and small (Fig. 24.3), but tumors may be parvilocular, or even a single large cyst. Necrosis and hemorrhage are mostly indications of previous torsion and are not worrisome gross features. Fibrous stroma varies in prominence but is usually inconspicuous. Mucinous adenofibromas (which differ from their serous counterparts only in the 'mucinous' feel to their cut surfaces) are distinctly uncommon lesions (Bell 1991b).

Neoplasms with low grade epithelial proliferation (Fig. 24.4) do not differ significantly from their benign counterparts, having an average diameter of 15–20 cm. There is, perhaps, a tendency to a finer honeycombing of the cut surface in higher grade proliferating tumors, but this may be only focal. Papillary areas, necrosis, and hemorrhage are noted only occasionally.

The frank mucinous carcinomas are predominantly multilocular cystic neoplasms averaging about 15–30 cm in diameter. Solid areas and luminal nodules are more common than in the less proliferative lesions, as are hemorrhage and

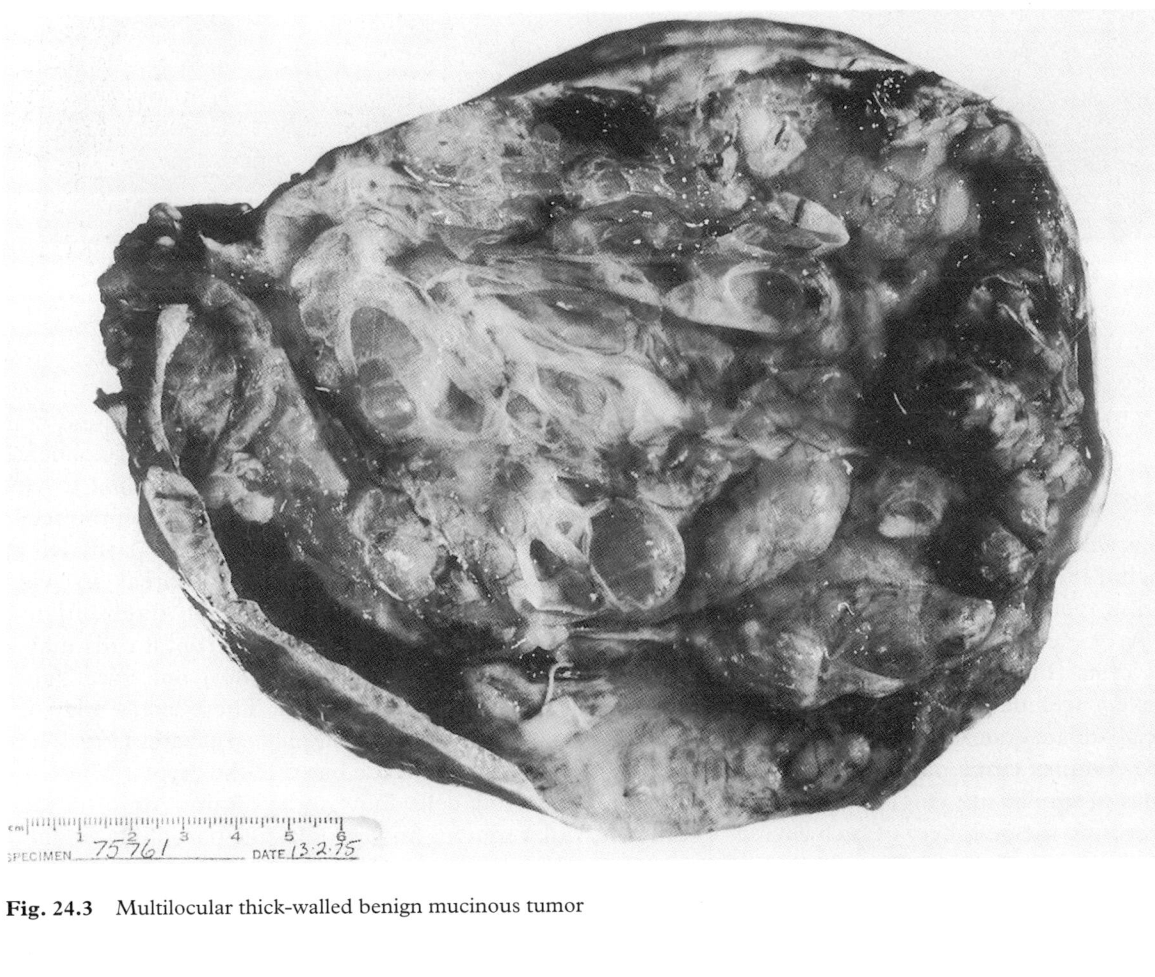

Fig. 24.3 Multilocular thick-walled benign mucinous tumor

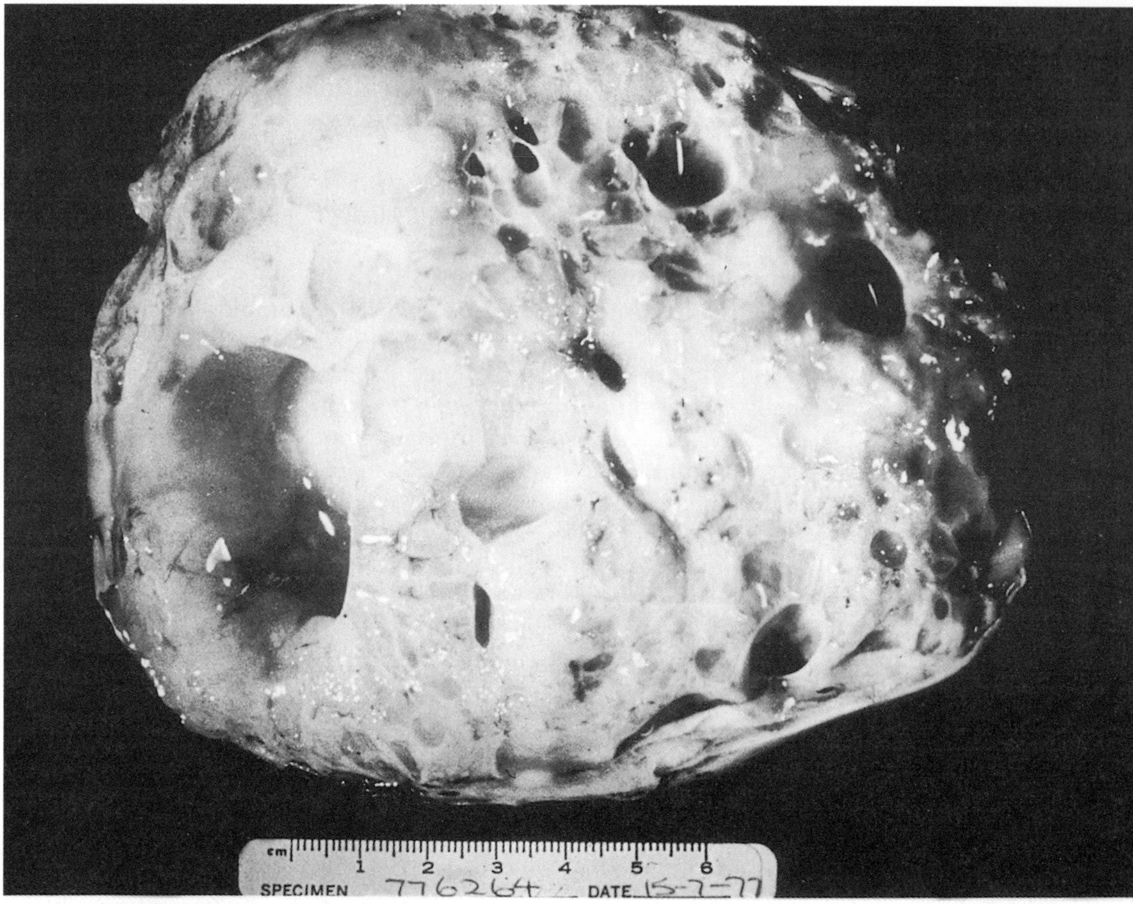

Fig. 24.4 Multilocular proliferating mucinous tumor

necrosis. Less commonly, the tumors are predominantly or entirely solid with a soft mucoid consistency to the cut surface (Fig. 24.5).

Microscopic features

The architecture of benign tumors in this group reflects the size and number of the cystic spaces and the relative prominence of intervening stroma. At one end of the spectrum are simple mucinous cysts (Fig. 24.6) with a thick, collagenous, relatively acellular outer wall, sometimes showing large spiculate deposits of dystrophic calcification. More complex cystic patterns are due to multiple locules of similar size (Fig. 24.7) or to a proliferation around the periphery of such cavities by small acini or 'daughter cysts' (Fig. 24.8) in a pseudoinvasive pattern (Fig. 24.9). Characteristically, mitotic activity is seen only in these actively growing areas.

The flat epithelium is single layered and composed of tall columnar cells with well-delineated cell margins and abundant eosinophilic to clear cytoplasm. The latter contains diffuse intracellular neutral and acid mucins. Basal nuclei are small and hyperchromatic. In areas in which goblet cells suggest intestinal differentiation, occasional argentaffin or argyrophil cells may be identified (Sasaki et al 1989), and rare Paneth cells may also be seen. These areas may also exhibit crypt-like epithelial structures (Fig. 24.10) with mitoses at the bases of the crypts. These proliferating cells show some diminution of intracellular mucins and cytoplasmic basophilia similar to the generative cells at the crypt bases in the normal colon. An apparently unique case of a benign

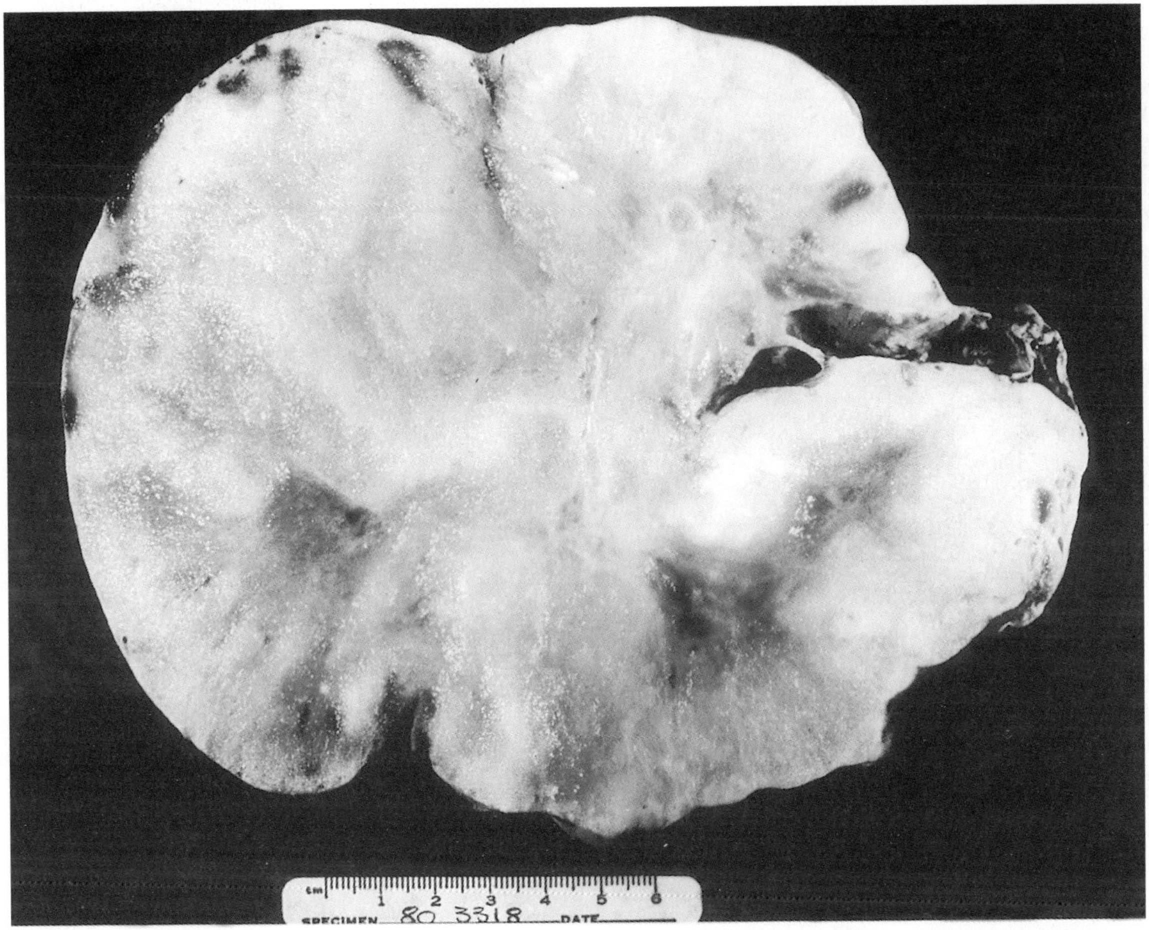

Fig. 24.5 An unusually solid mucinous carcinoma with central necrosis and no appreciable cystic component

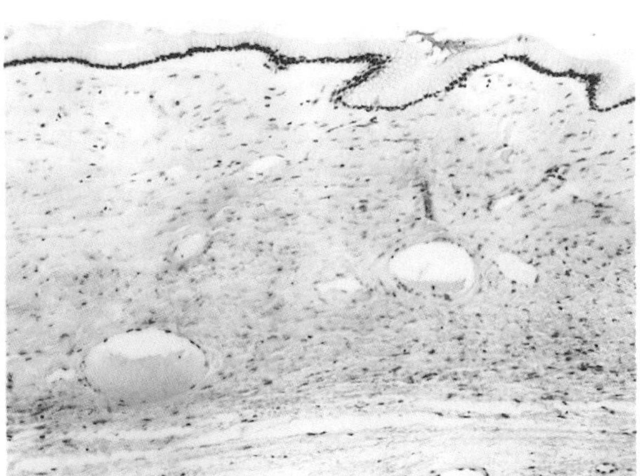

Fig. 24.6 Benign mucinous cyst with a typical 'picket fence' endocervical-type epithelium and a thick fibrous wall. H + E ×60

mucinous tumor has been reported showing atypia of the epithelium resembling the Arias–Stella reaction of gestational endometrium (Spaun & Toft 1986). Quite complex papillary areas (Fig. 24.11A), simple fronding (Fig. 24.11B), changes which resemble microglandular hyperplasia of the cervix (Fig. 24.11C), foci of squamous metaplasia (Fig. 24.12A) which may be quite exuberant (Mannion et al 1993), and bizarre degenerative nuclear atypia (Fig. 24.12B), but without other features of proliferation, are also observed from time to time. Pressure of accumulated secretion within cysts leads to attenuation of the epithelium. This may proceed to break down in its integrity, with leakage of the mucin into the surrounding stroma which then elicits focal stromal responses varying from very slight (as in

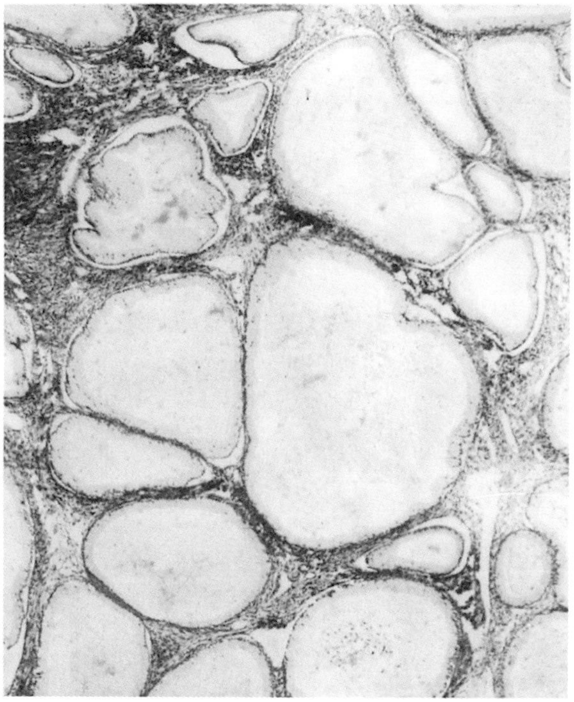

Fig. 24.7 Benign mucinous cystadenoma (same case as in Fig. 24.3) with a complex multilocular pattern. H + E ×35

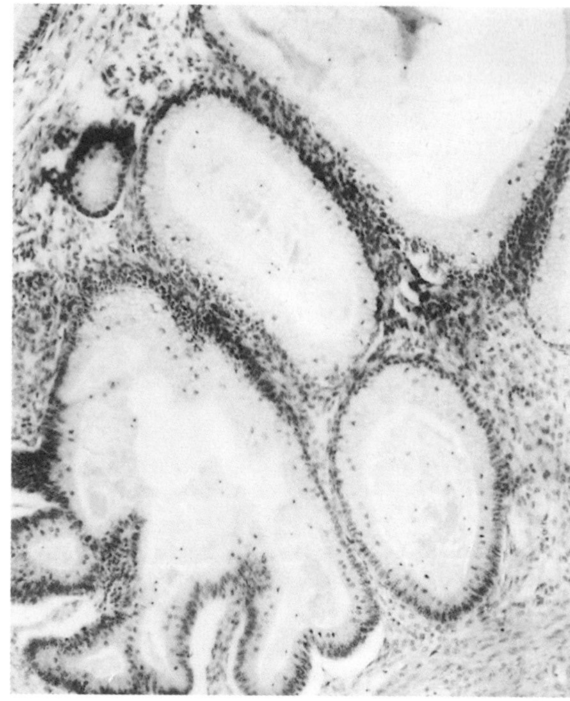

Fig. 24.8 Benign mucinous cystadenoma. There is apparent maturation of the intestinal-type epithelium from outer tumor margin (bottom – showing mitoses and decreased intracellular mucin) towards the tumor center (top – with mature epithelium and no mitoses). H + E ×90

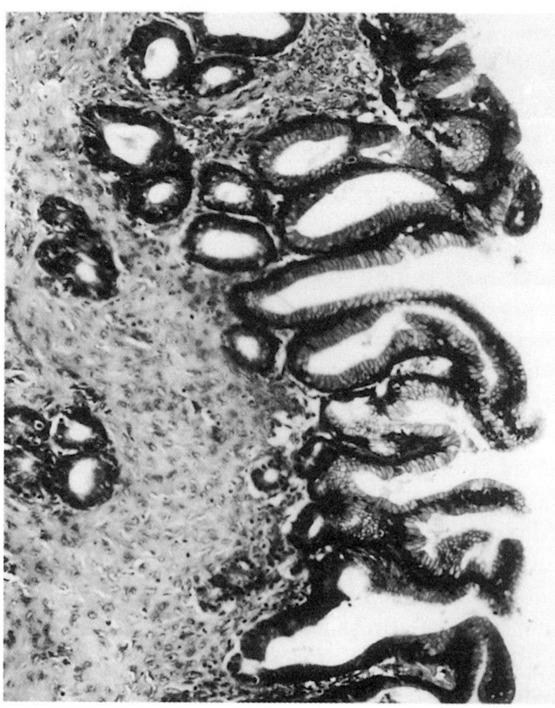

Fig. 24.9 Benign intrusion of glandular buds into the tumor stroma is one of the many patterns of pseudo-invasion which must be recognized. H + E ×90

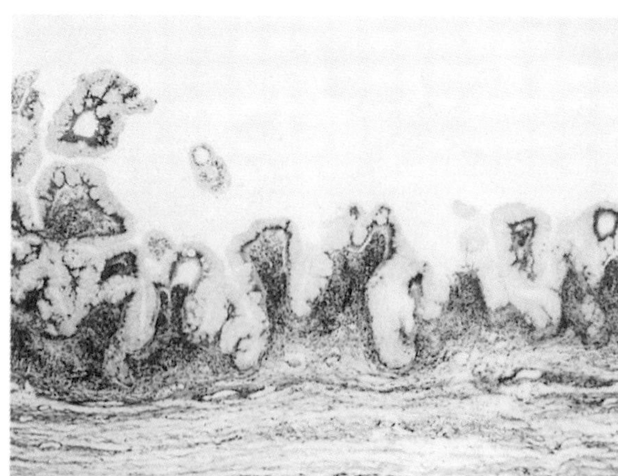

Fig. 24.10 The elaboration of intestinal crypt-like structures is another pattern of epithelial growth which is compatible with a diagnosis of benign mucinous cystadenoma and is not to be confused with atypical epithelial proliferation. H + E ×25

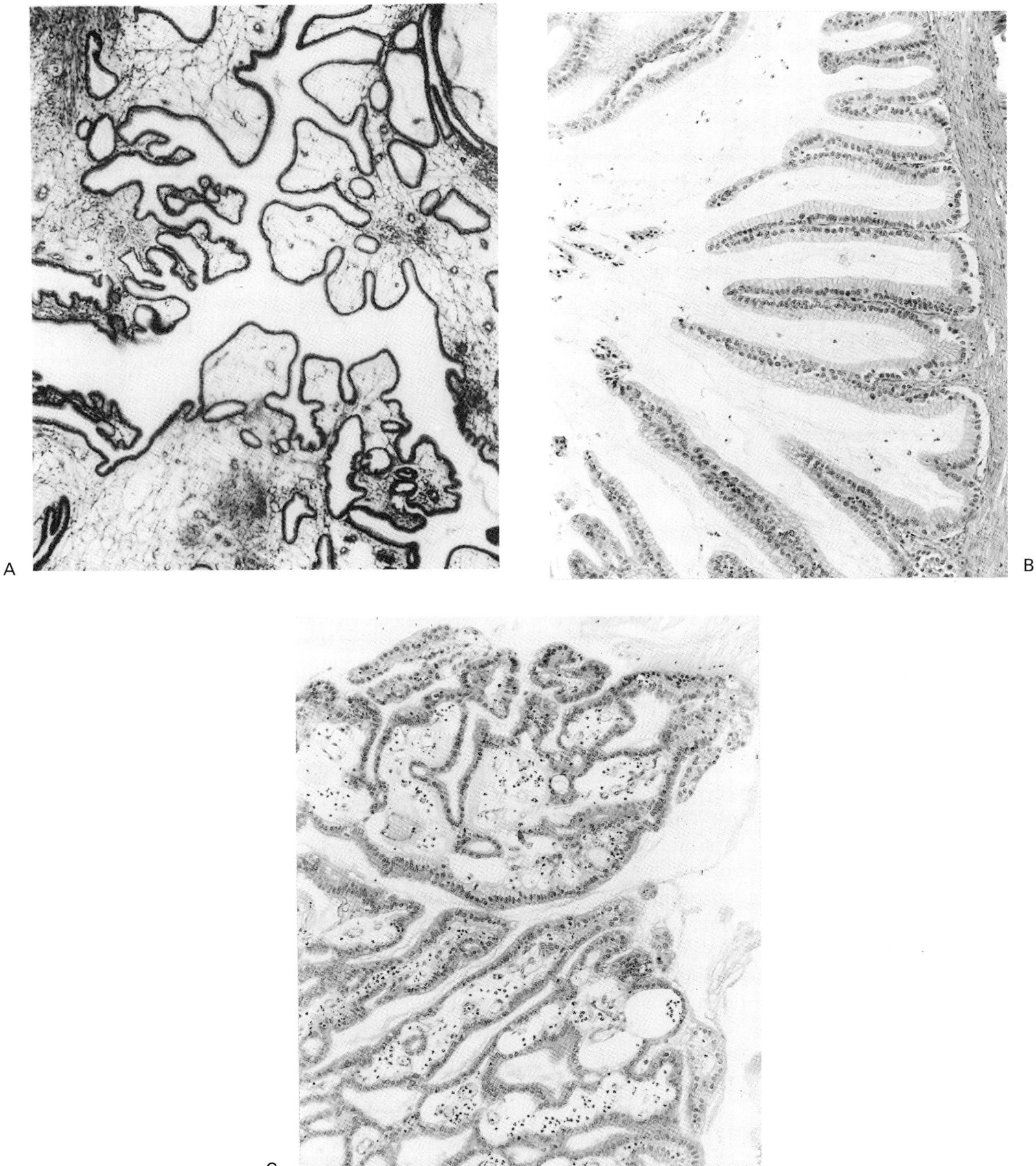

Fig. 24.11 Benign mucinous tumors with architectural features which should be differentiated from those of proliferating tumors. (A) A definite broad papillary pattern, each papilla lined by typical tall columnar mucus-secreting epithelium. H + E ×25. (B) Simple epithelial fronding. H + E ×60. (C) Relatively complex glands with features resembling those seen in microglandular hyperplasia of the endocervix. H + E ×60

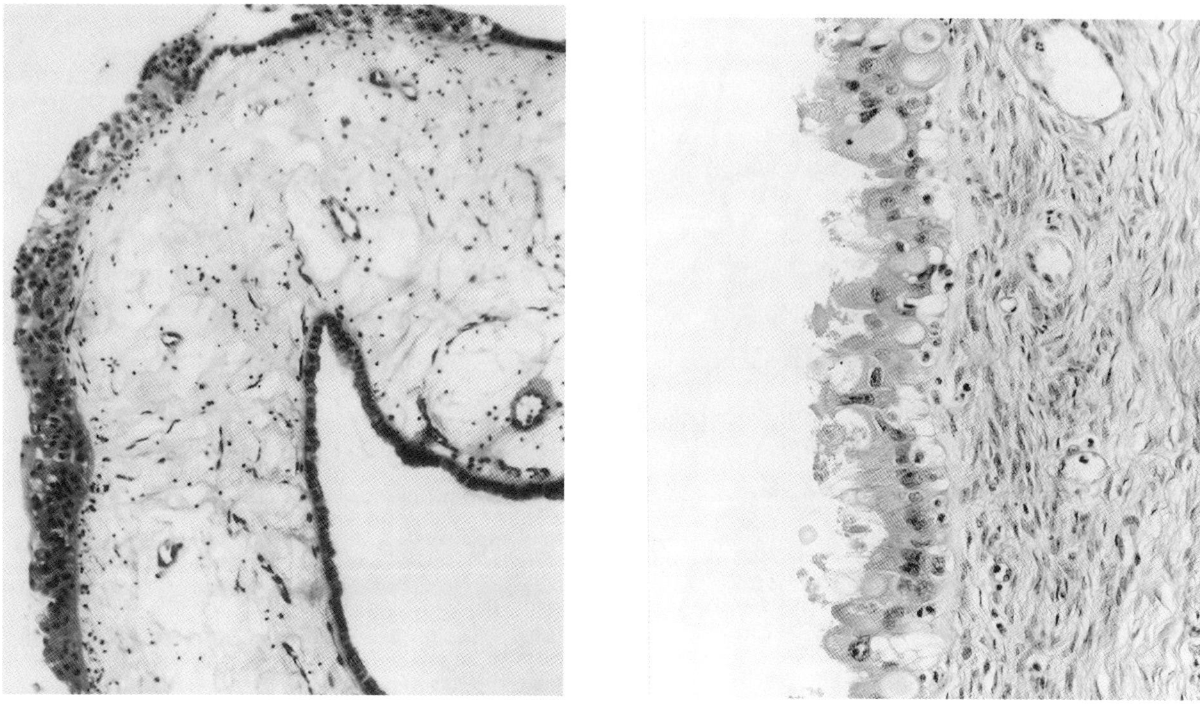

A B

Fig. 24.12 Benign endocervical type mucinous cystadenoma with cellular features which should be differentiated from those of proliferating tumors. (A) A mild chronic inflammatory infiltrate in the stroma and squamous metaplasia (left). H + E ×90. (B) Bizarre degenerative nuclear atypia with basal vacuolation of the epithelial cells. Such changes are more typical of endometrioid tumors. H + E ×116

pseudomyxoma ovarii) to quite florid foreign body inflammatory reactions (Fig. 24.13). An apparently unique case of mucinous cystadenoma coexisting with systemic sarcoidosis (White et al 1990) is differentiated by the discrete nature of the granulomas and their lack of tropism for exposed mucinous material. Acute inflammatory cells (polymorphs) may selectively infiltrate the epithelium and adjacent luminal mucin of benign or atypically proliferating mucinous tumors, without indicating infection. Such infiltrates may be quite severe yet very focal (Fig. 24.14), are almost always incidental findings in the tumors of afebrile patients, and the contents are sterile on routine microbiological culture.

The stroma is fibrocollagenous and the cellularity, although quite variable, rarely approaches that of the ovarian-like stroma of the serous tumors. Occasionally there is marked prominence of stroma between locules, giving rise to patterns of adenofibroma (Fig. 24.15). Stromal cellularity may be increased in the vicinity of the epithelium and in this zone lutein-like cells are seen in 25% of benign mucinous tumors. Rare benign tumors may show definite Leydig cells (with crystals) in the adjacent stroma (Fig. 24.16) without altering the diagnosis (Detre & Foldes 1984, Rutgers & Scully 1986, Pascal & Grecco 1988). Their presence, however, should alert one to the possibility that the tumor is a Sertoli–Leydig cell tumor with heterologous (i.e. mucinous) elements (see the section on composite tumors below, and Ch. 35), particularly if the mucinous epithelial elements appear intestinal in type. Indeed, minor Sertoli–Leydig cell tumor elements should be sought in patients with apparently pure mucinous cystic tumors in which there is clinical evidence of virilization. If found, such tumors are reclassified as Sertoli–Leydig cell tumors with heterologous elements (Roth et al 1974, Waxman et al 1981). Smooth muscle is noted sometimes in the stroma running parallel to the cyst linings (Scully 1979),

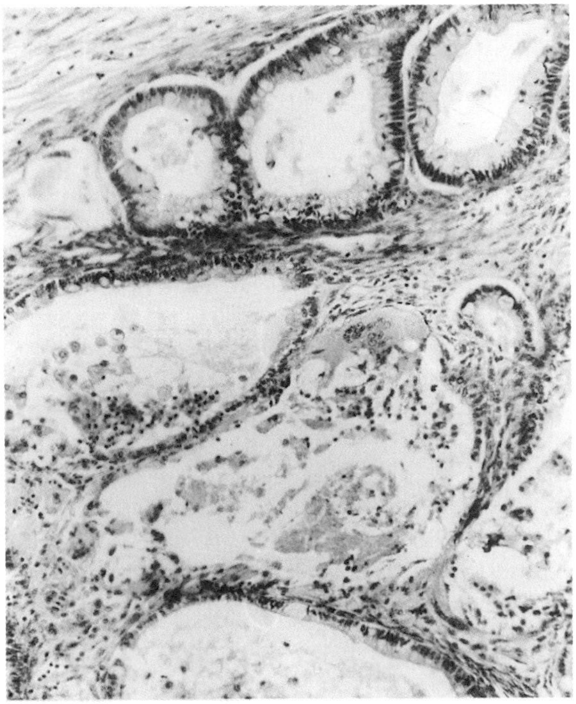

A

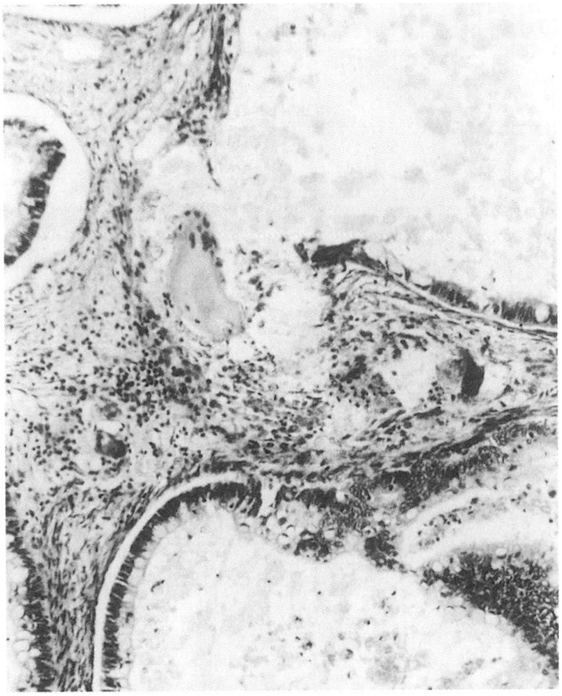

B

Fig. 24.13 Benign mucinous tumor with intestinal epithelium and focal breaches in the integrity of the glands/cysts. In some instances the giant cell and histiocytic infiltrate appears to be within the cyst space (a), while in others the giant cells are confined to the point of rupture (b). H + E ×90

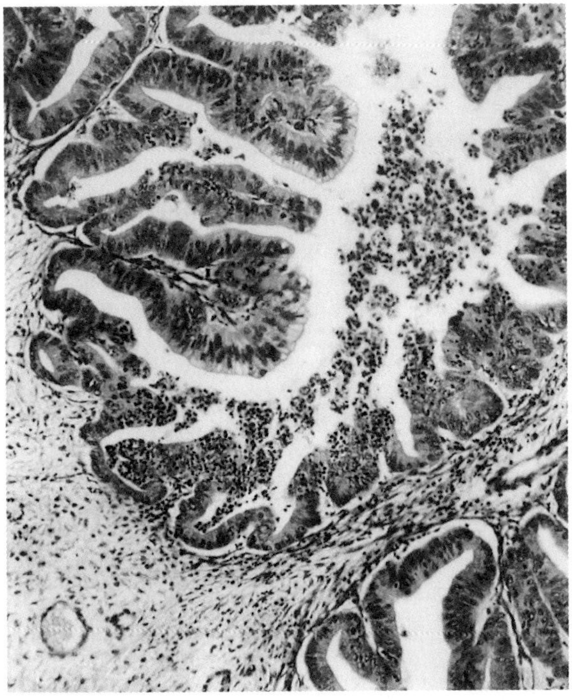

but never as prominently as in the rare cysts of the rete ovarii (see Ch. 31).

The architecture of mucinous tumors showing significant atypical epithelial proliferation (minimum of 10% of available tissue or about 1–2 low power fields per section) differs only in the exuberant growth of this component at the relative expense of stroma. Glandular buds and a microscopic filigree pattern (Fig. 24.17), similar to the tufting of proliferating serous tumors are characteristic of the corresponding cystic mucinous lesions. With increasingly atypical hyperplasia, more complex glandular/papillary patterns emerge (Figs 24.18–24.20) with epithelial multilayering and luminal reduplication (Figs 24.21, 24.22). Such changes may well vary considerably from field to field in the same tumor and it is common to find all grades of proliferation as well as benign

Fig. 24.14 An acute polymorph infiltrate in the epithelium and lumen of a proliferating mucinous tumor of mullerian or endocervical type. H + E ×90

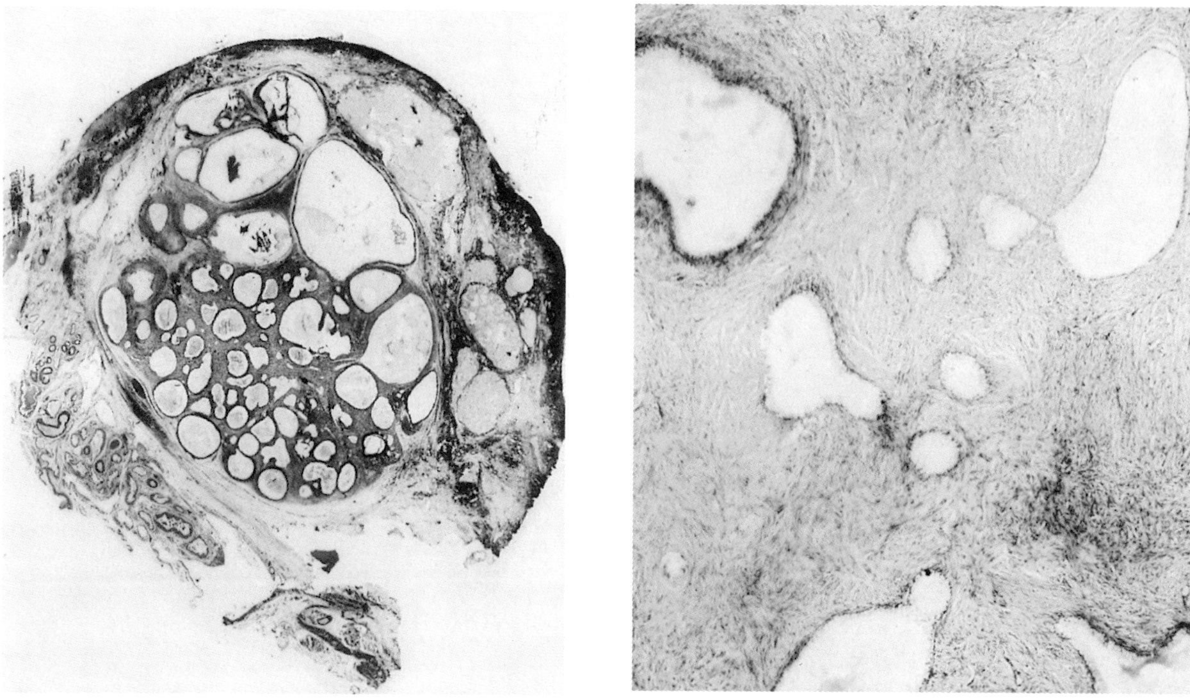

Fig. 24.15 Benign mucinous adenofibroma. (A) Low power showing the general architectural features. H + E ×5. (B) The blandness of the epithelium and relative acellularity of the stroma are conspicuous features. H + E ×35

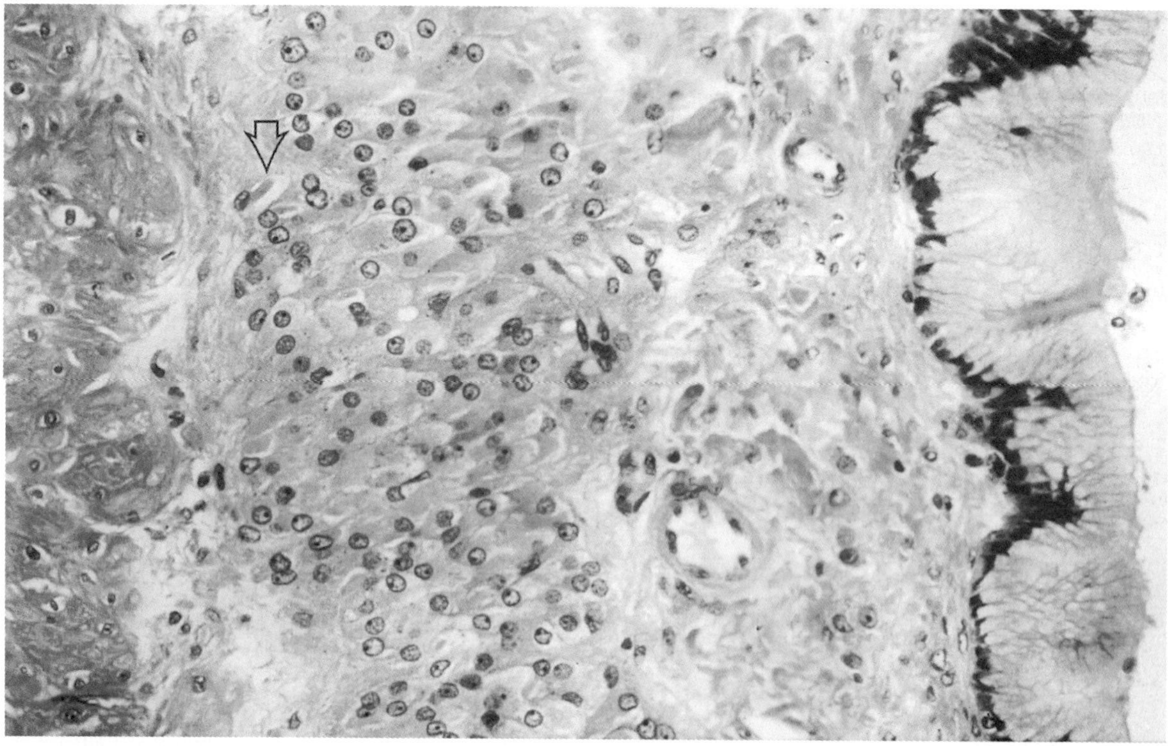

Fig. 24.16 A continuous zone of Leydig cells in the stroma of a benign mucinous tumor. Occasional Reinke crystals (arrow) are present. H + E ×250

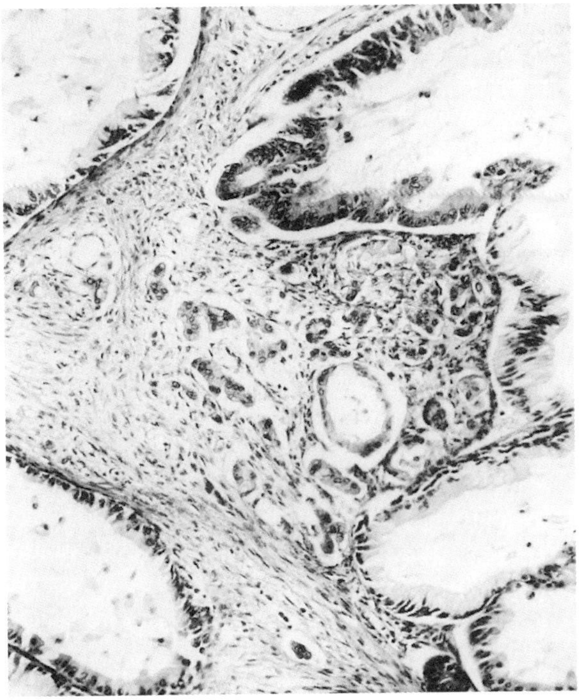

Fig. 24.24 An intestinal type proliferating mucinous tumor exhibiting a central microscopic focus of stromal invasion. Benign mucinous epithelium is present at top left. H + E ×90. (Reprinted, with permission, from Russell 1979c)

even benign areas. The invasive areas resemble mucin-secreting adenocarcinomas of intestinal origin and their architecture varies with the amounts of mucin produced, cellular differentiation, and prominence of stroma. Variation from area to area is common in mucinous tumors and occasional well-differentiated mucinous carcinomas have been described with focal mural nodules of anaplastic carcinoma (Prat et al 1982, Yamana et al 1984, Fujii et al 1985, Hayman & Östör 1985, Chan et al 1989, Sondergaard & Kaspersen 1991, Baergen & Rutgers 1994), and undifferentiated small cell carcinoma of neuroendocrine type (Eichhorn et al 1992).

Malignant adenofibromas (well-differentiated solid fibrous lesions) (Fig. 24.25) cause great difficulty in determining the presence of destructive stromal invasion. Subtle irregularities in gland contour and irregular budding may be the only pointers, little if any change in the character of the stroma being observed in these areas.

Fig. 24.25 Well-differentiated mucinous carcinoma. Irregular shaped and budding glands embedded in dense stroma. Other signs of stromal invasion (immaturity and inflammation) are absent. H + E ×125

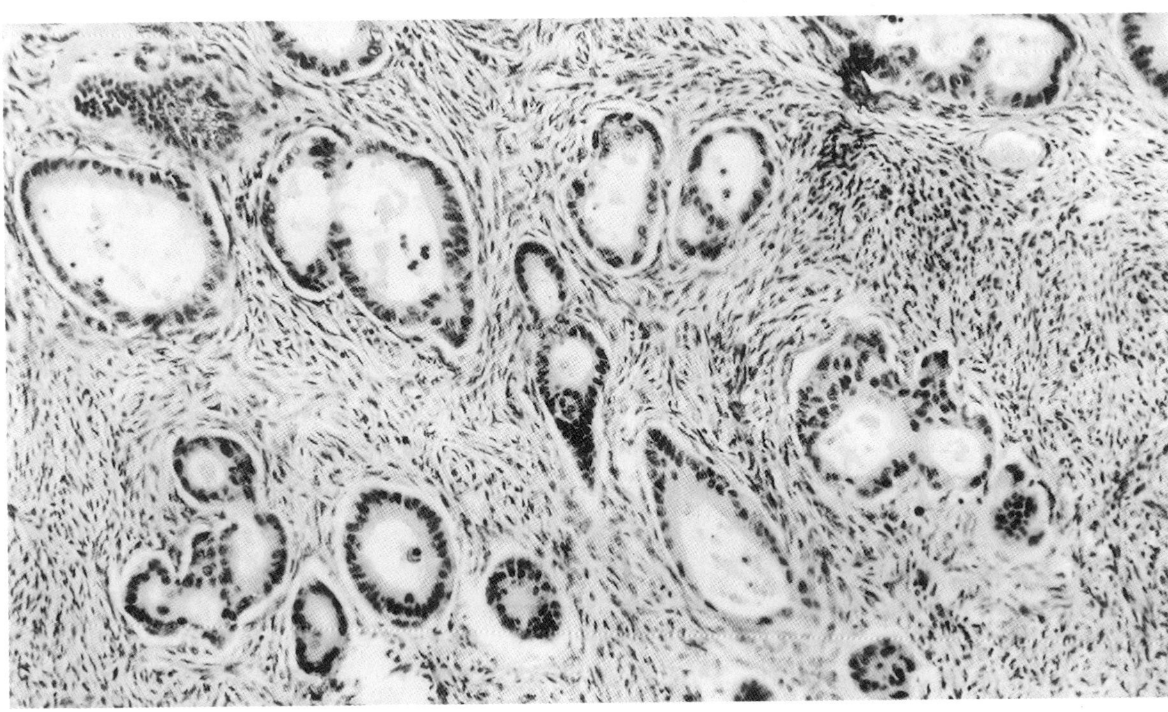

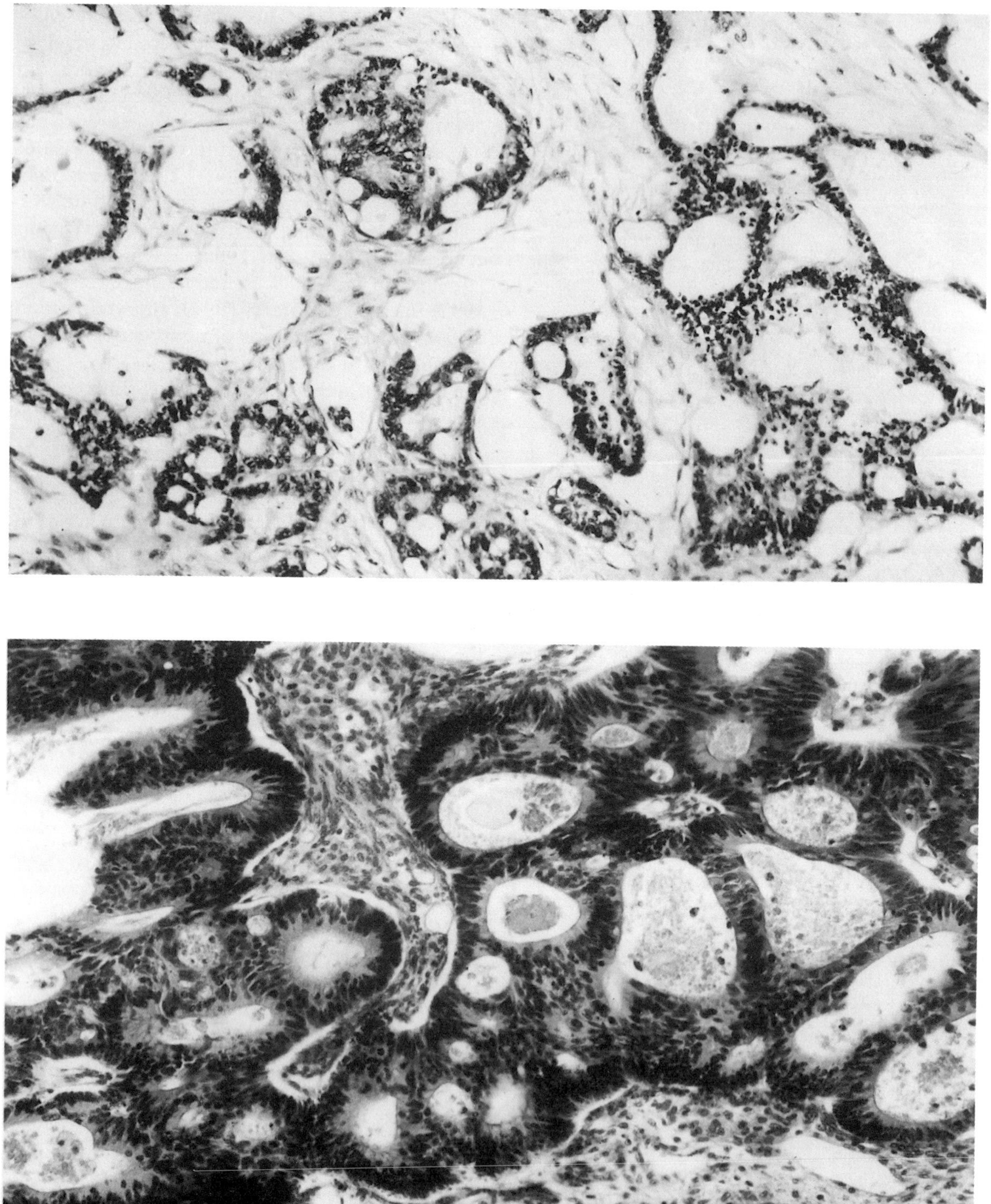

A

B

Fig. 24.26 Moderately differentiated mucinous carcinoma. (A) Cords and 'crescents' of atypical cells with much intra- and extracellular mucin. (B) Elsewhere this carcinoma exhibited a more cribriform pattern, although mucinous differentiation is still obvious. H + E ×125

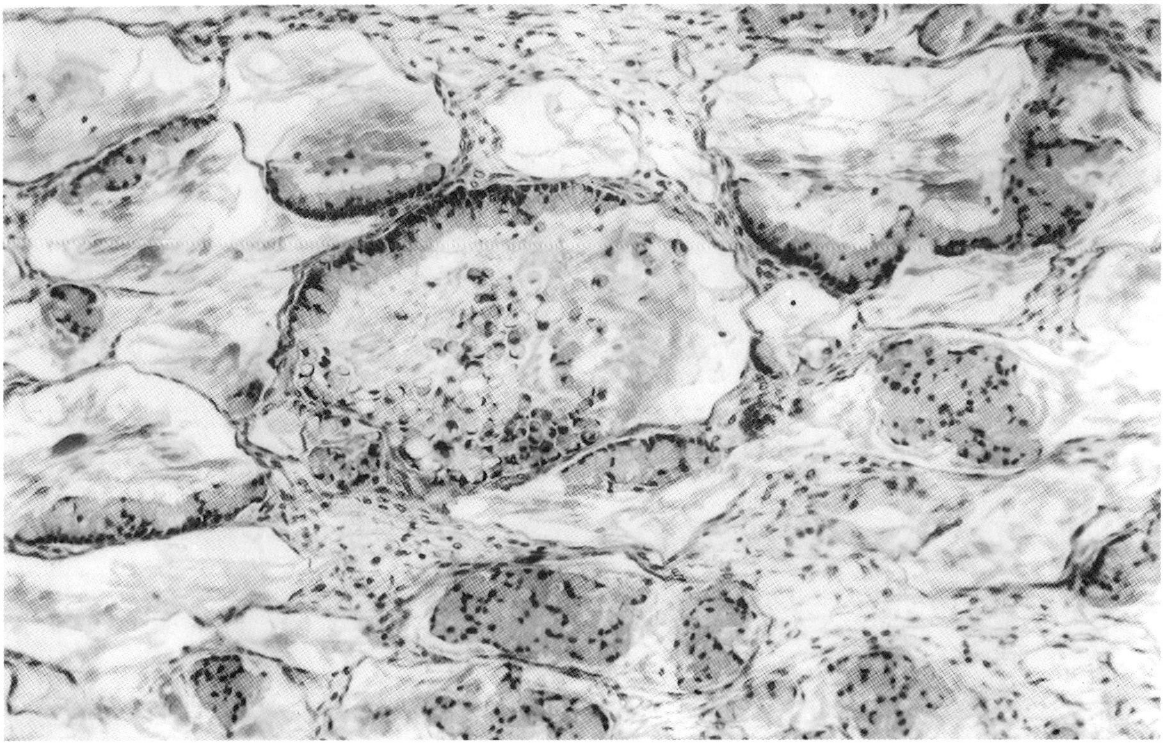

Fig. 24.27 Moderately differentiated mucinous carcinoma with large pools of mucin in the stroma (malignant pseudomyxoma), nests of tumor cells and signet-ring cells. H + E ×125

Moderately differentiated mucinous carcinomas (Fig. 24.26) create less difficulty in this regard. Pseudomyxomatous patterns in mucin-secreting carcinomas (Fig. 24.27) with a minor cellular component in large pools of mucin (like colloid carcinoma of colon) are sometimes seen. Pseudomyxoma peritonei associated with such tumors demonstrates the same cellular anaplasia as the 'primary' ovarian mass. Poorly differentiated mucinous carcinomas are very uncommonly encountered and show small clusters or singly infiltrating cells embedded in dense reactive ovarian stroma (Fig. 24.28). Signet-ring cells containing intracellular mucin are often noted, and the lesion may in parts resemble a Krukenberg tumor. Indeed rare instances have been reported of so-called 'primary Krukenberg tumor' of the ovary (Joshi 1968, Caballero et al 1991), but such a diagnosis should be made with extreme caution and perhaps only retrospectively after prolonged follow-up.

Mixed and composite mucinous tumors. Mullerian tumors of mixed epithelial differentiation (see Ch. 29) are relatively common lesions and, in these, mucinous elements are probably the most frequently encountered.

An obscure phenomenon, typically but not uniquely associated with ovarian mucinous neoplasms, is seen in a number of reported cases of osteoclastoma-like nodules in the walls of cystic ovarian mucinous tumors (Figs 24.29, 24.30). One such mucinous tumor seems to have been benign (Bettinger 1953), but the majority have been atypically proliferating or frankly malignant (Prat & Scully 1979b, Russell et al 1981, Czernobilsky et al 1983, Tsuruchi et al 1993, Verma et al 1993). These tumors have shown one or more quite discrete hemorrhagic mural nodules containing a heterogeneous population of benign osteoclast-like giant cells, mixed mononuclear inflammatory cells (Fig. 24.30A) and bizarre mononuclear giant cells (Fig. 24.30B). The latter

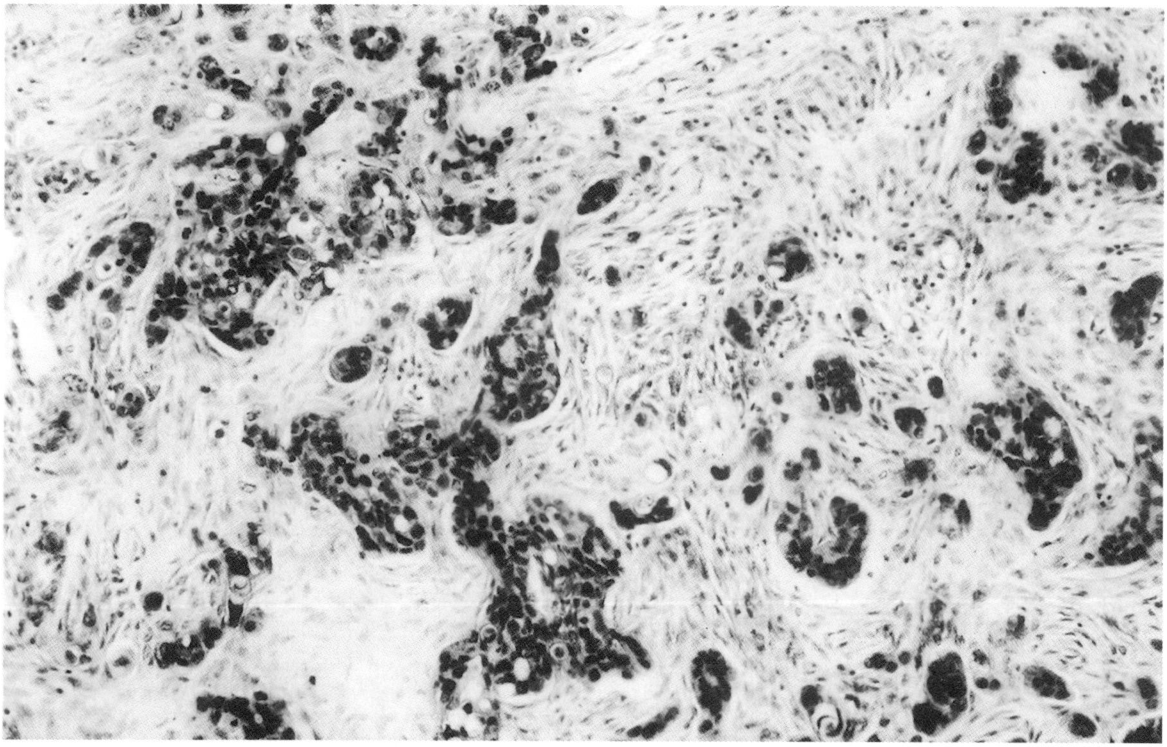

Fig. 24.28 Poorly differentiated mucinous carcinoma with abortive acini and signet-ring cells. H + E ×125

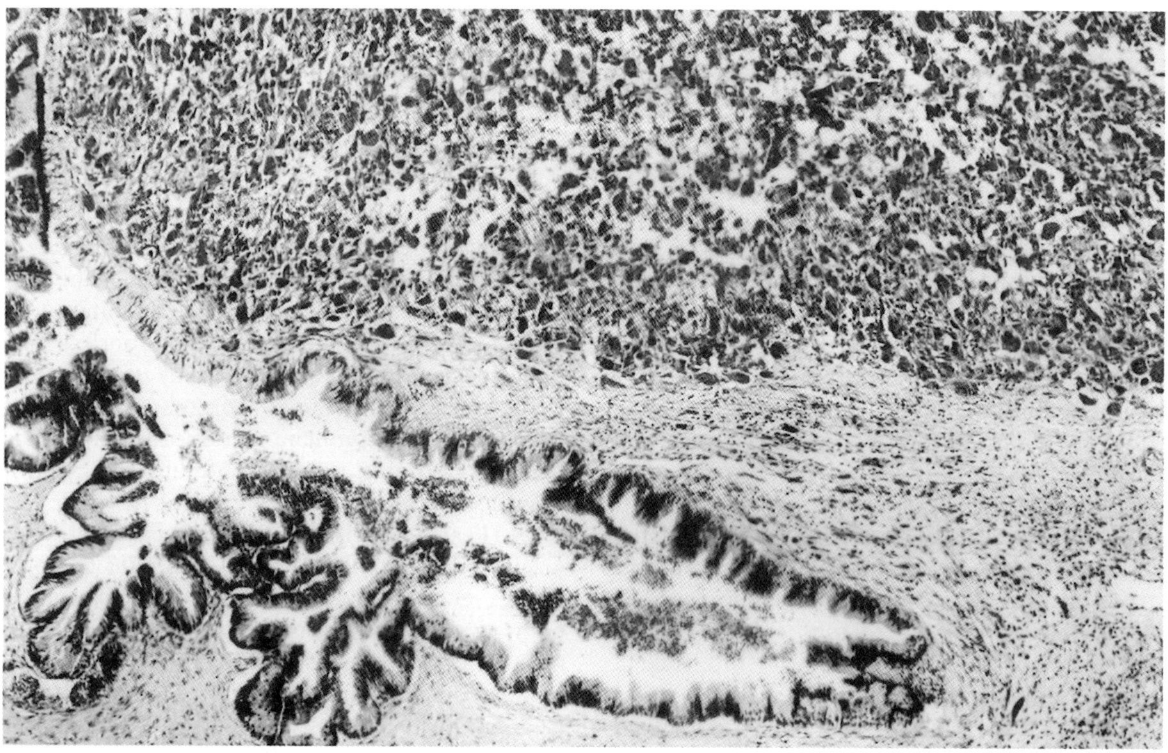

Fig. 24.29 Mucinous tumor showing atypical epithelial proliferation (bottom and left) associated with an adjacent giant cell 'mural nodule'. H + E ×50

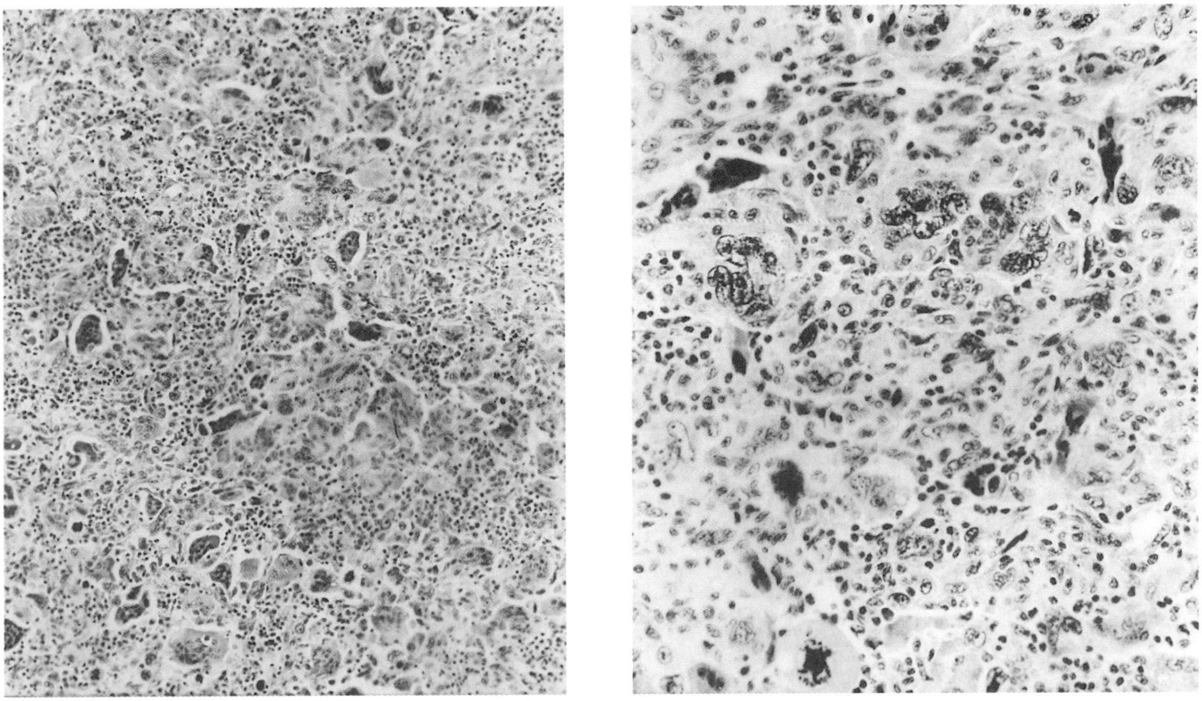

A B

Fig. 24.30 Giant cell 'mural nodules' from mucinous tumors. (A) A mixed inflammatory cell background is studded with multinuclear histiocytic giant cells. H + E ×90. (B) Higher power of a similar mural nodule in which bizarre mononuclear cells, multinuclear tumor giant cells, and atypical mitoses are present. H + E ×175

exhibit atypical mitoses and show electron microscopic and immunohistochemical evidence of epithelial differentiation (Russell et al 1981, Czernobilsky et al 1983, Kessler et al 1990, Nichols et al 1991, Matias-Guiu et al 1991). Extreme examples of this phenomenon may explain isolated reports of apparently pure osteoclastoma-like giant cell tumors of the ovary (Lorentzen 1980). The nature of the lesions is uncertain, but they do not appear to alter the behavior of the associated mucinous tumors or their prognosis (Bell 1991a). They must be distinguished from true sarcomas occurring in association with mucinous tumors (Prat & Scully 1979a, Bruijn et al 1987, Nichols et al 1991, Tsujimura & Kawano 1992; see Ch. 26), carcinosarcomas (Suurmeijer 1991) and anaplastic carcinomas (Fig. 24.31; see above), as each of these latter lesions does carry a much worse clinical prognosis.

Approximately 5% of benign mucinous ovarian tumors and rare examples of proliferating mucinous tumors (Hunter et al 1988) are found in juxtaposition to benign adult cystic teratomas; mucinous elements in such tumors are more likely to be intestinal rather than mullerian in differentiation (Russell 1979a) and may indeed be of teratomatous origin. Equally, other 'germ cell elements' such as yolk sac tumor (Mazur et al 1988), choriocarcinoma (Oliva et al 1993), carcinoid tumor (Waxman et al 1981, Alenghat et al 1986, Wolpert et al 1989), or high grade neuroendocrine carcinoma (Collins et al 1991) may be found in combination with mucinous neoplasms. Mucinous carcinomas may elaborate α-fetoprotein in the absence of yolk sac elements (Konishi et al 1988, Nomura et al 1992). Differing views exist as to their histogeneses.

More intriguing are the very rare composite mucinous and sex cord–stromal tumors. As noted earlier in this chapter, the sex cord–stromal element is most commonly Sertoli–Leydig cell in type and the mucinous epithelium intestinal in type (see Ch. 35). Two examples have been reported of mucinous tumors showing mullerian (endocervical) type epithelium combined with granulosa–theca cell differentiation in the sex cord–stromal elements (Price et al 1990, Chandran et al 1993) (see Figs 33.20, 33.21), and we have

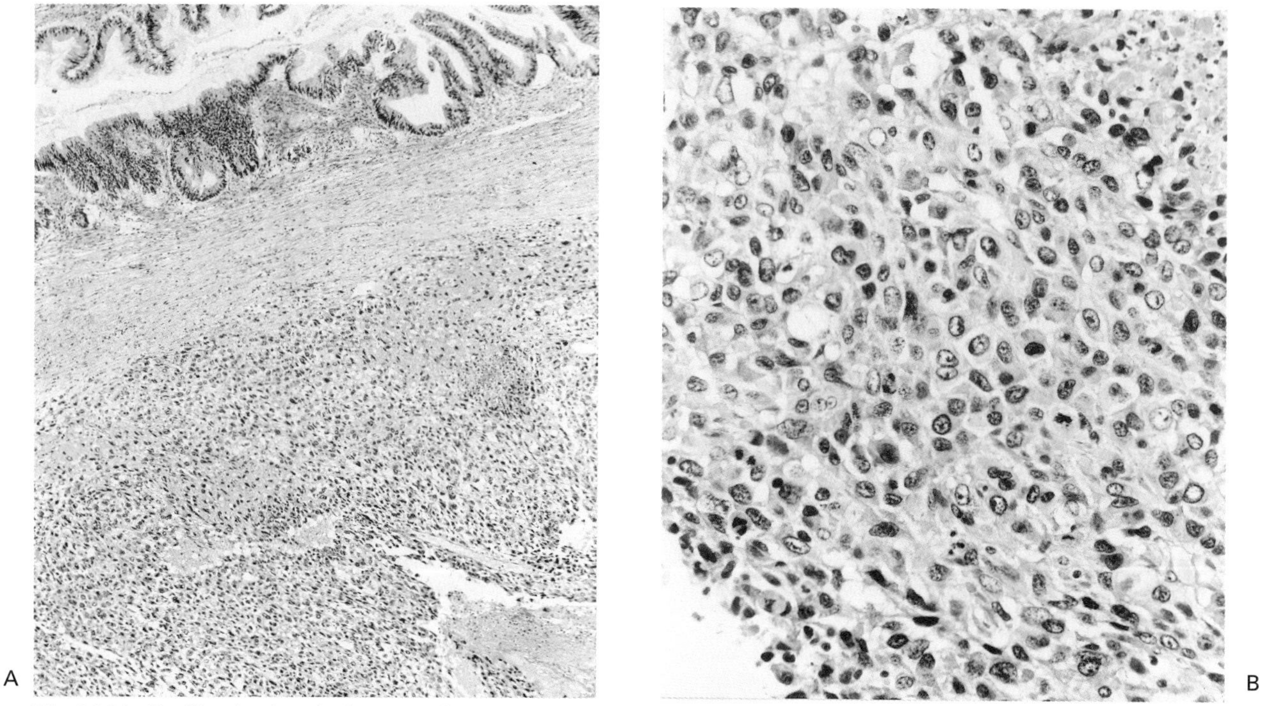

Fig. 24.31 Proliferating intestinal-type mucinous tumor with mural nodule of anaplastic carcinoma. (A) Low power showing both elements. H + E ×23. (B) High power of anaplastic carcinoma with coagulative necrosis at top right. H + E ×116

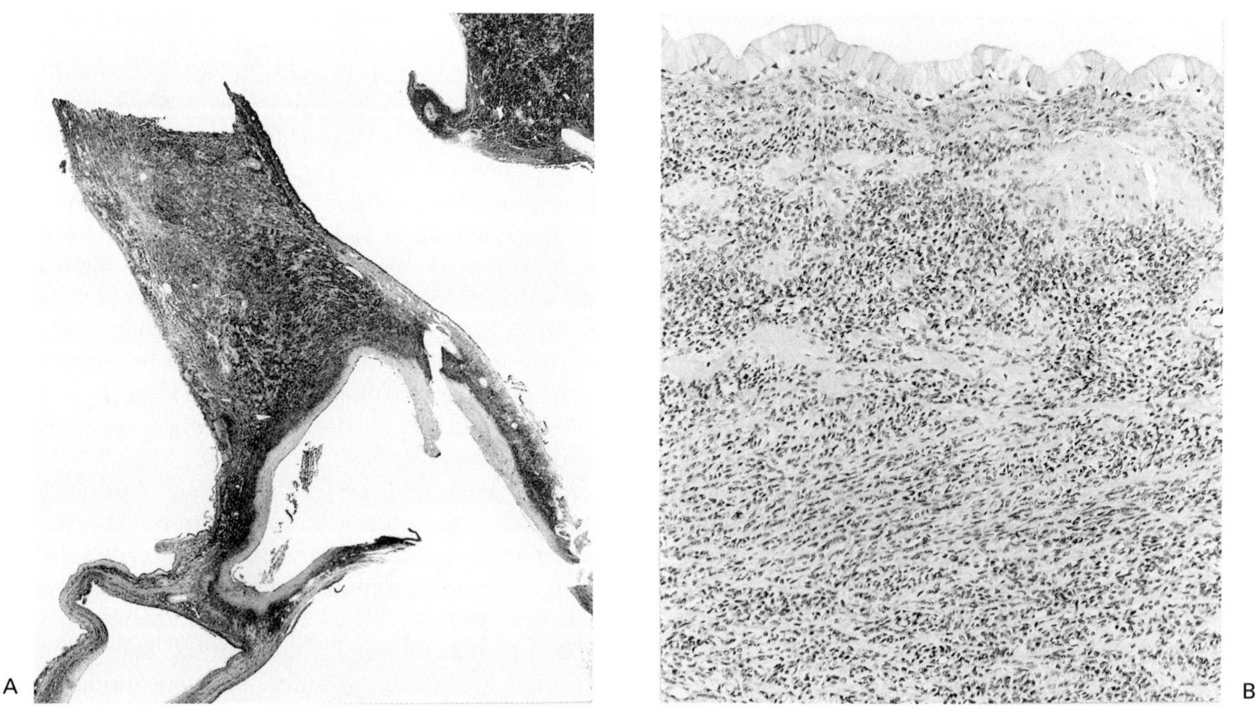

Fig. 24.32 Compound benign mucinous tumor (endocervical type) and sex cord–stromal tumor (cellular fibroma with minor sex cord elements). (A) Survey of multiloculated tumor with densely hypercellular tumor tissue between the cystic spaces. H + E ×3. (B) Higher power showing tall columnar mucin-secreting cells subtended by cellular spindle cell gonadal stromal tissue. Minor sex cord elements are present elsewhere. H + E ×59

seen a third in which the stromal component was a cellular fibroma with minor sex cord elements (Fig. 24.32).

Differential diagnosis

A difficult differential diagnosis is that between primary mucinous ovarian carcinomas and metastases of intestinal origin masquerading as primary neoplasms (Lash & Hart 1987). In practice, the latter are more commonly encountered and should be excluded as far as practicable each time. The clinical setting must be taken into account and the pathologist has to accept that in some cases it is impossible, on histological grounds alone, to make this distinction (see Table 55.1). The presence of pseudocystic change due to focal necrosis (Fig. 54.7), giving the so-called 'garland' pattern of Lash & Hart (1987), an inflammatory infiltrate in these necrotic areas ('dirty necrosis'), and an absence of evidence of a pre-existing benign or proliferating mucinous tumor are all features suggestive of an intestinal metastasis. Cytokeratin 7 has been suggested as an immunohistochemical discriminator between ovarian masses of mullerian type (positive) and intestinal type or derivation (negative) (Ueda et al 1993).

The discrimination between poorly differentiated primary mullerian carcinomas of serous/endometrioid types and mucinous carcinomas rests principally on the identification of intracellular mucins histochemically or ultrastructurally. Immunohistochemically, CEA is found in virtually all mucinous carcinomas, but only about 30% of endometrioid carcinomas and few serous tumors Table 24.1. CA-125 antigen and S-100 antigen, on the other hand, are positive in the vast majority of serous carcinomas, and 40–50% of endometrioid tumors, but are not present in mucinous carcinomas (Fleuren & Nap 1988, Lin et al 1991).

REFERENCES

Aguirre P, Daval Y, Scully R E, De Lellis R A 1984 Mucinous tumors of the ovary with argyrophil cells. An immunohistochemical analysis. American Journal of Surgical Pathology 8: 345–356

Alenghat E, Okagaki T, Talerman A 1986 Primary mucinous carcinoid tumor of the ovary. Cancer 58: 777–783

Aslani M, Scully R E 1989 Primary carcinoma of the broad ligament. Report of four cases and review of the literature. Cancer 64: 1540–1545

Azzopardi J G, Hou L T 1965 Intestinal metaplasia with argentaffin cells in cervical adenocarcinoma. Journal of Pathology and Bacteriology 90: 686–690

Baergen R N, Rutgers J L 1994 Mural nodules in common epithelial tumors of the ovary. International Journal of Gynecological Pathology 13: 62–72

Baird D B, Reddick R L 1991 Extraovarian mucinous metaplasia in a patient with bilateral mucinous borderline ovarian tumors: a case report. International Journal of Gynecological Pathology 10: 96–103

Ball N J, Robertson D I, Duggan M A, Snider D D 1990 Intestinal differentiation in ovarian mucinous tumors. Virchows Archiv [A] Pathological Anatomy and Histopathology 417: 197–201

Banerjee R, Gough J 1988 Cystic mucinous tumors of the mesentery and retroperitoneum: report of three cases. Histopathology 12: 527–532

Barnhill D, Heller P, Brzozowski P, Advani H, Gallup D, Park R 1985 Epithelial ovarian carcinoma of low malignant potential. Obstetrics and Gynecology 65: 53–59

Bell D A 1991a Ovarian surface epithelial–stromal tumors. Human Pathology 22: 750–762

Bell D A 1991b Mucinous adenofibromas of the ovary. A report of 10 cases. American Journal of Surgical Pathology 15: 227–232

Bettinger H F 1953 A giant cell tumor of bone in a pseudomucinous cystadenoma of the ovary. Journal of Obstetrics and Gynaecology of the British Empire 60: 230–232

Bostwick D G, Tazelaar H D, Ballon S C, Hendrickson M R, Kempson R L 1986 Ovarian epithelial tumors of borderline malignancy. A clinical and pathologic study of 109 cases. Cancer 58: 2052–2065

Bruijn J A, Smit V T H B M, Que D-Q, Fleuren G J 1987 Immunohistology of a sarcomatous mural nodule in an ovarian mucinous cystadenocarcinoma. International Journal of Gynecological Pathology 6: 287–293

Caballero J L, Neils A, Rios B 1991 Adenocarcinoma mucinoso primario de ovario con celulas en anillo de sello. Revue Medicino de Panama 16: 138–142

Campbell J S, Lou P, Ferguson J P, Kemeny T, Mitton D M, Allen N 1973 Pseudomyxoma peritonei et ovarii with occult neoplasms of appendix. Obstetrics and Gynecology 42: 897–902

Carter J, Carson L F, Moradi M M, Adcock L A, Twiggs L B 1991 Pseudomyxoma peritonei: a review. International Journal of Gynecologic Cancer 1: 243–247

Chaitin B A, Gershenson D M, Evans H L 1985 Mucinous tumors of the ovary: a clinicopathologic study of 70 cases. Cancer 55: 1958–1962

Chan Y-F, Ho H C, Yau S M, Ma L 1989 Ovarian mucinous tumor with mural nodules of anaplastic carcinoma. Gynecologic Oncology 35: 112–119

Chandran R, Rahman H, Gebbie D 1993 Composite mucinous and granulosa-theca-cell tumor of the ovary: an unusual neoplasm. Australian and New Zealand Journal of Obstetrics and Gynaecology 33: 437–439

Cohen I, Altaras M, Lew S, Jaffe R, Ben Aderet N 1988 Huge mesenteric mucinous cystadenoma in normal pregnancy. Obstetrics and Gynecology 71: 1030–1032

Collins R J, Cheung A, Ngan H Y, Wong L C, Chan S Y,

Ma H K 1991 Primary mixed neuroendocrine and mucinous carcinoma of the ovary. Archives of Gynecology and Obstetrics 248: 139–143
Czernobilsky B, Dgani R, Roth L 1983 Ovarian mucinous cystadenocarcinoma with mural nodule of carcinomatous derivation. Cancer 51: 141–148
de Boer W G R M, Ma J, Nayman J 1981 Intestine associated antigens in ovarian tumors: an immunohistological study. Pathology 13: 547–555
de Nictolis M, Montironi R, Tommasoni S et al 1994 Benign, borderline, and well differentiated malignant intestinal mucinous tumors of the ovary: a clinicopathologic, histochemical, immunohistochemical, and nuclear quantitative study of 57 cases. International Journal of Gynecological Pathology 13: 10–21
Deprest J, Moerman P, Corneillie P, Ide P 1992 Ovarian borderline mucinous tumor in a premenarchal girl: review on ovarian epithelial cancer in young girls. Gynecologic Oncology 45: 219–224
Detre Z, Foldes E 1984 Mucinous cystadenocarcinoma of ovary with Leydig cell hyperplasia. Pathology Research and Practice 178: 400–402
Eichhorn J H, Young R H, Scully R E 1992 Primary ovarian small cell carcinoma of pulmonary type. A clinicopathologic, immunohistologic, and flow cytometric analysis of 11 cases. American Journal of Surgical Pathology 16: 926–938
Fenoglio C M, Ferenczy A, Richart R M 1975 Mucinous tumors of the ovary. Ultrastructural studies of mucinous cystadenomas with histogenetic considerations. Cancer 36: 1709–1722
Fenoglio C M, Cottral G A, Ferenczy A, Richart R M 1976a Mucinous tumors of the ovary. III: Histochemical studies. Gynecologic Oncology 4: 151–157
Fenoglio C M, Ferenczy A, Richart R M 1976b Mucinous tumors of the ovary. II: Ultrastructural features of mucinous cystadenocarcinomas. American Journal of Obstetrics and Gynecology 125: 990–999
Fleuren G J, Nap M 1988 Carcinoembryonic antigen in primary and metastatic ovarian tumors. Gynecologic Oncology 30: 407–415
Fox H, Anderson M C, Beilby J O W et al 1983 Ovarian epithelial tumors of borderline malignancy: pathological features and current status. British Journal of Obstetrics and Gynaecology 90: 743–750
Fujii S, Konishi I, Kobayashi F, Okamura H, Yamabe H, Mori T 1985 Sarcoma-like mural nodules combined with a microfocus of anaplastic carcinoma in mucinous ovarian tumor. Gynecologic Oncology 20: 219–233
Fujii S, Konishi I, Okamura H, Mori T 1986 Mucinous cystadenocarcinoma of the retroperitoneum: a light and electron microscopic study. Gynecologic Oncology 24: 103–112
Fulcheri E, Baracchini P, Foglia G, Lapertosa G, Siciliano B, Ragni N 1990 Histochemical study of mucinous ovarian cystomas of intestinal and mixed types: O-acetylated sialomucin content in relation to biologic behaviour. Tumori 76: 73–76
Gotoh K, Konaga E, Arata A, Takeuchi H, Mano S 1992 A case of primary retroperitoneal mucinous cystadenocarcinoma. Acta Medica Okayama 46: 49–52
Gough D B, Donohue J H, Schutt A J et al 1994 Pseudomyxoma peritonei. Long-term patient survival with an aggressive regional approach. Annals of Surgery 219: 112–119
Graeme-Cook F, Mark E J 1991 Pulmonary mucinous cystic tumors of borderline malignancy. Human Pathology 22: 185–190
Griffiths A P, Cross D, Kingston R E, Harkin P, Wells M, Quirke P 1993 Flow cytometry and AgNORs in benign, borderline, and malignant mucinous and serous tumors of the ovary. International Journal of Gynecological Pathology 12: 307–314
Guerrieri C, Hogberg T, Wingren S, Fristedt S, Simonsen E, Boeryd B 1994 Mucinous borderline and malignant tumors of the ovary. Cancer 74: 2329–2340
Hart W R 1977 Ovarian epithelial tumors of borderline malignancy (carcinomas of low malignant potential). Human Pathology 8: 541–549
Hart W R, Norris H J 1973 Borderline and malignant mucinous tumors of the ovary. Cancer 31: 1031–1045
Hayman J A, Östör A G 1985 Ovarian mucinous tumor with a focus of anaplastic carcinoma: a case report. Pathology 17: 591–593
Hendrickson M R, Kempson R L 1993 In: Hendrickson M R (ed.) Surface epithelial neoplasms of the ovary. Hanley & Belfus, Philadelphia, PA, p 307–334
Higa E, Rosai J, Pizzimbono C A, Wise L 1973 Mucosal hyperplasia, mucinous cystadenoma, and mucinous cystadenocarcinoma of the appendix. Cancer 32: 1525–1541
Hunter V, Barnhill D, Jadwin D, Crooks L 1988 Ovarian mucinous cystadenocarcinoma of low malignant potential associated with a mature cystic teratoma. Gynecologic Oncology 29: 250–254
Jensen M L, Nielsen M N 1989 Broad ligament mucinous and serous cystadenomas of borderline malignancy. Acta Obstetricia et Gynecologica Scandinavica 68: 663–667
Joshi V V 1968 Primary Krukenberg tumor of the ovary. Review of literature and case report. Cancer 22: 1199–1207
Kahn M A, Demopoulos R I 1992 Mucinous ovarian tumors with pseudomyxoma peritonei: a clinicopathologic study. International Journal of Gynecological Pathology 11: 15–23
Kessler E, Halpern M, Koren R, Dekel A, Goldman J 1990 Sarcoma-like mural nodules with foci of anaplastic carcinoma in ovarian mucinous tumor: clinical, histological, and immunohistochemical study of a case and review of the literature. Surgical Pathology 3: 211–219
Klemi P J 1978 Pathology of mucinous ovarian cystadenomas. I: Argyrophil and argentaffin cells and epithelial mucosubstances. Acta Pathologica et Microbiologica Scandinavica A 86: 465–470
Klemi P J, Nevalainen T J 1978 Pathology of mucinous ovarian cystadenomas. II: Ultrastructural findings. Acta Pathologica et Microbiologica Scandinavica A 86: 471–481
Kliman L, Rome R M, Fortune D W 1986 Low malignant potential tumors of the ovary: a study of 76 cases. Obstetrics and Gynecology 68: 338–344
Konishi I, Fujii S, Kataoka N et al 1988 Ovarian mucinous cystadenocarcinoma producing alpha-fetoprotein. International Journal of Gynecological Pathology 7: 182–189
Kurita M, Komatsu H, Hata Y et al 1994 Pseudomyxoma peritonei due to adenocarcinoma of the lung: case report. Journal of Gastroenterology 29: 344–348
Langley F A, Cummins P A, Fox H 1972 An ultrastructural study of mucin secreting epithelia in ovarian neoplasms. Acta Pathologica et Microbiologica Scandinavica A 80 (suppl 233): 76–86
Lash R H, Hart W R 1987 Intestinal adenocarcinomas

metastatic to the ovaries. A clinicopathologic evaluation of 22 cases. American Journal of Surgical Pathology 11: 114–121

Lin M, Hanai J, Wada A et al 1991 S-100 protein in ovarian tumors. A comparative immunohistochemical study of 135 cases. Acta Pathologica Japonica 41: 233–239

Look K Y, Stehman F B, Moore D H, Sutton Gynecological Pathology 1995 Intraperitoneal 5-fluorouracil for pseudomyxoma peritonei. International Journal of Gynecological Cancer 5: 361–365

Lorentzen M 1980 Giant cell tumor of the ovary. Virchows Archiv [A] Pathological Anatomy and Histopathology 388: 113–122

Louwerens J K, Schaberg A, Bosman F T 1983 Neuroendocrine cells in cystic mucinous tumors of the ovary. Histopathology 7: 389–398

Mannion E, O'Grady J T, al Nafussi A I 1993 Metaplastic cystadenofibroma of the ovary. Histopathology 23: 581–584

Matias-Guiu X, Aranda I, Prat J 1991 Immunohistochemical study of sarcoma-like mural nodules in a mucinous cystadenocarcinoma of the ovary. Virchows Archiv [A] Pathological Anatomy and Histopathology 419: 89–92

Mazur M T, Talbot W H Jr, Talerman A 1988 Endodermal sinus tumor and mucinous cystadenofibroma of the ovary. Occurrence in an 82-year-old woman. Cancer 62: 2011–2015

Michael H, Sutton G, Roth L M 1987 Ovarian carcinoma with extracellular mucin production: reassessment of 'pseudomyxoma ovarii et peritonei'. International Journal of Gynecological Pathology 6: 298–312

Minguillon C, Friedmann W, Vogel M, Wessel J, Lichtenegger W 1992 Muzinose Metaplasie der Tubenschleimhaut als urasche eines Pseudomyxoma. Zentralblatt fur Pathologie 138: 363–365

Morigana S, Ohyama R, Koizumi J 1992 Low grade mucinous cystadenocarcinoma in the spleen. American Journal of Surgical Pathology 16: 903–908

Motoyama T, Chida T, Fujiwara T, Watanabe H 1994 Mucinous cystic tumor of the retroperitoneum. A report of two cases. Acta Cytologica 38: 261–266

Nation J G, Krepart G V 1986 Ovarian carcinomas of low malignant potential: staging and treatment. American Journal of Obstetrics and Gynecology 154: 290–293

Nelson H, Benjamin B, Alberty R 1988 Primary retroperitoneal mucinous cystadenocarcinoma. Cancer 61: 2117–2121

Nichols G E, Mills S E, Ulbright T M, Czernobilsky B, Roth L M 1991 Spindle cell mural nodules in cystic ovarian mucinous tumors. A clinicopathologic and immunohistochemical study of five cases. American Journal of Surgical Pathology 15: 1055–1062

Nogales F F, Caballero T, Fernandez P L, Linares J, Ruiz-Avila I 1991 Pseudomyxoma peritonei et ovarii associated with sequential ovarian and appendicular tumors and acromegaly. Gynecologic Oncology 40: 78–80

Nomura K, Miyasaka Y, Murae M, Terashima Y, Aizawa S 1992 Ovarian mucinous cystadenocarcinoma producing alpha-fetoprotein. A case report. Acta Pathologica Japonica 42: 372–375

O'Hanlan KA 1994 Resection of a 303.2-pound ovarian tumor. Gynecologic Oncology 54: 365–371

Oliva E, Andrada E, Pezzica E, Prat J 1993 Ovarian carcinomas with choriocarcinomatous differentiation. Cancer 72: 2441–2446

Pant K D, Fenoglio-Preiser C M, Berry C O A et al 1986 COTA (colon-ovarian tumor antigen). An immunohistochemical study. American Journal of Clinical Pathology 86: 1–9

Park U, Han K C, Chang H K, Huh M H 1991 A primary mucinous cystadenocarcinoma of the retroperitoneum. Gynecologic Oncology 42: 64–67

Pascal R R, Grecco L A 1988 Mucinous cystadenoma of the ovary with stromal luteinisation and hilar cell hyperplasia during pregnancy. Human Pathology 19: 179–180

Pejovic T, Heim S, Mandahl N et al 1990 Trisomy 12 is a consistent chromosomal aberration in benign ovarian tumors. Genes Chromosomes and Cancer 2: 48–52

Pelletier B, Dubigeon P, Despins P, de Lajartre A Y 1993 Tumeur kystique mucineuse pulmonaire de malignite frontiere. A propos d'un cas. Annales de Pathologie 13: 405–408

Pennell T C, Gusdon J P Jr 1989 Retroperitoneal mucinous cystadenoma. American Journal of Obstetrics and Gynecology 160: 1229–1231

Prat J, Scully R E 1979a Sarcomas in ovarian mucinous tumors. A report of two cases. Cancer 44: 1327–1331

Prat J, Scully R E 1979b Ovarian mucinous tumors with sarcoma-like mural nodules. A report of seven cases. Cancer 44: 1332–1344

Prat J, Young R H, Scully R E 1982 Ovarian mucinous tumor with foci of anaplastic carcinoma. Cancer 50: 300–304

Prayson R A, Hart W R, Petras R E 1994 Pseudomyxoma peritonei. A clinicopathologic study of 19 cases with emphasis on site of origin and nature of associated ovarian tumors. American Journal of Surgical Pathology 18: 591–603

Price A, Russell P, Elliott P, Bannatyne P 1990 Composite mucinous and granulosa cell tumor of ovary: a case report of a unique neoplasm. International Journal of Gynecological Pathology 9: 372–378

Puls L E, Powell D E, de Priest P D et al 1992 Transition from benign to malignant epithelium in mucinous and serous ovarian cystadenocarcinoma. Gynecologic Oncology 47: 53–57

Ronnett B M, Kurman R J, Zahn C M et al 1995a Pseudomyxoma peritonei in women: a clinicopathologic analysis of 30 cases with emphasis on site of origin, prognosis, and relationship to ovarian mucinous tumors of low malignant potential. Human Pathology 26: 509–524

Ronnett B M, Zahn C M, Kurman R J, Kass M E, Sugarbaker P H, Shmookler B M 1995b Disseminated peritoneal adenomucinosis and peritoneal mucinous carcinomatosis. A clinicopathologic analysis of 109 cases with emphasis on distinguishing pathologic features, site of origin, prognosis, and relationship to 'pseudomyxoma peritonei'. American Journal of Surgical Pathology 19: 1390–1408

Roth L M, Cleary R E, Rosenfield R L 1974 Sertoli–Leydig cell tumor of the ovary, with an associated mucinous cystadenoma: an ultrastructural and endocrine study. Laboratory Investigation 31: 648–657

Rothacker D, Knolle J, Stiller D, Borchard F 1993 Primary retroperitoneal mucinous cystadenomas with gastric epithelial differentiation. Pathology Research and Practice 189: 1195–1204

Russell P 1979a The pathological assessment of ovarian neoplasms. I: Introduction to the common 'epithelial' tumors and analysis of benign 'epithelial' tumors. Pathology 11: 5–26

Russell P 1979b The pathological assessment of ovarian neoplasms. II: The proliferating 'epithelial' tumors. Pathology 11: 251–282

Russell P 1979c The pathological assessment of ovarian neoplasms. III: The malignant 'epithelial' tumors. Pathology 11: 493–532

Russell P 1987 Common epithelial tumors of the ovary. In: Fox H (ed.) Haines & Taylor gynaecological and obstetrical pathology, 3rd edn. Churchill Livingstone, Edinburgh, ch. 19

Russell P 1992 Ovarian epithelial tumors with atypical proliferation. In: Lowe D, Fox H (eds) Advances in gynaecological pathology. Churchill Livingstone, Edinburgh, p 299–320

Russell P, Merkur H 1979 Proliferating ovarian 'epithelial' tumors: a clinicopathological analysis of 144 cases. Australian and New Zealand Journal of Obstetrics and Gynaecology 19: 45–51

Russell P, Wills E J, Schweitzer P, Bannatyne P M 1981 Mucinous ovarian tumors with giant cell mural nodules. Diagnostic Gynecology and Obstetrics 3: 233–249

Rutgers J L, Scully R E 1986 Functioning ovarian tumors with peripheral steroid cell proliferation: a report of twenty-four cases. International Journal of Gynecological Pathology 5: 319–337

Rutgers J L, Scully R E 1988 Ovarian mullerian mucinous papillary cystadenomas of borderline malignancy. a clinicopathologic analysis. Cancer 61: 340–348

Sandenbergh H A, Woodruff J D 1977 Histogenesis of pseudomyxoma peritonei. Review of nine cases. Obstetrics and Gynecology 49: 339–345

Sasaki E, Sasano N, Kimura N, Andoh N, Yajima A 1989 Demonstration of neuroendocrine cells in ovarian mucinous tumors. International Journal of Gynecological Pathology 8: 189–200

Scully R E 1979 Tumors of the ovary and maldeveloped gonads, AFIP fascicle 16, 2nd series. Armed Forces Institute of Pathology, Washington, DC, p 53–151

Scully R E 1982 Common epithelial tumors of borderline malignancy (carcinomas of low malignant potential). Bulletin du Cancer (Paris) 69: 228–238

Seidman J D, Elsayad A M, Sobin L H, Tavassoli F A 1993 Association of mucinous tumors of the ovary and appendix. American Journal of Surgical Pathology 17: 22–34

Shiozawa T, Tsukahara Y, Ishii K, Ota H, Nakayama J, Katsuyama T 1992 Histochemical demonstration of gastrointestinal mucins in ovarian mucinous cystadenoma. Acta Pathologica Japonica 42: 104–110

Siriaunkgul S, Robbins K M, McGowan L, Silverberg S G 1995 Ovarian mucinous tumors of low malignant potential: a clinicopathologic study of 54 tumors of intestinal and mullerian type. International Journal of Gynecological Pathology 14: 198–208

Sondergaard G, Kaspersen P 1991 Ovarian and extraovarian mucinous tumors with solid mural nodules. International Journal of Gynecological Pathology 10: 145–155

Spaun E, Toft B 1986 Epithelial atypia in ovarian mucinous cystadenoma during the puerperium. Acta Obstetricia et Gynecologica Scandinavica 65: 505–506

Sumithran E, Susil B J 1992 Concomitant mucinous tumors of the appendix and ovary. Result of a neoplastic field change? Cancer 70: 2980–2983

Sumithran E, Susil B J, Looi L-M. 1988 The prognostic significance of grading in borderline mucinous tumors of the ovary. Human Pathology 19: 15–18

Suurmeijer A J H 1991 Carcinosarcoma-like mural nodule in an ovarian mucinous tumor. Histopathology 18: 268–271

Szymanska K, Szamborski J, Miechowiecka N, Czerwinski W 1983 Malignant transformation of mucinous ovarian cystadenomas of intestinal type. Histopathology 7: 497–509

Tasker M, Langley F A 1985 The outlook for women with borderline epithelial tumors of the ovary. British Journal of Obstetrics and Gynaecology 92: 969–973

Tenti P, Aguzzi A, Riva C et al 1992 Ovarian mucinous tumors frequently express markers of gastric, intestinal, and pancreatobiliary epithelial cells. Cancer 69: 2131–2142

Tsujimura T, Kawano K 1992 Rhabdomyosarcoma coexistent with ovarian mucinous cystadenocarcinoma: a case report. International Journal of Gynecological Pathology 11: 58–62

Tsuruchi N, Kaku T, Kinoshita H et al 1993 Ovarian mucinous cystadenocarcinoma with sarcoma-appearing mural nodule of anaplastic carcinoma. Gynecologic Oncology 50: 259–263

Ueda G, Sawada M, Ogawa H, Tanizawa O, Tsujimoto M 1993 Immunohistochemical study of cytokeratin 7 for the differential diagnosis of adenocarcinomas in the ovary. Gynecologic Oncology 51: 219–223

Verma R N, Bhangui G R, Rao M K 1993 Sarcoma-like nodule in ovarian mucinous tumor (a case report). Indian Journal of Cancer 30: 38–41

Watkin W, Silva E G, Gershenson D M 1992 Mucinous carcinoma of the ovary. Pathologic prognostic factors. Cancer 69: 208–212

Waxman M, Damjanov I, Alpert L, Sardinsky T 1981 Composite mucinous ovarian neoplasms associated with Sertoli–Leydig and carcinoid tumors. Cancer 47: 2044–2052

Wertheim I, Fleischhacker D, McLachlin C M, Rice L W, Berkowitz R S, Goff B A 1994 Pseudomyxoma peritonei: a review of 23 cases. Obstetrics and Gynecology 84: 17–21

White A, Flaris N, Elmer D, Lui R, Fanburg B L 1990 Coexistence of mucinous cystadenoma of the ovary and ovarian sarcoidosis. American Journal of Obstetrics and Gynecology 162: 1284–1285

Wolpert H R, Fuller A F, Bell D A 1989 Primary mucinous carcinoid tumor of the ovary. A case report. International Journal of Gynecological Pathology 8: 156–162

Yamana K, Kinoshita T, Nakano R, Morimatsu M, Nakashima T 1984 Anaplastic giant cell tumor with mucinous cystadenocarcinoma of the ovary. Acta Pathologica Japan 34: 399–402

Young R H, Scully R E 1988 Mucinous ovarian tumors associated with mucinous adenocarcinomas of the cervix. A clinicopathological analysis of 16 cases. International Journal of Gynecological Pathology 7: 99–111

Young R H, Gilks C B, Scully R E 1991 Mucinous tumors of the appendix associated with mucinous tumors of the ovary and pseudomyxoma peritonei. A clinicopathological analysis of 22 cases supporting an origin in the appendix. American Journal of Surgical Pathology 15: 415–429

25

Endometrioid tumors

P. Russell A. Farnsworth

Endometrioid tumors are defined by 'the presence of epithelial elements, stromal elements, or a combination of the two, that resemble closely the components of typical tumors of the endometrium' (Scully 1979). While, by definition, they are homologous to *all* neoplasms arising in the endometrium, in practice this spectrum of tumors is restricted to only the more commonly occurring variants. To this group of carcinomas are added (by convention rather than rational argument) neoplasms containing a malignant stromal element – homologs of endometrial sarcomas (mullerian sarcomas, adenosarcomas, and malignant mixed mullerian tumors). It is our intention to discuss these separately (see Ch. 26), not only because their diagnosis can be independently based on pattern recognition alone, but also it is our feeling that, although they are mullerian in differentiation and perhaps origin, they need not necessarily be regarded as specifically endometrioid (see Ch. 27 on clear cell carcinomas).

The tumor cells of benign endometrioid neoplasms tend to resemble those of proliferative (preovulatory) endometrium (Fig. 25.1A), or of inactive endometrium (Fig. 25.1B). Staining by diastase-PAS and mucicarmine reveals some extracellular mucin plus staining of the luminal glycocalyx. The Grimelius technique (Ueda et al 1984) shows 45% of tumors to contain argyrophil cells. Ultrastructurally, some of the superficial argyrophil granules are mucin, while the basal and diffuse cytoplasmic granules are probably neurosecretory in type. Electron microscopic and histochemical studies have reinforced the homology between endometrioid ovarian carcinomas and tumors of the uterine corpus (Cummins et al 1974, Stenback & Kauppila 1981). Secretory changes similar to those seen in postovulatory endometrium are frequently seen in well-differentiated tumors with the attendant nuclear and cytoplasmic alterations (see Fig. 25.16) and squamoid elements are also often noted (see Figs 25.5, 25.9, 25.12, 25.14). In general, endometrioid ovarian carcinomas reported in the literature are moderately or well differentiated lesions, perhaps reflecting a reluctance to make the diagnosis in poorly differentiated cancers. It is our impression that the full 'endometrial spectrum' is reduplicated in the ovaries and, given always that truly undifferentiated or unclassifiable carcinomas will be encountered, poorly differentiated tumors should be designated endometrioid if and when minimum histological criteria supporting this diagnosis can be confidently identified (see Figs 25.19, 25.20). In establishing these criteria it is appropriate not only to consider the appearances of carcinomas occurring in the native endometrium, but also the clinical and pathological correlates of the ovarian tumors (e.g. site and stage of tumor, bilaterality, presence of other lesions such as endometriosis or a concomitant endometrial carcinoma).

Many endometrioid tumors are thought to derive from the surface epithelium of the ovary without the interposition of pre-existing endometriosis (Bell & Scully 1994), although 20–30% of such tumors are found in patients with endometriosis in the same ovary or elsewhere in the pelvis (Russell 1979a, Brescia et al 1989; see Ch. 21). Endometriosis lacks many of the features of neoplasia and has been classified by the World Health Organization (WHO) (Serov et al 1973) as a tumor-like condition. While there is lack of unanimity on this point (Fox et al 1983), the exclusion of endometriosis from the category of benign

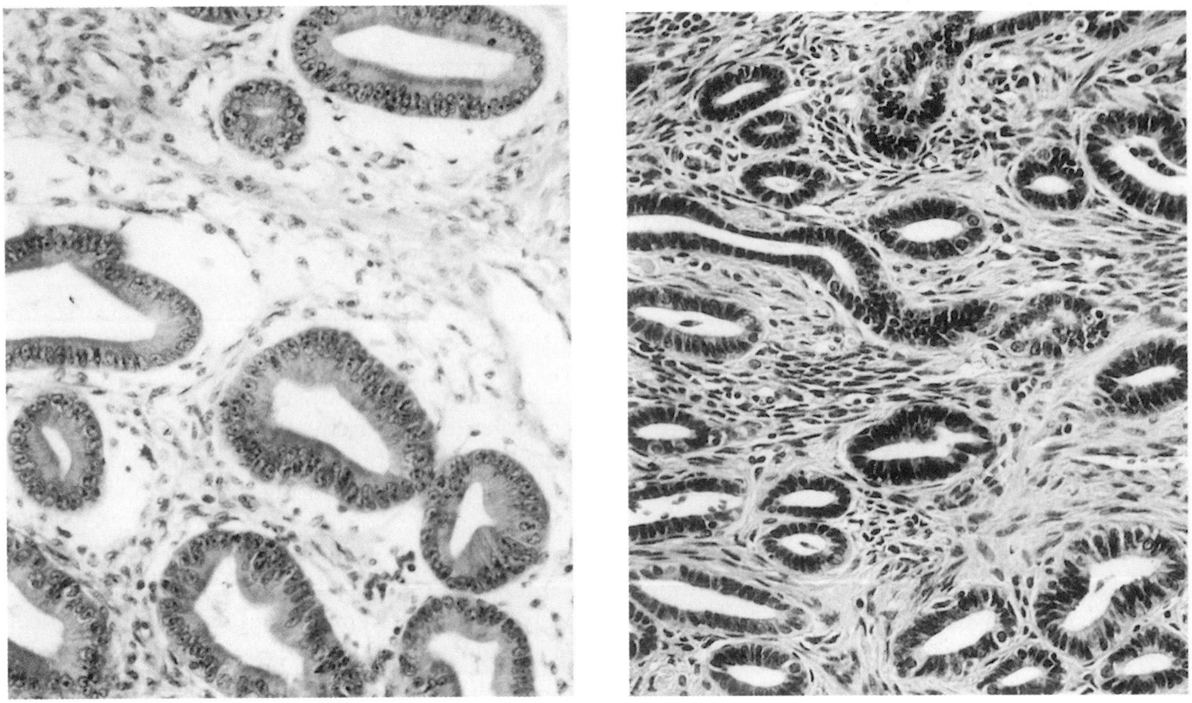

A B

Fig. 25.1 Benign ovarian endometrioid adenofibroma with typical endometrial-like glandular epithelial cells. H + E ×150

endometrioid tumors leaves the latter as very rare neoplasms. Some of this rarity also may be failure to recognize endometrioid epithelial differentiation in indolent tumors (Fig. 25.1b) (Hughesdon 1984). Such lesions occur as single case reports in the literature or as isolated examples in larger series. A series of 12 cases (Kao & Norris 1979) seems to confirm previous limited experience that they are mostly unilateral cystadenofibromas occurring in older women (median age 57 years). An architecturally and cytologically benign ovarian endometrioid adenofibroma, associated with omental lesions, has been described as malignant on the basis of 'metastatic disease' alone (Gaing et al 1988), and an apparently unique example of benign extraovarian endometrioid cystadenofibroma has been recorded arising from the posterior wall of the uterus (Ortega et al 1982).

Atypically proliferating endometrioid tumors are less rare, but the criteria for defining these lesions are less well established than for their serous or mucinous counterparts, particularly the dividing line between proliferating endometrioid tumors and invasive endometrioid carcinomas (Fox et al 1983, Snyder et al 1988, Norris 1993). Patients have a mean age at presentation of 55–60 years, and the common symptoms are abnormal vaginal bleeding, abdominal pain, and/or mass. These tumors may be associated with synchronous or metachronous hyperplasia or adenocarcinoma of the uterine endometrium (Russell 1979b, Bell & Scully 1985).

Endometrioid carcinomas, however, are the second most common form of ovarian epithelial malignancy. They are confined to the ovaries and adjacent pelvic structures in 70% of cases, and in such instances only 13% are bilateral (Kottmeier 1968), with an overall bilaterality rate of about 28%. They occur principally in the fifth and sixth decades, but also not infrequently in older women. Those cancers which can be shown to arise within an endometriotic cyst, on the other hand, present in women younger than the average by 10 years or more (Mostoufizadeh & Scully 1980). About 15–25% are associated with an histologically similar lesion in the endometrium; the latter are usually regarded as independent autochthonous neoplasms, although metastasis from one site to the other is theoretically difficult to exclude in some cases (Eifel et al 1982, Zaino et al 1984, Prat et al 1991, Pearl et al 1993, Martin-Jiminez et al 1994). Rare instances have been observed of synchronous or metachronous endometrioid carcinomas of the ovary and cervix (Kaminski & Norris 1984), and occasional primary extra-ovarian endometrioid carcinomas have been noted (Hyman 1977, Aslani & Scully 1989).

Cytogenetic and molecular genetic studies

Cytogenetic studies have identified, in a primary ovarian endometrioid carcinoma, three related near-haploid clones (Sreekantaiah et al 1990)

Macroscopic features

The mean size of benign tumors is about 10 cm in diameter with usually a smooth capsular surface and a firm, densely fibrous to honeycomb cut surface with multiple cysts of various sizes. The latter contain clear or straw colored watery fluid. Scully et al (1966) have described a polypoid nodule arising within an endometriotic cyst, but this appears to be a unique variant. Atypically proliferating endometrioid tumors exhibit two gross patterns. Many are multilocular cystadenofibromas (Fig. 25.2) with features indistinguishable from those of the benign lesions noted above (Kao & Norris 1978, Russell 1979b, Roth et al 1981, Bell & Scully 1985, Snyder et al 1988, Norris 1993). Papillary areas may also be noted. Less often the solid areas are softer in consistency and the cut surfaces show hemorrhage or necrosis. These tend to be the tumors with high grade epithelial proliferation and merge, in their gross appearances, with frankly invasive endometrioid carcinomas (Russell 1979b).

Malignant tumors are primarily cystic and usually measure 12–20 cm in diameter. The outer surfaces are generally smooth but sometimes bosselated. On section, friable soft masses or papillae partly fill the cyst lumens, which additionally

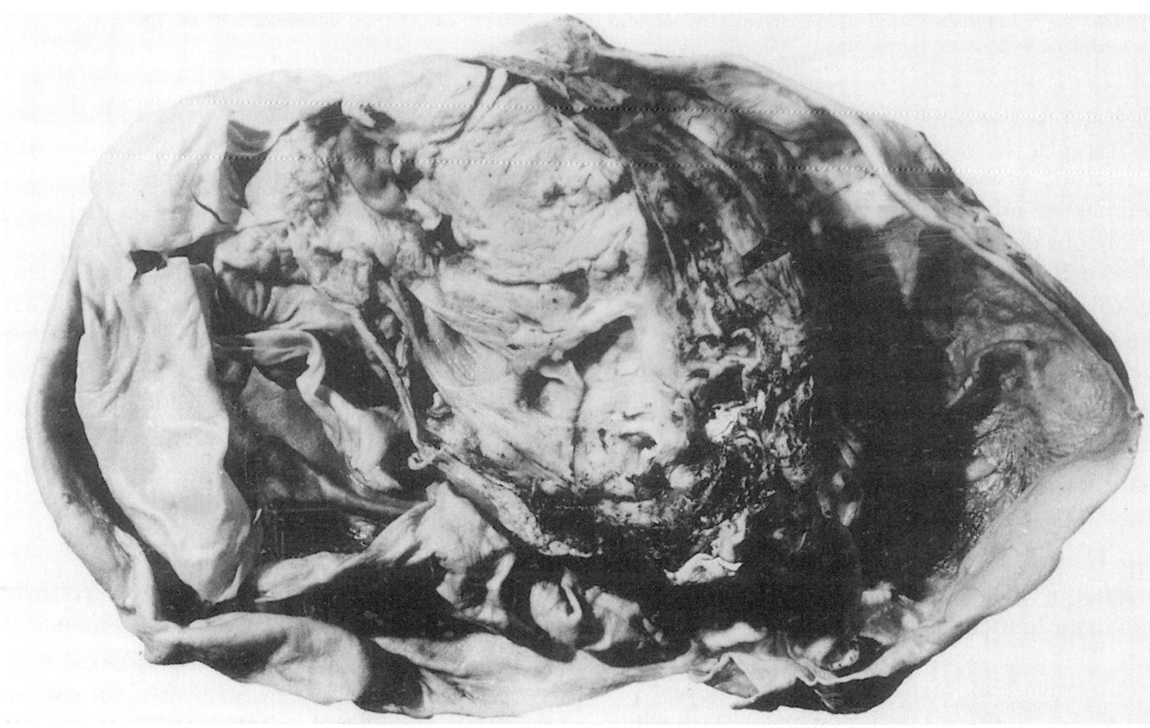

Fig. 25.2 Proliferating endometrioid tumor. Thick-walled multilocular cyst with a single firm fibrous intraluminal nodule. Areas softer in consistency are noted towards the top.

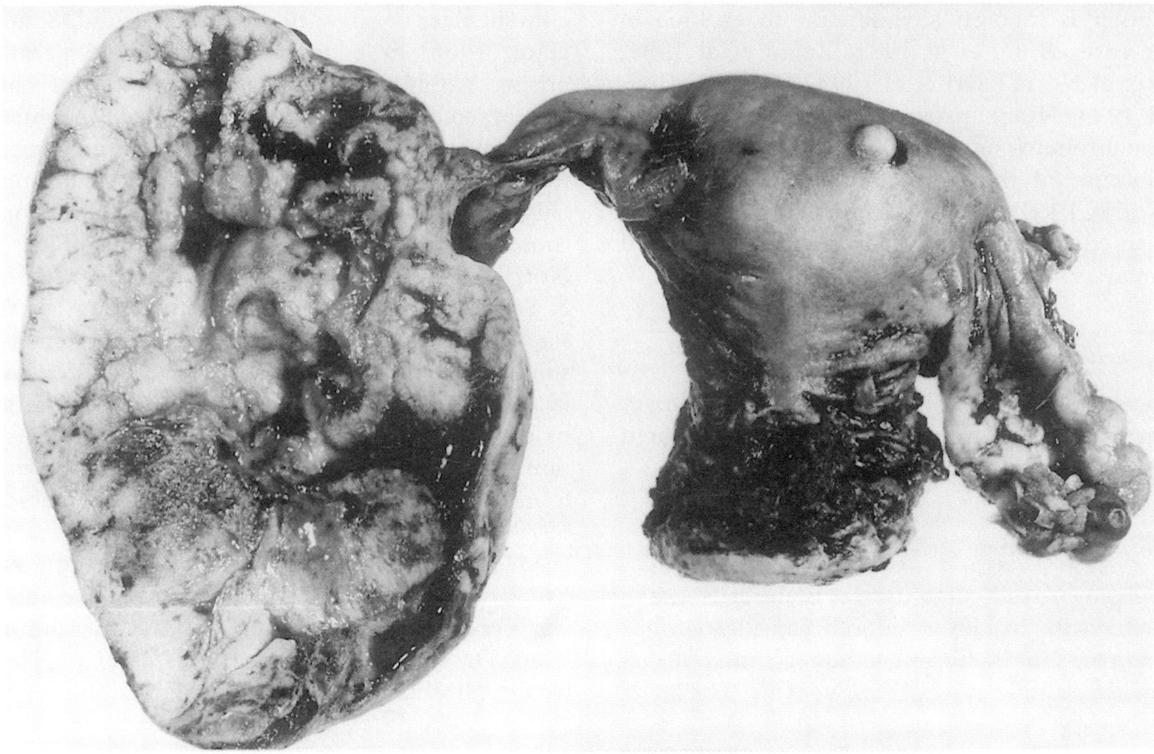

Fig. 25.3 A predominantly solid endometrioid carcinoma of the left ovary. Epithelial nodules protrude into the cystic spaces, which also contain altered blood

may contain bloodstained fluid (Fig. 25.3). Uncommonly, the neoplasms are completely solid with necrotic or hemorrhage areas. Mucus may sometimes be noted within the cysts, suggesting an erroneous diagnosis of mucinous carcinoma. If the tumor has arisen in an endometriotic cyst, it tends to be an exophytic polypoid lesion rather than a mural nodule, and if there is endometriosis in the adjacent uninvolved portion of ovary, the characteristic features of these non-neoplastic lesions will also be present (see Ch. 21).

Microscopic features

Benign tumors are adenofibromas (Fig. 25.4) or cystadenofibromas (Fig. 25.5). Epithelial components create branching tubular glands and cystic spaces. Tall columnar epithelium resembles that of proliferative endometrium, with basophilic to amphophilic cytoplasm and elongate nuclei with relatively coarse chromatin and small but obvious nucleoli, or inactive endometrium with uniform dark nuclei and scanty cytoplasm (see Fig. 25.1). Mitoses are rarely seen, in stark contrast to non-neoplastic proliferative endometrium (e.g. in endometriosis). Benign squamous metaplasia (Fig. 25.5B) has also been described (Scully et al 1966, Fox et al 1983), giving a picture of 'adeno-acanthofibroma'. The fibrovascular stroma resembles that of endometrial polyps or, less often, ovarian cortex. Smooth muscle may be prominent and stromal luteinization is occasionally observed (Chebrou et al 1993). The absence of typical endometrial-type stroma and lack of evidence of recurrent local hemorrhage (cyclical response) further differentiate these lesions from non-neoplastic endometriosis.

Minimum requirements for defining epithelial proliferation/atypia are not as well outlined in the literature as for serous or mucinous tumors (although the principles are the same – see Ch. 22). Low grade adenofibromatous and cystadenofibromatous variants of proliferating endometrioid lesions are characterized by crowded endometrial-

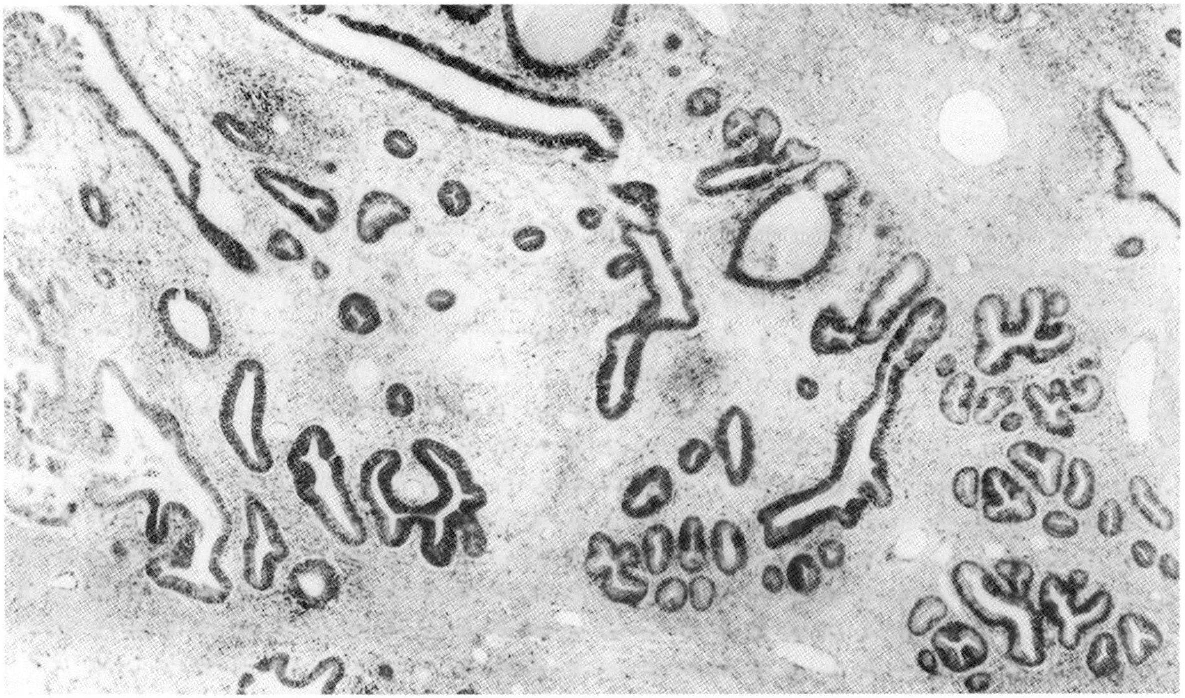

Fig. 25.4 Benign endometrioid adenofibroma. Simple tubular and cystic glands with focal branching in fibrous stroma. H + E ×50

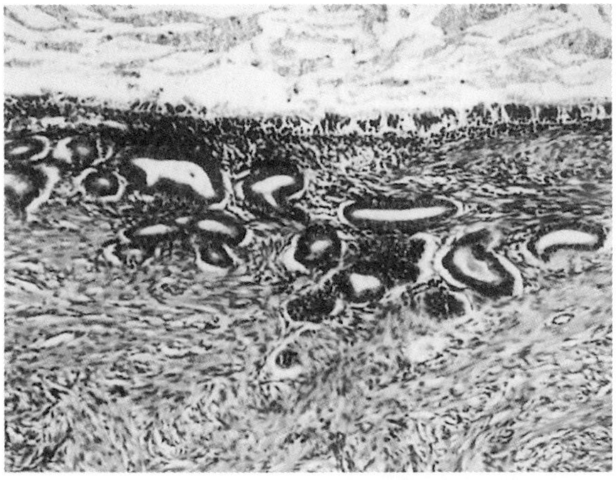

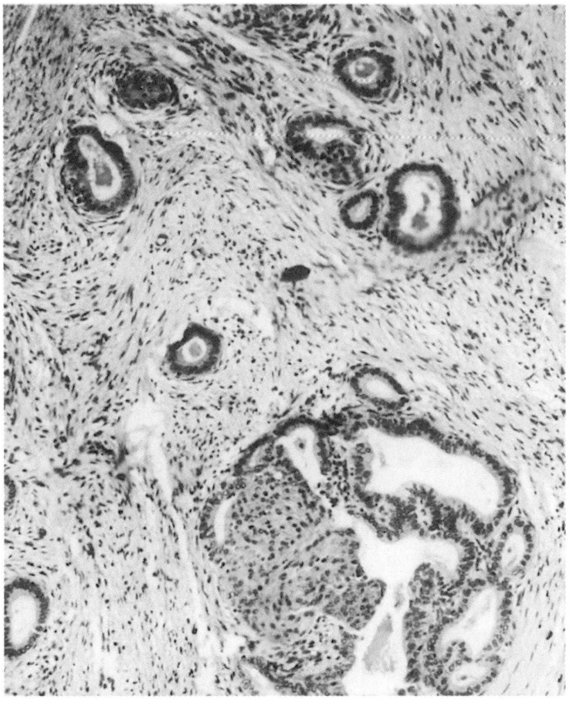

A B

Fig. 25.5 Benign endometrioid cystadenofibroma. (A) Degenerate epithelium lines the blood-filled cyst, and is subtended by clusters of endometrial-like glands. H + E ×60. (B) Focal benign squamous metaplasia. H + E ×75

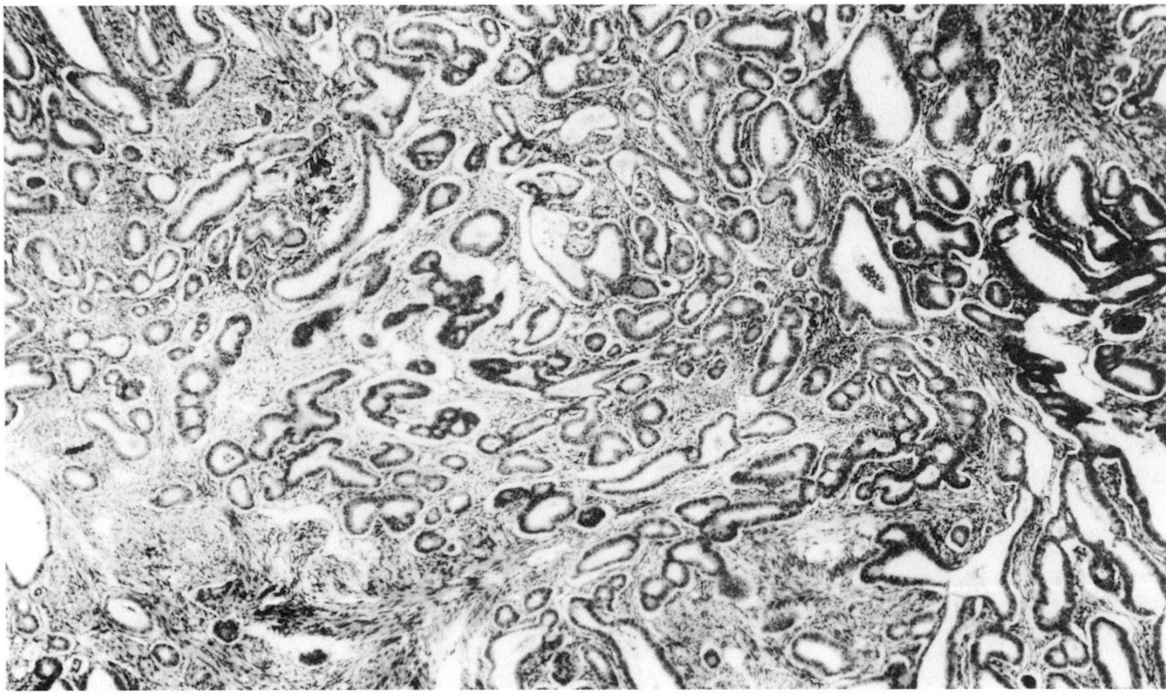

A

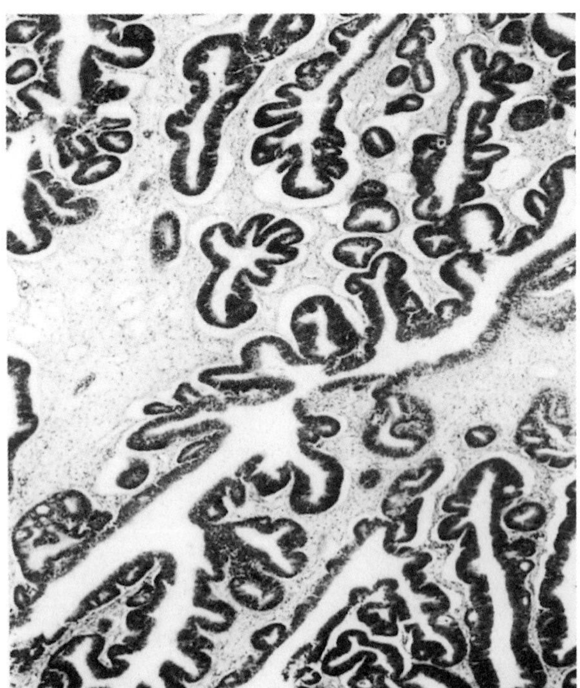

B

Fig. 25.6 Low grade proliferating endometrioid adenofibromas. (A) Mild atypical proliferation with irregular branching and budding glands in fibrous stroma. Note smooth muscle at bottom left. H + E ×50 (B) More complex but less crowded glandular elements. H + E ×30 (Reprinted, with permission, from Russell 1979b)

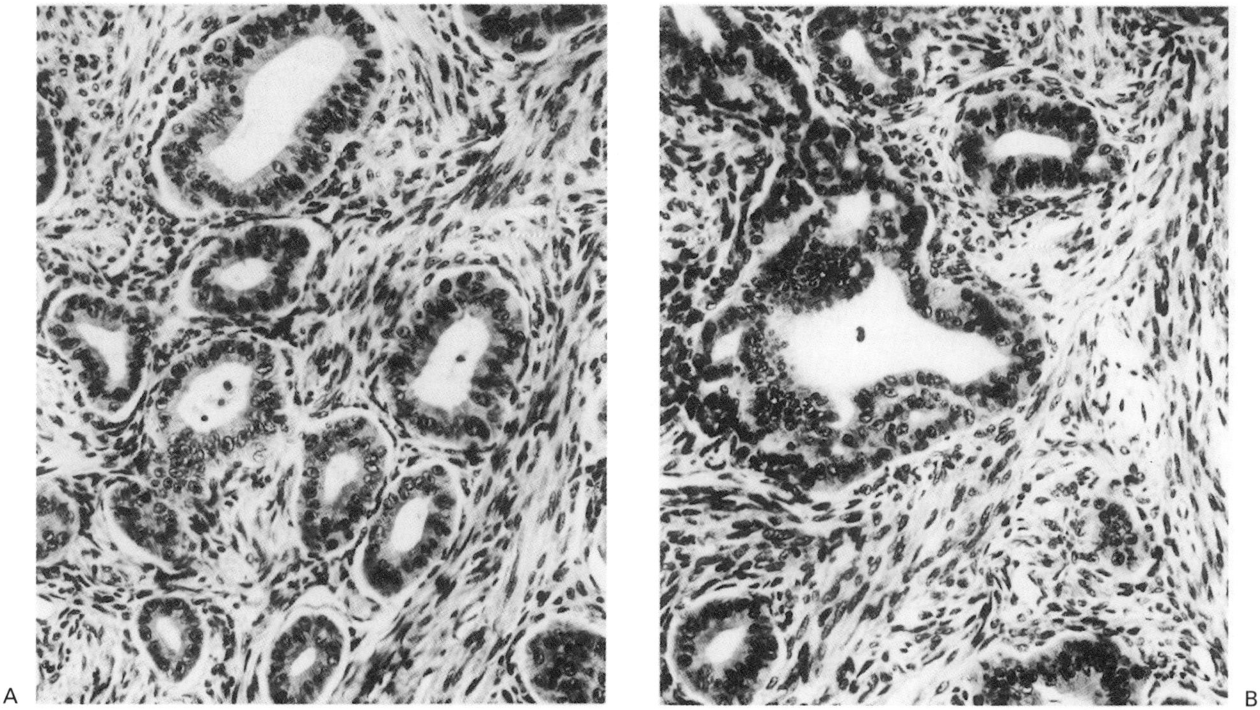

Fig. 25.7 Low grade proliferating endometrioid adenofibromas. High power showing glandular spaces with (A) cellular and nuclear atypia, and (B) epithelial bridging and stratification. Contrast cytological features with Fig. 25.1. H + E ×150

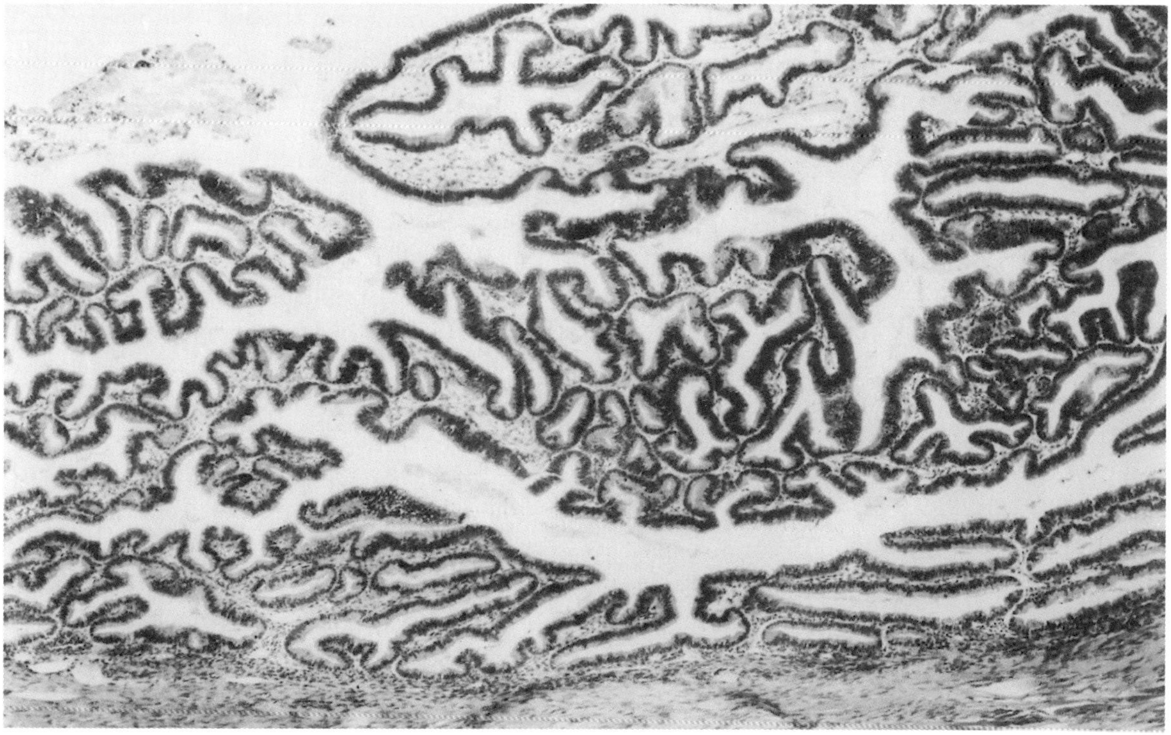

Fig. 25.8 High grade proliferating endometrioid tumor with an intracystic papillary pattern, but no significant cellular atypia. At base of the figure, a smooth stromal/epithelial interface is present. H + E ×50

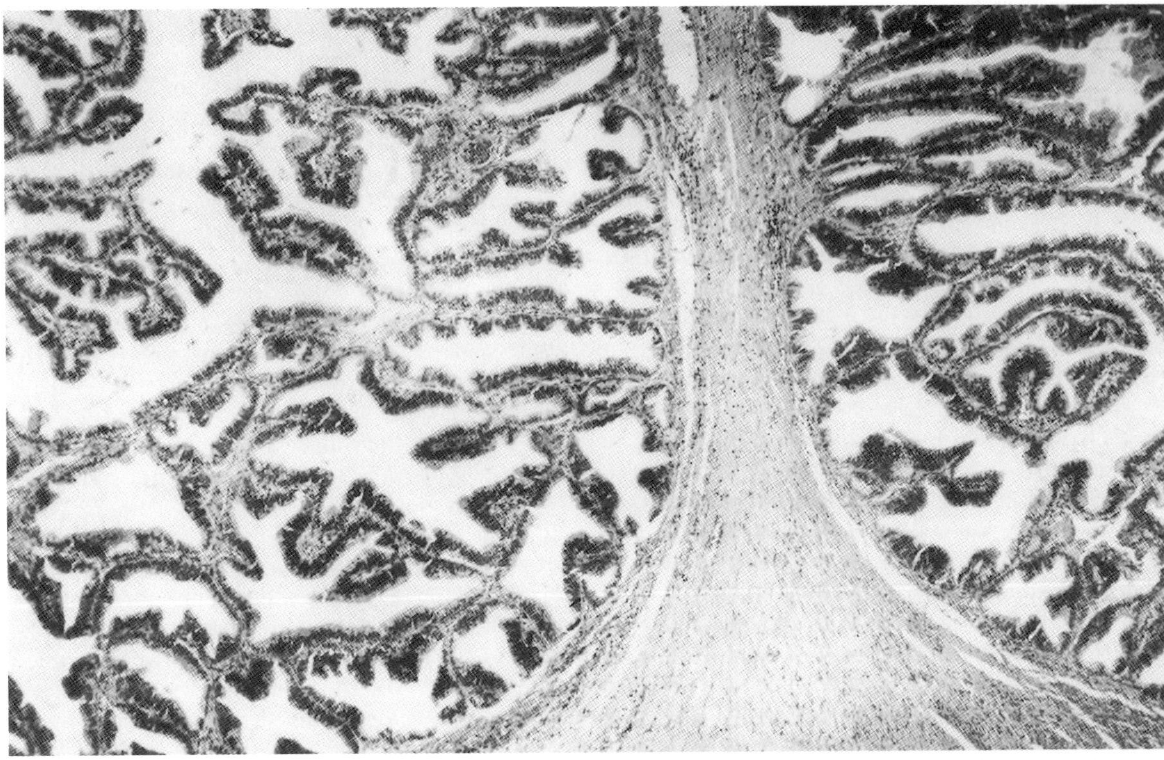

A

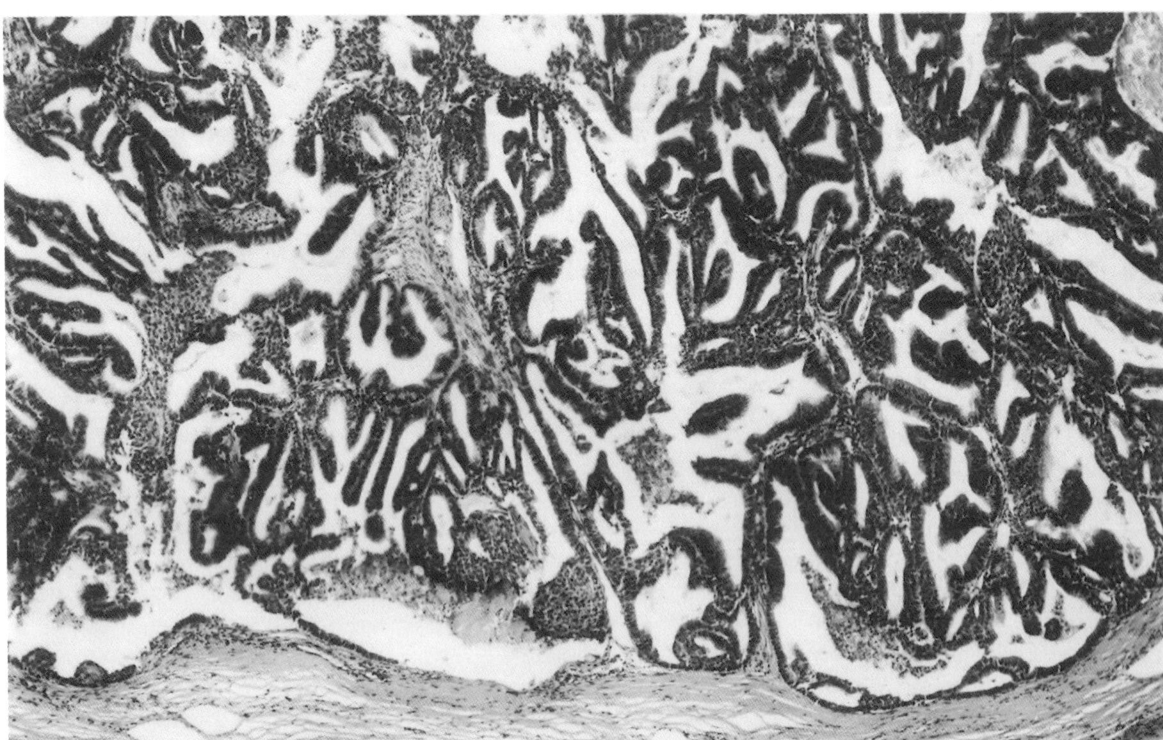

B

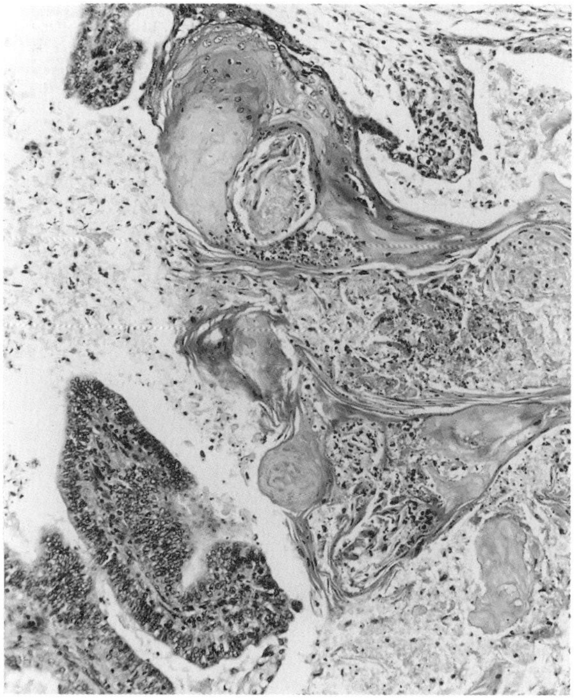

C

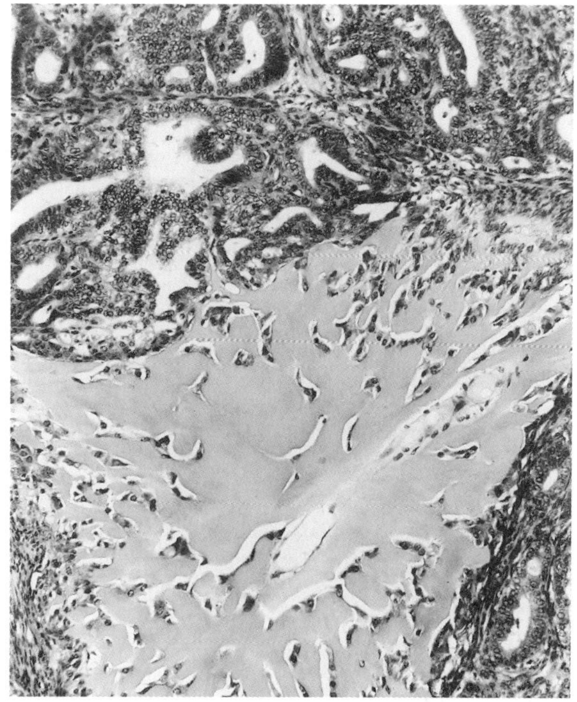

D

Fig. 25.9 High grade proliferating endometrioid tumors. (A) 'Back-to-back' appearance, but a smooth stromal/epithelial interface (i.e. no destructive stromal invasion). H + E ×50. (B) Features similar to those seen in (A), but with benign squamous metaplasia as well. H + E ×50. (C) Florid keratinizing squamous epithelial 'metaplasia' with degenerative changes and inflammatory infiltrates. H + E ×59. (D) Focal benign metaplastic bone formation in the tumor stroma. H + E ×59

like glands and cystic spaces embedded in stroma which varies from ovarian to hyaline or collagenous (Fig. 25.6). Patchy smooth muscle may be seen in the stroma (Fig. 25.6A). Glands are randomly oriented and show a similar range of epithelial proliferation to that seen in endometrial polyps with complex hyperplasia. Closer perusal reveals hallmarks of atypical proliferation, i.e. nuclear crowding and atypia (Fig. 25.7A), and epithelial stratification with tufting and bridging (Fig. 25.7B). This stratification is stressed as being important in differentiating borderline from benign endometrioid cystadenofibromas (Kao & Norris 1978, Roth et al 1981). Such tumors are termed 'atypical endometrioid adenofibromas' by Bell & Scully (1985), and 'proliferative endometrioid tumors' by Snyder et al (1988). Mitoses range up to 4/10HPF, but are rarely atypical. Stromal luteinization is occasionally noted. High grade proliferating endometrioid tumors show even less prominent stroma and more exuberant intracystic coarse papillary (Fig. 25.8) and glandular proliferation. They resemble somewhat the various patterns of complex endometrial hyperplasia with atypia, except for this tendency to papillation. They may show a back-to-back arrangement of glands (Russell 1979b, Bell & Scully 1985), giving a broad well-defined interface between the mature relatively acellular stroma and the intracystic epithelial compartment (Fig. 25.9), with an almost total lack of chronic inflammatory cells. In our material, and that of others (Bell & Scully 1985, Snyder et al 1988, Norris 1993), this is taken as the upper limit of noninvasive or preinvasive endometrioid neoplasia. Benign squamous metaplasia is present in about one-third to one-half of all cases (Fig. 25.9B), and may be occasionally both florid and keratinizing (Fig. 25.9C), and give rise to a foreign body giant cell reaction. Another uncommonly encountered stromal change is the presence of focal metaplastic benign bone formation (Fig. 25.9D). Rare high grade proliferating endometrioid tumors of the ovaries have been reported with extraovarian lesions or

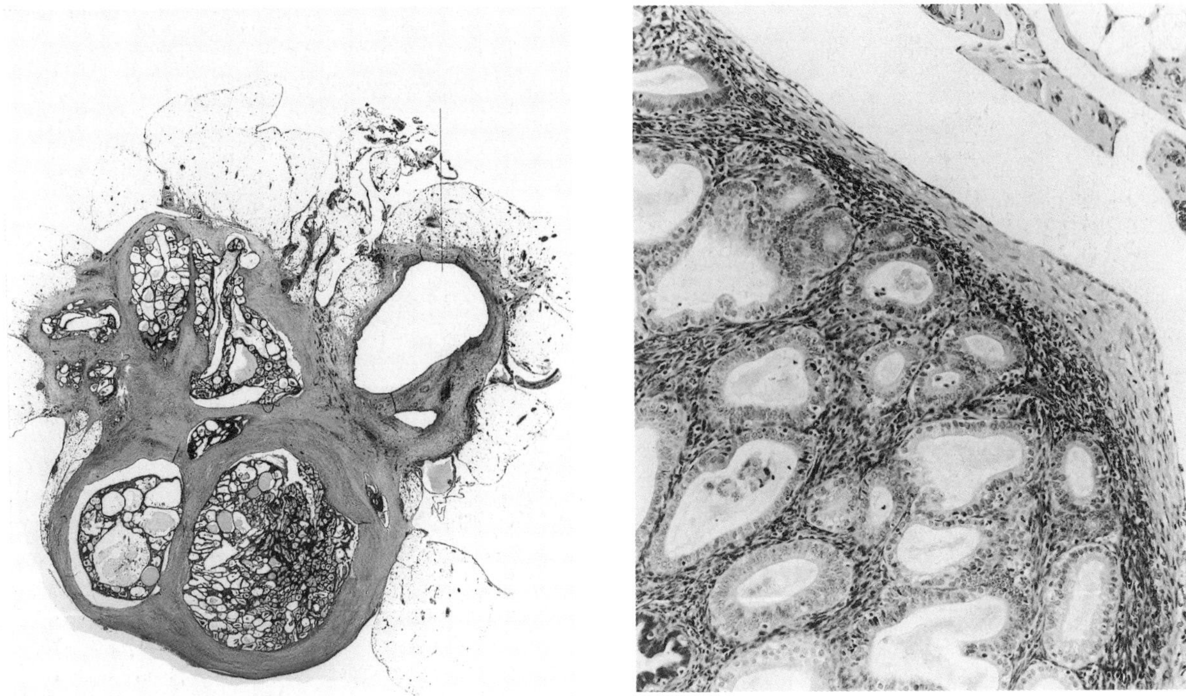

A B

Fig. 25.10 Omental nodule associated with a low grade proliferating endometrioid tumor. (A) Survey showing intracystic polypoid nodules separated from the omental fat by dense hyalinized connective tissue. H + E ×3.3. (B) Higher power of one of the 'polyp-like' nodules exhibiting endometrioid glands and dense hypercellular stroma. Architecturally and cytologically, this lesion in benign. H + E ×59

'implants' (Fig. 25.10) (Russell 1979b, Snyder et al 1988).

Occasional examples of proliferating endometrioid tumors with microinvasion have been documented (Snyder et al 1988, Norris 1993), typified by haphazard stromal infiltration by nests and cords of malignant epithelial cells.

All carcinoma subtypes documented in the uterine corpus have also been identified in the ovary, and cytologically, if not architecturally, these tumors closely resemble their uterine counterparts. The tendency for ovarian tumors to become cystic is accompanied by a coarse papillary pattern of growth more often than is encountered in the exophytic luminal component of the equivalent uterine tumors.

Well differentiated adenocarcinomas (Fig. 25.11) account for the majority and also are represented disproportionately amongst tumors seen to arise from endometriotic cysts. Predominantly, they have a glandular growth pattern with irregular budding and luminal reduplication. Tumor stroma resembles that of the ovary or is nonspecific and fibroblastic in appearance. The epithelium is tall columnar with pseudostratification or multilayering. Glandular buds have rounded contours. Mitoses range up to about 5/10HPF. Nuclear debris is occasionally present within gland-like spaces accompanied by histiocytic giant cells (Fig. 25.12). The character of this response is quite different, however, from that associated with ovarian mucinous tumors (Fig. 24.13). Squamous metaplasia is seen in about 30% (Fig. 25.13) and is usually cytologically benign, varying from small morules to large confluent sheets connecting the malignant glands. This squamous epithelium is mostly separated from stroma by the generative glandular epithelium. If, however, it is in direct contact with the stroma, and particularly if degenerate, a foreign body giant cell reaction may be seen. These 'keratin granulomas' may be identified in the peritoneal washings of such patients without necessarily implying intraperitoneal spread of carcinoma (Kim & Scully 1990). Sometimes the neoplastic squamous element is independently malignant and is then intimately

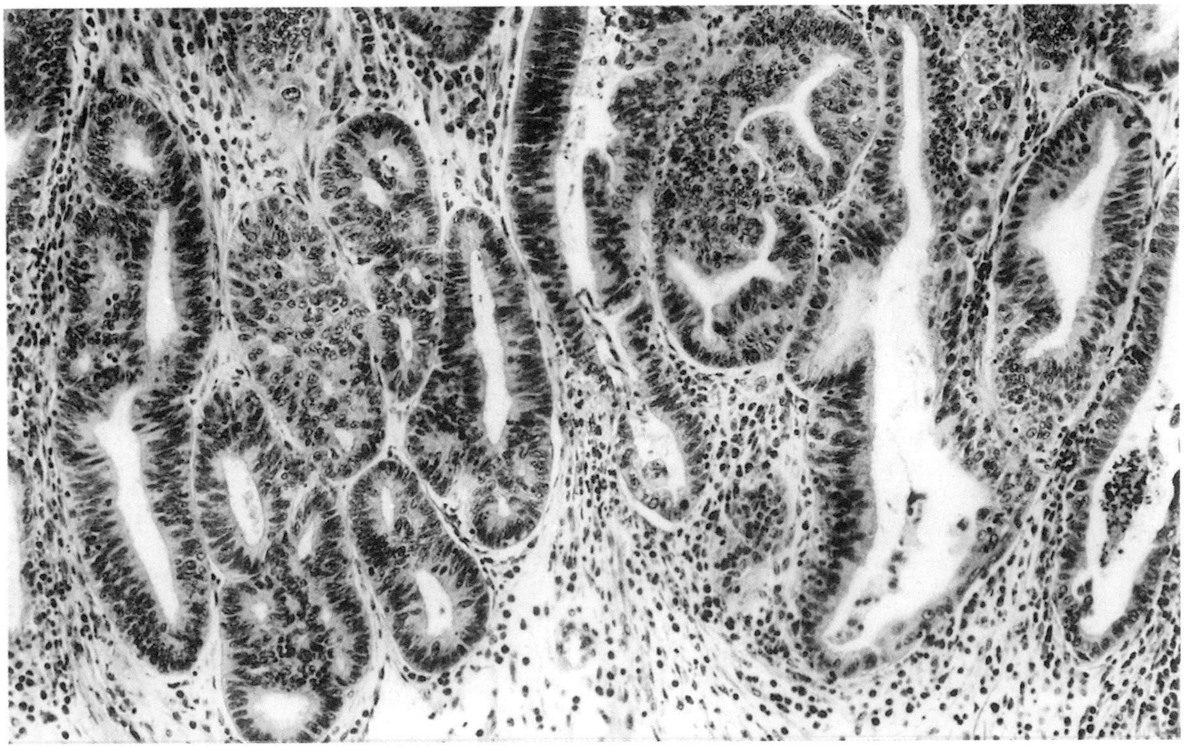

Fig. 25.11 Well-differentiated endometrioid carcinoma. H + E ×125

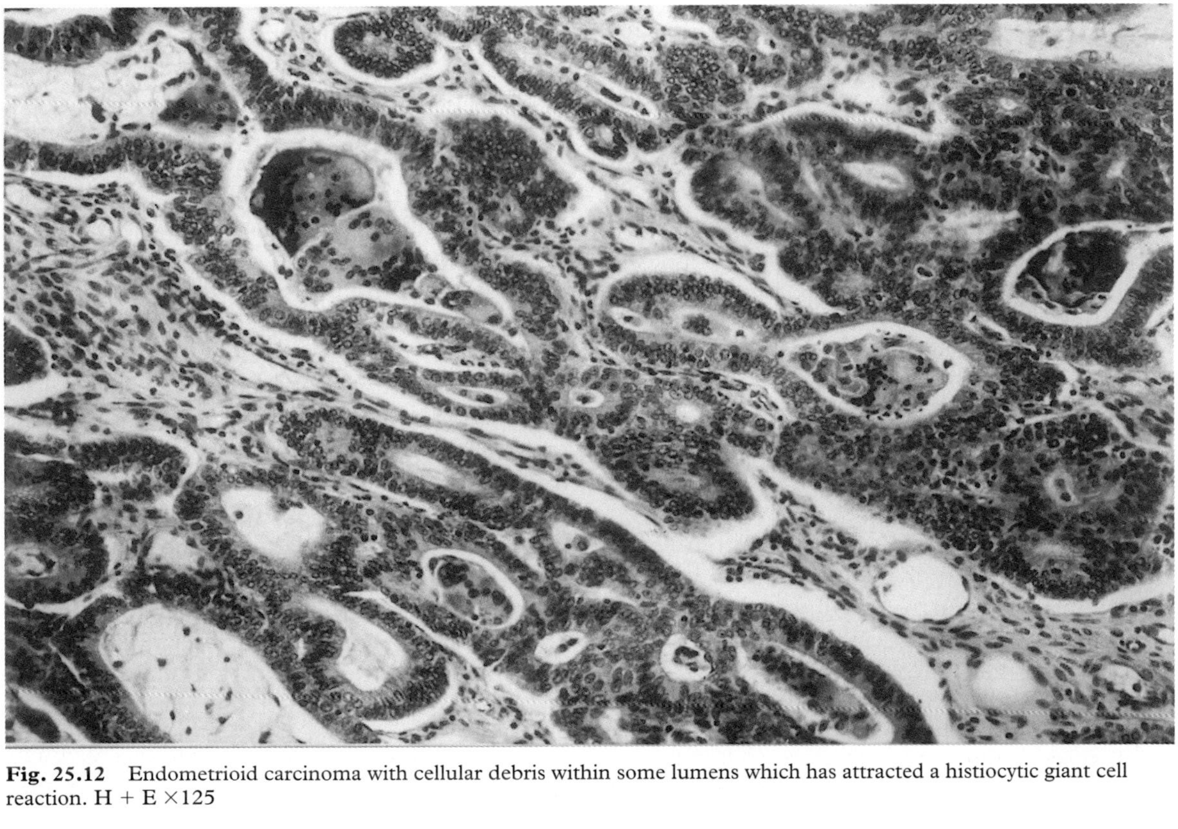

Fig. 25.12 Endometrioid carcinoma with cellular debris within some lumens which has attracted a histiocytic giant cell reaction. H + E ×125

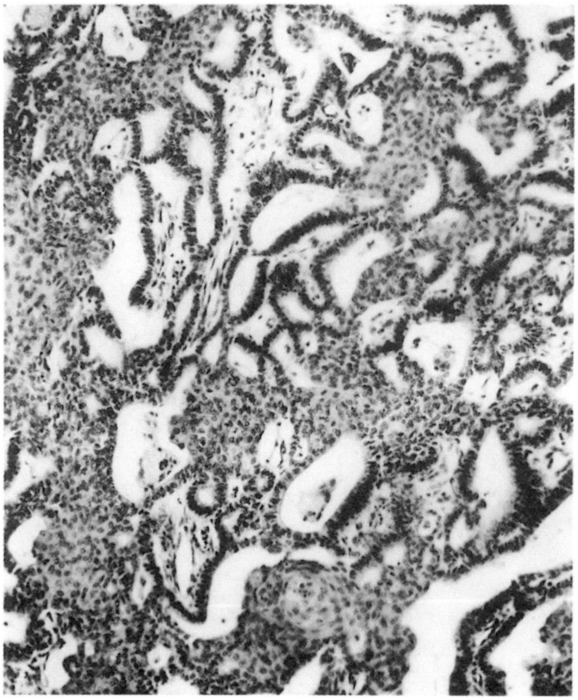

Fig. 25.13 Well-differentiated invasive endometrioid carcinomas with prominent benign squamous metaplasia. H + E ×75

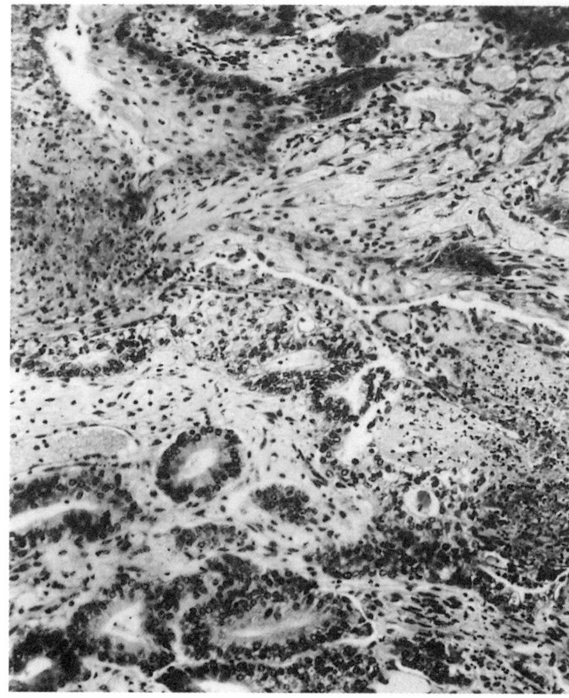

Fig. 25.14 Ovarian adenosquamous carcinoma with invasive squamous (top) and glandular (bottom) components and prominent necrosis. H + E ×75

admixed with the adenocarcinoma (Scully 1979) or produces quite separate zones of invasive squamous cell carcinoma and adenocarcinoma (Fig. 25.14). Secretory patterns (Fig. 25.15) differ from those of typical clear cell carcinoma in that the cells remain tall columnar and show supranuclear and/or subnuclear vacuoles (rather than diffuse cytoplasmic clearing around eccentric nuclei producing large pavement-like clear cells), this change being seen focally in approximately one-third of endometrioid ovarian carcinomas. Hobnail cells are not seen. Papillary areas are common, the papillae being broad, blunt structures with obvious connective tissue cores and differing markedly from the usually fine micropapillae of serous carcinomas. Psammoma bodies can also occasionally be present, but are never prominent. Extracellular mucin is sometimes focally prominent and may give rise to difficulty in differentiating endometrioid from mucinous cancers. Mucin stains (diastase-PAS, mucicarmine, alcian blue), however, will show only apical intracellular mucin in typical endometrioid tumor cells. Up to one-half of ovarian endometrioid carcinomas contain argyrophil cells without otherwise altering their classification (Klemi & Gronroos 1979, Ueda et al 1984). Occasional well-differentiated endometrioid carcinomas with prominent fibrous stroma have been described (Roth et al 1981, Moore et al 1991), usually with obvious benign squamous metaplasia. Stromal invasion in such tumors is difficult to document and inferred only by the extent, complexity and irregularity of the epithelial component, and the immature desmoplastic nature of the stroma (Bell & Scully 1985).

Moderately differentiated endometrioid adenocarcinomas show more complex glandular/microglandular patterns (Fig. 25.16). Epithelial multilayering is less prominent, but pleiomorphism, nuclear atypia, and mitotic activity (up to about 1/HPF) are all increased, and tumor giant cells may be seen. Necrosis and hemorrhage are also more obvious. Secretory change and squamous areas are noted with about the same frequency as in well-differentiated tumors, but some evidence suggests that the squamous component

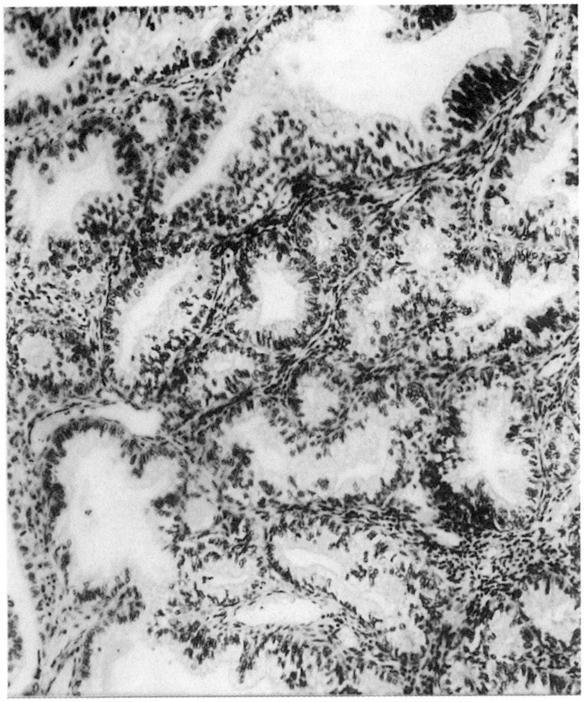

Fig. 25.15 Well-differentiated endometrioid carcinoma with tall columnar cells showing supranuclear vacuoles – so-called 'secretory' adenocarcinoma. H + E ×75

in such tumors is more likely to be malignant (Fu et al 1979). Occasional lesions superficially resemble sex cord–stromal tumors, either granulosa cell (Fig. 25.17) or Sertoli cell tumors (Fig. 25.18), because of trabecular/tubular areas or nests of microglandular pattern simulating Call–Exner bodies, or the intimate admixture of well-differentiated epithelial-lined tubules and spindled cells which simulate the lobular patterns of moderately differentiated Sertoli–Leydig cells (Tornos et al 1995). These latter spindled cells are strongly positive immunohistochemically for cytokeratins (spindle cell carcinoma). Luteinized stromal cells can, if present, further compound the interpretative problem. We do not feel that these tumors demonstrate sufficient clinical departure from the mainstream of endometrioid carcinomas to justify being separately designated as 'sertoliform variants' (Roth et al 1982) and suggest that their importance is only in the diagnostic difficulty they cause (Young et al 1982, Aguirre et al 1989). This

Fig. 25.16 Moderately differentiated endometrioid carcinoma with a typical microglandular pattern. H + E ×125

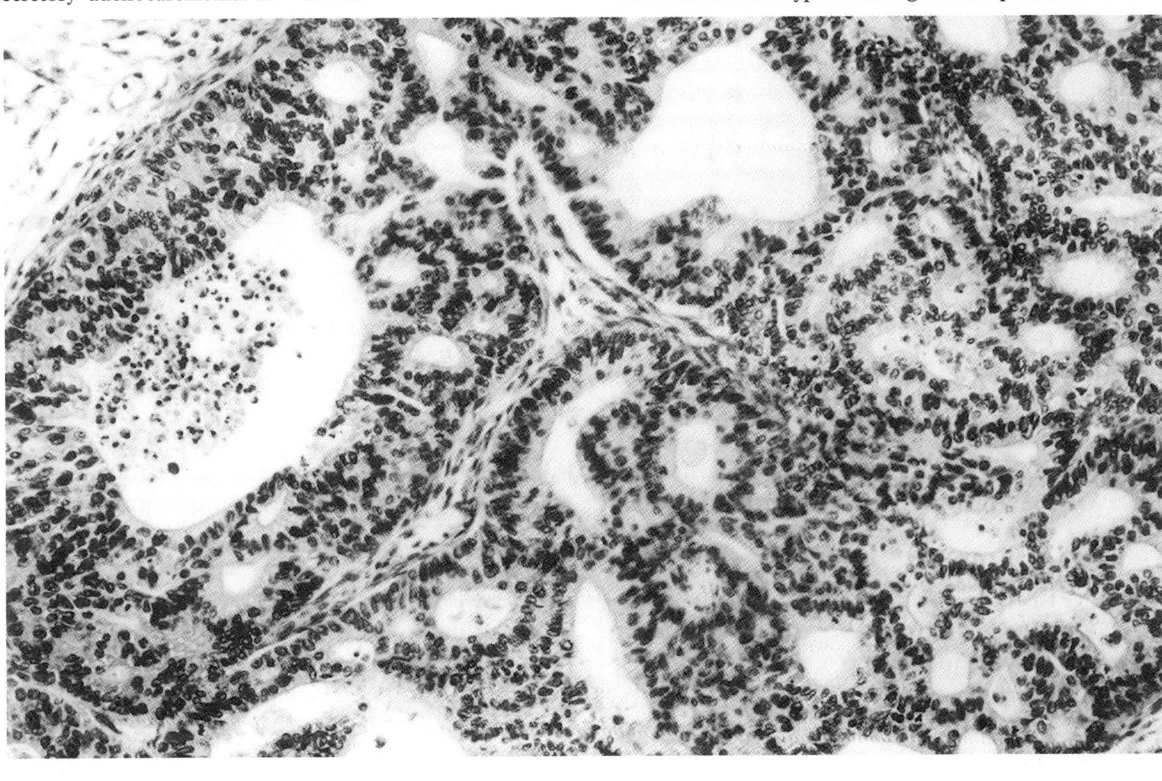

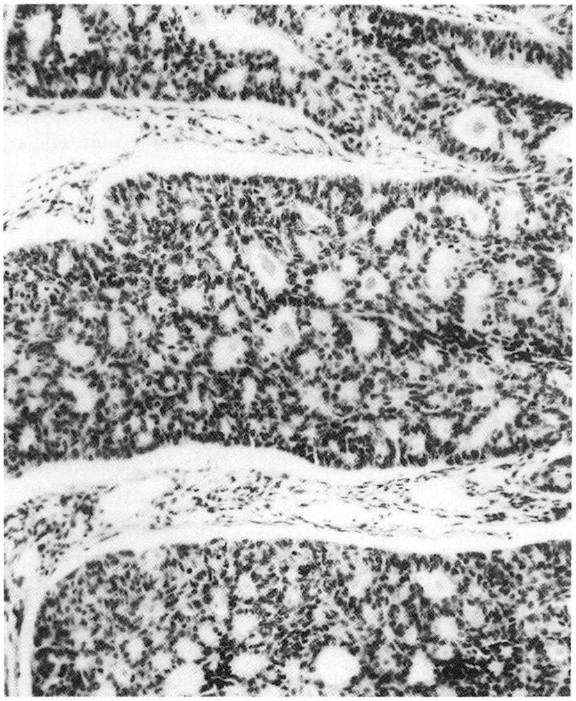

Fig. 25.17 Endometrioid carcinoma with a solid pattern resembling granulosa cell carcinoma. H + E ×75

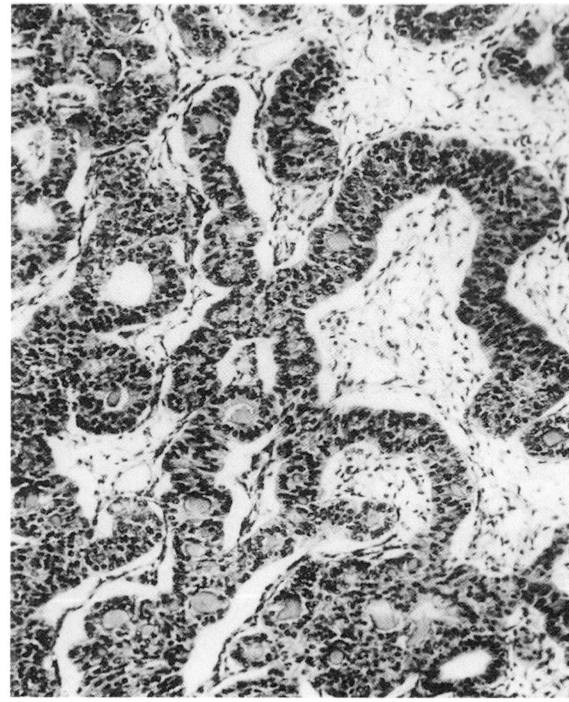

Fig. 25.18 Endometrioid carcinoma with a trabecular pattern resembling Sertoli cell tumor. H + E ×75

is usually successfully addressed by identifying the much greater pleiomorphism and mitotic activity, obvious true gland formation, and squamous differentiation in endometrioid carcinomas. Immunohistochemical presence of EMA and OM-1 may assist further (Table 25.1).

Poorly differentiated endometrioid carcinomas have a mainly solid pattern with residual microglandular areas (Fig. 25.19). Microglandular foci may be separate and distinct, or they may produce a peripheral cuff about islands of solid undifferentiated carcinoma. Mitotic activity is high (up to 5/HPF or more), but squamous or secretory change is rarely noted. Hemorrhage and/or necrosis are widespread (Fig. 25.20).

Differential diagnosis

Discrimination between moderately differentiated endometrioid and mucinous carcinomas with cribriform patterns may, on occasion, be difficult. Mucin stains (diastase-PAS, mucicarmine, alcian blue), however, should reveal only apical intracellular mucin in the endometrioid tumor cells; by contrast, many cells containing abundant intracellular mucin, goblet cells, pseudomyxoma ovarii, and/or 'mucoid degeneration' are strong pointers to the diagnosis of a mucinous carcinoma. Immunohistochemical staining reveals similar differential patterns as exist between mucinous and serous tumors (see Ch. 24).

Distinction between poorly differentiated endometrioid and serous carcinomas is usually

Table 25.1 Immunophenotype of endometrioid carcinomas

Antibody against	Expression (%)
Cytokeratins (AE1/AE3, CAM 5.2)	100
Epithelial membrane antigen (EMA)	100
OM-1	85
B72.3 antigen	75
Vimentin	70
CA 19.9	60
Carcinoembryonic antigen (CEA)	45
S100 protein	40
GFAP	35
CA-125 antigen	25

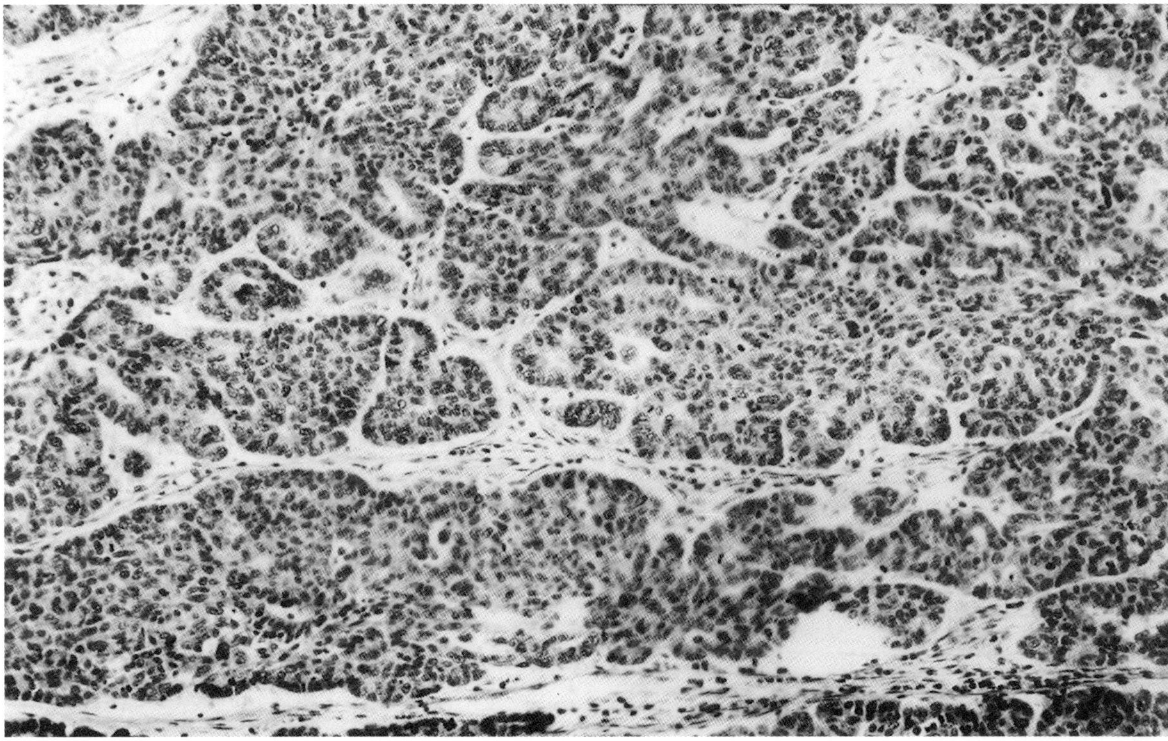

Fig. 25.19 Poorly differentiated endometrioid carcinoma. Discriminating such tumors from poorly differentiated serous carcinomas in particular is difficult. H + E ×125

possible by examining the character of the glandular spaces (when present), which tend to be elongate or slit-like and branching in serous tumors and microacinar in endometrioid lesions. Psammoma bodies are rarely helpful, being found only in better differentiated carcinomas. A further problem is encountered in some moderately differentiated endometrioid ovarian carcinomas, namely the focal presence of ciliated cells (Fig. 25.21), as has been well recognized in adenocarcinomas of the uterine endometrium. The pathologist has to be guided by overall architectural and cytological features of such tumors in determining their position in the classification.

Endometrial carcinomas have been estimated to account for up to one-third of tumors metastatic to the ovaries. Endometrial stromal sarcomas and malignant mixed mullerian tumors account for an additional few cases (Mazur et al 1984, Ulbright & Roth 1985). Ovarian tumors have been found at autopsy in 34–47% of women with endometrial carcinoma (Henriksen 1975) and in 2–12% of women undergoing surgery for endometrial malignancy (Scully 1979, Annegers & Malkasian 1981, Axelrod et al 1984). However, it is clear from survival studies of patients with simultaneous or metachronous uterine and ovarian carcinomas that, on the balance of probabilities, most of them do not represent metastases from one site to the other, but rather independent primary lesions, arising in response to the same carcinogenic influences (Russell 1979c, Scully 1979, Parker & Currie 1981, Eifel et al 1982, Woodruff et al 1985, Jambhekar & Sampat 1988, Eisner et al 1989, Montoya et al 1989, Prat et al 1991, Pearl et al 1993, Martin-Jiminez et al 1994). This is in accordance with the developing concept of multifocal tumorigenesis in the upper genital tract, ovaries, and pelvic peritoneum (Russell et al 1985). This point is important to recognize because of the implications for treat-

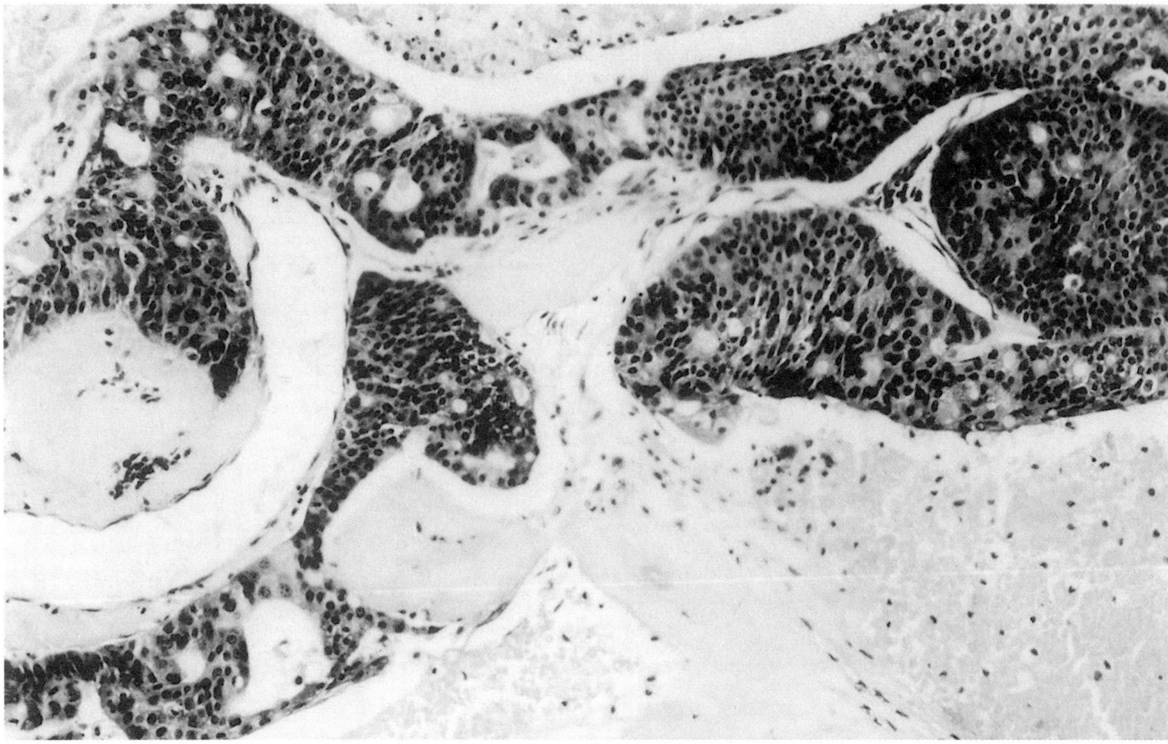

Fig. 25.20 Poorly differentiated endometrioid carcinoma. Solid carcinoma, but with still identifiable microglandular pattern. Necrosis is prominent. H + E ×125

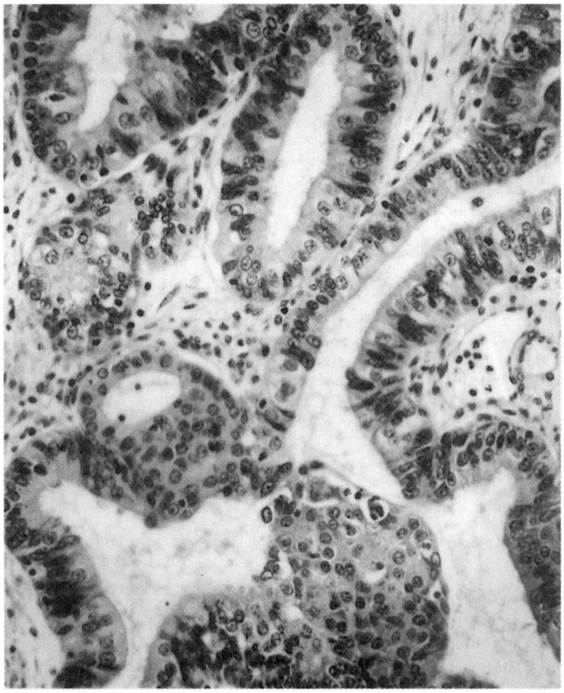

Fig. 25.21 Moderately well-differentiated ovarian endometrioid carcinoma showing focally prominent ciliated cells adjacent to benign squamous morules. H + E ×150

ment. Most simultaneous tumors are of similar histological type, i.e. predominantly endometrioid (Scully 1979, Choo & Naylor 1982, Zaino et al 1984, Ulbright & Roth 1985, Pearl et al 1993). A similar, but rare, problem exists with simultaneous endometrioid carcinomas in the ovaries and cervix (Kaminski & Norris 1984).

Recent attempts to differentiate morphologically as well as clinically between independent endometrial and ovarian primaries and metastases from one site to the other have been made (Scully 1979, Eifel et al 1982, Mazur et al 1984, Ulbright & Roth 1985). Metastatic spread from the endometrium to the ovaries is said to be very much more common than is the reverse (Ulbright & Roth 1985), although in our experience neither is

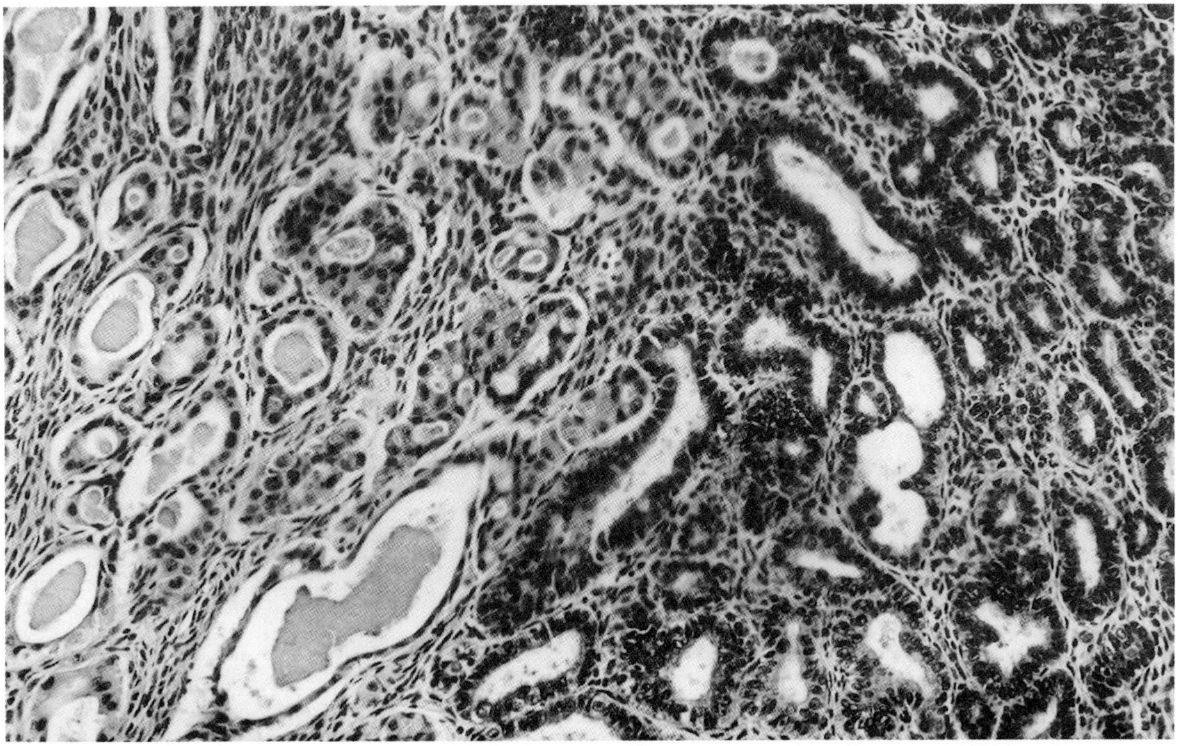

Fig. 25.22 Infiltrating ovarian endometrioid carcinoma (left) adjacent to proliferating but noninvasive endometrioid tumor (right), the latter being indicative of in situ genesis of the ovarian lesion. H + E ×125

common. As in many other organs, demonstration of recognized premalignant or noninvasive proliferative processes in close proximity to the carcinoma is strong evidence of an in situ genesis. In the uterus, this means identification of atypical endometrial hyperplasia. In the ovaries it requires demonstration of a pre-existing benign or proliferating tumor of similar histological type (Fig. 25.22) or origin in the wall of a non-neoplastic endometriotic cyst. Coexistence of endometriosis in the same ovary is insufficient. Disparate histological type (but not grade) of synchronous endometrial and ovarian tumors is good evidence of independent primaries. However, the converse, tumors of similar histological type, is not evidence of metastasis from one to the other. Points for and against a specific ovarian lesion being metastatic from the uterus are outlined in Table 25.2. Criteria for diagnosis of independent primaries are more likely to be found in endometrioid carcinomas and of metastatic tumors in

Table 25.2 Differential diagnosis of simultaneous endometrial and ovarian neoplasms: primary endometrioid ovarian carcinoma versus metastatic endometrial carcinoma

Primary endometrioid carcinoma	Metastatic endometrial carcinoma
Clinical/gross	
Cystic/solid mass	Multinodular solid mass
Mostly unilateral	Usually bilateral
Larger than uterine tumor	Smaller than uterine tumor
Spread beyond ovaries unlikely	Spread beyond ovaries likely
Pre-existing proliferating or benign lesions	No premalignant lesion
Possible origin in endometriosis	No origin in endometriosis
Histological	
Uterine tumor low grade with minimal myometrial penetration	Uterine tumor high grade with deep myometrial penetration
No evidence of mechanism of tumor spread	Evidence of mechanism of tumor spread (lymphatic permeation)

adenosquamous carcinomas, mixed mullerian tumors, and nonendometrioid carcinomas (e.g. serous and clear cell) (Eifel et al 1982, Ulbright & Roth 1985). However, the relationship between the two cancers cannot always be established by pathological examination alone, especially in patients with advanced disease. In these cases, it is advisable to follow FIGO recommendations of classifying the carcinomas according to their manner of presentation (Scully 1979).

Rare examples of yolk sac tumor may mimic moderately differentiated endometrioid carcinoma, particularly those with secretory activity (Clement et al 1987). These rare neoplasms will typically present in young women and be associated with greatly raised serum levels of α-fetoprotein. The clinical context, supported by immunohistochemical identification of α-fetoprotein, should suffice to distinguish them from mullerian malignancies of endometrioid type.

REFERENCES

Aguirre P, Thor A D, Scully R E 1989 Ovarian endometrioid carcinomas resembling sex cord–stromal tumors. An immunohistochemical study. International Journal of Gynecological Pathology 8: 364–373

Annegers J F, Malkasian G D 1981 Patterns of other neoplasia in patients with endometrial carcinoma. Cancer 48: 856–859

Aslani M, Scully R E 1989 Primary carcinoma of the broad ligament. Report of four cases and review of the literature. Cancer 64: 1540–1545

Axelrod J H, Fruchter R, Boyce J G 1984 Multiple primaries among gynecologic malignancies. Gynecologic Oncology 18: 359–372

Bell D A, Scully R E 1985 Atypical and borderline endometrioid adenofibromas of the ovary. American Journal of Surgical Pathology 9: 205–214

Bell D A, Scully R 1994 Early de novo ovarian carcinoma. A study of fourteen cases. Cancer 73: 1859–1864

Brescia R J, Dubin N, Demopoulos R I 1989 Endometrioid and clear cell carcinoma of the ovary. Factors affecting prognosis. International Journal of Gynecological Pathology 8: 132–138

Chebrou D M, Provendier B, Chebrou C, Fetissof F, Ledoux A 1993 Adenofibrome endometrioide de l'ovaire. A propos d'un cas anatomoclinique. Journal de Gynecologie Obstetrique et Biologie de la Reproduction (Paris) 22: 254–256

Choo Y C, Naylor B 1982 Multiple primary neoplasms of the ovary and uterus. International Journal of Gynaecology and Obstetrics 20: 327–334

Clement P B, Young R H, Scully R E 1987 Endometrioid-like variant of ovarian yolk sac tumor. A clinicopathologic analysis of eight cases. American Journal of Surgical Pathology 11: 767–778

Cummins P A, Fox H, Langley F A 1974 An electronmicroscopic study of the endometrioid adenocarcinoma of the ovary and a comparison of its fine structure with that of normal endometrium and of adenocarcinoma of the endometrium. Journal of Pathology 113: 165–173

Eifel P, Hendrickson M, Ross J, Ballon S, Martinez A, Kempson R 1982 Simultaneous presentation of carcinoma involving the ovary and the uterine corpus. Cancer 50: 163–170

Eisner R F, Nieberg R K, Berek J S 1989 Synchronous primary neoplasms of the female reproductive tract. Gynecologic Oncology 33: 335–339

Fox H, Anderson M C, Beilby J O W et al 1983 Ovarian epithelial tumors of borderline malignancy: pathological features and current status. British Journal of Obstetrics and Gynaecology 90: 743–750

Fu Y S, Stock R J, Reagan J W, Storaasli J P, Wentz W B 1979 Significance of squamous components in endometrioid carcinoma of the ovary. Cancer 44: 614–621

Gaing A A, Kimble C C, Belmonte A H, Agustin E, Tchertkoff V 1988 Invasive ovarian endometrioid adenofibroma with omental implants and collision with endometrial adenocarcinoma. Obstetrics and Gynecology 71: 440–444

Henriksen E 1975 The lymphatic dissemination in endometrial carcinoma. A study of 188 necropsies. American Journal of Obstetrics and Gynecology 123: 570–576

Hughesdon P E 1984 Benign endometrioid tumors of the ovary and the Mullerian concept of ovarian epithelial tumors. Histopathology 8: 977–990

Hyman M P 1977 Extraovarian endometrioid carcinoma. American Journal of Clinical Pathology 68: 522–526

Jambhekar N A, Sampat M B 1988 Simultaneous endometrioid carcinoma of the uterine corpus and ovary: a clinicopathologic study of 15 cases. Journal of Surgery and Oncology 37: 20–23

Kaminski P F, Norris H J 1984 Coexistence of ovarian neoplasms and endocervical adenocarcinoma. Obstetrics and Gynecology 64: 553–556

Kao G F, Norris H J 1978 Cystadenofibroma of the ovary with epithelial atypism. American Journal of Surgical Pathology 2: 357–363

Kao G F, Norris H J 1979 Unusual cystadenofibromas: endometrioid, mucinous and clear cell types. Obstetrics and Gynecology 54: 729–736

Kim K R, Scully R E 1990 Peritoneal keratin granulomas with carcinomas of endometrium and ovary and atypical polypoid adenomyoma of endometrium. A clinicopathologic analysis of 22 cases. American Journal of Surgical Pathology 14: 925–932

Klemi P J, Gronroos M 1979 Endometrioid carcinoma of the ovary. A clinicopathologic, histochemical and electron microscopic study. Obstetrics and Gynecology 53: 572–579

Kottmeier H L 1968 Surgical management – conservative surgery. Indications according to the type of tumor. In: Gentils F, Junqueira A C (eds) Ovarian cancer, UICC monograph series, vol 11. Springer-Verlag, New York, p 157–164

Martin-Jiminez A, Miralles-Pi R M, Gine-Martin L, Petit-Cabello J, Balaguero-Llado L 1994 Endometrioid carcinoma of the ovary. A clinicopathological study of

17 cases. European Journal of Gynaecological Oncology 15: 96–100

Mazur M T, Hsueh S, Gersell D J 1984 Metastases to the female genital tract: Analysis of 325 cases. Cancer 53: 1978–1984

Montoya F, Martin M, Schneider J, Matia J C, Rodriguez-Escudero F J Simultaneous appearance of ovarian and endometrial carcinoma: a therapeutic challenge 1989 European Journal of Gynaecological Oncology 10: 135–139

Moore D H, Fowler W C, Santrach P J 1991 Malignant endometrioid cystadenofibroma of the ovary. Archives of Gynecology and Obstetrics 249: 156

Mostoufizadeh M, Scully R E 1980 Malignant tumors arising in endometriosis. Clinical Obstetrics and Gynecology 23: 951–963

Norris H J 1993 Proliferative endometrioid tumors and endometrioid tumors of low malignant potential of the ovary. International Journal of Gynecological Pathology 12: 134–140

Ortega I, Nogales F, Gonzalez-Campora R, Matilla A, Galera H 1982 Extragenital endometrioid cystadenofibroma. Acta Obstetricia et Gynecologica Scandinavica 61: 283–284

Parker R T, Currie J L 1981 Metastatic tumors of the ovary. In: Coppleson M (ed) Gynecologic oncology. Churchill Livingstone, Edinburgh, p 731–742

Pearl M L, Johnston C M, Frank T S, Roberts J A 1993 Synchronous dual primary and endometrial carcinomas. International Journal of Gynaecology and Obstetrics 43: 305–312

Prat J, Matias-Guiu X, Barreto J 1991 Simultaneous carcinoma involving the endometrium and the ovary. A clinicopathologic, immunohistochemical, and DNA flow cytometric study of 18 cases. Cancer 68: 2455–2459

Roth L M, Czernobilsky B, Langley F A 1981 Ovarian endometrioid adenofibromatous and cystadenofibromatous tumors: benign, proliferating and malignant. Cancer 48: 1838–1845

Roth L M, Liban E, Czernobilsky B 1982 Ovarian endometrioid tumors mimicking Sertoli and Sertoli–Leydig cell tumors. Sertoliform variant of endometrioid carcinoma. Cancer 50: 1322–1331

Russell P 1979a The pathological assessment of ovarian neoplasms. I: Introduction to the common 'epithelial' tumors and analysis of benign 'epithelial' tumors. Pathology 11: 5–26

Russell P 1979b The pathological assessment of ovarian neoplasms. II: The proliferating 'epithelial' tumors. Pathology 11: 251–282

Russell P 1979c The pathological assessment of ovarian neoplasms. III: The malignant 'epithelial' tumors. Pathology 11: 493–532

Russell P, Bannatyne P M, Solomon H J, Stoddard L D, Tattersall M H N 1985 Multifocal tumorigenesis in the upper female genital tract – implications for staging and management. International Journal of Gynecological Pathology 4: 192–210

Scully R E 1979 Tumors of the ovary and maldeveloped gonads, AFIP fascicle 16, 2nd series. Armed Forces Institute of Pathology, Washington, DC, p 53–151

Scully R E, Richardson G S, Barlow J F 1966 The development of malignancy in endometriosis. Clinical Obstetrics and Gynecology 9: 384–411

Serov S F, Scully R E, Sobin L H 1973 Histological typing of ovarian tumors. International histological classification of tumors No. 9. World Health Organization, Geneva, p 17–54

Snyder R R, Norris H J, Tavassoli F 1988 Endometrioid proliferative and low malignant potential tumors of the ovary. A clinicopathologic study of 46 cases. American Journal of Surgical Pathology 12: 661–671

Sreekantaiah C, Crickard K, Crickard U, Yoonessi M, Sandberg A A 1990 Three related near-haploid clones in a primary endometrioid carcinoma of the ovary. Gynecologic Oncology 38: 282–285

Stenback F, Kauppila A 1981 Endometrioid ovarian tumors: Morphology and relation to other endometrial lesions. Gynecologic and Obstetrical Investigation 12: 57–70

Tornos C, Silva E G, Ordonez N G, Gershenson D M, Young R H, Scully R E 1995 Endometrioid carcinoma of the ovary with a prominent spindle-cell component, a source of diagnostic confusion. American Journal of Surgical Pathology 19: 1343–1353

Ueda G, Yamasaki M, Inoue M et al 1984 Argyrophil cells in the endometrioid carcinoma of the ovary. Cancer 54: 1569–1573

Ulbright T M, Roth L M 1985 Metastatic and independent cancers of the endometrium and ovary. A clinicopathologic study of 34 cases. Human Pathology 16: 28–34

Woodruff J D, Solomon D, Sullivant H 1985 Multifocal disease in the upper genital tract. Obstetrics and Gynecology 65: 695–698

Young R H, Prat J, Scully R E 1982 Ovarian endometrioid carcinomas resembling sex cord–stromal tumors. A clinicopathologic analysis of 13 cases. American Journal of Surgical Pathology 6: 513–522

Zaino R J, Unger E R, Whitney C 1984 Synchronous carcinomas of the uterine corpus and ovary. Gynecologic Oncology 19: 329–335

26

Mullerian mesenchymal tumors

P. Russell   A. Farnsworth

These lesions are uncommon in the ovary and are characterized by neoplastic stromal or mesenchymal cells exhibiting varying degrees of proliferation and malignant potential as well, as many patterns of mesenchymal differentiation. Many contain neoplastic epithelial elements as well, which may be benign or malignant. They all have more frequently observed homologs elsewhere in the female genital tract (particularly the uterus), and rarely beneath the pelvic and abdominal peritoneum or within the omentum (presumably from the same cells which give rise to endometriosis and endosalpingiosis). A comprehensive schema of classification is modified from that used by Hendrickson and Kempson (1980) for uterine mesenchymal tumors and outlined in Table 26.1.

Table 26.1 Classification of ovarian mullerian mesenchymal tumors

Benign tumors and tumor-like conditions
Leiomyomatosis peritonealis disseminata
Leiomyomas and histological variants
? Stromal endometriosis, deciduosis

Malignant tumors
Pure sarcomas:
  Homologous
  – leiomyosarcomas
  – low grade endometrioid stromal sarcomas ('endolymphatic stromal myosis', 'stromatosis')
  – high grade endometrioid stromal sarcomas
  Heterologous (? some nonmullerian, see Chs. 34, 52)
  – rhabdomyosarcomas
  – chondrosarcomas
  – osteogenic sarcomas
  – fibrosarcomas (? ovarian stromal sarcoma)
Mixed sarcomas – homologous or heterologous
Malignant mixed mullerian tumors:
  Low grade ('adenosarcomas')
  – homologous
  – heterologous
  High grade
  – homologous ('carcinosarcomas')
  – heterologous ('mixed mesodermal tumors')
Sarcomas, not otherwise unclassified

TUMORS AND TUMOR-LIKE CONDITIONS OF SMOOTH MUSCLE

Peritoneal leiomyomatosis

This rare disease entity (also known as leiomyomatosis peritonealis disseminata (LPD)) is typically a self-limiting tumor-like condition of the peritoneal subcoelomic mesenchyme, manifesting as myriad nodules of smooth muscle up to a centimeter or so in diameter. LPD affects the ovaries in about one-quarter of cases (Tavassoli & Norris 1982). It occurs mostly in young women with a median age of 30 years, and one-half are pregnant or immediately postpartum (of the 50 or so cases in the literature, only two have been reported in postmenopausal women (Kokcu et al 1994)). Many other women are taking oral contraceptive agents at the time of presentation. Spontaneous regression is the rule, while clinical recurrence may be observed with subsequent pregnancies. A single example of malignant LPD has been reported, but in this case the ovaries were not involved (Rubin et al 1986).

Macroscopic features

LPD is characterized grossly by tens to hundreds of firm rounded nodules, seldom exceeding 1 cm in diameter, distributed widely in the omentum and beneath the pelvic peritoneum. Less frequently, they are seen on the serosal surfaces of the ovaries, uterus, fallopian tubes, and bowel.

Microscopic features

LPD exhibits small subperitoneal nodules which cytologically and architecturally resemble small seedling myomas in the uterus. The typical spindled smooth muscle cells, often with prominent eosinophilic cytoplasm, may merge with the surrounding tissue or be sharply demarcated from it. Nuclear atypia is absent, but mitoses may be easily found. Decidual cells are prominent in pregnant or immediately postpartum patients. The intimate association of LPD with such cells, as well as with endometriosis (Kuo et al 1980) and benign serosal inclusions (Chen et al 1982), has led most investigators to favor a subcoelomic mesenchymal metaplastic origin of the disease (Tavassoli & Norris 1982, Walley 1983), a concept which is expanded upon in Chapter 20, and which is supported by the occasional exhibition of other types of mesenchymal differentiation such as myofibroblastic and adipocytic (Kitazawa et al 1992).

Leiomyomas

Although smooth muscle is sometimes seen as a minor component of benign or low grade ovarian mullerian epithelial tumors (particularly endometrioid and mucinous), and uncommonly as part of the cellular proliferation in stromal hyperplasia, true leiomyomas in the ovary are rare neoplasms (Fallahzadeh et al 1972, Matamala et al 1988, Sonobe et al 1989, Vierhout et al 1990, Prayson & Hart 1992, Prasad et al 1993, Randrianjafisamindrakotroka et al 1994). Reported cases have occurred in women aged 20–76 years (85% of cases occurring in premenopausal women), and usually present as an abdominal mass or as incidental findings at hysterectomy for uterine myomas. Synchronous tumors in the uterus are often present. Ascites may accompany the tumor, but pleural effusions have not been recorded (Tsalacopoulos & Tiltman 1981). Rare cases have presented with virilization due to associated hilus cell hyperplasia (Parish et al 1984) or stromal hyperthecosis (Mallya et al 1990).

Macroscopic features

Of examples reported in the literature or observed in our own hospital, most leiomyomas appear to occupy the hilus, suggesting an origin from preformed smooth muscle in this region. But, when large, it is difficult to be certain whether they are of ovarian or broad ligament origin. They are unilateral, pale, solid, rubbery tumors which vary greatly in size (mean diameter 4–5 cm); two reports have detailed massive bilateral lesions in young women (Kandalaft & Estaban 1992, Macri & Vasilev 1993). They have the familiar bulging, whorled cut surface with well-circumscribed margins (Fig. 26.1), which helps to distinguish them from the more common ovarian fibromas that merge with the surrounding ovarian parenchyma at their periphery (Fallahzadeh et al 1972). Cystic degeneration and dystrophic calcification may be present in larger examples.

Microscopic features

Leiomyomas are composed of elongate cells, with obvious eosinophilic cytoplasm and uniform, blunt-ended, cigar-shaped nuclei. The cells are arranged in swirling and intersecting bundles which also contain a variable amount of collagen. Nuclear distribution is usually orderly and palisading may be obvious. Mitoses are usually inconspicuous but, as in their uterine counterparts, may occasionally be numerous, giving rise to so-called 'mitotically active leiomyomas, (Prayson & Hart 1992). The tumors have broad pushing margins (Fig. 26.1), and only occasionally do the edges merge with the surrounding ovarian tissues. Larger leiomyomas often exhibit hyaline change, in which hyaline fibrillary material replaces smooth muscle cells and, when marked, leads to focal cystic degeneration. Focal zones of adipocytic differentiation (so-called 'lipoleiomyomas') have been described (Dodd et al 1989, Mira 1991).

Leiomyosarcomas

Leiomyosarcomas of teratomatous (see Ch. 48) and nonteratomatous origin (Azoury & Woodruff 1971, Shakfeh & Woodruff 1987, Friedman & Mazur 1991, Dixit et al 1993) have also been reported in the ovaries in elderly women and, even more rarely, in young women (Monk et al 1993).

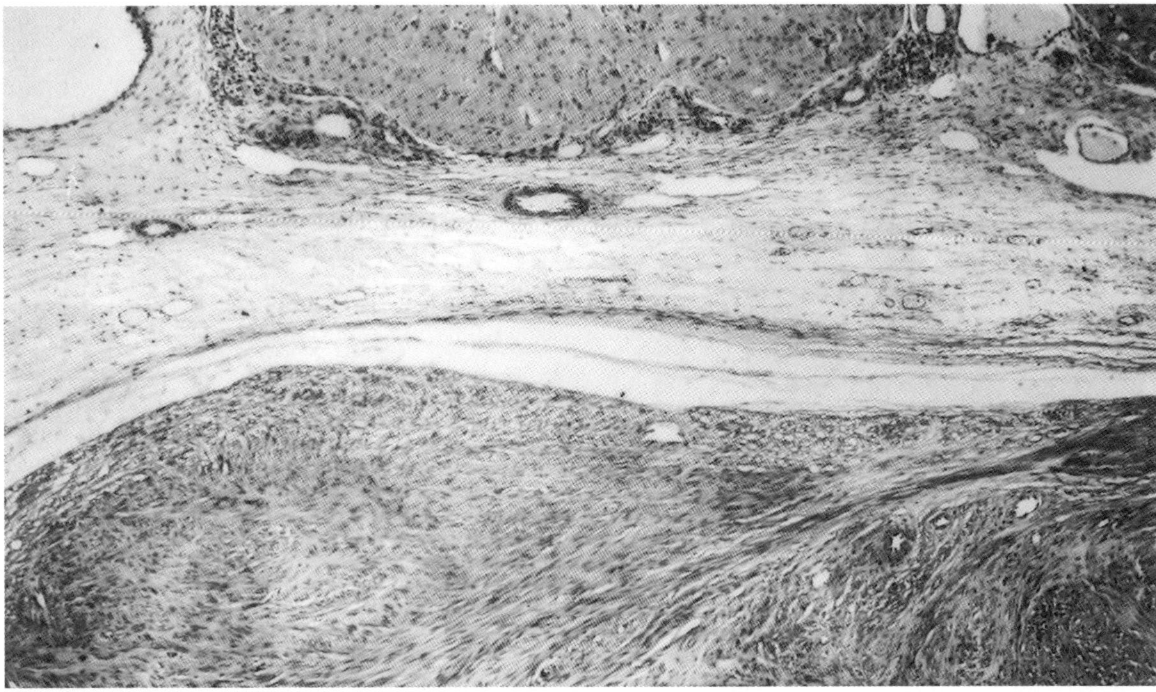

Fig. 26.1 Benign ovarian leiomyoma showing well circumscribed margin abutting adjacent ovarian stroma and a corpus luteum. H + E ×50

Macroscopic features

They are large, soft, pale, fleshy tumors indistinguishable from other ovarian sarcomas on naked eye examination. Cystic areas, degenerative in nature, are frequently seen. Myxoid variants have a gelatinous cut surface.

Microscopic features

Leiomyosarcomas differ from their benign counterparts in being hypercellular (Fig. 26.2A) and exhibiting a markedly increased mitotic rate (greater than 10 per 10HPF). Cells tend to be uniform and spindled, and organized in whorled, interwoven bundles with pleiomorphism prominent only in areas of ischemic degeneration. Nuclei are elongate and blunt ended. Myxoid leiomyosarcomas (Nogales et al 1991) show a reticular meshwork of elongate cells surrounded by basophilic material (Fig. 26.2B). Immunohistochemically, tumor cells stain for vimentin, desmin and muscle-specific actin.

Too few cases of leiomyosarcoma have been reported to test the sophisticated criteria of malignancy which have been applied to uterine smooth muscle neoplasms (Hendrickson & Kempson 1980), but our recommendations are that (a) they be utilized in the interim with the additional proviso that (b) consideration be given to the proclivity for smooth muscle tumors to increase their mitotic activity under conditions of ischemia, such as torsion, which not infrequently complicates ovarian neoplasms.

Differential diagnosis

Pleiomorphism is somewhat less marked in leiomyosarcomas than in malignant fibrous histiocytomas. The latter tumors have not been recorded in the ovaries, but we have encountered examples presenting as pelvic masses in which the ovaries could not be identified, requiring that ovarian mullerian sarcomas be excluded from the differential diagnosis. This differentiation may require a range of immunohistochemical stains for histiocytic and myocellular markers as well as

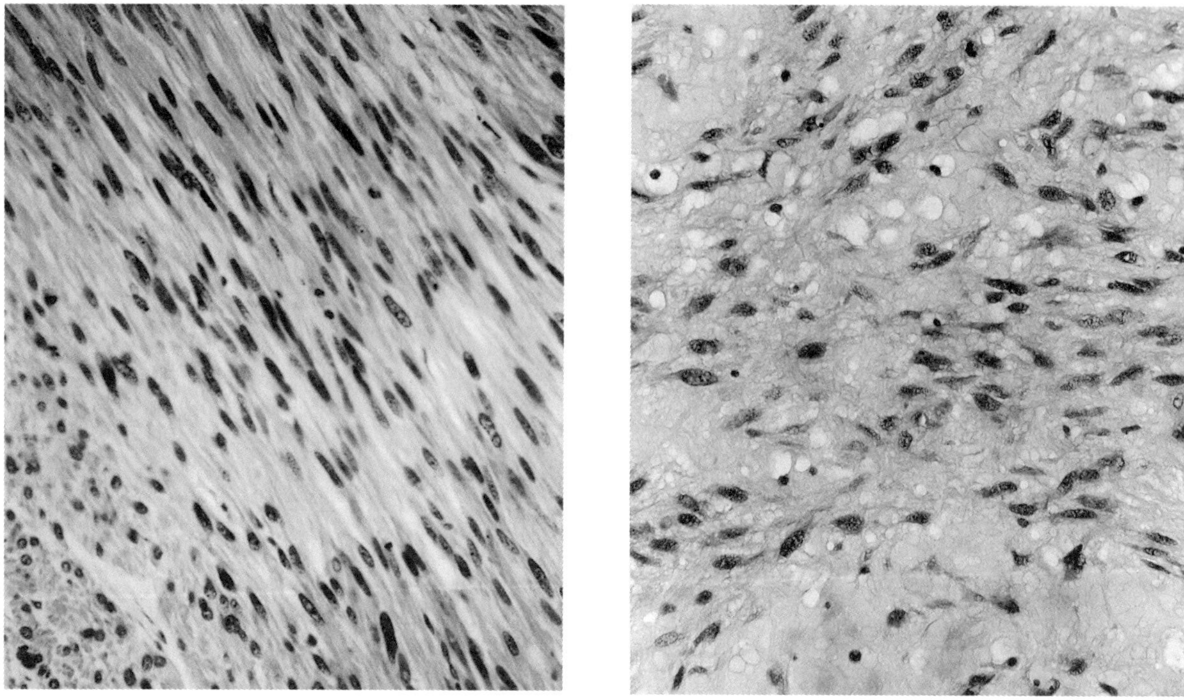

Fig. 26.2 Ovarian leiomyosarcomas. (A) Broad bundles of spindled cells with elongate, blunt-ended nuclei and prominent mitotic activity. H + E ×150. (B) Myxoid leiomyosarcoma with a reticular meshwork of spindle cells surrounded by abundant myxoid background material. H + E ×116

electron microscopy (Friedman & Mazur 1991). Myxoid variants need to be differentiated from myxomas and massive edema.

TUMORS OF ENDOMETRIOID STROMAL DIFFERENTIATION

Low and high grade endometrioid stromal sarcomas

Occasional reports of primary ovarian sarcomas of mullerian or endometrioid type have appeared in the literature, although clear interpretation of instances with synchronous or metachronous involvement of both uterus and ovary is seldom given (Young et al 1984). Some such lesions are high grade endometrioid stromal sarcomas, whilst most are cytologically less pleiomorphic and mitotically active and correspond to low grade endometrioid stromal sarcomas or endolymphatic stromal myosis ('stromatosis') (Shakfeh & Woodruff 1987). It is far from clear, however, whether this distinction has any prognostic significance for the patient (Chang et al 1993). Most of the latter lesions are thought to arise in pre-existing endometriosis, which is found in association with 50–85% of cases (Scully 1979, Silverberg & Fernandez 1981, Young et al 1984), are often bilateral and widespread within the abdomen at the time of diagnosis, and occur in women in their 5th and 6th decades.

Macroscopic features

Low grade endometrioid stromal sarcomas (endolymphatic stromal myosis) tend to appear as ill-defined and homogeneous ovarian enlargement with tumor extensions into adjacent tissues, and rather less commonly as multinodular fleshy tumors, although a cystic component may occasionally be prominent. Focal intracystic hemorrhage may be an indication of associated endometriosis. High grade sarcomas are usually discrete, white fleshy ovarian masses averaging 10 cm in diameter, with prominent necrosis and evidence of local invasion.

Microscopic features

Endometrioid stromal sarcomas, either low or high grade, show the same spectrum of change observed in the more common uterine lesions. Most often they are composed of closely packed sheets of small, round to oval cells, which are often whorled around a fine meshwork of small arteriolar vessels (Fig. 26.3). Reticulin fibers invest individual cells and accentuate the vascularity. Tongues of apparently intravascular tumor growth resembling endolymphatic stromal myosis may also be present (Fig. 26.4). Cytoplasm is scant, and the nuclei are round to oval with inapparent nucleoli (Fig. 26.5). Immunohistochemically, cells stain strongly for vimentin. Desmin positivity is occasional, focal, and weak.

A second distinct pattern is created by the deposition of intercellular hyaline material, which may be focally prominent (Fig. 26.6), and which separates clusters of small tumor cells. Thick-walled cleft-like vascular spaces are evident in this variant. Storiform patterns are sometimes seen, as are less cellular areas more closely resembling those of ovarian fibromas (Young et al 1984).

Nuclei in low grade lesions are bland and mitoses infrequent (by definition fewer than 10/10HPF) and always normal. Nuclear atypia is seen in high grade tumors (Figs 26.7, 26.8) with mitoses above 10 per 10HPF.

Differential diagnosis

Metastatic amelanotic malignant melanoma (see Ch. 54) may also produce sheets of uniform, spindled, sarcoma-like cells in H + E sections. However, even in the absence of pigment (which should be diligently sought), reticulin stains show a carcinoma-like pattern in melanoma, and immunohistochemical stains for S-100 protein and/or NKI/C-3 will, in our experience, always confirm this diagnosis.

Diffuse or sarcomatoid granulosa cell tumors (see Ch. 33) may also superficially resemble low

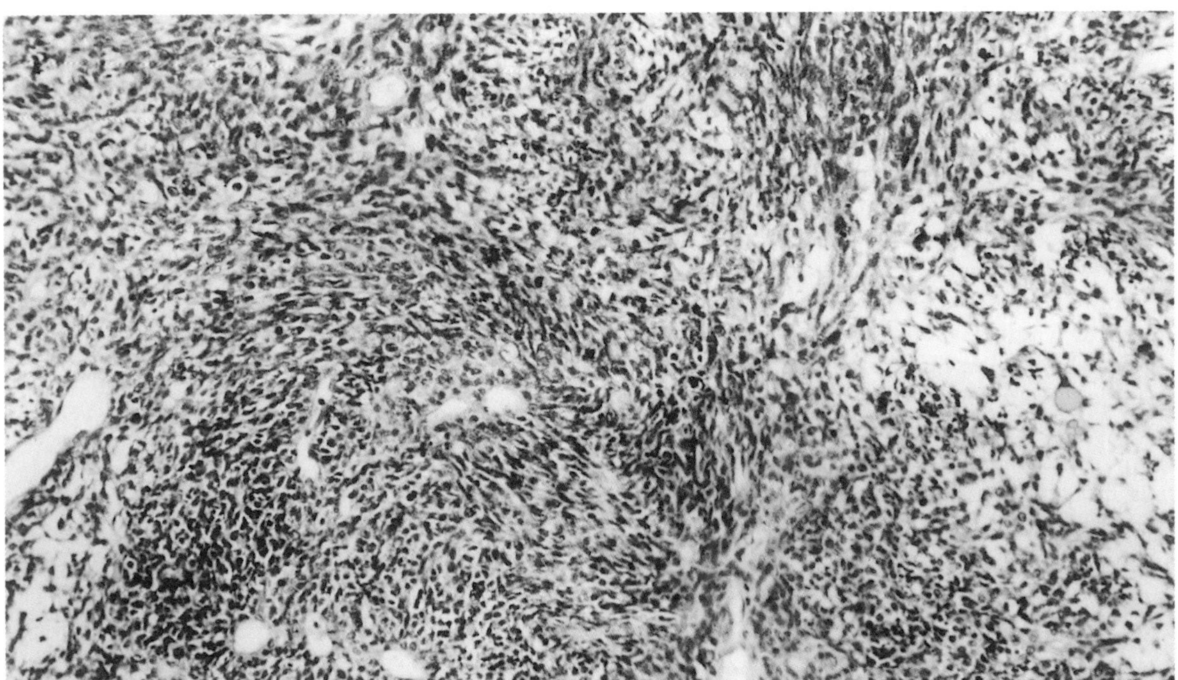

Fig. 26.3 Low grade endometrioid stromal sarcoma. Vascularity is prominent. Nuclear pleiomorphism and mitotic activity are minimal. H + E ×125

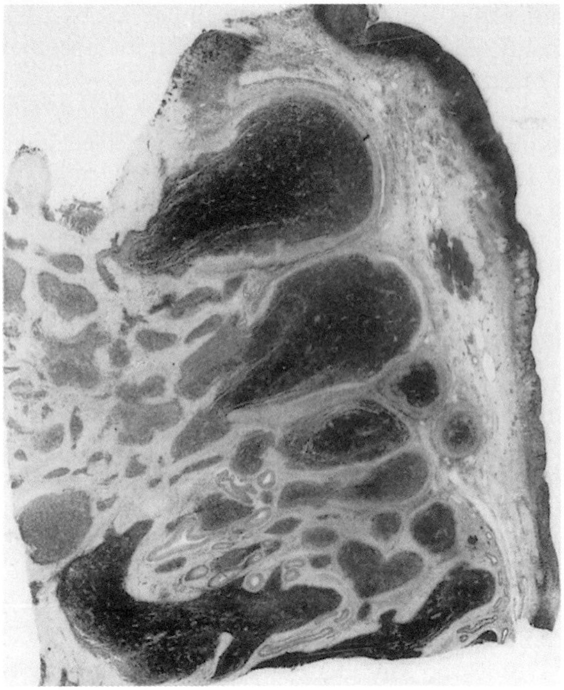

Fig. 26.4 Low grade endometrioid stromal sarcoma. Slug-like processes of hypercellular tumor infiltrate the ovarian medulla. The contralateral ovary was the site of a primary tumor mass 15 cm in diameter. H + E ×5

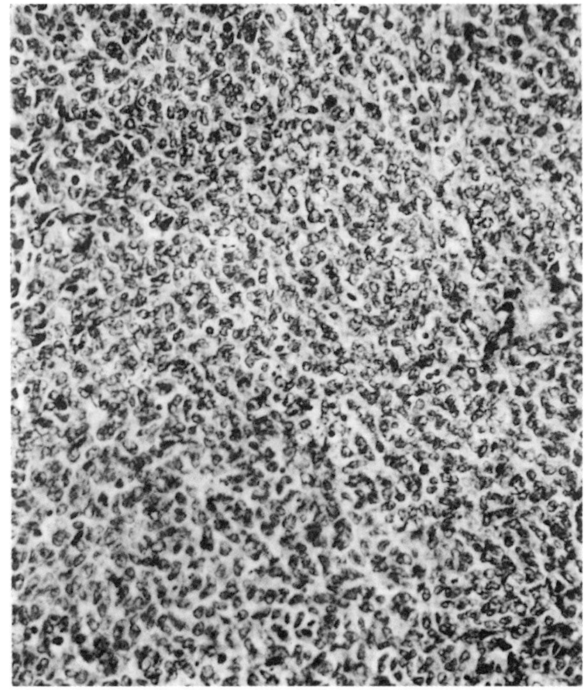

Fig. 26.5 Low grade endometrioid stromal sarcoma. Cells show scant cytoplasm, no appreciable mitotic activity, and little nuclear atypia. H + E ×150

grade endometrioid stromal sarcomas. This diagnostic difficulty is further increased by endometrioid stromal sarcomas occasionally exhibiting nests or cords of cells with nuclear palisading. Nuclear grooving is usually apparent in the granulosa cell tumors, while apparent endovascular extensions in endometrioid stromal sarcomas are useful distinguishing features, when present. Reticulin stains tend to exhibit sparse reticulin fibers in sarcoma-like areas of sex cord–stromal tumors, and rich fine networks in endometrioid stromal sarcomas. Immunohistochemical staining for inhibin is positive in most granulosa cell tumors, and negative in stromal sarcomas.

MALIGNANT MIXED MULLERIAN TUMORS

Low grade (mullerian adenosarcomas)

These differ from the sarcomas described above in that a benign epithelial component is also present. They differ from ordinary adenofibromas in that their stroma is hypercellular and often frankly sarcomatous. The term 'adenosarcoma' was used first by Clement & Scully (1974) to describe such tumors in the uterus, and has since been applied to adnexal neoplasms (Clement & Scully 1978, Kao & Norris 1978, Russell et al 1979, Kerner et al 1989). These tumors are unilateral and mostly confined to the ovaries at laparotomy. Their mean age of incidence is about 50 years.

Macroscopic features

Adenosarcomas measure about 10 cm in average diameter, some with smooth external surfaces and others with external papillary or polypoid excrescences. Their cut surfaces are spongy and multicystic (containing clear or yellowish fluid) with intervening tough fibrous tissue. Focal hemorrhage may be present in larger tumors.

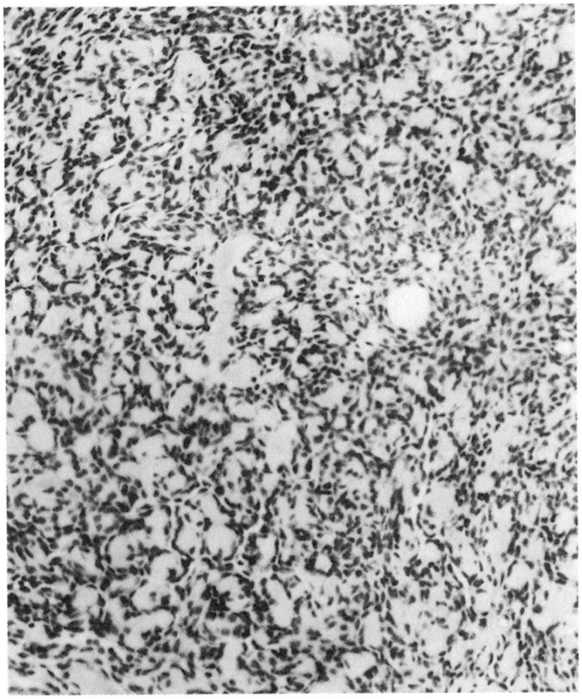

Fig. 26.6 Low grade endometrioid stromal sarcoma. Prominent deposition of intercellular hyaline material. H + E ×125

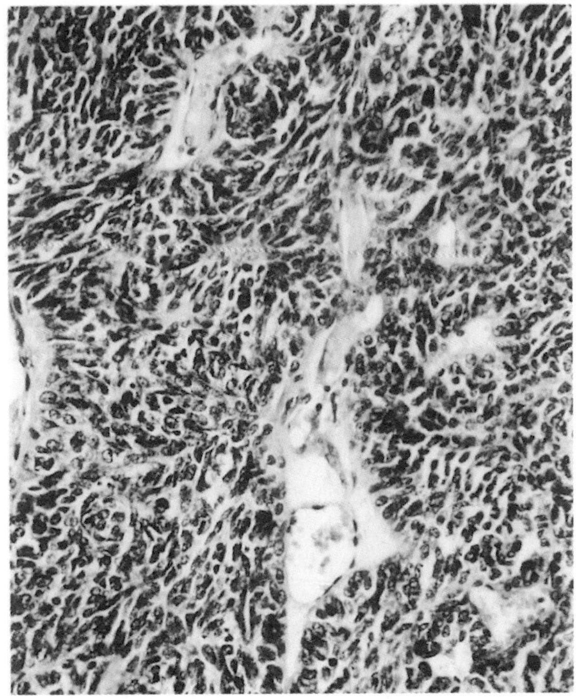

Fig. 26.7 High grade endometrioid stromal sarcoma with larger, more pleiomorphic, and densely hyperchromatic nuclei (contrast with Fig. 26.5). H + E ×150

Microscopic features

Adenosarcomas show an epithelial component which is usually endometrial in type and disposed in clefts or cystic spaces. Less often they exhibit a serous papillary pattern (Figs 26.9, 26.10). Pseudostratification and nuclear hyperchromatism are sometimes present. The stroma is usually most cellular immediately adjacent to the epithelium, but varies greatly within each tumor. Stromal cell nuclei are more pleiomorphic than in benign adenofibromas, and mitoses are increased up to 5 per 10HPF in tumors subcategorized as 'cellular adenofibromas', and 2–25 per 10HPF in those designated as 'adenosarcoma' by Kao & Norris (1978). Heterologous elements infrequently occur in the stroma of corresponding uterine lesions, for which reason Kao & Norris (1978) prefer to designate them as 'benign and low grade variants of mixed mesodermal tumors'. A solitary example of so-called 'benign mixed mullerian tumor' of the ovary has been reported (Flam & Silfversward 1992).

High grade (carcinosarcomas, mixed mesodermal tumors)

These comparatively rare tumors contain epithelial and mesenchymal elements, both of which are histologically malignant. The mesenchymal elements may, on the one hand, differentiate towards tissues 'homologous' to the mullerian tract (endometrial stroma, fibrous tissue, smooth muscle). On the other hand, they may show 'heterologous' tissues foreign to the mullerian tract (bone, cartilage, fat, skeletal muscle). Heterologous elements, such as rhabdomyoblasts, cartilage, osteoid, or fat, can be prominent and widespread, or limited to occasional small foci. Of the 300 or so cases in the English literature (Carlson et al 1983, Morrow et al 1984, Dictor 1985, Dinh et al 1988, Deligdisch et al 1988, Sahin & Benda 1988, Suggs et al 1988, Clarke 1990, Hano et al 1990, Pfeiffer et al 1991, Barakat et al 1992, Haba et al 1993, de Brito et al 1993, Boucher & Tetu 1994), one-third fall into the homologous group. Barwick & LiVolsi (1980) point out that all sarcomas

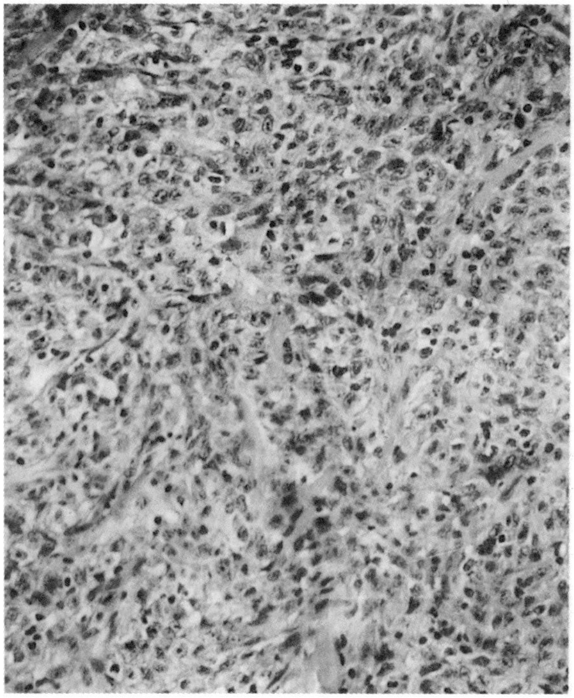

Fig. 26.8 High grade endometrioid stromal sarcoma. Cells exhibit pronounced nuclear pleiomorphism and prominent nucleoli. H + E ×150

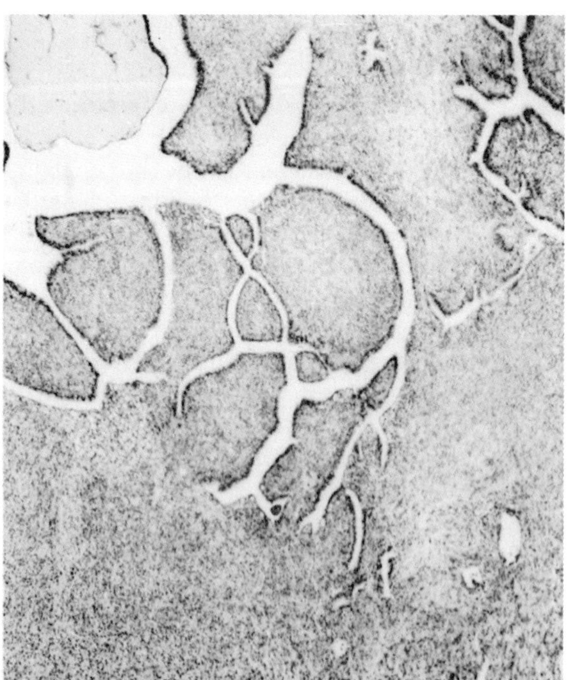

Fig. 26.9 Ovarian adenosarcoma. Low power showing a coarse papillary pattern and hypercellular stroma. H + E ×30

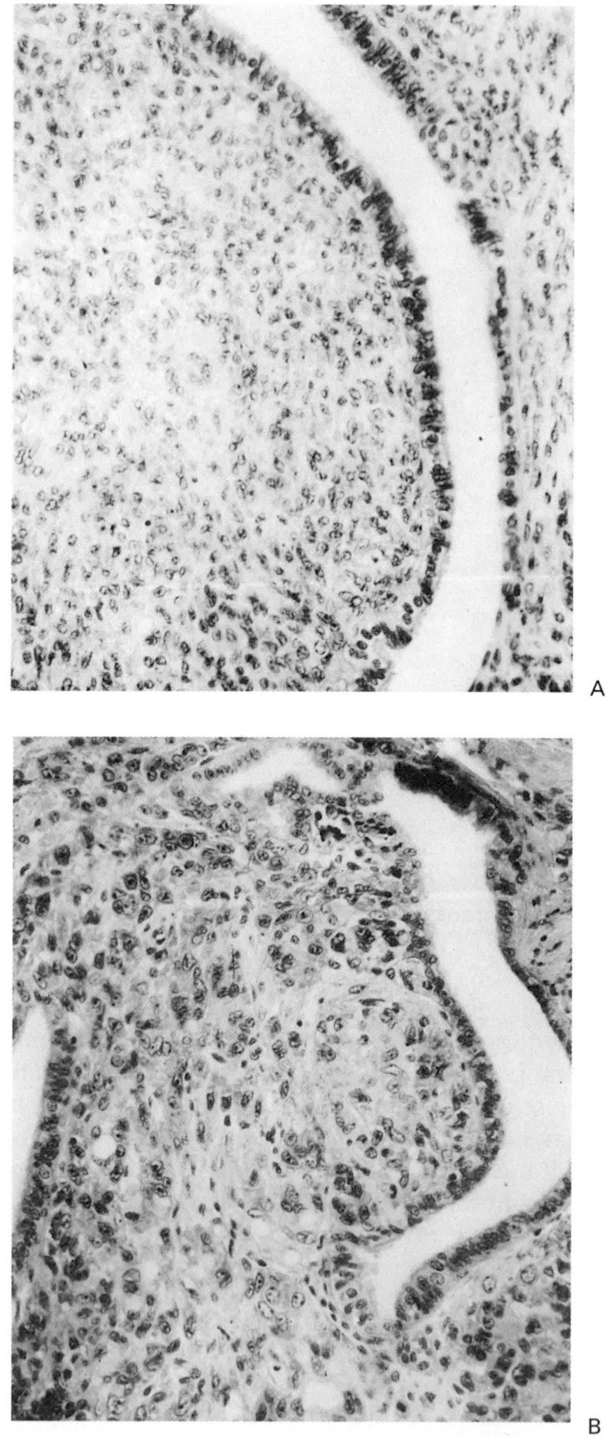

Fig. 26.10 Ovarian adenosarcoma. (A) Benign, ciliated, serous (tubal) type epithelium and atypical, hypercellular stroma. (B) Pelvic metastasis which developed 5 months after initial surgery. Nuclear changes in the stromal cells are more marked, but the epithelium is still cytologically benign. Reproduced, with permission, from Russell et al 1979). H + E ×150

(except fibrosarcoma) are heterologous to the ovary, and suggest that there is no justification for this distinction. There are conflicting views on the prognostic importance of various morphological features such as epithelial (Barakat et al 1992, Boucher & Tetu 1994) and mesenchymal elements (Dictor 1985). Recent immunohistochemical evidence has been published, both for (Masuda et al 1987, Hano et al 1990, de Brito et al 1993, Haba et al 1993) and against (Clarke 1990) the concept that the mesenchymal elements may arise by a process of metaplasia from the carcinoma (i.e. so-called 'metaplastic' carcinoma). Rarely, they are seen to arise in ovarian endometriosis.

They account for less than 1% of malignant ovarian neoplasms and are almost exclusively reported in postmenopausal women (often nulliparous), with a mean age of incidence of 60 years. They are bilateral in 10% of cases, and in over 85% of patients the tumor exhibits extraovarian abdominal spread at diagnosis. The progression of these tumors is rapid; only one-quarter of patients survive 2 years (with a median survival of 10 months), and examples of long-term survival are anecdotal, with poor results for combination chemotherapy (Carlson et al 1983, Terada et al 1989, Barakat et al 1992). Similar neoplasms are, of course, far more commonly seen in the uterus, but occasional extraovarian malignant mixed mullerian tumors may arise from the fallopian tubes (Imachi et al 1992) or from the pelvic or abdominal peritoneum (Garde et al 1991, Solis et al 1991, Nimaroff et al 1993, Chen 1996).

Cytogenetic and molecular genetic studies

Two case reports have been published that indicate, among other chromosomal abnormalities, a B-group isochromosome i(5p) (Pejovic et al 1990).

Macroscopic features

Carcinosarcomas and malignant mixed mesodermal tumors are large, averaging 15–20 cm in diameter, with bosselated outer surfaces showing prominent vessels and focal hemorrhage. Cut surfaces reveal yellow to brown friable fleshy nodules, soft in consistency and showing obvious

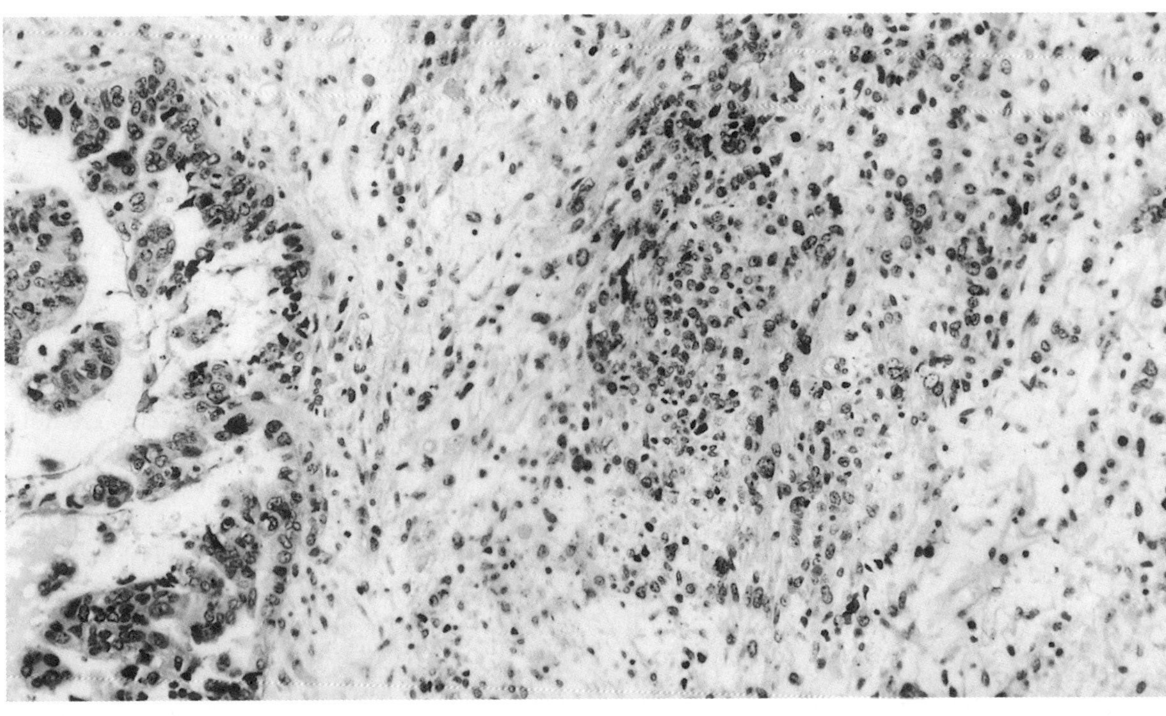

Fig. 26.11 Homologous malignant mixed mullerian tumor with typical high grade serous carcinoma (left) and a malignant stromal component of poorly defined and rather nondescript small cells with marked mitotic activity. H + E ×125

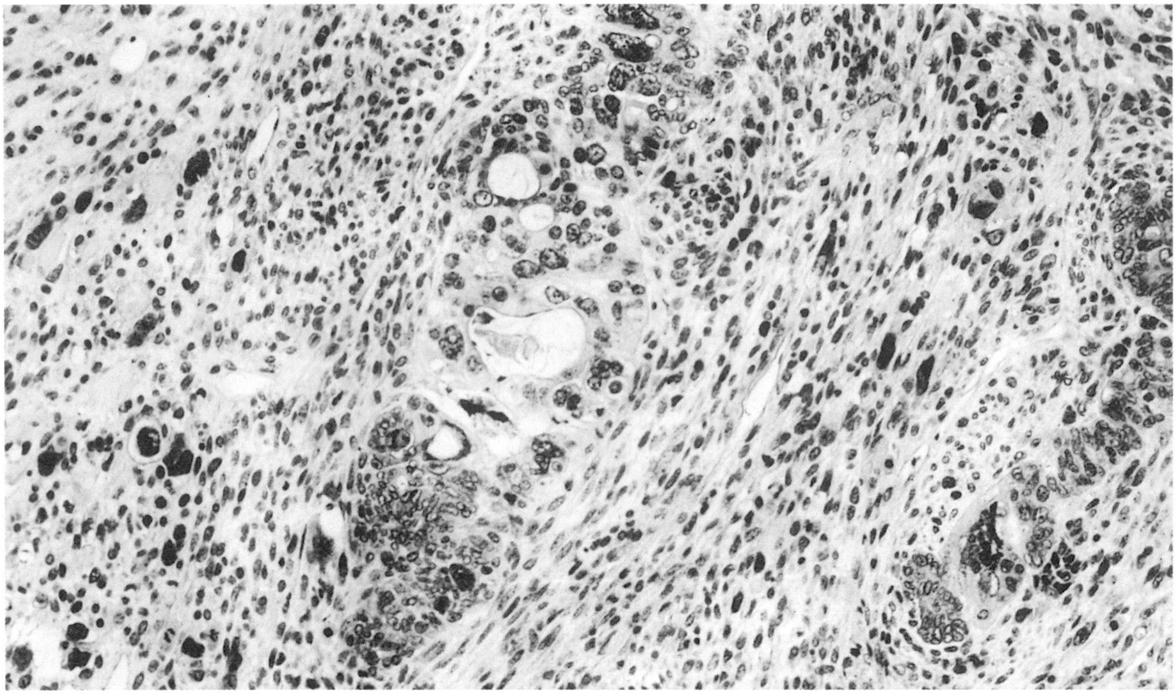

Fg. 26.12 Homologous malignant mixed mullerian tumor with poorly differentiated endometrioid carcinoma admixed with high grade 'spindle-cell' sarcoma. Cellular pleiomorphism is prominent in both components. H + E ×125

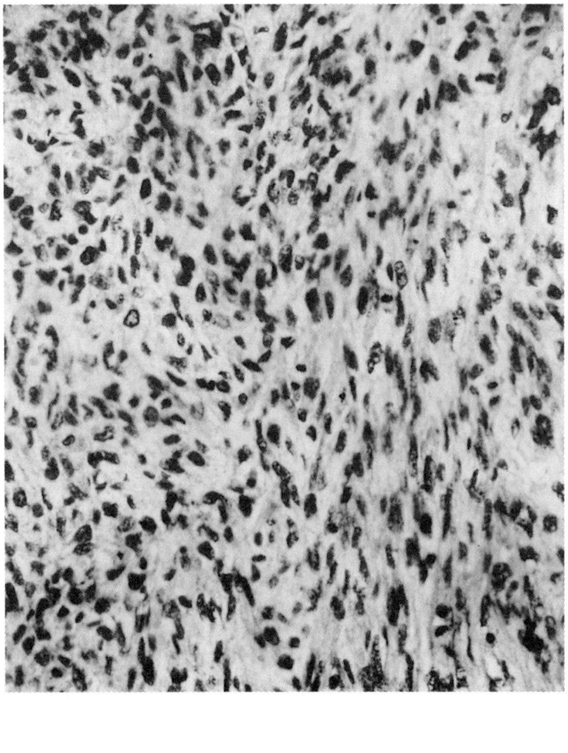

hemorrhage and necrosis. A variable cystic component usually contains polypoid excrescences and bloodstained fluid. Heterologous (mixed mesodermal) sarcomas and mixed tumors may show cartilage or bone.

Microscopic features

The epithelial element in high grade malignant mixed mullerian tumors is, in our experience, most commonly serous carcinoma (Fig. 26.11). Less frequently, endometrioid (Fig. 26.12), mucinous, clear cell, or squamous elements are noted. Other investigators have found endometrioid differentiation the most common (Morrow et al 1984, Dinh et al 1988). If the epithelium is mucinous, care should be taken to differentiate such

Fig. 26.13 True sarcomatous nodule, showing some features of smooth muscle differentiation, in the wall of an atypically proliferating mucinous tumor. It is arguable whether such tumors are best categorized here or with other mucinous neoplasms. H + E ×150

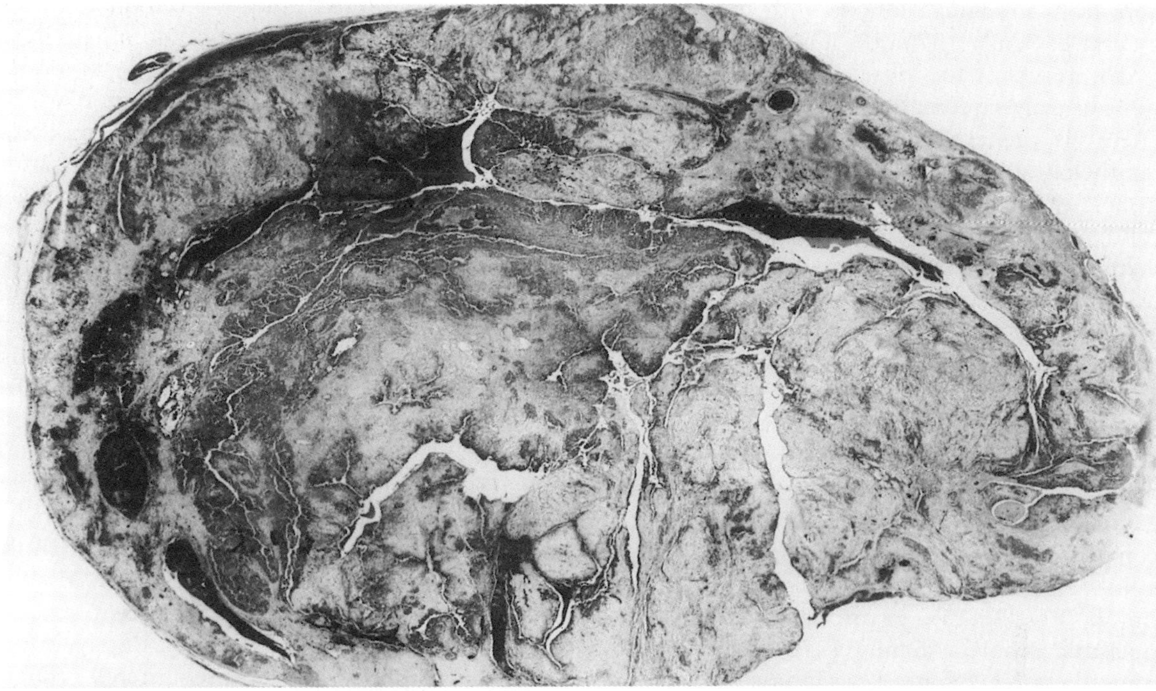

Fig. 26.14 Homologous malignant mixed mullerian tumor showing the variegated appearance occasioned by a complex admixture of epithelial and stromal elements. The fine slit-like spaces (center left) suggest serous epithelial differentiation. Pale myxoid stroma is noted to the lower right. H + E ×3

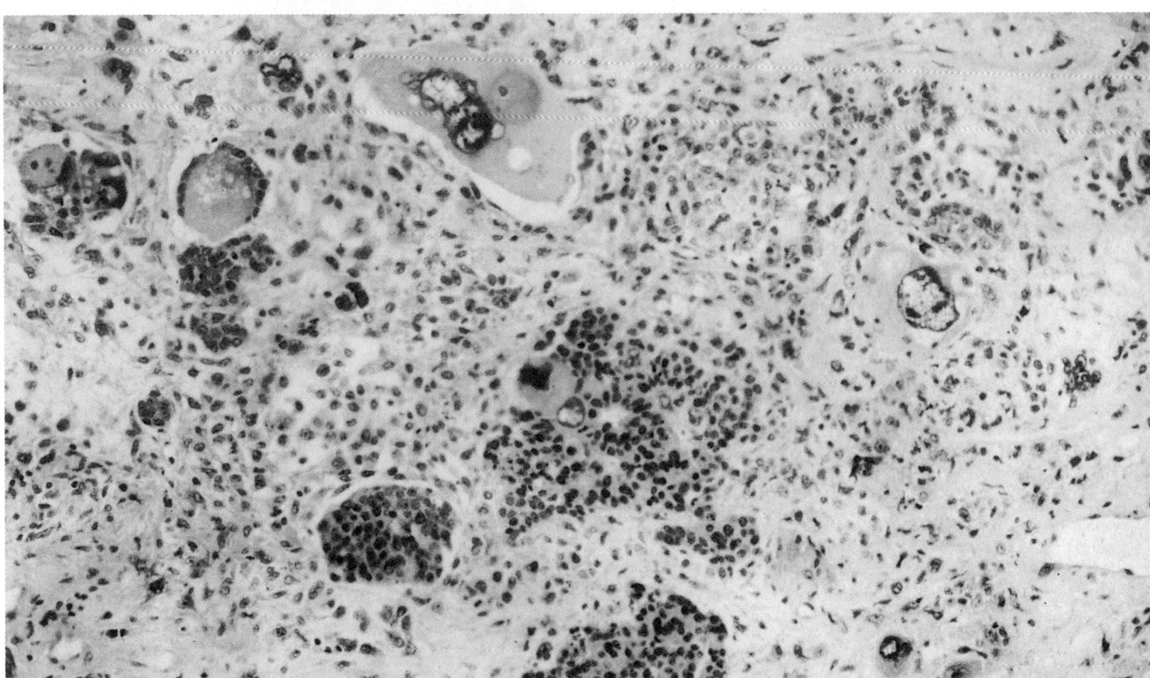

Fig. 26.15 Homologous malignant mixed mullerian tumor with much variability in the epithelial component. Clustered small uniform cells are seen, as well as bizarre giant cells – the latter identified only immunohistochemically as epithelial in nature. H + E ×125

tumors from mucinous lesions with mural nodules (Prat & Scully 1979a,b). The latter nodules may be reactive to invasive carcinoma (see Ch. 24) or truly sarcomatous (Fig. 26.13).

There is generally a complex admixture of epithelial and malignant stromal elements (Fig. 26.14), particularly if the latter is composed of undifferentiated or primitive myxoid mesenchyme; transitions, however, are uncommon. Reticulin-rich (sarcomatous areas) and reticulin-poor (carcinomatous areas) zones are typical, and positive immunohistochemical stains for EMA and cytokeratins (AE1/AE3 and CAM 5.2) and negative staining for vimentin assist in distinguishing poorly differentiated carcinoma from sarcoma, although focal coexpression of keratin and vimentin may be present in spindle cell sarcoma-like areas (Sahin & Benda 1988). Pleiomorphic and bizarre epithelial giant cells are common (Fig. 26.15), as are cells with hyaline cytoplasmic droplets (Scully 1979). Large fields composed entirely of either carcinoma or sarcoma may be encountered, and in occasional tumors one or other component may predominate in the tumor overall. However, the finding of even a small focus of sarcoma in a large tumor justifies the diagnosis of malignant mixed mullerian tumor, as the behavior of the lesion and its attendant prognosis are significantly and unfavorably altered in such cases.

Sarcomatous elements are predominantly hypercellular sheets of small hyperchromatic round to spindle cells, with a high mitotic rate and without apparent differentiation. In routine H + E sections, chondrosarcoma is the most frequently encountered heterologous stromal element (Fig. 26.16); less often, malignant osteoid (Fig. 26.17) and skeletal muscle (Fig. 26.18) may be seen. Recent use of immunohistochemical techniques to identify myoglobin (Mukai et al 1980) and desmin suggest that rhabdomyoblasts are more common than has previously been reported (Dehner et al 1971). Rarely, bizarre malignant lipoblasts are encountered (Dictor

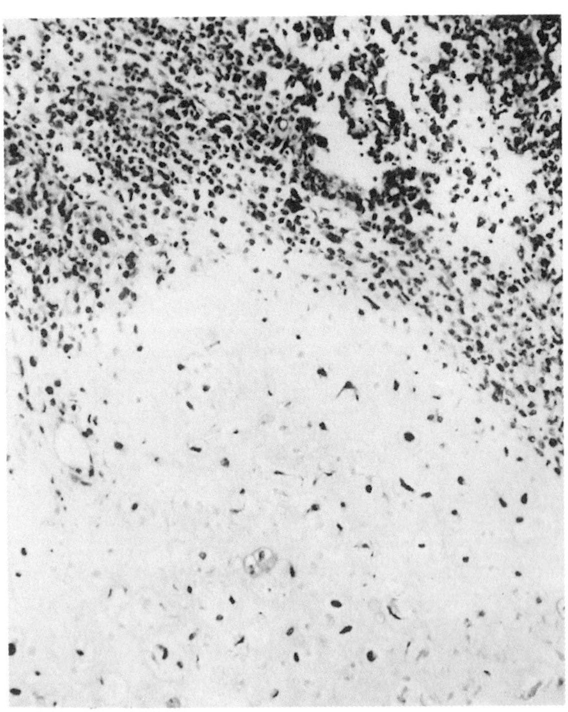

Fig. 26.16 Heterologous malignant mixed mullerian tumor with islands of malignant cartilage. H + E ×75

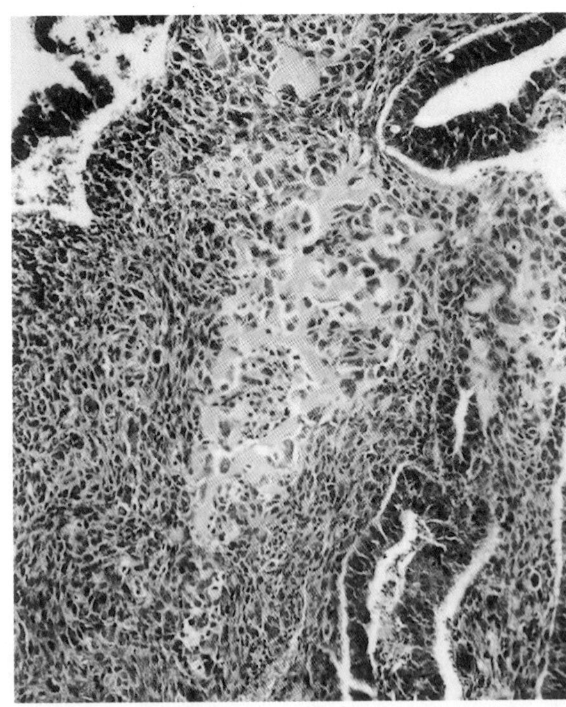

Fig. 26.17 Heterologous malignant mixed mullerian tumor with small discrete foci of malignant osteoid. The nearby epithelium is endometrioid in type. H + E ×75

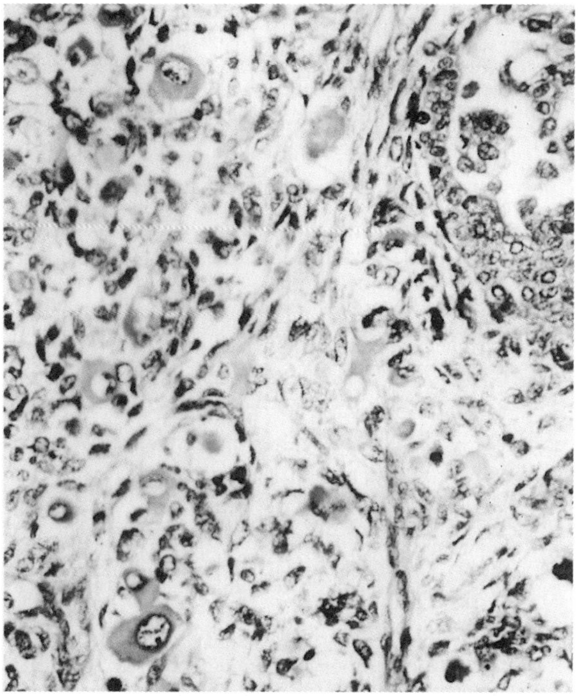

Fig. 26.18 Heterologous malignant mixed mullerian tumor with bizarre mononuclear cells having dense eosinophilic cytoplasm and resembling embryonal rhabdomyoblasts. Immunohistochemical stains for myoglobin or desmin should be positive to confirm skeletal muscle differentiation. H + E ×150

1985), and an apparently unique example showing trophoblastic differentiation has been reported (Barua & Richmond 1988).

Evidence of pelvic endometriosis is seen more frequently than would be expected by chance, and the tumors may rarely arise within ovarian endometriotic cysts.

Table 26.2 Differential diagnosis: malignant mixed mullerian tumors versus immature teratomas

Malignant mixed mullerian tumor	Immature teratoma
Clinical	
Mean age of incidence 60 years (rarely <40 years)	Mean age of incidence 16 years (rarely >40 years)
Histological	
Only mesodermally derived tissues present	Tissue elements from all three embryonic layers present
Neuroectoderm almost never present	Neuroectoderm virtually always present
Totally haphazard arrangement of epithelial and mesenchymal elements	Variably ordered arrangement of tissues, especially ectodermal and endodermal elements
Malignant tissues resemble adult carcinomas/sarcomas	Malignant tissues resemble immature fetal tissues

Differential diagnosis

Discrimination between malignant mixed mullerian tumors and immature teratomas (see Ch. 47) involves clinical and histological features (Table 26.2). Immature teratomas occur in young women (rarely over 40 years). Microscopically, the teratomas will show some orderly arrangement of the immature stromal and epithelial tissues with ectodermal (particularly neuroectoderm) and endodermal (gut, respiratory) as well as mesodermal elements present. Malignant mixed mullerian tumors occur in postmenopausal women, and feature gross disorganization of malignant adult tissues, with ectodermal and endodermal derivatives conspicuously absent in all but the rarest of instances (Fetissof et al 1989, Ehrmann et al 1990).

REFERENCES

Azoury R S, Woodruff J D 1971 Primary ovarian sarcomas. Report of 43 cases from the Emil Novak ovarian tumor registry. Obstetrics and Gynecology 37: 920–941

Barakat R R, Rubin S C, Wong G, Saigo P E, Markman M, Hoskins W J 1992 Mixed mesodermal tumor of the ovary: analysis of prognostic factors in 31 cases. Obstetrics and Gynecology 80: 660–664

Barua R, Richmond D 1988 Trophoblastic differentiation in a malignant mixed mesodermal tumor of the ovary. Human Pathology 19: 1235–1236

Barwick K W, LiVolsi V A 1980 Malignant mixed mesodermal tumors of the ovary. A clinicopathologic assessment of 12 cases. American Journal of Surgical Pathology 4: 37–42

Boucher D, Tetu B 1994 Morphologic prognostic factors of malignant mixed mullerian tumors of the ovary: a clinicopathologic study of 15 cases. International Journal of Gynecological Pathology 13: 22–28

Carlson J A Jr, Edwards C, Wharton J T, Gallager H S, Delclos L, Rutledge F 1983 Mixed mesodermal sarcoma of the ovary. Treatment with combination radiation therapy and chemotherapy. Cancer 52: 1473–1477

Chang K L, Crabtree G S, Lim-Tan S K, Kempson R L, Hendrickson M R 1993 Primary extrauterine endometrial stromal neoplasms: a clinicopathologic study of 20 cases and review of the literature. International Journal of Gynecological Pathology 12: 282–296

Chen K T K 1996 Malignant mixed müllerian tumor of the

peritoneum. International Journal of Surgical Pathology 3: 155–162

Chen K T K, Hendricks E J, Freeburg B 1982 Benign glandular inclusions of the peritoneum associated with leiomyomatosis peritonealis disseminata. Diagnostic Gynecology and Obstetrics 4: 41–44

Clarke T J 1990 Histogenesis of ovarian malignant mixed mesodermal tumors. Journal of Clinical Pathology 43: 287–290

Clement P B, Scully R E 1974 Mullerian adenosarcoma of the uterus. A clinicopathologic analysis of ten cases of a distinctive type of mullerian mixed tumor. Cancer 34: 1138–1149

Clement P B, Scully R E 1978 Extrauterine mesodermal (mullerian) adenosarcoma. American Journal of Clinical Pathology 69: 276–283

de Brito P A, Silverberg S G, Orenstein J M 1993 Carcinosarcoma (malignant mixed mullerian (mesodermal) tumor) of the female genital tract: immunohistochemical and ultrastructural analysis of 28 cases. Human Pathology 24: 132–142

Dehner L P, Norris H J, Taylor H B 1971 Carcinosarcomas and mixed mesodermal tumors of the ovary. Cancer 27: 207–216

Deligdisch L, Plaxe S, Cohen C J 1988 Extrauterine pelvic malignant mixed mesodermal tumors. A study of 10 cases with immunohistochemistry. International Journal of Gynecological Pathology 7: 361–372

Dictor M 1985 Malignant mixed mesodermal tumor of the ovary: A report of 22 cases. Obstetrics and Gynecology 65: 720–724

Dinh T V, Slavin R E, Bhagavan B S, Hannigan E V, Tiamson E M, Yandell R B 1988 Mixed mesodermal tumors of the ovary; a clinicopathologic study of 14 cases. Obstetrics and Gynecology 72: 409–412

Dixit S, Singhal S, Baboo H A et al 1993 Leiomyosarcoma of the ovary. Journal of Postgraduate Medicine 39: 151–153

Dodd G D 3rd, Lancaster K T, Moulton J S 1989 Ovarian lipoleiomyoma: a fat-containing mass in the female pelvis. American Journal of Radiology 153: 1007–1008

Ehrmann R L, Weidner N, Welch W R, Gleiberman I 1990 Malignant mixed mullerian tumor of the ovary with prominent neuroectodermal differentiation (teratoid carcinosarcoma). International Journal of Gynecological Pathology 9: 272–282

Fallahzadeh H, Dockerty M B, Lee R A 1972 Leiomyoma of the ovary: report of five cases and review of the literature. American Journal of Obstetrics and Gynecology 113: 394–398

Fetissof F, Arbeille B, Lansac J, Lhuintre Y 1989 Tumeur mixte mesodermique maligne de l'ovaire avec contingent neuro-ectodermique. Annals de Pathologie 9: 204–208

Flam F, Silfversward C 1992 Benign mixed mullerian tumor of the ovary. Acta Obstetricia et Gynecologica Scandinavica 71: 485–486

Friedman H D, Mazur M T 1991 Primary ovarian leiomyosarcoma. An immunohistochemical and ultrastructural study. Archives of Pathology and Laboratory Medicine 115: 941–945

Garde J R, Jones M A, McAfee R, Tarraza H M 1991 Extragenital malignant mixed mullerian tumor: review of the literature. Gynecologic Oncology 43: 186–190

Haba R, Kobayashi S, Miki H et al 1993 Mixed mesodermal tumor of the ovary: immunohistochemical study with histogenetic consideration. Acta Pathologica Japonica 43: 696–701

Hano H, Endo M, Sekino S, Takasaki S, Ushigome S 1990 Malignant mixed mullerian tumor of the ovary. Report of a case studied by immunohistochemistry. Acta Pathologica Japonica 40: 845–850

Hendrickson M R, Kempson R L 1980 Surgical pathology of the uterine corpus. W B Saunders, Philadelphia, p 389–529

Imachi M, Tsukamoto N, Shigematsu T et al 1992 Malignant mixed mullerian tumor of the fallopian tube: report of two cases and review of the literature. Gynecologic Oncology 47: 114–124

Kandalaft P L, Esteban J M 1992 Bilateral massive ovarian leiomyomata in a young woman: a case report with review of the literature. Modern Pathology 5: 586–589

Kao G F, Norris H J 1978 Benign and low grade variants of mixed mesodermal tumor (adenosarcoma) of the ovary and adnexal region. Cancer 42: 1314–1324

Kerner H, Lichtig C, Beck D 1989 Extrauterine mullerian adenosarcoma of the peritoneal mesothelium: a clinicopathologic and electron microscopic study. Obstetrics and Gynecology 73: 510–513

Kitazawa S, Shiraishi N, Maeda S 1992 Leiomyomatosis peritonealis disseminata with adipocytic differentiation. Acta Obstetricia et Gynecologica Scandinavica 71: 482–484

Kokcu A, Alvur Y, Baris Y S, Kuskonmaz I 1994 Leiomyomatosis peritonealis disseminata. Acta Obstetricia et Gynecologica Scandinavica 73: 81–83

Kuo T-T, London S N, Dinh T V 1980 Endometriosis occurring in leiomyomatosis peritonealis disseminata. Ultrastructural study and histogenetic consideration. American Journal of Surgical Pathology 4: 197–204

Macri C I, Vasilev S A 1993 Bilateral giant primary ovarian leiomyomas. A case report. Journal of Reproductive Medicine 38: 480–482

Mallya S, MacFarlane I A, Taylor W, van Heyningen C 1990 Thecal cell reaction associated with an ovarian leiomyoma and presenting with virilization. Gynecologic Endocrinology 4: 271–276

Masuda A, Takeda A, Fukami H, Yamada C, Matsuyama M 1987 Characteristics of cell lines established from a mixed mesodermal tumor of the human ovary. Carcinomatous cells are changeable to sarcomatous cells. Cancer 60: 2696–2703

Matamala M F, Nogales F F, Aneiros J, Herraiz M A, Caracuel M D 1988 International Journal of Gynecological Pathology 7: 190–196

Mira J L 1991 Lipoleiomyoma of the ovary: report of a case and review of the English literature. International Journal of Gynecological Pathology 10: 198–202

Monk B J, Nieberg R, Berek J S 1993 Primary leiomyosarcoma of the ovary in a perimenarchal female. Gynecologic Oncology 48: 389–393

Morrow C P, d'Ablaing G, Brady L W, Blessing J A, Hreshchyshyn M M 1984 A clinical and pathologic study of 30 cases of malignant mixed mullerian epithelial and mesenchymal ovarian tumors: A Gynecologic Oncology Group study. Gynecologic Oncology 18: 278–292

Mukai K, Varela-Duran J, Nochomovitz L E 1980 The rhabdomyoblast in mixed mullerian tumors of the uterus and ovary: an immunohistochemical study of myoglobin in 25 cases. American Journal of Clinical Pathology 74: 101–104

Nimaroff M, Gal D, Susin M, Lovecchio J 1993 Extragenital

malignant mixed mullerian tumor. European Journal of Gynaecological Oncology 14: 23–27
Nogales F F, Ayala A, Ruiz-Avila I, Sirvent J J 1991 Myxoid leiomyosarcoma of the ovary: analysis of three cases. Human Pathology 22: 1268–1273
Parish J M, Lufkin E G, Lee R A, Gaffey T A 1984 Ovarian leiomyoma with hilus cell hyperplasia that caused virilization. Mayo Clinic Proceedings 59: 275–277
Pejovic T, Heim S, Mandahl N, Floderus U M, Willwn H, Mitelman F 1990 Complex karyotypic anomalies, including an i(5p) marker chromosome, in malignant mixed mesodermal tumor of the ovary. Cancer Genetics and Cytogenetics 46: 65 69
Pfeiffer P, Hardt-Masden M, Rex S, Holund B, Bertelsen K 1991 Malignant mixed mullerian tumors of the ovary: report of 13 cases. Acta Obstetricia et Gynecologica Scandinavica 70: 179–180
Prasad K R, Aruna C, Saheb D A 1993 Primary leiomyoma of ovary. Indian Journal of Medical Science 47: 39–41
Prat J, Scully R E 1979a Ovarian mucinous tumors with sarcoma-like mural nodules. A report of seven cases. Cancer 44: 1332–1344
Prat J, Scully R E 1979b Sarcomas in ovarian mucinous tumors. A report of two cases. Cancer 44: 1321–1325
Prayson R A, Hart W R 1992 Primary smooth-muscle tumors of the ovary. A clinicopathologic study of four leiomyomas and two mitotically active leiomyomas. Archives of Pathology and Laboratory Medicine 116: 1068–1071
Randrianjafisamindrakotroka N S, Chadli-Debbiche A, Phillipe E 1994 Les leiomyomes de l'ovaire. A propos de douze cas. Archives de Anatomie Cytologie et Pathologie 42: 26–28
Rubin S C, Wheeler J E, Mikuta J J 1986 Malignant leiomyomatosis peritonealis disseminata. Obstetrics and Gynecology 68: 126–130
Russell P, Slavutin L, Laverty C R, Cooper-Booth J 1979 Extrauterine mesodermal (Mullerian) adenosarcoma. A case report. Pathology 11: 557–560
Sahin A, Benda J A 1988 An immunohistochemical study of primary ovarian sarcoma. An evaluation of nine tumors. International Journal of Gynecological Pathology 7: 268–279
Scully R E 1979 Tumors of the ovary and maldeveloped gonads, AFIP fascicle 16, 2nd series. Armed Forces Institute of Pathology, Washington, DC, p 53–151
Shakfeh S M, Woodruff J D 1987 Primary ovarian sarcomas: report of 46 cases and review of the literature. Obstetrical and Gynecological Survey 42: 331–349
Silverberg S G, Fernandez F N 1981 Endolymphatic stromal myosis of the ovary. A report of three cases and literature review. Gynecologic Oncology 12: 129–138
Solis O G, Bui H X, Malfetano J H, Ross J S 1991 Extragenital primary mixed malignant mesodermal tumor. Gynecologic Oncology 43: 182–185
Sonobe H, Hayashi K, Takahashi K, Ohtsuki Y, Okatani Y, Sagara Y 1989 A case of ovarian leiomyoma. Acta Medica Okayama 43: 131–134
Suggs C L 3rd, Lee J L Jr, Choi H, Lewis G C 1988 Malignant mixed mesodermal tumors of the ovary. A report of 13 cases. American Journal of Clinical Oncology 11: 12–15
Tavassoli F A, Norris H J 1982 Peritoneal leiomyomatosis (leiomyomatosis peritonealis disseminata): a clinicopathologic study of 20 cases with ultrastructural observations. International Journal of Gynecological Pathology 1: 59–74
Terada K Y, Johnson T L, Hopkins M, Roberts J A 1989 Clinicopathologic features of ovarian mixed mesodermal tumors and carcinosarcomas. Gynecologic Oncology 32: 228–232
Tsalacopoulos G, Tiltman A J 1981 Leiomyoma of the ovary. A report of 3 cases. South African Medical Journal 59: 574–575
Varma T R, Patal R H, Burke M 1988 Virilization due to a rare ovarian tumor in a postmenopausal woman. International Journal of Gynaecology and Obstetrics 27: 443–449
Vierhout M E, Pijpers L, Tham M N, Chadha-Ajwani S 1990 Leiomyoma of the ovary. Acta Obstetrica et Gynecologica Scandinavica 69: 445–447
Walley VM 1983 Leiomyomatosis peritonealis disseminata. International Journal of Gynecological Pathology 2: 222–223
Young R H, Prat J, Scully R E 1984 Endometrioid stromal sarcomas of the ovary. A clinicopathologic analysis of 23 cases. Cancer 53: 1143–1155

27

Clear cell tumors

P. Rusell A. Farnsworth

The hallmark of these tumors is the presence of either large polyhedral clear cells (resembling to a greater or lesser extent those found in the Arias–Stella reaction of gestational endometrium), similar cells with eosinophilic granular cytoplasm, or peg-like 'hobnail' cells with little cytoplasm and large nuclei that bulge towards the lumens of cystic spaces (Figs 27.1, 27.2). Mucicarmine and diastase-PAS stained material is sometimes present at the luminal border of the cells and commonly in the luminal secretions (Norris & Robinowitz 1971); immunohistochemically, cells stain diffusely for cytokeratins (AE1/AE3, CAM 5.2), B72.3, and Leu M1, and focally for CA-125 antigen and vimentin in 10% of tumors. Electron microscopically, clear cells have cytoplasm packed with glycogen granules which obscure other organelles. Occasional lipid

A 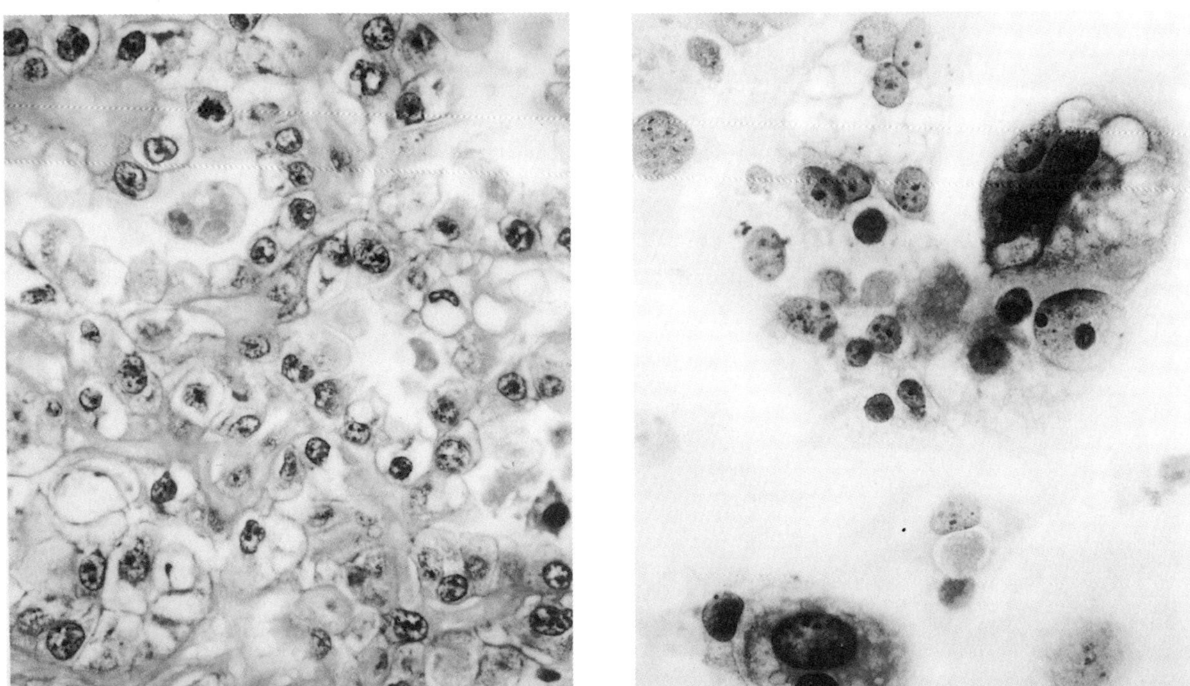 B

Fig. 27.1 Component cells of clear cell tumors. (A) Clear cell carcinoma showing large pavement-like cells with central nuclei and cytoplasm which varies from clear to eosinophilic and granular. H + E ×150. (B) Monolayer of an in vitro cell line derived from the tumor in (A). Prominently vacuolated cytoplasm and variably sized nuclei with multiple nucleoli remain characteristic of the derivative cells cultured in vitro. H + E ×300. (Material courtesy of Dr Carolien van Haaften-Day, Sydney).

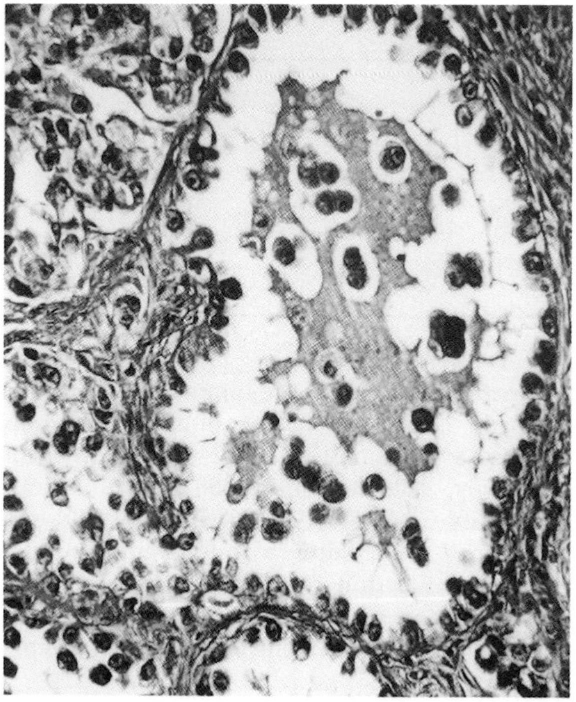

Fig. 27.2 Component cells of clear cell tumors. Cells in this field of a proliferating clear cell tumor are almost exclusively 'hobnail'. H + E ×150

droplets, lysosomal complexes, and characteristic dense bodies are noted. Apical cell surfaces exhibit short stubby microvilli. The nuclei are rounded to convoluted with variably prominent nucleoli which, electron microscopically, do not show the 'mesh-basket' pattern seen in endometrioid carcinomas (Okagaki & Richart 1970).

Clear cell tumors exhibit the same proliferative spectrum as other common epithelial tumors (Serov et al 1973), but the benign lesions rate only rare mention – only a dozen or so examples have been described in the literature (Kao & Norris 1979, Roth et al 1984, Bell & Scully 1985, Tsurunaga et al 1992) – and about 30 proliferating clear cell tumors (Russell 1979a, Roth et al 1984, Bell & Scully 1985, Katsube et al 1989). Parvilocular tumors of Schiller fit uneasily into the current taxonomic schema. Fox & Langley (1976) suggest classifying them as benign, and certainly some merge with those described by Kao & Norris (1979) and illustrated in Fig. 27.3. However,

Fig. 27.3 Parvilocular cystoma (benign clear cell adenofibroma). Cystic spaces lined by hobnail cells. H + E ×50

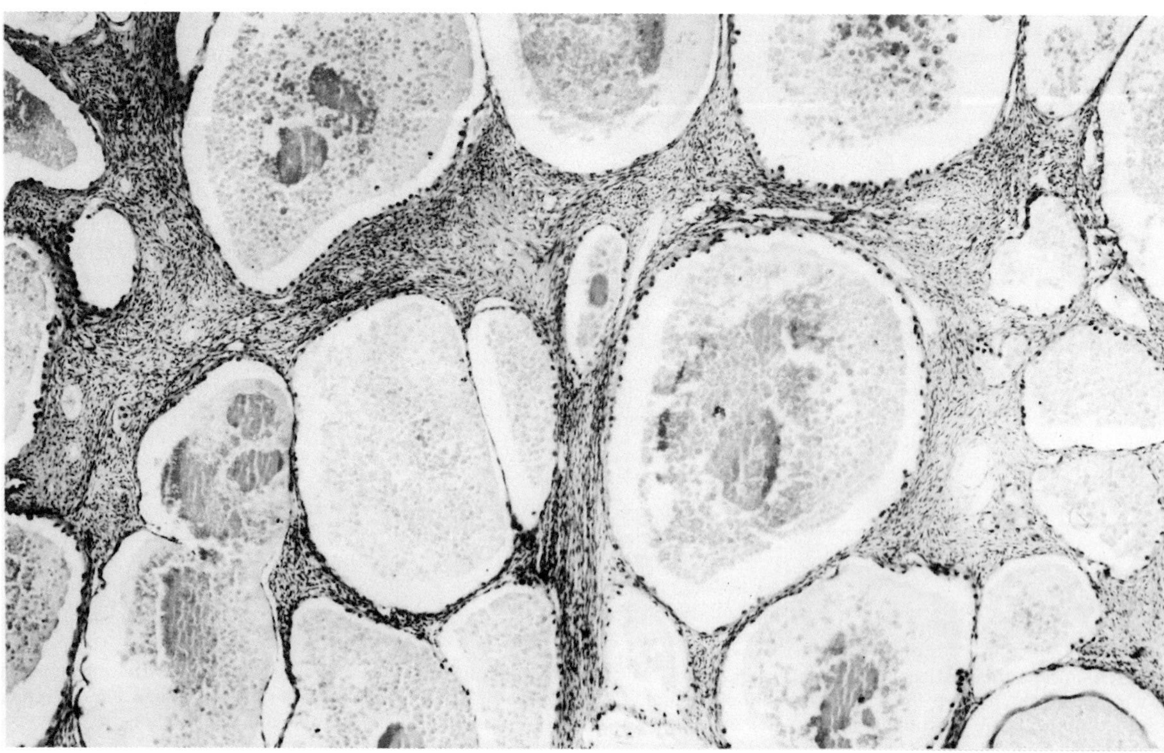

some show mitotic activity and cellular atypism; this is possibly sufficient to justify their designation as proliferating tumors (Roth et al 1984). The majority of clear cell tumors are, therefore, invasive clear cell carcinomas (Scully 1977, 1979, Brescia et al 1989, Crozier et al 1989, Jenison et al 1989, Montag et al 1989, Kennedy et al 1989, 1993), and these constitute about 5–10% of all primary ovarian malignancies.

These epithelial–stromal tumors have a greater frequency of associated pelvic endometriosis (60–65%) (Brescia et al 1989, Montag et al 1989) than any other (even endometrioid), and one-quarter can be shown to arise from the epithelial lining of endometriotic cysts (see Ch. 21). Occasional tumors have been shown to arise de novo from the ovarian serosa (Bell & Scully 1994). Mixtures of clear cell and endometrioid carcinomas are common both within the ovaries and the uterus. These observations have led to the view that clear cell carcinomas represent merely histological variants of endometrioid carcinomas (Shevchuk et al 1981). The very frequent concurrence of endometrial carcinoma and endometrioid ovarian carcinoma is not paralleled with clear cell ovarian cancer, although 40% or so of associated endometria show some estrogenic stimulation, and occasional instances of multifocal neoplasia of the female genital tract are recorded in association with ovarian clear cell carcinomas (Scharl et al 1990). Rare examples of extraovarian clear cell carcinoma are noted to have arisen from the uterine broad ligament (Aslani & Scully 1989), sigmoid mesocolon (Evans et al 1990) and pelvic and abdominal endometriosis (Hitti et al 1990).

The mean age of incidence for benign clear cell tumors is 45–46 years. In our experience, proliferating tumors occur in the same general age

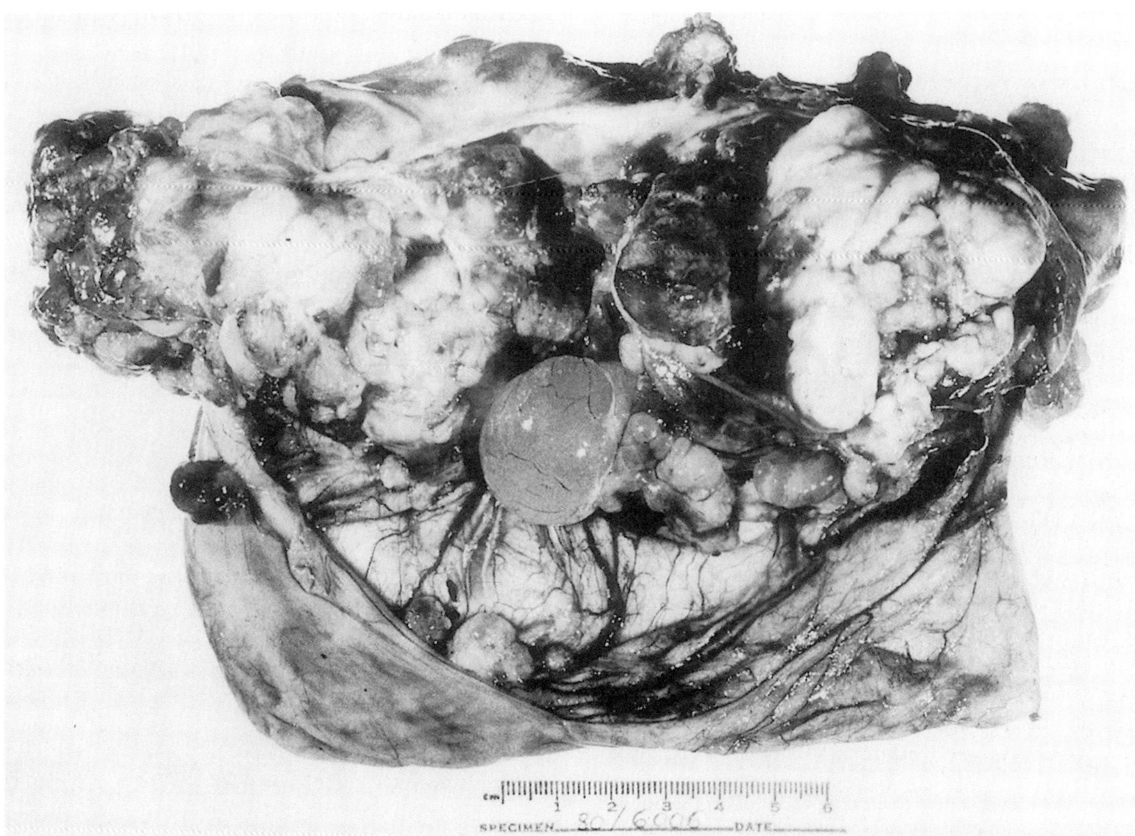

Fig. 27.4 Typical clear cell carcinoma. Cyst wall has been opened to expose solid tumor nodules protruding into the lumen

group, although the cases reported by Roth et al (1984) and Bell & Scully (1985) occurred at mean ages in the seventh decade, which is significantly older than the age for either benign or frankly malignant clear cell tumors. Extraovarian implants have not been recorded in association with clear cell tumors with this degree of proliferation, and only one case of possible distant (lung) metastasis is to be found in the literature (Bell & Scully 1985).

Typically, clear cell carcinomas occur in the fifth to seventh decades, with a peak age of incidence of about 52 years. One-half to two-thirds of women are nulliparous and the most common presenting symptoms relate to the presence of an enlarging, non-hormone-producing abdominal mass (Jenison et al 1989). Paraneoplastic hypercalcemia is an uncommon but recognized accompaniment of ovarian clear cell carcinoma (Kennedy et al 1989; see Appendix D). At laparotomy, 50% of clear cell carcinomas are confined to the ovaries, and of these stage I cases only 3% are bilateral (overall bilaterality rate of 10%). Some series have recorded a left-sided preponderance (Norris & Robinowitz 1971) amongst unilateral cases. The most sensitive prognostic index is the FIGO stage at laparotomy (Kennedy et al 1989, Montag et al 1989). The 5-year survival of patients with stage 1 tumors is about 85–93% (Shevchuk et al 1981, Brescia et al 1989), and the 5-year survival for patients in all stages is 40–50% (Crozier et al 1989, Jenison et al 1989). Follow-up data do not relate any single histological pattern or feature or clinical outcome, and grading of clear cell carcinomas is, in our view and that of others (Montag et al 1989, Kennedy et al 1993), not a productive exercise.

Macroscopic features

Benign clear cell tumors have smooth, somewhat lobulated external surfaces without adhesions. The median diameter is about 12 cm. Cut surfaces

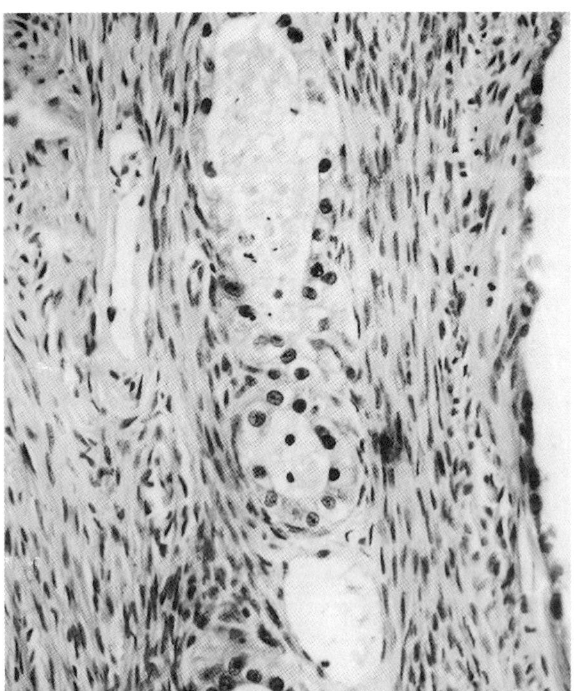

Fig. 27.5 Tubules of a benign clear cell adenofibroma lined by cuboidal cells with pale vacuolated cytoplasm. The larger cyst (right) is lined by poorly preserved hobnail cells. H + E ×150

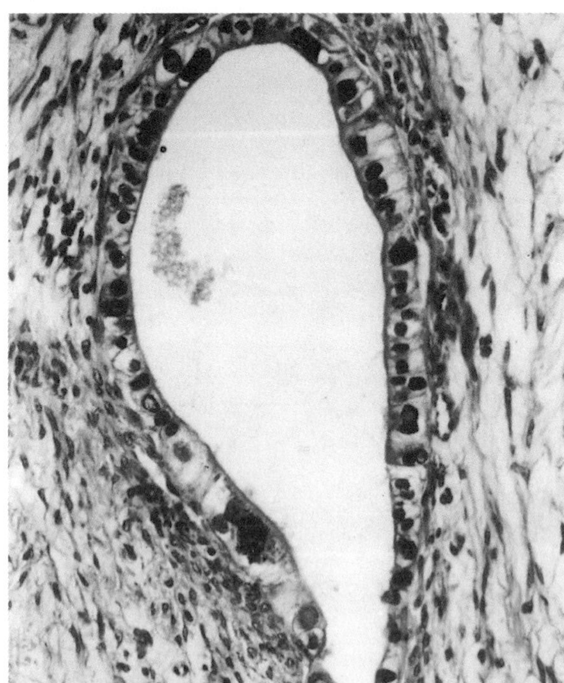

Fig. 27.6 Benign clear cell adenofibroma. Occasional glands may show mild nuclear atypia, but multilayering, luminal tufting, and increased mitotic activity are absent. H + E ×150

have a fine honeycomb of minute cysts embedded in firm rubbery stroma. Cyst fluid is clear and watery. Proliferating clear cell tumors vary up to 23 cm in diameter (mean diameter about 15 cm) and have smooth capsular surfaces. They are also unilateral adenofibromas with abundant stroma and various sized cystic spaces filled with watery fluid. Softer, more fleshy areas denote higher grade epithelial proliferation.

Invasive clear cell carcinomas vary greatly in size (up to 30 cm in diameter), with a mean size of about 15 cm. Surface adhesions are not uncommon but, in the majority of cases, these are inflammatory and do not denote extraovarian extension. The commonest gross appearance is of thick-walled unilocular cysts into which project several fleshy nodules (Fig. 27.4). The latter may be white on cut surface, but are often yellow-beige in color with focal necrosis and hemorrhage. Slightly less frequently, the cysts are multilocular, containing either watery or mucinous fluid. Rarely, the tumors are solid and fibrous.

Microscopic features

Benign clear cell tumors are adenofibromas with tubular spaces lined by one or, at most, two layers of hobnail cells (Fig. 27.3), clear cells or, less commonly, 'indifferent' cuboidal cells (Fig. 27.5). Nuclei tend to be regular in size and shape, and cellular atypia, if present, is only mild and focal (Fig. 27.6). Solid sheets of clear cells and luminal tufting are absent, and mitoses are rarely encountered. Cells contain intracytoplasmic glycogen. Mucin may be demonstrable within cystic spaces but not in cells. The intervening stroma is compact and fibrocollagenous, often being more cellular adjacent to the epithelial elements.

Atypically proliferating tumors have a similar architectural framework with fibrocollagenous or ovarian-like stroma. The cell types lining the cystic spaces are similar to those in benign tumors. Nuclear atypia (irregularity in size and shape, chromatin clumping, and prominent nucleoli) (Fig. 27.7A), epithelial budding (Fig. 27.2), and

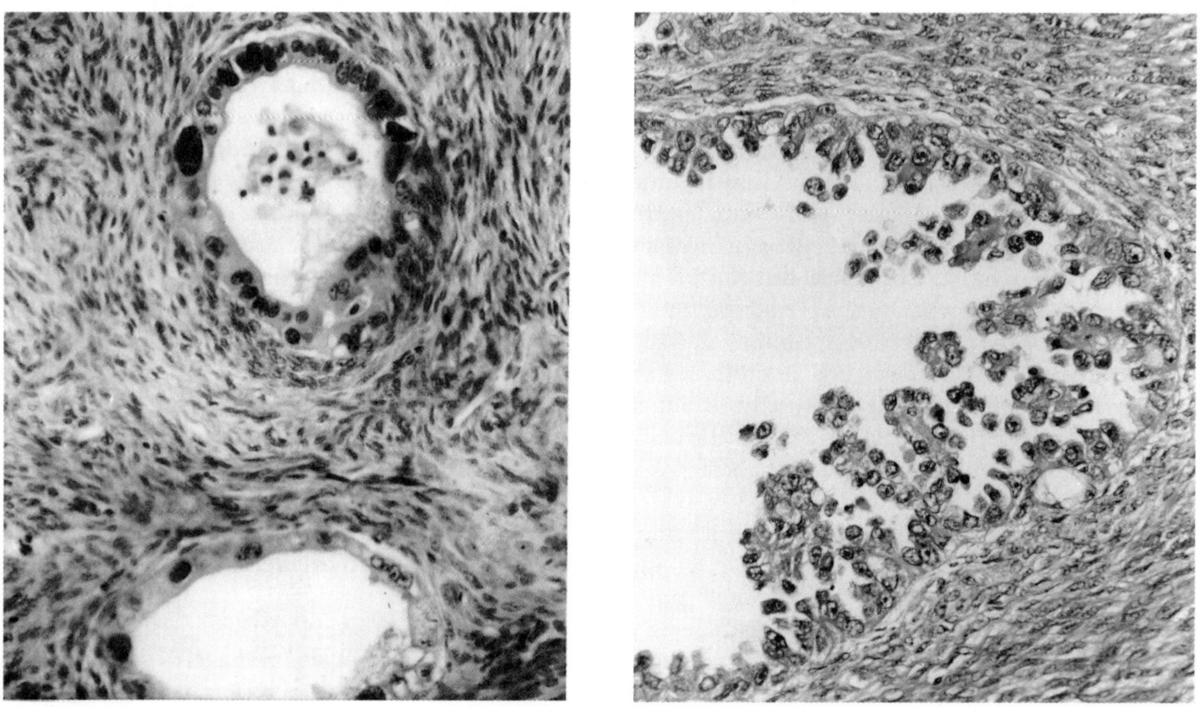

A B

Fig. 27.7 Low grade proliferating clear cell tumors. (A) With marked nuclear atypia and cellular variability. Most cells have eosinophilic granular cytoplasm in this field. H + E ×150. (B) With luminal budding and true papillary structures. H + E

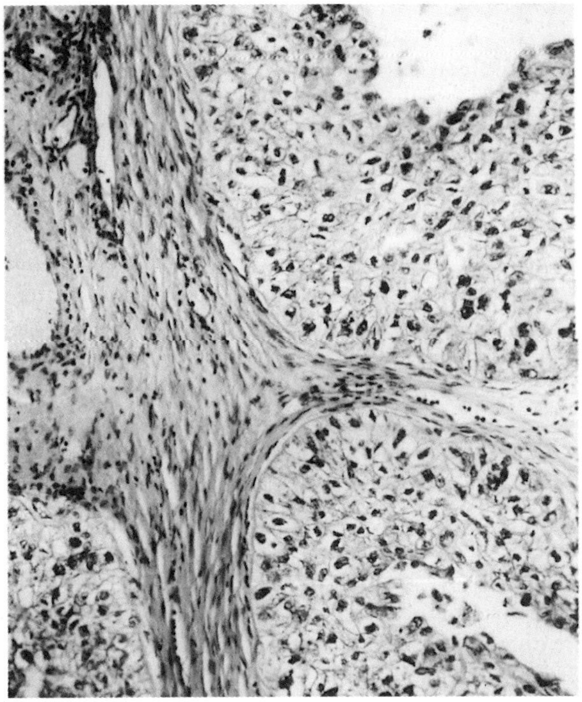

Fig. 27.8 High grade proliferating clear cell tumor. Small solid nests of clear cells are well circumscribed and have smooth epithelial/stromal interfaces. The adjacent stroma is mature and circumferentially laminated. H + E ×75. (Reprinted, with permission, from Russell 1979a)

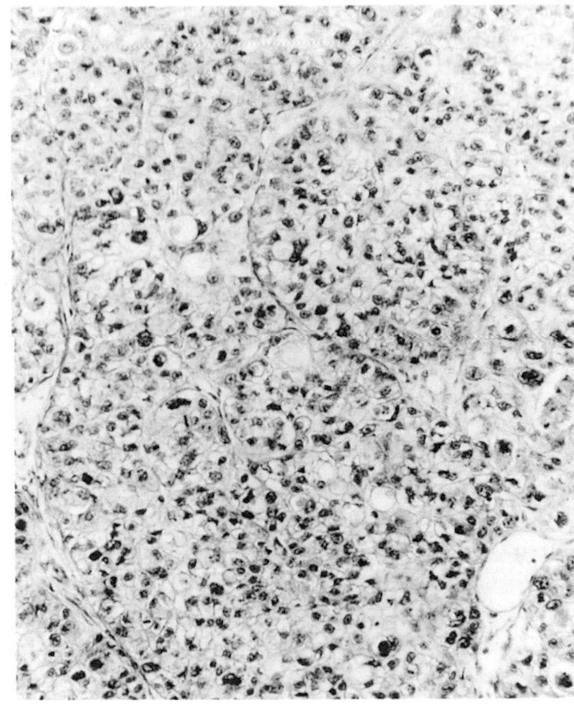

Fig. 27.9 Clear cell carcinoma with sheets of typical polyhedral clear cells and delicate connective tissue septa. H + E ×75

mitoses (up to 3 per 10HPF) (Russell 1979a) are present. True papillary structures are rarely seen (Fig. 27.7B). Epithelial proliferation may produce small solid morules of clear cells and, in the absence of obvious destructive stromal invasion (Fig. 27.8), separation from clear cell carcinomas is uncertain. The approach we have adopted here, as with other common epithelial tumors, is that if the stromal/epithelial interface is smooth and the stroma itself is 'inactive' or 'mature' without an inflammatory infiltrate, a diagnosis of noninvasive or proliferating tumor is favored and conservative management recommended.

Invasive clear cell carcinomas exhibit a variety of architectural patterns, any one or a combination of which may be found in an individual tumor. A common pattern is of small to large sheets of polyhedral clear cells separated by delicate fibrovascular septa (Fig. 27.9). The clear cells have distinct cell borders and eccentric rounded or slightly angular nuclei, often with prominent nucleoli. The cytoplasm is distended by abundant particulate glycogen, but not mucin, and may contain varied amounts of fat (Norris & Robinowitz 1971). Extracellular mucin may be present. Cells with eosinophilic granular cytoplasm may be admixed with typical clear cells (Fig. 27.10).

The second major pattern is tubulopapillary. The papillae are of the same order of dimension as in well-differentiated serous carcinoma, and may be either simple or quite complex. The connective tissue cores are composed of quite delicate immature mesenchymal tissue, which is occasionally hyalinized. Tubules and cystic structures also may be complex and are often separated by fibrous or hyaline stroma. The tubules and papillae are lined by typical clear, hobnail (Fig. 27.11) or eosinophilic cells (Fig. 27.12), or by columnar secretory cells. These latter have well defined vacuoles (so-called 'vacuolated cells') (Czernobilsky et al 1970), which are also seen in secretory serous or endometrioid carcinomas. These tall columnar secretory cells, when numerous, are responsible

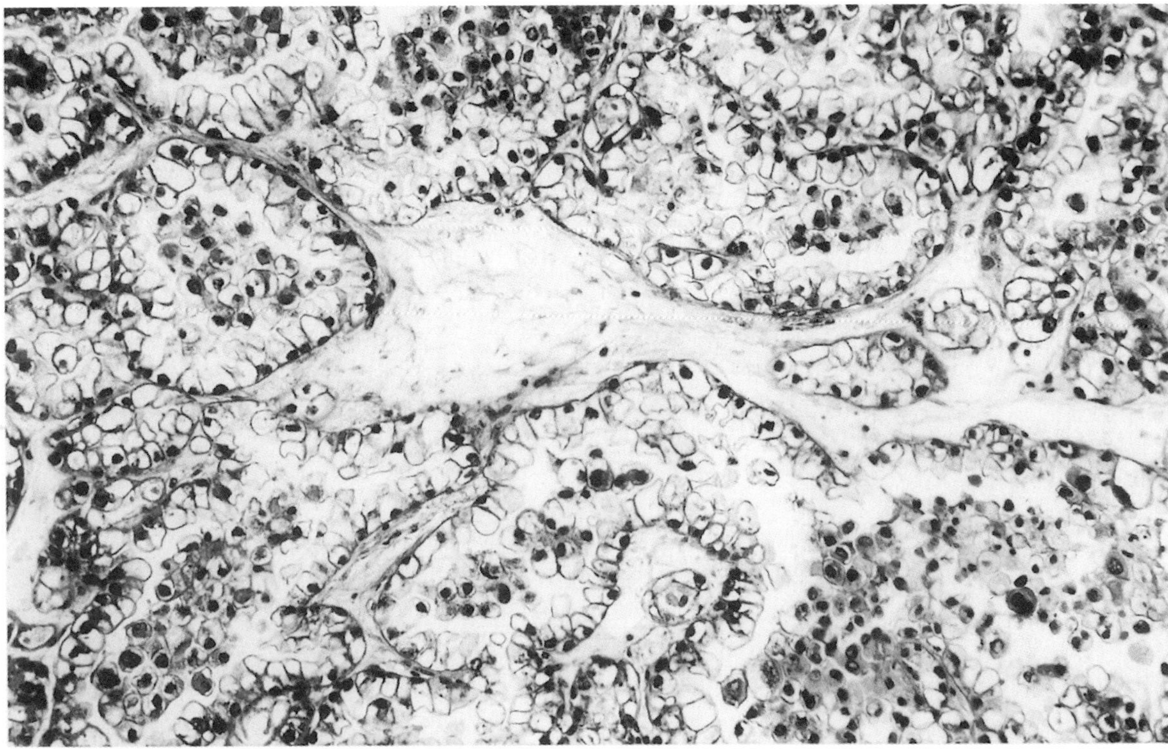

Fig. 27.10 A tubulocystic pattern with predominantly clear cells, but also clusters of cells with granular eosinophilic cytoplasm. H + E ×125

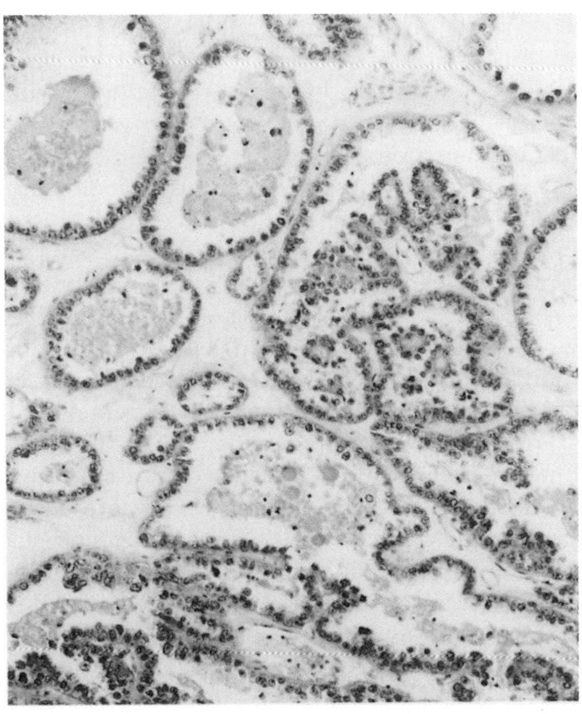

for considerable blurring of the distinction between mullerian clear cell carcinoma and both serous and endometrioid carcinomas, and are part of the interface in mixed epithelial malignancies. The diagnosis of clear cell carcinoma must be based on the identification of typical pavement-like clear or eosinophilic cells or hobnail cells.

With regard to general features, mitoses are not as numerous as in other primary epithelial carcinomas, and range up to only 2 per HPF in clear cell carcinomas. Indeed, a mitotic rate of only 6/10HPF or greater is regarded as an adverse prognostic variable (Kennedy et al 1993). The tumor stroma rarely resembles ovarian cortex and does not exhibit the periglandular hypercellularity of the benign and borderline clear cell tumors. Luteinized stromal cells are only occasionally noted. Microcalcification is seen in 10–30% of

Fig. 27.11 Clear cell carcinoma. Tubulopapillary pattern with prominent hobnail cells and somewhat hyalinized stroma. H + E ×75

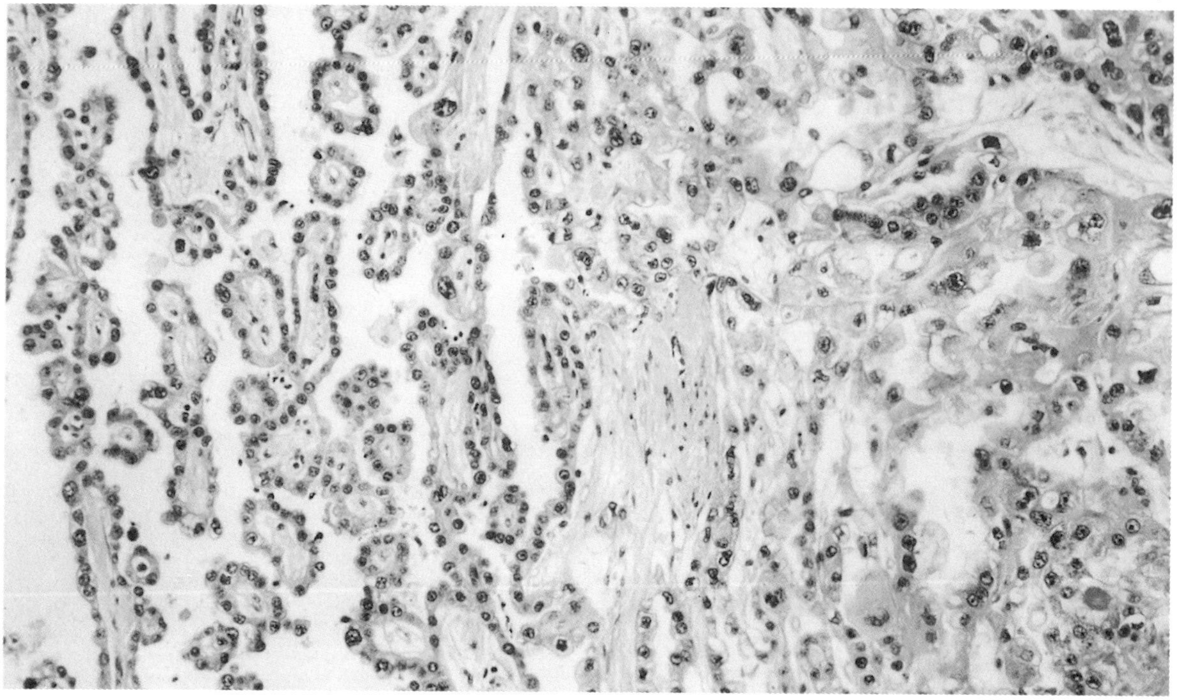

Fig. 27.12 Clear cell carcinoma with a papillary pattern (left) and solid pattern (right), both featuring cells with eosinophilic granular cytoplasm. H + E ×125

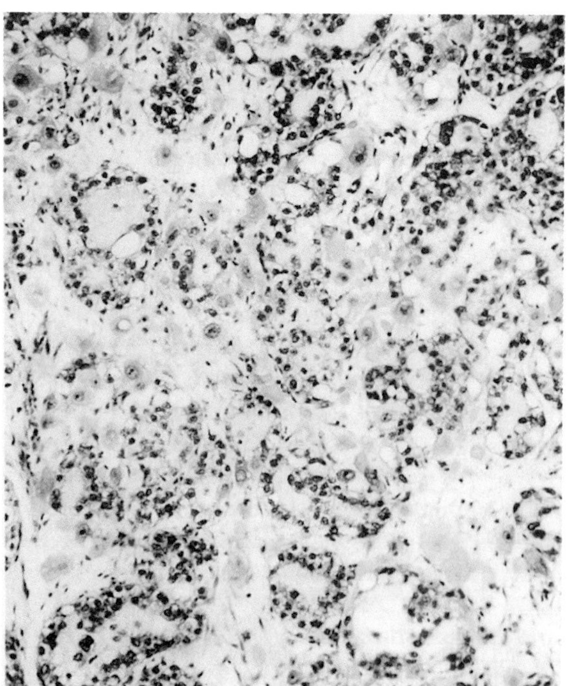

Fig. 27.13 Clear cell carcinoma in which bizarre eosinophilic giant cells are dispersed singly in the stroma amongst typical clear cell tubules. H + E ×75

cases, but is hardly ever prominent. Necrosis, hemorrhage and stromal lymphocytic infiltrates are inconstant. The various architectural and cytological features do not correlate well with prognosis, and we do not advocate grading of clear cell carcinomas.

Less frequently observed patterns include those in which eosinophilic granular cells are scattered singly amongst typical clear cells (Fig. 27.13) or form small clusters to give an organoid appearance to part of the tumor (Fig. 27.14), as well as the so-called 'oxyphilic clear cell carcinoma' of Young & Scully (1987). Degenerative changes in these eosinophilic cells may be extreme, and bizarre forms may predominate. Figure 27.15 shows an example, in which rims of bizarre surviving eosinophilic cells surround islands of flocculent necrotic cellular debris. Clear cell carcinomas containing β-human chorionic gonadotrophin

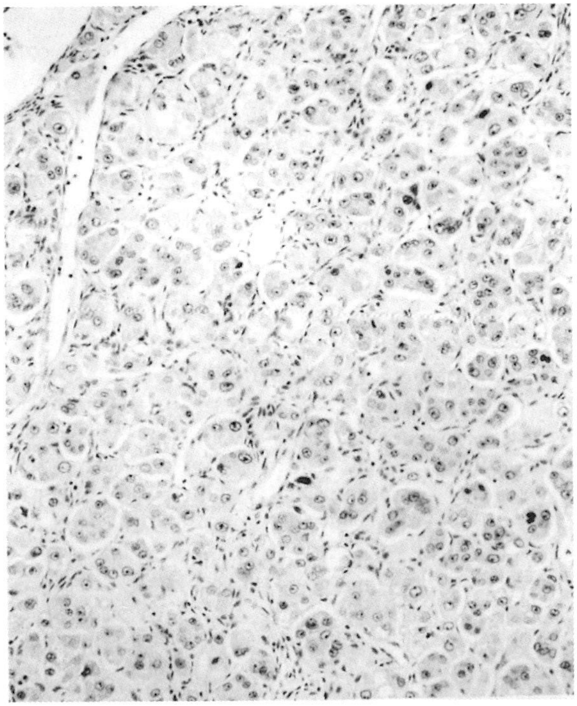

Fig. 27.14 Eosinophilic cells arranged in an organoid pattern resembling a lipid cell tumor. H + E ×75

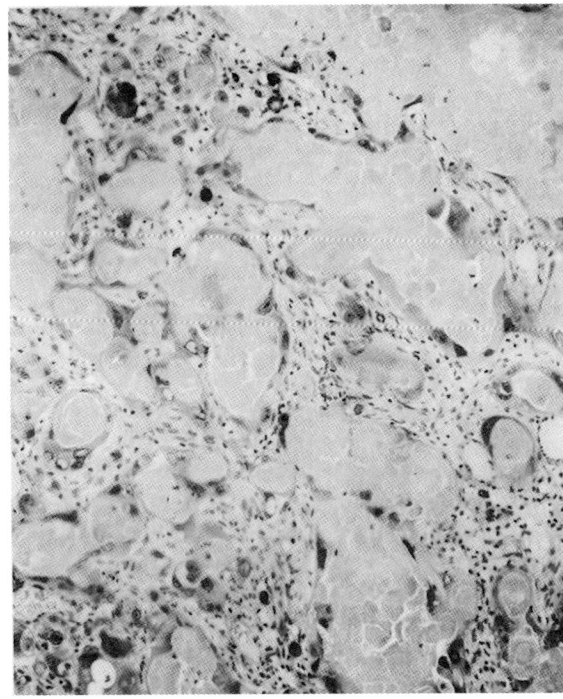

Fig. 27.15 An area in an otherwise typical clear cell carcinoma in which extremely bizarre eosinophilic cells surround necrotic cellular debris. The extreme pleiomorphism of these granular eosinophilic cells is a useful pointer to clear cell differentiation in some anaplastic carcinomas. H + E ×75

(β-hCG) negative giant cells are rarely seen (Betta et al 1988); paradoxically, examples which elaborate β-hCG in the absence of syncytiotrophoblast-like giant cells have also been reported (Kobayashi et al 1990). Clear cells with coalescent vacuoles containing targetoid eosinophilic PTAH-positive and PAS-positive globules (Fig. 27.16), which may stain for α_1-antitrypsin but not α-fetoprotein, produce another cell variant. Such 'targetoid' cells are seen in other mullerian epithelial carcinomas, but far less frequently than in clear cell carcinomas (al-Nafussi et al 1993). Areas of typical parvilocular pattern may be seen in otherwise unremarkable clear cell carcinomas (Fig. 27.17), and rare solid tumors have been observed with a pattern best designated as malignant adenofibroma (Fig. 27.18). Destructive stromal invasion is not obvious, yet the striking prominence and the cellular atypia of the epithelial (particularly hobnail) cells serve to differentiate it from the parvilocular pattern of proliferating and benign clear cell tumors (see Fig. 27.3). An uncommonly encountered but important pattern to recognize is one in which single or small clusters of cells are scattered in loose edematous stroma and resemble Krukenberg tumors (Fig. 27.19). Such a pattern is, in our experience, usually only a minor part of otherwise typical clear cell carcinomas, but may be a dominant component leading to diagnostic difficulty.

Differential diagnosis

The presence of typical hobnail cells, luminal mucin, and occasionally cellular apical mucin, and a relative lack of tumor vascularity, all help distinguish primary ovarian clear cell carcinomas from much rarer renal cell carcinomas metastatic to the ovaries. Useful immunohistochemical markers include B72.3 (present in 100% of clear cell carcinomas but only 10% of renal cell carcinomas) and COTA (absent in all renal cell carcinomas) (Loy & Darkow 1993).

The papillary structures of clear cell carcinomas are more complex than those seen in the 'festoon'

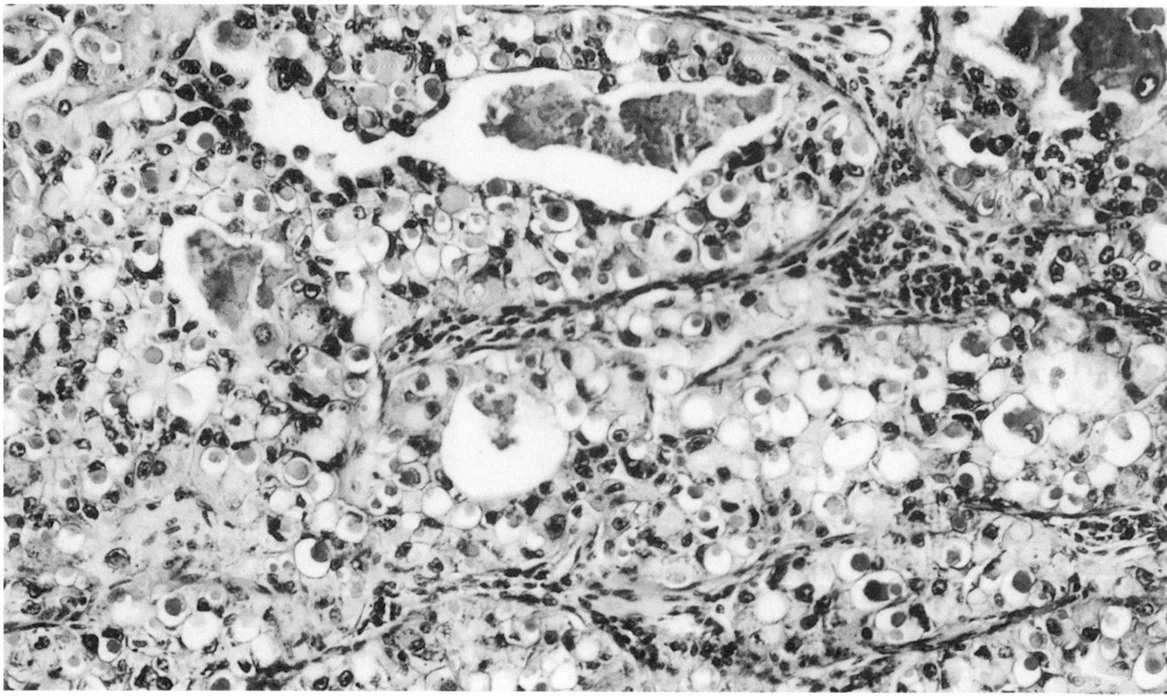

Fig. 27.16 Clear cell carcinoma. Vacuolated cells containing 'targetoid' amorphous eosinophilic inclusions. H + E ×125

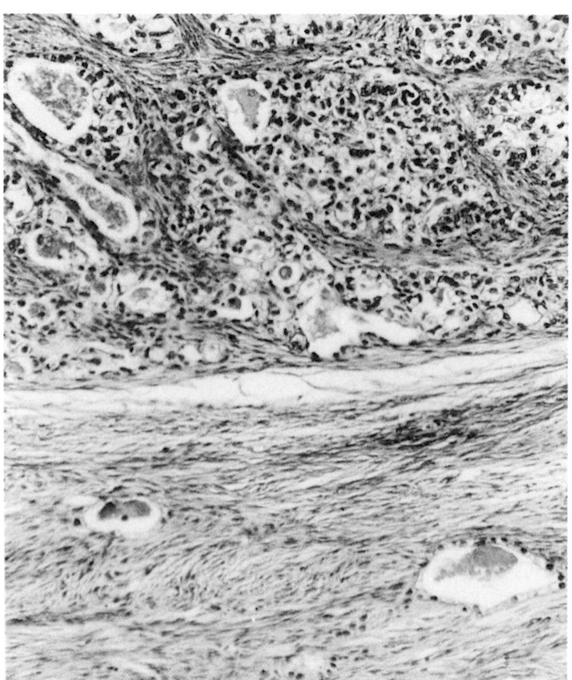

Fig. 27.17 Clear cell carcinoma with adjacent parvilocular area. H + E ×75. (Reprinted, with permission, from Russell 1979b)

pattern of endodermal sinus tumors (see Ch. 42) and may be distinguished by both the character of the epithelial lining cells as well as the absence of typical Schiller–Duval bodies (Table 42.1). Clear cells with a 'targetoid' appearance also need to be distinguished from the cells with hyaline droplets seen in endodermal sinus tumors. Endodermal sinus tumors typically occur at a much younger age than clear cell carcinomas, and are always associated with raised serum α-fetoprotein levels, this tumor-associated antigen (as well as α1-antitrypsin) being readily demonstrable immunohistochemically within tumor cells of the former but only the latter in the targetoid cells of clear cell carcinomas. Additionally, it has been claimed that the *combination* of positivity for Leu M1 and negativity for α-fetoprotein is diagnostic of clear cell carcinoma, while the converse of negativity for Leu M1 and positivity for α-fetoprotein is diagnostic of yolk sac tumor (Zirker et al 1989).

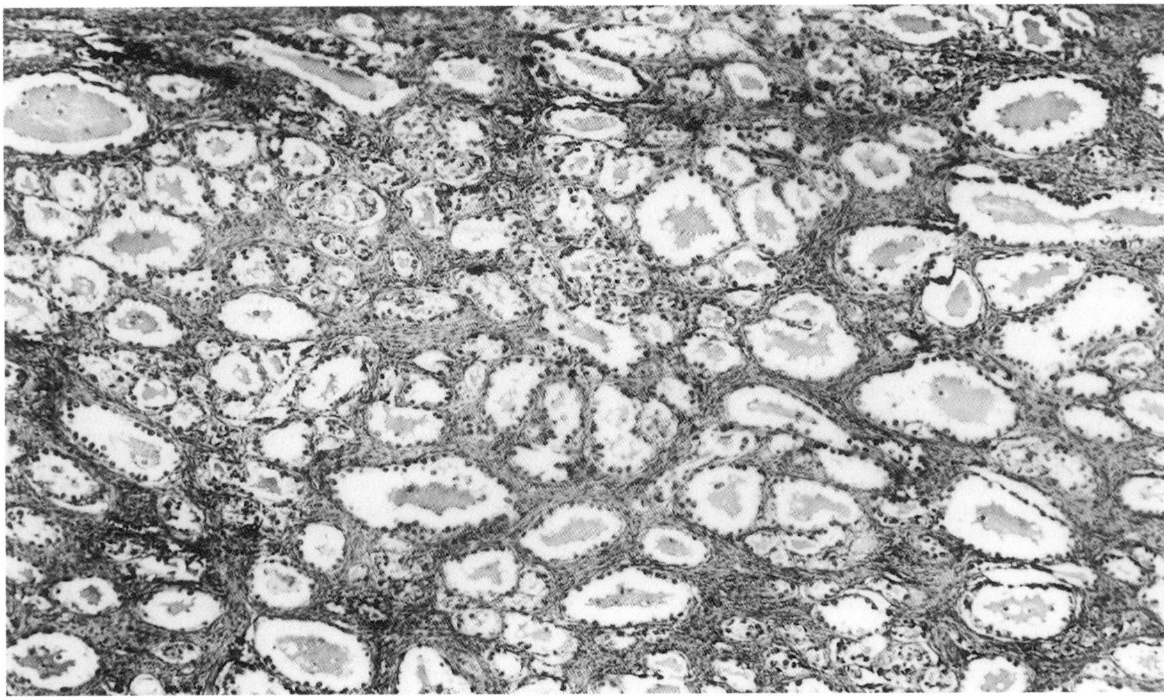

Fig. 27.18 Malignant clear cell adenofibroma. Contrast with benign lesion in Fig. 27.3. H + E ×50

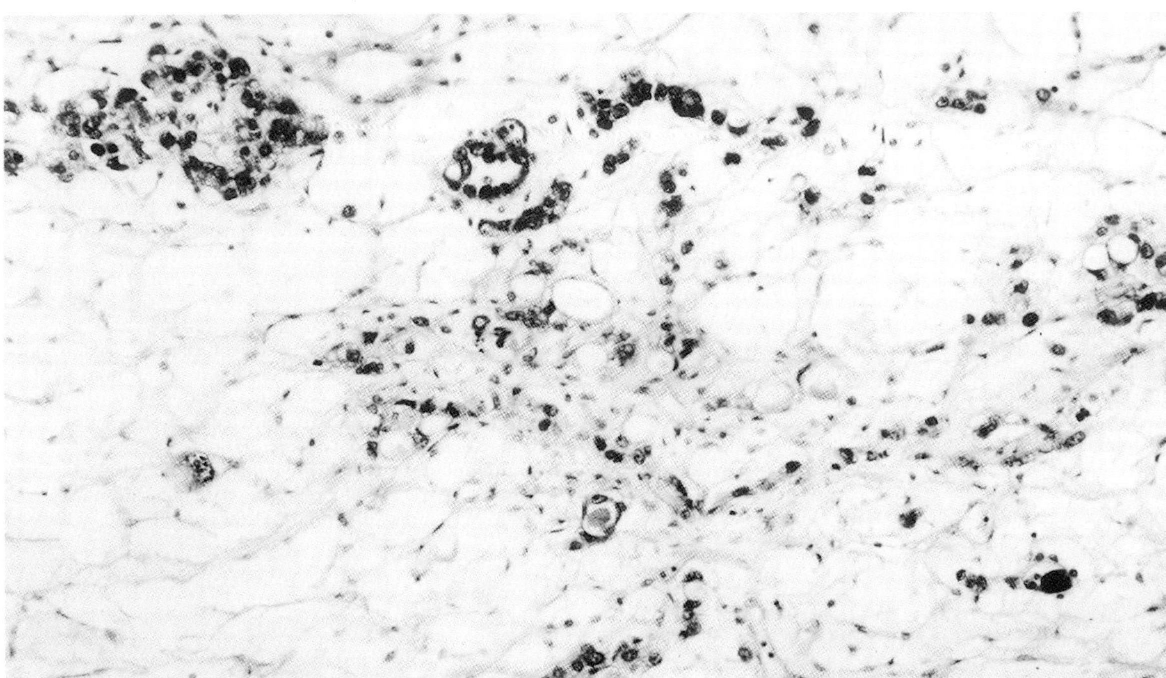

Fig. 27.19 Clear cell carcinoma. Loose edematous stroma with small clusters of epithelial cells. Negative mucin stains readily distinguish this from mucinous carcinoma (primary or secondary). H + E ×125

REFERENCES

al-Nafussi A I, Hughes D E, Williams A R 1993 Hyaline globules in ovarian tumors. Histopathology 23: 563–566

Aslani M, Scully R E 1989 Primary carcinoma of the broad ligament. Report of four cases and review of the literature. Cancer 64: 1540–1545

Bell D A, Scully R E 1985 Benign and borderline clear cell adenofibromas of the ovary. Cancer 56: 2911–2931

Bell D A, Scully R E 1994 Early de novo ovarian carcinoma. A study of fourteen cases. Cancer 73: 1859–1864

Betta P G, Robutti F, Spinoglio G, Bottero G 1988 Uncommon histological variants of clear cell carcinoma of the ovary. Report of two cases with immunohistochemical and ploidy studies. European Journal of Gynaecological Oncology 9: 431–434

Brescia R J, Dubin N, Demopoulos R I 1989 Endometrioid and clear cell carcinoma of the ovary. Factors affecting survival. International Journal of Gynecological Pathology 8: 132–138

Crozier M A, Copeland L J, Silva E G, Gershenson D M, Stringer C A 1989 Clear cell carcinoma of the ovary: a study of 59 cases. Gynecologic Oncology 35: 199–203

Czernobilsky B, Silverman B B, Enterline H T 1970 Clear-cell carcinoma of the ovary. Cancer 25: 762–772

Evans H, Yates W A, Palmer W E, Cartwright R L, Antemann R W 1990 Clear cell carcinoma of the sigmoid mesocolon: a tumor of the secondary mullerian system. American Journal of Obstetrics and Gynecology 162: 161–163

Fox H, Langley F A 1976 Tumours of the ovary. Heinemann, London, p 74–118

Hitti I F, Glasberg S S, Lubicz S 1990 Clear cell carcinoma arising in extraovarian endometriosis: report of three cases and review of the literature. Gynecologic Oncology 39: 314–320

Jenison E L, Montag A G, Griffiths C T et al 1989 Clear cell adenocarcinoma of the ovary: a clinical analysis and comparison with serous carcinoma. Gynecologic Oncology 32: 65–71

Kao G F, Norris H J 1979 Unusual cystadenofibromas: endometrioid, mucinous and clear cell types. Obstetrics and Gynecology 54: 729–736

Katsube Y, Fujiwara H, Tanioka Y, Imajo M, Fujiwara A 1989 Ovarian clear cell adenofibroma of borderline malignancy. A case report. Hiroshima Journal of Medical Science 38: 87–90

Kennedy A W, Biscotti C V, Hart W R, Webster K D 1989 Ovarian clear cell adenocarcinoma. Gynecologic Oncology 32: 342–349

Kennedy A W, Biscotti C V, Hart W R, Tuason L J 1993 Histologic correlates of progression-free interval and survival in ovarian clear cell adenocarcinoma. Gynecologic Oncology 50: 334–338

Kobayashi M, Hamada H, Yamoto M, Nakano R 1990 Ovarian clear cell carcinoma producing estradiol and human chorionic gonadotropin. Acta Obstetricia et Gynecologica Scandinavica 69: 183–185

Loy T S, Darkow G V 1993 Distribution of colon-ovarian tumor antigen in adenocarcinoma. An immunohistochemical study of 501 cases. American Journal of Clinical Pathology 99: 207–210

Montag A G, Jenison E L, Griffiths C T, Welch W R, Lavin P T, Knapp R C 1989 Ovarian clear cell carcinoma. A clinicopathologic analysis of 44 cases. International Journal of Gynecological Pathology 8: 85–96

Norris H J, Robinowitz M 1971 Ovarian adenocarcinoma of mesonephric type. Cancer 28: 1074–1081

Okagaki T, Richart R M 1970 Mesonephroma ovarii (hypernephroid carcinoma). Light microscopic and ultrastructural study of a case. Cancer 26: 453–461

Roth L M, Langley F A, Fox H, Wheeler J E, Czernobilsky B 1984 Ovarian clear cell adenofibromatous tumors: benign, of low malignant potential, and associated with invasive clear cell carcinoma. Cancer 53: 1156–1163

Russell P 1979a The pathological assessment of ovarian neoplasms. II: The proliferating 'epithelial' tumors. Pathology 11: 251–282

Russell P 1979b The pathological assessment of ovarian neoplasms. III: The malignant 'epithelial' tumors. Pathology 11: 493–532

Scharl A, Gunther M, Gohring U J, Bolte A, Fischer R 1990 Multifokale Karzinome des oberen weiblichen Genitaltrakts: Diffuse Mullersche Neoplasie. Geburtshilfe und Frauenheilkind 50: 158–160

Scully R E 1977 Ovarian tumors. A review. American Journal of Pathology 87: 686–720

Scully R E 1979 Tumors of the ovary and maldeveloped gonads. AFIP fascicle 16, 2nd series. Armed Forces Institute of Pathology, Washington, DC, p 53–151

Serov S F, Scully R E, Sobin L H 1973 Histological typing of ovarian tumors. International histological classification of tumors No. 9. World Health Organization, Geneva, p 17–54

Shevchuk M M, Winkler-Monsanto B, Fenoglio C M, Richart R M 1981 Clear cell carcinoma of the ovary: a clinicopathologic study with review of the literature. Cancer 47: 1344–1351

Tsurunaga T, Iwai E, Okamoto Y et al 1992 Ovarian clear cell adenofibromatous tumor: report of 2 cases. Nippon Sanka Fujinka Gakkai Zasshi 44: 105–108

Young R H, Scully R E 1987 Oxyphilic clear cell carcinoma of the ovary. Report of nine cases. American Journal of Surgical Pathology 11: 661–667

Zirker T A, Silva E G, Morris M, Ordonez N G 1989 Immunohistochemical differentiation of clear-cell carcinoma of the female genital tract and endodermal sinus tumor with the use of alpha-fetoprotein and Leu M1. American Journal of Clinical Pathology 91: 511–514

28

Transitional cell (Brenner) tumors

P. Russell A. Farnsworth

Most transitional cell tumors appear to derive directly from the surface epithelium of the ovary, which undergoes metaplasia to form the urothelial-like components of these neoplasms. The cytological features of these tumors are similar to those of Walthard's rests, epithelial inclusions found most commonly beneath the serosa of the fallopian tubes but also occasionally in the hilar regions of the ovaries. It is this, along with a frequent mixture of other mullerian epithelial elements (mucinous, serous) in the tumors (Fig. 28.1), which prompts grouping of such lesions with the other 'epithelial–stromal tumors'. Although 'urothelial' is the term most frequently used to characterize Brenner (transitional cell) epithelium, and cytologically and immunohistochemically there are similarities

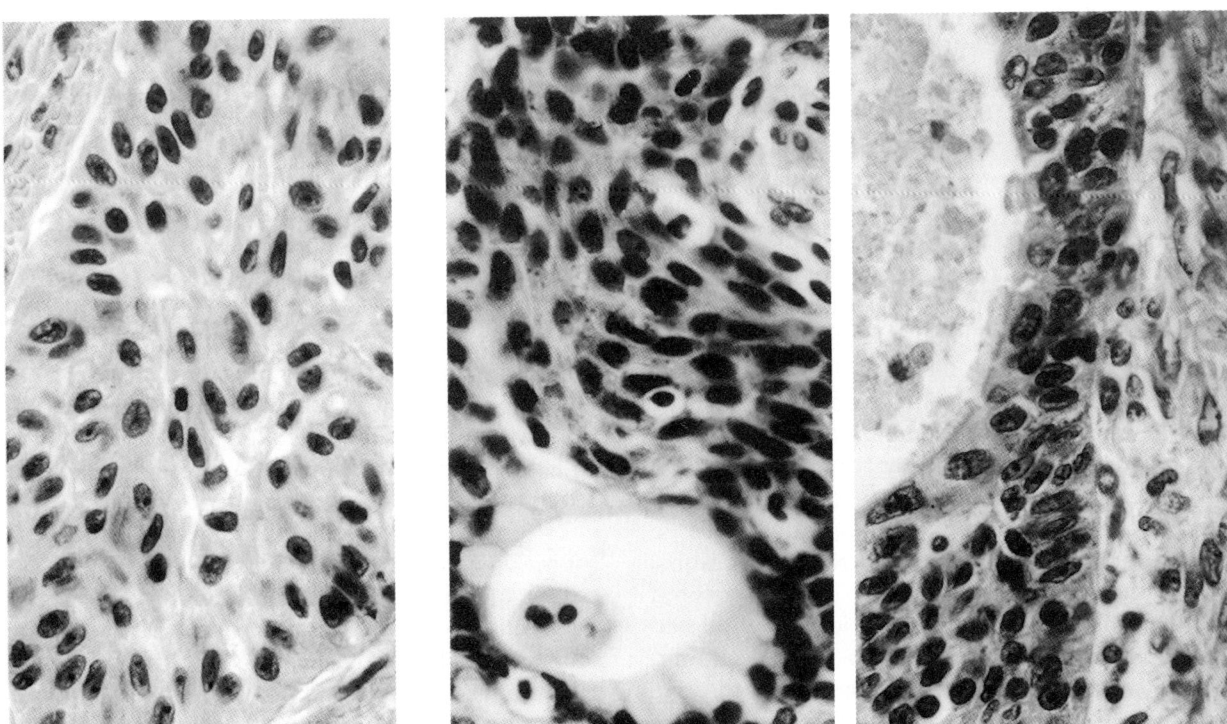

A B C

Fig. 28.1 Characteristic cell types in benign transitional cell epithelial nests. (A) Typical transitional cell epithelial cells with elongate, longitudinally folded, (so-called 'coffee-bean') nuclei. (B) Mucinous cells lining a small central cystic space. (C) Serous ciliated cells lining a similar cystic space. H + E ×500 with the epithelium lining the urinary tract (Seldenrijk et al 1986, Lifschitz-Mercer et al 1988, Santini et al 1989), we have occasionally observed metaplastic transitional cell epithelium at various sites in mullerian duct derivatives (fallopian tubes, ecto- and endocervix, vagina) (Egan & Russell 1996a,b) and support the view of Woodruff and coworkers (Genadry et al 1979, Woodruff et al 1981) that benign transitional cell epithelium has much more in common with epithelia of mullerian type than has hitherto been claimed. Other possible histogeneses (such as origin from rete structures) are suggested by the hilar position of some small transitional cell tumors, as well as the testis and epididymis in the male (Caccamo et al 1991).

The epithelial cells are polyhedral to elongate and, electron microscopically, separated by wide intercellular spaces into which project villiform cytoplasmic processes. Mitochondria, free ribosomes, and lysosomal structures are plentiful, but Golgi bodies and granular endoplasmic reticulum are inconspicuous. Some cells contain variable, but occasionally abundant, glycogen (Roth 1971, Silverberg & Wilson 1972, Cummins et al 1973). The nuclei are ovoid and often deeply grooved longitudinally ('coffee-bean' nuclei) with fine, evenly dispersed chromatin and prominent nucleoli. While most of the transitional cell nests are composed exclusively of cells of this type (Fig. 28.1A), others have central cystic or gland-like spaces lined by mucinous epithelium of endocervical type (Fig. 28.1B), or, uncommonly, pseudostratified ciliated epithelium of serous (tubal) type (Fig. 28.1C). The vast majority of transitional cell tumors have a major stromal component and are therefore designated as adenofibromas.

Transitional cell tumors constitute about 2% of all primary ovarian neoplasms (Russell 1979a) and are almost always benign. Some benign transitional cell tumors are microscopic lesions, while most of the remainder are discovered incidentally at surgical intervention for unrelated pelvic conditions, ranging from uterine leiomyomas to endometrial hyperplasias. Rare massive transitional tumors may be capable of androgenic or estrogenic activity (Sasano et al 1989, de Lima et al 1989). They are found in patients mostly in the fourth to eighth decades, with a mean age of incidence of about 50 years. They are bilateral in 6–7% of instances, while unilateral lesions may be more commonly found in the left ovary (Silverberg 1971).

In 1971, Roth and Sternberg described three unusual transitional cell tumors which, on the basis of histological characteristics, they termed 'proliferating' and placed as intermediate between benign and carcinomatous forms. Since then, other authors have also preferred the term 'proliferating' (Miles & Norris 1972, Woodruff et al 1981) to 'borderline' (Hallgrimsson & Scully 1972), implying an essentially benign clinical course. Roth et al (1985) have expanded the spectrum by differentiating between proliferating transitional cell tumors and those 'of low malignant potential'. Of the 50 or so proliferating transitional cell tumors in the literature (Roth & Sternberg 1971, Hallgrimsson & Scully 1972, Miles & Norris 1972, McKenna & Ansford 1976, Pratt-Thomas et al 1976, Chang et al 1977, Klemi & Nevalainen 1977, Russell 1979b, Woodruff et al 1981, Genton 1984, Roth et al 1985), only one has not behaved in an entirely benign fashion (McKenna & Ansford 1976), leading to local recurrence. The case report by Pratt-Thomas et al (1976) documenting liver metastases has been reviewed and reinterpreted as an example of frankly malignant Brenner tumor (Czernobilsky 1985). These neoplasms appear to occur at an older age than their benign counterparts (with a mean age of 60 years) and, because of their size, tend to present with symptoms referable to the ovarian mass. Rarely, proliferating transitional cell tumors are associated with synchronous or metachronous transitional cell carcinomas in the urinary bladder (Colgan & Norris 1983, Kunze et al 1983, Svenes & Eide 1984, Young & Scully 1988).

The true incidence of malignant Brenner/transitional cell tumors is difficult to establish, as criteria for histological identification have not been fully delineated. Many earlier reports such as that of Idelson (1963) would, using current World Health Organization (WHO) criteria (Serov et al 1973), be reinterpreted as atypically proliferating rather than frankly malignant neoplasms. The malignant epithelial component is broadly similar to transitional cell carcinoma of the urinary tract in architectural arrangement and character, but may have minor squamous or glandular elements. How prominent these latter components may be, yet still be compatible with a diagnosis of malignant transitional cell tumor, is open to debate. It is recommended that a careful search, in suspected cases, be made for typical areas of benign or proliferating transitional cell tumor, with some authorities recommending avoidance of the diagnosis of malignant Brenner tumor in the absence of these additional findings (Scully 1979, Roth & Czernobilsky 1985). Austin & Norris (1987) and others (Robey et al 1989, Silva et al 1990, Gershenson et al 1993) have championed the concept of 'transitional cell carcinomas' of the ovary (without associated benign transitional cell elements) and differentiating such tumors from malignant Brenner tumors (with these 'precursor' components), noting significant differences between the two tumor subgroups in both histological features and clinical course (specifically an increased responsiveness to chemotherapy of the 'transitional cell' tumor group) to justify this distinction. It may well be that the category of malignant Brenner tumors is not homogeneous. It is further recommended that mucinous or serous carcinomas found in association with benign transitional cell tumor should be so classified (Roth & Czernobilsky 1985) and excluded from this category. Applying these restrictions, many cases in the literature are unacceptable, leaving a residuum of about 100 examples (Rybak et al 1981, Woodruff et al 1981, Roth & Czernobilsky 1985, Austin & Norris 1987, Silva et al 1990). The mean age of patients presenting with malignant transitional cell tumors is 60 years. Abdominal pain and swelling are the most common presenting symptoms, with abnormal uterine bleeding occurring in about 20% of cases. Associated endometrial hyperplasia is seen in 15% of patients (Fox & Langley 1976), and occasional tumors have been documented to be estrogen secreting (Kuhnel et al 1987). FIGO stage at presentation is the major correlate of patient survival; 5-year survival for stage 1a cases is 50%, and for stage 1b–4 cases is less than 10% (Woodruff et al 1981), irrespective of the mode of therapy. Roth & Czernobilsky (1985) have reported a relationship between survival and tumor differentiation in early (stage 1) cases.

Cytogenetic and molecular genetic studies

In the study by Martin et al (1992), all assessable benign transitional cell tumors were diploid. One of four proliferating transitional cell tumors was tetraploid, the others diploid. Four of five malignant Brenner tumors and all transitional cell carcinomas were aneuploid.

Macroscopic features

Although occasional benign tumors may reach considerable size (Hoffman et al 1989), few exceed 10 cm and most are less than 2 cm in diameter. Only rare examples are bilateral (Conforti et al 1989). The majority are well circumscribed (although unencapsulated) and solid with a smooth or slightly bosselated external surface. They have a firm rubbery consistency and the cut surface is whorled and sometimes faintly lobulated (Fig. 28.2). They are usually grey-white in color, but may have a yellowish hue. Flecks of calcification are sometimes felt on cutting the tumor. These are usually cortical in

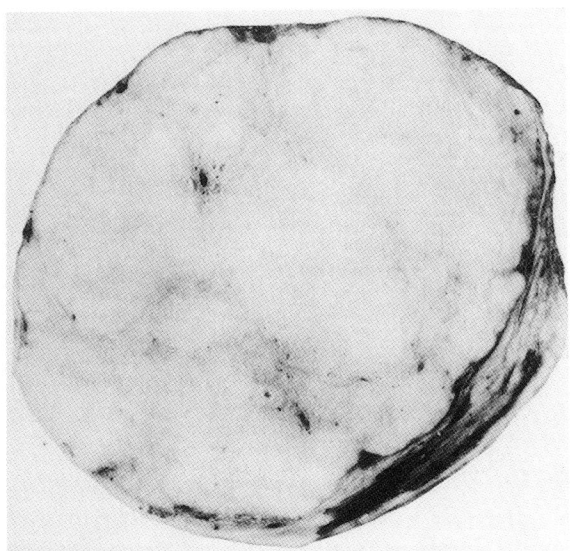

Fig. 28.2 A 7 cm benign transitional cell tumor with a faintly lobulated cut surface and compression of surrounding ovarian tissue

position, but hilar lesions may occasionally be encountered. Less commonly, these tumors have a significant cystic component (many of these cysts will be lined by mucinous epithelium; see Ch. 29). Coexistent benign transitional cell tumors and struma ovarii have been reported (Elemenoglou et al 1994), but the significance of this association is unclear.

Proliferating transitional cell tumors are usually unilateral and multilocular cysts, measuring 10–25 cm in diameter. A small percentage of cases are bilateral. Characteristically, papillary or polypoid masses project into the cyst lumens (Fig. 28.3). These masses tend to be somewhat friable in contrast to the tough fibrous consistency of areas of benign transitional cell tumor, which are often found nearby. Rare examples may show a surface papillary component.

Malignant transitional cell tumors are usually partly cystic tumors with a diameter of 10–30 cm (average 20 cm). They are rarely bilateral (Hayden 1981). The cysts frequently have a shaggy lining and contain friable, polypoid masses projecting from the walls (Fig. 28.4). Cyst fluid is watery or mucinous in consistency. Areas of hemorrhage and necrosis may be prominent and there is grossly evident gritty calcification in 50%. Tough fibrous tumors indistinguishable from benign transitional cell tumors are less frequently found.

Microscopic features

Benign transitional cell tumors are typified by sharply demarcated epithelial nests set in fibrous stroma (Fig. 28.5). Cell nests vary in size as well as prominence from tumor to tumor. The epithelial cells are round to polygonal, with clear margins and eosinophilic to clear cytoplasm (see Fig. 28.1A). The oval nuclei have obvious nucleoli and often longitudinal grooving (so-called 'coffee-bean' appearance). This latter feature is not always prominent, and is to some extent

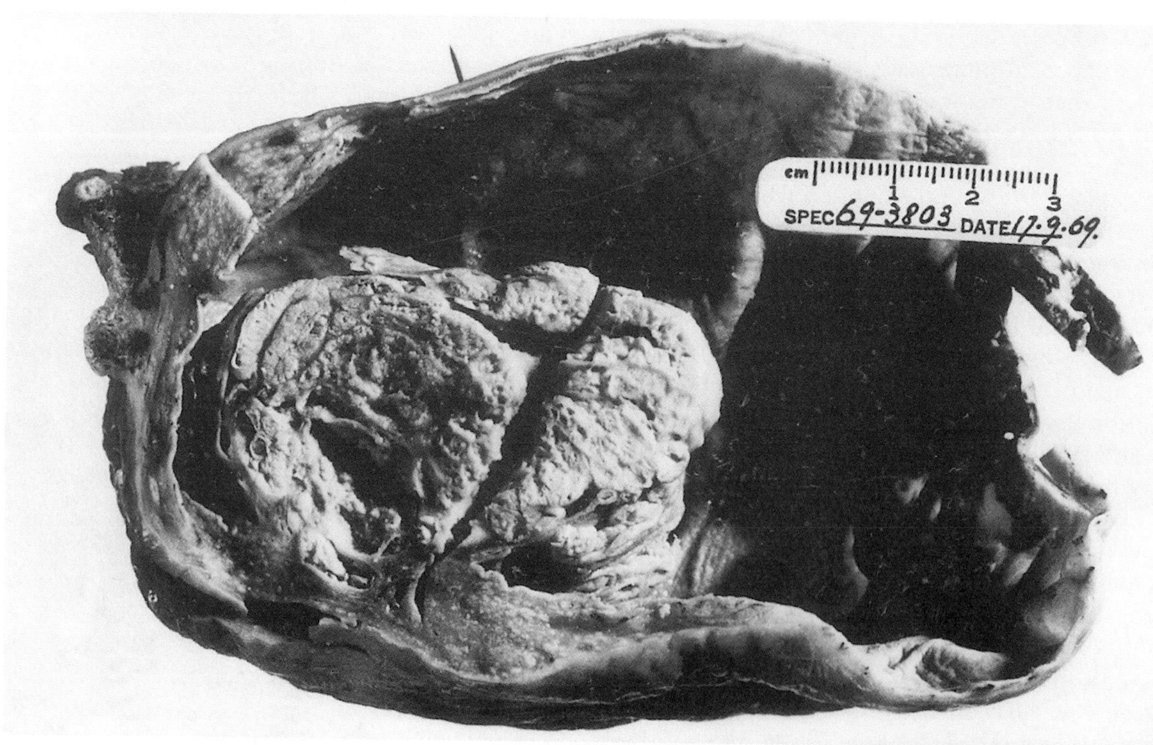

Fig. 28.3 Proliferating transitional cell tumor. Large cyst with nodular masses projecting into the lumen. Stippled fibrous tissue (top left, bottom center) in the cyst wall are areas of benign transitional cell tumor

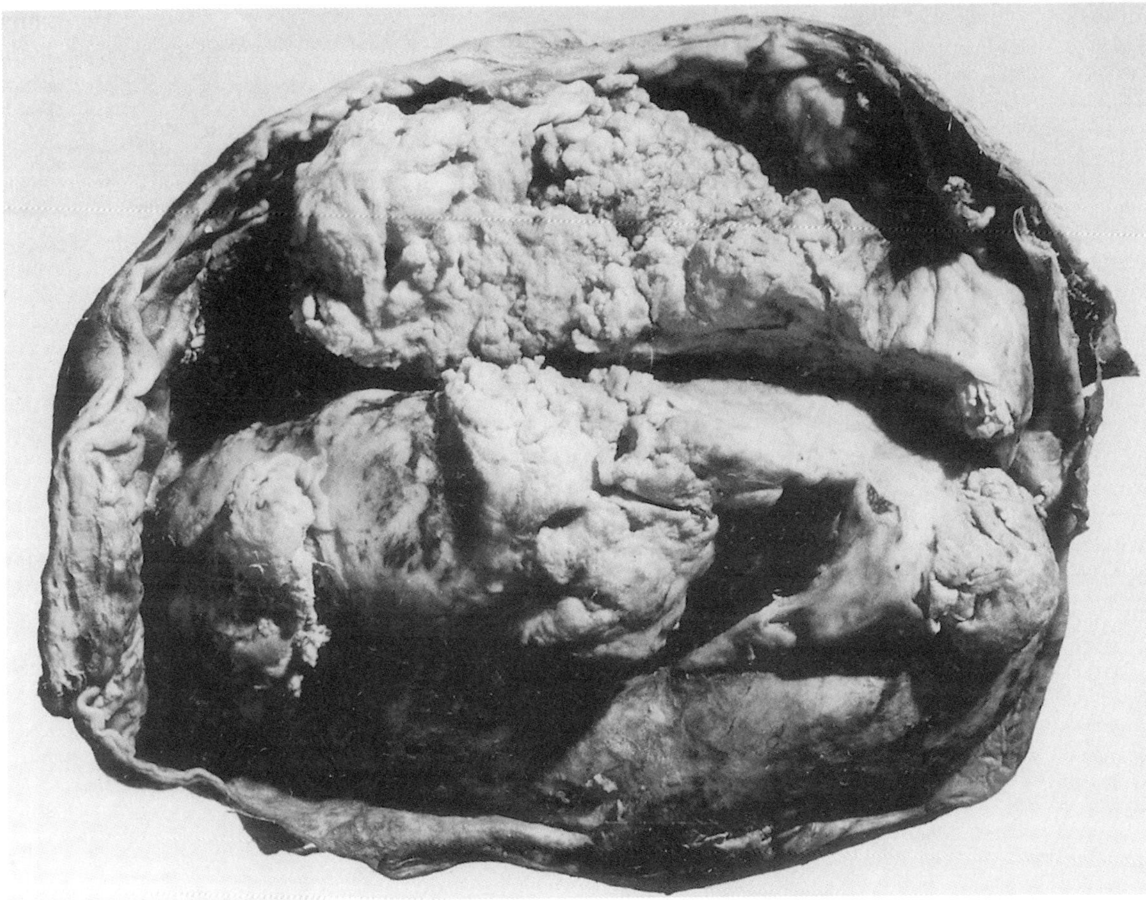

Fig. 28.4 Malignant Brenner tumor. A large, partly cystic tumor with the solid polypoid masses composed of soft friable and partly necrotic tumor tissue

nonspecific, being observed in other cells of 'epithelial' and sex cord derivation. Epithelial atypia is rare and mitoses are fewer than 1 per 10HPF. These cells contain abundant diffuse glycogen, acidic sialomucins at their apical borders and both sialomucins and neutral mucins in luminal secretions. Immunohistochemically, the cells elaborate various cytokeratins (Lifschitz-Mercer et al 1988). Argyrophilic cells, exhibiting serotonin, chromogranin and neuron-specific enolase, are regularly seen in many tumors (Aguirre et al 1984, Santini et al 1989). Often the cell nests become cystic, and these microcysts (containing eosinophilic debris or mucin) are mostly lined by otherwise unremarkable transitional cells. Less commonly, cervical type mucinous (see Fig. 28.1B) and, rarely, ciliated cells (see Fig. 28.1C) are seen in this situation. Cystic change may be more prominent (Fig. 28.6), to the point of having macroscopically visible cysts forming a significant portion of the tumor. These cysts are lined by typical transitional cell epithelium or by the same epithelium showing varying degrees of mucinous metaplasia. Roth et al (1985, 1993) have designated such neoplasms 'metaplastic transitional cell tumors'. Without intending to negate metaplasia as a likely explanation for the array of epithelia present, we prefer to classify such tumors among those of mixed epithelial differentiation (see Ch. 29). The histological patterns of these tumors may appear complex, but features of atypical epithelial proliferation are absent. The extreme end of this spectrum is for a small nodule of transitional cell tumor to be found in the wall of

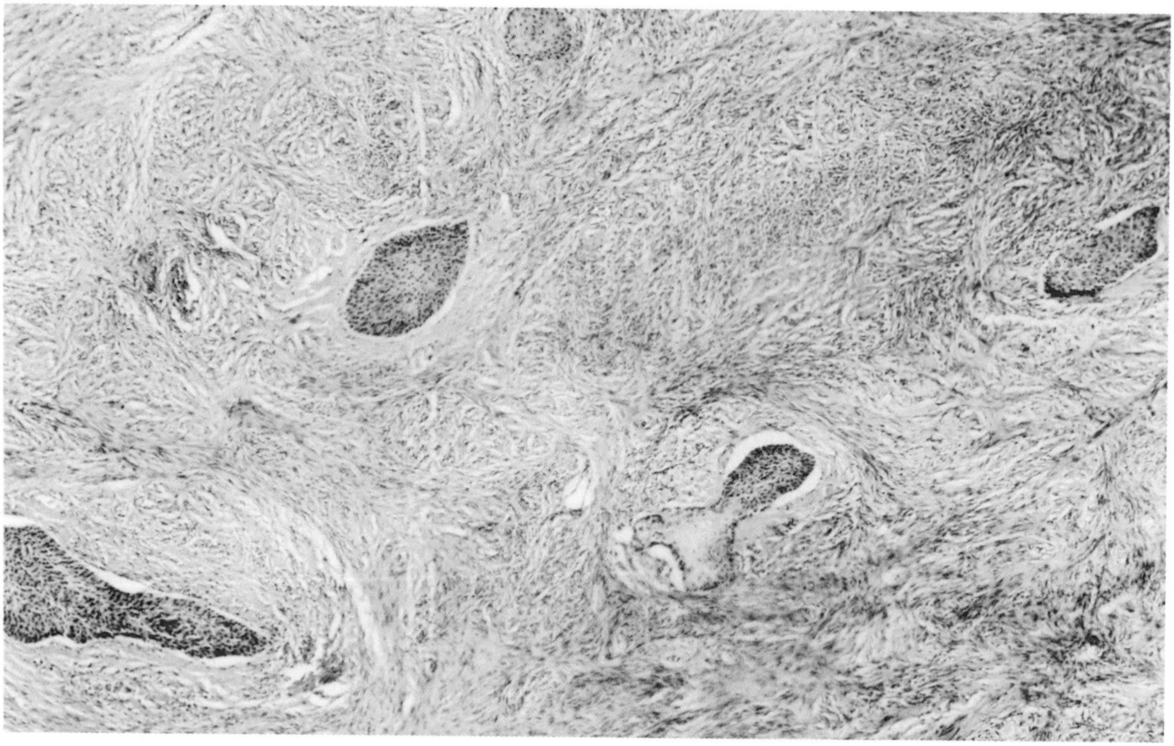

Fig. 28.5 Benign transitional cell adenofibroma. Circumscribed epithelial nests embedded in fibromatous stroma. H + E ×50

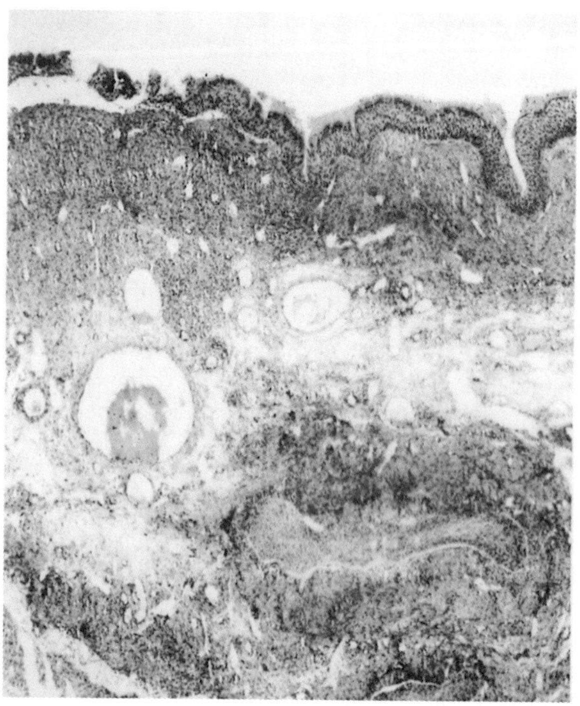

an otherwise typical benign mucinous cystadenoma.

The stroma is formed by spindled cells and generally differs little from that of other common epithelial adenofibromas. There is much variation in cellularity, which is inversely proportional to collagen formation and hyalinization; the latter most often being prominent around, or in juxtaposition to, epithelial nests. Dystrophic spiculate calcification (in one-half of benign transitional cell tumors (Russell 1979a)) is frequently present in such sites (Fig. 28.7A). New bone formation and marked stromal edema (Fig. 28.7B,C) may rarely be noted. Stromal luteinization is seen in 10–15% of tumors, even to the extent of appearing thecomatous (Fig. 28.7D) (Morimura et al 1994). Rare reports claim to show malignant stroma (?adenosarcoma) but documentation is not con-

Fig. 28.6 Cystic benign transitional cell tumor. H + E ×30

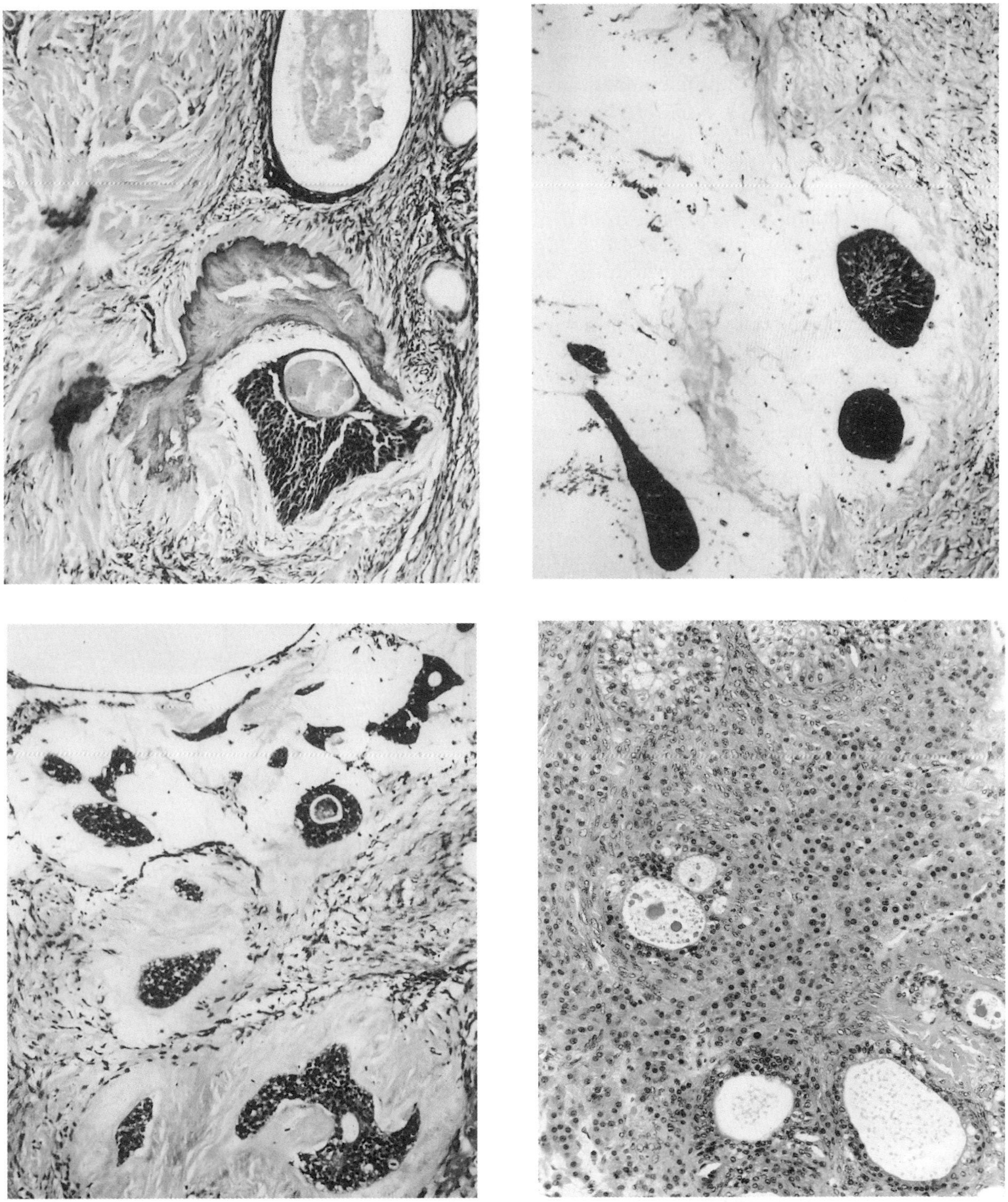

A B C D

Fig. 28.7 Benign transitional cell tumor. (A) Stromal hyalinization and dystrophic calcification. H + E ×75. (B) Grossly edematous, myxoid stroma surrounds epithelial cell nests. H + E ×75. (C) Adjacent field in which edematous stroma has become more hyalinized. H + E ×75. (D) Prominent 'thecoma-like' proliferation and luteinization of the stromal cells. H + E ×59 clusive (Behrens 1953, Bamforth et al 1956) and they more likely represent pseudosarcomatous alteration of benign stroma.

Coarse papillary portions of proliferating transitional cell tumors, as well as cysts, are lined by multilayered atypical epithelium, which has been likened by some authors (Roth et al 1985) to that of low grade transitional cell carcinomas of the bladder, and to squamous carcinoma in situ of the cervix by others (Woodruff et al 1981). In deeper portions of these proliferative nodules, the papillary pattern merges with that of closely packed sheets of transitional cell epithelium with little intervening stroma (Fig. 28.8A). Cellular details do not differ significantly from those described for benign transitional cell tumors, prominent nucleoli and nuclear grooving both being features. Mitoses occur (up to 1 per HPF) and there is, by definition, no stromal invasion (Fig. 28.8B). Mucus-secreting cells, ciliated cells, and squamous metaplasia are sometimes seen, disposed as in benign tumors. Luteinization of the stroma is occasionally noted (Miles & Norris 1972, Genton 1984). Adjacent zones of typical benign transitional cell tumor are seen in almost all cases. Focal necrosis is uncommonly observed.

Most frankly malignant Brenner tumors show a heterogeneous solid carcinomatous proliferation (Figs 28.9–28.11), with a variable amount of intervening stroma. Cysts are lined by multilayered epithelium featuring hyperchromatic and pleiomorphic nuclei and prominent mitotic activity. Occasional bizarre giant cells are seen. Similar features of malignancy are present in the underlying sheets of usually transitional-like cells (Fig. 28.10). Squamoid areas (Fig. 28.11A) or attempts at glandular differentiation (Fig. 28.11B) are commonly encountered. Discrete nests of carcinoma cells may undergo central necrosis producing a 'comedo carcinoma' pattern. The often sparse intervening stroma is usually immature and shows a variable inflammatory infiltrate consistent with invasion. Focal necrosis is demonstrable in

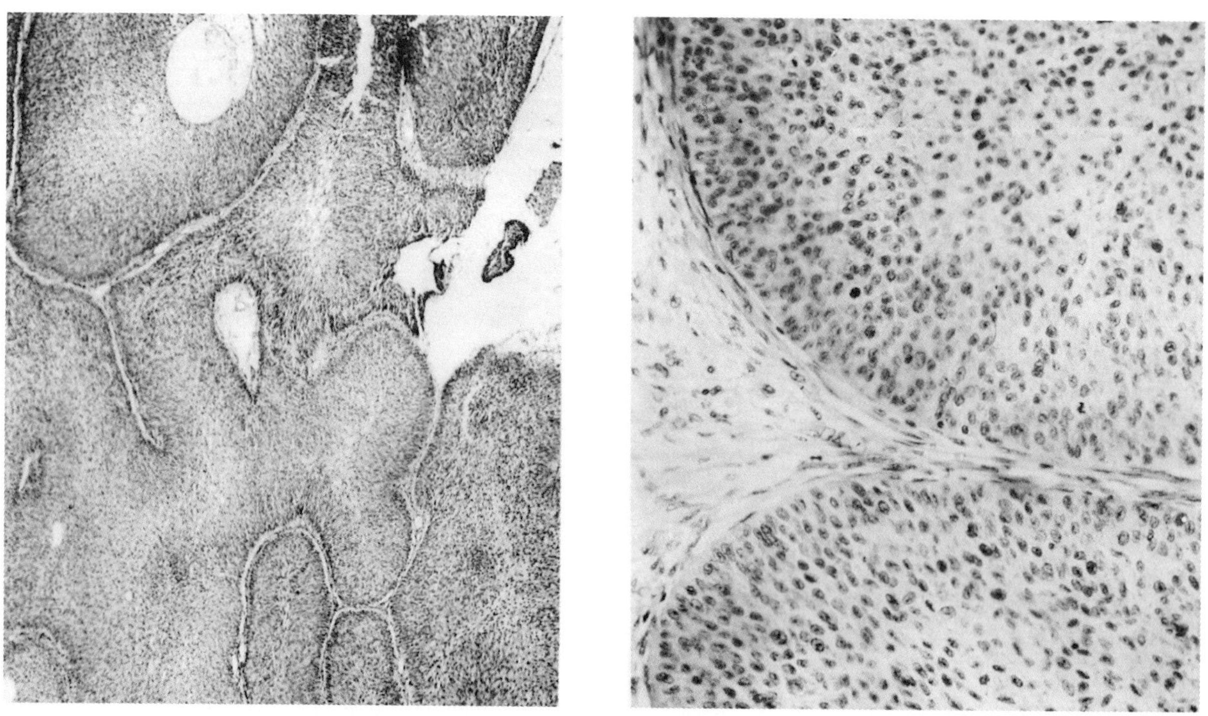

A B

Fig. 28.8 Proliferating transitional cell tumor. (A) Solid sheets of epithelial cells separated by sparse intervening stroma. H + E ×30. (B) Smooth epithelial/stromal interface with transitional cells and occasional mitoses, but no invasion. H + E ×150. (Reprinted, with permission, from Russell 1979b)

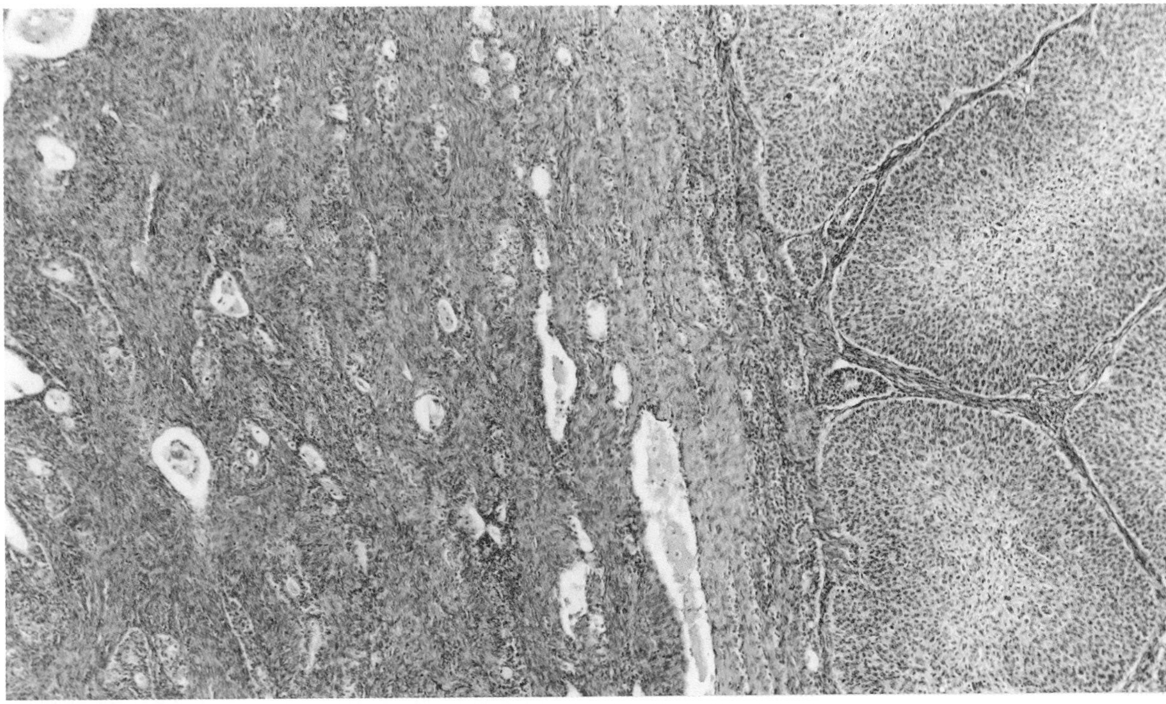

Fig. 28.9 Survey of malignant Brenner tumor with biphasic differentiation towards transitional cell carcinoma (right) and adenocarcinoma (left). H + E ×33

A

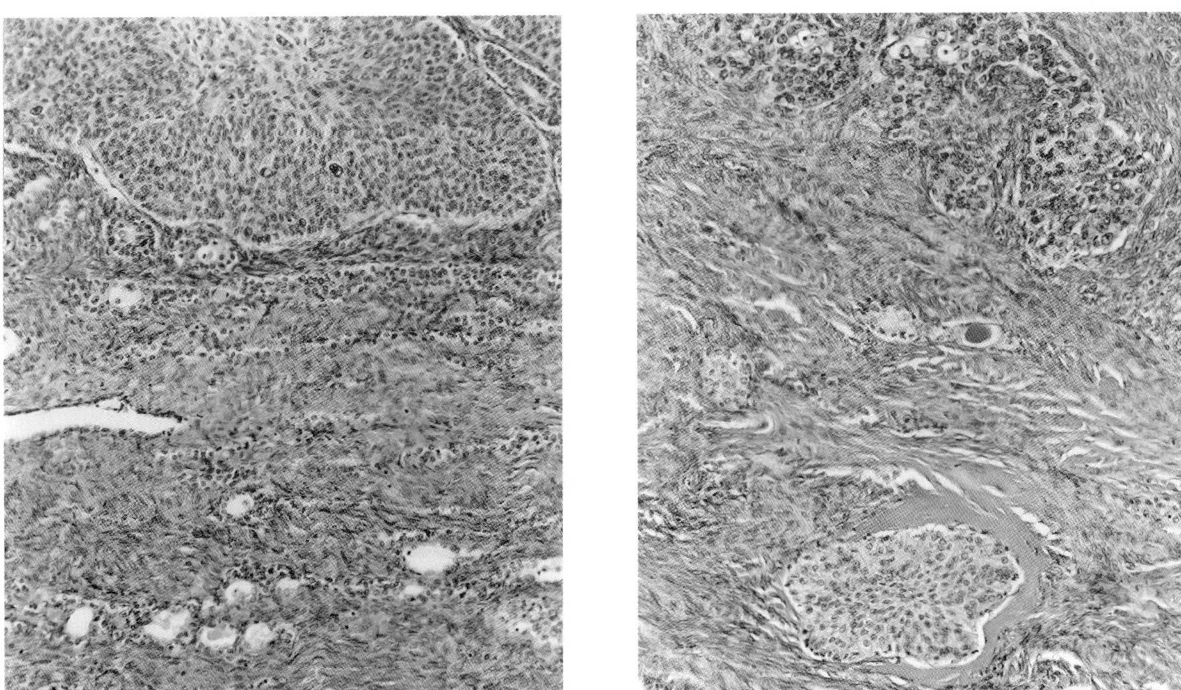

B

Fig. 28.10 Malignant Brenner tumor (same tumor as in Fig. 28.9). (A) Interface between grade 2 transitional cell carcinoma and adenocarcinoma. H + E ×59. (B) Juxtaposition between adenocarcinoma and benign transitional cell elements. H + E ×59

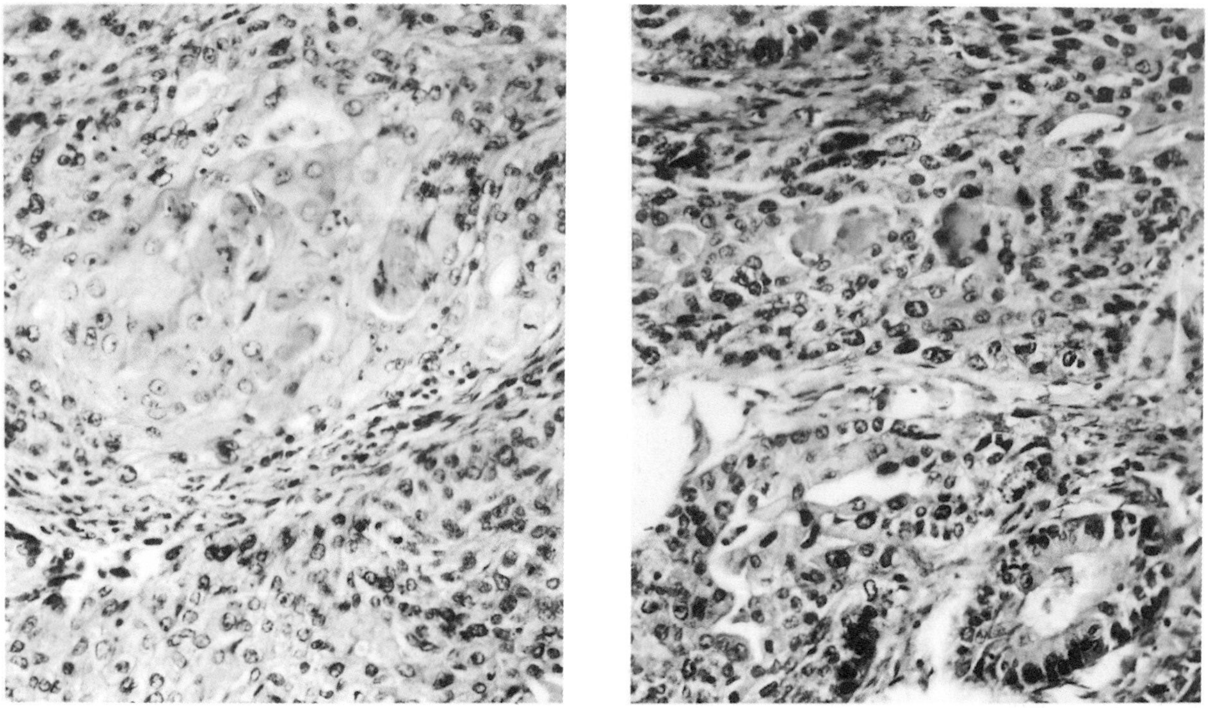

A B

Fig. 28.11 Malignant Brenner tumor. (A) Solid area of carcinoma with undifferentiated or transitional cell area (bottom) and squamous differentiation (center). (B) Focus from same tumor with glandular differentiation. H + E ×150

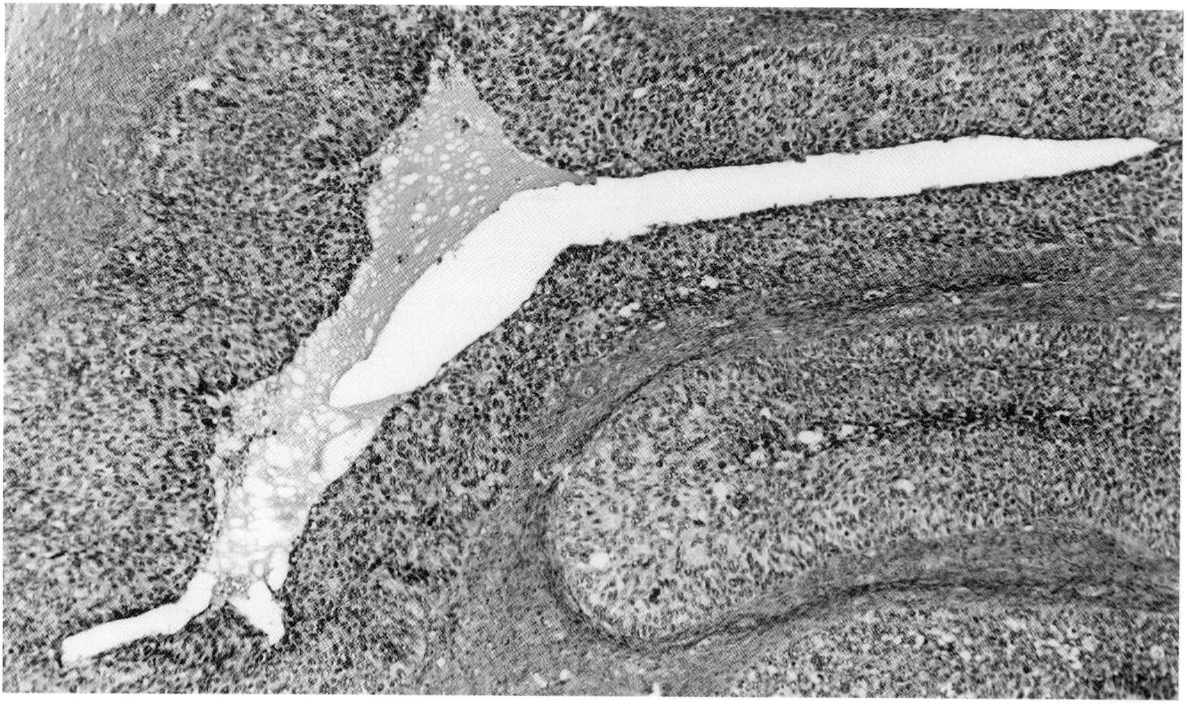

Fig. 28.12 'Pure' transitional cell carcinoma of ovary. H + E ×33

most tumors, as is dystrophic spiculate calcification (Austin & Norris 1987).

Less frequently, the stromal component is more prominent and the tumor architecture more 'adenofibromatous' in pattern (Figs 28.9, 28.10). Epithelial nests show cytological evidence of malignancy but, as in other malignant epithelial adenofibromas, the demonstration of clear-cut stromal invasion required for the diagnosis of malignant Brenner tumor is quite subjective and may necessitate extensive sampling of the neoplasm. Irregularity, branching, and confluence of epithelial nests, depletion of stroma by crowded epithelial masses, and desmoplastic stromal reactions (Roth & Czernobilsky 1985) are useful features to identify.

Foci of benign or proliferating transitional cell tumor nearby (in over half of cases) are important to identify (Fig. 28.10B). Some investigators (Roth & Czernobilsky 1985, Austin & Norris 1987, Silva et al 1990) regard their presence as definitional and, in their absence, recommend a diagnosis of 'transitional cell carcinoma' of the ovary (Fig. 28.12). Austin & Norris (1987) describe small areas of squamous or glandular differentiation in over one-third of their cases of transitional cell carcinoma; calcification is absent and mitoses average almost 3 per HPF. In the absence of a benign or proliferating transitional cell component, the discrimination between malignant Brenner tumors and some other poorly differentiated ovarian carcinomas (such as adenosquamous carcinomas of endometrioid type) may be difficult. Identification of a mucus-secreting adenocarcinomatous component, if present, would strongly favor the former diagnosis, while origin from or juxtaposition to an endometriotic cyst would favor the latter. Differentiating between primary transitional cell carcinoma and transitional cell carcinoma metastatic to the ovaries from the urinary tract is heavily dependent upon clinical features (Young & Scully 1988).

REFERENCES

Aguirre P, Daval Y, Scully R E, de Lellis R A 1984 Mucinous tumors of the ovary with argyrophil cells. An immunohistochemical analysis. American Journal of Surgical Pathology 8: 345–356

Austin R M, Norris H J 1987 Malignant Brenner tumors and transitional cell carcinoma of the ovary. International Journal of Gynecological Pathology 6: 29–39

Bamforth J, Dempster K R, Garland G W 1956 Brenner tumor of the ovary. A report of 2 cases presenting unusual features. Journal of Obstetrics and Gynaecology of the British Empire 63: 344–348

Behrens H 1953 Ein Brennertumorahnliches Sarkom des Ovars. Archiv fur Geschwulstforschung 5: 212–215

Caccamo D, Socias M, Truchet C 1991 Malignant Brenner tumor of the testis and epididymis. Archives of Pathology and Laboratory Medicine 115: 524–527

Chang S H, Roberts J M, Homesley H D 1977 Proliferating Brenner tumor. Obstetrics and Gynecology 49: 489–493

Colgan T J, Norris H J 1983 Ovarian epithelial tumors of low malignant potential: a review. International Journal of Gynecological Pathology 2: 367–382

Conforti S, di Serio C, Donofrio V, Mastrantonio P 1989 Bilateral Brenner tumor. European Journal of Gynaecological Oncology 10: 438–441

Cummins P A, Fox H, Langley F A 1973 An ultrastructural study of the nature and origin of the Brenner tumor of the ovary. Journal of Pathology 110: 167–176

Czernobilsky B 1985 Common epithelial tumors of the ovary. In: Roth L M, Czernobilsky B (eds) Tumors and tumorlike conditions of the ovary. Churchill Livingstone, New York, p 11–43

de Lima G R, de Lima O A, Baracat E C, Vasserman J, Burnier M Jr 1989 Virilizing Brenner tumor of the ovary: case report. Obstetrics and Gynecology 73: 895–898

Egan M, Russell P 1996a Transitional (urothelial) metaplasia of the fallopian tube mucosa. Morphological assessment of three cases. International Journal of Gynecological Pathology 15: 72–76

Egan M, Russell P 1996b Transitional (urothelial) metaplasia of the uterine cervix. Morphological assessment of 31 cases. International Journal of Gynecologic Pathology (in press)

Elemenoglou A, Zizi-Serbetzoglou A, Trihia H, Vasilakaki T, Bournia E 1994 Mixed ovarian neoplasm composed of struma ovarii and Brenner tumor. Report of a case. European Journal of Gynaecological Oncology 15: 138–141

Fox H, Langley F A 1976 Tumours of the ovary. Heinemann, London, p 74–118

Genadry R, Parmley T, Woodruff J D 1979 Simultaneous malignant squamous metaplasia of the cervix and ovary. Gynecologic Oncology 8: 87–91

Genton C Y 1984 An unusual tumor of the ovary. Pathology Research and Practice 179: 110–112

Gershenson D M, Silva E G, Mitchell M F, Atkinson E N, Wharton J T 1993 Transitional cell carcinoma of the ovary: a matched control study of advanced-stage patients treated with cisplatin-based chemotherapy. American Journal of Obstetrics and Gynecology 168: 1178–1185

Hallgrimsson J, Scully R E 1972 Borderline and malignant Brenner tumors of the ovary. A report of 15 cases. Acta Pathologica Microbiologica et Immunologica Scandinavica (A) 80 (suppl 233): 56–66

Hayden M T 1981 Bilateral malignant Brenner tumor. Report of a case with ultrastructural study. Human Pathology 12: 89–92

Hoffman M, Ruffulo E H, Harris W 1989 Giant Brenner tumor. Case report. Journal of Florida Medical Association 76: 772–773
Idelson M G 1963 Malignancy in Brenner tumors of the ovary with comments on histogenesis and possible estrogen production. Obstetrical and Gynecological Survey 18: 246–267
Klemi P J, Nevalainen T J 1977 Ultrastructure of the benign and borderline Brenner tumors. Acta Pathologica et Microbiologica Scandinavica (A) 85: 826–835
Kuhnel R, Rao B R, Stolk J G, van Kessel H, Seldenrijk C A, Willig A P 1987 Estrogen synthesizing rare malignant Brenner tumor of the ovary with the presence of progesterone and androgen receptors in the absence of estrogen receptors. Gynecologic Oncology 26: 263–269
Kunze E, Schauer A, Schmitt M 1983 Histology and histogenesis of two different types of inverted urothelial papillomas. Cancer 51: 348–358
Lifschitz-Mercer B, Czernobilsky B, Shezen E, Dgani R, Leitner O, Geiger B 1988 Selective expression of cytokeratin polypeptides in various epithelia of human Brenner tumor. Human Pathology 19: 640–650
McKenna H, Ansford A 1976 Malignant Brenner tumor. Australian and New Zealand Journal of Obstetrics and Gynaecology 16: 244–248
Martin A R, Kotylo P K, Kennedy J C, Fineberg N S, Roth L M 1992 International Journal of Gynecological Pathology 11: 188–196
Miles P A, Norris H J 1972 Proliferative and malignant Brenner tumors of the ovary. Cancer 30: 174–186
Morimura Y, Ohishi M, Hoshi K, Sato A, Munakata S, Azuma T 1994 A case of ovarian Brenner tumor with stromal estrogenic activity. Asia Oceania Journal of Obstetrics and Gynaecology 20: 165–171
Pratt-Thomas H R, Kreutner A Jr, Underwood P B, Dowdeswell R H 1976 Proliferative and malignant Brenner tumors of the ovary. Report of 2 cases, one with Meigs' syndrome, review of the literature and ultrastructural comparisons. Gynecologic Oncology 4: 176–193
Robey S S, Silva E G, Gershenson D M, McLemore D, el-Naggar A, Ordonez N G 1989 Transitional cell carcinoma in high-grade high-stage ovarian carcinoma. An indicator of favorable response to chemotherapy. Cancer 63: 839–847
Roth L M 1971 Fine structure of the Brenner tumor. Cancer 27: 1482–1488
Roth L M, Czernobilsky B 1985 Ovarian Brenner tumors. II: Malignant. Cancer 56: 592–601
Roth L M, Sternberg W H 1971 Proliferating Brenner tumors. Cancer 27: 687–693
Roth L M, Dallenbach-Hellweg G, Czernobilsky B 1985 Ovarian Brenner tumors. I: Metaplastic, proliferating and of low malignant potential. Cancer 56: 582–591
Roth L M, Gersell D J, Ulbright T M 1993 Ovarian Brenner tumors and transitional cell carcinoma: recent developments. International Journal of Gynecological Pathology 12: 128–133
Russell P 1979a The pathological assessment of ovarian neoplasms. I: Introduction to the common 'epithelial' tumors and analysis of benign 'epithelial' tumors. Pathology 11: 5–26
Russell P 1979b The pathological assessment of ovarian neoplasms. II: The proliferating 'epithelial' tumors. Pathology 11: 251–282
Rybak B J, Ober W B, Bernacki E G 1981 Malignant Brenner tumor of the ovary. Diagnostic Gynecology and Obstetrics 3: 61–74
Santini D, Gelli M G, Mazzoleni G et al 1989 Brenner tumor of the ovary: a correlative histologic, histochemical, immunohistochemical, and ultrastructural investigation. Human Pathology 20: 787–795
Sasano H, Wargotz E S, Silverberg S G, Mason J I, Simpson E R 1989 Brenner tumor of the ovary: immunoanalysis of steroidogenic enzymes in 23 cases. Human Pathology 20: 1103–1107
Scully R E 1979 Tumors of the ovary and maldeveloped gonads. AFIP fascicle 16, 2nd series. Armed Forces Institute of Pathology, Washington, DC, p 53–151
Seldenrijk C A, Willig A P, Baak J P A et al 1986 Malignant Brenner tumor: a histologic, morphometrical, immunohistochemical and ultrastructural study. Cancer 58: 754–760
Serov S F, Scully R E, Sobin L H 1973 Histological typing of ovarian tumors. International histological classification of tumors No. 9. World Health Organization, Geneva, p 17–54
Silva E G, Robey-Cafferty S S, Smith T L, Gershenson D M 1990 Ovarian carcinomas with transitional cell carcinoma pattern. American Journal of Clinical Pathology 93: 457–465
Silverberg S G 1971 Brenner tumor of the ovary. A clinicopathologic study of 60 tumors in 54 women. Cancer 28: 588–596
Silverberg S G, Wilson M A 1972 Ultrastructure of the Brenner tumor. American Journal of Obstetrics and Gynecology 112: 91–100
Svenes K B, Eide J 1984 Proliferative Brenner tumor or ovarian metastases? A case report. Cancer 53: 2692–2697
Woodruff J D, Dietrich D, Genadry R, Parmley T H 1981 Proliferative and malignant Brenner tumors. Review of 47 cases. American Journal of Obstetrics and Gynecology 141: 118–125
Young R H, Scully R E 1988 Urothelial and ovarian carcinomas of identical cell types: problems in interpretation. A report of three cases and review of the literature. International Journal of Gynecological Pathology 7: 197–211

29

Mixed epithelial tumors

P. Russell A. Farnsworth

No generally accepted criteria exist for defining or classifying these tumors. Their origin is equally poorly understood, but is most likely to be the result of biphasic or multiphasic differentiation within the neoplastic state. Malignant epithelial tumors of mixed differentiation are not uncommon elsewhere in the female genital tract, expressing much the same spectrum as is observed in the ovaries. They are defined by the exhibition of two or more of the epithelial elements described in the preceding six chapters, present in variable proportions, intimately mixed or producing discrete areas (Fig. 29.1) and occupying the full proliferative spectrum from benign to invasive carcinoma. By convention, minor components (isolated fields or cellular aggregates) of a second or third epithelial tissue type should be disregarded in mullerian tumors for the purposes of tumor classification (Serov et al 1973, Russell 1979a), and such neoplasms are best categorized in accordance with

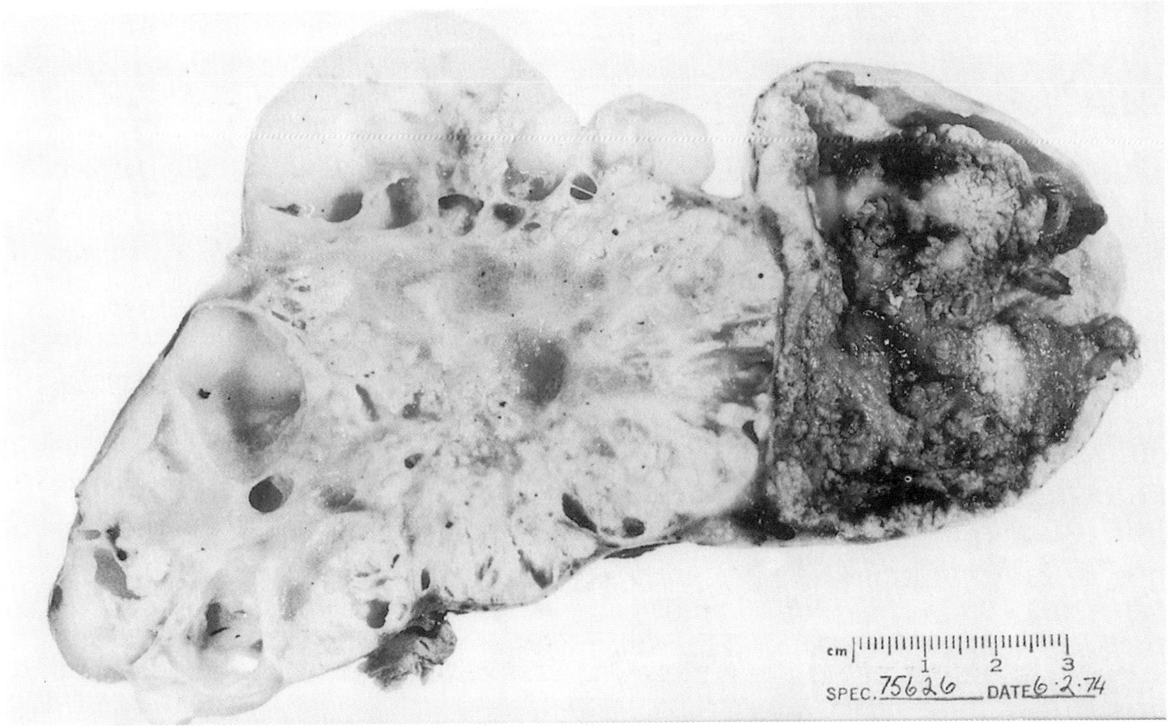

Fig. 29.1 Mixed endometrioid and serous carcinoma of the ovary. The former component (left) predominates, while the serous carcinoma has formed a discrete cystic mass at one pole of the neoplasm

the differentiation of the dominant epithelial element. Examples of this would include typical endometrioid carcinomas with focal areas of ciliated cells (see Fig. 25.21), the latter not qualifying as significant serous differentiation, or Brenner tumors with occasional microcysts lined by mucinous epithelium. Another convention dictates that mucinous carcinomas arising in association with benign Brenner tumors (see Ch. 28) be classified as mixed epithelial carcinomas rather than malignant Brenner tumors. The arbitrary minimum criterion we have adopted for inclusion of tumors in this category is a 10% representation of minor epithelial elements in the tissue sections (Russell 1979a, Scully 1982). In our material, this results in about 2–3% of benign tumors, a similar percentage of those showing atypical proliferation, and 1–2% of invasive malignant epithelial tumors being categorized as mixed (Russell 1979a–c).

The diagnosis may be difficult, not only in the carcinoma group where a relative lack of epithelial differentiation may be expected to compromise assessment, but also in benign tumors in which intermediate or 'indifferent' epithelial elements may be present. At each point in the proliferative spectrum it appears that epithelial combinations reflect, to some extent, the relative frequencies with which the different 'pure' types occur. Thus, of benign mixed epithelial tumors (Table 29.1), serous–mucinous (Fig. 29.2) and mucinous–Brenner (Fig. 29.3) are the commonly observed associations. Roth et al (1985) proposed that

Table 29.1 Approximate percentage concurrence of the different mullerian epithelial types based on an analysis of 558 benign epithelial tumors (Russell 1979a).

Example: of all benign mucinous tumors, 2% have an associated Brenner component. Conversely, of all benign Brenner tumors, 25% will have an appreciable benign mucinous element

Dominant component	Minor component			
	Serous	Mucinous	Endometrioid	Brenner
Serous		1	1	1
Mucinous	3			2
Endometrioid	50			
Brenner	10	25		

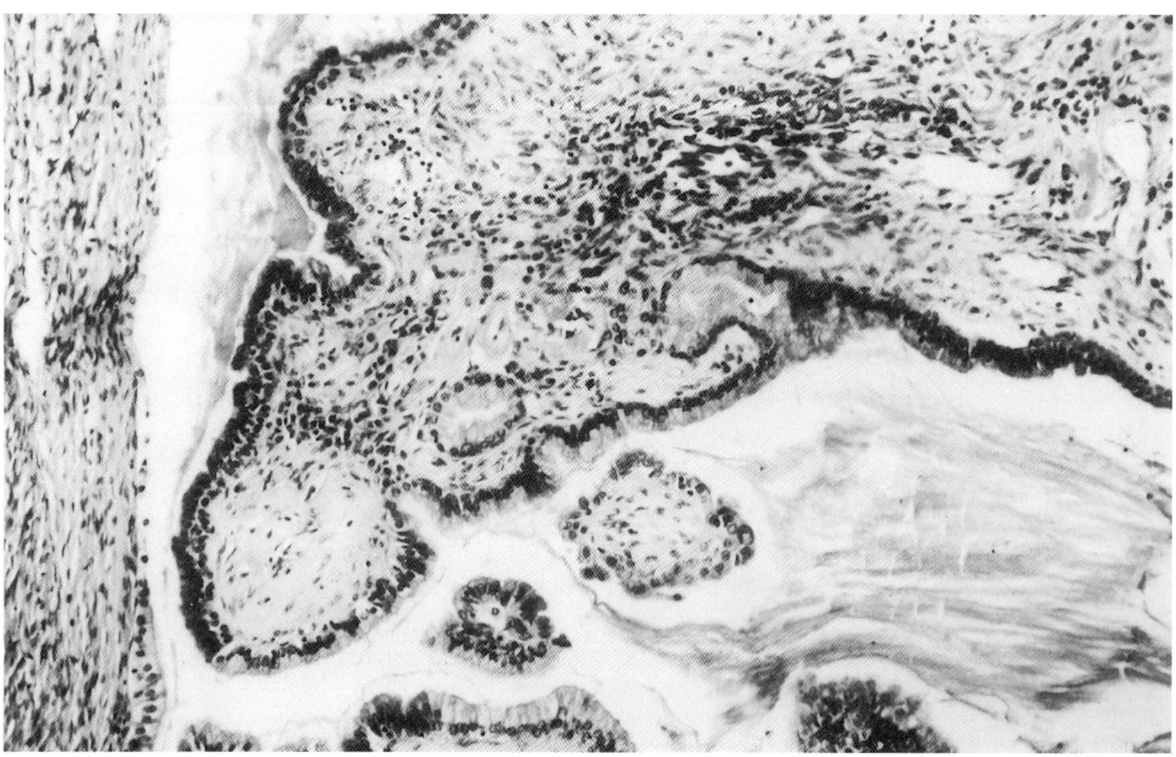

Fig. 29.2 Benign mixed serous and mucinous cystadenoma with an intimate admixture of the epithelial subtypes. H + E ×125. (Reprinted, with permission, from Russell 1979a)

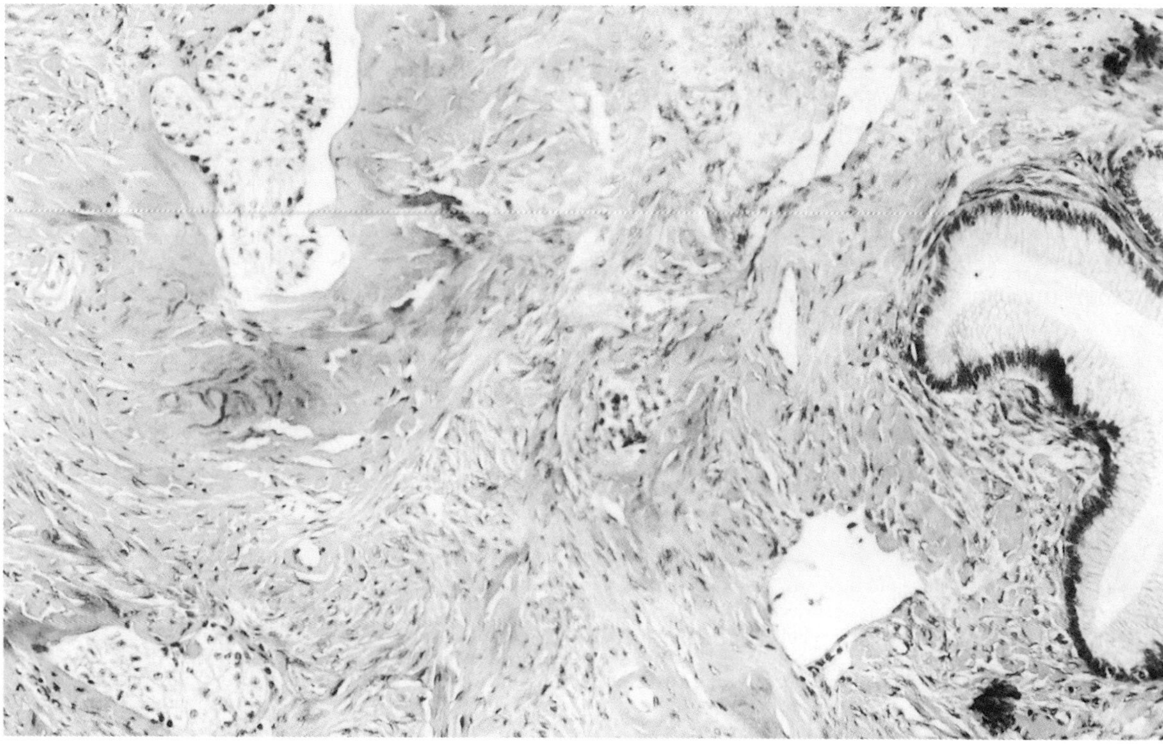

Fig. 29.3 Benign mixed mucinous and Brenner tumor. H + E ×125

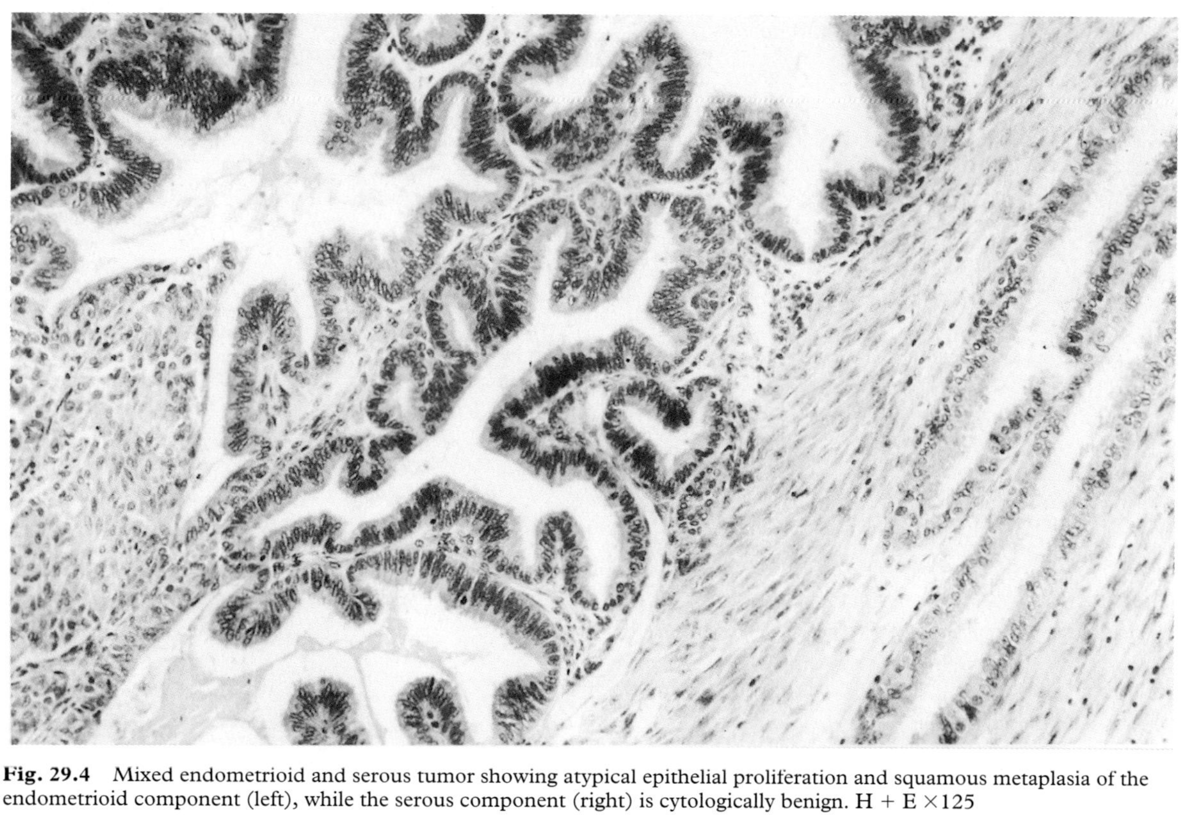

Fig. 29.4 Mixed endometrioid and serous tumor showing atypical epithelial proliferation and squamous metaplasia of the endometrioid component (left), while the serous component (right) is cytologically benign. H + E ×125

mixed Brenner–mucinous tumors be classified as 'metaplastic Brenner tumors', a concept with which we disagree. Mixed epithelial tumors with atypical proliferation are rare and show various combinations of serous, mucinous, and/or endometrioid epithelia (Fig. 29.4). The largest published series of atypically proliferating ovarian tumors of mixed serous and mucinous differentiation (Rutgers & Scully 1988) stresses the mullerian rather than intestinal differentiation of the mucinous component, the high association (53%) of pelvic endometriosis, and occasional local recurrences, presumably due to unrecognized 'implants' at the time of original surgery. Not all epithelial elements need be atypically proliferating to so categorize a tumor (Anderson 1972). Within the malignant mixed epithelial subgroup, serous–endometrioid and endometrioid–clear cell are the most commonly encountered (Tornos et al 1994).

There is some evidence to suggest that these tumors behave similarly to the 'pure' counterpart of their dominant epithelial element, both with respect to patterns of pathogenesis and clinical outcome for the patient – e.g. a predominantly serous tumor is more likely to have extraovarian manifestations at laparotomy, and a predominantly endometrioid tumor is more likely to be associated with pelvic endometriosis (Russell 1979a–c, Rutgers & Scully 1988).

REFERENCES

Anderson M C 1972 Endometrioid tumor of the ovary with mucinous and serous components. American Journal of Obstetrics and Gynecology 113: 686–690

Roth L M, Dallenbach-Hellweg G, Czernobilsky B 1985 Ovarian Brenner tumors. I: Metaplastic, proliferating and of low malignant potential. Cancer 56: 582–591

Russell P 1979a The pathological assessment of ovarian neoplasms. I: Introduction to the common 'epithelial' tumors and analysis of benign 'epithelial' tumors. Pathology 11: 5–26

Russell P 1979b The pathological assessment of ovarian neoplasms. II: The proliferating 'epithelial' tumors. Pathology 11: 251–282

Russell P 1979c The pathological assessment of ovarian neoplasms. III: The malignant 'epithelial' tumors. Pathology 11: 493–532

Rutgers J L, Scully R E 1988 Ovarian mixed-epithelial papillary cystadenomas of borderline malignancy of mullerian type. A clinicopathologic analysis. Cancer 61: 546–554

Scully R E 1982 Common epithelial tumors of borderline malignancy (carcinomas of low malignant potential). Bulletin du Cancer (Paris) 69: 228–238

Serov S F, Scully R E, Sobin L H 1973 Histological typing of ovarian tumors. International histological classification of tumors No. 9. World Health Organization, Geneva, p 17–54

Tornos C, Silva E G, Khorana S M, Burke T W 1994 High-stage endometrioid carcinoma of the ovary. Prognostic significance of pure versus mixed histologic types. American Journal of Surgical Pathology 18: 687–693

30

Undifferentiated carcinomas

P. Russell A. Farnsworth

In the World Health Organization (WHO) classification (Serov et al 1973), 'undifferentiated carcinomas' are defined as including tumors with minimal differentiation such as occasional endometrial-like glands, psammoma bodies, and droplets or pools of mucin. From a strictly semantic standpoint, therefore, the term 'undifferentiated' is incorrect, and a more accurate interpretation of the intended definition would be given by the phrase 'poorly differentiated carcinomas not otherwise classifiable'. Indeed, the only truly undifferentiated carcinomas (unilateral tumors in young women and often associated with hypercalcemia) are quite specifically excluded from this category, and are discussed in Chapter 31. Furthermore, the concept of 'minimal differentiation' is difficult to quantitate and, for example, precludes any real reproducibility in separating such carcinomas from poorly differentiated serous or endometrioid carcinomas. This is indicated by the great dispari-

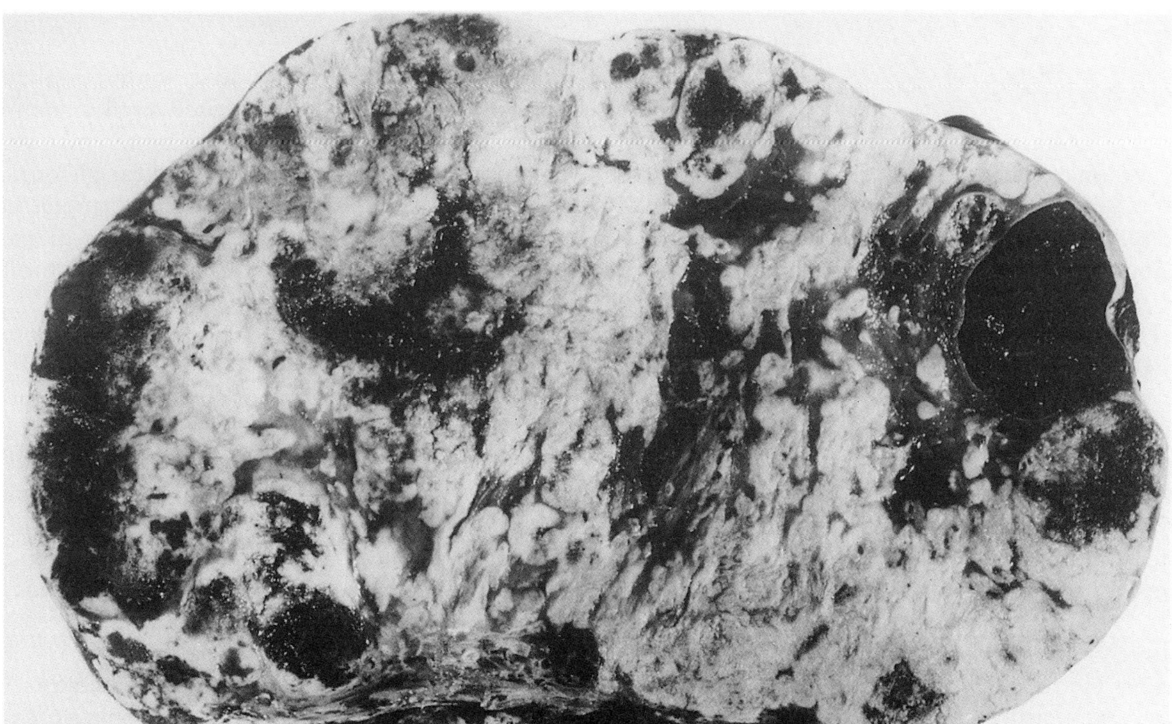

Fig. 30.1 A 15 cm solid undifferentiated carcinoma of the ovary with obvious widespread necrosis and hemorrhage

ty in their reported incidence of 5–15% of all primary ovarian malignancies (Scully 1977). Their mean age of incidence is about 55 years. They are bilateral in over 50% of cases and disseminated at the time of laparotomy in over 80% of cases. Prognosis, as might be expected, is poor, with Silva et al (1991) giving a 5-year survival rate of only 11%. A specific subtype of undifferentiated small cell carcinoma, resembling the more common small cell carcinomas of the lung, has recently been described (Eichhorn et al 1992). These 11 examples occurred in women with a mean age of 59 years, were large tumors, bilateral in one-half of cases, and had a poor clinical outcome.

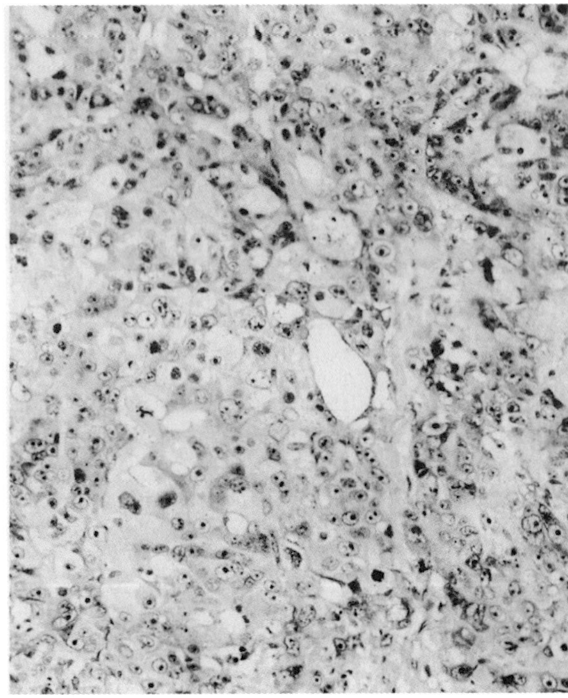

Fig. 30.2 Undifferentiated carcinoma composed of sheets of anaplastic epithelial cells. H + E ×125

Macroscopic features

Distinctive macroscopic features are absent in these tumors. The tumors tend to be large, mostly solid masses, and often show necrosis and hemorrhage (Fig. 30.1). Surface adhesions and rupture of the capsule are frequently present. Less commonly, the tumors may be partly cystic, usually with hemorrhage into the cysts.

Microscopic features

Several histological patterns are observed, based largely on variation in cell size and the relative prominence of stroma. The epithelial nature of the cells is confirmed by the sparseness of the reticulin fibers and immunohistochemical staining for epithelial cell markers (e.g. EMA, cytokeratins, CA-125 antigen, B72.3).

Many such tumors are composed of solid sheets of anaplastic epithelial cells (Fig. 30.2), which may have a vaguely squamoid or transitional appearance (Silva et al 1991); the dividing line between such examples and adenosquamous carcinomas or malignant Brenner tumors is blurred. The cell size and shape may suggest to the experienced observer poorly differentiated serous (Fig. 30.3) or endometrioid carcinomas, and it is generally accepted that the majority of these tumors are probably at the end of one or other of these neoplastic spectra (Czernobilsky 1977, Scully 1979). Bizarre eosinophilic mononuclear giant cells are frequently encountered in typical clear cell carcinomas, so that undifferentiated epithelial malignancies composed predominantly or exclusively of such cells (Fig. 30.4B) may well belong to this tumor category. Nuclear pleiomorphism and the absence of coarse cytoplasmic granularity would distinguish these carcinomas from the recently described ovarian oncocytomas (see Ch. 31).

Other examples have rather more stroma intervening between nests and cords of undifferentiated cells. The stroma is generally immature, but may be quite desmoplastic and often contains a variable inflammatory infiltrate (usually lymphoplasmacytic, but occasionally with many eosinophils).

Undifferentiated small cell carcinomas of 'pulmonary' or neuroendocrine type (so termed to distinguish them from those associated with hypercalcemia in young women; see Ch. 31) are characterized by patternless sheets and nests of small to medium sized rounded or spindle cells with sparse cytoplasm and focal streaming of hematoxyphilic material (Fig. 30.5A). Tumor

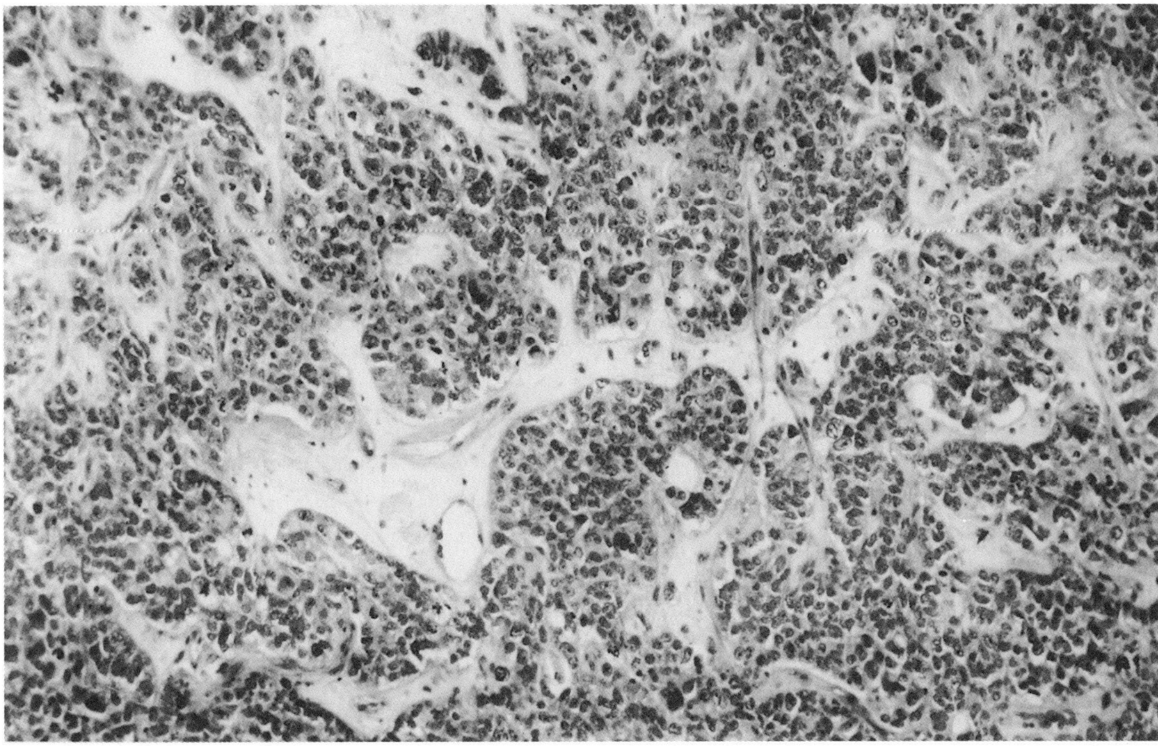

Fig. 30.3 Undifferentiated carcinoma composed of uniform small cells, possibly of serous differentiation. H + E ×125

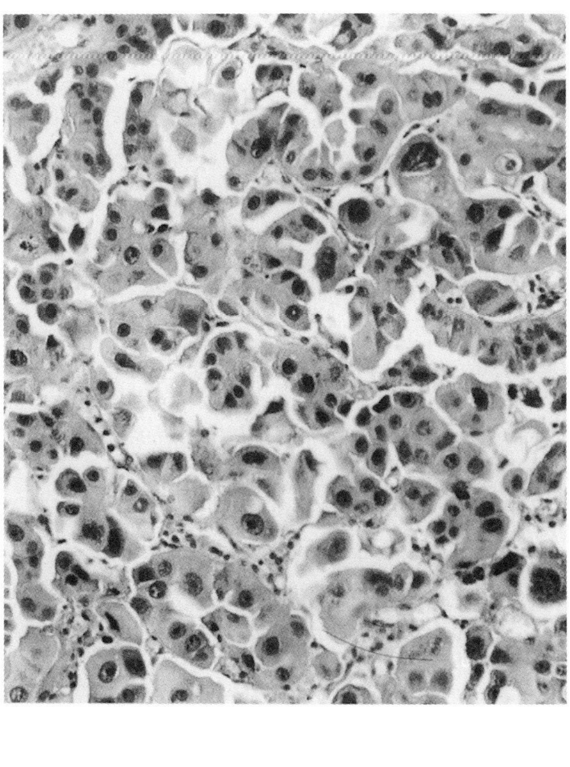

cells have rounded to oval hyperchromatic nuclei with evenly dispersed chromatin, indistinct nuclear membranes, and inapparent nucleoli (Fig. 30.5B). Mitoses are numerous and atypical. Apoptosis and focal coagulative necrosis are also common features. In the series of Eichhorn et al (1992), evidence of coexistent transitional cell (Brenner), endometrioid, or mucinous neoplasia was found in most lesions, suggesting origin from these surface epithelial–stromal tumors. Immunostaining the small cell carcinomatous component of these neoplasms frequently (but not always) revealed cytokeratin intermediate filaments, NSE, and EMA, but all tumors were all negative for vimentin.

Differential diagnosis

Care should be taken to distinguish these poorly

Fig. 30.4 Undifferentiated adenocarcinoma composed exclusively of pleiomorphic cells with abundant eosinophilic cytoplasm, possibly of clear cell origin. H + E ×125

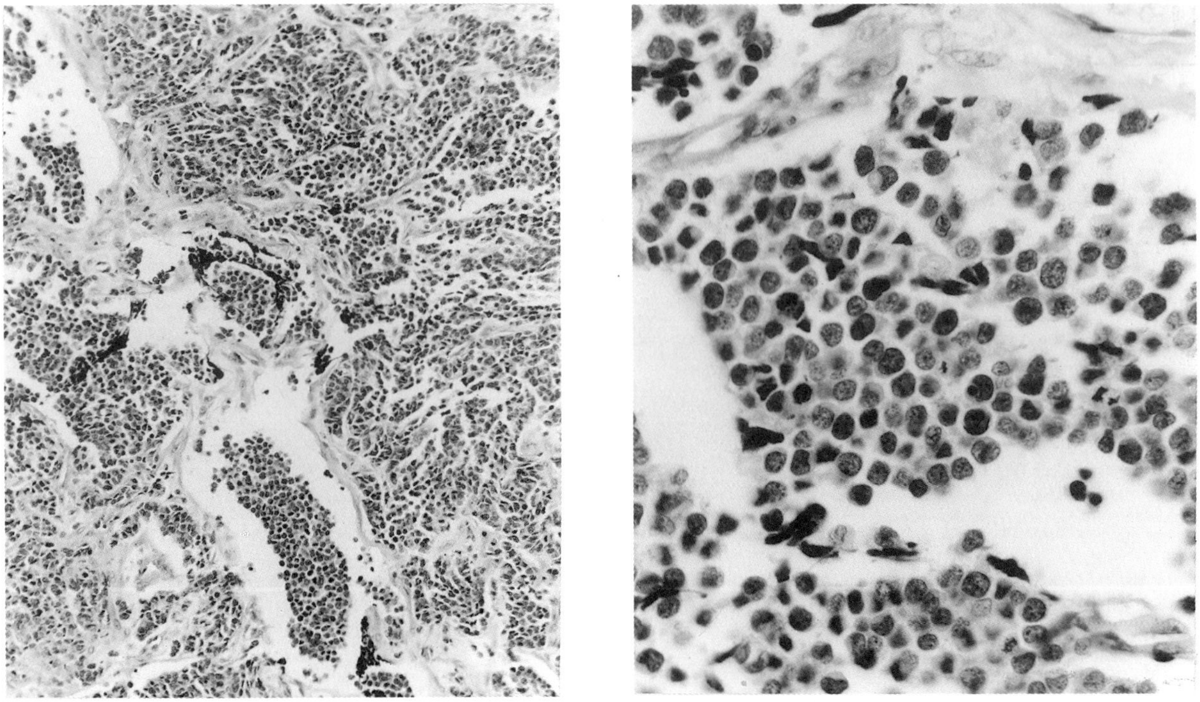

Fig. 30.5 Undifferentiated small cell carcinoma of 'pulmonary' or neuroendocrine type. (A) Patternless sheets and nests of small 'oat cells' with prominent vascular permeation and streaming of hematoxylinophilic debris. H + E ×59. (B) Cellular detail showing scanty cytoplasm, finely stippled chromatin and inapparent nucleoli. H + E ×231

differentiated epithelial malignancies from diffuse variants of granulosa cell tumors. The latter are unilateral and exhibit much less nuclear pleiomorphism, mitotic activity, and tumor necrosis. With the exception of weak focal immunostaining for cytokeratin intermediate filaments, cell markers usually associated with poorly differentiated ovarian carcinomas (EMA, CA-125 antigen, CA19-9, B72.3) are negative in granulosa cell tumors (Gitsch et al 1991, 1992, Silva et al 1991).

Discrimination between undifferentiated small cell carcinomas and metastases of pulmonary origin is achieved largely on clinical grounds, unless adjacent fields of primary ovarian mullerian carcinoma are found, with transitions between the two patterns.

REFERENCES

Czernobilsky B 1977 Primary epithelial tumors of the ovary. In: Blaustein A (ed) Pathology of the female genital tract, Springer-Verlag, New York, p 453–504

Eichhorn J H, Young R H, Scully R E 1992 Primary ovarian small cell carcinoma of pulmonary type. A clinicopathologic, immunohistologic, and flow cytometric analysis of 11 cases. American Journal of Surgical Pathology 16: 926–938

Gitsch G, Kohlenberger P, Hanzal E, Kolbl H, Breitenecker G 1991 Immunohistochemical differentiation between ovarian granulosa cell tumors and ovarian carcinomas. Archives of Gynecology and Obstetrics 249: 173–177

Gitsch G, Kohlenberger P, Steiner A, Neumeister B, Breitenecker G 1992 Expression of cytokeratins in granulosa cell tumors and ovarian carcinomas. Archives of Gynecology and Obstetrics 251: 193–197

Scully R E 1977 Ovarian tumors. A review. American Journal of Pathology 87: 686–720

Scully R E 1979 Tumors of the ovary and maldeveloped gonads. AFIP fascicle 16, 2nd series. Armed Forces Institute of Pathology, Washington, DC, p 53–151

Serov S F, Scully R E, Sobin L H 1973 Histological typing of ovarian tumors. International histological classification of tumours No. 9. World Health Organization, Geneva, p 17–54

Silva E G, Tornos C, Bailey M A, Morris M 1991 Undifferentiated carcinoma of the ovary. Archives of Pathology and Laboratory Medicine 115: 377–381

31

Unclassified and miscellaneous cysts and tumors

P. Russell *A. Farnsworth*

UNCLASSIFIED EPITHELIAL TUMORS

At every level of experience with ovarian neoplasms there seems to be a residuum of tumors in which the epithelial component fails to demonstrate features sufficiently characteristic to allow

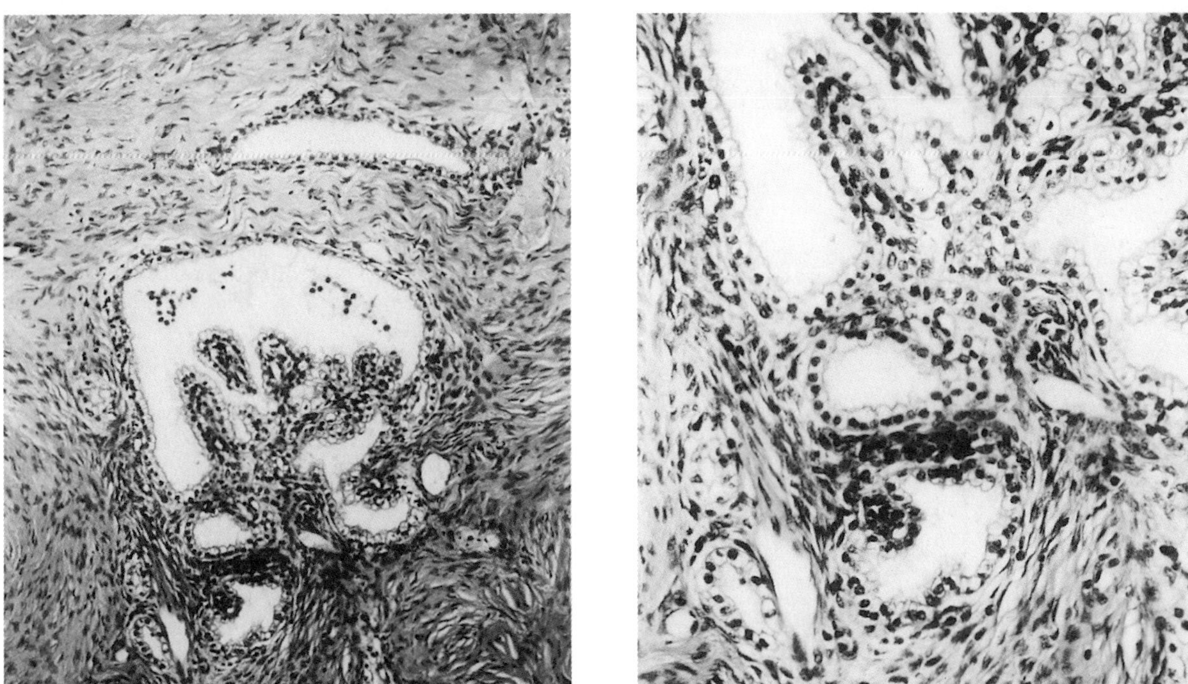

A B

Fig. 31.1 A 4 cm solid papillary adenofibroma. (A) The architectural features are typical of a serous adenofibroma. H + E ×75. (B) The scattered epithelial elements have cytological features intermediate between mesothelial and either secretory serous or clear cell. H + E ×150.

its classification into one of the previously described groups, even though it is clearly not an undifferentiated carcinoma. For example, interpretation of tumors with features intermediate between serous and endometrioid differentiation can be extremely difficult, and such lesions account for many examples in this category. This difficulty is present at both ends of the neoplastic spectrum, both in adenofibromas with ill-defined epithelial components as well as carcinomas with intermediate features. Subjectivity clearly plays a part in their assessment, but there is some merit in placing as few tumors as practicable into this unclassified category. Figures 31.1–31.4 give examples of the diagnostic difficulties encountered and the types of tumor appropriately placed here.

Two examples of primary so-called 'oncocytic tumors of the ovaries' merit comment (Takeda et al 1983, Yoshida et al 1984). The first of these tumors was a 15 cm unilocular cystic tumor occurring in a 39-year-old woman. Histologically it was a well differentiated adenocarcinoma with a papillary pattern of growth. The second tumor was an 11 cm solid tumor, with a lobulated cut surface, occurring in a 22-year-old woman. This lesion had a solid pattern of growth histologically. Both tumors were composed uniformly of typical oncocytes with small round uniform vesicular nuclei, and abundant eosinophilic granular cytoplasm which ultrastructurally was filled with mitochondria. Neither tumor has pursued a malignant course.

OVARIAN MESOTHELIOMAS

Tumors arise from the ovarian surface which morphologically, histochemically, and ultrastruc-

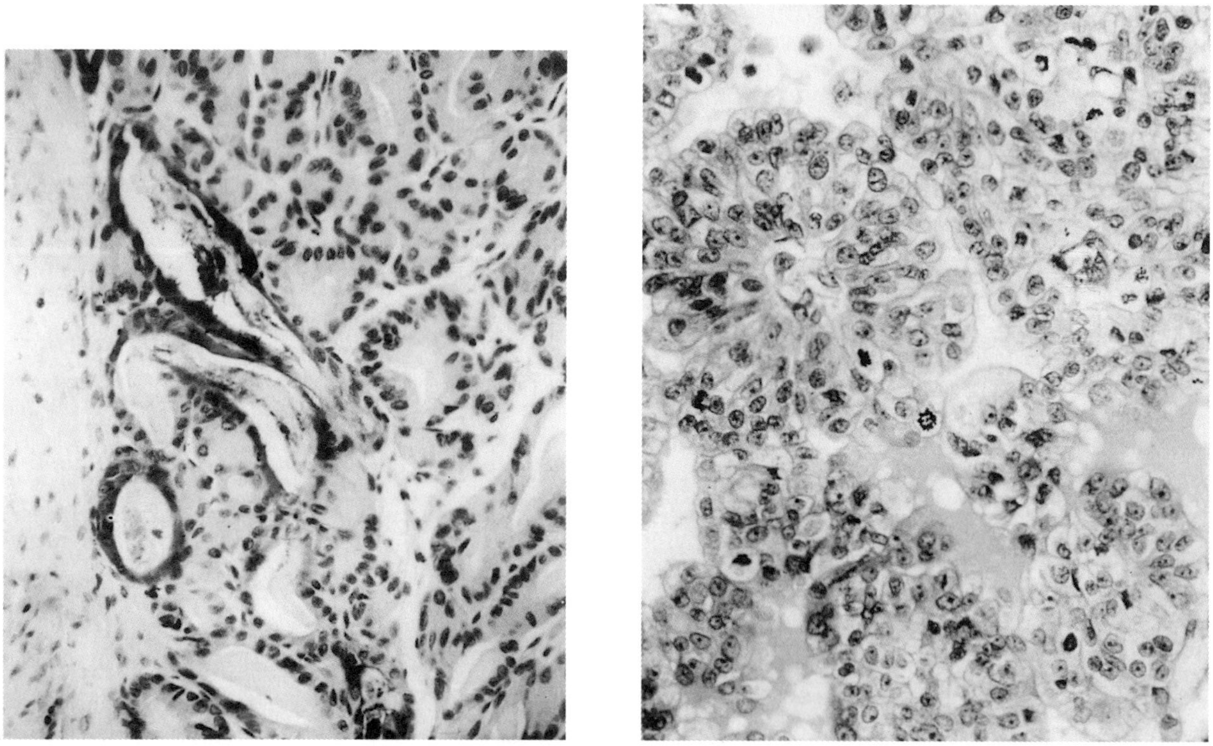

A B

Fig. 31.2 (A) A 6 cm cystic tumor with a small mural nodule. The cyst wall was lined by typical serous epithelium of a low grade proliferating tumor. The mural nodule is characterized by uniform tubules lined by columnar cells with brightly eosinophilic cytoplasm which immunostains focally for CEA (center left), and oval, longitudinally grooved nuclei (top). Immunostain for CEA ×150. (B) A solid–cystic ovarian mass with a papillary pattern of growth. Histologically, the papillae are covered by multilayered epithelium, with cytoplasmic features suggesting clear cell differentiation and nuclear features (high mitotic rate, small uniform round nuclei) of serous differentiation. H + E ×250

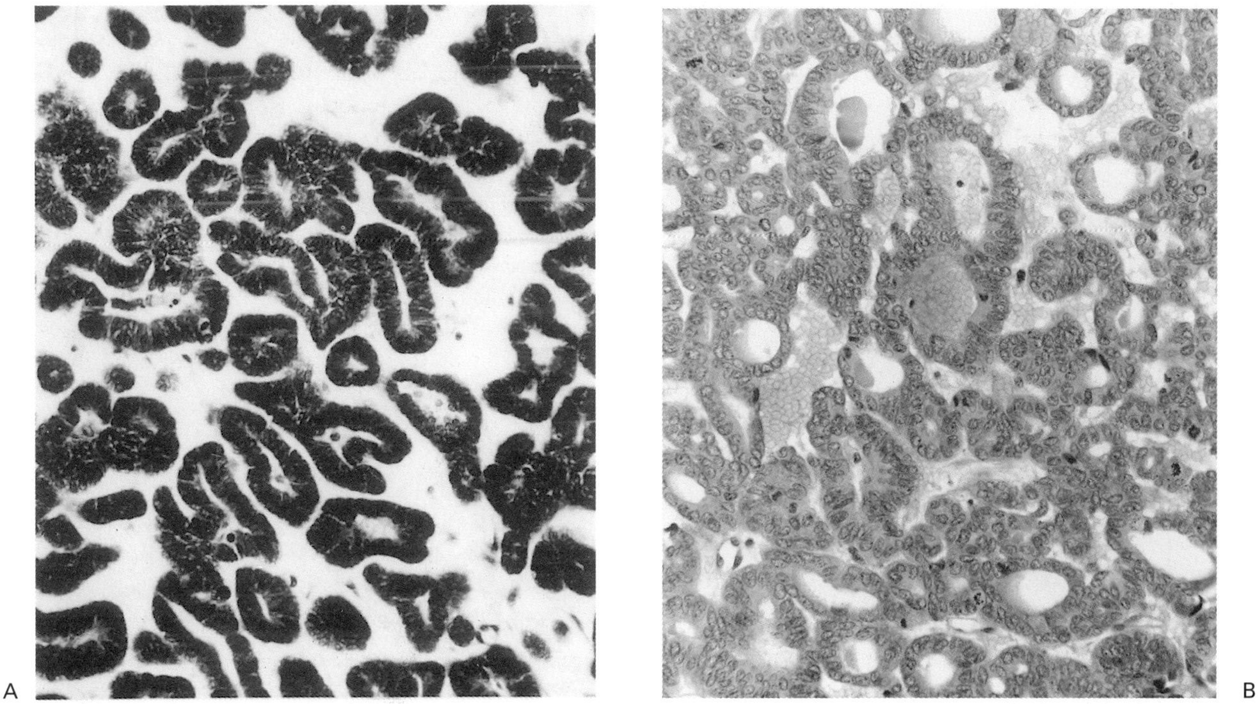

Fig. 31.3 (A) A 12 cm cystic–solid ovarian tumor with omental metastases, in a 76-year-old woman. Both primary and secondary tumor deposits are characterized by uniform tubules composed of tall columnar cells with elongate, densely hyperchromatic nuclei and scanty cytoplasm. Mucin stains are negative, but immunostains for epithelial differentiation (EMA, cytokeratins) are strongly positive. Intervening stroma is acellular and myxoid in type. H + E ×150. (B) A similar ovarian tumor mass in a 64-year-old woman, exhibiting discrete and separate tubular and follicular structures in loose myxoid stroma. Some resemblance to endometrioid carcinoma is apparent in the cellular detail, but more typical patterns were absent from the tumor. H + E ×116

turally resemble mesotheliomas originating elsewhere in the serous cavities. We do not subscribe to the idea that such ovarian mesotheliomas are undifferentiated neoplasms, but rather that they represent another specific path of neoplastic differentiation analogous to the various mullerian types seen in the common 'epithelial' tumor group (see Table 20.1). Although Parmley & Woodruff (1974) have put forward the concept that all the ovarian common 'epithelial' tumors are basically mesotheliomas, showing patterns of mullerian differentiation to a variable extent, their view has not been generally accepted and, irrespective of the supposed ultimate cell of origin, there are important clinical and epidemiological reasons for separating these two groups of tumors – whether of ovarian or extraovarian origin (Kannerstein et al 1977, Foyle et al 1981). Of some interest, with regard to the histogenetic considerations which they raise, are the occasional tumors which show histological characteristics intermediate between mesotheliomas and mullerian tumors (Foyle et al 1981).

Peritoneal mesotheliomas exhibit a range of clinical behavior not always predictable from their morphology (Kannerstein & Churg 1977, Addis & Fox 1983). At one end of the spectrum are the malignant, usually fatal, tumors, which involve the peritoneal cavity diffusely, and at the other are the benign so-called adenomatoid tumors, which are circumscribed lesions with no untoward clinical sequelae. The behavior of well differentiated papillary tumors is less predictable. Localized lesions are usually benign, but the diffuse or multifocal lesions may pursue an indolent course. Benign cystic mesotheliomas have a tendency to recur. Only the diffuse malignant mesotheliomas are associated with asbestos exposure.

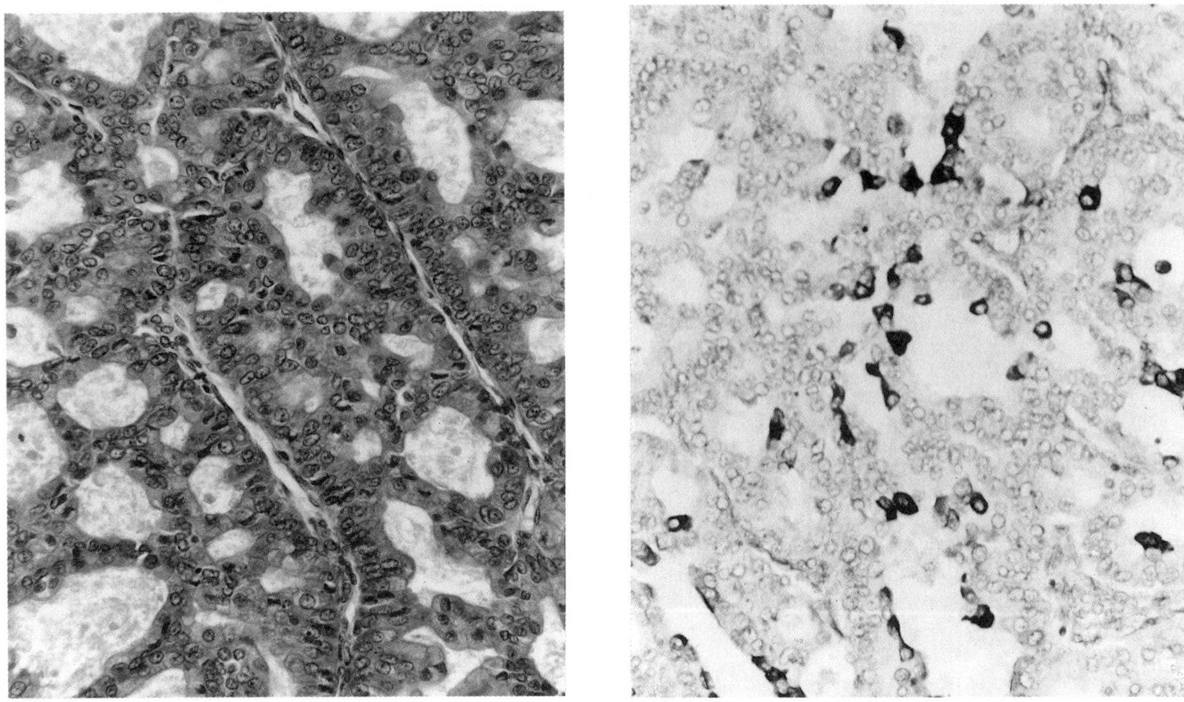

A B

Fig. 31.4 A 10 cm hemorrhagic and partly necrotic right ovarian tumor with a distinctly 'mucoid' character to the cyst contents and cut surface. (A) The epithelial lining of most cystic spaces and glands is composed of large mucin-containing polyhedral or columnar cells resembling endocervical rather than intestinal cell type. A second population of single epithelial cells is scattered over the luminal surface of the mucin-secreting cells. These have more densely eosinophilic and a syncytial character to their cytoplasm. These cells do not contain mucin. H + E ×116. (B) The differentiation between the two populations of cells is highlighted by strong immunostaining for cytokeratin-7 (CK7) in the scattered single superficial cells. It is not clear whether such a tumor should be regarded as a mullerian adenocarcinoma of mucinous or of indeterminate differentiation. Immunostain for CK7 ×116.

Adenomatoid tumors

These tumors are not uncommonly encountered, as incidental findings, in the uterus and fallopian tubes, but are rarely reported in the ovaries (Ferenczy et al 1972, Fox & Langley 1976, Hirawaki et al 1988, Young et al 1991). A solitary report notes their presence in both uterus and ovary in the same patient (Kupryjanczyk 1989).

Macroscopic features

They occur in the hilar region, forming well circumscribed grey-white or yellowish nodules 1–1.5 cm in diameter. A honeycomb pattern of tiny cystic spaces may be evident macroscopically.

Microscopic features

Vascular-like spaces are lined by flattened or cuboidal cells, in turn surrounded by stroma rich in elastic, collagen and smooth muscle fibers. Cords and small clusters of vacuolated cells may also be present (Fig. 31.5). The tumor cells have eosinophilic or vacuolated cytoplasm which is alcian blue positive at pH 2.5; this reaction, including the nonspecific stromal staining, can be eliminated by prior incubation with hyaluronidase. The mucicarmine stain is negative, but PAS after diastase digestion may be focally positive. Glycogen is sometimes demonstrable. The round or bean-shaped nuclei have finely dispersed chromatin with well defined nuclear membranes but inconspicuous nucleoli. Nuclear atypia is minimal or absent, and mitoses are infrequent. Immunohistochemically, mesothelial tumor cells are cytokeratin and epithelial membrane antigen (EMA) positive, but CEA and factor-VIII-related antigen negative (Battifora & Kopinski 1985,

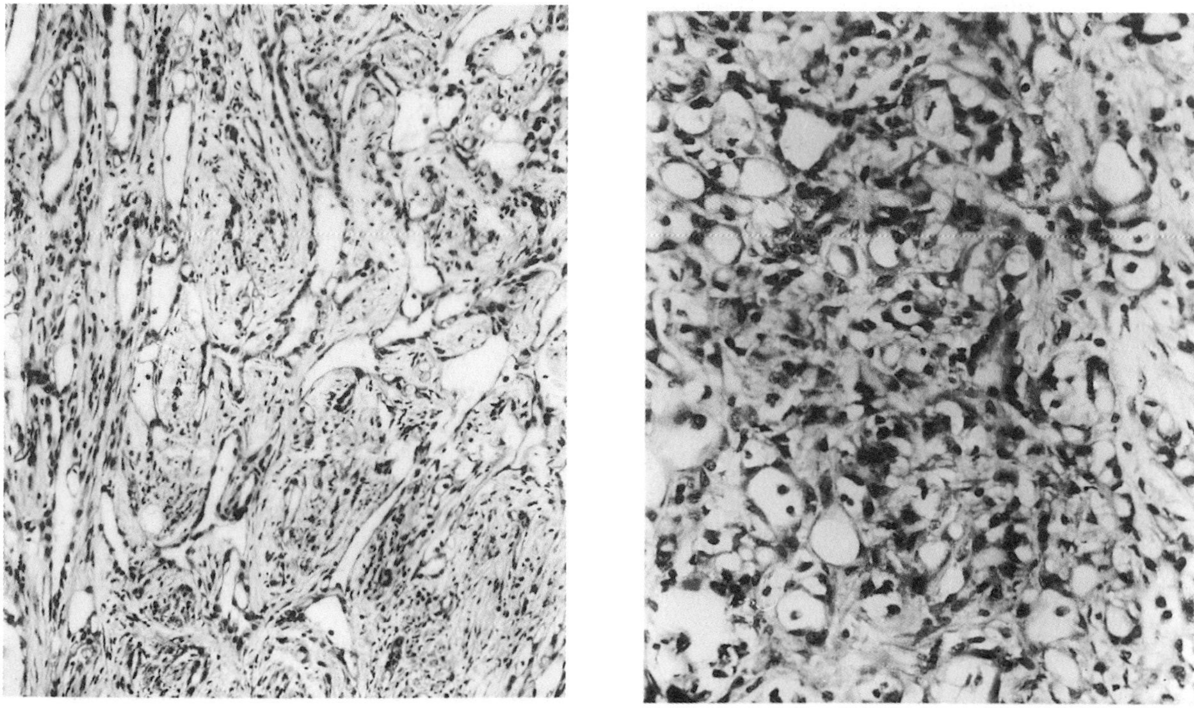

A B

Fig. 31.5 Adenomatoid tumor. (A) Slit-like spaces lined by flattened or cuboidal cells. Intervening stroma includes smooth muscle fibers. H + E ×90. (B) Different area from same tumor showing small cystic spaces and groups of mesothelial cells, some vacuolated, which may mimic signet ring cells. The oval or bean-shaped nuclei are cytologically benign. H + E ×200

Urdiales-Viedma et al 1985, Sienkowski et al 1986). Electron microscopy demonstrates the characteristic features of mesothelial cells, i.e. abundant elongate microvilli, numerous cytoplasmic tonofilaments, intracytoplasmic lumens, and dilated intercellular spaces, the latter two features correlating with the vacuoles that are evident light microscopically (Stephenson & Mills 1986).

Differential diagnosis

The differential diagnosis most often considered is lymphangioma, because of the frequent prominence of cystic spaces lined by flattened cells resembling endothelium. However, in lymphangiomas the cells lining the spaces are uniformly flattened rather than focally cuboidal and are factor-VIII-related antigen positive; cords of vacuolated cells are not seen (Table 31.1). Prominence of vacuolated cells may raise the suspicion of metastatic signet-ring cell carcinoma (Krukenberg tumor), but histochemistry will resolve this problem. Young et al (1991) have drawn attention to some shared features with ovarian yolk sac tumors which may cause a problem in a young patient.

Table 31.1 Differential diagnosis: mesothelioma (cystic and adenomatoid) versus lymphangioma

Mesothelioma	Lymphangioma
Cells flat and cuboidal	Flat cells only
Exfoliated cell clusters (C)	None
Lymphocytes sparse	Lymphocytes plentiful
Acid mucins present	None
Cords of vacuolated cells (A)	Absent
Smooth muscle absent (C)	Always present
Factor VIII negative (IP)	Factor VIII positive

(A) Adenomatoid tumor; (C) benign cystic mesothelioma; (IP) immunoperoxidase method.

Cystic mesotheliomas

These lesions are sometimes referred to as 'peritoneal inclusion cysts', since there is some doubt as to whether they are true tumors (McFadden &

Clement 1986). Characteristics of cystic mesotheliomas which support their neoplastic, rather than reactive, nature include spontaneous development in most cases, i.e. no history of previous surgery or PID, formation of tumor-like masses, clinical behavior, which often involves recurrences, and histological features which overlap with other types of mesotheliomas, especially adenomatoid tumors.

Cystic mesotheliomas appear to have a predilection for the female pelvis and occur mostly in younger women (Menneyer & Smith 1979, Katsube et al 1982, Carpenter et al 1982, Schneider et al 1983, Nirodi et al 1984, Philip & Reilly 1984). There is no known association with asbestos exposure. Presentation is usually with abdominal pain and a mass, or as an incidental finding at surgery. One-quarter to one-half recur locally, but spread beyond the peritoneal cavity has not been reported.

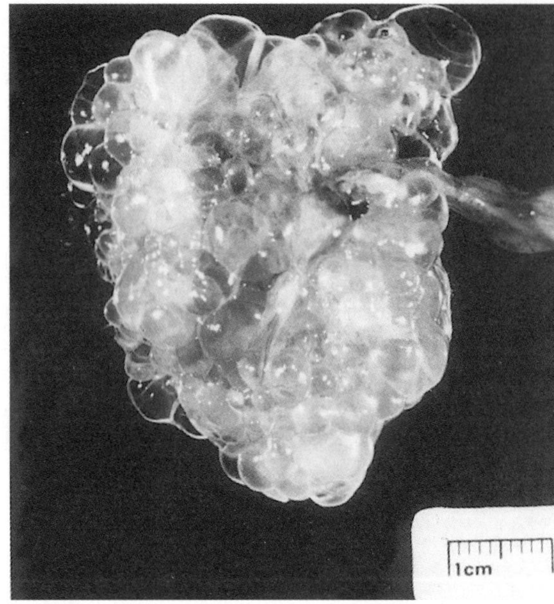

Fig. 31.6 Cystic mesothelioma. Small pedunculated lesion attached to fallopian tube. Mass consists of thin-walled cysts containing clear fluid

Macroscopic features

At surgery, the lesions are typically multicystic pelvic or abdominal masses 10–15 cm in diameter, but occasionally larger (Fig. 31.6). Cysts may fill the pouch of Douglas and also lie free in the peritoneal cavity. The ovarian surfaces may be involved but, as with other viscera, there is no invasion of underlying parenchyma (Menneyer & Smith 1979, Farhi & Silverberg 1982, Katsube et al 1982, Schneider et al 1983, Philip & Reilly 1984). The omentum is the most commonly involved intra-abdominal structure. Adhesions are frequent. Individual cysts are mostly in the size range 0.5–1.5 cm, but have been reported up to 7 cm. They are filled with clear, sometimes mucoid, material.

Microscopic features

The cysts are lined by flattened or cuboidal cells, with focal tufting, and some lumens contain exfoliated cell clusters (Figs 31.7, 31.8). Groups of very small cysts, reminiscent of adenomatoid tumors, are sometimes observed, but tubulopapillary patterns are not seen. The scanty but vascular stroma is loose and myxoid, but may be focally hyalinized. There is often a sprinkling of inflammatory cells, especially lymphocytes. The cytological features of the cyst lining cells are bland; nucleoli are generally inconspicuous, but sometimes 'hobnail' cells with mild nuclear pleiomorphism are present. Their histochemical and ultrastructural characteristics are typical of mesothelial cells, as described above (Menneyer & Smith 1979, Moore et al 1980, Katsube et al 1982, Schneider et al 1983, Dumke et al 1983).

Differential diagnosis

Distinction from reactive mesothelial proliferations, e.g. peritoneal inclusion cysts (see Ch. 20), can be very difficult, or impossible, unless obvious tumor masses are present. Diagnosis can sometimes only be confirmed by documentation of recurrences or continued tumor growth (Moore et al 1980).

Many cystic mesotheliomas have probably been misdiagnosed as lymphangiomas in the past. These latter tumors usually occur in the abdominal mesentery rather than the pelvic peritoneal

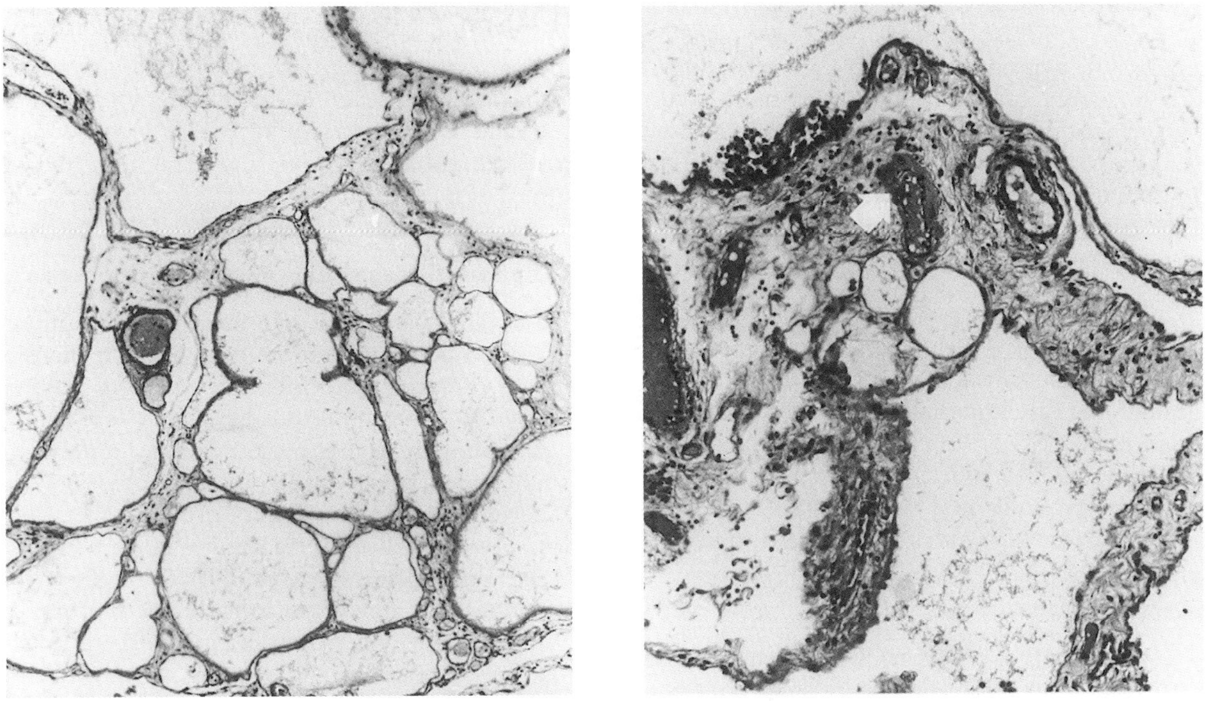

A B

Fig. 31.7 Cystic mesothelioma from omentum, resected at caesarean section. (A) Small and larger cysts are lined by very attenuated mesothelial cells. Sparse loose vascular stroma. H + E ×50. (B) Cystic spaces lined by more conspicuous mesothelial cells, forming a tuft at top left. Stroma contains a few lymphocytes, and some decidualized cells are present around blood vessel (arrow). H + E ×80

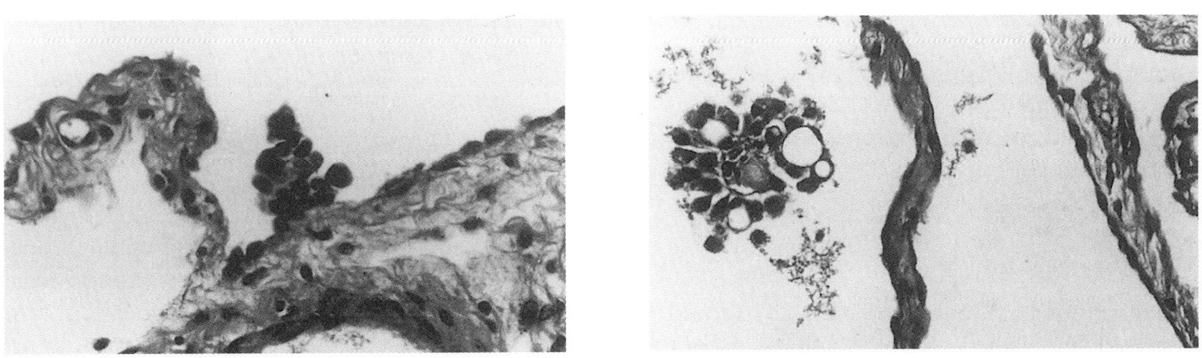

A B

Fig. 31.8 Cystic mesothelioma – detail of mesothelial cells. (A) Tuft of cells with regular round to oval nuclei and prominent nucleoli. H + E ×640. (B) Exfoliated cell cluster in lumen of cyst. Note abundant cytoplasm and some vacuolation. H + E ×400

cavity. The cyst fluid may be chylous and contain numerous lymphocytes. The cysts are lined by a uniformly flattened endothelium, with no exfoliated cell clusters. The walls frequently contain smooth muscle, and lymphoid tissue is often conspicuous (Table 31.1).

Papillary mesotheliomas

Peritoneal papillary mesotheliomas may be associated with a range of clinical behaviors, as alluded to above. The more common localized forms are benign and are usually encountered incidentally at laparotomy. The clinical course of the rarer multifocal or diffuse papillary peritoneal mesotheliomas is less predictable, and can be indolent, with a history of recurrences over many years. Involvement of the ovaries by either type is, however, unusual (Russell & Laverty 1978, Russell 1979, Scully 1979, Foyle et al 1981, Addis & Fox 1983, Alicantara-Vazquez et al 1989).

Macroscopic features

These are similar to those of extraovarian peritoneal papillary mesotheliomas (Goepel 1981), although the case reported by Addis & Fox (1983) was unusually large (9 cm maximum diameter) and displayed solid as well as papillary components. They are typically grey-white papillary tumors, 1–3 cm in diameter, with no visceral invasion.

Microscopic features

A very orderly pattern with finely branched papillae around a thicker central stalk is evident (Fig. 31.9A). Sometimes there is a tubular component within the papillary cores (Fig. 31.9B). The sparsely cellular stroma may be focally hyalinized; blood vessels are scanty and tend to be centrally located (Figs 31.9A,C). Small numbers of inflammatory cells, especially lymphocytes, may be present. Psammoma bodies are uncommonly encountered. The papillae are covered by a single layer of cuboidal cells, with cytological and histochemical features typical of mesothelial cells, as described above (Fig. 31.9C).

Differential diagnosis

Benign serous papillomas (see Ch. 23) should be clearly distinguished from papillary mesotheliomas. These show a less orderly architecture and the stromal blood vessels tend to be located peripherally in the papillary cores. The connective tissue of even small papillae may be hyalinized. The epithelial cells range from cuboidal to columnar, and ciliated cells may be present. Apical neutral mucin is usually demonstrable. Psammoma bodies are more commonly encountered than in mesothelioma (Table 31.2).

Reactive mesothelial proliferations may be difficult or impossible to distinguish from small papillary mesotheliomas (Foyle et al 1981). These are most commonly associated with pelvic inflammatory disease or tubal ectopic pregnancies, and show heterogeneous histological patterns rather than the very orderly, purely papillary pattern of mesotheliomas.

Malignant diffuse peritoneal mesotheliomas

These tumors are rarer than their pleural counterparts, and occur more frequently in men than in women. A high percentage of patients have a history of asbestos exposure. They are more aggressive than pleural mesotheliomas, and death usually occurs within 12 months of diagnosis (Moertel 1972). The tumors grow in sheet-like fashion with peritoneal thickening up to 6 cm, or form multiple plaques and nodules. Tumor growth and adhesions may result in extensive matting of the abdominal and pelvic organs. Visceral invasion, most often of liver and gut, may occur. Sometimes there is a very large dominant tumor mass; this is most often in omentum, low abdominal cavity or pelvis. Tumor may involve the surfaces of the ovaries (Russell 1979, Falkson 1985).

Microscopically, malignant peritoneal mesotheliomas are predominantly tubulopapillary (Fig. 31.10) with only minor (see pleural tumors) sarcomatoid components. A detailed description of these tumors is given by Kannerstein & Churg (1977).

As mentioned above, there are cogent clinical (especially therapeutic) and epidemiological reasons for separating common 'epithelial' ovarian tumors from mesotheliomas. This applies especially to peritoneal serous carcinomas and malignant peritoneal mesotheliomas (Kannerstein et al 1977), for which therapy and prognosis are quite different. The distinguishing features are presented in Table 31.3.

Foyle et al (1981) have described atypical diffuse mesotheliomas with morphology and behavior intermediate between benign localized papillary mesotheliomas and papillary serous carcinomas. All four tumors were multifocal and, in two cases involved the ovarian surfaces. The general histological pattern was similar to that of benign localized papillary mesotheliomas, but there were

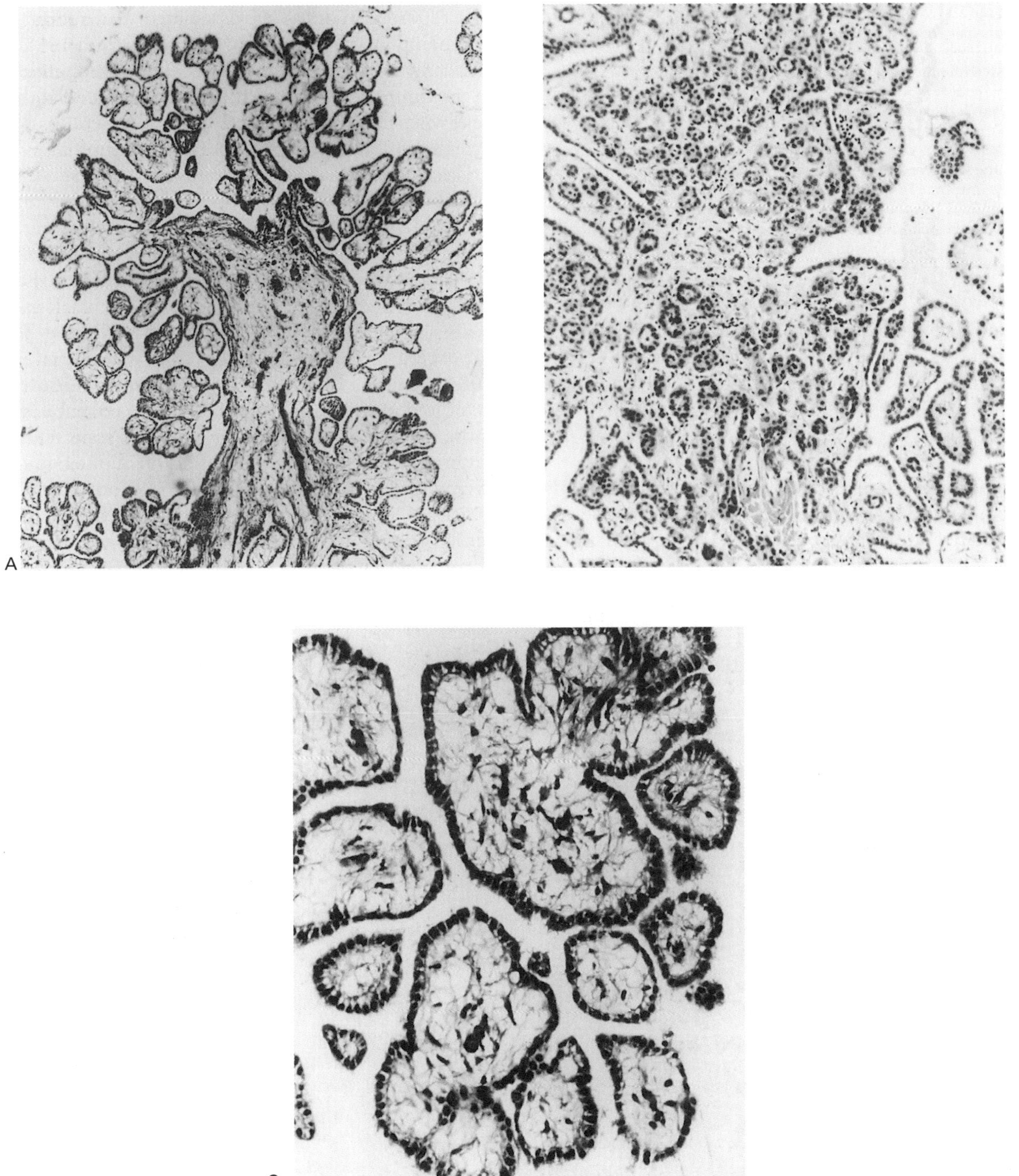

Fig. 31.9 Benign peritoneal papillary mesothelioma. (A) Branching papillae with centrally located blood vessels in the cores of loose connective tissue. H + E ×50. (B) Papillae which include small tubular structures lined by similar cells to those covering the surface. H + E ×90. (C) Detail of Fig. 31.9a. Papillae covered by regular small cuboidal cells. Loose connective tissue cores contain small centrally located capillaries. H + E ×200

Table 31.2 Differential diagnosis: papillary mesothelioma versus benign serous papilloma

Mesothelioma	Serous papilloma
Papillary pattern uniform	Architecture diverse
Vessels central	Vessels peripheral
Cells flat to cuboidal	Cells cuboidal to columnar
One cell type, no cilia	Ciliated and secretory cells
Psammoma bodies rare	Psammoma bodies common
Stromal lymphocytes	No inflammatory cells
Cytoplasmic acid mucin	Apical neutral mucin (scanty)
Glycogen vacuoles sometimes	Glycogen vacuoles absent

cellular pleiomorphism, focal epithelial tufting, and psammoma bodies – features more in keeping with serous carcinomas.

EPIDERMOID CYSTS

These rare lesions are defined as cysts lined by epidermis unaccompanied by skin appendages or other teratomatous elements. The small cysts are usually incidental findings, but the larger examples reported to date were associated with abdominal pain and swelling (Carinelli & Senzani 1985, Pezzica et al 1991). The lesions are located either in the hilus, medulla, or cortex, and are filled with yellowish creamy material (Fig. 31.11). The cysts are generally considered to be of teratomatous origin (ectodermal or endodermal) and are still classified as such in the World Health Organization (WHO) classification (see Appendix B). However, other histogenetic possibilities have been suggested, such as squamous metaplasia of endometriotic cysts, rete ovarii, mesonephric tubules, or coelomically derived epithelium (More 1967, Nogales & Silverberg 1976, Young et al 1980, Wheeler et al 1984, Carinelli & Senzani 1985). Some cysts have exhibited mural nests of epithelial cells resembling those of Walthard's rests or Brenner tumors, a finding which supports the theory of coelomic origin (Nogales & Silverberg 1976, Young et al 1980). It is possible that not all cysts share the same origin, and that histogenesis may vary according to location.

A 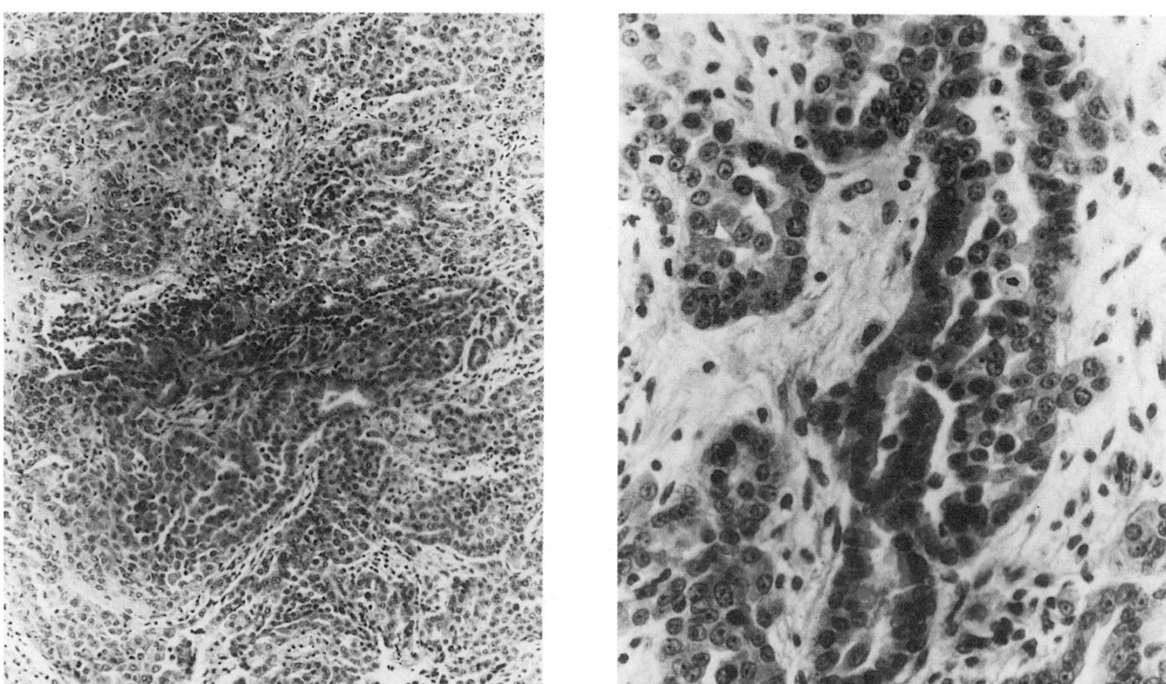 B

Fig. 31.10 Malignant peritoneal mesothelioma. (A) Tubulopapillary pattern with foci of necrosis. H + E ×80. (B) Fairly uniform malignant mesothelial cells with focally abundant cytoplasm. Some nuclei show irregularly dispersed chromatin or mitotic activity. Nucleoli are very conspicuous in most cells. H + E ×250

Table 31.3 Differential diagnosis: malignant mesothelioma versus serous carcinoma

Malignant mesothelioma	Serous carcinoma
Clinical	
History of asbestos exposure	No history of asbestos exposure
Diffuse peritoneal tumor	Usually dominant ovarian mass
Rapidly fatal, unresponsive to all treatments	Some response to surgery and chemotherapy
Histological	
Sarcomatoid and adenomatoid foci	Absent
Columnar cells rare	Columnar cells numerous
Psammoma bodies rare	Psammoma bodies not uncommon
Nuclei round	Nuclei oval or elongate
Cytoplasmic acid mucin	Apical neutral mucin (scanty)
*Ultrastructural**	
Abundant tonofilaments	Tonofilaments usually sparse
Cilia never numerous	Cilia often numerous
Intracytoplasmic lumina common	Intracytoplasmic lumina uncommon
Apical 'snouts' rare common	Apical 'snouts'

*Warhol et al (1982).

SQUAMOUS CELL CARCINOMAS

In addition to the benign squamous ovarian lesions, epidermoid cysts (described above), examples of squamous carcinoma in situ (Black & Benitez 1964, Motoyama & Watanabe 1988, McGrady et al 1993) and invasive carcinoma (Shingleton et al 1974, Macko & Johnson 1983, Ben-Baruch et al 1988, Yetman & Dudzinski 1989, Radhi & Awad 1990) have been reported. In some cases it is particularly difficult to exclude a coexisting teratoma, which may have been overrun by expanding carcinoma (see Ch. 48). Other possible origins should be explored histologically. This may require extensive sampling of the ovarian mass. Focal glandular differentiation might be evidence for an endometrioid (adenosquamous) carcinoma, and sampling of cyst walls, if present, may reveal evidence of a pre-existing endometriotic cyst (Lele et al 1978, Naresh et al 1991). Glandular differentiation or areas resembling transitional cell carcinoma also raise the possibility of malignant Brenner tumor, which requires (by convention) confirmation by finding areas of typical benign (solid fibrous areas) or atypically proliferating Brenner tumor (see Ch. 28). Squamous carcinoma metastatic to the ovaries is rare (see Ch. 53) and we have not encountered, for example, a case of occult cervical carcinoma which has presented as an adnexal tumor. Scully (1979) has observed three ovarian pure squamous carcinomas (two in situ, one in situ and invasive) and made the interesting observation that two of these had coexistent squamous carcinoma in situ of the uterine cervix. This has also been the experience of others (Motoyama & Watanabe 1988, Yetman & Dudzinski 1989, McGrady et al 1993). Histologically, ovarian squamous carcinoma in situ is usually identified as atypical squamous epithelium lining a cyst (Fig. 31.12) or, rarely, as an extension onto the ovarian serosa of widespread squamous carcinoma in situ involving the mullerian duct derivatives (Willis (1967), as cited by Kanbour & Stock (1978)). Infiltrating squamous carcinoma (well differentiated keratinizing squamous carcinoma in the only examples we have encountered) (Fig. 31.13), occurs as mural nodules in epidermoid cysts or, less commonly, as solid masses.

TUMORS OF PROBABLE WOLFFIAN ORIGIN

Following the characterization of 'tumors of probable wolffian origin' arising in the juxta-ovarian region (Kariminejad & Scully 1973), similar tumors were identified in the ovary itself (Hughesdon 1982, Young & Scully 1983). The basis for considering these tumors to be of wolffian or mesonephric origin, derived from vestigial embryonic remnants in the broad ligaments or ovarian hilus, is the similarity, especially the presence of conspicuous basement membranes, to normal wolffian duct remnants, which are frequently identified in the anatomical sites where these tumors have been discovered, and the lack of similarity to any currently recognized mullerian tumors (Young & Scully 1983). The tumors also resemble, in some aspects, the rare cervical adenocarcinomas acknowledged to be of wolffian derivation (McGee et al 1962). Continuity between wolffian vestiges and a hamartomatous

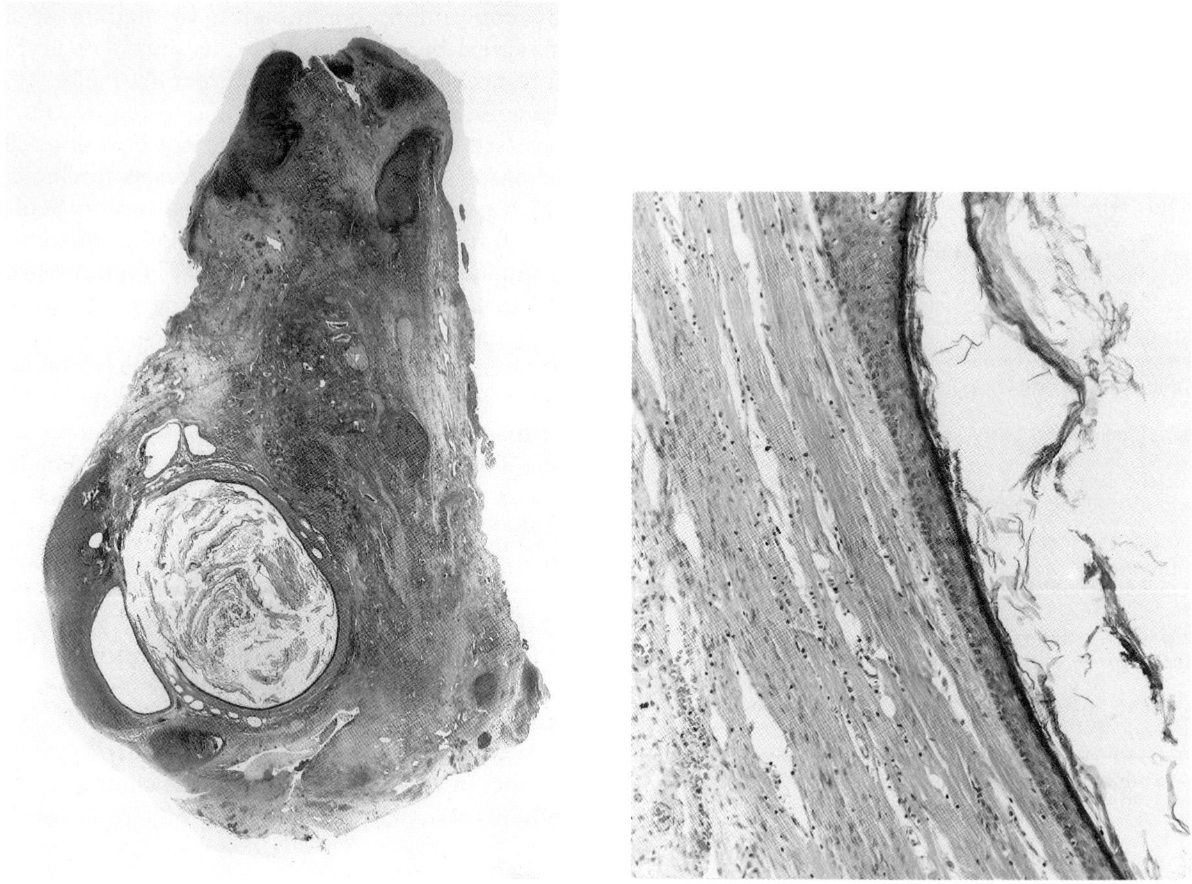

A B

Fig. 31.11 Epidermoid cyst of ovary. (A) Survey of lesion, indicating its medullary position and showing thick keratinous debris in the lumen. H + E ×3.3. (B) High power of benign squamous epithelial lining of the cyst wall. H + E ×59

parovarian nodule, resembling a tumor of probable wolffian origin, in a female fetus, further supports the concept (Sivathondan et al 1979). Electron microscopic studies have not elucidated the histogenesis of these tumors, but have not excluded the current hypothesis. It is difficult to establish ultrastructural analogy between the tumors and physiological wolffian remnants because, in the limited studies available, the morphology of the latter appears to vary according to their position in the duct system. In addition, many of the observed differences, both ultrastructural, light microscopic, and histochemical, between wolffian derived structures and the diverse mullerian tumors with which they are being contrasted are quantitative only (Taxy & Battifora 1976, Demopoulos et al 1980). However, one clear-cut difference is the virtual absence of mucin in tumors of probable wolffian origin.

In order to benefit from the analysis of a larger number of cases, the clinicopathologic features, as gleaned from the literature, of both ovarian (13 cases) and juxtaovarian (14 cases) tumors of probable wolffian origin (assumed to differ only in their location) will be presented (Kariminejad & Scully 1973, Taxy & Battifora 1976, Sivathondan et al 1979, Demopoulos et al 1980, Abbot et al 1981, Hughesdon 1982, Young & Scully 1983, Delaloye et al 1993, Daya 1994). The age ranges from 18 to 81 years, with most cases occurring in the fifth decade. Patients present with abdominal enlargement, pain, or unrelated gynecological symptoms which draw attention to an adnexal mass. There is no evidence that the tumors are endocrinologically active, but some have been

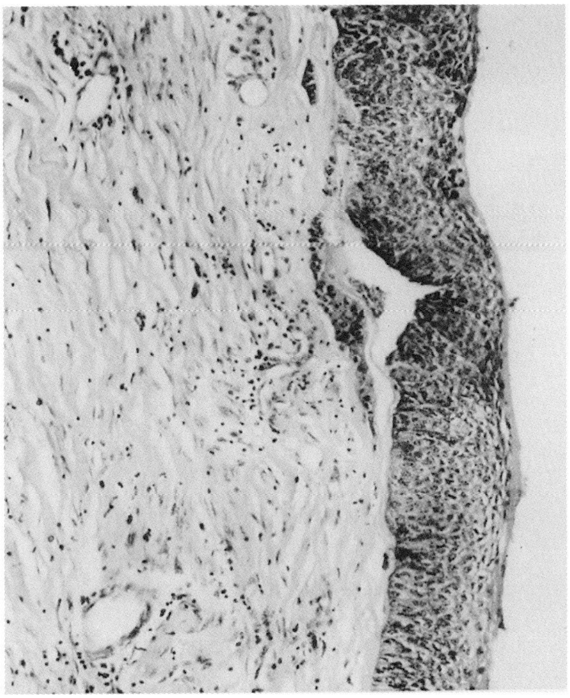

Fig. 31.12 Epidermoid cyst of the ovary lined by markedly atypical squamous epithelium (squamous carcinoma in situ). A mild chronic inflammatory cell infiltrate is present in the fibrous stroma beneath the abnormal 'epidermis', but there is no invasion. H + E ×75

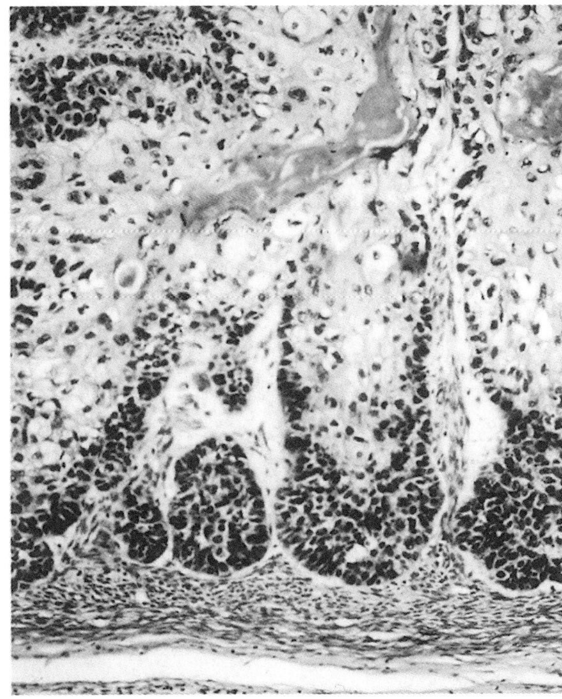

Fig. 31.13 Primary well differentiated keratinizing squamous cell carcinoma of the ovary, with tumor tissue abutting ovarian stroma at the lower margin. H + E ×75

associated with endometrial hyperplasia, a not uncommon finding in the age group involved and not necessarily causally related (Sivathondan et al 1979). Three ovarian and three juxtaovarian tumors metastasized to abdominopelvic peritoneum (four instances), lung, pleura, and liver. In three of these cases, metastases did not become apparent until 6–8 years after initial surgical excision of the tumor. Tumor caused the deaths of three patients within the follow-up period.

A unique benign parovarian fibroma with heterotopic bone formation has been described by Terada et al (1993), and a wolffian origin suggested.

Macroscopic features

The tumors are unilateral and range in size from 2 to 20 cm, with most being 8–12 cm in diameter. They have smooth lobulated surfaces. The cut surfaces show a solid or mixed solid and cystic pattern with locules, usually small, but sometimes up to 11 cm in diameter, containing clear yellow or hemorrhagic fluid. The solid tissue is gray-white or tan, and rubbery or firm in texture. Necrosis and hemorrhage are unusual.

Microscopic features

A variety of patterns of epithelial proliferation are observed, often within the same tumor. The most common are tubular, microcystic (sieve-like), or solid (diffuse), and one of these usually predominates (Fig. 31.14). The prototypical tubular pattern consists of cuboidal or columnar epithelial cells arranged in closely packed glands and anastomosing cords delineated by prominent basement membranes which can be highlighted by PAS or reticulin stains (Fig. 31.15). Another common pattern is that of microcysts dispersed in a solid background; the component cells are again cuboidal, but sometimes 'hobnailed'. The diffuse pattern consists of sheets of oval or spindle cells

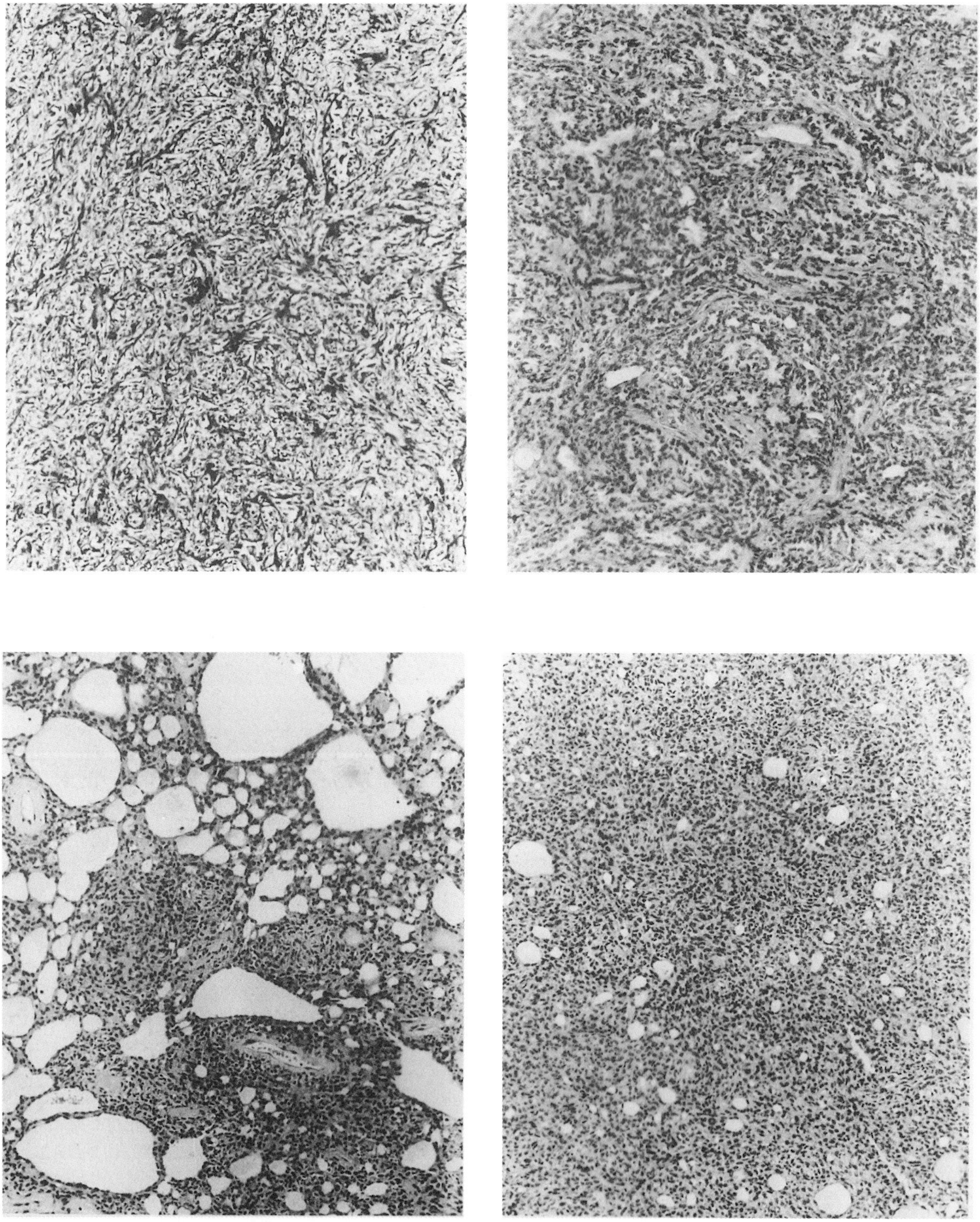

Fig. 31.14 Ovarian tumor of probable wolffian origin; patterns of epithelial proliferation. (A) Closely packed anastomosing cords. H + E ×80. (B) Branching tubules, separated by prominent basement membranes. H + E ×100. (C) Microcystic. H + E ×80. (D) Solid or diffuse. H + E ×100

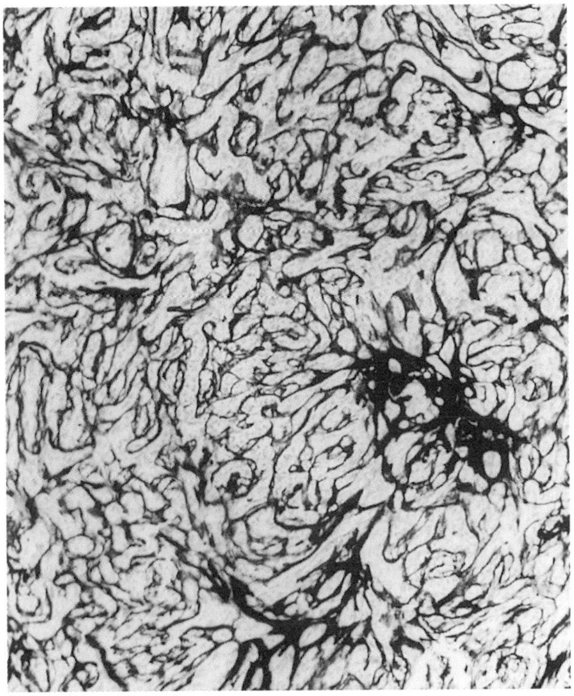

Fig. 31.15 Ovarian tumor of probable wolffian origin. Anastomosing cords highlighted by reticulin stain (similar field to Fig. 31.14A). H + E ×80

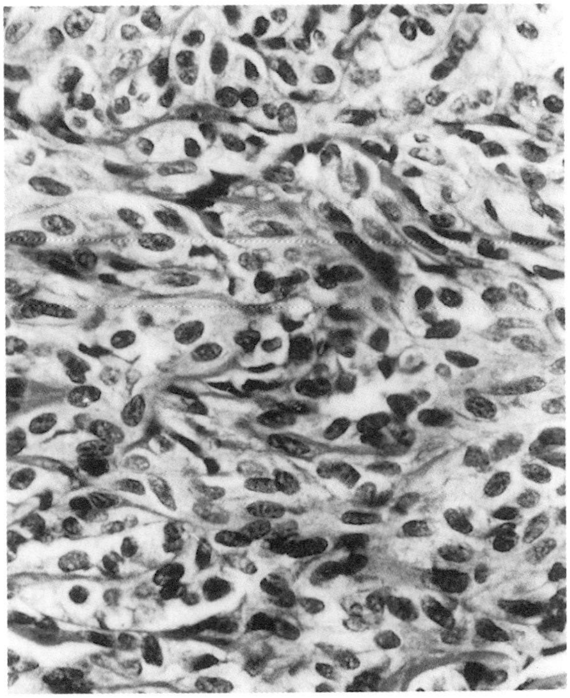

Fig. 31.16 Cytological detail of tumor of probable wolffian origin. Regular oval nuclei with dispersed chromatin and inconspicuous nucleoli. Cytoplasm is clear. H + E ×400. (Courtesy of Dr A. Östör, Melbourne)

resembling mesenchyme. Papillary foci are also described.

The cells have indistinct margins and vacuolated, clear, or eosinophilic cytoplasm which is free of stainable mucin but may include a very small amount of glycogen. Some tumors exhibit a trace of luminal mucin. The round to oval nuclei are vesicular or show finely dispersed chromatin and nucleoli are inconspicuous (Fig. 31.16). The mitotic activity is low (usually less than 2 per 10HPF) and nuclear pleiomorphism is unusual. Necrosis and hemorrhage are usually minimal. Fibrous stroma is not usually conspicuous, but sometimes it breaks up the tumor into lobules (Fig. 31.17). Calcification is rare. The tumor margin may be irregular microscopically, with 'invasion' of the capsule by tongues of tumor.

All the five tumors which metastasized have

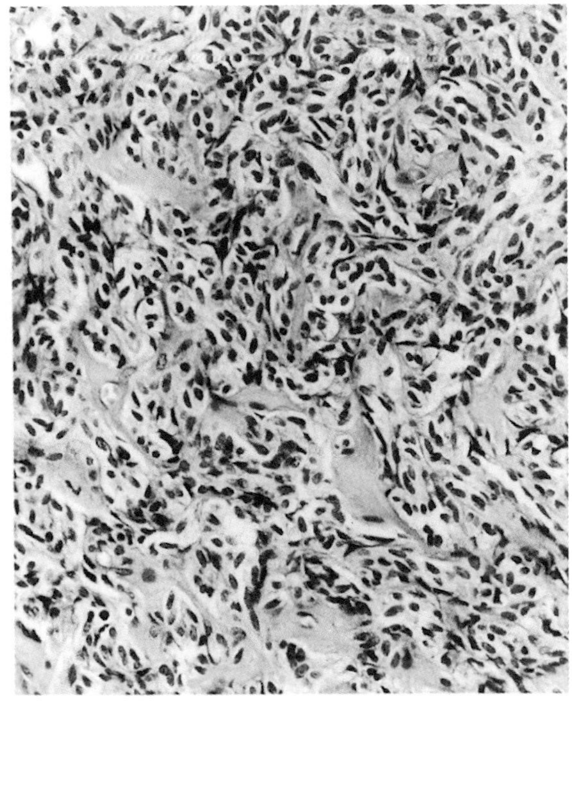

Fig. 31.17 Ovarian tumor of probable wolffian origin. Hyalinized stroma separates some epithelial cords. H + E ×200

exhibited one or more atypical features, including an unusual degree of epithelial pleiomorphism or cytological atypia, a very prominent hypercellular spindle cell diffuse pattern, increased mitotic activity (5 and 13 per 10HPF), lymphatic permeation, and a focus of undifferentiated carcinoma. It seems that tumors conforming to the typical appearance and with a low mitotic rate can be expected to behave in a benign fashion, but those with atypical features may metastasize, sometimes after a lengthy disease-free interval.

Differential diagnosis

There are several ovarian neoplasms which superficially resemble one or more of the histological patterns observed in tumors of probable wolffian origin. However, none (except perhaps clear cell carcinomas) show the diversity of patterns within a single tumor, and none show the characteristic prominent basement membranes.

Androblastomas (see Ch. 35), the neoplasms most often confused with tumors of probable wolffian origin, commonly exhibit closely packed epithelial tubules and cords with focally vacuolated cytoplasm, but the other patterns (cystic and diffuse) typical of tumors of probable wolffian origin are absent. Except in the rare pure Sertoli cell type, tumors in this group contain clusters of Leydig cells, and endocrine manifestations (usually androgenic) are common.

Granulosa cell tumors (see Ch. 33) may occasionally mimic the diffuse and some of the tubular patterns of tumors of probable wolffian origin. However, the other patterns typical of the latter are absent. Grooved nuclei are often present; cytoplasm is scanty (except in luteinized variants) and reticulin fibers are sparse. Endocrine manifestations (usually estrogenic) are common.

Endometrioid adenocarcinomas (see Ch. 25) may focally resemble the tubular patterns of tumors of probable wolffian origin, but sieve-like and diffuse spindle cell areas are absent. Apical and luminal mucin are often present, but are rare in tumors of probable wolffian origin. Mitotic activity is usually in excess of the low rate (less than 2 per 10HPF) found in nonmetastasizing tumors of probable wolffian origin.

Mullerian clear cell carcinomas (see Ch. 27) are pleiomorphic tumors, the appearance of which may overlap with the cystic and papillary areas of tumors of probable wolffian origin. However, closely packed tubules and cords and spindle cell foci are absent. The cytoplasm contains abundant glycogen, some mucin, and occasionally lipid, as well as the characteristic diastase-resistant PAS-positive eosinophilic globules (see Fig. 27.16).

Adenomatoid tumors (see above), with their closely packed cords and tubules, which may include vacuolated cells, can mimic the tubular areas of tumors of probable wolffian origin. However, cystic and spindle cell areas are not present. The cells may contain some glycogen, but cytoplasmic acid mucin (hyaluronic acid) is also demonstrable. The tumors are small, usually less than 1.5 cm, and are incidental findings only.

CYSTS AND ADENOMAS OF THE RETE OVARII

Rete ovarii tubules may become dilated to form cysts. These are usually only small hilar lesions, but substantial cysts up to 12 cm in diameter also occur. Some have been associated with virilization in postmenopausal women (Rutgers & Scully 1986, 1988, Robinson et al 1988). The cysts are lined by nonciliated cuboidal or, less commonly, ciliated columnar epithelium, and their fibrous wall includes bundles of smooth muscle (Fig. 31.18) and often peripheral Leydig cell hyperplasia. The epithelial lining may undergo squamous metaplasia, and this represents one possible origin of ovarian epidermoid cysts (see above). Adenomas (Rutgers & Scully 1988) are composed of cords and tubules lined by cells similar to those seen in the normal rete.

SMALL CELL CARCINOMAS ASSOCIATED WITH HYPERCALCEMIA

These tumors, first described by Dickersin et al (1982), are discussed here, although their origin is far from established (Aguirre et al 1989, Lifschitz-Mercer et al 1992, Dickersin & Scully 1993). Their epithelial nature, on the one hand, is suggested by ultrastructural features such as the presence of desmosomes, tight junction complexes,

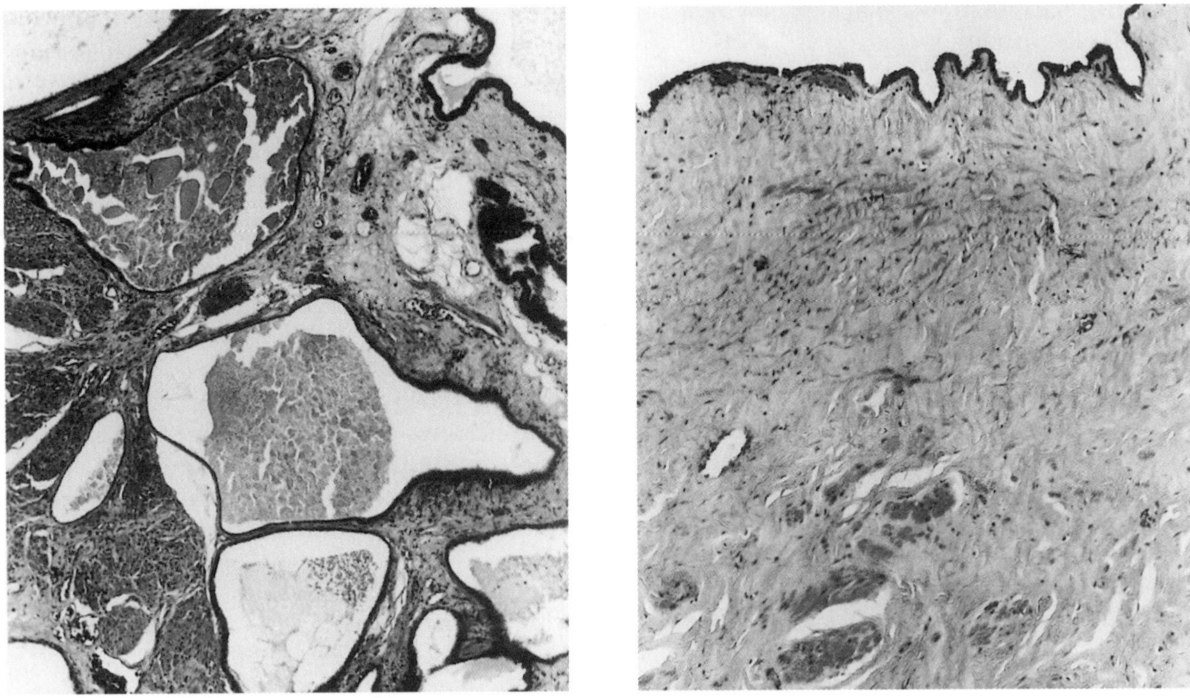

Fig. 31.18 (A) Cyst of rete ovarii in virilized postmenopausal woman. Lining of simple cuboidal cells with wall of fibrous tissue and some strands of smooth muscle. Peripheral hilus cell hyperplasia not illustrated. H + E ×80. (B) Adjacent dilated rete ovarii; some tubules are lined by ciliated epithelium. H + E ×50. (Courtesy of Dr R. Eckstein, Sydney)

cytoplasmic interdigitations, and partial investment with basal lamina (Patsner et al 1985). Dense-core neurosecretory granules have been observed by some investigators (Abeler et al 1988), but not others (McMahon & Hart 1988). On the other hand, Ulbright et al (1987) have suggested a germ cell origin and favor these tumors being variants of yolk sac tumors (showing parietal yolk sac differentiation). These undifferentiated small cell carcinomas account for a little over one-half of reported cases of paraneoplastic hypercalcemia due to ovarian malignancy (see Appendix D); raised serum calcium levels are found in about two-thirds of patients (Young et al 1987, Aguirre et al 1989, Taraszewski et al 1991). The mechanism of the hypercalcemia, which spontaneously regresses after removal of the tumor, is thought to be associated with 'parathyroid-hormone-related protein' (PTHrp) in many cases (Matias-Guiu et al 1994).

These small cell carcinomas represent the major proportion of 'undifferentiated' ovarian carcinomas encountered in women under the age of 40 years, and they rarely present above that age (mean age 23 years). The youngest patient was a prepubertal girl aged 10 years (Ulbright et al 1987). The most common presenting symptoms are abdominal pain and swelling. They may rarely present in pregnancy (Jensen et al 1991). Tumours are almost always unilateral at surgery (unlike the poorly differentiated mullerian carcinomas more commonly encountered in the older age group; see Ch. 30), although recurrences sometimes manifest first in the residual ovary, suggesting that bilaterality (at least at a microscopic level) is understated in the literature. Despite tumors being apparently limited to stage 1 in two-thirds of cases, small cell carcinomas tend to progress rapidly (Peccatori et al 1993), with an overall 5-year survival rate of only 10% (Young et al 1987) and 30% survival for patients with stage 1a disease (Scully 1993).

Cytogenetic and molecular genetic studies

The tumors are almost always diploid on flow

cytometric analysis of cellular DNA content (Eichhorn et al 1992).

Macroscopic features

They are large solid tumors, usually measuring 15–20 cm in diameter. The cut surface tends to be pale and featureless, frequently with areas of hemorrhage, cystic degeneration, and necrosis.

Microscopic features

Characteristically, they show sheets of small densely packed epithelial cells with small hyperchromatic nuclei and inapparent cytoplasm (Fig. 31.19). Cells with rather more prominent and eosinophilic cytoplasm (Dickersin & Scully 1993) are seen in 40% of tumors, and in some tumors these cells predominate (Fig. 31.20). The nuclei may contain a single prominent nucleolus, and mitoses are very numerous. The cells are typically arranged diffusely, but may also form insular or anastomosing trabecular patterns. Islands of cells may be well circumscribed (Fig. 31.21), or show peripheral neoplastic spindle cells producing a 'sarcomatoid' appearance. Single cell necrosis (apoptosis) is common, particularly in the centers of the cellular islands. The presence of 'follicle-like' structures, seen in most examples, is regarded as typical of these tumors (Figs 31.19, 31.21). Eosinophilic intracellular hyaline globules may be evident (Ulbright et al 1987).

Mucin stains are largely negative, although a few mucinous glands have been seen in 9% of tumors in the large series of Young et al (1987). Immunohistochemically, tumors almost always exhibit cytokeratin, often vimentin intermediate filaments, and occasionally epithelial membrane antigen. The hyaline globules do not stain for α-fetoprotein. No argyrophilia is demonstrable by

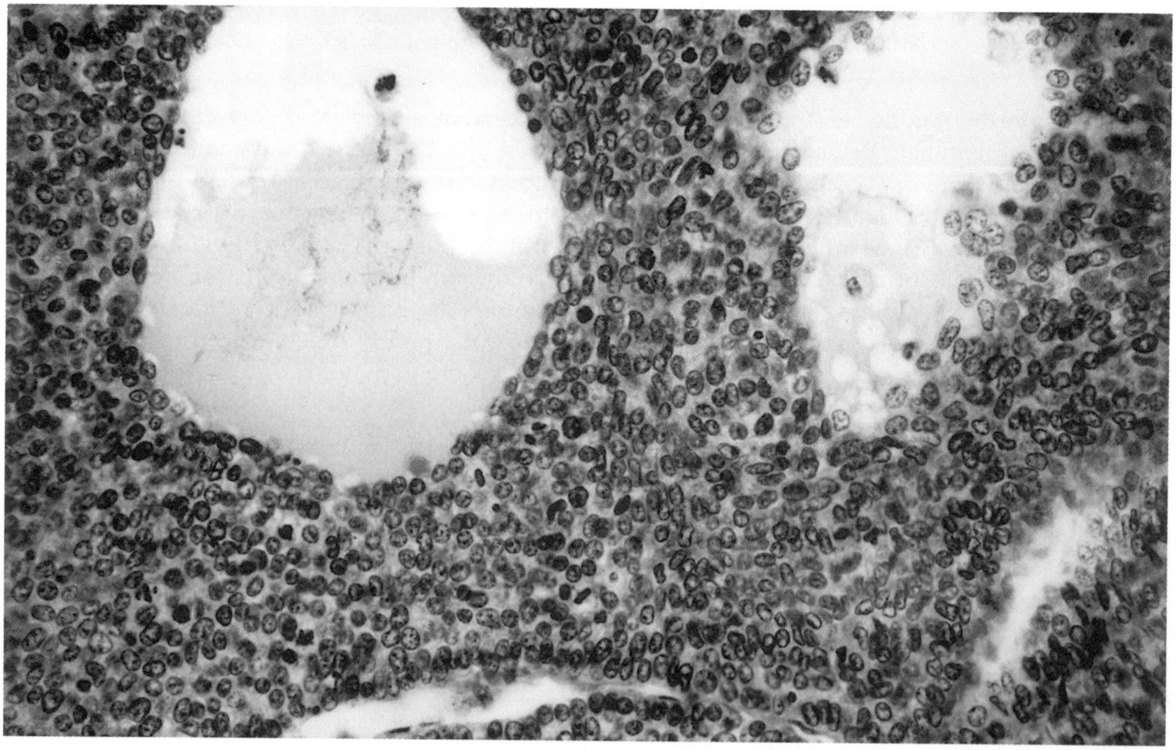

Fig. 31.19 Undifferentiated small cell carcinoma of ovary associated with hypercalcemia. Typical example exhibiting sheets of small uniform cells with rounded, hyperchromatic nuclei, inapparent cytoplasm, and 'follicle-like' spaces filled with proteinaceous fluid. H + E ×250

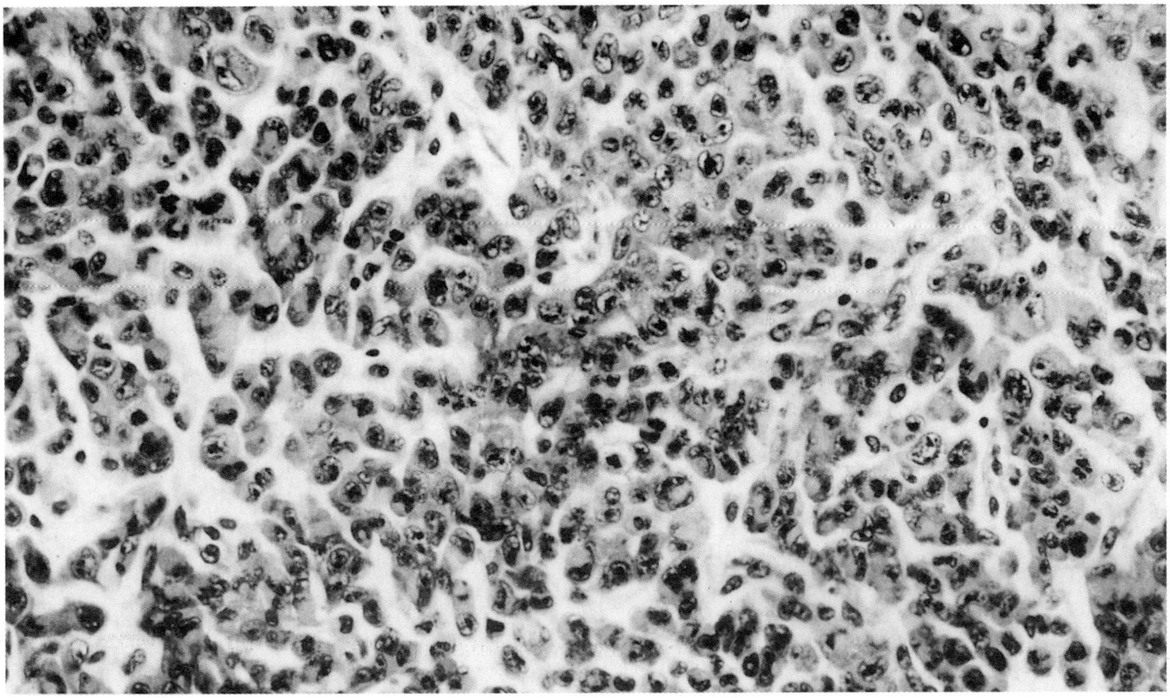

Fig. 31.20 Undifferentiated small cell carcinoma of the ovary from a 23-year-old woman with paraneoplastic hypercalcemia. Cytoplasm is more prominent and eosinophilic in this example. H + E ×250

the Grimelius technique. The pattern of reticulin fibers varies from scant fibrils surrounding large masses of cells to rich networks enveloping small groups or even single cells (Dickersin et al 1982).

Differential diagnosis

Given the clinical context in which these malignant neoplasms occur, the tumors with which they are most likely to be confused are granulosa cell tumors, of both adult and juvenile types. The differentiating features are discussed in Chapter 33 (see Table 33.2).

Metastases from typical oat-cell carcinomas of pulmonary or, more locally, endometrial origin (Kristensen & Paulsen 1985) are usually distinguishable from primary undifferentiated small cell carcinomas of ovary on clinical grounds. Grimelius stains for argyrophilia and immunohistochemical stains for neuroendocrine differentiation (neuron-specific enolase, bombesin, chromogranin) may aid in this confirmation. Similar clinical and histological profiles clearly distinguish these small cell carcinomas of hypercalcemic type, occurring in young women, from primary ovarian small cell carcinomas of so-called 'pulmonary' type, which are related to the mullerian spectrum of malignancies, and occur in women in the usual cancer age group (see Ch. 30).

DESMOPLASTIC SMALL CELL TUMORS OF CHILDHOOD

These rare tumors have a distinctive clinical presentation as well as characteristic morphological features and immunophenotype. They were first described by Gerald & Rosai (1989) as occurring in young patients (mean age of incidence: 20 years in males, 15 years in females), with symptoms of short duration, and operative findings of widely disseminated intra-abdominal tumor, but without an identifiable parenchymal primary neoplasm. The postoperative course usually includes an initial response to chemotherapy followed by early clinical relapse and tumor progression (Zaloudek et al 1995). Only a minority of cases occur in

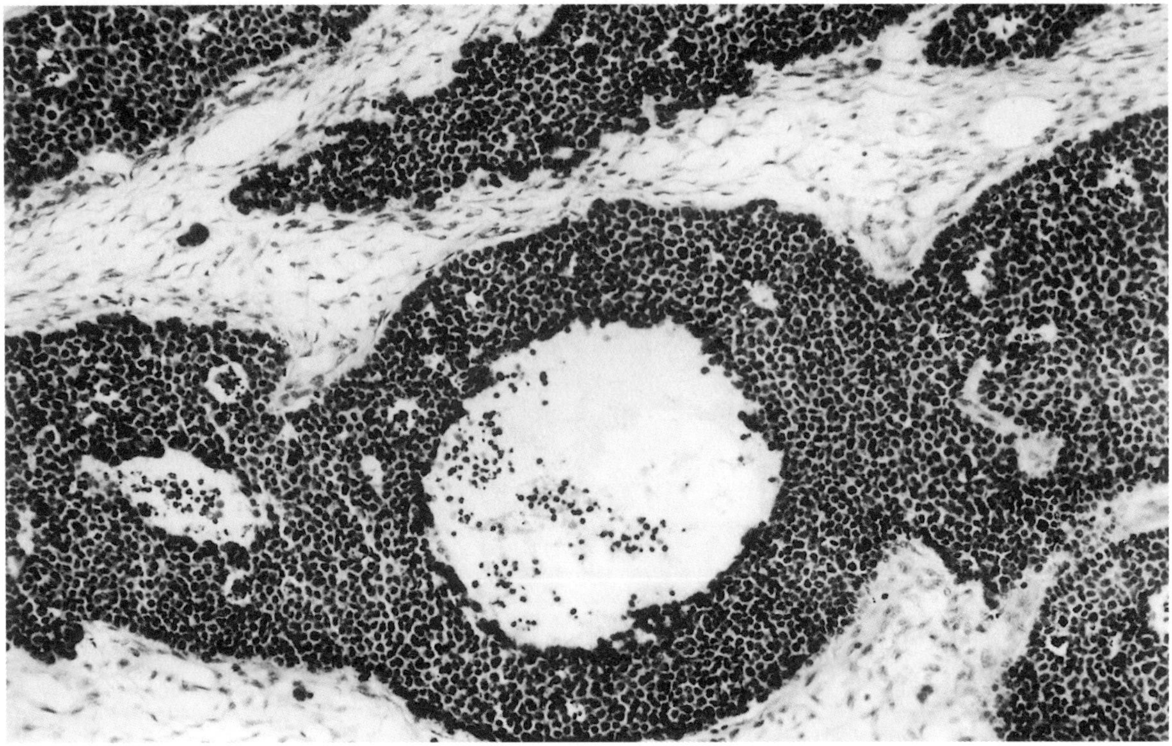

Fig. 31.21 Undifferentiated small cell carcinoma of ovary associated with hypercalcemia. Histological similarities to so-called 'oat-cell' carcinoma are striking in this case, although cohesion of tumor cells is a more consistent feature of the 'hypercalcemic' than 'pulmonary' type of small cell carcinoma of ovary. Apoptosis, peripheral palisading of nuclei, and the presence of 'follicle-like' structures are obvious features. H + E ×125

females (Gerald et al 1991, Ordóñez et al 1993, Yeoh et al 1993), but of these a disproportionate number (30%) involve the ovaries (Young et al 1992, Zaloudek et al 1995).

Macroscopic

The ovaries, if involved, are replaced by firm, pale tan to gray tumor tissue masses ranging up to 15 cm in diameter. Necrosis and hemorrhage are usually not prominent on gross examination. Similar masses are characteristically seen in the pelvis and abdominal cavity.

Microscopic

The tumor cells are seen in well-circumscribed but variably sized sheets, nests, and trabeculae, most commonly separated by broad bands of eosinophilic, collagenous stroma with focal areas of cystic or myxoid change (Fig. 31.22). Microfoci of necrosis are noted histologically within the epithelial sheets, but broader zones of necrosis are uncommon. Tumor cells are characterized by uniform, small, round to oval, hyperchromatic nuclei with finely granular chromatin and absent or inconspicuous nucleoli (Fig. 31.22B). Rosettes and gland-like structures are typically absent. Mitoses are numerous (often >2 per HPF). Cell cytoplasm is scanty to moderate, and cell borders are poorly defined. Patchy spindling of the tumor cells is occasionally seen, as are small aggregates of larger, more polyhedral cells with eosinophilic cytoplasm (Zaloudek et al 1995). The immunophenotye of the small dark cells is characteristic, showing strong diffuse cytoplasmic positivity for low molecular weight cytokeratins (AE1/AE3, CAM 5.2), EMA, and punctate juxtanuclear staining for desmin in all cases, as well as vimentin in about 80% of tumors. Infrequently,

ovary. A report of three cases with comments on histogenesis. American Journal of Clinical Pathology 73: 272–276

Young R H, Dickersin G R, Scully R E 1987 Small cell carcinoma of the ovary. An analysis of 75 cases of a distinctive ovarian tumor commonly associated with hypercalcemia [abstract]. Laboratory Investigation 56: 89a

Young R H, Silva E G, Scully R E 1991 Ovarian and juxtaovarian adenomatoid tumors: a report of six cases. International Journal of Gynecological Pathology 10: 364–371

Young R H, Eichhorn J H, Dickersin G R, Scully R E 1992 Ovarian involvement by the intra-abdominal desmoplastic small round cell tumor with divergent differentiation: a report of three cases. Human Pathology 23: 454–464

Zaloudek C, Miller T R, Stern J L 1995 Desmoplastic small cell tumor of the ovary: a unique polyphenotypic tumor with an unfavorable prognosis. International Journal of Gynecological Pathology 14: 260–265

SECTION 6

Sex cord–stromal tumors

32

Introduction, clinical perspective, and principles of management

A. Ferrier

Controversy still exists as to the embryological cells of origin of the ovarian cortical and medullary parenchymal tissues. Yet there is merit in identifying and delineating that range of ovarian neoplasms which, by virtue of their cytological and architectural features and their frequent ability to elaborate a range of steroidal hormones, are considered to arise from the cells which are the adult derivatives of the primitive gonadal sex cords or cortical lobules and interstitium or mesenchyme (see Ch. 1). Such tumors are variously termed 'gonadal stromal tumors', 'mesenchymomas', or 'sex cord–stromal tumors' to reflect the histogenetic perceptions of the particular authors (Morris & Scully 1958, Norris & Taylor 1968, Serov et al 1973, Norris & Chorlton 1974, Scully 1979). The term we favor for these lesions is 'sex cord–stromal tumors', in general acknowledgment of the World Health Organization (WHO) recommendation (Serov et al 1973), and reflecting the weight of embryological evidence supporting the coelomic sex cord origin of the granulosa and Sertoli cells of the primitive gonads and the mesenchymal or stromal origin of the intervening cellular stroma, including those cells showing specific differentiation (i.e. Leydig and theca cells).

Sex cord–stromal tumors are difficult to classify precisely as they exhibit overlapping and multidirectional spectra of histological differentiation as well as a variety of endocrine profiles and degrees of malignancy. The great majority are composed of cells of which the non-neoplastic analogs are seen in the normal adult ovaries (granulosa and/or theca cells), while only occasional lesions show predominantly, or exclusively, cells considered testicular in differentiation (Sertoli and/or Leydig cells). Very rare tumors showing an apparent mixture of cells differentiated in an ovarian direction and in a testicular direction may also be encountered (designated 'gynandroblastoma'), as may examples in which a lack of adequate differentiation precludes assignment to a particular category.

The cellular components may resemble any of these cell types or their luteinized variants (i.e. cells that have accumulated abundant cytoplasm so that they resemble cells of a corpus luteum) to a greater or lesser extent, depending on the level of differentiation and the architectural configuration of the tumors. The stromal elements may be fibroblastic rather than resembling steroid hormone secreting cells. Either the sex cord *or* stromal components of the tumors may be poorly differentiated. The WHO classification (see Appendix B) is thus purely morphological, implying neither potential hormonal activity nor a specific histogenesis. This is equally true of sex cord–stromal tumors showing evidence of 'male' or 'female' differentiation. Moderately and poorly differentiated Sertoli–Leydig cell tumors (androblastomas), for example, may resemble early stages of testicular development, for which reason the terms 'arrhenoblastoma' and 'androblastoma' have been used synonymously. However, the first of these terms carries the misleading connotation that they are uniformly masculinizing; in fact some are either endocrinologically inactive or, rarely, estrogenic. The second of these terms is our preferred generic term for all such lesions. As there are no Sertoli cells in the normal adult ovary, the histogenesis is presumed to be from ovarian cells of sex cord origin which, in the neoplastic state, manifest a capacity for male or testicular differentiation. Leydig cells are present in the ovarian hilus, and their presence is disclosed in

Table 32.1 Relative percentage histological distribution of sex cord–stromal tumors seen at King George V Hospital

Granulosa–stromal cell tumors	99
Granulosa cell tumors	
Adult type	12.0
Juvenile type	_*
Thecoma–fibroma group	
Thecoma:	
–typical thecoma	7.0
–luteinized thecoma	_*
Thecafibroma	13.0
Fibroma–fibrosarcoma:	
–fibroma	64.5
–cellular fibroma	_*
–fibrosarcoma	_*
Sclerosing stromal tumors	2.5
Unclassified	_*
Androblastomas	1
Well differentiated	_*
Of intermediate differentiation	_*
Poorly differentiated (sarcomatoid)	_*
With heterologous elements	_*
Gynandroblastoma	_*
Sex cord tumor with annular tubules	_*
Unclassified	_*
Total	100

*Rarely encountered tumors.

the medullary and cortical stroma in hyperplastic and neoplastic conditions. Morphological resemblances between these Leydig cells and the cells comprising both luteomas and ovarian 'adrenal-like' tumors have, on the one hand, influenced some authors to place hilus cell (Leydig cell, interstitial cell) tumors in the generic group of 'steroid cell tumors' (see Ch. 39). On the other hand, homology with Leydig cell tumors of the testis and the fact that the cells found in this type of neoplasm are identical with those seen in ovarian Sertoli–Leydig cell tumors are persuasive of its appropriate position being amongst the group of androblastomas.

Although the stromal tumors in this group are almost always 'pure', those notionally designated as being of sex cord origin usually contain mixed cell populations. For example, stromal tumors in the thecoma–fibroma group may, on rare occasions, contain scattered cellular aggregates of sex cord derivation. These latter may resemble granulosa or Sertoli cells, and tumors in which they are found have been named thecomas or fibromas 'with minor sex cord elements' (Young & Scully 1983). By way of contrast, most granulosa cell tumors exhibit variable numbers of theca cells, and this has led to such lesions being generically referred to as 'granulosa–theca cell tumors'. Although such an appellation details the cell types present in many neoplasms, the simpler term 'granulosa cell tumors' is more widely accepted. It is, of course, possible that the theca cell component is sometimes a response of the ovarian stroma to the neoplastic granulosa cells rather than being an integral part of the neoplasms. Supporting such an interpretation is the presence of theca-like cells in a wide spectrum of ovarian tumors, both benign and malignant, primary and secondary, and also the fact that these cells may not be present in extraovarian deposits of granulosa cell tumor, and that granulosa cell tumors which recur outside the ovary are typically not estrogenic (Fathalla 1967). It seems probable, however, that those tumors in which the theca cell component is prominent or even dominant are truly mixed neoplasms (Scully 1982). No such controversy surrounds androblastomas in which Leydig cells may be found in the metastatic deposits, confirming that they are an integral part of the neoplastic process (Fig. 32.1), although it must be said that the recent claim that the Sertoli cell component of such tumors may be of stromal or mesonephric rather than sex cord origin (Park & Kim 1994) raises another and separate controversy.

Given the age distribution of sex cord–stromal tumors, it is not surprising that they comprise less than 1% of primary ovarian neoplasms associated with pregnancy (Young et al 1989) while comprising about 10% of all ovarian tumors. However, unlike other groups of ovarian tumors, they present specific diagnostic traps when encountered in pregnant women. Alterations in their histology and a lesser association with 'endocrine symptoms' often misdirect the pathologist, resulting in an incorrect diagnosis. These issues are dealt with in sections relating to the specific tumor types.

Granulosa cell tumors are the most commonly encountered malignant sex cord–stromal neoplasm. The average age at diagnosis is 52 years (Hoskins & Rubin 1992). The rarer juvenile variant is seen most commonly in prepubertal girls

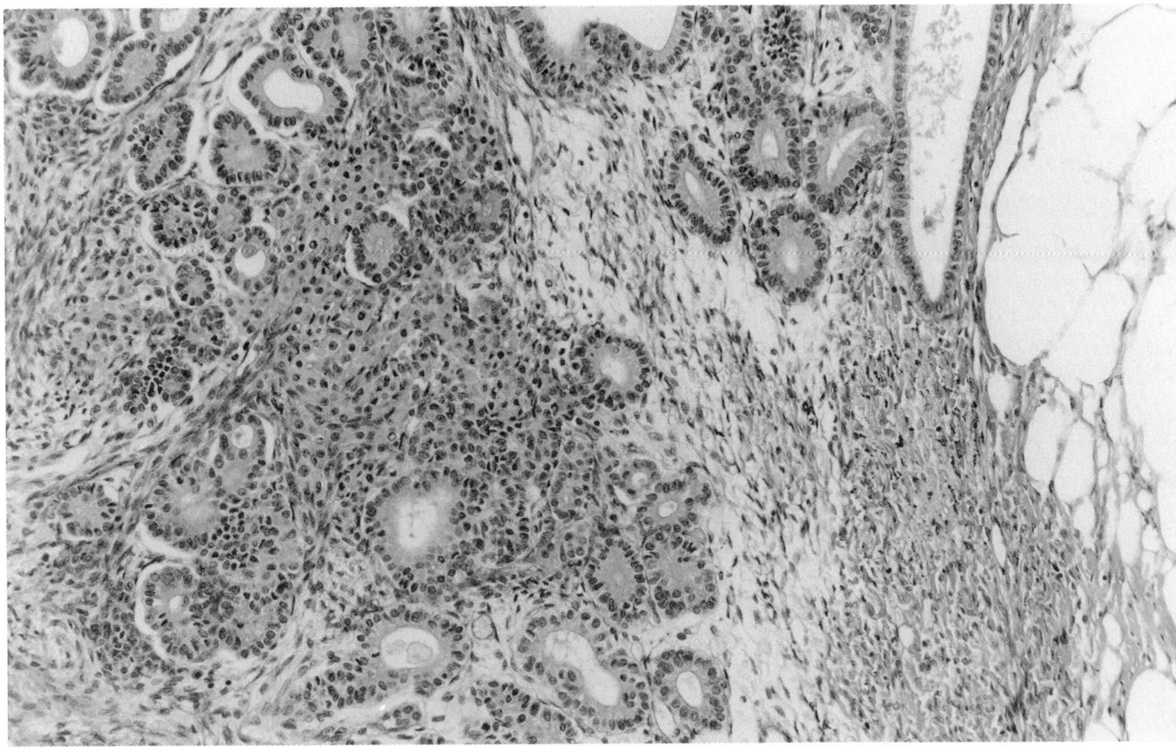

Fig. 32.1 A well differentiated focus in an otherwise poorly differentiated Sertoli–Leydig cell tumor metastatic to the omentum. Sertoli cell tubules are prominent, as are sheets of Leydig cells with eosinophilic cytoplasm and rounded nuclei (center). H + E ×99

(Young et al 1984b). Common presenting symptoms include amenorrhea, menorrhagia, oligomenorrhea, or postmenopausal bleeding. Isosexual pseudoprecosity is associated with 80% of juvenile granulosa cell tumors. Granulosa cell tumors are frequently associated with elevated serum levels of estradiol and estrone. More recently, serum inhibin, a polypeptide secreted by granulosa cells to regulate follicle stimulating hormone secretion from the pituitary, has been proposed as a tumor marker (Lappöhn et al 1989). The perimenopausal clustering of cases of granulosa cell tumor suggests a role for pituitary trophins in their genesis, and a recent report of 12 cases occurring in women who had recently been subjected to clomiphene citrate or gonadotrophin therapy for ovarian stimulation lends support to this concept (Willemsen et al 1993). At a time when follicular structures are, by definition, almost exhausted, it is interesting to speculate about the cells of origin of such tumors. The occasional 'emergence' of sex-cord-like elements out of fields of hyperplastic ovarian cortical stroma (Fig. 32.2) highlights a potential pathogenetic mechanism.

The effect of high, frequently unopposed estrogen results in endometrial hyperplasia in approximately 50% of patients with frank adenocarcinoma in 13% of cases (Evans et al 1980). An endometrial biopsy should always be part of the assessment of a patient with granulosa cell tumor. At laparotomy, the tumors are unilateral and International Federation of Gynecology and Obstetrics FIGO stage 1 in 90% of cases (Bjorkholm & Silfversward 1981). When metastatic disease is present, coleomic spread is the commonest route of dissemination. Lymphatic and hematogenous spread also occur. With this in mind, the same surgical approach employed with epithelial–stromal ovarian tumors is applied to granulosa cell tumors. Where fertility is an issue in management, unilateral salpingo-oophorectomy,

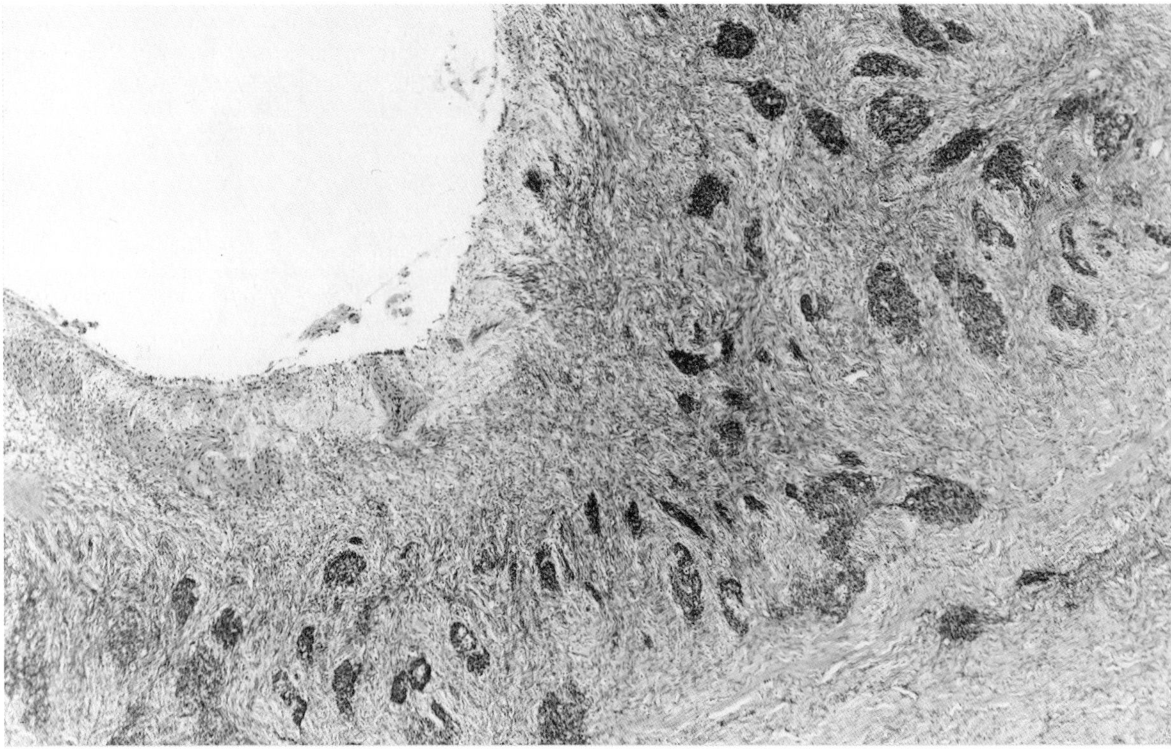

Fig. 32.2 The wall of a chronic ovarian endometriotic cyst. The hyperplastic cortical stroma, beyond the fibrocollagenous cyst wall, is remarkable for the emergence of numerous focal aggregates of cells of sex cord type. H + E ×99

peritoneal biopsies with an ipsilateral pelvic and para-aortic lymph node dissection is the recommended surgical procedure. Recognition of the juvenile-type granulosa cell tumor is particularly important to avoid overzealous surgery. With advanced disease, radical cytoreductive surgery is undertaken. Unlike their epithelial counterparts, granulosa cell tumors may recur late, with one series reporting a mean time to recurrence of 9 years (Stenwig et al 1979), while other series describe most recurrences within 2 years of diagnosis (Fox et al 1975). The pattern of recurrence is probably most dependent on the extent of disease at diagnosis and the duration of follow-up. Although several case series describing adjuvant treatment have been published, there are no convincing data to support any modality of treatment in an adjuvant setting. The results of chemotherapy and radiotherapy in cases of advanced disease are also disappointing. A complete response rate of 55% using cisplatin, vinblastine, and bleomycin in a small series is yet to be corroborated (Colombo et al 1986). The cornerstone of a sustained progression-free interval would appear to be radical cytoreductive surgery.

Sertoli–Leydig cell tumors constitute the other major group of malignant neoplasms within the sex cord–stromal classification. In contrast to the granulosa cell tumors, the average age at diagnosis is 28 years (Scully 1979). The neoplasms present with symptoms of a pelvic mass, androgen excess, or a menstrual disturbance, usually amenorrhea. Endocrine studies evaluating clinical signs of virilization may demonstrate elevated free serum testosterone, low serum estradiol, and normal dehydroepiandrosterone sulphate DHEAS. At laparotomy, these tumors are almost always unilateral. Unilateral adnexectomy is the recommended surgical procedure when fertility is a management issue. When childbearing is complete, a total abdominal hysterectomy and bilateral salpingo-oophorectomy is performed. More than 97% of patients will have stage 1 disease (Young & Scully).

Prognosis is dependent on stage and tumor grade. All patients with advanced disease have a poor prognosis, regardless of therapy. In patients with early stage disease and well differentiated tumors, recurrence is rare. Moderate and poorly differentiated tumors are associated with a recurrence rate of 7% (Young & Scully 1985).

REFERENCES

Bjorkholm E, Silfversward C 1981 Prognostic factors in granulosa-cell tumors. Gynecologic Oncology 11: 261–274

Colombo N, Sessa C, Landoni F, Sartori E, Pecorelli S, Mangioni C 1986 Cisplatin, vinblastine and bleomycin combination chemotherapy in metastatic granulosa cell tumor of the ovary. Obstetrics and Gynecology 67: 265–268

Evans A T, Gaffey T A, Malkasian G D, Annegers J F 1980 Clinicopathologic review of 118 and 82 theca cell tumors. Obstetrics and Gynecology 55: 231–238

Fathalla M F 1967 The occurrence of granulosa and theca tumors in clinically normal ovaries. A study of 25 cases. Journal of Obstetrics and Gynaecology of the British Commonwealth 74: 279–282

Fox H, Agrawai M B, Langley F A 1975 A clinicopathologic study of 92 cases of granulosa cell tumor of the ovary with special reference to the factors influencing prognosis. Cancer 35: 231–241

Hoskins W J, Rubin S C 1992 Malignant gonadal stromal tumors of the ovary: clinical features and management. In: Coppleson M (ed) Gynecologic oncology: fundamental principles and clinical practice, 2nd edn. Churchill Livingstone, Edinburgh, p 961–970

Lappöhn R E, Burger H G, Bouma J, Bangah M, Krans M, de-Bruijn H W 1989 Inhibin as a marker for granulosa cell tumors. New England Journal of Medicine 321: 790–793

Morris J McL, Scully R E 1958 Endocrine pathology of the ovary. Mosby, St Louis

Norris H J, Chorlton I 1974 Functioning tumors of the ovary. Clinical Obstetrics and Gynecology 17: 189–228

Norris H J, Taylor H B 1968 Prognosis of granulosa–theca tumors of the ovary. Cancer 21: 255–263

Park S H, Kim I 1994 Histogenetic consideration of ovarian sex cord–stromal tumors analyzed by expression pattern of cytokeratins, vimentin, and laminin: correlation studies with human gonads. Pathology Research and Practice 190: 449–456

Scully R E 1979 Tumors of the ovary and maldeveloped gonads. AFIP fascicle No. 16, 2nd series. Armed Forces Institute of Pathology, Bethesda, MD, p 152–153

Scully R E 1982 Sex cord–stromal tumors. In: Blaustein A (ed) Pathology of the female genital tract, 2nd edn. Springer-Verlag, New York, p 581–601

Serov S F, Scully R E, Sobin L H 1973 Histological typing of ovarian tumors. International histological classification of tumors No. 9. World Health Organization, Geneva, p 17–54

Stenwig J T, Hazekamp J T, Beecham J B 1979 Granulosa cell tumors of the ovary. Gynecologic Oncology 7: 136–152

Willemsen W, Kruitwagen R, Bastiaans B, Hanselaar T, Rolland R 1993 Ovarian stimulation and granulosa cell tumor. Lancet 341: 986–988

Young R H, Scully R E 1983 Ovarian stromal tumors with minor sex cord elements: a report of seven cases. International Journal of Gynecological Pathology 2: 227–234

Young R H, Scully R E 1985 Ovarian Sertoli–Leydig cell tumors: a clinicopathological analysis of 207 cases. American Journal of Surgical Pathology 9: 543–569

Young R H, Dudley A G, Scully R E 1984 a Granulosa cell, Sertoli–Leydig cell, and unclassified sex cord–stromal tumors associated with pregnancy: a clinicopathologic analysis of 36 cases. Gynecologic Oncology 18: 181–205

Young R H, Dickersin G R, Scully R E 1984b Juvenile granulosa cell tumor of the ovary. American Journal of Surgical Pathology 8: 575–596

33

Granulosa cell tumors

P. Rusell A. Farnsworth

The hallmark of these tumors is the conspicuous presence of cells which resemble those of the follicular granulosa or their luteinized variants. What exactly constitutes 'conspicuous' is still open to debate, but a useful guideline is at least a 10% representation in the material examined; tumors with a lesser granulosa cell component may be designated as 'fibromas with minor sex cord elements' (Young & Scully 1983a). Granulosa cells are small, usually round to polygonal, but may be spindle shaped with scanty amphophilic cytoplasm, usually containing only occasional small lipid droplets, and having indistinct cell borders. Their bland round, oval, or angular nuclei often show a deep longitudinal groove and may exhibit a small, variably prominent nucleolus (Fig. 33.1). The nuclear chromatin may be compact and dense, or loose and vesicular. The luteinized

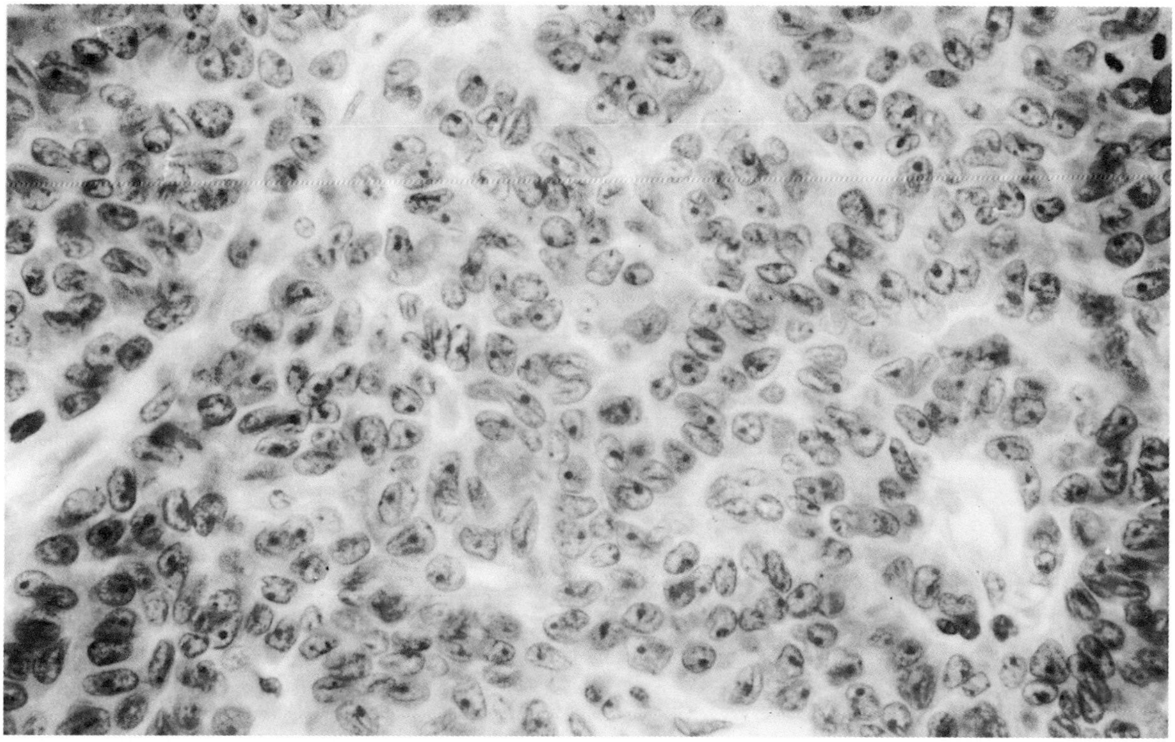

Fig. 33.1 Well differentiated granulosa cell tumor. Cells are typically crowded with scanty cytoplasm and bland, elongate, longitudinally grooved nuclei. H + E ×500

granulosa cells, seen particularly in the diffuse, multicystic and 'juvenile' types of granulosa cell tumors, have larger, more rounded, and generally ungrooved nuclei of similar general appearance, and abundant pale eosinophilic lipid-laden cytoplasm. Granulosa cells regularly contain vimentin and smooth muscle actin intermediate filaments and, less commonly cytokeratins (Table 33.1).

Although such tumors may, on occasion, appear to be composed almost exclusively of granulosa cells, other cells (of ovarian stromal origin, and similar to those in the theca interna or externa of the developing follicle or their luteinized variants) commonly accompany them, and these latter cells may indeed be a dominant component without negating the diagnosis (Scully 1979). It is not known whether this variable ovarian stromal element is reactive to the presence of the neoplastic granulosa cells or is an integral part of the tumor (see Ch. 32). The fact that theca cells can be found also in the stromal component of common epithelial tumors is not a convincing argument in favor of either theory (Fox & Langley 1976), but it is perhaps a good reason why their presence should not unduly influence the classification within the granulosa cell tumor group. While there is clear demarcation between sex cord and stromal elements in the better differentiated granulosa cell tumors, this distinction is blurred in poorly differentiated lesions, particularly those with a diffuse or so-called 'sarcomatoid' pattern. A reticulin stain may be of particular use in such tumors, the granulosa cell component showing only sparse fibrils except around small blood vessels, while the theca cells are individually invested by reticulin fibrils (Fig. 33.2). Intermediate reticulin patterns are occasionally encountered (Scully 1982).

The vast majority of granulosa cell tumors occur in adult women (with a peak incidence at about 45–55 years) and, of these, somewhat more than one-half occur after the menopause. Patients present with nonspecific abdominal symptoms (20%), complaints suggesting an endocrinological disturbance (50%), or both (30%). Abdominal pain and swelling, backache, dysuria, or dyspareunia are noted in one-third of patients, and the abdominal distension is due to either tumor mass or ascites, which accompanies nearly 10% of granulosa cell tumors, and rarely Meigs' syndrome is diagnosed. Occasionally, patients complain of acute abdominal pain due to hemorrhage into the tumor or rupture of a cystic neoplasm with hemoperitoneum, particularly in young women and in those presenting in pregnancy. In

Table 33.1 Immunophenotype of granulosa cell tumors

Antibody	Presence %
α- and β-inhibin	100
CD 99	100
Vimentin	95
Smooth muscle actin	90
S-100 protein	50
35BH11	40
AE1/AE3	40
CAM 5.2	20
Desmin	10
CA-125 antigen	–
CA 19-9	–
EMA	–
OM-1	–
B72.3	–
CEA	–

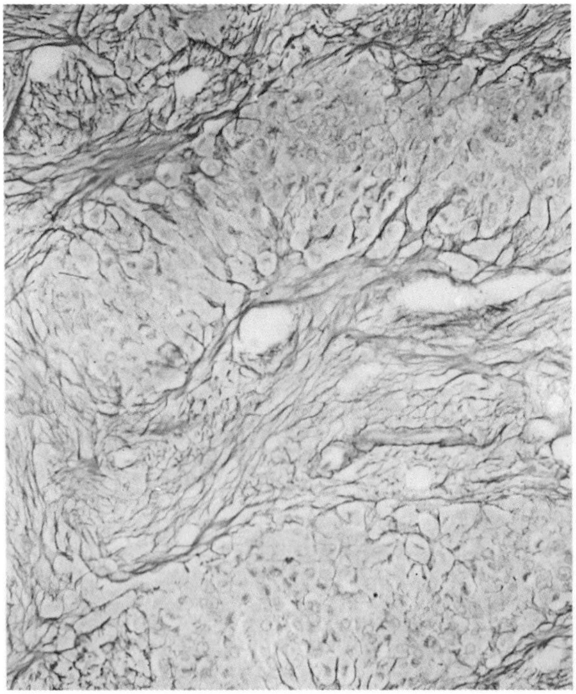

Fig. 33.2 Granulosa–theca cell tumor showing reticulin-poor granulosa cell areas and intervening zones of theca cells densely enmeshed by reticulin fibers. Reticulin stain ×150

premenopausal women the commonest 'endocrine' symptoms are irregular menstruation or menorrhagia, and less frequently prolonged anemorrhea or painful enlargement of the breasts. In postmenopausal women there is usually vaginal bleeding, and breast enlargement may also be noticed. As may be inferred from these data, there is a variable but high proportion of granulosa cell tumors associated with endometrial hyperplasias (50%) (Gusberg & Kardon 1971, Evans et al 1980) and carcinomas (5–13%) (Stenwig et al 1979, Evans et al 1980). Occasional reports of granulosa cell tumors presenting with symptoms suggesting virilization (amenorrhea, hirsutes, acne, breast atrophy) have documented partial or complete regression of the symptoms following removal of the tumor (Norris & Taylor 1969, Nakashima et al 1984). Sporadic reports of granulosa cell tumors occurring in pregnancy have appeared in the literature. While they may be producing large amounts of hormone, appreciable estrogenic manifestations are not a feature of granulosa cell tumors in this clinical situation, whereas occasionally they are associated with symptoms suggesting virilization (Young et al 1984b) (see also Ch. 10). Unilocular cystic adult granulosa cell tumors and 'juvenile' granulosa cell tumors are disproportionately represented among the latter. Uncommonly, and in our opinion coincidentally, other primary ovarian tumors will be found in the same ovaries as granulosa cell tumors, both of germ cell and epithelial type (Evans et al 1980, Bichel 1985, Dgani et al 1993).

A small but definable subset of granulosa cell tumors, which includes the vast majority (90%) of neoplasms in prepubertal girls as well as many occurring in adolescents and only very infrequently occurring in adult women (Biscotti & Hart 1989), have a distinctive histological appearance which has been designated 'juvenile' granulosa cell tumor (Young et al 1984a). In over 80% of juvenile granulosa cell tumors occurring in prepubertal girls, an anovulatory form of isosexual precocious pseudopuberty is the presenting complaint, although more acute thoracoabdominal symptoms may be present (Imai et al 1992). The majority of granulosa cell tumors removed or diagnosed during pregnancy belong to this histological group (Young et al 1984b). There has been documented an infrequent association with multiple enchondromatosis (Ollier's disease) or enchondromatosis with hemangiomas (Maffucci's syndrome) (Tamini & Bolan 1984, Young et al 1984a, Pounder et al 1985, Tanaka et al 1992), and rarely with leprechaunism (Brisigotti et al 1993). They may occur in dysgenetic gonads (Young et al 1985, Tanaka et al 1994).

Rare examples of extraovarian granulosa cell tumors in women have been reported in the broad ligament (Powell & Black 1940, Ragins & Frankel 1940, Reddy et al 1963), adrenal gland (Orselli & Bassler 1973), myometrium (Langley et al 1953), endometrium (Fox & Langley 1975), and the adult testis (Nistal et al 1992, Jiminez-Quintero et al 1993).

Irrespective of the particular microscopic pattern observed, granulosa cell tumors should all be considered as low grade malignancies. The spectrum of differentiation described below correlates poorly with the patient's clinical outcome. For example, juvenile granulosa cell tumors, although appearing poorly differentiated and pleiomorphic, are associated with a high cure rate, except in high stage cases which recur early and progress rapidly (Powell et al 1993). Fox et al (1975) point out that most of the reported prognostic criteria are functions of the size of these slow growing tumors, and the stage as determined by laparotomy and clinical findings. Any granulosa cell tumor may extend beyond the ovary or recur after surgery. Spread is mostly within the pelvic or lower abdominal cavities, and uncommonly to the retroperitoneal nodes. Distant metastases are rare, but have been reported in lungs, brain, bones, and liver (Margolin et al 1985, Davidson et al 1990, Ebel et al 1993). Although recurrent disease may present within 5 years of removal of the primary tumor, quite commonly it is not evident until much later (Norris & Taylor 1968, Fox et al 1975, Evans et al 1980). It is accepted that one-third of recurrences occur after 5 years and 20% after 10 years, and some investigators have reported a corrected death rate from granulosa cell tumor of 30–50% at 20 years (Fox et al 1975). It is apparent, in our present state of knowledge, that clinical factors are as important as pathological features of the tumor in identifying those granulosa cell tumors that are likely to progress or recur. A list of the more widely accepted features considered to indicate a likely poor clinical outcome for the patient is given below (Fox & Langley 1975, Stenwig et al 1979, Evans et al 1980, Bjorkholm & Silfversward 1981, Scharl et al 1988, Malmstrom et al 1994, Piura et al 1994):

- extraovarian spread at laparotomy (i.e. stage 2–4)
- rupture of tumor in stage 1a cases
- tumor diameter greater than 5 cm (this may not be independent of stage)
- numerous mitotic figures (5 or more per 10HPF).

Cytogenetic and molecular genetic studies

Flow cytometric studies (Hitchcock et al 1989, Chadha et al 1990, Klemi et al 1990, Suh et al 1990, Haba et al 1993) have indicated that 75–90% of adult granulosa cell tumors have a diploid cellular DNA content. These may be associated with a somewhat more favorable clinical outlook than aneuploid tumors; similarly, tumors with a high S-phase fraction had a poorer clinical outcome than those with a lower S-phase fraction at discriminatory levels of 6% (Klemi et al 1990) or 10% (Haba et al 1993). Parallel studies of juvenile granulosa cell tumors (Swanson et al

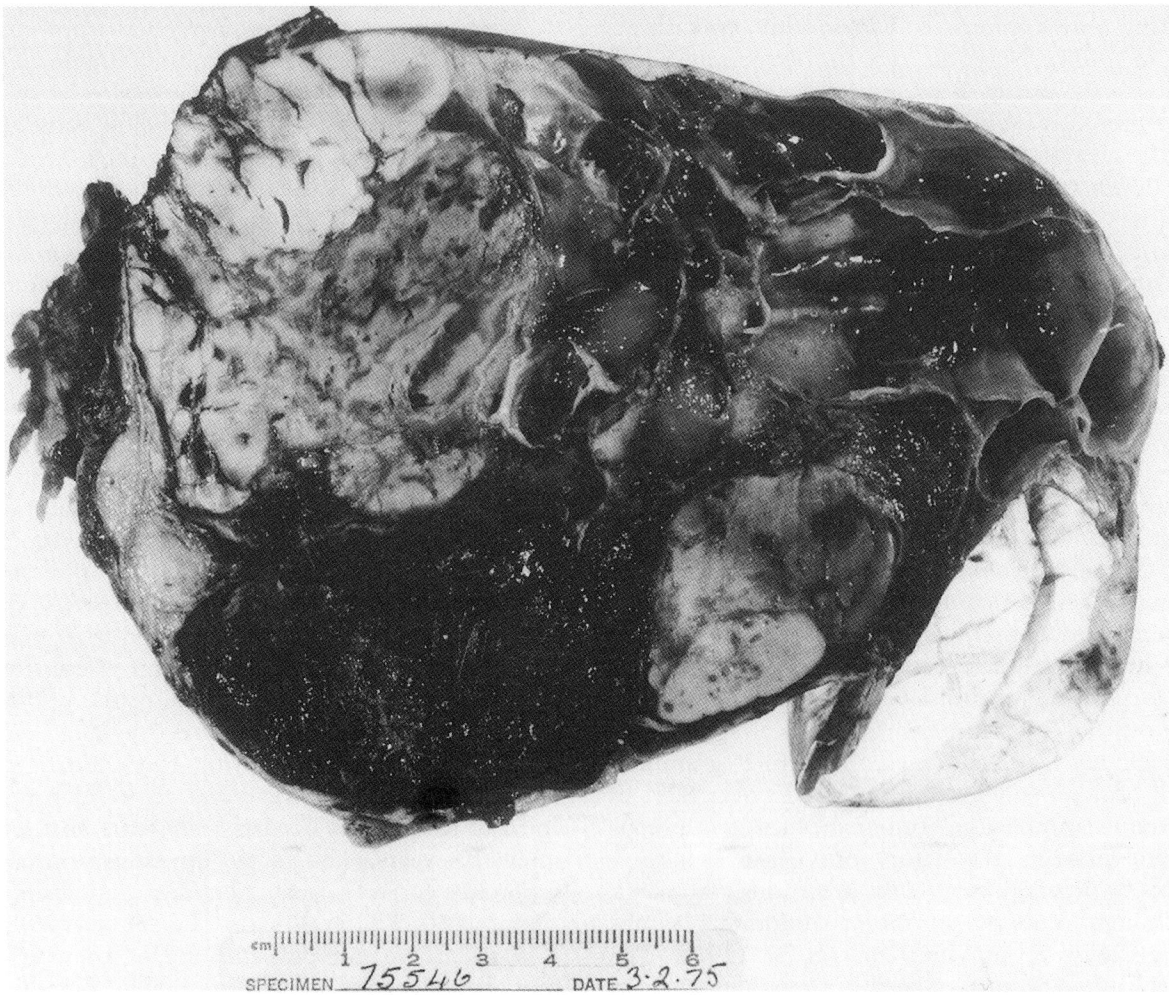

Fig. 33.3 Cut surface of a typical granulosa cell tumor. Solid areas are pale and featureless, but with focal necrosis. Areas of cystic degeneration are filled with proteinaceous fluid or old blood clot

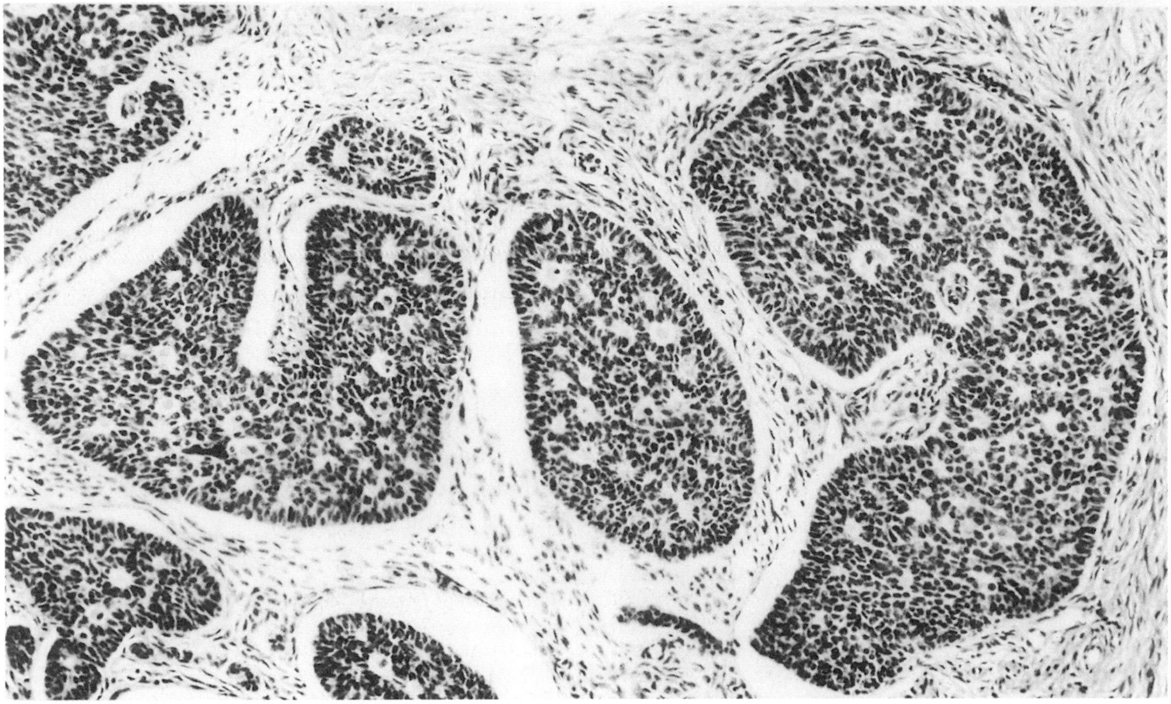

Fig. 33.4 Well differentiated granulosa cell tumor with a microfollicular pattern. Cells show some palisading around the periphery of cell masses, but rarely more pronounced than illustrated here. Call–Exner bodies are numerous. H + E ×125

1990, Jacoby et al 1992) have shown that approximately 55% are diploid but that ploidy does not impact materially upon prognosis.

Cytogenetic studies of adult granulosa cell tumors have identified structural changes to chromosome 6 leading to loss of 6q material (Verhest et al 1992), trisomy 12 in both juvenile and adult granulosa cell tumors (Fletcher et al 1991, Schofield & Fletcher 1992, Halperin et al 1995), and complex chromosomal changes in an additional case of juvenile granulosa cell tumor (Rodriguez et al 1992).

Macroscopic features

These tumors vary in size from tiny subclinical lesions to quite extraordinary masses filling the abdomen (Choi & Pritchard 1990) with a mean diameter in reported series of about 13 cm. The external surface may be smooth or bosselated. The cut surface of granulosa cell tumors is characteristically partly solid and partly cystic (in well over one-half of cases), while the remaining tumors are either completely solid or totally cystic. Solid areas may be hard and rubbery or soft in consistency and tend to be yellowish or gray in color, while cystic spaces contain proteinaceous

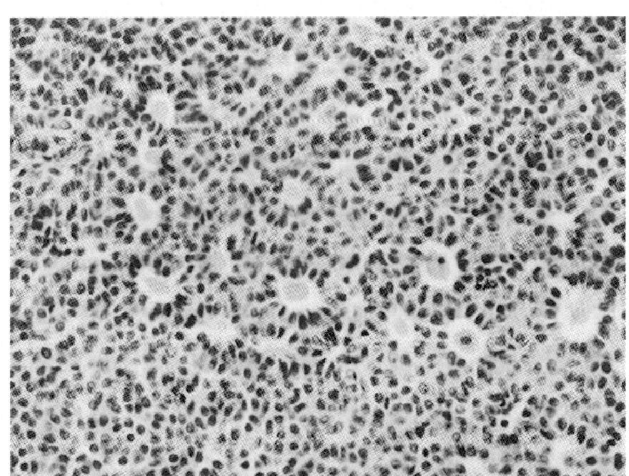

Fig. 33.5 Well differentiated granulosa cell tumor – microfollicular pattern. Numerous Call–Exner bodies containing hyaline material and cellular debris. H + E ×150

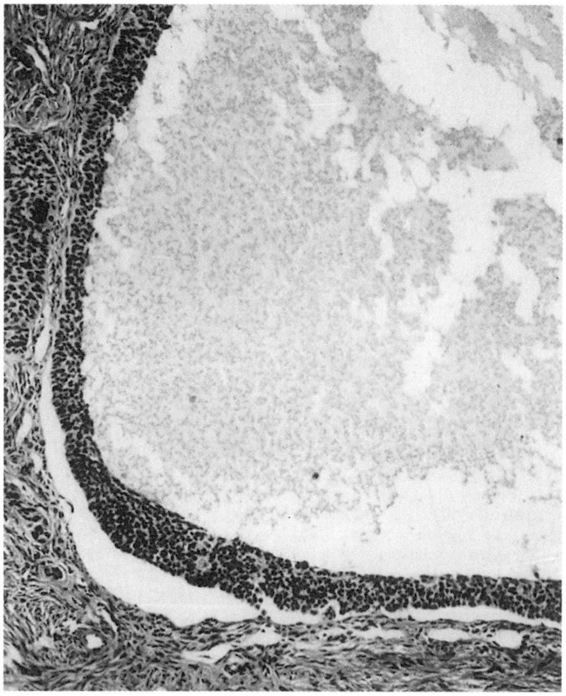

Fig. 33.6 Well differentiated granulosa cell tumor – macrofollicular pattern. Lining cells closely resemble those of normal preovulatory follicles. No thecal layer is present in this example. H + E ×75

fluid or old altered blood (Fig. 33.3). Thin-walled parvilocular cystic granulosa cell tumors may be mistaken grossly for benign serous tumors (Palladino et al 1965, Norris & Taylor 1969). Foci of hemorrhage and necrosis are quite common. At laparotomy, granulosa cell tumors are confined to the ovaries in 90% of patients (Bjorkholm & Silfversward 1981) and are bilateral in only 2%. In many of these latter cases, the poor clinical outcome suggests that they represent examples of a primary tumor in one ovary and a metastatic deposit in the other.

Microscopic features

Although one particular pattern of growth may be

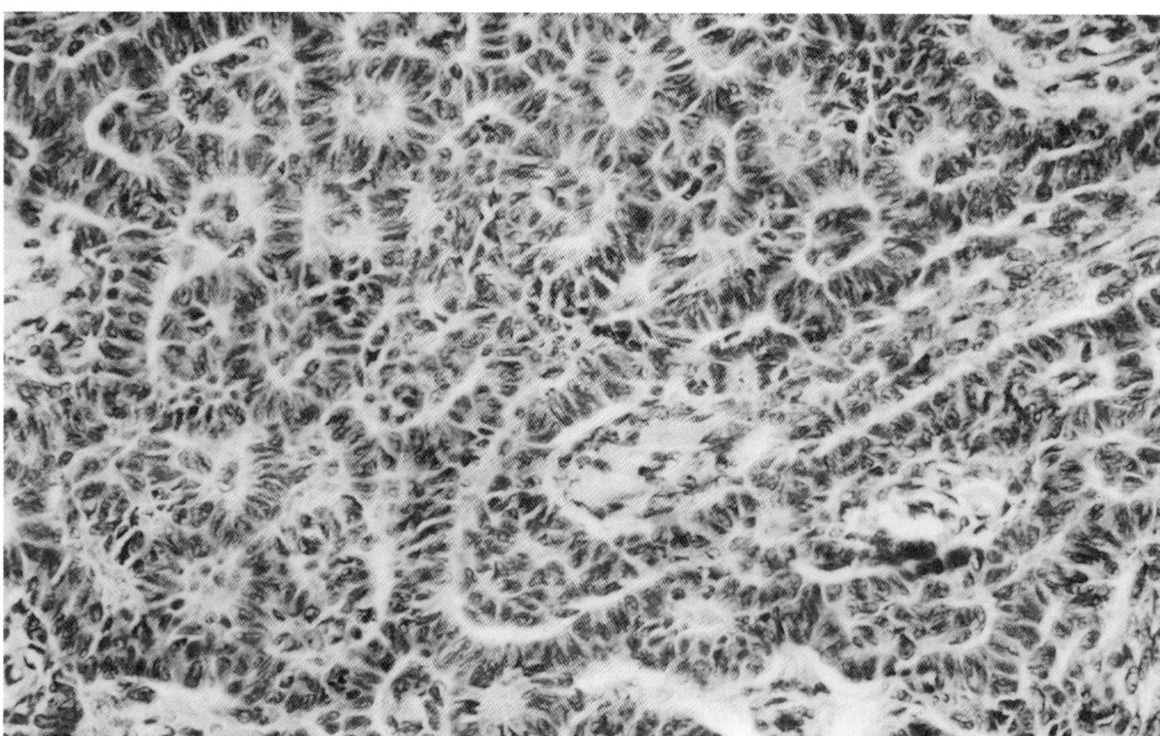

Fig. 33.7 Well differentiated granulosa cell tumor – trabecular pattern. Cords of cells vary from one to two cells thick with oval nuclei oriented perpendicularly. H + E ×250

dominant, variation in the histological appearance from area to area in any given tumor is more common.

Well differentiated granulosa cell tumors exhibit one or more of so-called microfollicular, macrofollicular, trabecular, or insular patterns. The microfollicular variant (Fig. 33.4), the most easily recognized, is characterized by multiple small rounded spaces formed by cystic degeneration in small aggregates of granulosa cells, and containing eosinophilic PAS-positive material (chondroitin 6-sulfate) and often fragments of nuclear debris or pyknotic nuclei. These spaces are known as Call–Exner bodies, but are found in only about one-third to one-half of all granulosa cell tumors. The granulosa cell nuclei are oriented somewhat radially around these structures (Fig. 33.5), although not with the same precision as are adenocarcinoma cells around an acinus. The macrofollicular variant (Fig. 33.6) comprises cysts of differing sizes lined by multilayered well differentiated granulosa cells, often cuffed by a layer of theca-like cells, and apparently also formed by cystic degeneration in large masses of granulosa cells. Either or both of these cell layers may be luteinized. In the uncommon totally cystic granulosa cell tumors, the lining cells of the cysts may so closely resemble those of non-neoplastic ovarian follicle cysts that differentiation on purely histological criteria presents a problem. In the trabecular variant the cellular arrangement gives rise to anastomosing ribbons or cords which may be one (Fig. 33.7) to several cells wide (Fig. 33.8). The granulosa cell cords are set in a background of stromal cells and show variable peripheral nuclear palisading. They may rarely produce true tubules, but the conspicuous presence of these should arouse suspicion of Sertoli cell differentiation. A trabecular pattern with hyaline or mucoid change (hyaluronic acid and chondroitin 6-sulfate) in the stroma gives rise to the so-called cylindromatous form of granulosa cell tumor (Fig. 33.9). Insular variants exhibit masses or islands of polyhedral granulosa cells with

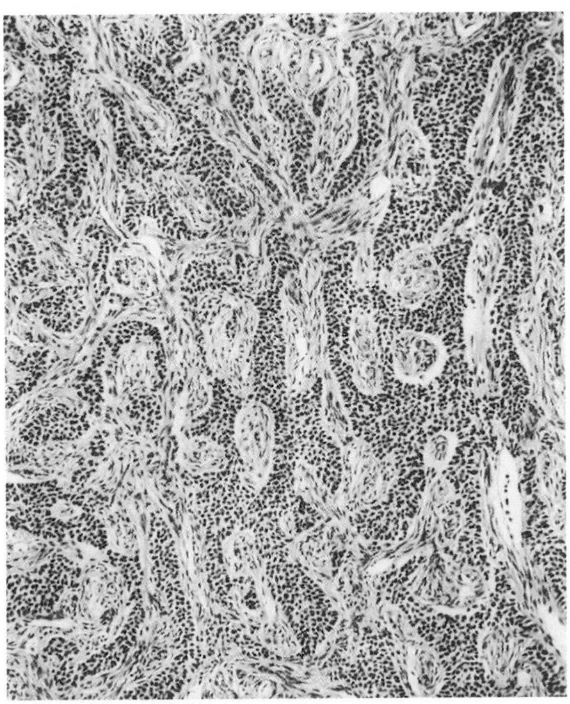

Fig. 33.8 Well differentiated granulosa cell tumor – trabecular pattern. Cords of cells are much thicker than in the previous variant (Fig. 33.7) and are interposed by prominent fibrothecoma-like stroma. H + E ×75

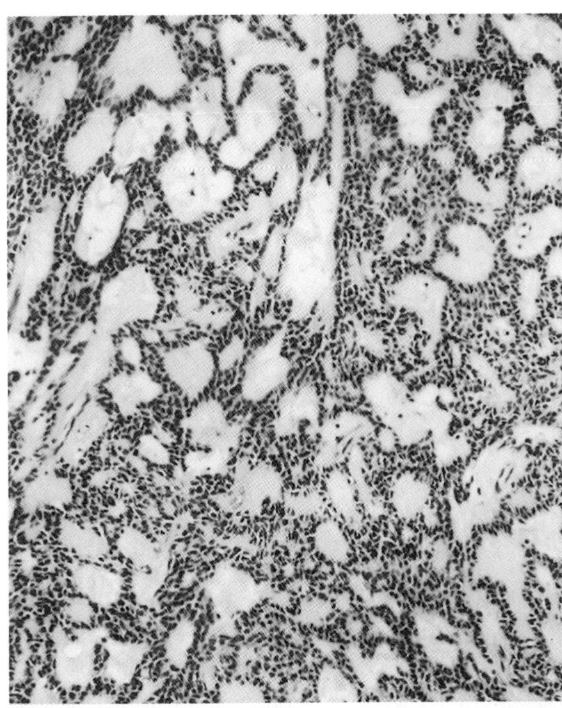

Fig. 33.9 Well differentiated granulosa cell tumor. With the addition of hyaline change to the stroma, the tumor acquires a 'cylindromatous' appearance. H + E ×75

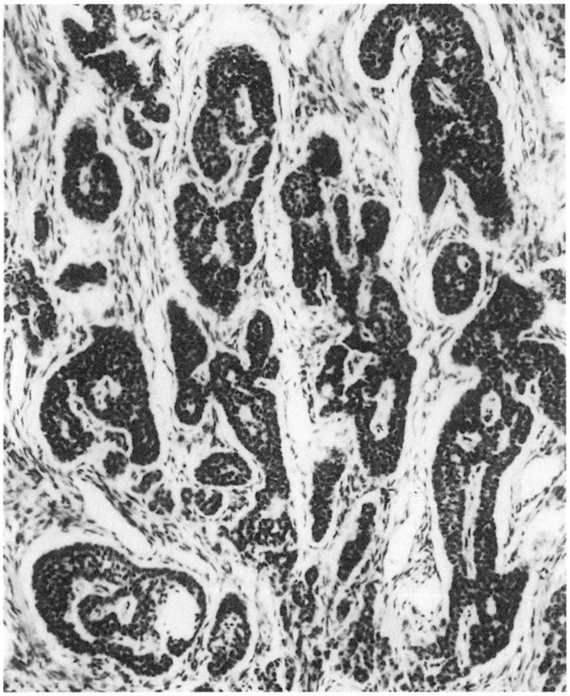

Fig. 33.10 So-called 'insular' variant of microfollicular granulosa cell tumor, important only in the difficulty it may present in being distinguished from ovarian carcinoid tumors. H + E ×75

peripherally palisaded nuclei separated by a fibroma-like or thecoma-like stroma (Fig. 33.10). Call–Exner bodies are common in this variant and there is overlap with the microfollicular pattern described above. Occasional, otherwise unremarkable, well differentiated granulosa cell tumors exhibit small foci where cells have enlarged bizarre nuclei (Fig. 33.11) and/or multinucleated giant cells (Young & Scully 1983b). These foci appear to be degenerative in nature and in no way alter the classification, typing, or grading of the tumor in which they are found. Another unusual degenerative phenomenon is central sclerosis within islands or masses of granulosa cells, again probably ischemic in nature (Fig. 33.12). A unique case has been reported of a granulosa cell tumor with scattered eosinophilic polygonal cells in the stroma showing an immunophenotype of true hepatic cell differentiation (Nogales et al 1993).

In moderately differentiated forms, the trabecular pattern is more complex and is composed of fine narrow undulating cords of granulosa cells

A 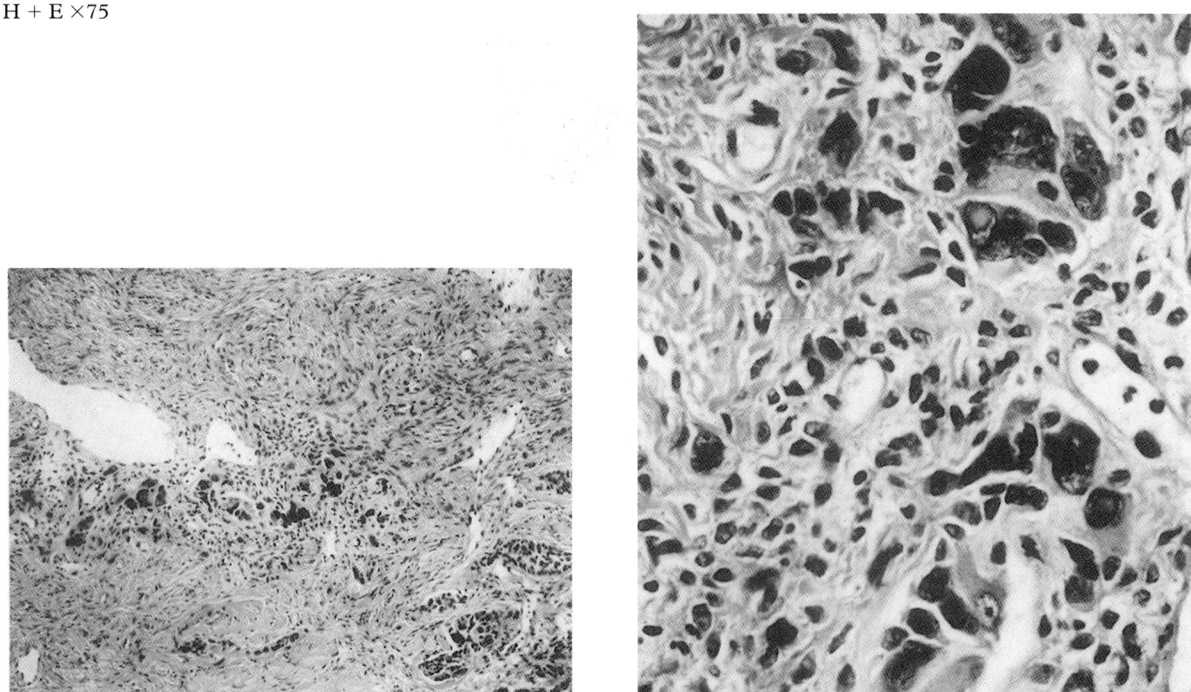 B

Fig. 33.11 Well differentiated granulosa cell tumor with focally bizarre nuclei. They may occur in any of the histological variants of this tumor. (A) H + E ×60. (B) Higher power of same cells. H + E ×300

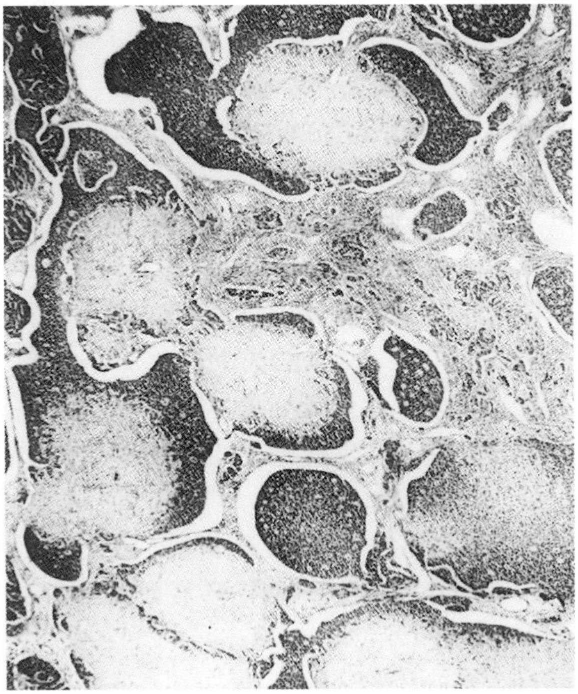

Fig. 33.12 Microfollicular tumor with pronounced central sclerosis in large islands of granulosa cells. H + E ×30

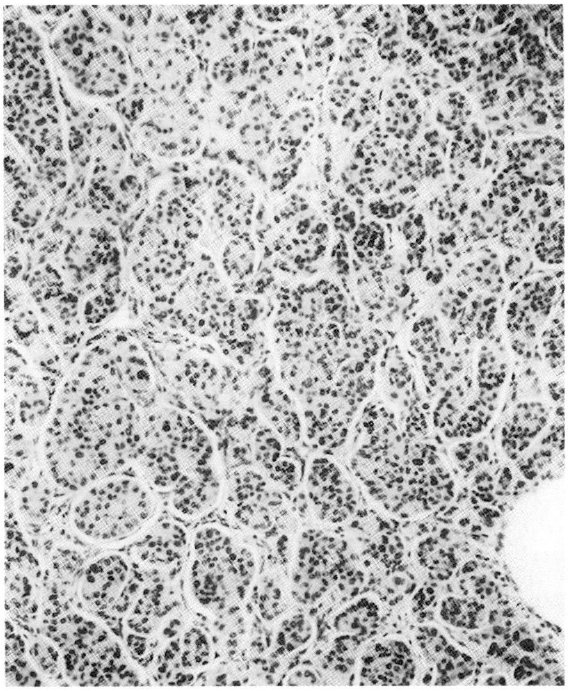

Fig. 33.14 Moderately differentiated granulosa cell tumor. A complex insular pattern with a scanty stromal component. H + E ×75

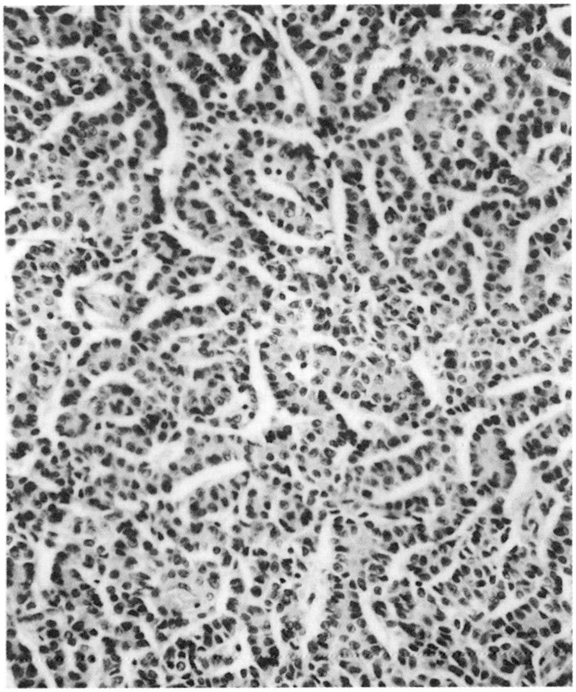

with little intervening stroma, producing so-called watered-silk (moiré-silk) or gyriform appearances (Fig. 33.13). Insular patterns also become increasingly complex with diminution in the intervening stroma (Fig. 33.14).

Poorly differentiated diffuse or 'sarcomatoid' forms produce monotonous cellular growth resembling a low grade round cell (Fig. 33.15) or spindle cell sarcoma (Fig. 33.16). The uniform cells are closely packed and arranged in poorly circumscribed sheets, which often appear to merge at their periphery with nearby acellular areas or the surrounding normal ovarian stroma. Luteinization further effaces the architecture (Fig. 33.17). The cells contain regular and relatively bland nuclei and, although mitoses may at times be numerous, they do not approach the high counts observed in the undifferentiated carcinomas or sarcomas

Fig. 33.13 Moderately differentiated granulosa cell tumor – gyriform or 'moiré-silk' pattern. Nuclei are still uniform and bland, with few mitoses. H + E ×150

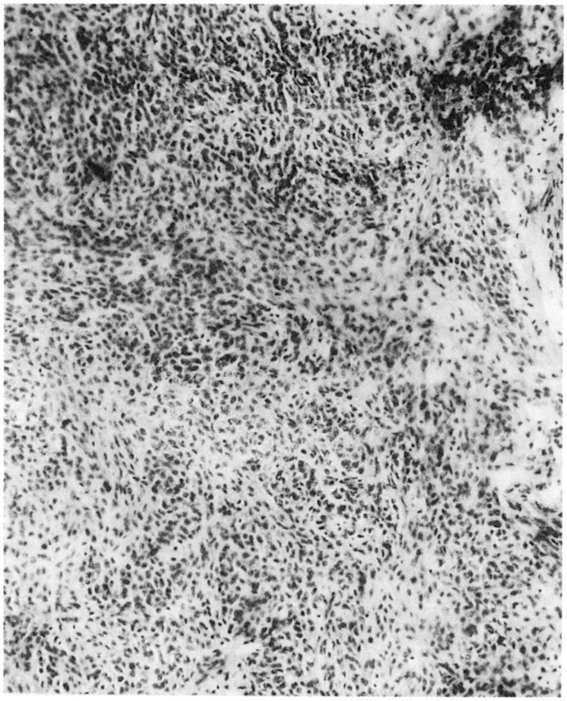

Fig. 33.15 Poorly differentiated diffuse granulosa cell tumor. Solid sheets of uniform small round cells. H + E ×75

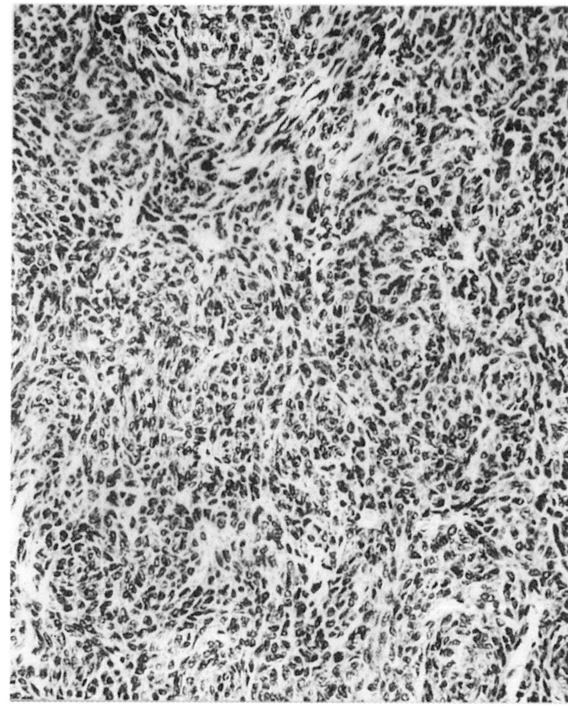

Fig. 33.16 Poorly differentiated diffuse granulosa cell tumor. Solid sheets of small spindled cells. Vascular spaces are relatively infrequent compared to low grade endometrioid stromal sarcoma. H + E ×150

forming the differential diagnosis of this variant of granulosa cell tumor. Fewer than 10% of granulosa cell tumors exhibit mitoses over 5 per 10HPF. Diffuse granulosa cell tumors contain variable amounts of reticulin fibrils, depending on the relative presence of a stromal (theca cell) component, and such reticulin as is present tends to outline groups rather than individual cells, this being of some help in differentiating them from low grade endometrioid sarcomas.

Juvenile granulosa cell tumor occurs mostly in the first two decades and only occasionally in women over the age of 30 years. This type of granulosa cell tumor is characterized by partially coalescing solid nodules of proliferating granulosa cells arranged randomly in sheets or around irregular follicle-like spaces (Fig. 33.18). Intersecting fibrous bands accentuate this nodularity, occasionally (when marked) producing a superficial resemblance to sclerosing stromal tumors (see Ch. 34). Intercellular edema may be quite pronounced, particularly if the patient is pregnant. The thick-walled follicles and cavities are smaller than those seen in adult macrofollicular granulosa cell tumors, and may contain mucicarmine-positive material in over one-half of cases. Solid tubular patterns are sometimes seen (Young et al 1984a). Theca cells are often prominent, particularly at the periphery of the nodules, but may be intimately admixed with the granulosa cells. Reticulin stains can be employed to highlight the relative proportions of these two cellular elements. Cytologically, both cell types appear less 'mature' than their equivalents in other types of granulosa cell tumor. The nuclei are larger and more hyperchromatic, and the granulosa cells rarely show nuclear grooving (Fig. 33.19). Mitoses, occasionally atypical, are often prominent, and average about 7 per 10HPF (Young et al 1984a). Luteinization is also a common feature of both granulosa and theca cell elements. Table 33.2 outlines histological differentiation between juvenile and 'adult' granulosa cell tumors. Rare and isolated examples of juvenile granulosa cell

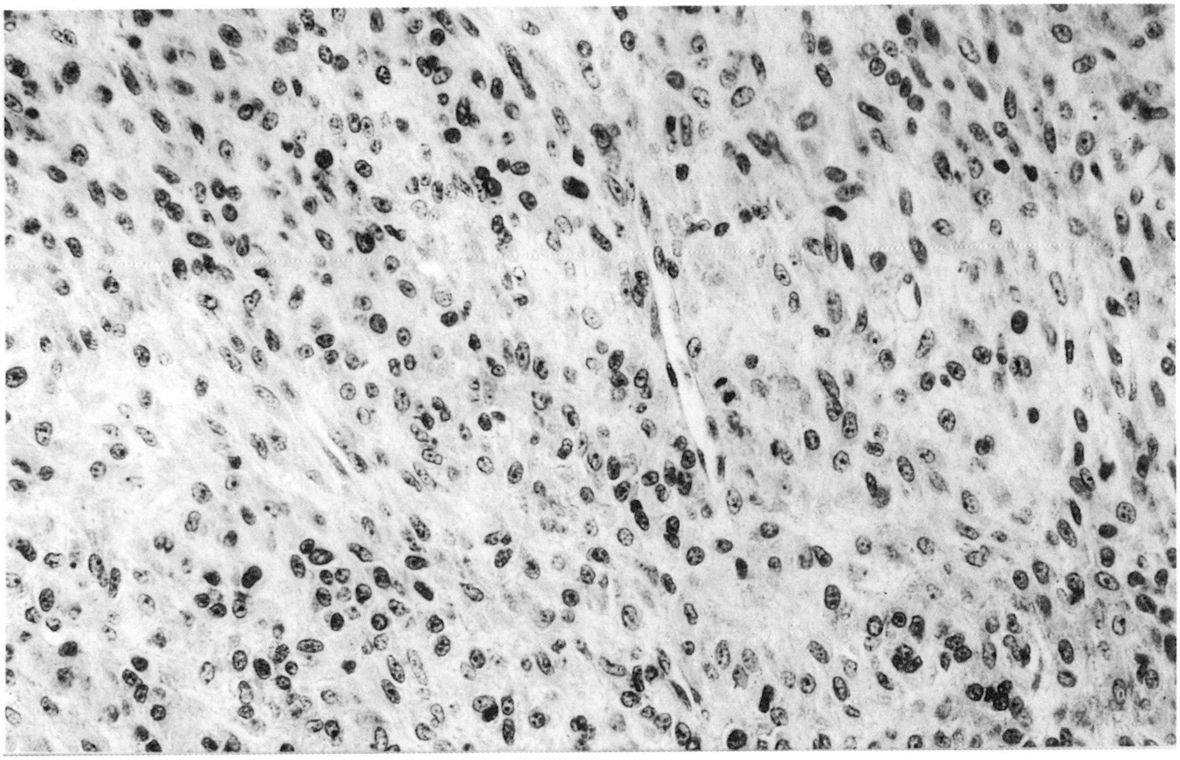

Fig. 33.17 Poorly differentiated and luteinized granulosa cell tumor. Nuclei are bland and uniform. Occasional mitoses are present. H + E ×250

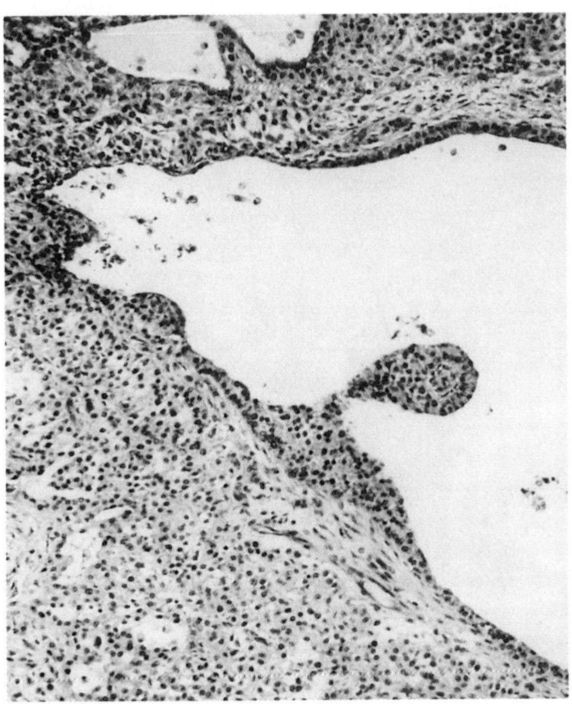

tumors showing focal specific mesenchymal differentiation towards skeletal muscle (Raafat et al 1990) or Wilms' tumor (O'Dowd & Ismail 1990) have been reported.

While isolated case reports detail the coincidence of granulosa cell tumor and ovarian tumors of epithelial (Bichel 1985) or germ cell type (Gee & Russell 1981, Dgani et al 1993), true combined neoplasms are rarely documented. We have encountered a combined granulosa cell and benign mucinous tumor (Figs. 33.20, 33.21) (Price et al 1990), which appears to be analogous to the Sertoli–Leydig cell tumors with heterologous elements (see Ch. 35). A second composite granulosa–theca cell and mucinous

Fig. 33.18 Juvenile granulosa cell tumor with an irregular follicle-like structure, lined by a variably thickened granulosa, in a solid nodule of pale eosinophilic cells with rounded nuclei. H + E ×75. (Material by courtesy of Dr R. E. Scully, Boston)

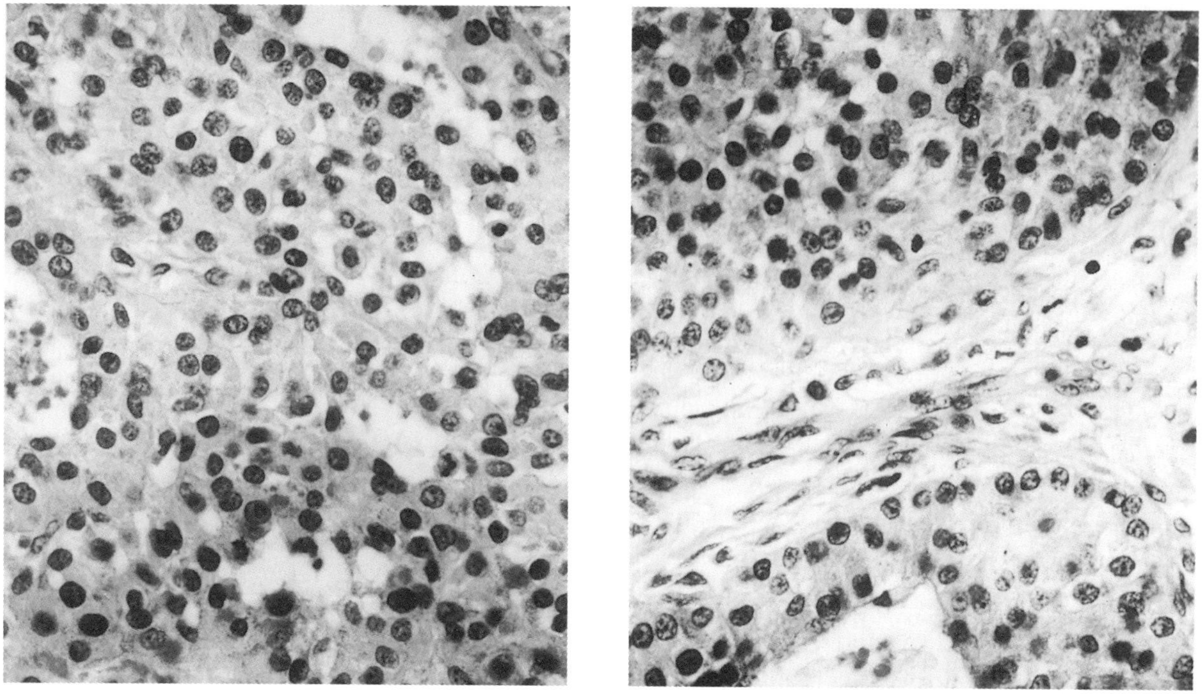

A B

Fig. 33.19 Juvenile granulosa cell tumor. Polyhedral cells, separated by intercellular edema, with eosinophilic cytoplasm and rounded, 'immature', nongrooved nuclei. Mitoses are focally numerous. Solid nodule (A) with an adjacent follicle-like structure (B). H + E ×300. (Material by courtesy of Dr R. E. Scully, Boston)

Table 33.2 Differential diagnosis: adult versus juvenile granulosa cell tumor of ovary

Juvenile granulosa cell tumor	Adult granulosa cell tumor
Clinical	
50% prepubertal, rare after the age of 30 years	50% postmenopausal, uncommon before the age of 30 years
Rarely malignant	Indolent course if malignant
Histological	
Predominantly solid pattern	Various patterns
Immature follicles with mucinous contents	Mature follicles with Call–Exner bodies
Cytoplasm usually abundant	Cytoplasm scanty
Luteinization common	Luteinization infrequent
Nuclei dark, ungrooved and often pleiomorphic	Nuclei pale and bland, often grooved
Mitoses common	Mitoses variable

tumor has been described with a malignant mucinous epithelial element (Chandran et al 1993).

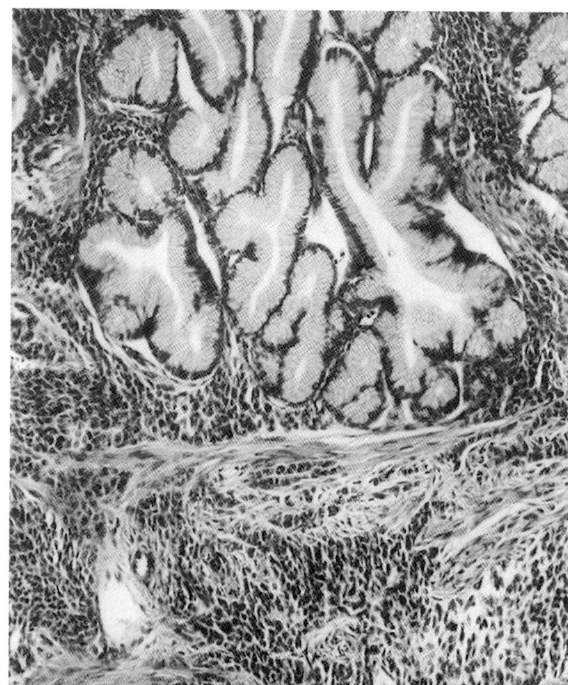

Fig. 33.20 Combined granulosa cell/benign mucinous tumor with densely hypercellular cyst wall due to granulosa cells proliferating around mucinous glands. H + E ×75

Differential diagnosis

The discrimination between an undifferentiated

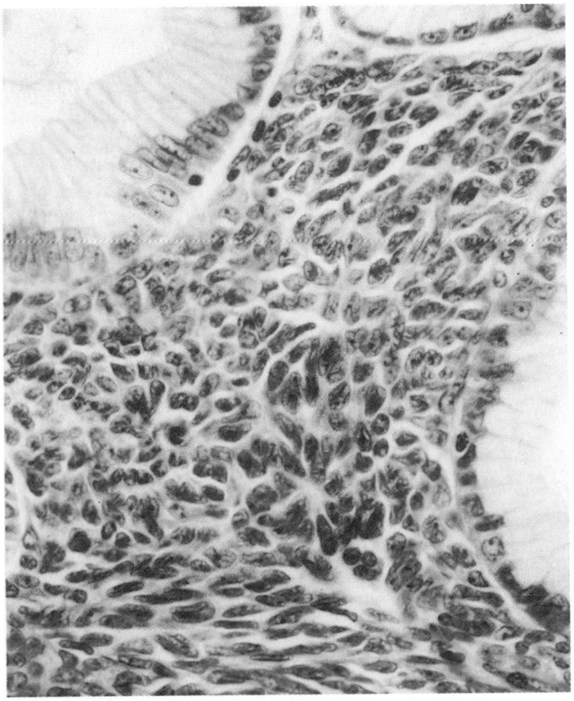

Fig. 33.21 Combined granulosa cell/benign mucinous tumor. Benign mullerian (endocervical) mucinous glands intimately mixed with typical granulosa cells. H + E ×300

small cell carcinoma of the ovary (see Ch. 31) and a granulosa cell tumor is one of the most important in ovarian tumor pathology. If a tumor is behaving in an unexpectedly aggressive fashion for one originally diagnosed as granulosa cell tumor, the possibility of such a misdiagnosis must be considered. The growth patterns, including the presence of cystic spaces, and the monotonous uniformity of the constituent cells can be quite similar in these two entities. Distinguishing criteria are outlined in Table 33.3, but the most readily appreciable criterion for distinguishing these two tumors is the appearance of the nuclei, which are typically bland and often grooved in granulosa cell tumors and have few mitoses, but show variation in size and shape, marked hyperchromatism, and are rarely grooved in undifferentiated small cell carcinomas. Numerous mitoses, frequently atypical, are often also found in the latter.

Granulosa cell tumors may be readily confused with carcinoid tumors, particularly those which have an insular pattern. The cells in an insular carcinoid tumor, however, usually have well defined cell margins, obvious eosinophilic granular cytoplasm, and more regular and rounded nuclei than those in granulosa cell tumors (Table 33.4). A Grimelius stain regularly identifies large numbers of argyrophil cells, and chromogranin will be

Table 33.3 Differential diagnosis: granulosa cell tumor versus undifferentiated small cell carcinoma

Undifferentiated small cell carcinoma	Adult granulosa cell tumor
Clinical	
Always premenopausal (always under 40 years of age)	50% postmenopausal (80% over 40 years of age)
Rapid progression	Indolent course if malignant
Poor prognosis	Good prognosis
60% in stage I	90% in stage I
60% have clinical or biochemical hypercalcemia	80% show evidence of estrogenic or androgenic activity
Histological	
Nuclei hyperchromatic, often bizarre; prominent nucleoli	Nuclei bland, uniform, may be grooved; inconspicuous nucleoli
Mitoses numerous and may be atypical	Mitoses variable, but usually infrequent
Apoptosis and tumor necrosis common	Tissue and cellular necrosis uncommon

Table 33.4 Differential diagnosis: granulosa cell tumor versus insular carcinoid

Insular carcinoid tumor	Granulosa cell tumor
Histological	
Islands and rounded acini	Various histological patterns
Small uniform acini with dense contents; sometimes calcified	Call–Exner bodies with watery to dense eosinophilic content, and occasionally nuclear debris
Obvious eosinophilic cytoplasm, usually with basal granules	Scanty amphophilic cytoplasm, no granules
Many argyrophil cells and some argentaffin cells	Occasional argyrophil cells and no argentaffin cells
Round nuclei, coarse chromatin, very regular orientation	Round or angular bland nuclei, often grooved, little discernible orientation
Fibromatous or hyaline stroma	Thecomatous stroma common
May be associated with other teratomatous elements	No teratomatous elements
Immunohistochemical	
Neuron-specific enolase, chromogranin	Vimentin, inhibin

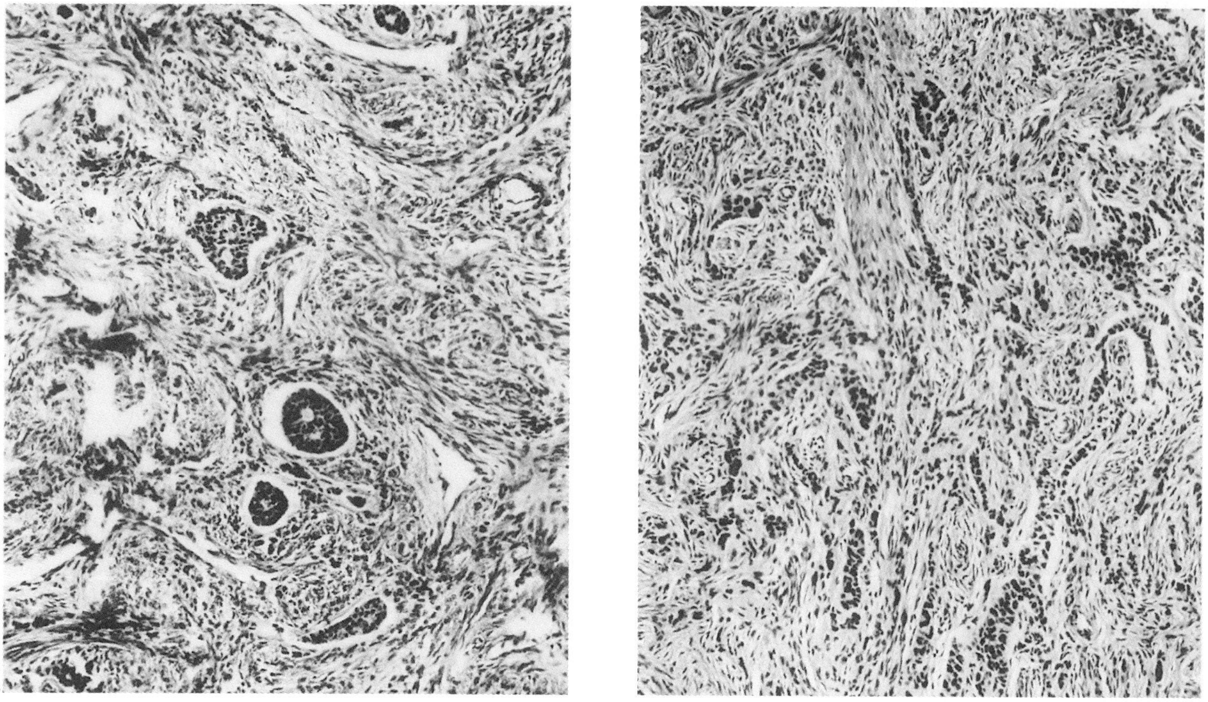

Fig. 33.22 Granulosa cell tumors with only minor sex cord components. (A) Insular pattern. (B) Trabecular pattern. H + E ×75

demonstrable immunohistochemically in carcinoid tumors.

It is necessary to distinguish the Call–Exner bodies of granulosa cell tumors from the glands of adenocarcinomas and the hyaline bodies of similar size observed in gonadoblastomas (see Ch. 51) and sex cord tumors with annular tubules (see Ch. 37). The acini of adenocarcinomas are often filled with thick mucin, and the nuclei are usually more pleiomorphic than those of the granulosa cell tumor. The hyaline bodies in gonadoblastoma and sex cord tumor with annular tubules are denser than Call–Exner bodies and can sometimes be observed to be continuous with hyaline basement membrane material around the periphery of the tumor cell nests. These bodies may also be calcified.

Formerly, extensively luteinized diffuse granulosa cell tumors were likely to be called 'malignant thecomas'. However, there is considerable doubt that such an entity exists. Norris & Taylor (1968) described one such case, but by their own diagnostic criteria some doubt exists as to whether or not the tumor was an ovarian or retroperitoneal fibrosarcoma (see Ch. 34). Most granulosa cell tumors can be easily distinguished from androblastoma, but this distinction may be impossible in very poorly differentiated cases, and in difficult cases we consider it appropriate to assign such lesions to the category of sex cord–stromal tumor of indeterminate differentiation. As noted in the introduction, the granulosa cell component may only be a minor one. The watershed between such tumors and the so-called 'fibromas with minor sex cord elements' (Young & Scully 1983a) is arbitrarily set at about 10% representation by the sex cord (granulosa cell) components (Fig. 33.22).

REFERENCES

Bichel P 1985 Simultaneous occurrence of a granulosa cell tumor and a serous papillary cystadenocarcinoma in the same ovary. Acta Pathologica Microbiologica et Immunologica Scandinavica 93: 175–181

Biscotti C V, Hart W R 1989 Juvenile granulosa cell tumors of the ovary. Archives of Pathology and Laboratory Medicine 113: 40–46

Bjorkholm E, Silfversward C 1981 Prognostic factors in

granulosa cell tumors. Gynecologic Oncology 11: 261–274

Brisigotti M, Fabbretti G, Pesce F et al 1993 Congenital bilateral juvenile granulosa cell tumor of the ovary in leprechaunism: a case report. Pediatric Pathology 13: 549–558

Chadha S, Cornelisse C J, Schaberg A 1990 Flow cytometric DNA ploidy analysis of ovarian granulosa cell tumors. Gynecologic Oncology 36: 240–245

Chandran R, Rahman H, Gebbie D 1993 Composite mucinous and granulosa–theca-cell tumor of the ovary: an unusual neoplasm. Australian and New Zealand Journal of Obstetrics and Gynaecology 33: 437–439

Choi C H, Pritchard J R 1990 Large cystic granulosa cell tumor: case report. American Journal of Obstetrics and Gynecology 163: 74–76

Davidson P G, McGinn J T Jr, Goldberg S L 1990 Bilateral spontaneous pneumothoraces caused by metastatic ovarian granulosa cell tumor. Chest 98: 503–505

Dgani R, Rozenman D, Lifschitz-Mercer B 1993 Granulosa cell tumor arising in an ovary with mature cystic teratoma. International Journal of Gynaecology and Obstetrics 41: 287–289

Ebel H, Villagran R, Conzen M, Schnabel R, Oppel F 1993 Solitare intrakranielle Spatmetastase eines Granulosazelltumors des Ovars. Neurochirurgia Stuttgart 36: 131–134

Evans A T, Gaffey T A, Malkasian G D, Annegers J F 1980 Clinicopathologic review of 118 granulosa and 82 theca cell tumors. Obstetrics and Gynecology 55: 231–238

Fletcher J A, Gibas Z, Donovan K, Perez-Atayde A, Genest D, Morton C C 1991 Ovarian granulosa–stromal cell tumors are characterized by trisomy 12. American Journal of Pathology 138: 515–520

Fox H, Langley F A 1975 Tumours of the ovary. Heinemann, London, p 119–137

Fox H, Agrawal K, Langley F A 1975 A clinicopathological study of 92 cases of granulosa cell tumor of the ovary with special reference to the factors influencing prognosis. Cancer 35: 231–241

Gee D C, Russell P 1981 The pathological assessment of ovarian neoplasms. IV: The sex cord–stromal tumors. Pathology 13: 235–255

Gusberg S B, Kardon P 1971 Proliferative endometrial response to theca–granulosa cell tumors. American Journal of Obstetrics and Gynecology 111: 633–643

Haba R, Miki H, Kobayashi S, Ohmori M 1993 Combined analysis of flow cytometry and morphometry of ovarian granulosa cell tumor. Cancer 72: 3258–3262

Halperin D, Visscher D W, Wallis T, Lawrence W D 1995 Evaluation of chromosome 12 copy number in ovarian granulosa cell tumors using interphase cytogenetics. International Journal of Gynecological Pathology 14: 319–323

Hitchcock C L, Norris H J, Khalifa M A, Wargotz E S 1989 Flow cytometric analysis of granulosa tumors. Cancer 64: 2127–2132

Imai A, Furui T, Shimokawa K, Tamaya T 1992 Juvenile granulosa cell tumor in a 2-year-old infant: report of a case complicated with ascites and acute respiratory distress. Gynecologic Oncology 46: 397–400

Jacoby A F, Young R H, Colvin R B et al 1992 DNA content in juvenile granulosa cell tumors of the ovary: a study of early- and advanced-stage disease. Gynecologic Oncology 46: 97–103

Jiminez-Quintero L P, Ro J Y, Zavala-Pompa A et al 1993 Granulosa cell tumor of the adult testis: a clinicopathologic study of seven cases and a review of the literature. Human Pathology 24: 1120–1125

Klemi P J, Joensuu H, Salmi T 1990 Prognostic value of flow cytometric DNA content analysis in granulosa cell tumor of the ovary. Cancer 65: 1189–1193

Langley F A, Smith J P, Woodcock A S 1953 Debatable uterine tumors. Acta Obstetricia et Gynecologica Scandinavica 32: 143–169

Margolin K A, Pak H Y, Esensten M L, Doroshow J H 1985 Hepatic metastases in granulosa cell tumor of the ovary. Cancer 56: 691–695

Malmstrom H, Hogberg T, Risberg B, Simonsen E 1994 Granulosa cell tumors of the ovary: prognostic factors and outcome. Gynecologic Oncology 52: 50–55

Nakashima N, Young R H, Scully R E 1984 Androgenic granulosa cell tumors of the ovary: a clinicopathologic analysis of 17 cases and review of the literature. Archives of Pathology and Laboratory Medicine 108: 786–791

Nistal M, Lazaro R, Garcia J, Paniagua R 1992 Testicular granulosa cell tumor of the adult type. Archives of Pathology and Laboratory Medicine 116: 284–287

Nogales F F, Concha A, Plata C, Ruiz-Avila I 1993 Granulosa cell tumor of the ovary with diffuse true hepatic differentiation simulating stromal luteinisation. American Journal of Surgical Pathology 17: 85–90

Norris H J, Taylor H B 1968 Prognosis of granulosa–theca tumors of the ovary. Cancer 21: 255–263

Norris H J, Taylor H B 1969 Virilization associated with cystic granulosa tumors. Obstetrics and Gynecology 34: 629–635

O'Dowd J, Ismail S M 1990 Juvenile granulosa cell tumor of the ovary containing a nodule of Wilms' tumor. Histopathology 17: 468–470

Orselli R C, Bassler T J 1973 Theca granulosa cell tumor arising in the adrenal. Cancer 31: 474–477

Palladino V S, Duffy J L, Bures G J 1965 Probable true cystic granulosa cell tumor. Obstetrics and Gynecology 25: 729–733

Piura B, Nemet D, Yanai-Inbar I, Cohen Y, Glezerman M 1994 Granulosa cell tumor of the ovary: a study of 18 cases. Journal of Surgical Oncology 55: 71–77

Pounder D J, Iyer P V, Davy M L J 1985 Bilateral juvenile granulosa cell tumors associated with skeletal enchondromas. Australian and New Zealand Journal of Obstetrics and Gynaecology 25: 123–126

Powell C, Black W C 1940 Extra-ovarian granulosa cell tumor. American Journal of Obstetrics and Gynecology 40: 318–323

Powell J L, Johnson N A, Bailey C L, Otis C N 1993 Management of advanced juvenile granulosa cell tumor of the ovary. Gynecologic Oncology 48: 119–123

Price A, Russell P, Elliott P, Bannatyne P 1990 Composite mucinous and granulosa cell tumor of ovary: a case report of a unique neoplasm. International Journal of Gynecological Pathology 9: 372–378

Raafat F, Klys H, Rylance G 1990 Juvenile granulosa cell tumor. Pediatric Pathology 10: 617–623

Ragins A B, Frankel L 1940 Intraligamentous granulosa cell tumor. American Journal of Obstetrics and Gynecology 40: 302–306

Reddy D B, Rao D B, Sarojini J S 1963 Extra-ovarian granulosa cell tumor. Journal of the Indian Medical Association. 41: 254

Rodriguez E, Rao P H, Reuter V 1992 Cytogenetic analysis of a juvenile granulosa cell tumor. Cancer Genetics and Cytogenetics 61: 207–209

Scharl A, Vierbuchen M, Kusche M, Bolte A 1988 Zür Klinik und Prognose von Granulosazelltumoren des Ovars. Geburtshilfe und Frauenheilkind 48: 567–573

Schofield D E, Fletcher J A 1992 Trisomy 12 in pediatric granulosa–stromal cell tumors. Demonstration by a modified method of fluorescence in situ hybridization on paraffin-embedded material. American Journal of Pathology 141: 1265–1269

Scully R E 1979 Tumors of the ovary and maldeveloped gonads. AFIP fascicle 16, 2nd series. Armed Forces Institute of Pathology, Washington, DC, p 152–173

Scully R E 1982 Sex cord–stromal tumors. In: Blaustein A (ed) Pathology of the female genital tract, 2nd edn. Springer-Verlag, New York, p 581–601

Stenwig J T, Hazekamp J T, Beecham J B 1979 Granulosa cell tumors of the ovary. A clinicopathological study of 118 cases with long-term follow-up. Gynecologic Oncology 7: 136–152

Suh K S, Silverberg S G, Rhame J G, Wilkinson D S 1990 Granulosa cell tumor of the ovary. Histopathologic and flow cytometric analysis with clinical correlation. Archives of Pathology and Laboratory Medicine 114: 496–501

Swanson S A, Norris H J, Kelsten M L, Wheeler J E 1990 DNA content of juvenile granulosa tumors determined by flow cytometry. International Journal of Gynecological Pathology 9: 101–109

Tamini H K, Bolan J W 1984 Enchondromatosis (Ollier's disease) and ovarian juvenile granulosa cell tumor. A case report and review of the literature. Cancer 53: 1605–1608

Tanaka Y, Sasaki Y, Nishihira H, Izawa T, Nishi T 1992 Ovarian juvenile granulosa cell tumor associated with Maffucci's syndrome. American Journal of Clinical Pathology 97: 523–527

Tanaka Y, Sasaki Y, Tachibana K, Suwa S, Terashima K, Nakatani Y 1994 Testicular juvenile granulosa cell tumor in an infant with X/XY mosaicism clinically diagnosed as true hermaphroditism. American Journal of Surgical Pathology 18: 316–322

Verhest A, Nedoszytko B, Noel J C, Dangou J M, Simon P, Limon J 1992 Translocation (6;16) in a case of granulosa cell tumor of the ovary. Cancer Genetics and Cytogenetics 60: 41–44

Young R H, Scully R E 1983a Ovarian stromal tumors with minor sex cord elements: a report of seven cases. International Journal of Gynecological Pathology 2: 227–234

Young R H, Scully R E 1983b Ovarian sex cord–stromal tumors with bizarre nuclei: a clinicopathologic analysis of 17 cases. International Journal of Gynecological Pathology 1: 325–335

Young R H, Dickersin G R, Scully R E 1984a Juvenile granulosa cell tumor. A clinicopathologic analysis of 125 cases. American Journal of Surgical Pathology 8: 575–596

Young R H, Dudley A G, Scully R E 1984b Granulosa cell, Sertoli–Leydig cell, and unclassified sex cord–stromal tumors associated with pregnancy: a clinicopathologic analysis of 36 cases. Gynecologic Oncology 18: 181–205

Young R H, Lawrence W D, Scully R E 1985 Juvenile granulosa cell tumor – another neoplasm associated with abnormal chromosomes and ambiguous genitalia. Report of three cases. American Journal of Surgical Pathology 9: 737–743

34

Thecoma–fibroma group of tumors

P. Russell A. Farnsworth

These neoplasms arise from the ovarian stroma and exhibit a spectrum of histological appearances which includes, at one end, simple fibromas and, at the other end, tumors showing distinct differentiation to specialized perifollicular or follicular theca cells. Implicit in this continuous spectrum is some variability in the reported relative frequencies of the different subtypes. Thecomas are defined by the World Health Organization (WHO) (Serov et al 1973) as 'stromal tumors, many cells of which contain abundant lipid-rich cytoplasm and resemble theca cells'. Varying numbers of fibroblasts may also be present in these tumors (Scully 1982). However, according to Scully (1979), the term 'luteinization' is applied to a distinct subtype of thecal cell implying that the lipid-rich cells of thecal appearance in most thecomas are not in fact luteinized. Partially or completely luteinized theca cell tumors have special names – 'luteinized thecoma', 'luteothecoma' (Hughesdon 1966), 'stromal luteoma' (Scully 1964), 'lipid cell thecoma' (Hughesdon 1983) – such tumors exhibiting a range of histological changes intermediate between typical thecomas and lipid cell tumors (Ch. 39). Young & Scully (1982) apply the term 'thecoma' to stromal tumors associated with some clinical evidence of steroid hormone production, and concede that morphological criteria alone may not be sufficiently exact to distinguish them from other ovarian stromal tumors. Diagnostic difficulty occasioned by those tumors which lie morphologically between typical thecomas and fibromas, and usually containing some lipid, is more apparent than real. Of the terms applied to such tumors (fibrothecoma, thecafibroma), the latter is our preference (Gee & Russell 1981). In our experience, such tumors appear to be clinically and histologically much closer to the fibroma end of the spectrum and can be readily distinguished from typical thecomas.

Tumors in the thecoma–fibroma group vary from microscopic to very large, and fibromas in particular are frequently quite small and picked up as incidental findings at operation. Scully (1982) has advocated that fibromas smaller than 3 cm in diameter be ignored for statistical purposes. We feel this is unacceptably restrictive and, for consistency, have chosen the 1 cm limit widely adopted for the benign surface epithelial–stromal tumors (Ch. 22). This nevertheless introduces yet another variable into figures purporting to indicate relative frequencies of such lesions.

The presence of occasional small aggregates of cells of sex cord type is acceptable without altering the primary diagnosis. It is recommended by Young & Scully (1983a) that such tumors be classified according to the dominant histological pattern, but with the rider 'with minor sex cord elements' added for descriptive accuracy.

Employing these general guidelines, ovarian fibromas are by far the commonest ovarian neoplasms of sex cord–stromal origin (see Ch. 32) and account for 6% of all primary ovarian tumors. Typical thecomas, on the other hand, are uncommon lesions, while tumors with features intermediate between these histological extremes are only somewhat more frequently encountered.

THECOMAS

These essentially always benign tumors may occur at any age, but predominantly above age 40 years and rarely in children (Evans et al 1980). The mean age of incidence is about 55 years, and three-quarters occur after the menopause. Luteinized variants (see below) are more likely to occur in younger women. Estrogenic manifestations are by far the commonest mode of clinical presentation, and usually take the form of menstrual irregularities or postmenopausal bleeding (Barrenetxea et al 1990). Androgenic thecomas are rare but well documented (Givens et al 1975, Longscope & Robboy 1980). Nonspecific abdominal symptoms relating to the tumor itself are uncommon, although abdominal pain and swelling and even Meigs' syndrome have been reported (Faber 1962). A case has been reported in a patient with Maffucci's syndrome (Hamdoun et al 1993).

Cytogenetic and molecular genetic studies

As with other sex cord–stromal tumors, trisomy 12 is an emerging karyotypic aberration in ovarian thecomas (Mrozek et al 1990, 1992).

Macroscopic features

They range in size from small subclinical nodules to large, firm, solid rubbery tumors several centimeters in diameter. The cut surface characteristically is bright yellow to orange, although many appear paler in hue. They are almost always unilateral. The remainder of the ovary, and indeed the contralateral ovary, may show diffuse or nodular hyperplasia.

Microscopic features

Most tumors conform to one of two patterns. Typical thecomas consist of large, ill-defined, somewhat nodular masses of plump eosinophilic or vacuolated cells interspersed by relatively less conspicuous bands of fibrous connective tissue (Fig. 34.1). The fibrous bands are composed mostly of tight bundles of elongated fibroblastic cells, but often exhibit plaques of hyalinization (Fig. 34.2). The theca cells are uniformly spindle

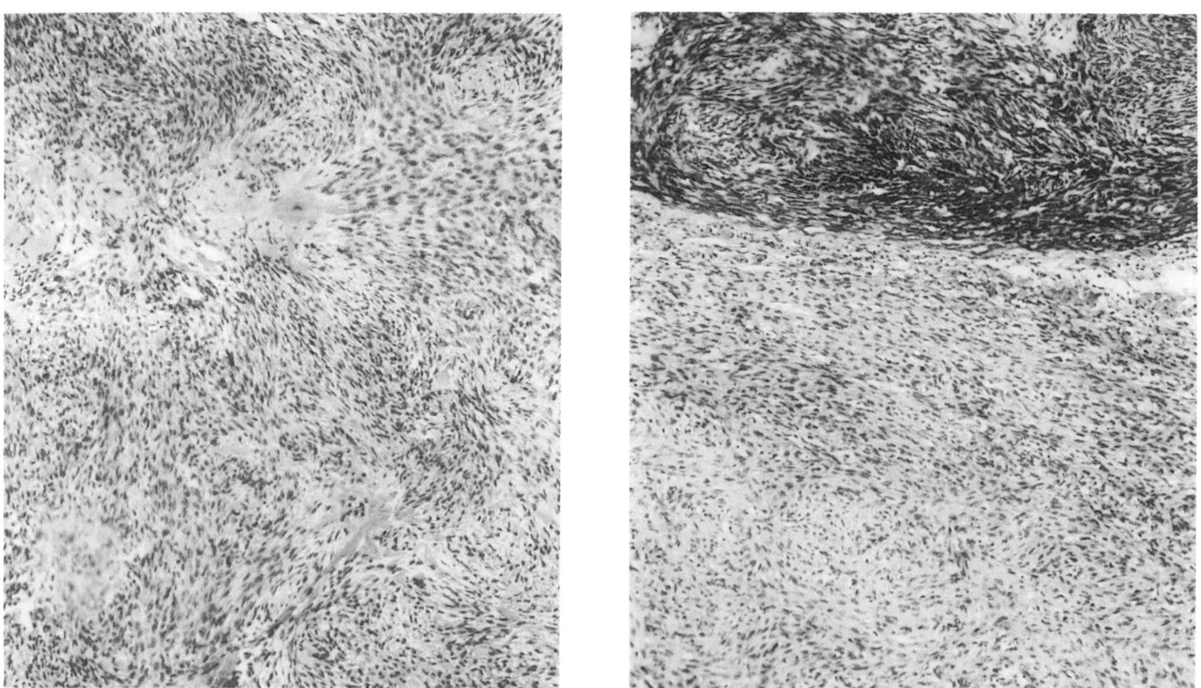

A

B

Fig. 34.1 Ovarian thecoma. (A) Swathes and bundles of plump spindle cells intermixed with bands of smaller cells with small elongate nuclei. Note focal stellate hyalinization of the stroma. H + E ×75. (B) Broad bands of typical, plump theca-like cells in the tumor. Contrast with the marked hypercellularity of adjacent ovarian cortical stromal hyperplasia (top). H + E ×75

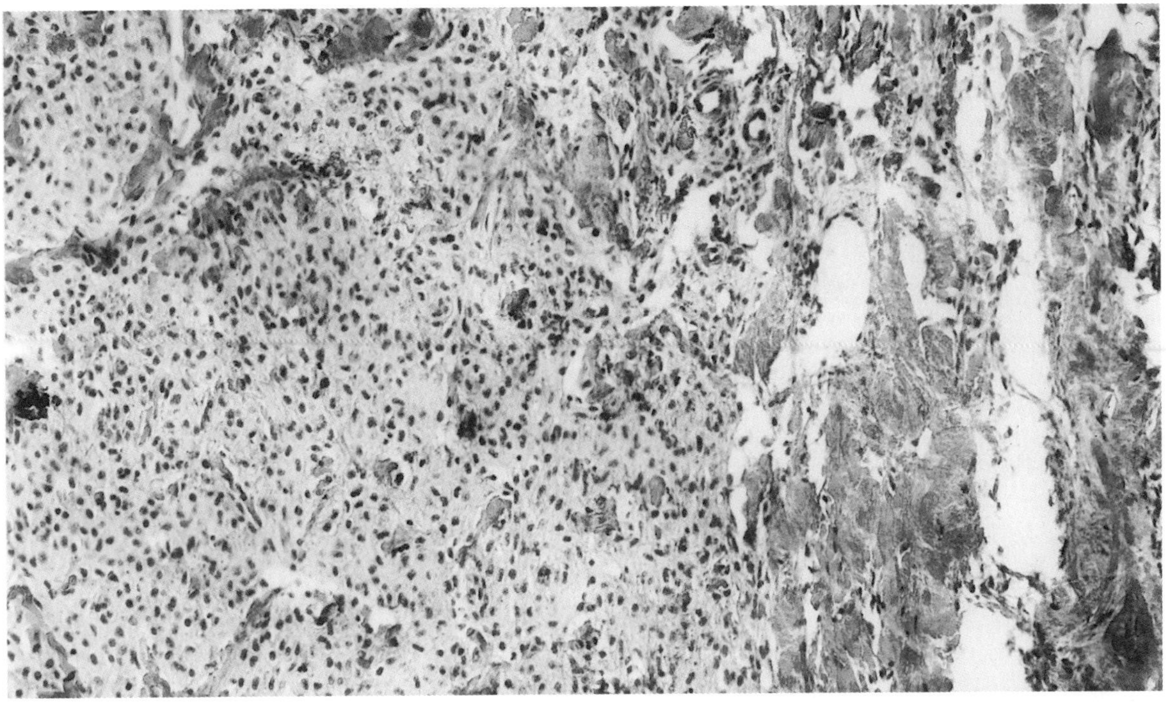

Fig. 34.2 Ovarian thecoma. Lipid-rich theca-like cells with pale vacuolated cytoplasm and round to oval nuclei. Patchy hyalinization of the stroma is prominent. A small focus of dystrophic calcification is seen at the left margin. H + E ×125

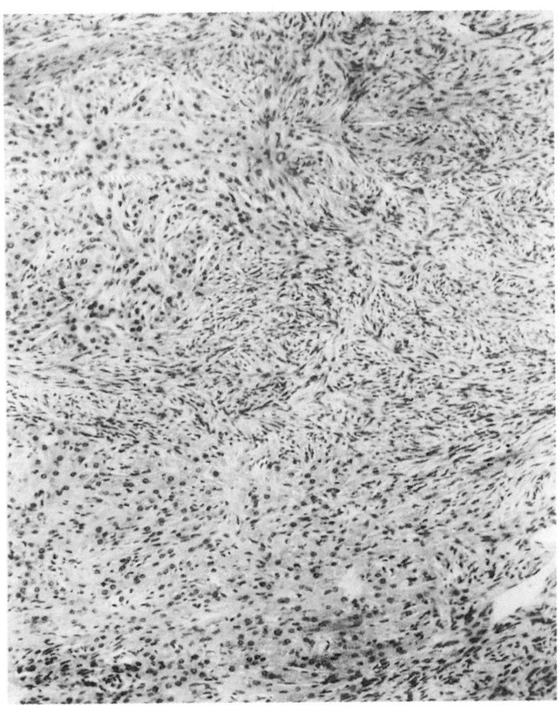

Fig. 34.3 Luteinized thecoma. Large masses of clearly luteinized theca cells (abundant eosinophilic cytoplasm, round, slightly hyperchromatic, vesicular nuclei) interposed by bands of smaller spindled cells. H + E ×75

shaped with small, pale, round, or ovoid, central, nongrooved nuclei (Fig. 34.2). Reticulin stains show a fine meshwork of fibrils about individual cells. Mitoses are occasionally noted (up to 1 per 10HPF in some tumors). Edema or myxoid change is often prominent, and some tumors show an occasional focus of stromal dystrophic calcification. A particular subtype characterized by extensive calcification has been occasionally noted in young women (Young et al 1988). Occasional small nests of granulosa cells are found; such tumors are called 'thecomas with minor sex cord elements' (Young & Scully 1983a). Over 50% of thecomas are associated with stromal hyperplasia (Fig. 34.1B) in the same and/or contralateral ovary, which may be diffuse or nodular (including nodular thecal hyperplasia). These hyperplastic ovaries fre-

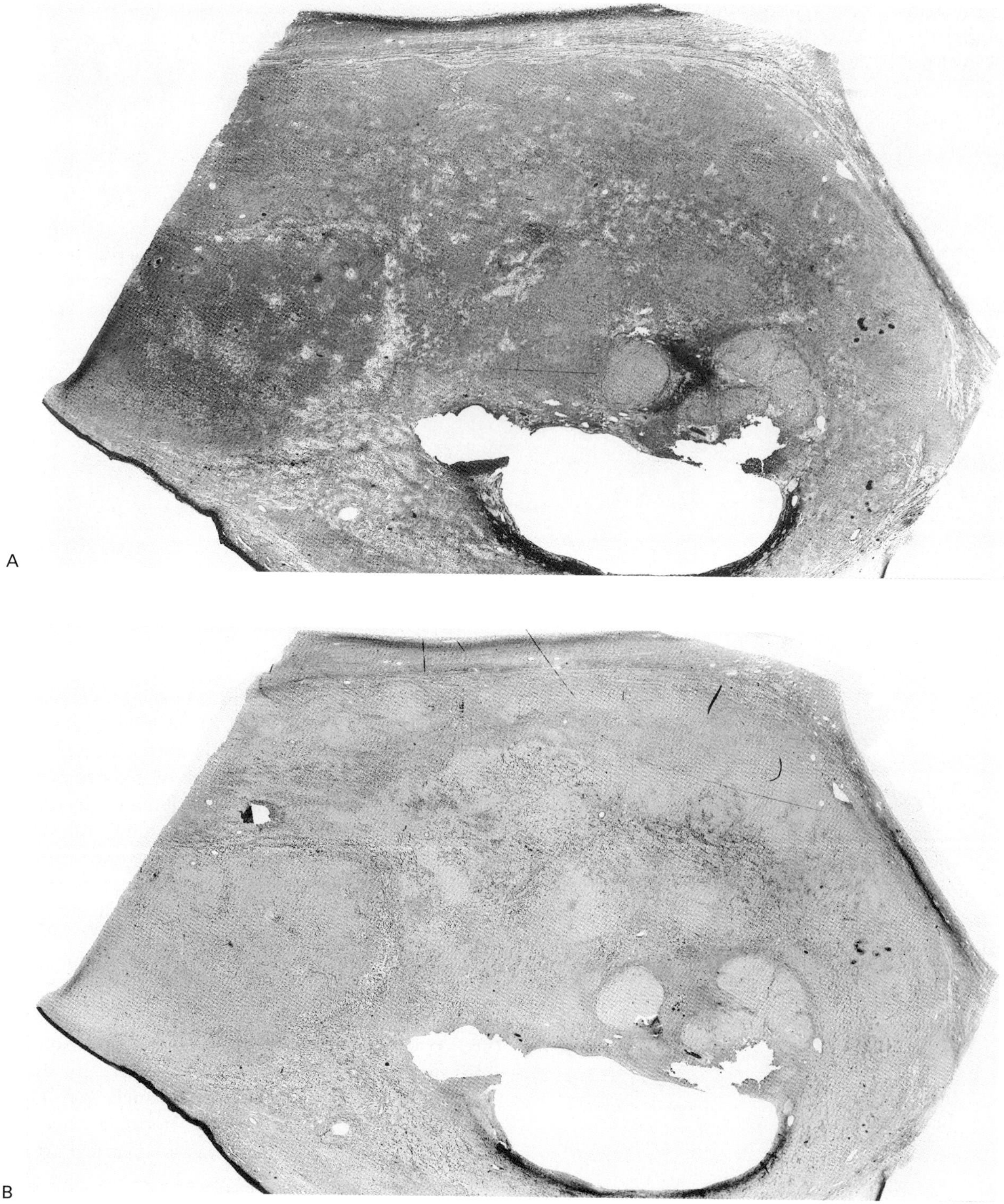

Fig. 34.4 Luteinized thecoma. An otherwise typical thecoma with small, irregularly scattered nodules of large eosinophilic lutein cells. (A) Survey showing ill-defined nodules of various sizes, but particularly noticeable above the large follicular cyst to center right. Note the attenuated (i.e. not hyperplastic) cortical stroma at the top and right. H + E ×3.3. (B) The nodularity of the tumor is accentuated by a reticulin stain. Reticulin ×3.3

quently show focal luteinization, justifying the designation of thecosis or thecomatosis (Novak & Woodruff 1979), and raising the old question of focal nodular hyperplasia versus neoplasia with respect to some thecal tumors, a problem elegantly addressed by Sternberg & Dhurandhar (1977).

The second defined histological pattern is of otherwise typical thecomas or perhaps more fibromatous tumors throughout which clusters of large eosinophilic lipid-laden lutein cells are scattered (Fig. 34.3), an appearance which has been designated 'luteinized thecoma' (Roth & Sternberg 1983). These lesions can only be distinguished from the very rare so-called 'stromal Leydig cell tumors' of Sternberg & Roth (1973) by the absence of Reinke crystals, although these latter tumors often arise in an older age group and may have a variegated gross appearance. It is doubtful whether such a distinction is always possible or indeed valid (Zhang et al 1982), and over 10% of such luteinized thecomas are androgenic. Luteinized thecomas do tend, however, to be solitary lesions, occur more frequently in younger women, are unassociated with a background of stromal hyperplasia (Fig. 34.4), and are therefore distinguishable from stromal luteomas (Scully 1964) which are regarded by some as completely luteinized thecomas and by others as lipid cell tumors (see Ch. 39). Stromal luteomas, however, are almost always seen as dominant nodules in a background of nodular thecal hyperplasia (stromal hyperplasia with focal luteinization), and we regard them as hyperplastic or tumor like in nature and have discussed them in Chapter 14.

The existence of malignant thecomas has been challenged by some investigators but, given that many of the reported examples are better reinterpreted as fibrosarcomas, luteinized diffuse granulosa cell tumors, or fibromatosis (see Ch. 16), a residuum of apparently genuine examples remains (Waxman et al 1979, Karck et al 1991). In the absence of established criteria, thecomatous tumors exhibiting hypercellularity and four or more mitoses per 10HPF should be treated as malignant. Nuclear atypia per se is not an indication of malignancy, and rare thecomas or luteinized thecomas may contain focal aggregates of bizarre nuclei without compromising the patient's prognosis (Young & Scully 1983b).

THECAFIBROMAS

These tumors exhibit a much lower frequency of associated endometrial pathology and evidence of endocrine disturbance than do the 'pure' thecomas, and in this respect more closely resemble the largely hormonally inactive fibromas and sclerosing stromal tumors. The general age at presentation and clinical findings are also very similar to those outlined below for ovarian fibromas. It is relevant to note here that the existence of tumors intermediate between thecomas and fibromas is evidence of the specialized ovarian stromal origin of most, if not all, ovarian fibromas. For all practical purposes, these tumors are benign. As with thecomas, rare cases reported as malignant fibrothecoma (Halalau et al 1982), based on the presence of intracytoplasmic lipid in spindle cell

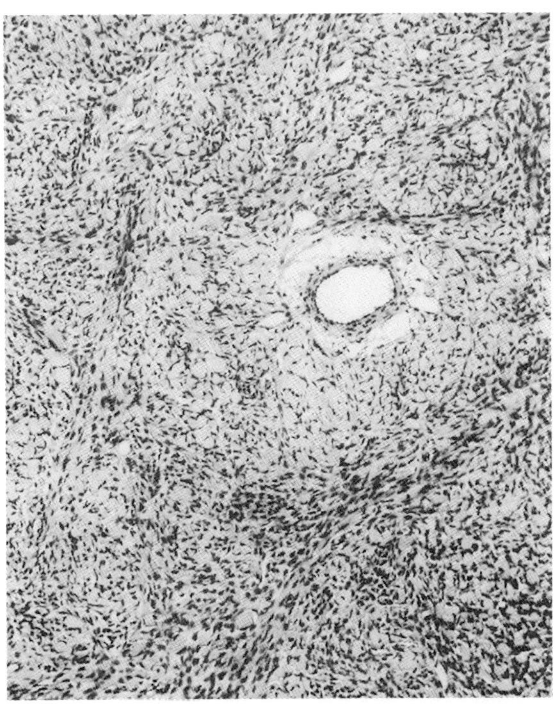

Fig. 34.5 Thecafibroma showing the dominant fibromatous pattern. Stromal hyalinization with perivascular accentuation is present. H + E ×75

sarcomas, are also best reinterpreted as fibrosarcomas in which intracytoplasmic lipid may be found (Prat & Scully 1981).

Macroscopic features

Thecafibromas are solid rubbery tumors showing gross features indistinguishable from those of ovarian fibromas.

Microscopic features

The basic architecture of these tumors is that of a cellular fibroma with variably interlaced bundles of thin spindle cells producing collagen, in some areas quite prominently (Fig. 34.5). Edema is present in half and is often pronounced. The collagenous component is usually fibrillary in appearance, but hyalinization is sometimes seen (Fig. 34.5). The latter is often accentuated perivascularly.

Theca cells are present in variable numbers, but are usually seen in small clusters, often observed only on close examination of several sections, or as larger but isolated fields in fibrous tumors (Fig. 34.6). By convention, luteinized theca cells are not seen, as their presence alters the diagnosis to luteinized thecoma.

SCLEROSING STROMAL TUMORS

Sclerosing stromal tumors were first differentiated from other sex cord–stromal tumors by Chalvardjian & Scully (1973) and later by Damjanov et al (1975), who convincingly demonstrated their origin from ovarian stroma but

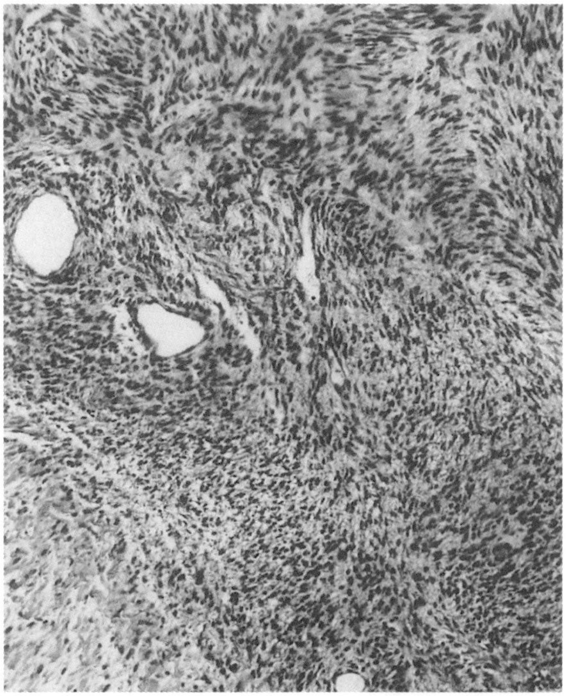

Fig. 34.6 Thecafibroma. An adjacent field from the same tumor as in Figure 34.5. Thecal cell differentiation can be seen in the upper portion of the figure. H + E ×75

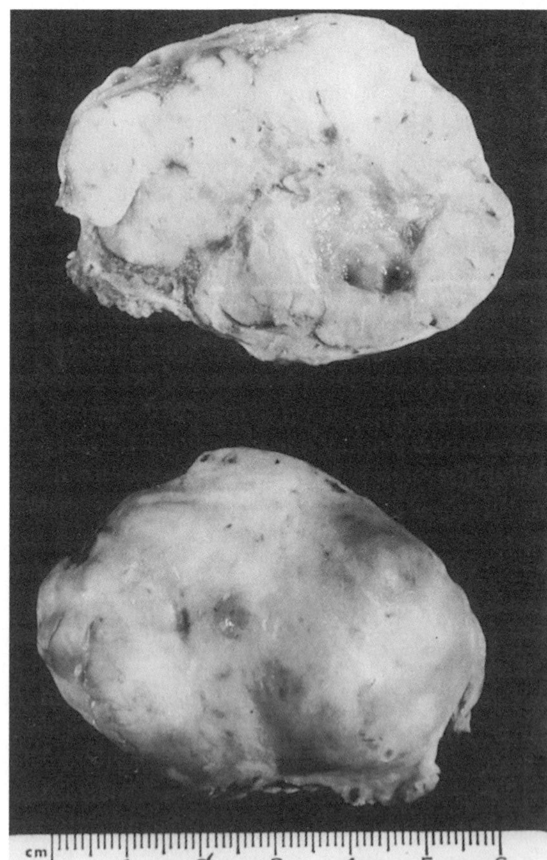

Fig. 34.7 Sclerosing stromal tumor. Cystic degeneration and vague pseudolobulation are apparent in the cut surface. (Reproduced, by permission, from Gee & Russell 1979)

justified their separation on the basis of an unusual clinical setting (80% occur below 30 years of age) and a surprising lack (given the histological features) of hormonally related abnormalities. It is suggested that they arise from perifollicular myoid stromal cells, a population of muscle-specific, actin-positive cells in the theca externa (Shaw et al 1992). We feel that the clinical distinction is perhaps not as clear-cut as initially indicated (Gee & Russell 1979, Quinn et al 1981, Ho Yuen et al 1982), but there is no doubting the validity of classifying sclerosing stromal tumors as a distinct and definable entity on histological and histogenetic grounds. A number of patients have presented with anovulation, due to the secretion of estrogen, progesterone, and testosterone (Ho Yuen et al 1982), or masculinization (Cashell & Cohen 1991), which resolved spontaneously after removal of the tumor. Ascites and abnormal uterine bleeding in elderly patients are rare presenting symptoms, and a solitary case has been documented in association with endometrial carcinoma (Katsube et al 1988). Rare lesions may be incidental findings at laparotomy for other ovarian neoplasms (Valente et al 1985), and a solitary case has been found in a patient with Gorlin's syndrome (Ismail & Walker 1990). All sclerosing stromal tumors have, to date, pursued a benign course. Local excision is adequate therapy.

Cytogenetic and molecular genetic studies

A solitary case of sclerosing stromal tumor exhibiting monosomy 16 and histological features suggesting 'low grade malignancy' has been reported (Lopes et al 1990).

Macroscopic features

They are unilateral, solid, distinctly lobulated, firm tumors, averaging 3–5 cm in diameter, which are sharply circumscribed from the adjacent ovarian parenchyma. The cut surface is pale, 'fleshy',

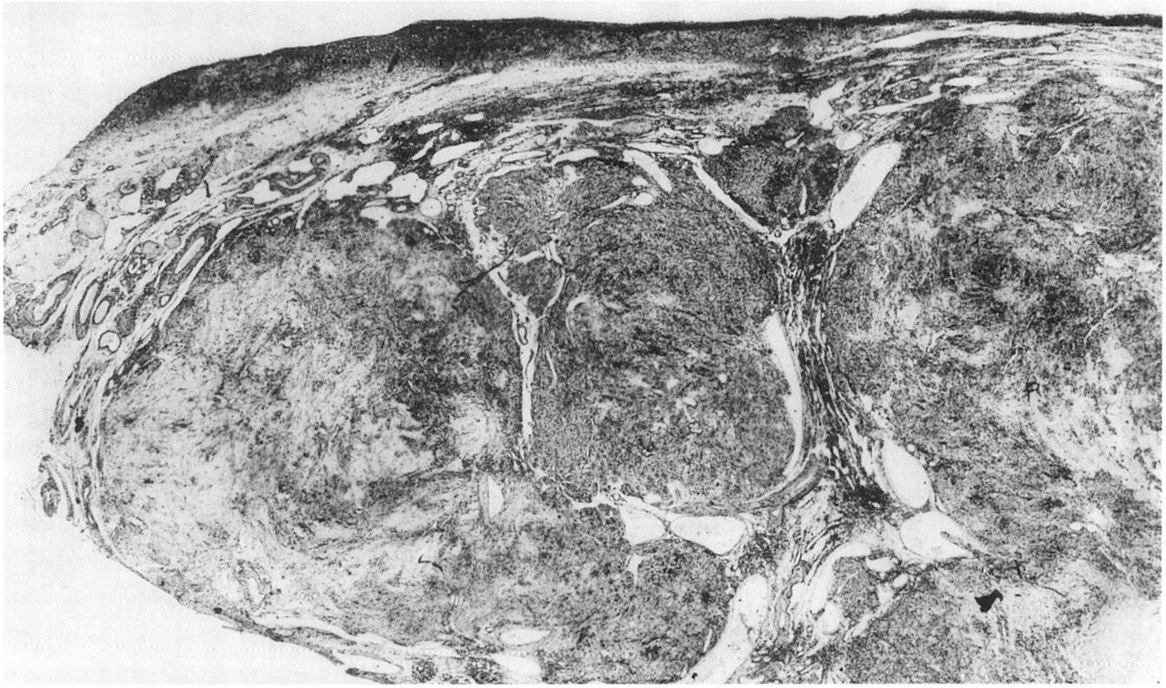

Fig. 34.8 Sclerosing stromal tumor. Pseudolobulation is marked with clear division into cellular and fibrous zones. H + E ×5. (Reproduced, by permission, from Gee & Russell 1979)

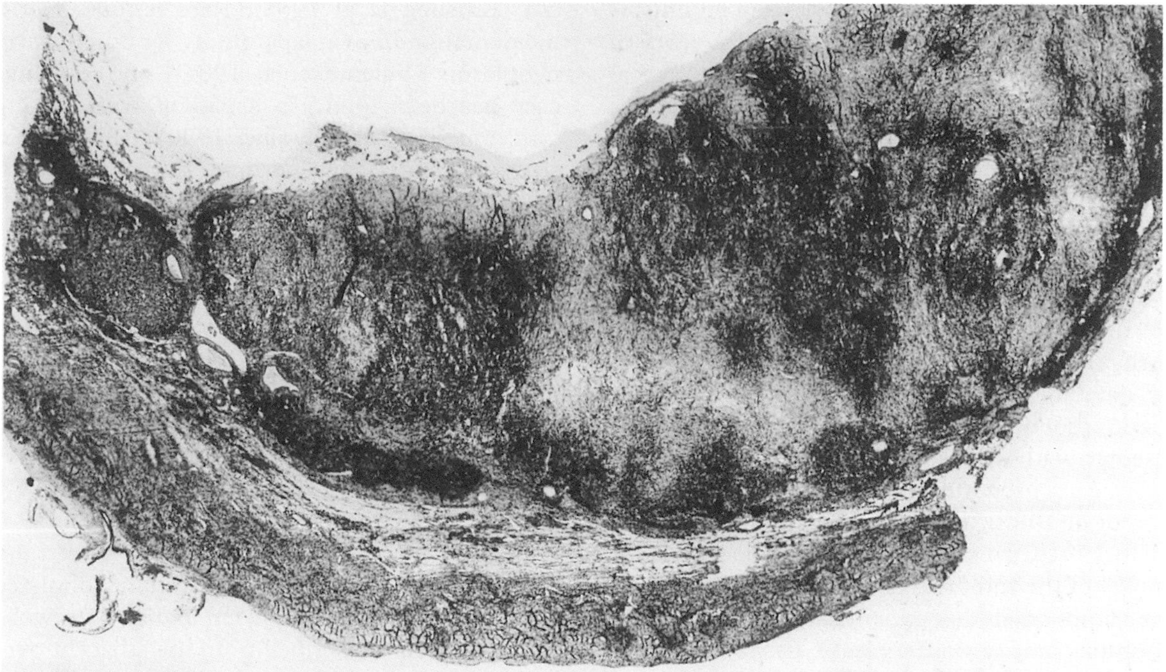

Fig. 34.9 Sclerosing stromal tumor. Section from lower right corner of the tumor shown in Figure 34.7. Cellular and stromal zones are apparent, as is cystic degeneration at top. H + E ×5. (Reproduced, by permission, from Gee & Russell 1979)

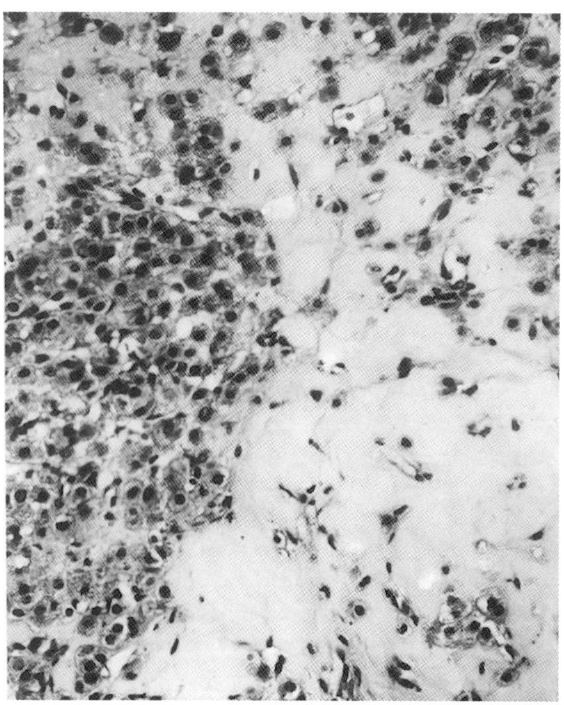

Fig. 34.10 Cellular area of a sclerosing stromal tumor showing encroachment of hyalinized connective tissue between nests and individual polyhedral lutein-like tumor cells. H + E ×150

and variegated, with focal yellowish areas and sometimes patchy cystic degeneration (Fig. 34.7). Rarely, they form a single large cyst (Chalvardjian & Scully 1973, Hsu et al 1983).

Microscopic features

They are characterized by a pseudolobular pattern of cellular zones separated by broad swathes of acellular sclerotic or edematous connective tissue (Figs 34.8, 34.9). Within the cellular nodules, fine strands of this sclerotic stroma also interdigitate randomly between individual cells and small groups of cells (Fig. 34.10). Numerous branching vascular spaces of various sizes are present in the cellular areas. The cells are typically rounded to polyhedral with vacuolated (Fig. 34.11) or eosinophilic cytoplasm (Fig. 34.10), or are

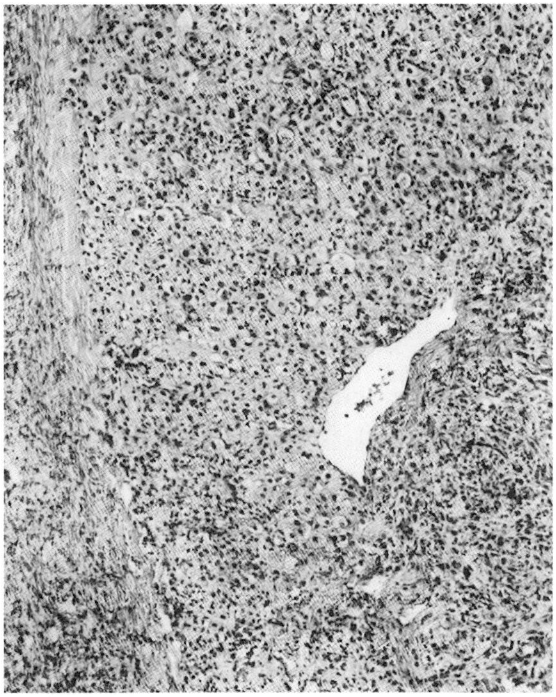

Fig. 34.11 Sharply circumscribed cellular area composed of large polyhedral cells with eosinophilic or vacuolated cytoplasm. H + E ×75

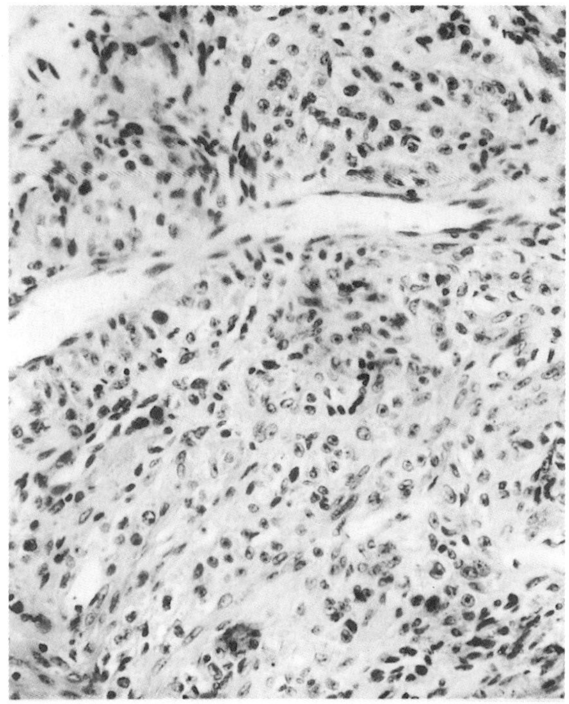

Fig. 34.12 Cellular area of sclerosing stromal tumor with an admixture of polyhedral and spindled tumor cells. Tumor cells have rather more vesicular nuclei and obvious nucleoli. H + E ×150. (Reproduced, by permission, from Gee & Russell 1979)

spindle-shaped fibroblasts (Fig. 34.12). It is this variety of cell types which is distinctive of sclerosing stromal tumors. Component cells have small, dark, nongrooved nuclei, sometimes with a prominent nucleolus. Mitoses are very infrequent. Individual cells are surrounded by a fine meshwork of reticulin fibers. Isolated spindle cells in the cellular areas stain immunohistochemically for desmin and smooth muscle actin (Saitoh et al 1989, Shaw et al 1992). Mast cells may be seen in the stroma (Ho Yuen et al 1982). Occasional vacuolated cells have crescentic nuclei resembling signet-ring cells and, when embedded in dense stroma, may suggest a diagnosis of Krukenberg tumor (Fig. 34.13). Ramzy (1976, 1977) and others (Suarez et al 1993) have described such tumors as 'signet-ring stromal tumors of the ovary'.

The sclerotic and edematous stromal changes are constant features of these tumors (Fig. 34.14). The edema is zonal, in contrast to that seen in massive ovarian edema (see Ch. 16) or an edematous fibroma (see Fig. 34.18). Dystrophic calcification is rarely present (Fig. 34.15).

Differential diagnosis

It is the histological pattern of stromal sclerosis (particularly the transition from dense acellular hyaline connective tissue, through broad bands of similar stroma to fine tentacles interposed between the theca-like cells in the cellular nodules) which allows differentiation of sclerosing stromal tumors from 'luteinized thecoma' (Table 34.1) and from other various forms of thecafibroma.

While the presence of 'signet-ring' cells in association with edematous stroma may raise the possibility of Krukenberg tumor, these latter malignant neoplasms occur typically in women in the sixth and seventh decades, are mostly bilateral, and do not have the pseudolobulated pattern of sclerosing stromal tumors on cut surfaces. Furthermore, signet-ring cells of Krukenberg tumors contain

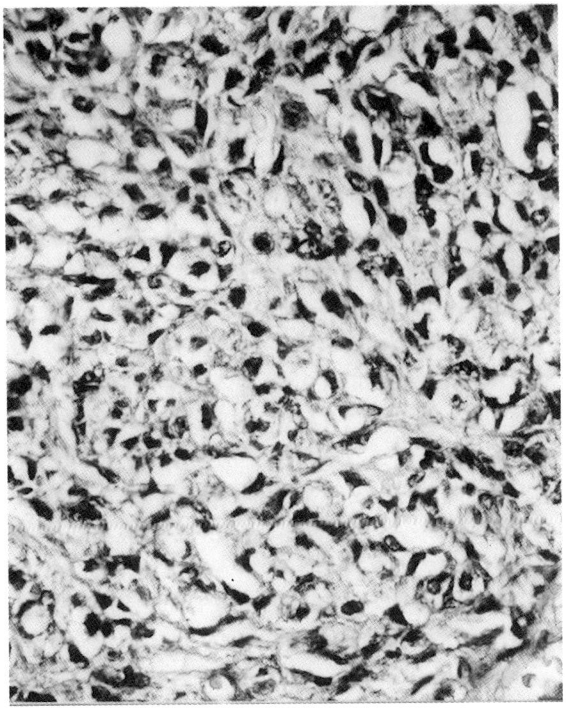

Fig. 34.13 Cellular area of a sclerosing stromal tumor in which many of the tumor cells resemble signet-ring cells. H + E ×300

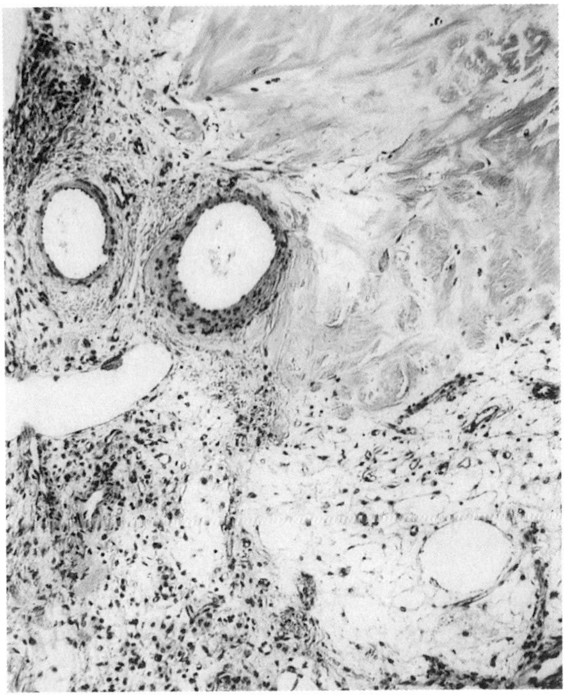

Fig. 34.14 Margin between cellular and acellular zones of a sclerosing stromal tumor, the latter showing both hyaline collagenous connective tissue and marked edema. H + E ×75

mucin rather than lipid and they may exhibit mitotic activity.

FIBROMAS

Fibromas are, by far, the most commonly encountered subtype of the sex cord–stromal tumors, accounting for almost two-thirds of neoplasms in this group. The mean age of incidence is about 48 years and 90% or more occur in women over the age of 30 years. Although some ovarian fibromas may be found in patients with clinical manifestations of hyperestrogenism, this appears not to be more common than expected by mere chance, and may in turn be consequent upon ovarian stromal hyperplasia, which sometimes accompanies these tumors. Of the general abdominal symptoms associated with ovarian fibromas, ascites is one of the commonest, being present in over 10% of cases (Samanth & Black 1970, Gee & Russell 1981, Sivanesaratnam et al 1990). Size of the tumor is an important (though not the sole) determinant of the presence of ascites (fibromas over 10 cm in diameter are associated with ascites in 40% of cases) and appears also to correlate with the presence of Meigs' syndrome (Meigs 1954).

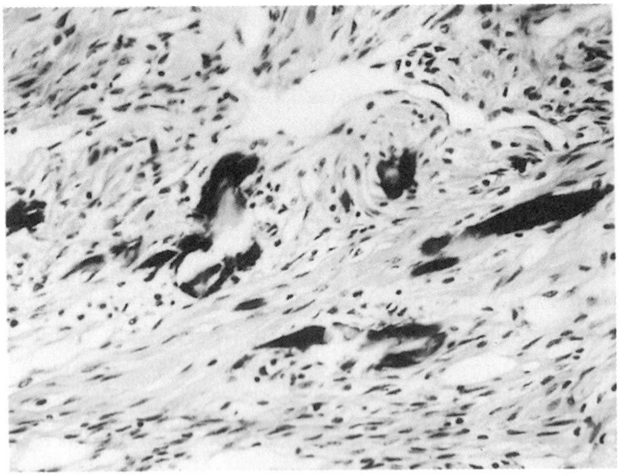

Fig. 34.15 Sclerosing stromal tumor. An area of spiculate dystrophic calcification. H + E ×125

Table 34.1 Differential diagnosis: sclerosing stromal tumor versus luteinized thecoma of ovary

Sclerosing stromal tumor	Luteinized thecoma
Clinical	
75% under age 30 years (mean age 25 years)	90% over age 30 years (mean age 48 years)
Mostly hormonally inactive	Typically oestrogenic
Histological	
Marked pseudolobulation	Uniform architecture
Prominent sclerosis around clusters and individual cells	No sclerosis
Prominent vasculature	Inapparent vasculature
No perivascular hyaline plaques	Perivascular hyaline plaques
Adjacent ovary normal	Adjacent ovary may be hyperplastic

The only clinical condition statistically associated with an increased risk of ovarian fibroma is the hereditary 'basal cell naevus syndrome' (Berlin et al 1966, Bosch-Banyeras et al 1989, Howell et al 1990), although a solitary example has been reported in a patient with Maffucci's syndrome (Christman & Ballon 1990).

Fibromatous tumors of the ovary are almost always benign, but occasional cellular and mitotically active tumors are seen, which behave in a locally aggressive fashion or pursue a frankly malignant course. Fibrosarcomas of the ovary are still classified amongst the nonspecific stromal tumors by some authors (Fox & Langley 1976), but are equally legitimately grouped with the sex cord–stromal neoplasms. A solitary example has been reported as part of the basal cell naevus syndrome (Kraemer et al 1984).

Cytogenetic and molecular genetic studies

Trisomy 12 has been identified cytogenetically in two benign ovarian fibromas (Pejovic et al 1990).

Macroscopic features

One-third of fibromas are 3 cm in diameter or smaller, but they commonly exceed 15 cm in maximum dimension. Fibromas are bilateral in only about 5% of cases. Larger tumors have a smooth or slightly bosselated serosal surface and are hard and rubbery in consistency. Smaller lesions may appear as polypoid nodules on the ovarian surface, or as poorly circumscribed nodules within the ovary. The cut surface is white and faintly whorled, often with areas of cystic degeneration (Fig. 34.16); in extreme cases, this gives rise to large ragged-walled cysts filled with protein-rich serous fluid. Other degenerative phenomena such as calcification are occasionally present, particularly in fibromas occurring as part of the basal cell naevus syndrome. The rare cellular fibromas and fibrosarcomas tend to be large and friable, attached to pelvic structures and to exhibit hemorrhage and necrosis.

Microscopic features

The basic architectural pattern of fibromas comprises variably cellular bundles and intersecting swathes of collagenous fibrous tissue, occasionally

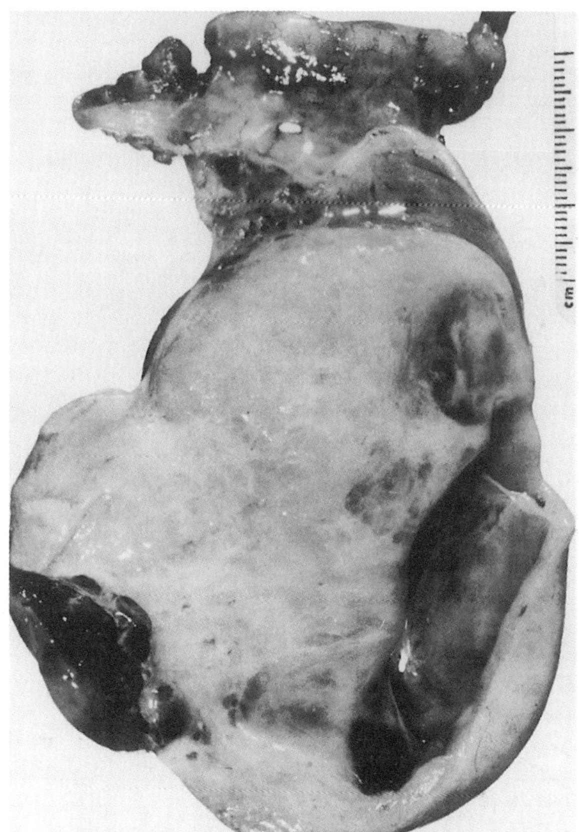

Fig. 34.16 Ovarian fibroma. Grey-white cut surface, featureless apart from areas of cystic degeneration.

A 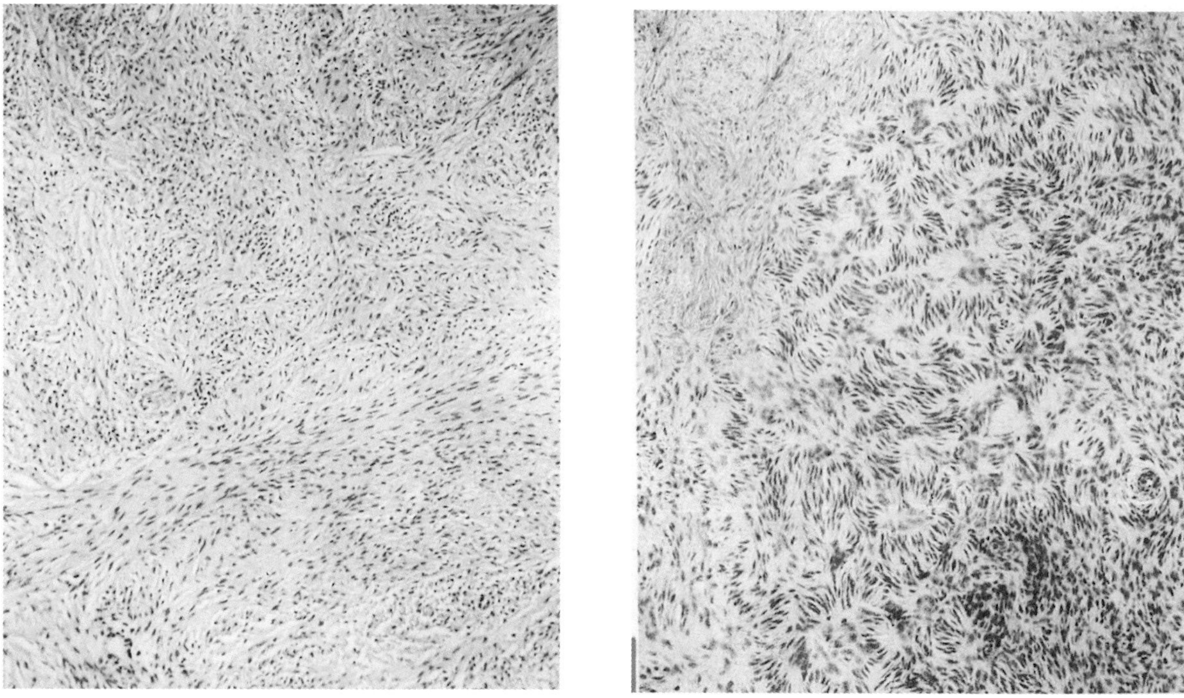 B

Fig. 34.17 Ovarian fibroma. (A) Typical lesion showing woven bundles of relatively hypocellular collagenous connective tissue. (B) Tightly whorled 'storiform' pattern of small spindled cells more closely resembling normal ovarian cortical stroma. H + E ×75

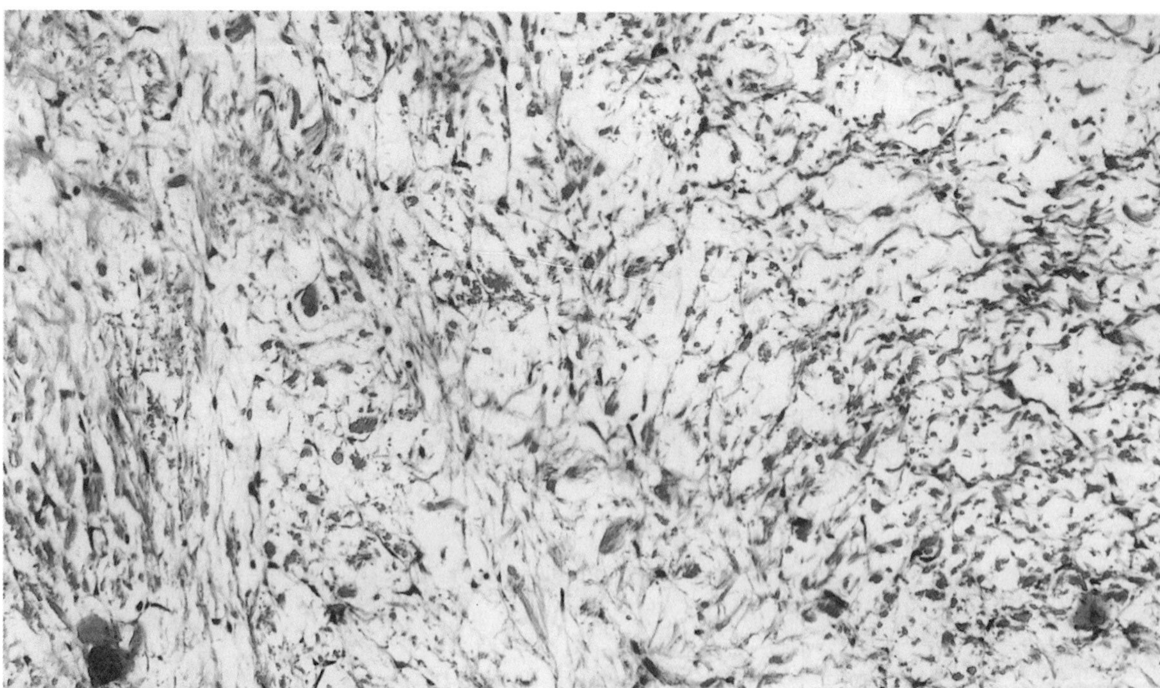

Fig. 34.18 Edematous ovarian fibroma. Acellular collagenous connective tissue dispersed by intercellular edema fluid. H + E ×125

with a striking storiform pattern resembling ovarian cortex (Fig. 34.17). The elongate fibroblastic tumor cells have spindle-shaped nuclei and may contain small amounts of lipid in their otherwise inapparent cytoplasm. The collagen is usually hyaline in appearance or somewhat wavy. The cellularity of the tumors varies inversely with both collagen production and stromal edema, both of which may be quite marked (Fig. 34.18). An interesting aside to this observation is the suggestion that pure ovarian myxomas (see Ch. 52) are variants of the tumors in the thecafibroma spectrum, on the basis of a continuum of edema–myxoid change seen in these groups of neoplasms (Costa et al 1993), a position with which we disagree. Edematous fibromas are more likely to be associated with ascites than are those with sclerotic or cellular stroma (Samanth & Black 1970). A sometimes difficult histological distinction is between an edematous ovarian fibroma and massive ovarian edema (Table 34.2). Dystrophic spic-

Table 34.2 Differential diagnosis: edematous ovarian fibroma versus massive edema of ovary

Edematous fibroma	Massive edema
Clinical	
90% over age 30 years (mean age 48 years)	Almost all below age 30 years (mean age 20 years)
Abdominal mass and ascites	Abdominal pain
Hormonally inactive	Often masculinizing (clinical background of polycystic ovary syndrome frequently present)
Histological	
Displaces ovarian structures	Incorporates ovarian structures
Focal/nodular lesion	Involves ovary uniformly
No luteinized cells	Luteinized stromal cells
Adjacent ovary may be hyperplastic	

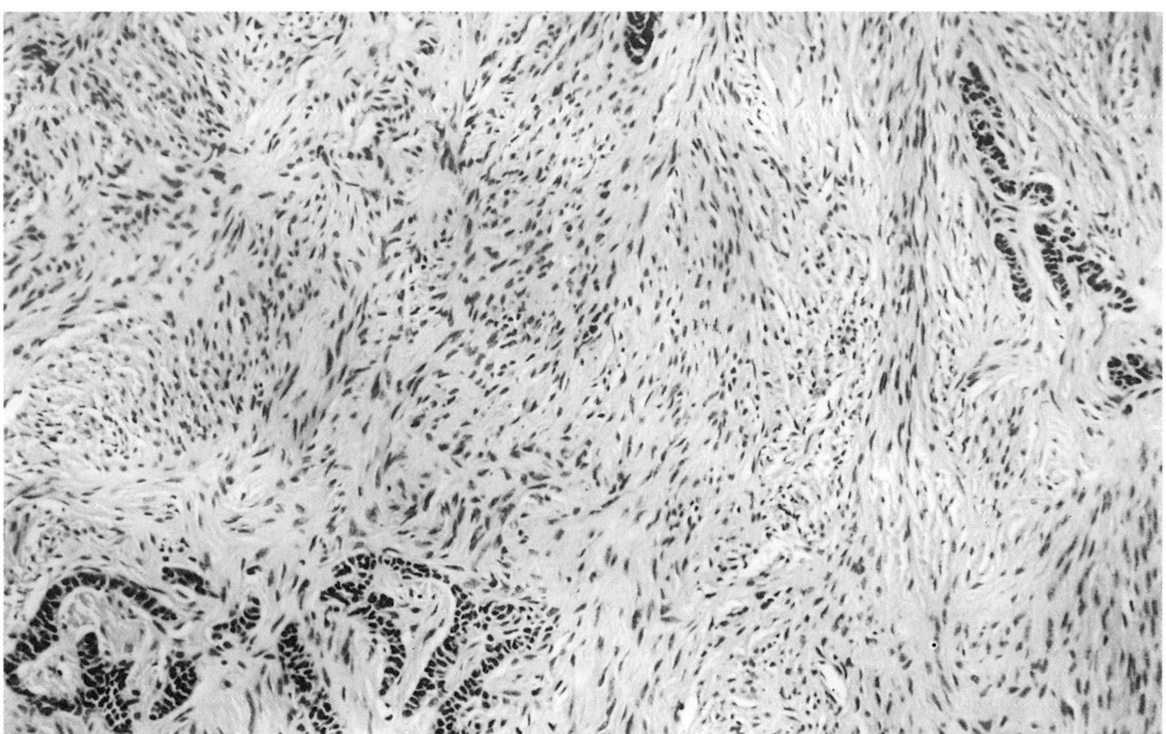

Fig. 34.19 Fibroma with minor sex cord element. Occasional small cords or tubule-like structures of ill defined sex cord cells set in an otherwise unremarkable fibroma. H + E ×125

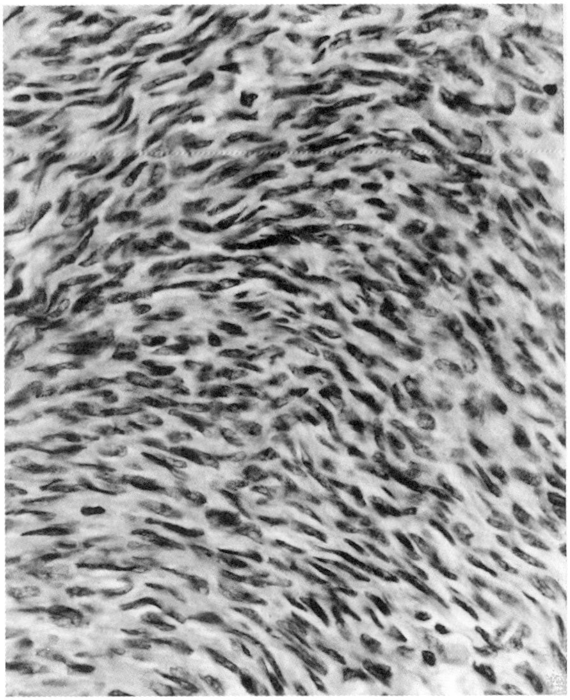

Fig. 34.20 Benign cellular fibroma. Woven bundles or fascicles of ill-defined spindle cells separated by wavy collagen. Cells have thin, elongate, tapered nuclei and few, if any, mitoses. H + E ×198

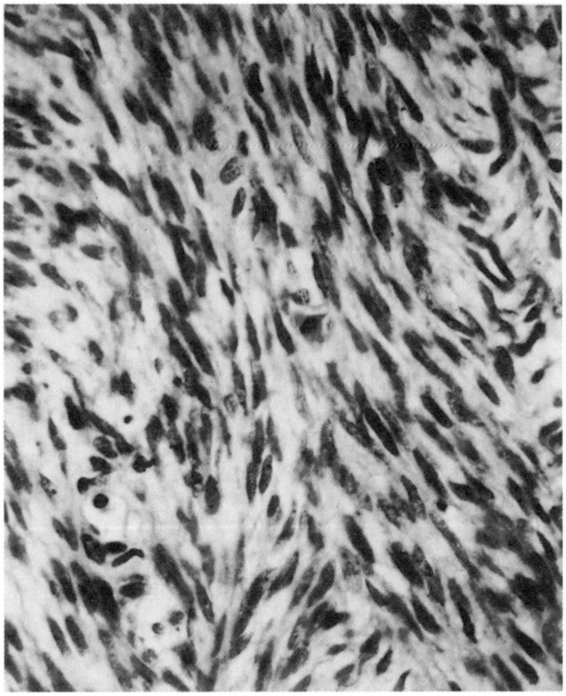

Fig. 34.21 Ovarian fibrosarcoma. Marked hypercellularity, nuclear hyperchromatism and mitotic activity (center) are characteristic of this lesion. H + E ×300

ulate calcification is occasionally seen, as are focal necrosis and hemorrhage. Nuclear atypia and mitoses are rarely seen. The uninvolved portion of the ovary and/or the contralateral ovary sometimes show nodular or diffuse stromal hyperplasia.

Rare, otherwise typical, fibromas contain sparse, poorly formed tubular structures composed of Sertoli-like cells or nests of cells resembling granulosa cells. These have been referred to as 'fibromas with minor sex cord elements' (Young & Scully 1983a) and, by definition, the sex cord elements must amount to less than 10% of the tumor in the tissue reviewed (Fig. 34.19). Fibromas which exhibit aggregates of lipid-laden, lutein-like cells are termed 'luteinized thecomas'.

Occasional fibromatous tumors are hypercellular and/or show appreciable mitotic activity. Criteria have been suggested to separate out those tumors designated as cellular fibromas and fibrosarcomas. Cellular fibromas contain 1–3 mitoses per 10HPF (Fig. 34.20) and usually behave in a benign fashion, although they may occasionally recur locally (Lyday 1952, Prat & Scully 1981). Fibrosarcomas are defined as having a mitotic rate of 4/10HPF or more (Fig. 34.21), and these tumors almost always pursue a frankly malignant course (Miles et al 1985). Intracytoplasmic lipid may be demonstrated by fat stains, particularly in the cellular fibromas, and such examples may be an explanation for the rarely reported malignant thecomas and fibrothecomas. With regard to highly cellular, mitotically active, spindle cell tumors of the ovary, an alternative way of thinking of them is as *ovarian stromal sarcomas* (Fig. 34.22). Arbitrary differentiation from fibrosarcomas, more apparent than real, is suggested only by a slight storiform pattern of tumor cells and blunt-ended elongate or oval nuclei. Discrimination from poorly differentiated sex cord–stromal tumors, particularly Sertoli–Leydig cell tumors, is on the basis of total absence of even poorly formed epithelial-like structures or identifiable intracytoplasmic lipid.

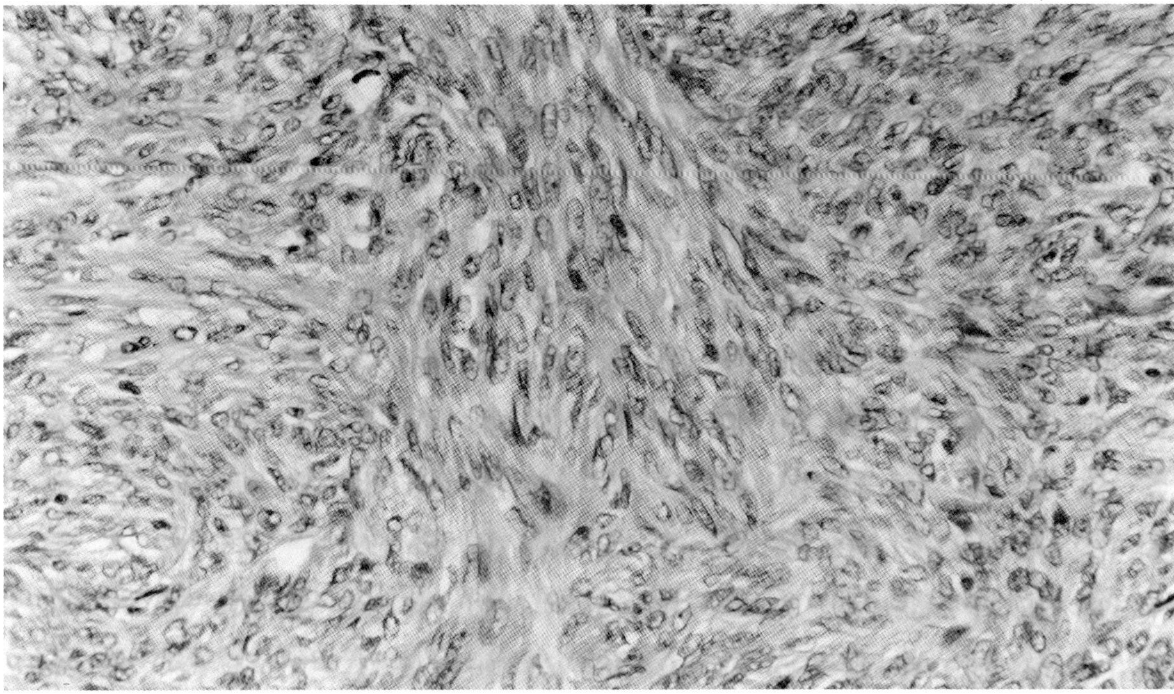

A

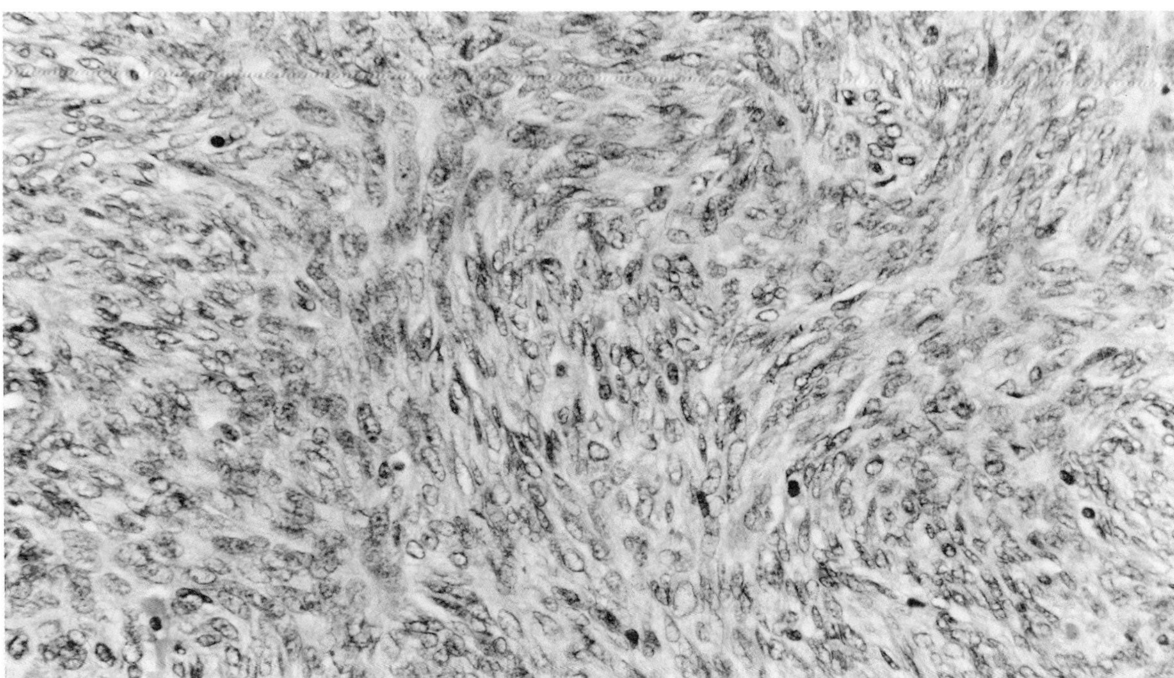

B

Fig. 34.22 'Ovarian stromal sarcoma'. An alternative concept for the high grade malignant end of the 'fibroma' spectrum. Tumor cells have elongate but blunt-ended or oval nuclei and an ill-defined storiform architectural pattern. (A) Fibrous area. H + E ×165. (B) Densely hypercellular area. H + E ×165

REFERENCES

Barrenetxea G, Schneider J, Centeno M M et al 1990 Pure theca cell tumors. A clinicopathologic study of 29 cases. European Journal of Gynaecological Oncology 11: 429–432

Berlin N I, Van Scott E J, Clendenning W E et al 1966 Basal cell nevus syndrome. Annals of Internal Medicine 64: 403–422

Bosch-Banyeras J M, Lucaya X, Bernet M et al 1989 Calcified ovarian fibromas in prepubertal girls. European Journal of Pediatrics 148: 749–750

Cashell A W, Cohen M L 1991 Masculinizing sclerosing stromal tumor of the ovary during pregnancy. Gynecologic Oncology 43: 281–285

Chalvardjian A, Scully R E 1973 Sclerosing stromal tumors of the ovary. Cancer 31: 664–670

Christman J E, Ballon S C 1990 Ovarian fibrosarcoma associated with Maffucci's syndrome. Gynecologic Oncology 37: 290–291

Costa M J, Morris R, de Rose P B, Cohen C 1993 Histologic and immunohistochemical evidence for considering ovarian myxoma as a variant of the thecoma-fibroma group of ovarian tumors. Archives of Pathology and Laboratory Medicine 117: 802–808

Damjanov I, Drobnjak P, Grizelj V, Longhino N 1975 Sclerosing stromal tumors of the ovary. Obstetrics and Gynecology 45: 675–679

Evans A T, Gaffey T A, Malkasian G D Jr, Annegers J F 1980 Clinicopathologic review of 118 granulosa and 82 theca cell tumors. Obstetrics and Gynecology 55: 231–238

Faber H K 1962 Meigs' syndrome with thecoma of both ovaries in a 4 year old girl. Journal of Pediatrics 61: 769–773

Fox H, Langley F A 1976 Tumours of the ovary. Heinemann, London, p 129–292

Gee D C, Russell P 1979 Sclerosing stromal tumors of the ovary. Histopathology 3: 367–376

Gee D C, Russell P 1981 The pathological assessment of ovarian neoplasms. IV: The sex cord–stromal tumors. Pathology 13: 235–255

Givens J R, Andersen R N, Wiser W L, Donelson A J, Coleman S A 1975 A testosterone-secreting gonadotropin-responsive, pure thecoma and polycystic ovarian disease. Journal of Clinical Endocrinology and Metabolism 41: 845–853

Halalau F L, Laky D, Ardeleanu C, Alexa-Dogaru M 1982 Malignant fibrothecoma: pathomorphological comments. Morphology and Embryology 28: 173–175

Hamdoun L, Mouelhi C, Zhioua F, Jedoui A, Meriah S, Houet S 1993 Syndrome de Maffucci et tumeur ovarienne. Bulletin du Cancer (Paris) 80: 816–819

Howell C G Jr, Rogers D A, Gable D S, Falls G D 1990 Bilateral ovarian fibromas in children. Journal of Pediatric Surgery 25: 690–691

Ho Yuen B, Robertson I, Clement P B, Mincey E K 1982 Sclerosing stromal tumor of the ovary. Obstetrics and Gynecology 60: 252–256

Hsu C, Ma L, Mak L 1983 Sclerosing stromal tumor of the ovary: case report and review of the literature. International Journal of Gynecological Pathology 2: 192–200

Hughesdon P E 1966 Ovarian lipoid and theca cell tumors: their origins and interrelations. Obstetrical and Gynecological Survey 21: 245–288

Hughesdon P E 1983 Lipid cell thecomas of the ovary. Histopathology 7: 681–692

Ismail S M, Walker S M 1990 Bilateral virilizing sclerosing stromal tumors of the ovary in a pregnant woman with Gorlin's syndrome: implications for pathogenesis of ovarian stromal neoplasms. Histopathology 17: 159–163

Karck U, Kommoss F, Henne K, Runge M, Pfleiderer A 1991 Rezidivierender Thekazell-Tumor. Geburtshilfe und Frauenheilkind 51: 577–579

Katsube Y, Iwaoki Y, Silverberg S G, Fujiwara A 1988 Sclerosing stromal tumor of the ovary associated with endometrial adenocarcinoma. A case report. Gynecologic Oncology 29: 392–398

Kraemar B B, Silva E G, Sneige N 1984 Fibrosarcoma of ovary. A new component in the nevoid basal-cell carcinoma syndrome. American Journal of Surgical Pathology 8: 231–236

Longscope C, Robboy S J 1980 Case records of the Massachussetts General Hospital (case 10–1980). New England Journal of Medicine 302: 621–626

Lopes J M, Seruca R, Hall A P, Branco P, Castedo S M 1990 Cytogenetic study of a sclerosing stromal tumor of the ovary. Cancer Genetics and Cytogenetics 49: 103–106

Lyday R O 1952 Fibroma of the ovary with abdominal implants. American Journal of Surgery 84: 737–738

Meigs J V 1954 Fibroma of the ovary with ascites and hydrothorax. Meigs' syndrome. American Journal of Obstetrics and Gynecology 67: 962–987

Miles P A, Kiley K C, Mena H 1985 Giant fibrosarcoma of the ovary. International Journal of Gynecological Pathology 4: 83–87

Mrozek K, Nedoszytko B, Babinska M et al 1990 Trisomy of chromosome 12 in a case of thecoma of the ovary. Gynecologic Oncology 36: 413–416

Mrozek K, Limon J, Debniak J, Emerich J 1992 Trisomy 12 and 4 in a thecoma of the ovary. Gynecologic Oncology 45: 66–68

Novak E R, Woodruff J D 1979 Gynecologic and obstetric pathology, 8th edn. W B Saunders, Philadelphia, p 512

Pejovic T, Heim S, Mandahl N et al 1990 Trisomy 12 is a consistent chromosomal aberration in benign ovarian tumors. Genes Chromosomes and Cancer 2: 48–52

Prat J, Scully R E 1981 Cellular fibromas and fibrosarcomas of the ovary: a comparative clinicopathologic analysis of seventeen cases. Cancer 47: 2663–2670

Quinn M A, Östör A A, Fortune D 1981 Sclerosing stromal tumor. Case report with endocrine studies. British Journal of Obstetrics and Gynaecology 3: 155–159

Ramzy I 1976 Signet-ring stromal tumor of the ovary: histochemical light and electronmicroscopic study. Cancer 38: 166–172

Ramzy I 1977 Signet-ring stromal tumor of the ovary: cytologic appearances of fine needle aspiration biopsy. Acta Cytologica 21: 14–17

Roth L M, Sternberg W H 1983 Partly luteinized theca cell tumor of the ovary. Cancer 51: 1697–1704

Saitoh A, Tsutsumi Y, Osamura R Y, Watanabe K 1989 Sclerosing stromal tumor of the ovary. Immunohistochemical and electron-microscopic demonstration of smooth-muscle differentiation. Archives of Pathology and Laboratory Medicine 113: 372–376

Samanth K K, Black W C 1970 Benign ovarian stromal

tumors associated with free peritoneal fluid. American Journal of Obstetrics and Gynecology 107: 538–545

Scully R E 1964 Stromal luteoma of the ovary. A distinctive type of lipid-cell tumor. Cancer 17: 769–778

Scully R E 1979 Tumors of the ovary and maldeveloped gonads. AFIP fascicle 16, 2nd series. Armed Forces Institute of Pathology, Washington, DC, p 174–189

Scully R E 1982 Sex cord–stromal tumors. In: Blaustein A (ed) Pathology of the female genital tract, 2nd edn. Springer-Verlag, New York, p 587–601

Serov S F, Scully R E, Sobin L H 1973 Histological typing of ovarian tumours. International histological classification of tumors No. 9. World Health Organization, Geneva, p 17–54

Shaw J A, Dabbs D J, Geisinger K R 1992 Sclerosing stromal tumor of the ovary: an ultrastructural and immunohistochemical analysis with histogenetic considerations. Ultrastructural Pathology 16: 363–377

Sivanesaratnam V, Dutta R, Jayalakshmi P 1990 Ovarian fibroma – clinical and histopathological characteristics. International Journal of Gynaecology and Obstetrics 33: 243–247

Sternberg W H, Dhurandhar H M 1977 Functional ovarian tumors of stromal and sex cord origin. Human Pathology 8: 565–582

Sternberg W H, Roth L M 1973 Ovarian stromal tumors containing Leydig cells. I: Stromal–Leydig cell tumor and non-neoplastic transformation of ovarian stroma. Cancer 32: 940–951

Suarez A, Palacios J, Burgos E, Gamallo C 1993 Signet-ring stromal tumor of the ovary: a histochemical, immunohistochemical and ultrastructural study. Virchows Archiv [A] Pathological Anatomy and Histopathology 422: 333–336

Valente P T, Carr R F, Hanjani P 1985 Sclerosing stromal tumor and bilateral teratomas: an unusual association. Gynecologic Oncology 21: 252–259

Waxman M, Vuletin J C, Ureuyo R, Belling C G 1979 Ovarian low-grade stromal sarcoma with thecomatous features. A critical re-appraisal of the so-called 'malignant thecoma'. Cancer 44: 2206–2217

Young R H, Scully R E 1983a Ovarian stromal tumors with minor sex cord elements: a report of seven cases. International Journal of Gynecological Pathology 2: 227–234

Young R H, Scully R E 1982 Ovarian sex cord–stromal tumors: recent progress. International Journal of Gynaecological Pathology 1: 101–123

Young R H, Scully R E 1983b Ovarian sex cord–stromal tumors with bizarre nuclei: a clinicopathologic analysis of 17 cases. International Journal of Gynecological Pathology 1: 325–335

Young R H, Clement P B, Scully R E 1988 Calcified thecomas in young women. A report of four cases. International Journal of Gynecological Pathology 7: 343–350

Zhang J, Young R H, Arseneau J, Scully R E 1982 Ovarian stromal tumors containing lutein or Leydig cells (luteinised thecoma and stromal Leydig cell tumor). A clinicopathologic analysis of 50 cases. International Journal of Gynecological Pathology 1: 270–285

35

Androblastomas

P. Russell   A. Farnsworth

Androblastomas are characterized by the presence of Sertoli cells, Leydig cells, and/or fibroblastic cells in differing relative proportions and at various levels of differentiation. Synonyms are arrhenoblastoma and Sertoli–Leydig cell tumor, the latter term holding the imprimatur of the World Health Organization (Serov et al 1973). Some semantic argument revolves around whether tumor terminology should carry histogenetic and/or clinical connotations, or should be purely histological. We see 'androblastoma' as neutral in this regard and prefer it as the generic term for these tumors, which show a wide range of differentiation, provided that individual variants are characterized strictly according to morphological features. It is therefore an arbitrary decision to discuss Leydig cell tumors in this chapter, separately from other 'steroid cell' tumors with which they share many common features, particularly as classification is based principally on the finding of Reinke's crystals, which are ephemeral structures at best and are seen in typical testicular Leydig cell tumors in only 40% of cases (see below).

They are extremely uncommon neoplasms, accounting for only about 1% of sex cord–stromal tumors (see Ch. 32) and, therefore, between 0.1% and 0.5% of all primary ovarian neoplasms. They are bilateral in less than 2%, and confined to the ovaries in over 95% of cases (Young & Scully 1985). The majority (about two-thirds) of the reported cases are moderately or poorly differentiated combined Sertoli–Leydig cell tumors.

As a group, androblastomas occur predominantly in the second and third decades (mean age about 25 years) (Roth et al 1981, Zaloudek & Norris 1984, Young & Scully 1985), rarely before puberty (Kawagoe & Yoshiro 1989), and fewer than 10% after the menopause (Hansen & Sorensen 1993). Individual subtypes deviate a little from this general pattern; pure Sertoli cell tumors and, to a lesser extent, pure Leydig cell tumors, have bimodal age distributions with peaks of incidence in the third and seventh decades. In 40–50% of patients, the presenting symptoms relate to clinical signs of androgenic activity, while most of the remainder are nonspecific abdominal symptoms referable to the physical presence of a tumor mass. Occasionally, androblastomas are incidental findings at hysterectomy for unrelated pathology (Fig. 35.1). Pure, well differentiated, Sertoli cell tumors are mostly estrogenic (Tavassoli & Norris 1980, Young & Scully 1984a, Young 1993), and in prepubertal girls they may even be associated with isosexual precocious pseudopuberty (Ehrlich et al 1963) or Peutz–Jeghers syndrome (Young & Scully 1984a). Well differentiated Sertoli–Leydig cell tumors are often endocrinologically inactive, but may be androgenic or sometimes feminizing. By contrast, pure Leydig cell tumors and poorly differentiated Sertoli–Leydig cell tumors may also be feminizing (Ichinohasama et al 1989), but at least half are clinically androgenic. Patients complain of progressive oligomenorrhea and amenorrhea, breast atrophy, hirsutism, male pattern baldness, deepening of the voice, changes in body musculature, and clitoromegaly. Virilizing symptoms may rarely persist after removal of the tumor (Paraskevas & Scully 1989). A familial incidence has been rarely observed for moderately and poorly differentiated Sertoli–Leydig cell tumors (Murad et al 1973), and a solitary example has been reported in a 15-year-old girl with Ollier's disease (Weyl Ben Arush & Oslander 1991), an association more

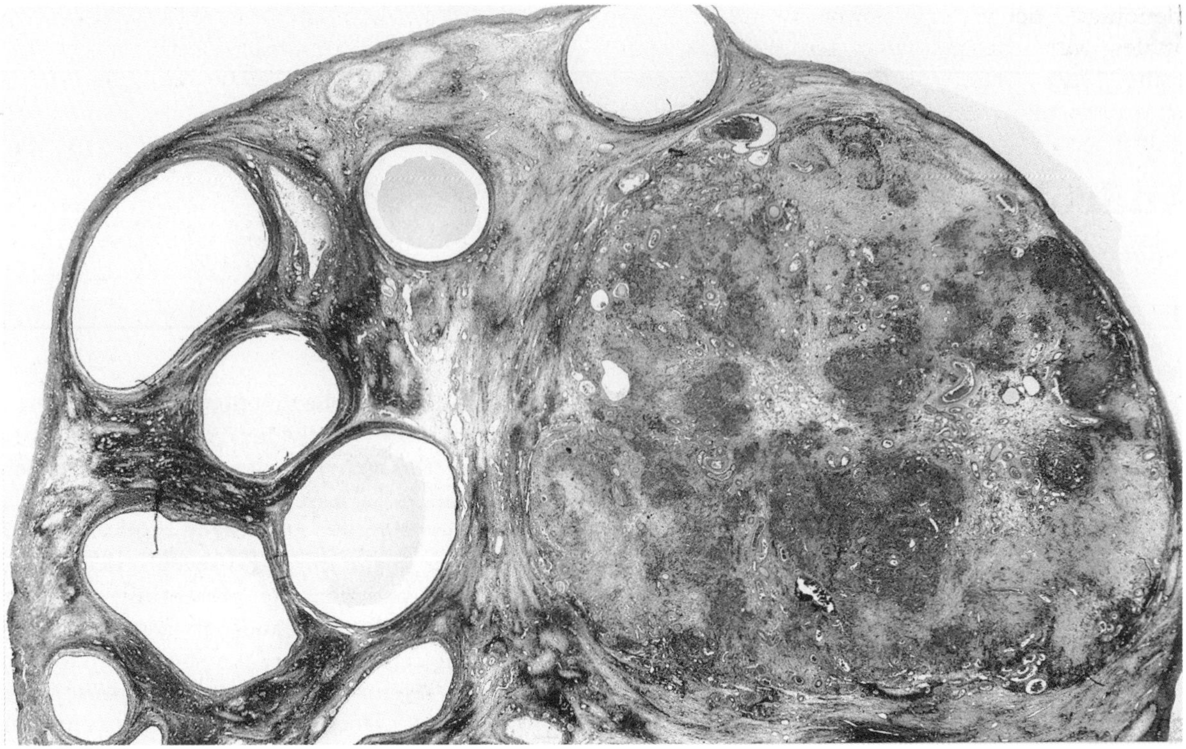

Fig. 35.1 A small moderately differentiated Sertoli–Leydig cell tumor found incidentally in the left ovary of a patient undergoing hysterectomy for unrelated pathology. H + E ×4

typical of juvenile granulosa tumor (see Ch. 33). Estrogenic manifestations may be explained either by direct estrogen production by the tumor (Gabrilove et al 1975, Costa et al 1994) or, more probably, by peripheral conversion to estrogens of androgenic secretions from the tumor (MacDonald et al 1967). Sertoli–Leydig cell tumors may be associated with raised serum levels of α-fetoprotein, but rarely to the levels seen with yolk sac tumors. Immunohistochemical studies indicate that the origin of this oncoprotein is in the Leydig cells, the Sertoli cells, and/or heterologous hepatocytes (Chadha et al 1987, Gagnon et al 1989, Motoyama et al 1989, Larsen et al 1992).

It is relevant to note that androblastomas presenting during pregnancy are much less likely to exhibit androgenic manifestations than are equivalent tumors occurring in nonpregnant women, presumably due to the ability of the placenta to aromatize androgens into estrogens (Hensleigh et al 1975), and that virilization during pregnancy, although occasionally due to such a tumor (Barkan et al 1984), is much more likely to be due to primary or secondary epithelial tumors with functioning stroma, steroid cell tumors (see Ch. 39), pregnancy luteomas (see Ch. 10), and hyperreactio luteinalis (see Ch. 10).

WELL DIFFERENTIATED SERTOLI CELL TUMORS

Well differentiated ovarian Sertoli cell tumors ('tubular androblastomas') are histologically indistinguishable from their homologs within the testis (Teilum 1976). They are mostly estrogenic, as are testicular Sertoli cell tumors (irrespective of the presence or absence of intracellular lipid storage; see below). They are associated unduly frequently with anomalies of the internal genitalia in women. An isochromosome 1q has been identified as a sole karyotypic anomaly in a Sertoli cell tumor (Pejovic et al 1993). Sertoli cell congeries and 'adenomas' occur commonly in phenotypic females with the testicular feminization syndrome. These data, taken in concert, suggest that a proportion of Sertoli cell tumors (but certainly not all) are hamartomas rather than true neoplasms (Fox & Langley 1976). In any event, well differentiated Sertoli cell tumors appear to be invariably benign, and simple oophorectomy is curative.

Macroscopic features

Sertoli cell tumors vary markedly in size, but the majority are smaller than 10 cm in diameter. They tend to be solid, unilateral, firm, encapsulated, and lobulated masses, typically yellow or tan in color. Small cystic areas are infrequently present.

Microscopic features

Well differentiated Sertoli cell tumors are composed of lobules of uniform, tortuous, solid, or hollow tubules, filled with or lined by one or more layers of cuboidal to columnar benign-appearing cells with eosinophilic or vacuolated cytoplasm and dark, oval, basal nuclei (Fig. 35.2A). Mitoses are rarely seen, and nucleoli are not prominent. In some tumors, these Sertoli cells have well defined cell borders and apical surfaces. More frequently, however, the apical margins of the cells are quite indistinct and the lateral cell boundaries less well defined. The Sertoli cells usually contain lipid droplets but, in some tumors they are grossly vacuolated (Fig. 35.2B) and distended by fat, giving rise to the so-called 'Sertoli cell tumor with lipid storage' or 'lipid-rich Sertoli cell tumor'. The tubules in this type of tumor tend to be solid, and larger discrete masses or nodules of the polyhedral vacuolated cells are also noted. Luminal mucin (stained by mucicarmine) is occasionally present. Ferry et al (1994) have reported three cases of Sertoli cell tumor with abundant eosinophilic cytoplasm.

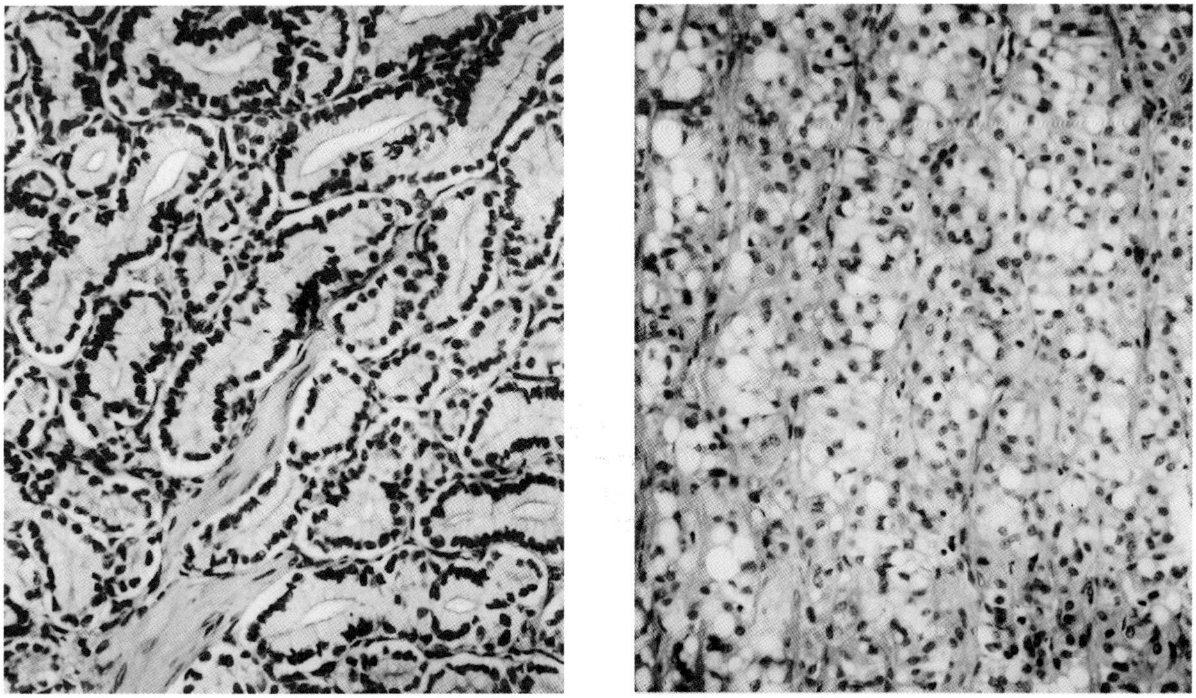

A B

Fig. 35.2 Well differentiated Sertoli cell tumor (tubular androblastoma). (a) With characteristic hollow tubules lined by tall columnar cells with basal nuclei and clear or vacuolated cytoplasm. H + E ×150. (b) With lipid storage in the tumor cells, obscuring to some extent the tubular architecture. H + E ×150

Intervening stroma is usually represented by a few bands of acellular connective tissue, which is either edematous or hyalinized and contains (by definition) few or no Leydig cells. Less commonly, the hyalinized stroma is more prominent, and, rarely, the stroma is the dominant component with the tumors then resembling ovarian fibromas with only a minor tubular element. Such lesions have been reclassified as 'fibromas with minor sex cord elements' (see Ch. 34). Pure Sertoli cell tumors with marked nuclear atypia and mitotic activity have been reported as Sertoli cell carcinomas (see below).

WELL DIFFERENTIATED SERTOLI–LEYDIG CELL TUMORS

These very uncommon tumors, occurring in women with a mean age in the mid-thirties, differ from the well differentiated Sertoli cell tumors described above only in the presence of an obvious Leydig cell component. In one large series (Young & Scully 1985), they account for 11% of all Sertoli–Leydig cell tumors. As with pure Sertoli cell tumors, there is a statistical association with congenital anomalies of the internal genitalia and the testicular feminization syndrome (Fox & Langley 1976). With the exception of a single case which recurred after 12 years (Dockerty & MacCarty 1939), well differentiated Sertoli–Leydig cell tumors reported in the literature have been benign.

Macroscopic features

Well differentiated Sertoli–Leydig cell tumors are almost always unilateral, and appear as well circumscribed, solitary, firm tumor masses in the ovary. They range in size up to 20 cm in diameter, with average tumors measuring 5–6 cm across. In occasional small lesions, their hilar location is still apparent. The cut surface is yellow and characteristically lobulated. Small cysts may be present and there is often focal hemorrhage.

Microscopic features

Histologically, they are formed of uniform solid or hollow tubular structures lined by Sertoli-type cells (Fig. 35.3) and showing the features outlined in the previous section. Tubules may contain eosinophilic secretion, but are more frequently empty. The intervening stroma contains a variable number of Leydig cells. These tend to be packed in ribbons or nests between the Sertoli cell tubules, but may form more solid sheets in some tumors (Fig. 35.3A). The cytological details of these cells are given in the next section dealing with pure Leydig cell tumors. Mitoses are rare in these tumors. An interesting histological feature of some tumors in this group is the coarse architectural arrangement into cellular and acellular areas, reminiscent of the nodular or pseudolobular pattern of sclerosing stromal tumors (Fig. 35.4). The acellular areas have the same dense hyaline and collagenous tissue background, with dilated sinusoidal vessels also prominent (Gee & Russell 1981). An unusual variant we have observed is a large unilocular cyst lined by fibrous connective tissue, in which are scattered tubules and cystic spaces lined by typical Sertoli cells as well as clusters of Leydig-like cells (Fig. 35.5).

The adjacent ovarian parenchyma is usually unremarkable, although both stromal hyperplasia and polycystic change have been noted.

LEYDIG (HILUS) CELL TUMORS

Leydig cell neoplasms of the ovary are formed exclusively of large eosinophilic cells similar to those usually present in the ovarian hilus. They are most uncommon lesions, and are thought to derive directly from hilus cells, or as one-sided development of a Sertoli–Leydig cell tumor (Scully 1979), or rarely from the ovarian stromal cells (Roth & Sternberg 1973, Paoletti et al 1987). For all practical purposes they should be regarded as benign, although rare cases of metastasizing Leydig cell tumor have been reported (Echt & Hadd 1968). Most are masculinizing, but about 10–20% are associated with some degree of estrogenic effect, most readily recognized in the endometrium (hyperplasia or carcinoma). The very rare 'stromal Leydig cell tumors' are either estrogenic or androgenic, occurring in approximately equal numbers.

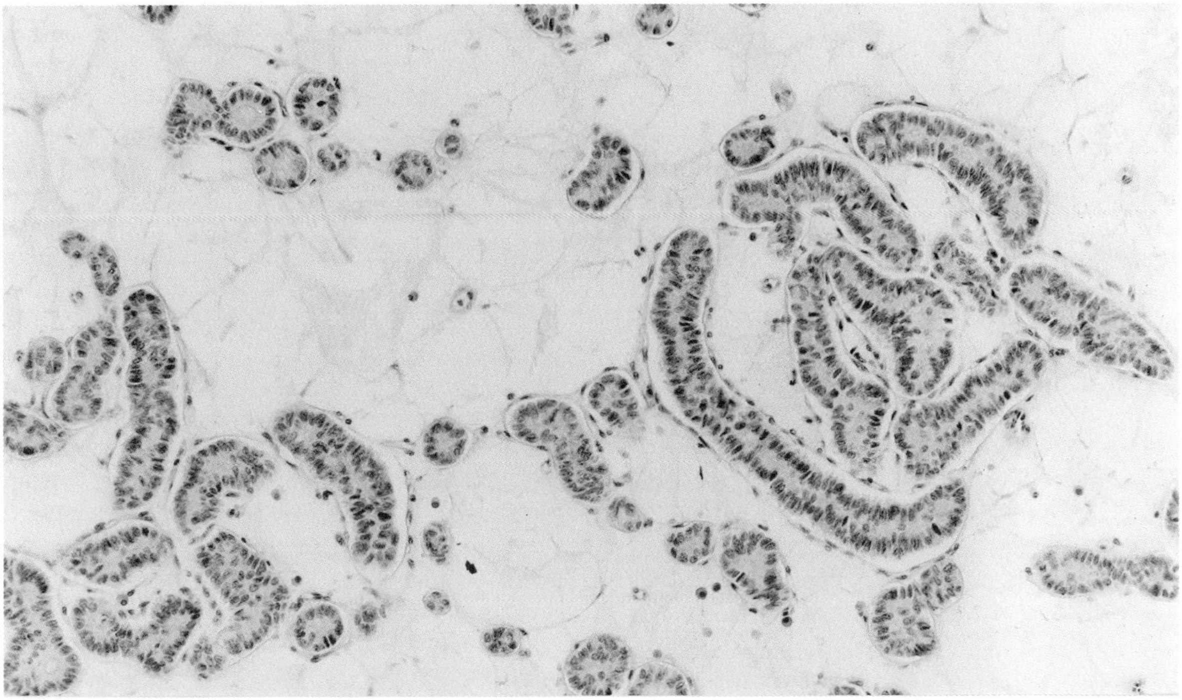

A

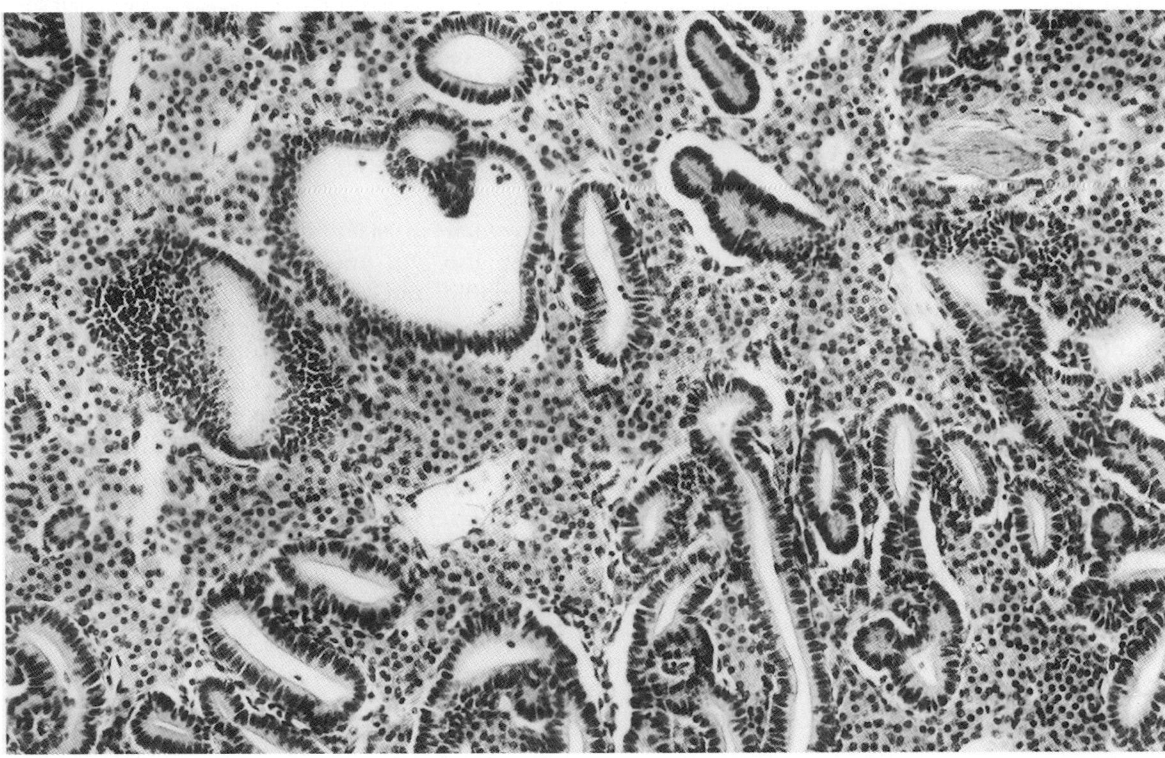

B

Fig. 35.3 Well differentiated Sertoli–Leydig cell tumor. (A) Edematous areas with widely separated Sertoli cell tubules. Leydig cells are present only at the periphery of such areas. H + E ×83. (B) Tubular and cystic spaces lined by Sertoli cells, separated by sheets of uniform eosinophilic Leydig cells with regular rounded nuclei. H + E ×125

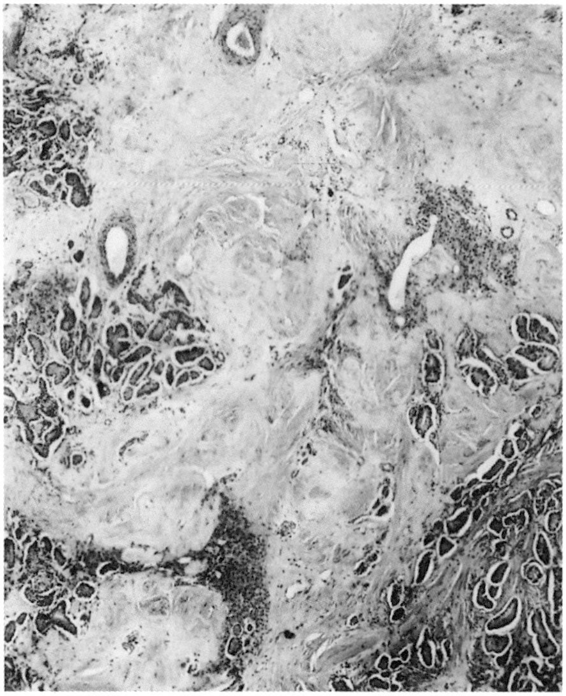

Fig. 35.4 Well differentiated Sertoli–Leydig cell tumor. This field shows an interface between acellular sclerotic zones with dilated vascular spaces and more cellular zones at the periphery. Small aggregates of Leydig cells are seen (bottom center and center right). H + E ×30

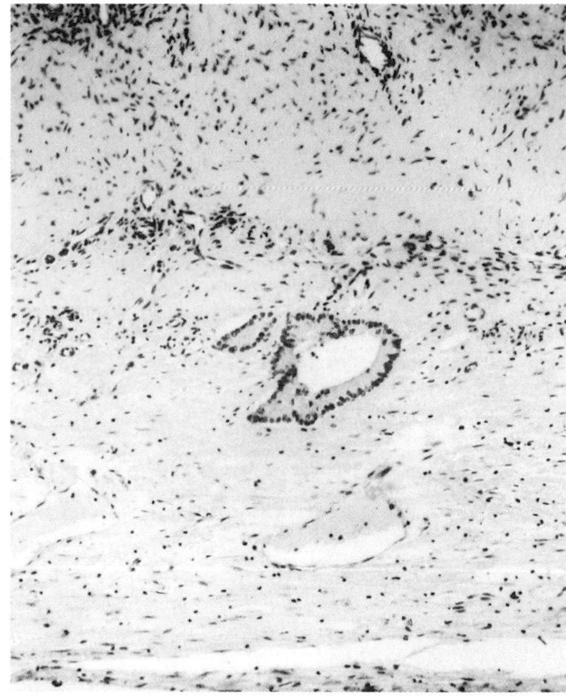

Fig. 35.5 A totally cystic well differentiated Sertoli–Leydig cell tumor (lumen at top). The cyst wall is composed of fibrous tissue and contains numerous scattered Sertoli cell tubules. H + E ×75

Macroscopic features

Leydig cell tumors are unilateral (only a handful of bilateral hilus cell or stromal Leydig cell tumors have been described) (Sternberg 1949, Baramki et al 1983, Bohm et al 1991, Luton et al 1991, Duun 1994) and vary in size, although uncommonly exceed 5 cm in diameter and are rarely large enough to produce symptoms relating to their size (Paoletti et al 1987). They usually occupy the hilar region of the ovary (Fig. 35.6) and adjacent mesovarium. They are well circumscribed, soft, fleshy, olive to tan nodules, in which focal hemorrhage is common (Fig. 35.7).

Microscopic features

Leydig cell tumors are composed of closely packed sheets or solid cords of uniform, polyhedral, eosinophilic cells measuring about 20 μm across. Nuclei are round, central, and vary somewhat in size. They have relatively sparse chromatin and one or more small but intensely basophilic nucleoli. Cytoplasmic pseudoinclusions may be noted. They frequently give an appearance of being unevenly distributed in the tumor with 'nuclear-rich' and 'nuclear-poor' zones, a feature we regard as being almost pathognomonic of Leydig cell differentiation, even in the absence of Reinke's crystals. Mitoses are rare (Fig. 35.8). Leydig cell cytoplasm is densely eosinophilic and finely granular with small sudanophilic lipid-containing cytoplasmic vacuoles. PAS-positive, yellow-brown lipochrome pigment is seen in many cells. Reinke's crystals (see Ch. 3) are slender birefringent rods with square or tapered ends, within an incomplete 'halo', and best seen when stained bright red with Mallory's trichrome stain. They are found in just over 50% of these tumors (Paraskevas & Scully 1989), but are often dissolved out in routine pro-

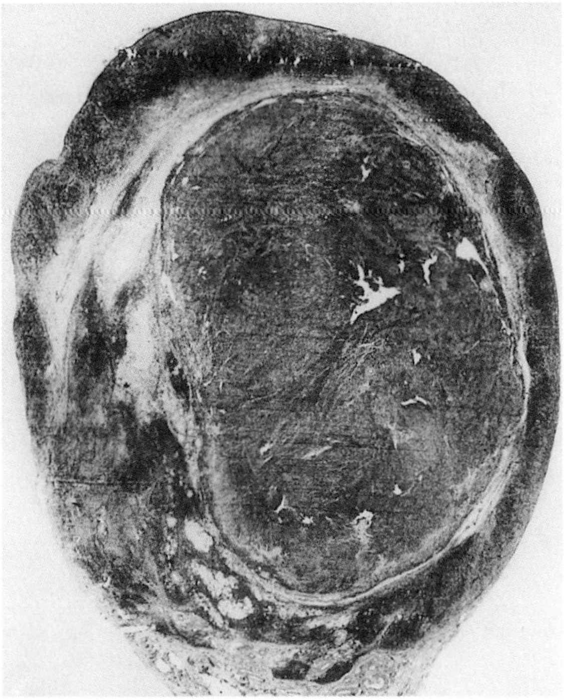

Fig. 35.6 Leydig (hilus) cell tumor. Note the clearly defined margins and the hilar position. H + E ×6

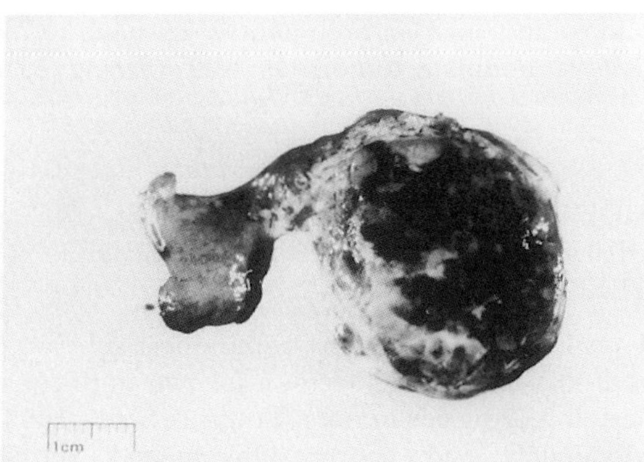

Fig. 35.7 Small Leydig (hilus) cell tumor, the cut surface of which demonstrated nodules of orange-brown tissue separated by hemorrhage.

cessing, are irregularly distributed in the tumor, and thus may require extensive searching to locate. While generally regarded pathognomonic of Leydig cell differentiation, Reinke's crystals may rarely be found in tumors of adrenal origin (Vasiloff et al 1986). Variably sized rounded colloid bodies may be seen in some cells. These are thought to be precursors of Reinke's crystals (Fox & Langley 1976).

At the tumor margins, the Leydig cells sometimes become more spindle shaped (Fig. 35.9), tending to merge with the adjacent stromal cells. Reticulin stains show a fine meshwork of fibrils and accentuate the marked vascularity which, in a hematoxylin and eosin stained section (see Fig. 35.8), often imparts an 'organoid' appearance. Collagen is rarely conspicuous (Fig. 35.10). Fibrinoid change in the walls of moderately sized vessels is noted in about 39% of tumors (Paraskevas & Scully 1989). The adjacent compressed ovarian tissue shows stromal hyperplasia, focal luteinization or hilus cell hyperplasia in a percentage of cases. Differentiation between Leydig cell tumors and Leydig cell hyperplasias may, on occasion, be difficult, and careful attention to histological detail is needed (Table 35.1). A solitary case has been reported with minor sex cord elements (Young & Scully 1983a).

In many Leydig cell tumors, there is a conspicuous admixture of large vacuolated cells similar to those in the adrenal cortex. A diagnosis of mixed Leydig cell–adrenal cell tumor suggests itself in some of these tumors, but has little to commend it other than the morphological variability of the component cells. Differentiation between Leydig cell tumors and the nonspecific 'steroid cell tumors' is usually achieved by identifying the features outlined in Table 35.2. However, there is definite histological and histogenetic justification to support the rare 'stromal Leydig cell tumors' as discrete and valid variants (Roth & Sternberg 1973, Sternberg & Roth 1973). In these tumors, nondescript ovarian stromal cells comprise the bulk, with focal single or clustered Leydig-like cells. These cells contain Reinke's crystals by definition, their presence being the only distinguishing feature between stromal Leydig cell tumors and the much less rare luteinized thecomas (see Ch. 34). It has been pointed out above that this single criterion may not be absolute in confirming or excluding a diagnosis of Leydig (hilus) cell

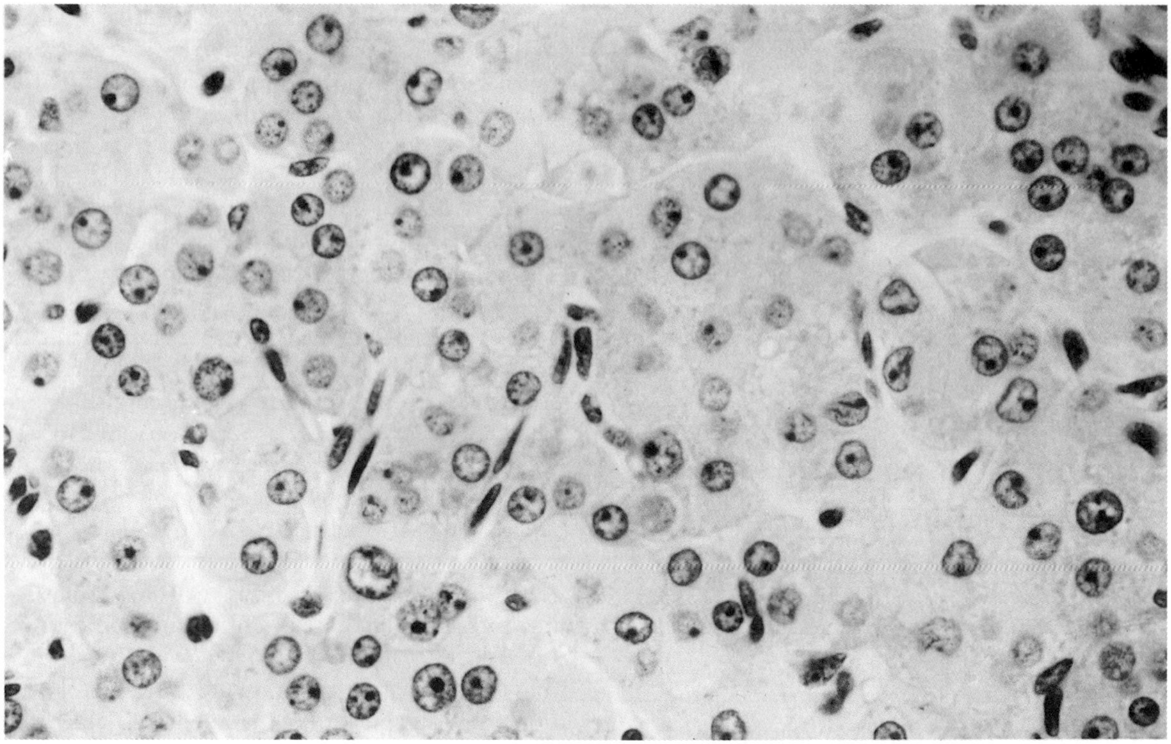

Fig. 35.8 Leydig cell tumor. Irregularity of distribution of nuclei is due to cellular orientation to the fine network of capillary vessels. Nuclei are round with one or more prominent nucleoli. H + E ×500

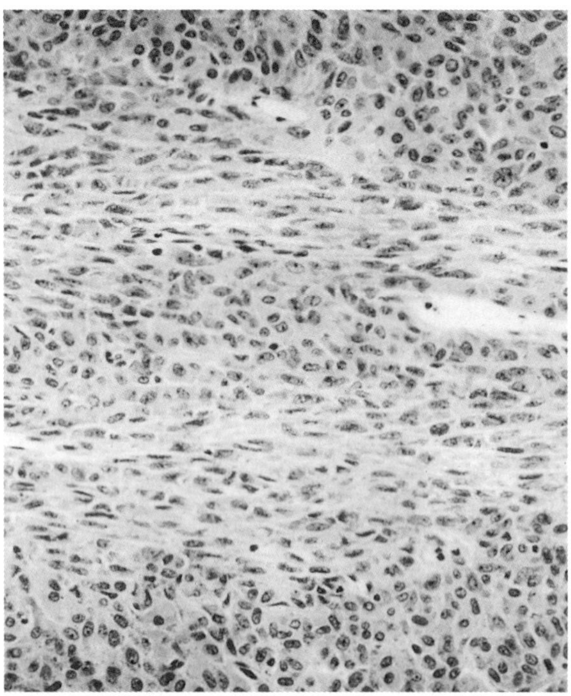

tumor, and such an argument is germane to this pair of nonhilar tumors as well (Zhang et al 1982).

MODERATELY AND POORLY DIFFERENTIATED SERTOLI–LEYDIG CELL TUMORS

Together, these form the commonest subtype of androblastomas, and account for two-thirds of all Sertoli–Leydig cell tumors (Young & Scully 1985). Moderately and poorly differentiated Sertoli–Leydig cell tumors are part of a histological continuum, and frequently particular tumors will show poor differentiation in one area and moderate differentiation in another. The Sertoli and Leydig cells may vary independently in their degree of maturity or differentiation.

Fig. 35.9 Leydig cell tumor with alternating zones of spindle-shaped and polyhedral cells. H + E ×150

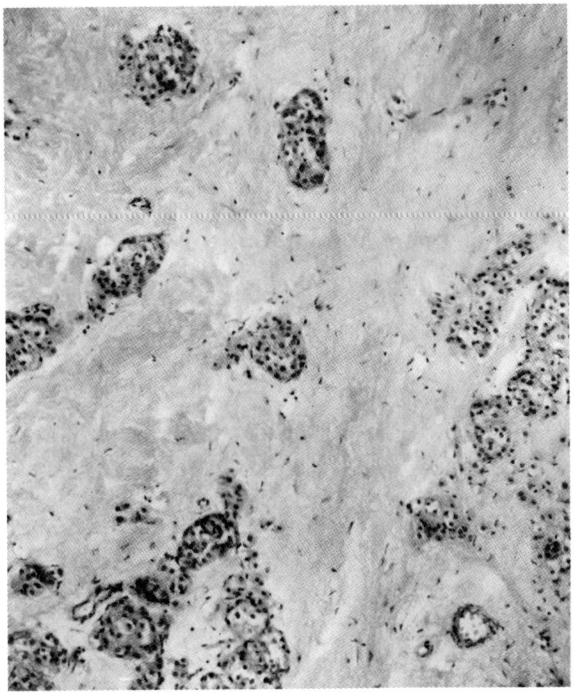

Fig. 35.10 Leydig cell tumor with pronounced stromal hyalinization. H + E ×75

Table 35.1 Differential diagnosis: Leydig cell tumor versus Leydig (hilus) cell hyperplasia

Leydig cell tumor	Leydig cell hyperplasia
Clinical	
Almost always unilateral	Typically bilateral
Macroscopically visible tumor	No discrete tumor mass
Histological	
Large solid sheet of cells	Fascicles or nodules of cells
Compresses surrounding ovarian tissue	Normal relationship to medullary nerves, ovary not otherwise affected

The incidence of malignancy in these tumors has variously been estimated at between 10% and 30% (Zaloudek & Norris 1984, Young & Scully 1985). The most reliable indication of malignancy is evidence of local extraovarian spread or of metastatic deposits at the time of staging laparotomy, all such tumors pursuing an aggressive and usually fatal course. Histological grade correlates to some extent with the likely clinical outcome; 11% of 'moderately' well differentiated tumors are malignant, while 20% of those with heterologous mesenchymal elements (see below) and 60% of poorly differentiated tumors are also likely to progress clinically (Zaloudek & Norris 1984, Young & Scully 1985). Recurrences or metastases in apparently early stage disease are usually apparent within 12 months (often before 6 months), and are commonly preceded by an exacerbation of the patient's virilization. Metastases occur in the omentum, abdominal lymph nodes or the liver, but have also been reported in lungs, bones, intestine, kidney, mediastinum, and brain.

Table 35.2 Differential diagnosis: Leydig cell tumor versus steroid cell tumor

Leydig cell tumor	Steroid cell tumor
Clinical	
Often mild and protracted virilization	Virilization early and rapidly progressing
Rarely larger than 5 cm	Often large and lobulated
Almost always benign	Over 20% malignant
Normal urinary 17-ketosteroids	Raised urinary 17-ketosteroids
Histological	
Usually eosinophilic cells	Typically large lipid-rich cells
Nonuniform distribution of nuclei	Uniform distribution of nuclei
Solid sheets of cells	Fascicles or 'organoid' pattern
Reinke's crystals in 50%	No Reinke's crystals

Macroscopic features

These tumors are bilateral in less than 2% of cases. They tend to be large, having a mean diameter of about 15 cm, are usually well circumscribed and have bosselated outer surfaces. The cut surfaces are typically partly solid, partly cystic; in general, smooth-walled cysts are more frequently present in larger neoplasms and those with a 'retiform' pattern (see below). Cysts most often contain clear yellow fluid and, unlike granulosa cell tumors, only occasionally contain altered blood clot. Polypoid masses may project into the cystic spaces. Solid portions of the tumor are lobulated, firm or fleshy in consistency (Fig. 35.11) and usually yellow-gray in color.

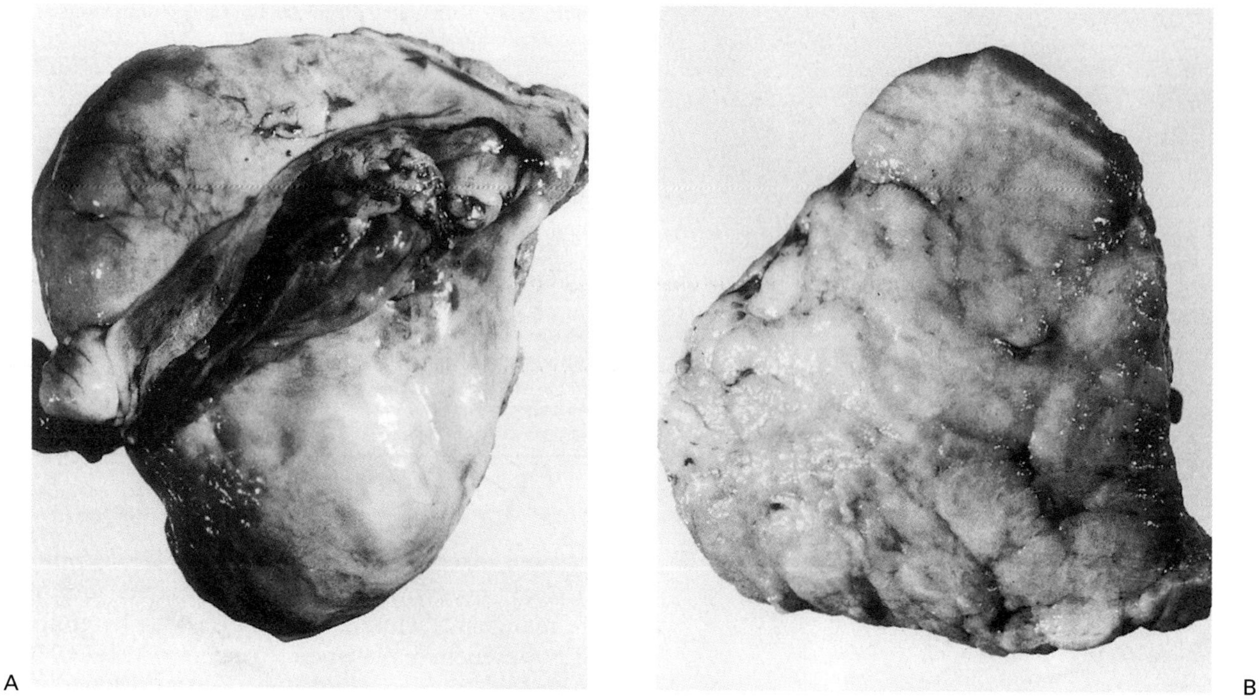

Fig. 35.11 A solid poorly differentiated Sertoli–Leydig cell tumor, 15 cm in diameter. The external surface (A) is slightly bosselated. The cut surface (B) is lobulated and fleshy in appearance.

Necrosis and hemorrhage are frequently prominent.

Microscopic features

Moderately differentiated Sertoli–Leydig cell tumors exhibit cellular nodules or 'lobules' of readily apparent epithelial cells separated by zones of loose fibrous or fibromyxoid mesenchymal stroma. Immature Sertoli-type cells, with small oval or angular nuclei and either scanty (Fig. 35.12) or rather more obvious pale cytoplasm (Fig. 35.13) are arranged in short, thin cords (resembling the sex cords of the immature testes and having double rows of cells with nuclei arranged antipodally), true hollow tubules or poorly circumscribed cell nests, and sheets. Such cells form the major components of the cellular lobules, while tubules or cords extend irregularly into the surrounding fibrous or fibromyxoid zones. Nuclei are relatively bland and mitoses infrequent (average about 5 per 10HPF). Rarely, thin walled cysts lined by flattened Sertoli cells (Fig. 35.14) create a sieve-like pattern. In 14% of moderately differentiated Sertoli–Leydig cell tumors a 'retiform' pattern is present (Young & Scully 1988). The indifferent fibrous mesenchyme is relatively abundant and consists of closely packed spindle-shaped cells (Fig. 35.15) associated with a very variable amount of collagen, which may be hyalinized. Mature Leydig cells are usually apparent in this stroma, particularly around the perimeter of the tumor or at the margins of cellular nodules, as sheets, clusters, or single cells, and less commonly within the cellular zones. In some instances the stromal (Leydig cell) component may also appear densely cellular. Sertoli and/or Leydig cell elements may contain varying amounts of lipid in the form of cytoplasmic vacuolation (Fig. 35.15) and, on rare occasions, show foci of bizarre nuclei as an isolated phenomenon (Young & Scully 1983b).

Poorly differentiated Sertoli–Leydig cell tumors consist largely (over 50%) (Roth et al 1981) of sheets of spindle-shaped cells in which occasional thin cord-like structures or tubules are noted

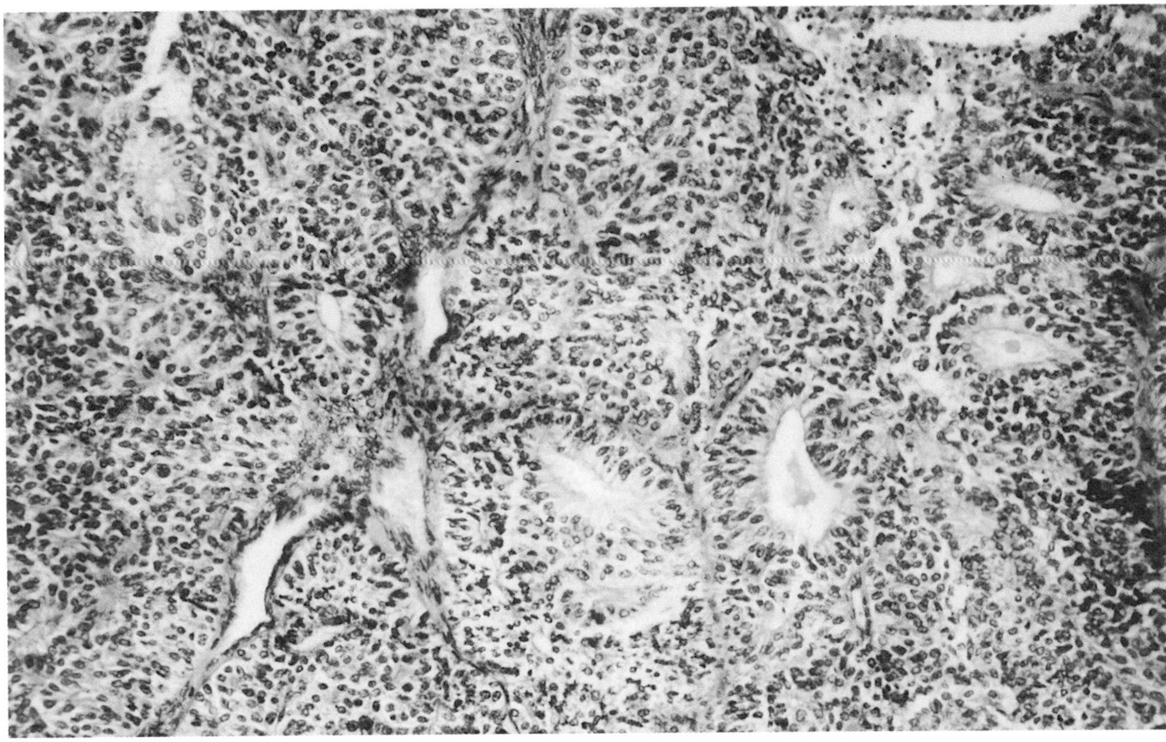

Fig. 35.12 Moderately differentiated Sertoli–Leydig cell tumor with hollow tubules. The immature Sertoli cells, here, have scant cytoplasm. H + E ×125

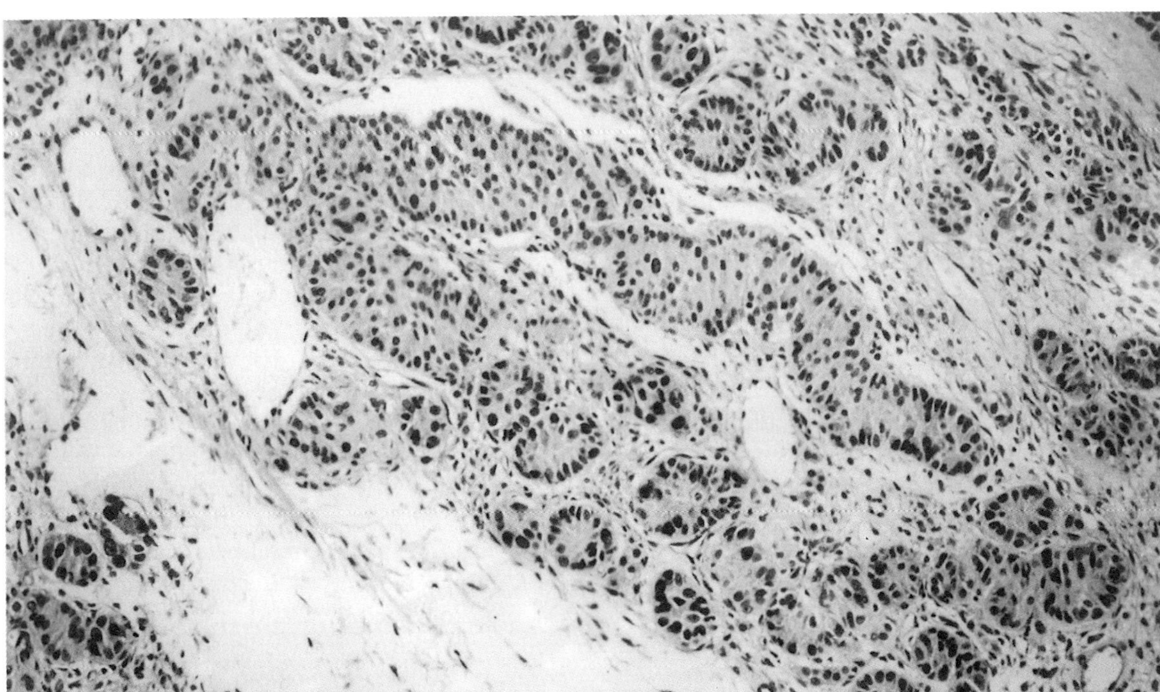

Fig. 35.13 Moderately differentiated Sertoli–Leydig cell tumor with solid tubules. Cytoplasm is more obvious than in Figure 35.12. H + E ×125

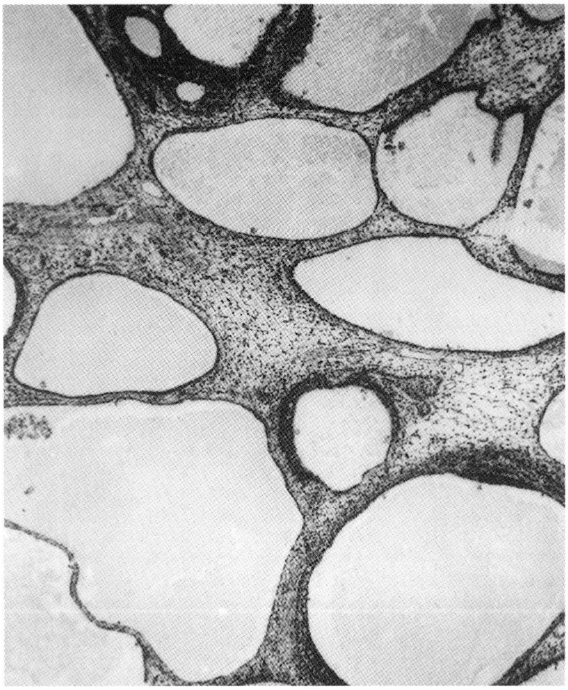

Fig. 35.14 Moderately differentiated Sertoli–Leydig cell tumor with a sieve-like pattern due to the aggregation of thin-walled cysts lined by Sertoli cells. H + E ×30

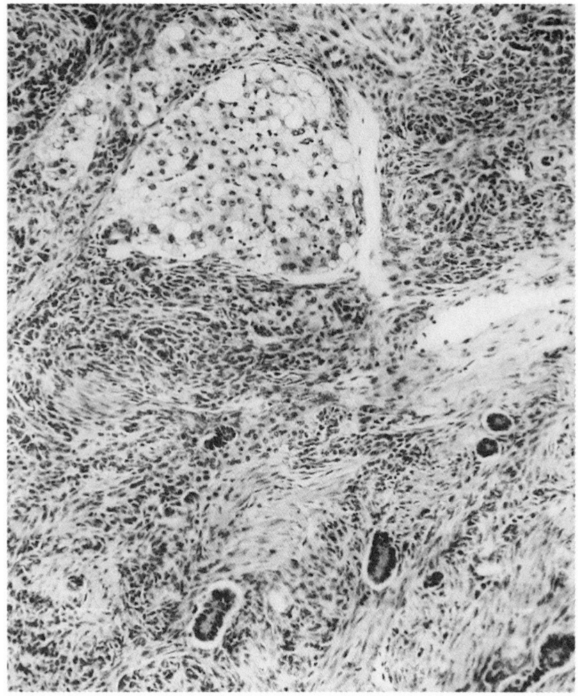

Fig. 35.15 Moderately differentiated Sertoli–Leydig cell tumor composed predominantly of indifferent mesenchyme with occasional well differentiated Sertoli cell tubules (lower right) and nests of lipid-laden Leydig cells (upper left). H + E ×75

(Fig. 35.16). These sarcoma-like areas (Fig. 35.17) may contain numerous mitoses (nearly always over 1 per HPF). Cribriform, trabecular, and 'moiré-silk' areas (Fig. 35.18) simulating granulosa cell tumors may rarely be seen, and thought must be given to applying rigid criteria before diagnosing gynandroblastoma (see Ch. 36). Focal variations in otherwise typical tumors may lead to 'organoid' or solid trabecular patterns (Fig. 35.19). Leydig cells may also be seen, but these are usually infrequent and require extensive searching to locate. As in moderately differentiated Sertoli–Leydig cell tumors, they are most readily found in loose mesenchyme adjacent to cellular nodules, and may have eosinophilic or foamy amphophilic cytoplasm (Fig. 35.20). The very rare pure Sertoli cell carcinomas with hollow or solid tubular architecture (Fig. 35.21) also belong in the poorly differentiated group (Young & Scully 1984b).

'Retiform' foci, so-called because of a resemblance to the rete testis, are found in 14% of moderately and 30% of poorly differentiated ovarian Sertoli–Leydig cell tumors (Young & Scully 1983c, 1985, Zaloudek & Norris 1984, Roth et al 1985). Tumors with this pattern occur at a slightly younger age than those without (mean age 17 years) and are also less likely to produce clinical signs of virilization (Young 1993). The retiform pattern, which may be represented by minor foci (Fig. 35.22) or large fields (Fig. 35.23), is typified by an irregular network of slit-like spaces and cysts, often containing papillae of various shapes. The cystic and compressed tubular spaces and the papillae are lined by flattened or cuboidal cells with the same general cytological features as the immature Sertoli cells described above. Papillae may be short and rounded with hyalinized cores, large and bulbous with edematous cores, or more complex and branched, occasionally simulating those of serous or endometrioid epithelial carcinomas.

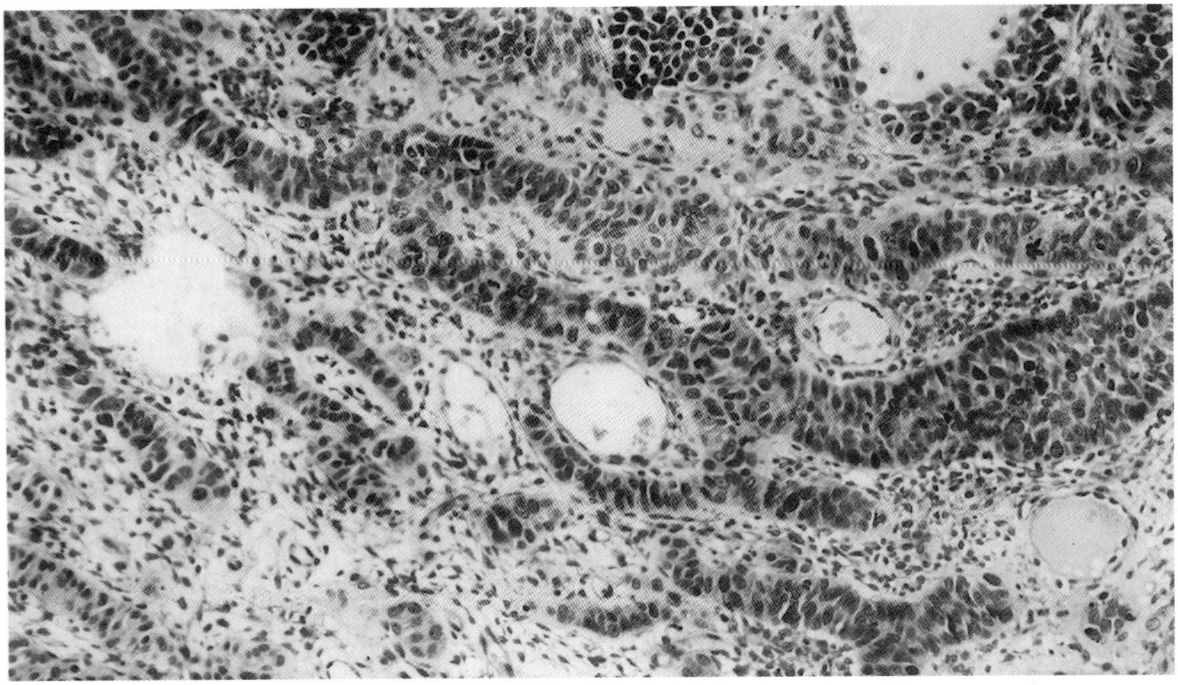

Fig. 35.16 Poorly differentiated Sertoli–Leydig cell tumor. An area showing primitive solid cords of cells with oval nuclei, scanty cytoplasm and numerous mitoses. H + E ×125

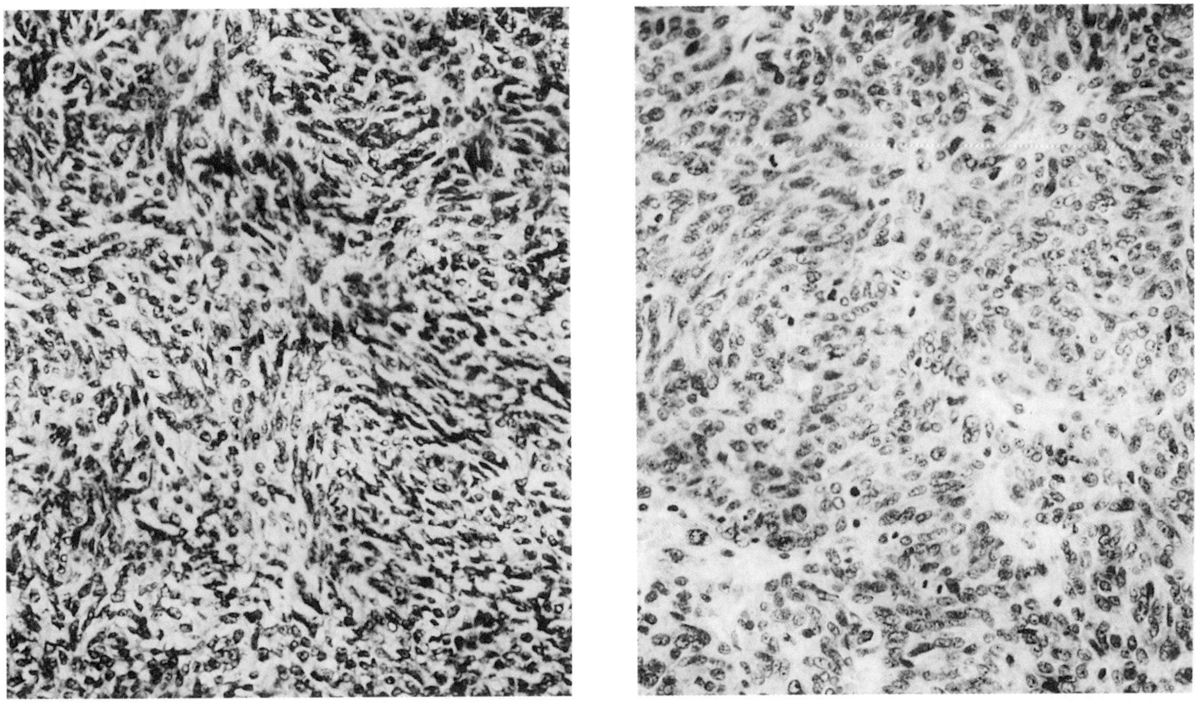

A B

Fig. 35.17 Poorly differentiated Sertoli–Leydig cell tumor. Sarcoma-like area of indifferent spindle cells (a) and showing conspicuous mitotic activity (b). H + E ×150

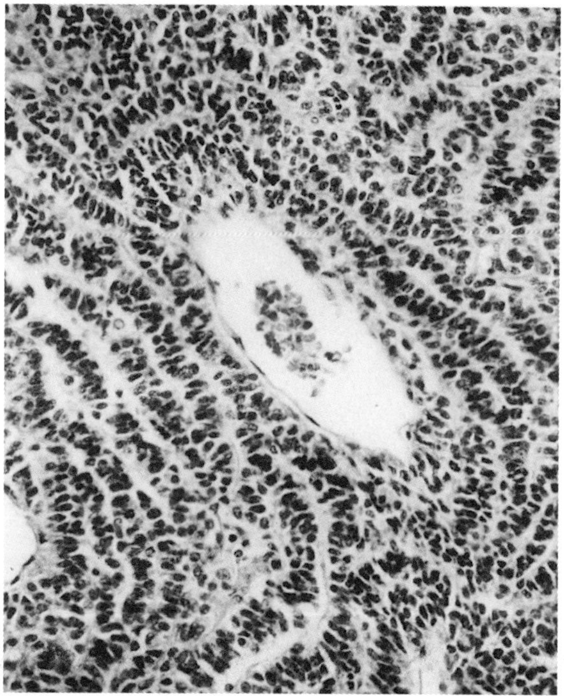

A

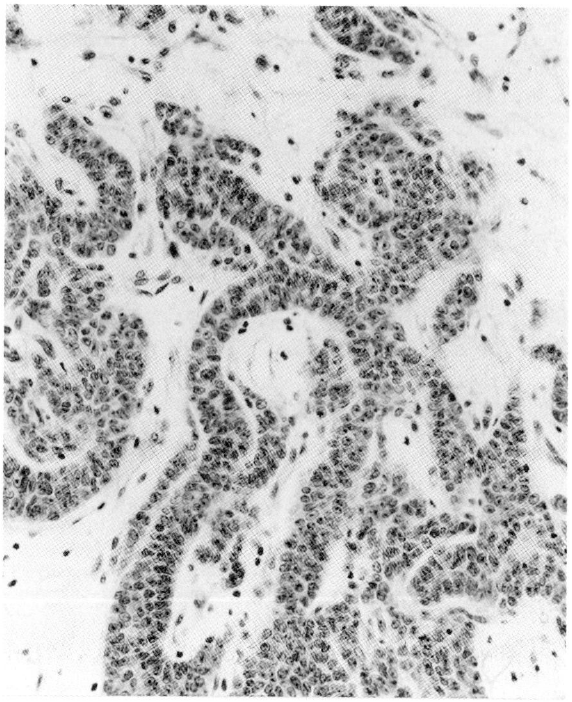

B

Fig. 35.18 Poorly differentiated Sertoli–Leydig cell tumor. (A) Fine trabecular or 'moiré-silk' area simulating patterns seen in granulosa cell tumors. H + E ×150. (B) More edematous area of same tumor, accentuating the trabecular pattern. H + E ×99

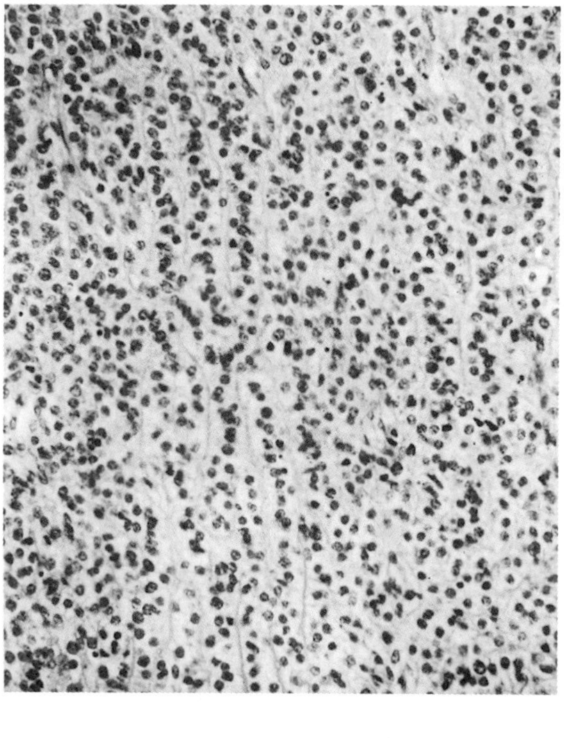

Fig. 35.19 Poorly differentiated Sertoli–Leydig cell tumor. Solid area of cords of immature Sertoli cells with rounded nuclei and clear or vacuolated cytoplasm. H + E ×150

Heterologous elements, such as intestinal-type mucinous epithelium, fat, cartilage, muscle, bone, etc., are found in over 20% of moderately differentiated and a smaller proportion of poorly differentiated Sertoli–Leydig cell tumors (in 40% of those with a retiform pattern) (Young & Scully 1983c); such tumors are described in the next section of this chapter.

The adjacent ovarian tissue is usually unremarkable, although it may be distinctly edematous if removed during pregnancy and rare instances have been reported of moderately and poorly differentiated Sertoli–Leydig cell tumors being associated with the morphological changes of the Stein–Leventhal syndrome in the affected or contralateral ovary (Zourlas & Jones 1969, Zaloudek & Norris 1984). There is also a known association with coexisting discrete benign adult cystic

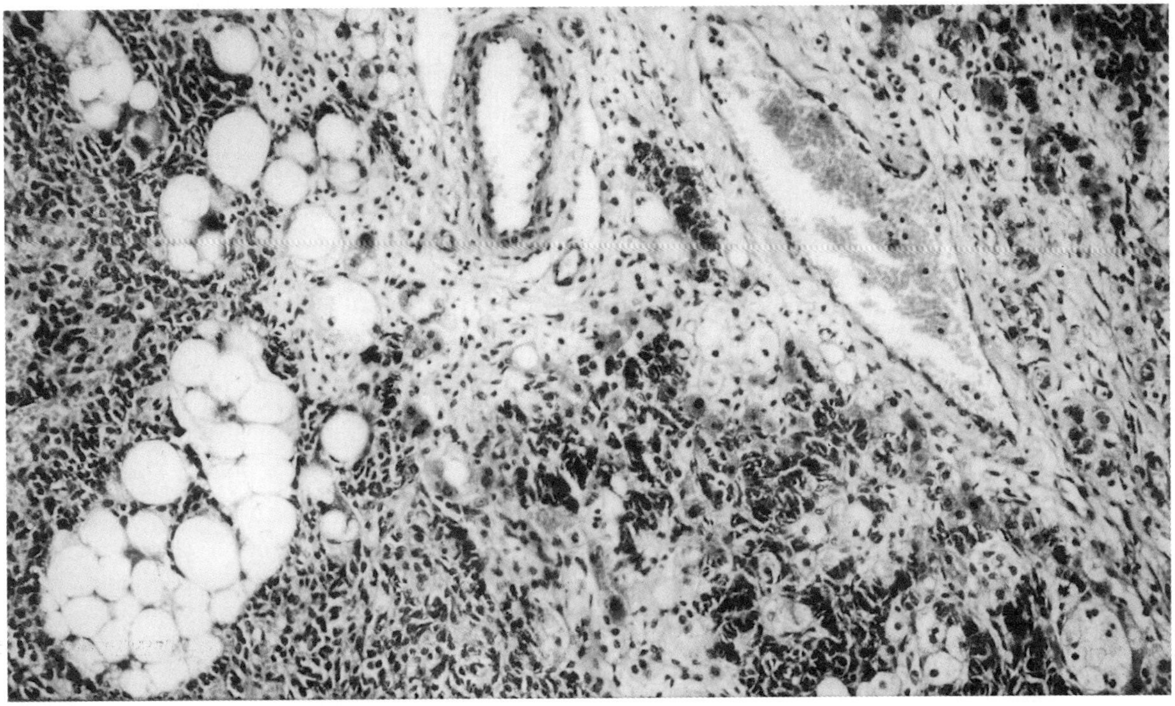

Fig. 35.20 Poorly differentiated Sertoli–Leydig cell tumor. Edge of cellular area with obvious Leydig cells. Those scattered near the center have dense eosinophilic cytoplasm, while those aggregated towards the left have grossly vacuolated cytoplasm. H + E ×125

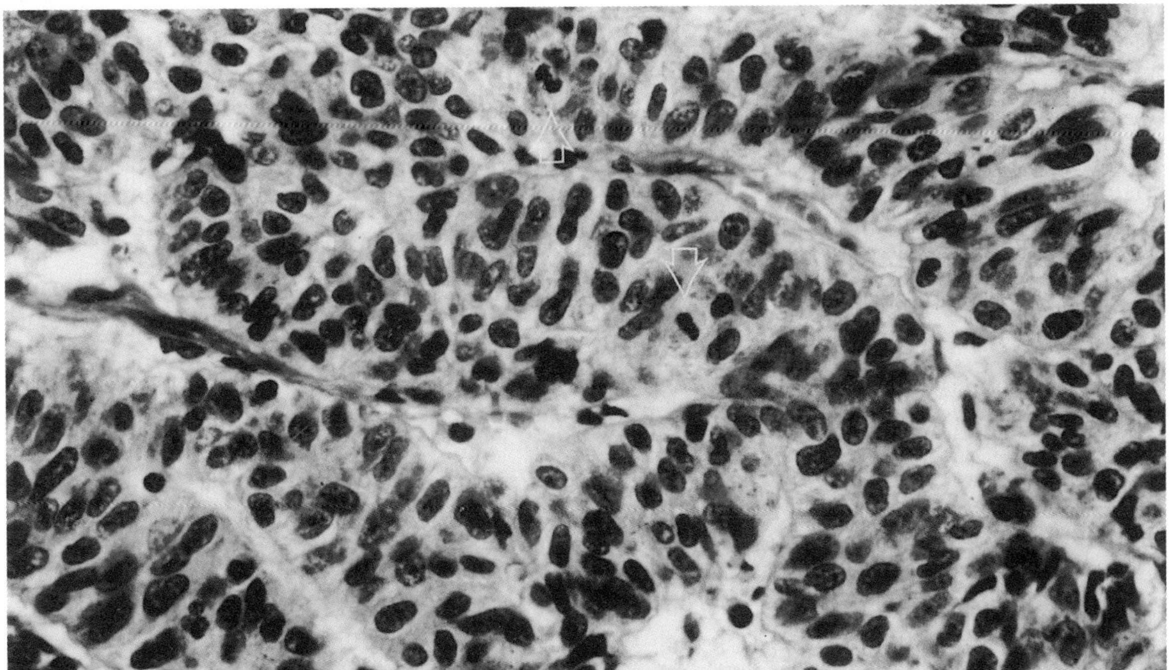

Fig. 35.21 Malignant, pure Sertoli cell tumor composed of solid gyriform tubules and cords of cells with ovoid nuclei and numerous mitoses (arrows). H + E ×500

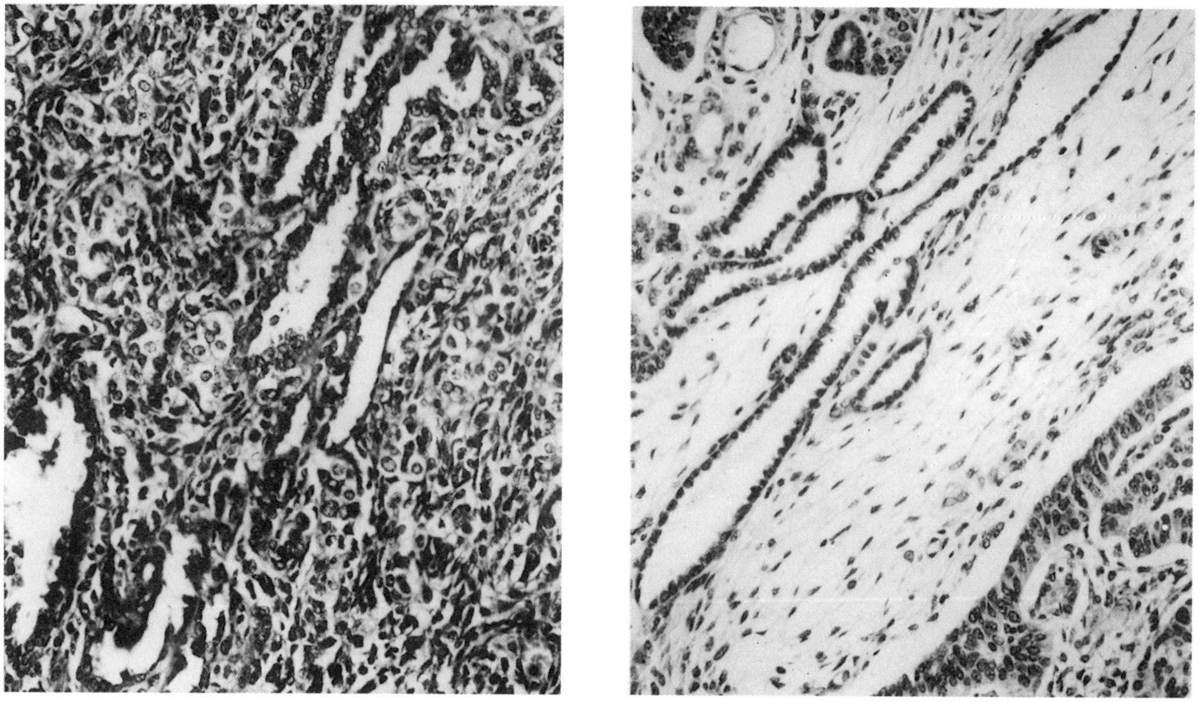

A B

Fig. 35.22 Small 'retiform' foci in poorly differentiated Sertoli–Leydig cell tumors. (A) Angular, branching, slit-like spaces lined by cuboidal epithelial cells are noted centrally. (B) Better defined cuboidal epithelial cells ('hobnail-like') lining the irregularly shaped retiform spaces. H + E ×150

teratoma (4%) (Seidman et al 1989) and benign mucinous cysts (3%) in either the same or contralateral ovary. In our experience, however, these are the most commonly encountered ovarian neoplasms in the age group in which Sertoli–Leydig cell tumors occur, and we are not convinced that this represents a statistically greater than expected association.

Differential diagnosis

The differentiation between granulosa and Sertoli–Leydig cell tumors may be impossible in the least differentiated forms, and a history of virilization is insufficient to justify attaching this diagnostic label to a neoplasm which would be better categorized as a sex cord–stromal tumor of indeterminate type. However, in relatively more mature tumors, although the basic histological architecture may be similar in some cases, the Sertoli cells do show appreciable differences from granulosa cells; Call–Exner bodies are not found in androblastomas, and Leydig cells are not present in granulosa cell tumors (Table 35.3).

Carcinomas, primary or metastatic, with imperfectly formed acini, may be mistaken for a moderately well differentiated Sertoli–Leydig cell tumors, especially if the stromal cells undergo luteinization and thus come to resemble Leydig cells. This is particularly so for moderately differentiated ovarian endometrioid carcinomas, some of which show a marked superficial resemblance to either granulosa cell tumors or Sertoli–Leydig cell tumors (so-called 'sertoliform' variants) (Roth et al 1982, Young et al 1982a). The age ranges of occurrence and the clinical settings of these tumors, as well as specific architectural features noted in Table 35.4, should facilitate their differentiation. Mucicarmine stains may be helpful in doubtful cases. Immunohistochemically, broad spectrum and low molecular weight cytokeratins (AE1/AE3 and CAM 5.2) are usually positive in epithelial-like areas of Sertoli–Leydig cell tumors but, unlike epithelial malignancies, such areas are

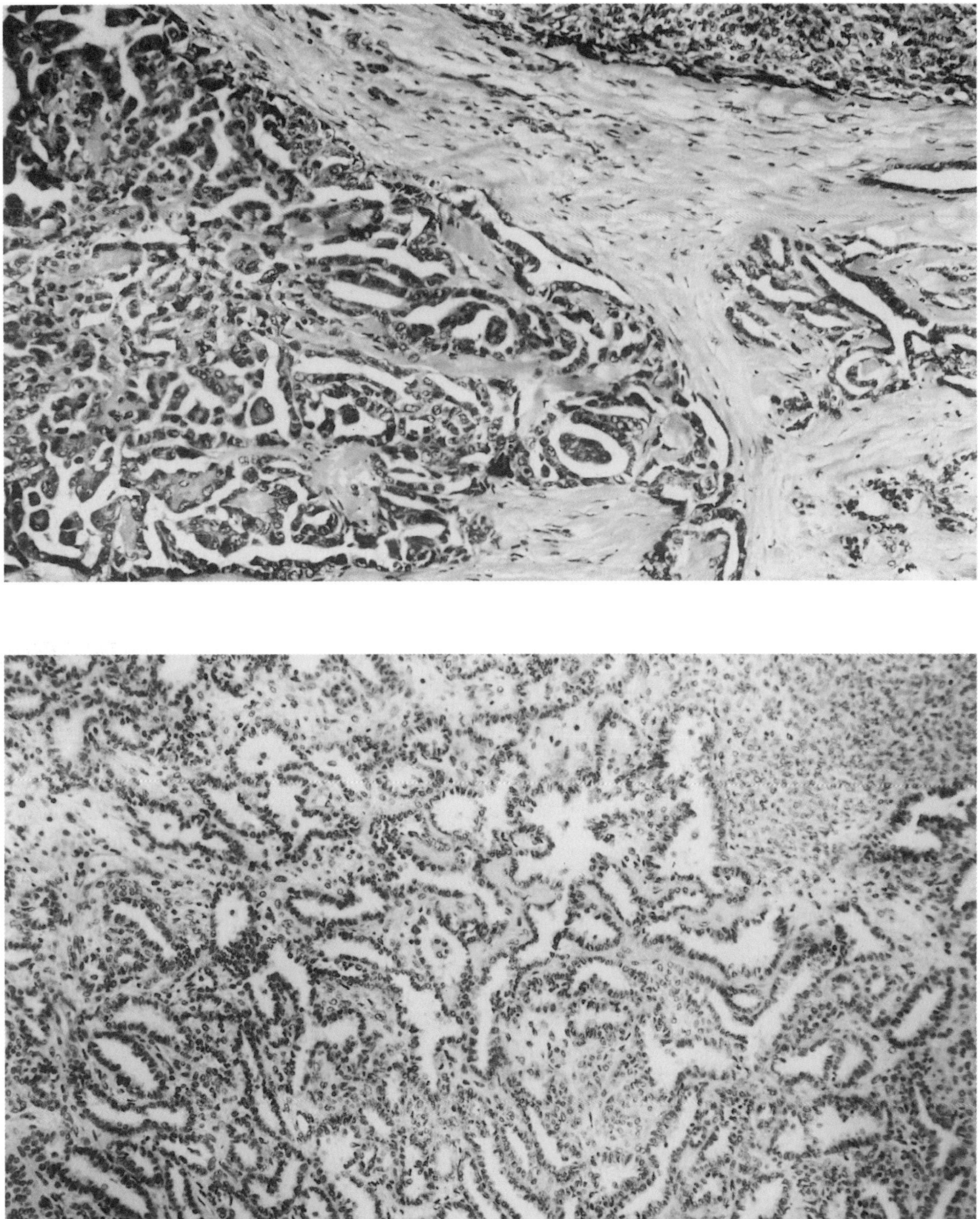

A

B

Fig. 35.23 Large fields with 'retiform' patterns in otherwise typical poorly differentiated Sertoli–Leydig cell tumors. (A) Branching, slit-like tubular spaces contain small papillary processes with hyalinized connective tissue cores. Epithelial cells are cuboidal. (B) The retiform character of the slit-like spaces is particularly striking in this field. H + E ×125

Table 35.3 Differential diagnosis: Sertoli–Leydig cell tumor versus granulosa cell tumor

Sertoli–Leydig cell tumor	Granulosa cell tumor
Clinical	
Mean age 25 years, <10% after menopause	Uncommon before the age of 30 years, 50% postmenopausal
Typically masculinizing	Typically feminizing
Histological	
Solid cords or hollow tubules, diffuse patterns which merge with stroma	Microfollicular, trabecular, insular, diffuse patterns
No Call–Exner bodies	Call–Exner bodies
Sertoli cells commonly immature with dark nuclei	Granulosa cells usually mature with pale, grooved nuclei
Fibromatous stroma between cellular nodules	Fibromatous stroma common
Clustered Leydig cells (may contain Reinke's crystals)	Lutein cells not prominent, do not form conspicuous groups
Heterologous elements in >20%	Heterologous elements not seen

Table 35.4 Differential diagnosis: Sertoli–Leydig cell tumor versus 'sertoliform' endometrioid carcinoma

Sertoli–Leydig cell tumor	Sertoliform endometrioid carcinoma
Clinical	
Mean age 25 years, <10% after menopause	Mean age 68 years, almost all postmenopausal
Typically masculinizing	Usually hormonally inactive
Bilateral in <2% of cases	Bilateral in 15% of cases
No characteristic pattern of associated pathology	Pelvic endometriosis in 25% and endometrial carcinoma in 25%
Histological	
Fibromatous stroma between cellular nodules	Adenofibromatous element common
No squamous metaplasia	Squamous metaplasia in one-third
Heterologous elements in >20%	Heterologous elements not seen; typical endometrioid carcinoma seen elsewhere
Luminal and cytoplasmic mucin associated only with heterologous elements	Conspicuous focal luminal mucin in most cases, no cytoplasmic mucin
Immunohistochemical	
Epithelial membrane antigen negative	Epithelial membrane antigen positive
Peanut agglutinin negative	Peanut agglutinin positive
Ulex europaeus negative	*Ulex europaeus* positive
Steroid hormone producing cells	
Leydig cells, some contain Reinke's crystals and/or lipochrome pigment	Lutein cells, may be prominent, no Reinke's crystals or lipochrome pigment

consistently negative for EMA (Aguirre et al 1989) and various lectins (peanut agglutinin and *Ulex europaeus*) (Bychkov et al 1992). Though it must be noted that heterologous mucinous epithelium is found in 20% of all androblastomas, such epithelium will show intracellular as well as luminal mucin. The so-called 'tubular Krukenberg tumors' (see Ch. 55) may be mistaken for moderately differentiated Sertoli–Leydig cell tumors, particularly if there is prominent stromal luteinization and clinical androgenization. The majority of these former tumors, however, are bilateral, and a mucicarmine stain will reveal typical signet-ring cells in all cases. The retiform variant may be confused with endodermal sinus tumors (see Ch. 42), serous epithelial carcinomas (see Ch. 23), or malignant mixed mullerian tumors, either homologous or heterologous (see Ch. 26).

ANDROBLASTOMAS WITH HETEROLOGOUS ELEMENTS

These tumors are separable from other moderately and poorly differentiated Sertoli–Leydig cell tumors on purely histological grounds; namely, the presence of heterologous elements, the most common of which is gastrointestinal mucin-secreting epithelium. Based on a review of the literature and their own large series, Young and coworkers estimate that 18% of Sertoli–Leydig cell tumors contain cystic or acinar structures lined by this type of epithelium, while about 5% contain immature skeletal muscle and/or cartilaginous elements (Prat et al 1982, Young et al 1982b, Young & Scully 1985, Young 1993). Rarely, they exhibit neuroblastoma (Scully 1979), fat (Novak 1938), carcinoid (Waxman et al 1981), smooth muscle, bone (Tragerman 1935), hepatocytes (Young et al 1984), endometrium (Stefanelli 1958), or endometrioid adenofibroma (Dardi et al 1982).

The origin of these neoplasms has not been settled. Androblastomatous tissue has been identified in a cystic teratoma (Bulwa & Lewis 1971), and Fox & Langley (1976) take the view that a small proportion (perhaps 5%) of androblastomas are of teratomatous origin. There does not, however, appear to be sufficient overlap of the most

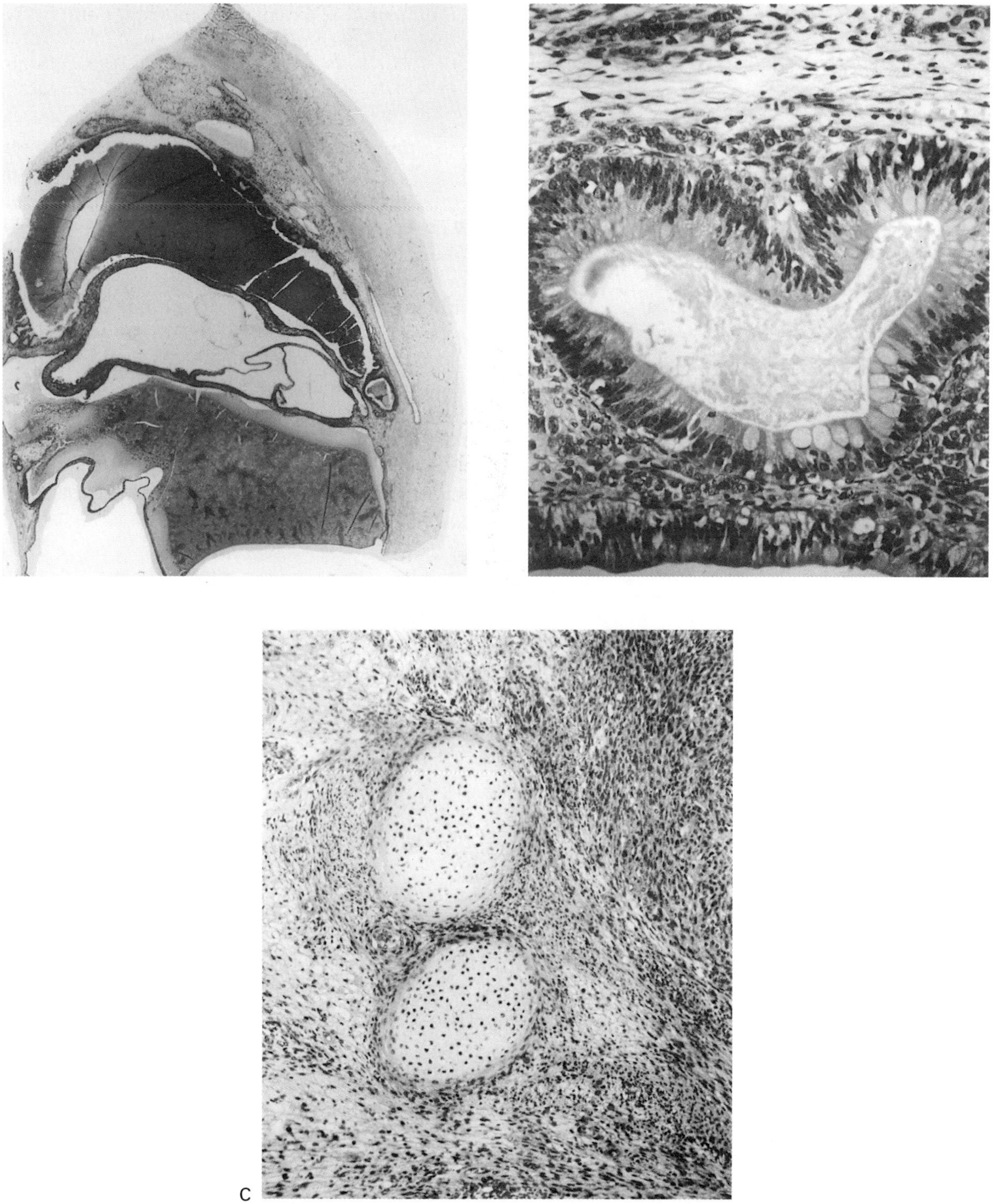

A B C

Fig. 35.24 Poorly differentiated androblastoma with heterologous elements. (A) Whole section mount demonstrating cystic spaces containing eosinophilic mucinous material. H + E ×5. (B) High power of the epithelial lining (bottom) and a subjacent glandular space of a cyst from this tumor. Goblet cells are a prominent feature of the enteric epithelium. H + E ×150. (C) Two circumscribed nodules of relatively bland hyaline cartilage adjacent to a sarcoma-like area (top right). H + E ×75 frequently observed elements of Sertoli–Leydig cell tumors and teratomas to make this likely, and we are in agreement with Young & Scully (1982), who prefer 'neometaplasia of the mesodermal neoplastic element' as their most acceptable explanation.

The clinical and endocrinological profiles of these neoplasms are the same as those of Sertoli–Leydig cell tumors without heterologous elements. About 20% pursue a malignant course.

Macroscopic features

These bosselated tumors tend to be of greater size than Sertoli–Leydig cell tumors in which heterologous elements are not found, and some show grossly visible mucin-filled cysts on the cut surfaces. Solid areas of friable yellow-gray tissue are comparable to solid areas in 'pure' Sertoli–Leydig cell tumors, and extensive hemorrhage and necrosis may be observed here.

Microscopic features

The mucinous epithelium in these tumors (Fig. 35.24B) is usually benign (but may be malignant) and is clearly enteric in type (Langley et al 1972, Hayes & Hunter 1973, Aguirre et al 1986); columnar cells being identical to those of normal small intestine and being commonly interspersed with goblet cells, Paneth cells, and basally situated argentaffin cells or other NSE-immunoreactive cells (Arai et al 1988). The latter may give rise to carcinoid or adenocarcinoid foci (Waxman et al 1981, Young et al 1982b, Sweeney et al 1983, Aguirre et al 1986). Further evidence of the endodermal nature of these heterologous elements is provided by rare examples featuring hepatocytic

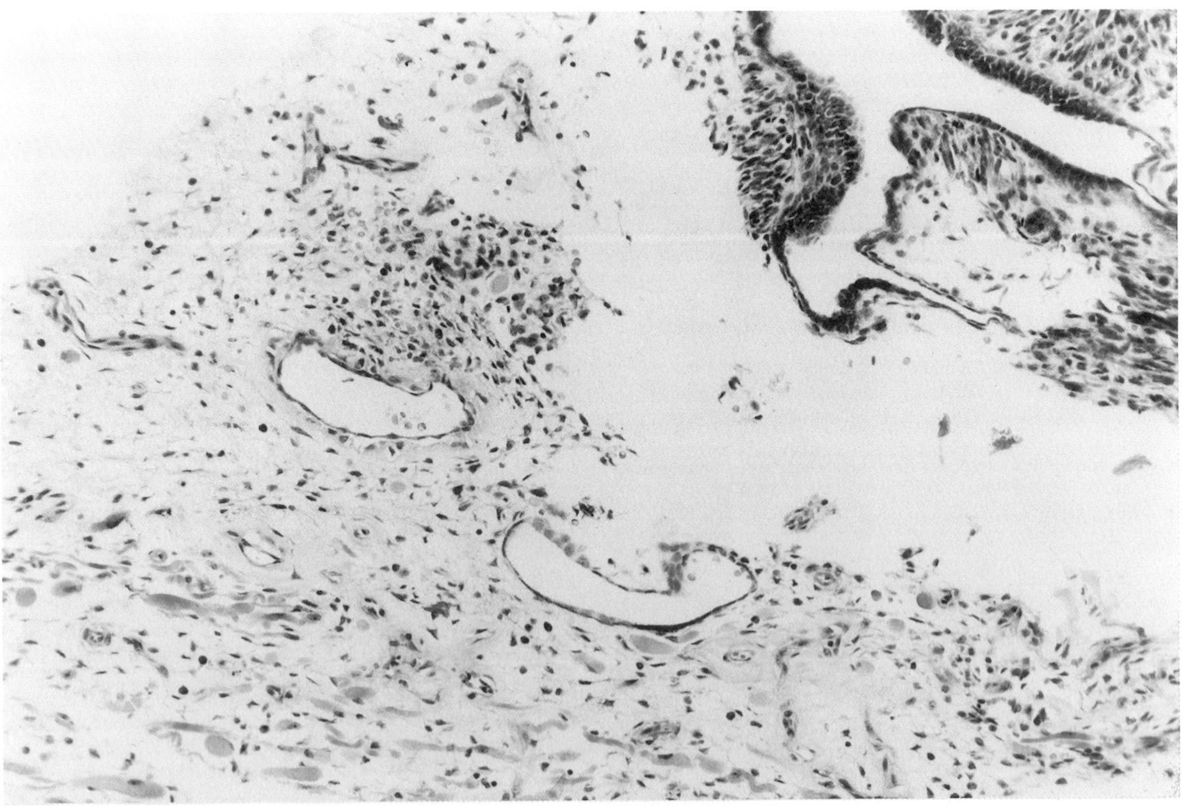

Fig. 35.25 Poorly differentiated retiform Sertoli–Leydig cell tumor with heterologous elements. Obvious rhabdomyoblasts, with strap-like eosinophilic cytoplasm, are seen at lower portion of the figure, with an irregular glandular structure at top right. H + E ×83

differentiation (Young et al 1984, Chadha et al 1987). The mucinous component varies from a minor element up to and including almost pure mucinous cystadenomas, with only microscopic evidence of Sertoli–Leydig cell differentiation. Similarly, mesenchymal elements vary enormously in their relative prominence and their degree of differentiation. Relatively banal immature cartilaginous islands (Fig. 35.24C) are readily apparent, but skeletal muscular components (Fig. 35.25) are frequently admixed with densely cellular spindle-cell tissue and easily missed. The wide range of tissue types seen in immature teratomas is characteristically absent, thus distinguishing these two entities (Prat et al 1982). If the Sertoli–Leydig cell component is small and overlooked, the tumor may be mistyped as a pure sarcoma. This has been proposed as an alternative explanation for the genesis of some pure chondrosarcomas and rhabdomyosarcomas of the ovary rather than monophasic malignant mixed mullerian tumor (see Ch. 52).

The androblastomatous components of these tumors are indistinguishable morphologically from those of Sertoli–Leydig cell tumors without heterologous elements; they are predominantly moderately differentiated in association with mucinous cysts and almost always poorly differentiated when mesenchymal elements or sarcoma are present. While the degree of differentiation of the Sertoli–Leydig cell tumor is probably of greater importance than the presence of unexpected heterologous tissue elements in determining prognosis, evidence does point to an unfavorable effect on clinical outcome occasioned by the presence of the latter (such as cartilage and striated muscle) (Prat et al 1982).

REFERENCES

Aguirre P, Scully R E, De Lellis R A 1986 Ovarian heterologous Sertoli–Leydig cell tumors with gastrointestinal-type epithelium. Archives of Pathology and Laboratory Medicine 110: 528–533

Aguirre P, Thor A D, Scully R E 1989 Ovarian endometrioid carcinomas resembling sex cord–stromal tumors: an immunohistochemical study. International Journal of Gynecological Pathology 8: 364–373

Arai N, Misugi K, Kamiya T, Shima S 1988 An ovarian Sertoli–Leydig cell tumor with heterologous mucinous gland and NSE-immunoreactive cell. Archives of Gynecology and Obstetrics 243: 55–60

Baramki T A, Leddy A L, Woodruff J D 1983 Bilateral hilus cell tumors of the ovary. Obstetrics and Gynecology 62: 128–131

Barkan A, Cassorla F, Loriaux D L, Marshall J C 1984 Pregnancy in a patient with virilizing arrhenoblastoma. American Journal of Obstetrics and Gynecology 149: 909–910

Bohm J, Roder-Weber M, Hofler H, Kolben M 1991 Bilateral stromal Leydig cell tumor of the ovary. Case report and literature review. Pathology Research and Practice 187: 348–352

Bulwa F L, Lewis M G 1971 Ovarian teratoma containing arrhenoblastic tissue. Journal of Obstetrics and Gynaecology of the British Commonwealth 78: 759–761

Bychkov V, Deligdisch L, Talerman A, Reddy V B 1992 Lectin histochemistry of sex cord–stromal tumors and small cell carcinoma of the ovaries. Gynecological and Obstetrical Investigation 34: 115–118

Chadha S, Honnebier W J, Schaberg A 1987 Raised serum α-fetoprotein in Sertoli–Leydig cell tumor (androblastoma) of ovary: report of two cases. International Journal of Gynecological Pathology 6: 82–88

Costa M J, Morris R, Sasano H 1994 Sex steroid biosynthesis enzymes in ovarian sex cord–stromal tumors. International Journal of Gynecological Pathology 13: 109–119

Dardi L E, Miller A W, Gould V E 1982 Sertoli–Leydig cell tumor with endometrioid differentiation. Case report and discussion of histogenesis. Diagnostic Gynecology and Obstetrics 4: 227–234

Dockerty M B, MacCarty W C 1939 Arrhenoblastoma. Surgery Gynecology and Obstetrics 68: 767–773

Duun S 1994 Bilateral virilizing hilus (Leydig) cell tumors of the ovary. Acta Obstetricia et Gynaecologica Scandinavica 73: 76–77

Echt C R, Hadd H E 1968 Androgen excretion patterns in a patient with a metastatic hilus cell tumor of the ovary. American Journal of Obstetrics and Gynecology 100: 1055–1061

Ehrlich E N, Dominguez O V, Samuels L T, Lynch D, Oberhelman H, Warner N E 1963 Aldosteronism and precocious puberty due to an ovarian androblastoma (Sertoli cell tumor). Journal of Clinical Endocrinology 23: 358–367

Ferry J A, Young R H, Engel G, Scully R E 1994 Oxyphil Sertoli cell tumor of the ovary. Report of three cases, two in patients with the Peutz–Jeghers syndrome. International Journal of Gynecological Pathology 13: 259–266

Fox H, Langley F A 1976 Tumours of the ovary. Heinemann, London, p 74–137

Gabrilove J L, Nicolis G L, Mitty H A, Sohval A R 1975 Feminising interstitial cell tumor of the testis. Personal observations and a review of the literature. Cancer 35: 1184–1202

Gagnon S, Tetu B, Silva E G, McCaughey W T 1989 Frequency of α-fetoprotein production by Sertoli–Leydig cell tumors of the ovary: an immunohistochemical study of eight cases. Modern Pathology 2: 63–67

Gee D C, Russell P 1981 The pathological assessment of ovarian neoplasms. IV: The sex cord–stromal tumors. Pathology 13: 235–255

Hansen T P, Sorensen B 1993 Sertoli–Leydig cell tumor of the ovary – a rare cause of virilization after menopause.

Acta Pathologica Microbiologica et Immunologica Scandinavica 101: 663–666

Hayes D M, Hunter R J 1973 Androblastoma of the ovary with heterotopic elements. Journal of Pathology 100: 267–270

Hensleigh P A, Carter R P, Grotan H E 1975 Fetal protection against masculinization with hyperreactio luteinalis and virilization. Journal of Clinical Endocrinology and Metabolism 40: 816–823

Ichinohasama R, Teshima S, Kishi K, Tsunematsu R, Ishii-Ohba H 1989 Leydig cell tumor of the ovary associated with endometrial carcinoma and containing 17-β-hydroxysteroid dehydrogenase. International Journal of Gynecological Pathology 8: 64–71

Kawagoe K, Yoshiro F 1989 Androblastoma in a five-year-old girl. Japanese Journal of Clinical Oncology 19: 149–152

Langley F A, Cummins P A, Fox H 1972 An ultrastructural study of mucin secreting epithelia in ovarian neoplasms. Acta Pathologica et Microbiologica Scandinavica A 80 (suppl 233): 76–86

Larsen W G, Felmar E A, Wallace M E, Frieder R 1992 Sertoli–Leydig cell tumor of the ovary: a rare cause of amenorrhea. Obstetrics and Gynecology 79: 831–833

Luton J P, Clerc J, Paoli V, Bonnin A, Dumez Y, Vacher-Lavenu M C 1991 Tumeur ovarienne bilaterale a cellules de Leydig–Berger chez une femme ayant une hyperplasie congenitale des surrenales. Le premier cas rapporte. Presse Medicale 20: 109–112

MacDonald P C, Rombaut R P, Siiteri P K 1967 Plasma precursors of estrogen. I: Extent of conversion of plasma γ^4-androstenedione to estrone in normal males and non-pregnant normal, castrated and adrenalectomised females. Journal of Clinical Endocrinology 27: 1103–1111

Motoyama I, Watanabe H, Gotoh A, Takeuchi S, Tanabe N, Nashimoto I 1989 Ovarian Sertoli–Leydig cell tumor with elevated serum α-fetoprotein. Cancer 63: 2047–2053

Murad T M, Mancini R, George J 1973 Ultrastructure of a virilizing ovarian Sertoli–Leydig cell tumor with familial incidence. Cancer 31: 1440–1450

Novak E 1938 Masculinising tumors of the ovary (arrhenoblastoma, adrenal ovarian tumors) with report of six additional cases of arrhenoblastoma. American Journal of Obstetrics and Gynecology 36: 840–858

Paoletti M, Pridjian G, Pkagaki T, Talerman A 1987 A stromal Leydig cell tumor of the ovary occurring in a pregnant 15-year-old girl. Ultrastructural findings. Cancer 60: 2806–2810

Paraskevas M, Scully R E 1989 Hilus cell tumor of the ovary. A clinicopathological analysis of 12 Reinke crystal-positive and nine crystal-negative cases. International Journal of Gynecological Pathology 8: 299–310

Pejovic T, Heim S, Alm P et al 1993 Isochromosome 1q as the sole karyotypic abnormality in a Sertoli cell tumor. Cancer Genetics and Cytogenetics 65: 79–80

Prat J, Young R H, Scully R E 1982 Ovarian Sertoli-Leydig cell tumors with heterologous elements. II: Cartilage and skeletal muscle: a clinicopathologic analysis of twelve cases. Cancer 50: 2465–2475

Roth L M, Sternberg W H 1973 Ovarian stromal tumors containing Leydig cells. II: Pure Leydig cell tumor, non-hilar type. Cancer 32: 952–960

Roth L M, Anderson M C, Govan A D T, Langley F A, Gowing N F C, Woodcock A S 1981 Sertoli-Leydig cell tumors: a clinicopathologic study of 34 cases. Cancer 48: 187–197

Roth L M, Liban E, Czernobilsky B 1982 Ovarian endometrioid tumors mimicking Sertoli and Sertoli–Leydig cell tumors. Sertoliform variant of endometrioid carcinoma. Cancer 50: 1322–1331

Roth L M, Slayton R E, Brady L W, Blessing J A, Johnson G 1985 Retiform differentiation in ovarian Sertoli–Leydig cell tumors. A clinicopathologic study of six cases from a Gynecologic Oncology Group study. Cancer 95: 1093–1098

Scully R E 1979 Tumors of the ovary and maldeveloped gonads. AFIP fascicle 16, 2nd series. Armed Forces Institute of Pathology, Washington, DC

Seidman J D, Patterson J A, Bitterman P 1989 Sertoli–Leydig cell tumor associated with a mature cystic teratoma in a single ovary. Modern Pathology 2: 687–692

Serov S F, Scully R E, Sobin L H 1973 Histological typing of ovarian tumours. International histological classification of tumors No. 9. World Health Organization, Geneva, p 17–54

Stefanelli S 1958 Raro caso di arrenoblastoma ovarico con aspetti teratomatosi e zone di endometriosi. Annals Ostetrica Ginecologica 80: 275–281

Sternberg W H 1949 The morphology, androgenic function, hyperplasia, and tumors of the human ovarian hilus cell. American Journal of Pathology 25: 493–521

Sternberg W H, Roth L M 1973 Ovarian stromal tumors containing Leydig cells. I: Stromal–Leydig cell tumor and non-neoplastic transformation of ovarian stroma. Cancer 32: 940–951

Sweeney E C, Barry-Walsh C, Robinson A 1983 Sertoli–Leydig cell tumor of the ovary with heterologous elements and carcinoid: an immunohistochemical and ultrastructural study. Ultrastructural Pathology 5: 185–194

Tavassoli F A, Norris H J 1980 Sertoli tumors of the ovary. A clinicopathologic study of 28 cases with ultrastructural observations. Cancer 46: 2281–2297

Teilum G 1976 Special tumors of ovary and testis and related extragonadal lesions, 2nd edn. Munksgaard, Copenhagen

Tragerman J L 1935 Arrhenoblastoma of the ovary. Archives of Pathology 19: 907–908

Vasiloff J, Chideckel E W, Boyd C B, Foshag L J 1986 Testosterone-secreting adrenal adenoma containing crystalloids characteristic of Leydig cells [abstract]. Journal of Urology 135: 1338

Waxman M, Damjanov I, Alpert L, Sardinsky T 1981 Composite mucinous ovarian neoplasms associated with Sertoli–Leydig and carcinoid tumors. Cancer 47: 2044–2052

Weyl Ben Arush M, Oslander L 1991 Ollier's disease associated with ovarian Sertoli–Leydig cell tumor and breast adenoma. American Journal of Pediatric Hematology and Oncology 13: 49–51

Young R H 1993 Sertoli–Leydig cell tumors of the ovary: review with emphasis on historical aspects and unusual variants. International Journal of Gynecological Pathology 12: 141–147

Young R H, Scully R E 1983a Ovarian stromal tumors with minor sex cord elements: a report of seven cases. International Journal of Gynecological Pathology 2: 227–234

Young R H, Scully R E 1983b Ovarian sex cord–stromal tumors with bizarre nuclei: a clinicopathologic analysis of 17 cases. International Journal of Gynecological Pathology 1: 325–335

Young R H, Scully R E 1983c Ovarian Sertoli–Leydig cell tumors with a retiform pattern: a problem in histopathologic diagnosis. A report of 25 cases. American Journal of Surgical Pathology 7: 755–771

Young R H, Scully R E 1984a Ovarian Sertoli cell tumors. A report of ten cases. International Journal of Gynecological Pathology 2: 349–363

Young R H, Scully R E 1984b Ovarian sex cord–stromal tumors: Recent advances and current status. Clinics in Obstetrics and Gynaecology 11: 93–134

Young R H, Scully R E 1985 Sertoli–Leydig cell tumors. A clinicopathologic analysis of 207 cases. American Journal of Surgical Pathology 9: 543–569

Young R H, Scully R E 1988 Ovarian sex cord-stromal tumors. Problems in differential diagnosis. Pathology Annual 23 (1): 237–296

Young R H, Prat J, Scully R E 1982a Ovarian endometrioid carcinomas resembling sex cord–stromal tumors. A clinicopathologic analysis of 13 cases. American Journal of Surgical Pathology 6: 513–522

Young R H, Prat J, Scully R E 1982b Ovarian Sertoli–Leydig cell tumors with heterologous elements. I: Gastrointestinal epithelium and carcinoid: a clinicopathologic analysis of 36 cases. Cancer 50: 2448–2456

Young R H, Perez-Atayde A R, Scully R E 1984 Ovarian Sertoli–Leydig cell tumor with retiform and heterologous components. Report of a case with hepatocytic differentiation and elevated serum α-fetoprotein. American Journal of Surgical Pathology 8: 709–718

Zaloudek C, Norris H J 1984 Sertoli–Leydig tumors of the ovary. A clinicopathologic study of 64 intermediate and poorly differentiated neoplasms. American Journal of Surgical Pathology 8: 405–418

Zhang J, Young R H, Arseneau J, Scully R E 1982 Ovarian stromal tumors containing lutein or Leydig cells (luteinised thecoma and stromal Leydig cell tumor). A clinicopathologic analysis of 50 cases. International Journal of Gynecological Pathology 1: 270–285

Zourlas P A, Jones H W Jr 1969 Stein–Leventhal syndrome and masculinizing ovarian tumors. Report of three cases. Obstetrics and Gynecology 34: 861–866

36

Gynandroblastomas

P. Russell   A. Farnsworth

These extremely rare neoplasms have been greatly overdiagnosed in the past, and a little over a dozen acceptable examples have been reported (Anderson & Rees 1975, Chalvardjian & Derzko 1982, Jaworski et al 1986, Yamada et al 1991, Zhang 1991, Martin-Jimenez et al 1994, Guo & Liu 1995). As discussed in the previous chapters, androblastomas occasionally exhibit small focal areas simulating granulosa cell differentiation and, on the other hand, rare hollow tubules lined by typical Sertoli cells may also be encountered in otherwise unremarkable granulosa cell tumors. The term 'gynandroblastoma', therefore, should be used only for those tumors which show intermingling of prominent amounts of well differentiated ovarian and testicular elements (Serov et al 1973), the importance of the 'intermingling' being to exclude rare cases of collision tumor such as that described by Dougherty et al (1958). It is axiomatic that the nature of the steroidal secretory product plays no part in the diagnostic process, and hormonal activity apparently inappropriate

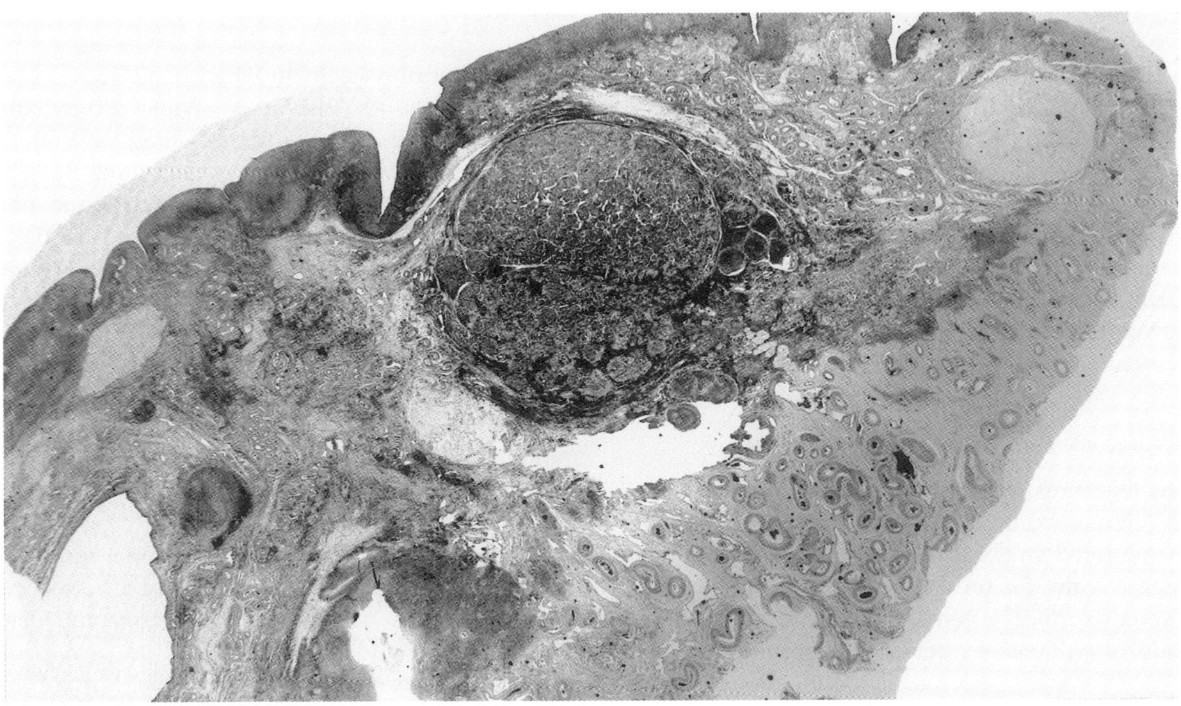

Fig. 36.1 A small gynandroblastoma identified in the medulla of an ovary removed from a 45-year-old woman with uterine fibroids. The rounded central nodule shows Sertoli cell differentiation only. The adjacent tumor is characterized by irregularly scattered small micronodules showing granulosa cell differentiation. H + E ×4

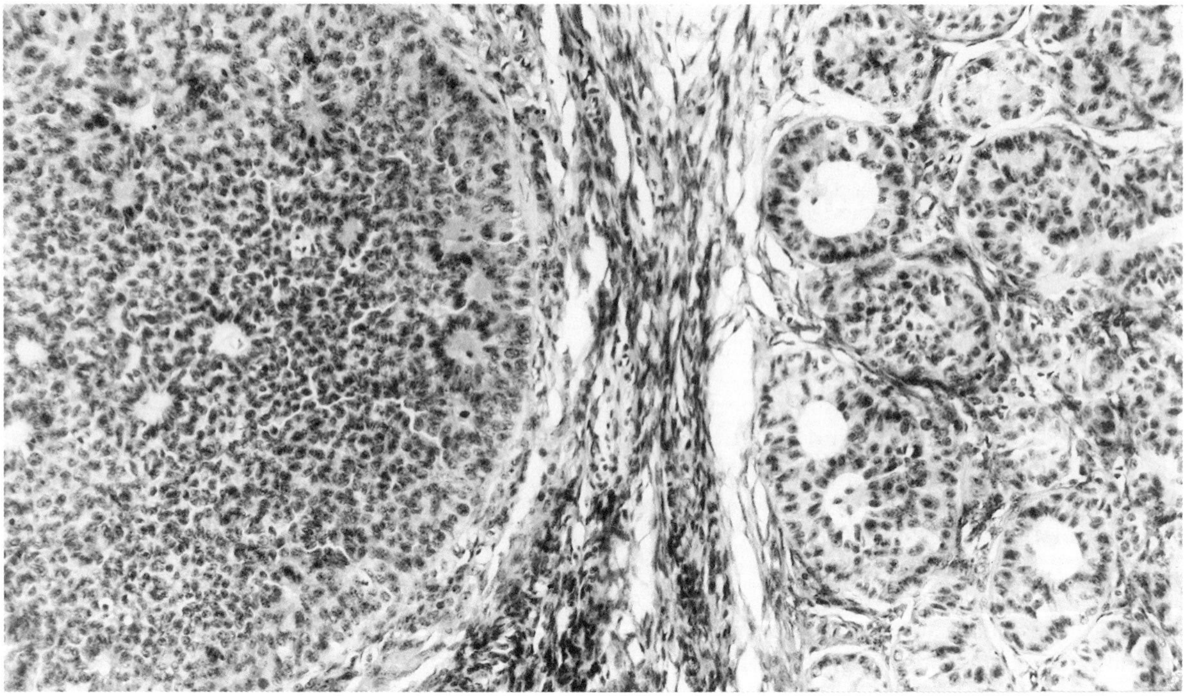

Fig. 36.2 High power image of Figure 36.1. The interface between the Sertoli cell nodule (right) with hollow tubules lined by tall columnar cells and an adjacent granulosa cell nest with a microfollicular pattern and typical Call–Exner bodies. H + E ×83

for the histological features present has been the basis for misdiagnosis in the past.

The majority of well documented cases have been virilizing and have presented in women with a mean age of 31 years (range 15–65 years), although a solitary case has presented with post-menopausal bleeding (Yamada et al 1991). To date, no case has pursued a malignant course (Jaworski et al 1986), but follow-up prior to case reporting has frequently been short.

Macroscopic features

The few cases reported have been unilateral, small (2–6 cm in diameter), solid, pale tumors. We have encountered an example as an incidental finding at hysterectomy for unrelated pathology (Fig. 36.1). The cut surfaces often show pink to yellow fleshy nodules with coarse intervening fibrous septa.

Microscopic features

The ovarian elements are represented by nests of mature granulosa cells in which Call–Exner bodies can be found (Fig. 36.2). Male or testicular components may be tubules lined by typical Sertoli cells and/or Leydig cells containing Reinke's crystals (Leydig cells have been described in only four cases). The residual rims of ovarian tissue and the contralateral ovaries have shown no noteworthy abnormalities. At the ultrastructural level, the tubular elements of gynandroblastomas more closely resemble the 'retiform' variant of Sertoli–Leydig cell tumors, while the Call–Exner bodies tend to be of the 'hyaline' rather than 'spongiform' type more commonly identified in granulosa cell tumors (Chalvardjian & Derzko 1982, Jaworski et al 1986).

Poorly differentiated sex cord–stromal tumors in which less than definite granulosa and Sertoli cell differentiation is seen are excluded from this diagnosis and should be categorized as sex cord–stromal tumors of indeterminate type. Using these strict criteria, almost all cases reported to date as gynandroblastomas are better placed amongst other subgroups of the sex cord–stromal tumors.

REFERENCES

Anderson M C, Rees D A 1975 Gynandroblastoma of the ovary. British Journal of Obstetrics and Gynaecology 82: 68–73

Chalvardjian A, Derzko C 1982 Gynandroblastoma: its ultrastructure. Cancer 50: 710–721

Dougherty C M, Thompson W B, McCall M L 1958 Hilus cell and granulosa tumors in the same ovary. American Journal of Obstetrics and Gynecology 76: 653–657

Guo L, Liu T 1995 Gynandroblastoma of the ovary. International Journal of Surgical Pathology 3: 137–140

Jaworski R, Fryatt J J, Turner T B, Osborn R A 1986 Gynandroblastoma of the ovary. Pathology 18: 348–351

Martin-Jimenez A, Condom-Munro E, Valls-Porcel M, Gine-Martin L, del Amo E, Balaguero-Llado L 1994 Gynandroblastome de l'ovaire. Revue de la litterature. Journal de Gynecologie Obstetrique et Biologie de la Reproduction (Paris) 23: 391–394

Serov S F, Scully R E, Sobin L H 1973 Histological typing of ovarian tumors. International histological classification of tumors No. 9. World Health Organization, Geneva

Yamada Y, Ohmi K, Tsunematu R et al 1991 Gynandroblastoma of the ovary having a typical morphological appearance: a case study. Japanese Journal of Clinical Oncology 21: 62–68

Zhang S Q 1991 Gynandroblastoma of the ovary. A case report. Chinese Medical Journal 104: 75–77

37

Sex cord tumors with annular tubules (SCTATs)

P. Russell   A. Farnsworth

Separation of sex cord tumors with annular tubules (SCTATs) from otherwise unclassified sex cord stromal tumors appears warranted on both morphological and clinical grounds. SCTATs were described in 1970 by Scully, who initially maintained that they arose from granulosa cells but gave rise to a growth pattern more consistent with Sertoli cells. They occur in two clinical settings.

First, they occur in almost all female patients with the Peutz–Jeghers syndrome (generalized hamartomatous intestinal polyposis and melanin spots of the oral mucosa, lips, and digits), such cases accounting for about one-third of reported examples of ovarian SCTATs (Young et al 1982, Benagiano et al 1988). In such examples, the tumors may occur at almost any age, but the mean age at presentation is 27 years; they are small lesions and are associated with menstrual irregularities in about 40% of instances. They are characteristically bilateral, multifocal, calcified, and very small (frequently microscopic), and are probably hamartomatous tumorlets rather than neoplasms. This concept would appear to be supported by the finding of similar structures of dysgenetic follicular origin in the ovaries of normal fetuses, infants, children, and adults (Safneck & de Sa 1986, Delides et al 1988) and in ovarian dysgenesis (see Ch. 8) and failure (see Ch. 9). All SCTATs associated with the Peutz–Jeghers syndrome have pursued a benign course, although they may rarely be associated with so-called 'adenoma malignum of the uterine cervix' (Young et al 1982) and other genital tract neoplasms and metaplasias (Chen 1986, Matseoane et al 1991, Podczaski et al 1991) and this former small risk should always be borne in mind in the postoperative management and follow-up of these women (Young et al 1982, Podczaski et al 1991).

Secondly, unassociated with the Peutz–Jeghers syndrome, SCTATs have almost always been large and unilateral, and should be regarded as true neoplasms, with at least 20% pursuing a malignant course (Hart et al 1980, Young et al 1982, Fox 1985, Ahn et al 1986, Shen et al 1993). Serum inhibin, mullerian-inhibiting substance (MIS) and progesterone levels may all be used as tumor markers in such patients (Gustafson et al 1992, Puls et al 1994). The mean age at presentation for those patients with SCTATs, unassociated with the Peutz–Jeghers syndrome is 34 years (Young et al 1982). Over one-half of patients give a history of postmenopausal bleeding, menstrual irregularities, or isosexual pseudopuberty, suggesting hyperestrogenism (Fox 1985), and rare case reports of SCTAT have been associated with a gestagen-like effect on the endometrium (Czernobilsky et al 1985, Shen et al 1993), these hormonal effects being thought to derive from the tumor cells themselves rather than from endocrinologically active stromal cells (Dolan et al 1986). A single instance has been reported of a patient with SCTAT, in whom the stigmata of the Peutz–Jeghers syndrome were not present, who developed an adenoma malignum of the cervix (Dolan et al 1986); a single case has been documented of SCTAT complicated by the supervention of a dysgerminoma (Hart et al 1980). Solitary extraovarian examples have been reported in the fallopian tube (Griffith & Carcangiu 1991) and umbilicus (Baron et al 1988). Divergent histogenetic views have continued to be promoted, particularly concerning those SCTATs unassociated with the Peutz–Jeghers syndrome, claiming granulosa cell (Anderson et al 1980, Hart et al 1980, Crissman & Hart 1981) or Sertoli cell origin (Tavassoli & Norris 1980, Astengo-Osuno 1984, Ahn et al 1986), the latter principally on ultrastructural evidence. Ahn et al (1986) have proposed 'Sertoli cell tumor, annular tubular type' as an alternative name for SCTATs.

Macroscopic features

Those examples occurring in conjunction with the Peutz–Jeghers syndrome are usually multifocal, bilateral, and are almost always very small tumorlets found incidentally in ovaries removed for reasons other than their presence. They frequently have a yellow cut surface. Focal calcification is occasionally obvious.

In patients without the Peutz–Jeghers syndrome, SCTATs are almost always unilateral and present as a solitary, large solid mass (up to 20 cm in diameter), although Young & Scully (1982) have reported occasional patients with microscopic multifocal SCTATs who did not exhibit the stigmata of the Peutz–Jeghers syndrome. They are commonly described as having nodules of firm yellow to tan tissue, occasionally with cysts and areas of hemorrhage and necrosis. Adhesions to adjacent pelvic organs, when present, are usually associated with local capsular infiltration by tumor.

Microscopic features

SCTATs typically exhibit well circumscribed, rounded or oval, epithelial islands made up of ring-shaped, lumenless tubules encircling glassy, acidophilic, PAS-positive, basement membrane-like material, and set in fibrous ovarian stroma (Fig. 37.1). This stroma may contain foci of luteinized cells and show focal hyalinization (Fox 1985). The stroma regularly condenses around the perimeter of cell nests to form thick hyaline

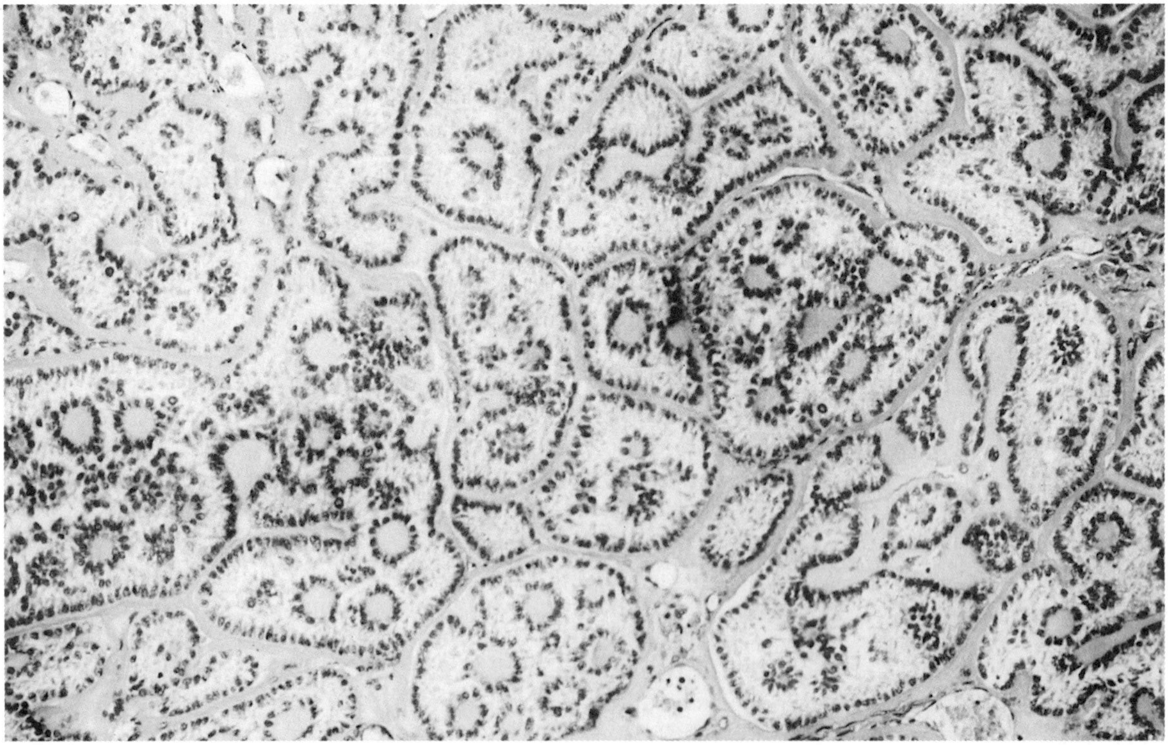

Fig. 37.1 Sex cord tumor with annular tubules. Clustered nests of columnar cells arranged in a complex ring-like or annular fashion around hyaline deposits. H + E ×125. (Material courtesy of Dr Robert Scully, Boston)

basement membranes (showing immunoreactivity for type IV collagen) (Takeshima & Inai 1992), which can be seen to be in continuity with the blunt-ended ellipsoid deposits of hyaline material within the cell nests. Sometimes simple annular cords envelop single deposits of hyaline material (Fig. 37.2) but, more commonly, a network of complex tubules encompasses and interdigitates with many such deposits (Fig. 37.3). The tubular cell cytoplasm is abundant, pale, and vacuolated or slightly granular. Regular, rounded, occasionally grooved nuclei, often with a single small nucleolus, are generally arranged in a double row, one row at the periphery of the cell nests and the second around the hyaline deposits. They may also proliferate towards the centers of the tubules to a variable degree. Microscopic focal calcification has been observed in over one-half of cases (Young & Scully 1984). Mitoses are rarely seen.

Tumours occurring in patients without Peutz–Jeghers syndrome differ somewhat from those in women with this syndrome, insofar as focal differentiation towards microfollicular granulosa cell tumor and/or areas indistinguishable from Sertoli cell tumor with elongated solid tubules (ultrastructurally confirmed by finding Charcot-Bottcher crystals in the neoplastic cells) (Tavassoli & Norris 1980, Ahn et al 1986) are commonly observed. Calcification is rarely seen. The immunophenotype of the tumor cells includes strong positivity for vimentin intermediate filaments (Nomura et al 1991). Hyalinization of the stroma may occasionally be profound, associated with degenerative changes in the tubular epithelial cells (Nakagawa et al 1982); coagulative necrosis may be present (Ahn et al 1986). Mitoses are uncommon (fewer than 1 per 10 HPF), while vascular permeation and destructive stromal invasion are not obvious, even in clinically malignant examples. A solitary case

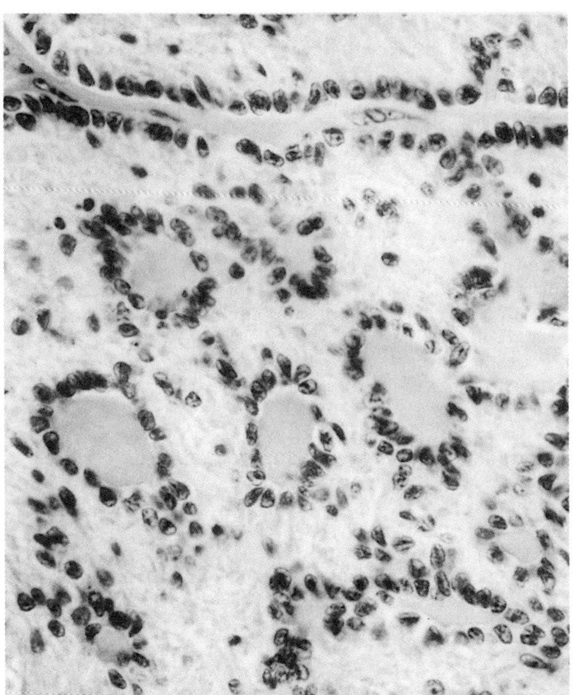

Fig. 37.2 Sex cord tumor with annular tubules featuring simple annular cords or lumenless tubules. Central hyaline material is similar to the thickened basement membrane around the perimeter of the cell nests. H + E ×300. (Material courtesy of Dr Robert Scully, Boston)

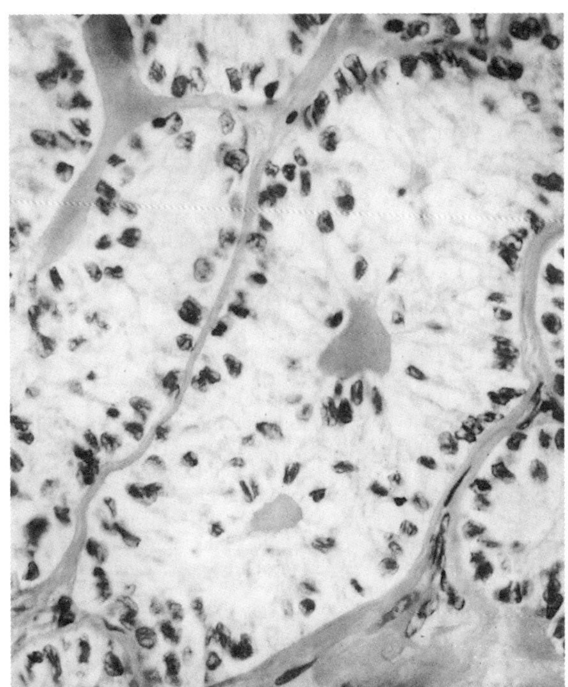

Fig. 37.3 Sex cord tumor with annular tubules. Area of the same tumor as in Figure 37.2, with a more complex pattern. Epithelial nuclei are ovoid and occasionally longitudinally grooved (lower right). H + E ×300. (Material courtesy of Dr Robert Scully, Boston)

of SCTAT has been documented (Czernobilsky et al 1985) in which a transition from typical SCTAT, through sertoliform tubular areas, to well differentiated endometrioid carcinoma was present. This may be analogous to the rare occurrence of so-called 'endometrioid' areas in Sertoli–Leydig cell tumors (see Ch. 35).

Differential diagnosis

SCTATs must be discriminated from microfollicular granulosa cell tumors, well differentiated Sertoli cell tumors, and gonadoblastomas. The cells of SCTATs tend to be larger, with more obvious and paler (or clear) cytoplasm than in granulosa cell tumors. The hyaline acidophilic deposits in the center of the cell nests are larger than the Call–Exner bodies of granulosa cell tumors, are frequently complex, and do not contain cellular debris. Nuclear palisading, prominent in SCTATs, is not a feature of granulosa cell tumors.

The cell morphology of SCTATs is very similar to that of well differentiated Sertoli cell tumors (see Ch. 35). The latter tumors, however, are composed predominantly of aggregates of hollow, simple tubules not seen in SCTAT.

SCTATs may superficially resemble gonadoblastomas in the patterns of cell nests, stromal calcification and stromal Leydig cells. Gonadoblastomas are composed of two cell types: large germ cells and smaller dark cells of sex cord origin. The smaller cells may produce rosettes resembling Call–Exner bodies, or be radially oriented around individual germ cells. They do not, however, produce annular tubules or cords with antipodally disposed nuclei as seen in SCTATs.

REFERENCES

Ahn H G, Chi J G, Lee S K 1986 Ovarian sex cord tumor with annular tubules. Cancer 57: 1066–1073

Anderson M C, Govan A D T, Langley F A, Woodcock A S, Tyagi S P 1980 Ovarian sex cord tumors with annular tubules. Histopathology 4: 137–145

Astengo-Osuna C 1984 Ovarian sex cord tumor with annular tubules: case report with ultrastructural findings. Cancer 54: 1070–1075

Baron B W, Schraut W H, Azizi F, Talerman A 1988 Extragonadal sex cord tumor with annular tubules in an umbilical hernia sac: a unique presentation with implications for histogenesis. Gynecologic Oncology 30: 71–75

Benagiano G, Bigotti G, Buzzi M et al 1988 Endocrine and morphological study of case of ovarian sex-cord tumor with annular tubules in a woman with Peutz–Jeghers syndrome. International Journal of Gynecology and Obstetrics 26: 441–452

Chen K T K 1986 Female genital tract tumors in Peutz–Jeghers syndrome. Human Pathology 17: 858–861

Crissman J D, Hart W R 1981 Ovarian sex cord tumors with annular tubules: an ultrastructural study of three cases. American Journal of Clinical Pathology 75: 11–17

Czernobilsky B, Gaedcke G, Dallenbach-Hellweg G 1985 Endometrioid differentiation in ovarian sex cord tumor with annular tubules accompanied by gestational effect. Cancer 55: 738–744

Delides G S, Elemenoglou J, Garas G 1988 Sex cord nests with annular tubules. The incidence of identifying them in normal ovaries. Acta Morphologica Hungarica 36: 3–6

Dolan J, Al-Timimi A H, Richards S M et al 1986 Does ovarian sex cord tumor with annular tubules produce progesterone? Journal of Clinical Pathology 39: 29–35

Fox H 1985 Sex cord–stromal tumors of the ovary. Journal of Pathology 145: 127–148

Griffith L M, Carcangiu M L 1991 Sex cord tumor with annular tubules associated with endometriosis of the fallopian tube. American Journal of Clinical Pathology 96: 259–262

Gustafson M L, Lee M M, Scully R E et al 1992 Mullerian inhibiting substance as a marker for ovarian sex-cord tumor. New England Journal of Medicine 326: 466–471

Hart W R, Kumar N, Crissman J D 1980 Ovarian neoplasms resembling sex cord tumors with annular tubules. Cancer 45: 2352–2363

Matseoane S, Moscovic E, Williams S, Huang J C 1991 Mucinous neoplasm in the cervix associated with a mucinous neoplasm in the ovary and concurrent bilateral sex cord tumors with annular tubules: immunohistochemical study. Gynecologic Oncology 43: 300–304

Nakagawa Y, Miyamoto H, Miyamoto M, Morino H, Taki I 1982 Ovarian sex cord tumor with annular tubules. Gynecologic Oncology 13: 129–135

Nomura K, Furusato M, Nikaido T, Aizawa S 1991 Ovarian sex cord tumor with annular tubules. Report of a case. Acta Pathologica Japonica 41: 701–706

Podczaski E, Kaminski P F, Pees R C, Singapuri K, Sorosky J I 1991 Peutz–Jeghers syndrome with ovarian sex cord tumor with annular tubules and cervical adenoma malignum. Gynecologic Oncology 42: 74–78

Puls L E, Hamous J, Morrow M S, Schneyer A, MacLaughlin D T, Castracane V D 1994 Recurrent ovarian sex cord tumor with annular tubules: tumor marker and chemotherapy experience. Gynecologic Oncology 54: 396–401

Safneck J R S, de Sa D J 1986 Structures mimicking sex cord–stromal tumors and gonadoblastomas in the ovaries of normal infants and children. Histopathology 10: 909–920

Scully R E 1970 Sex cord tumor with annular tubules. A distinctive ovarian tumor of the Peutz–Jeghers syndrome. Cancer 25: 1107–1121

Shen K, Wu P C, Lang J H, Huang R L, Tang M T, Lian L J 1993 Ovarian sex cord tumor with annular tubules: a report of six cases. Gynecologic Oncology 48: 180–184

Takeshima Y, Inai K 1992 Ovarian sex cord tumor with annular tubules – a case report and review of the literature in Japanese. Hiroshima Journal of Medical Science 41: 37–42

Tavassoli F A, Norris H J 1980 Sertoli tumors of the ovary. A clinicopathologic study of 28 cases with ultrastructural observations. Cancer 46: 2281–2297

Young R H, Scully R E 1982 Ovarian sex cord–stromal tumors. Recent progress. International Journal of Gynecological Pathology 1: 101–123

Young R H, Scully R E 1984 Ovarian sex cord–stromal tumors: recent advances and current status. Clinics in Obstetrics and Gynaecology 11: 93–134

Young R H, Welch W R, Dickersin G R, Scully R E 1982 Ovarian sex cord tumor with annular tubules: review of 74 cases including 27 with Peutz–Jeghers syndrome and 4 with adenoma malignum of the cervix. Cancer 50: 1384–1402

38

Unclassified sex cord–stromal tumors

P. Russell *A. Farnsworth*

Occasional ovarian neoplasms are associated with clinical or histological features which suggest sex cord or gonadal stromal origin yet do not conveniently conform to any of the previously described tumor types. This is largely a function of their rarity and the precision with which established subgroups of tumors are defined. As experience accumulates and patterns of incidence, clinical correlates, and morphological features emerge, some will undoubtedly be removed to new categories and thus expand further the established classification. Young & Scully (1984) place approximately 10% of all sex cord–stromal tumors (with 'patterns and cell types intermediate between those of a Sertoli–Leydig cell tumor and a granulosa cell tumor') in this group. Our approach is to attempt to restrict this category of tumors largely to those very uncommon poorly differentiated diffuse or

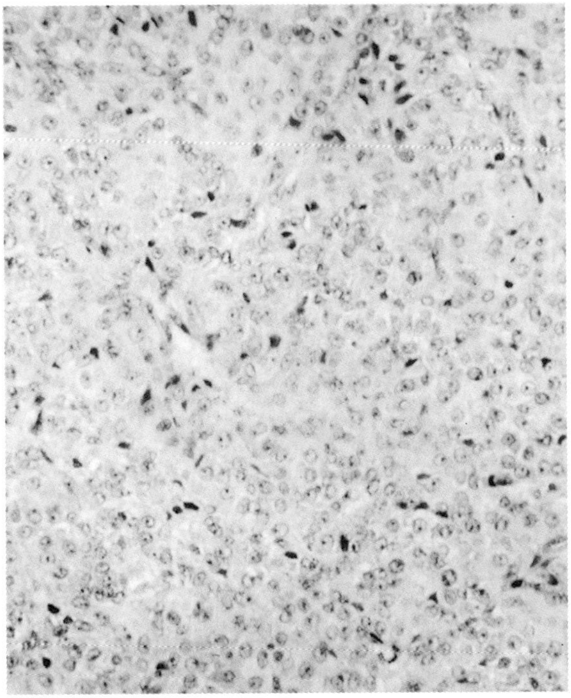

Fig. 38.1 Poorly differentiated sex cord–stromal tumor composed of sheets of uniform round to slightly spindled cells with central vesicular nuclei. H + E ×150

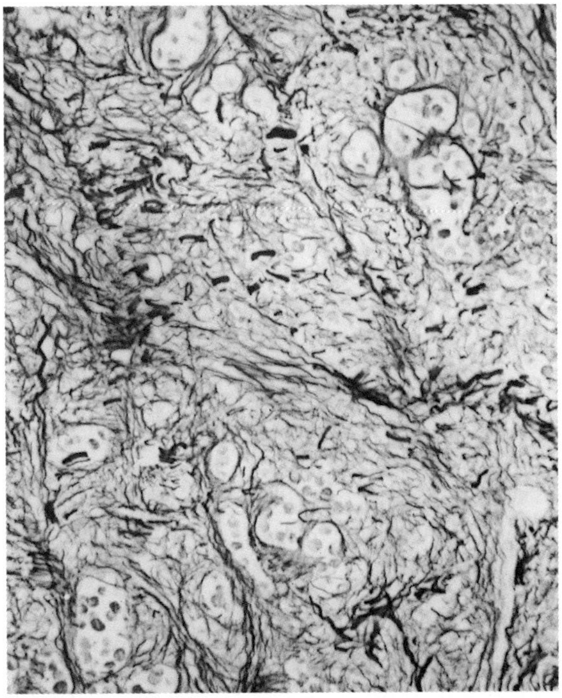

Fig. 38.2 Same tumor as shown in Figure 38.1. The distinction between sex cord and stromal elements is highlighted by staining for reticulin fibers, but further classification according to the nature of the sex cord elements is not possible. Reticulin ×150

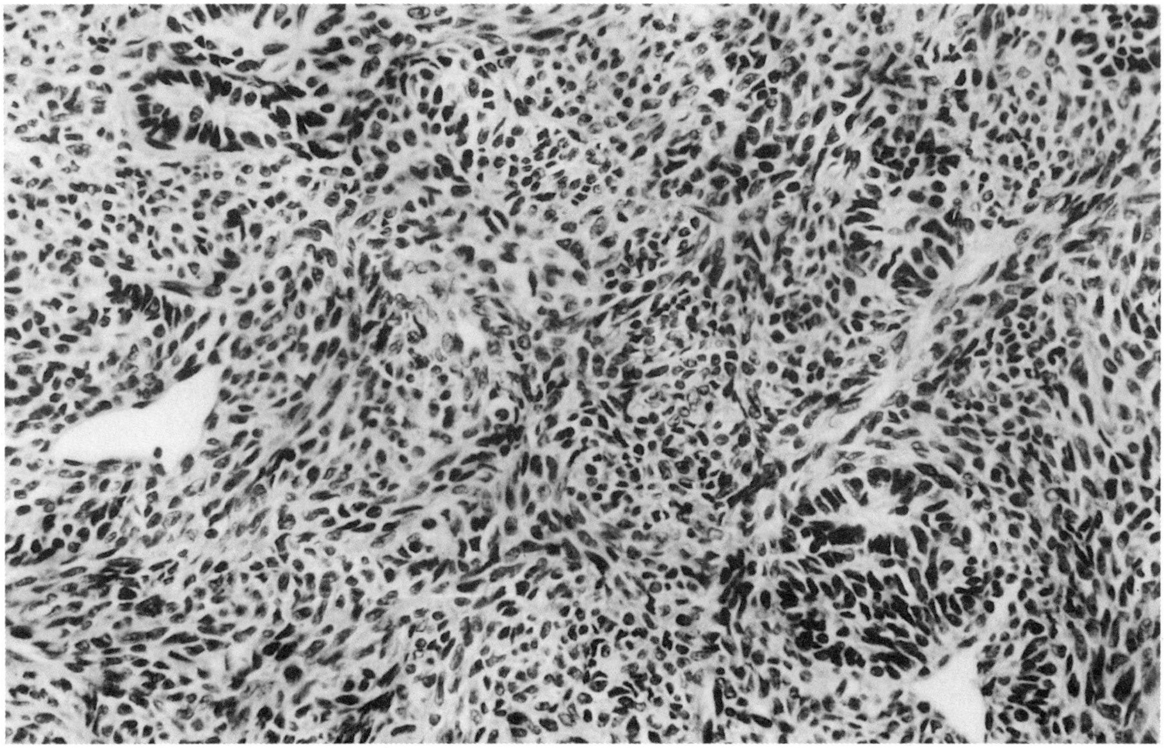

Fig. 38.3 Cellular fibroma with minor and poorly formed sex cord elements. Cellular anaplasia and nuclear atypia are absent, and this tumor behaved in a benign fashion. H + E ×250

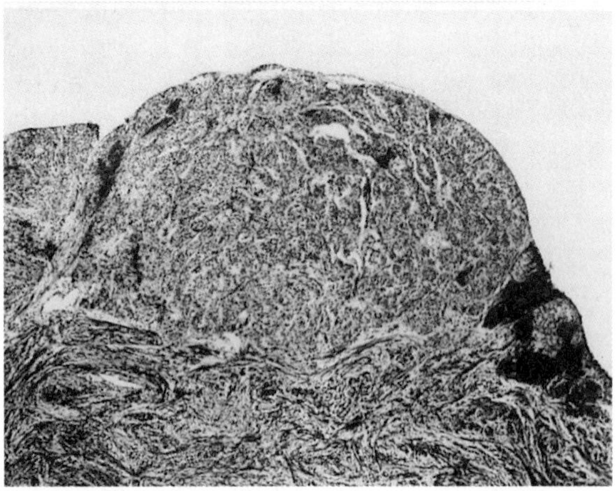

Fig. 38.4 Unclassified sex cord–stromal tumor. Several small nodules, varying from one to several millimeters across, were present beneath the serosa of the right ovary. Elsewhere there was marked stromal hyperthecosis. H + E ×25

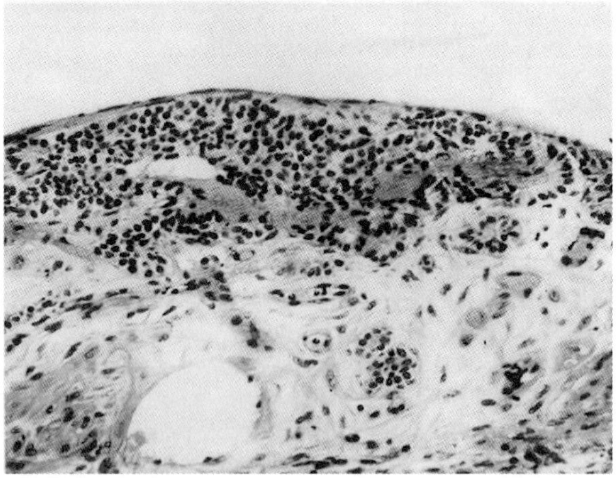

Fig. 38.5 Unclassified sex cord–stromal tumor (same tumor as shown in Fig. 38.4). Microscopic aggregate of cords of granulosa-like cells beneath the ovarian serosa. The histological absence of any stromal response and prolonged follow-up without clinical declaration of tumor recurrence were against these lesions being metastatic from some other site. H + E ×125

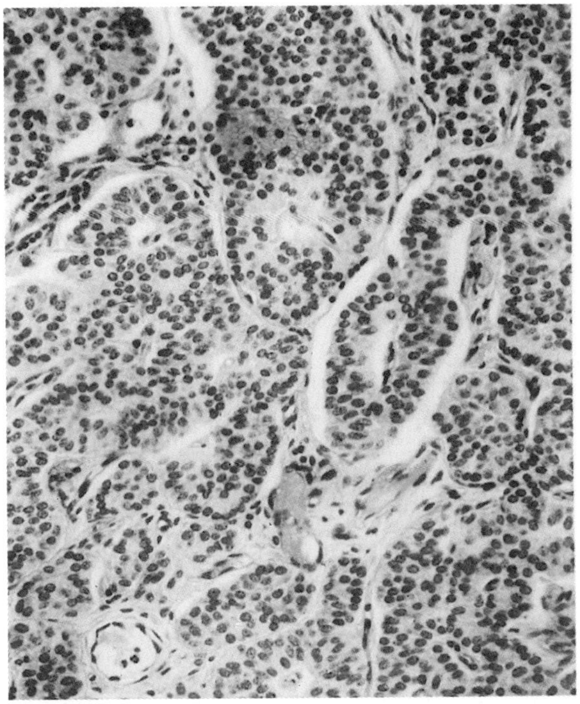

Fig. 38.6 Unclassified sex cord–stromal tumor (same tumor as shown in Fig. 38.4). Solid cords and ribbons of small granulosa-like cells. Immunohistochemical stains excluded carcinoid tumor. H + E ×150

spindle cell tumors with occasional tubular or cord-like structures which are impossible to categorize further (Figs 38.1, 38.2). Two small series (Morris & Scully 1958, Fox & Langley 1976) indicate a clinical course not appreciably different from that of granulosa cell tumors or Sertoli–Leydig cell tumors. It is important to stress that diagnosis is based on morphological features alone, and clinical evidence of hormonal activity plays no part in classification.

Well differentiated stromal tumors (fibromas) with minor sex cord elements (Fig. 38.3) represent another rare category of tumors which, until recently, we would have placed in this unclassified group (see Ch. 34). Tumors which are intermediate between thecomas and fibromas (and these, by contrast, are frequently observed) are placed in an 'unclassified' subgroup of the thecoma–fibroma group in the World Health Organization classification, but are termed 'thecafibromas' in our schema (see Ch. 34). By convention, steroid cell tumors are also discussed separately, although generically they belong to this group.

The distinctive morphology and clinical correlates justify separation of sex cord tumors with annular tubules (see Ch. 37) from this group of unclassified sex cord–stromal tumors. However, two examples of a perhaps related but distinct tumor associated with isosexual pseudoprecocity and occurring in girls with the Peutz–Jeghers syndrome (Young et al 1983) remain. Not having encountered a similar neoplasm in patients without this disorder, Young et al have suggested that this type of tumor may be an additional manifestation of Peutz–Jeghers syndrome, a concept supported by the unique concurrence of microscopic appearances in these tumors (diffuse areas, tubular differentiation, microcysts and papillae, and at least two distinctive cell types). Both tumors were benign, although follow-up in one case was short.

Other unusual lesions, such as those illustrated in Figures 38.4–38.6, are also best placed in this category to await further documentation.

REFERENCES

Fox H, Langley F A 1976 Tumours of the ovary. Heinemann, London

Morris J McL, Scully R E 1958 Endocrine pathology of the ovary, Mosby, St Louis, MI

Young R H, Scully R E 1984 Ovarian sex cord–stromal tumors: recent advances and current status. Clinics in Obstetrics and Gynaecology 11: 93–134

Young R H, Dickersin G R, Scully R E 1983 A distinctive ovarian sex cord–stromal tumor causing sexual precocity in the Peutz–Jeghers syndrome. American Journal of Surgical Pathology 7: 233–243

39

Steroid (lipid) cell tumors

P. Russell   A. Farnsworth

Steroid (lipid) cell tumors, not otherwise specified, are infrequently encountered ovarian neoplasms which exhibit an organoid or diffuse arrangement of large, rounded, or polygonal cells which resemble Leydig, stromal lutein, or adrenal cortical cells. The term 'lipid or lipoid cell tumors', suffering the disadvantages of encompassing a group of lesions of largely unknown origin, some of which contain little or no lipid, has been supplanted, in the revised World Health Organization classification of ovarian tumors by the term 'steroid cell tumors'. By convention, neoplasms with cellular features pathognomonic of a particular tumor type are excluded, although this is not a position endorsed by all (Fox & Langley 1976). Hilus or Leydig cells derived from the ovarian stroma (Sternberg & Roth 1973), indeed, are a suggested source for some steroid cell tumors. As Leydig cells can only be identified positively by finding Reinke's crystals, and these structures are often sparse in typical Leydig cell tumors of the ovary (see Ch. 35), it is highly likely that some steroid cell tumors are unidentifiable Leydig cell tumors.

The likely cells of origin of many of these tumors are theca–lutein or stromal–lutein cells. Evidence supporting this includes a marked resemblance of tumor cells to stromal–lutein cells and the demonstrable origin of occasional small discrete lesions, indistinguishable from typical steroid cell tumors, within the ovarian stroma. These nodules, associated often with stromal hyperthecosis (nodules of lutein cells in the neighboring stroma), have been designated as stromal luteomas (Scully 1964, Sternberg & Dhurandhar 1977), although in our view it is debatable whether such lesions are true neoplasms, and they are therefore discussed in Chapter 14. Pregnancy luteomas, or nodular theca–lutein hyperplasia of pregnancy (see Ch. 10), are histologically very similar to the steroid cell group of tumors and demonstrate the proliferative potential of the ovarian stroma. The differentiation of pregnancy luteomas from steroid cell tumors, not otherwise specified, is given in Table 39.1.

Although the lipid-rich cells of many of these tumors bear a close resemblance to the adrenocortical cells, this similarity cannot, in itself, be regarded as a serious basis for tumor classification. Adrenal cortical rests in the vicinity of the ovary have also, therefore, been proposed as a possible origin for some of these lesions. However, while such rests are common (see Ch. 3), they occur in the broad ligament, mesosalpinx, fallopian tube wall, and mesovarium rather than within the

Table 39.1 Differential diagnosis: steroid cell tumor versus pregnancy luteoma

Steroid cell tumor	Pregnancy luteoma
Clinical	
Mean age 47 years	Mean age 26 years
No relationship to pregnancy; no racial tendency	Diagnosed at or near term, or in puerperium; 80% in black women
Almost always unilateral	Often bilateral and multicentric
75% of women virilized	Asymptomatic
Histological	
Abundant intracellular lipid	Relatively little or no lipid
Necrosis, if present, only focal	Diffuse acute regressive changes if removed in puerperium
No pregnancy changes in adjacent uninvolved ovary	Pregnancy changes in adjacent ovary (deciduosis, hyperthecosis)

ovarian stroma (Symonds & Driscoll 1973); steroid cell tumors, by contrast, occur in the cortical and medullary stroma of the ovaries, and only isolated reports exist of steroid cell tumors located outside the ovaries (Klaiber et al 1987).

About 150 or so acceptable cases have been reported. Most frequently they occur in women of reproductive age, particularly during the third and fourth decades, and rarely in postmenopausal women or children (Harris et al 1991). They are clinically androgenic in 40% of cases (Hayes & Scully 1987) and regularly secrete androstenedione (Bonaventura et al 1978), α-hydroxyprogesterone, testosterone, and dehydroepiandrosterone (Scully 1979). The onset of virilization tends to be gradual rather than abrupt, and is usually preceded by amenorrhea and loss of female body contour. Also, a further 7% of cases have been associated with Cushing-like syndromes (Hayes & Scully 1987), with elevated serum cortisol levels. Biochemical profiles of these tumors, such as responses to adrenocortico trophic hormone (ACTH) stimulation and dexamethasone or prednisone suppression tests, are noted in Chapter 5. Nonspecific symptoms referable to the physical presence of the tumor, abdominal pain, and swelling occur in relatively few patients. A 'collision' tumor between a serous carcinoma and a steroid cell tumor has been reported (Nirenberg et al 1992).

Over 30% of steroid cell tumors in the largest reported series (Hayes & Scully 1987) have pursued a malignant clinical course, with spread within the abdomen and occasional distant metastases. In this series tumor size (7 cm in diameter or larger), 2 or more mitoses per 10 HPF, necrosis and hemorrhage, and marked nuclear atypia were adverse correlates of prognosis. Fox & Langley (1976), by contrast, have noted a benign course in 95% of adrenal-like tumors, which form the bulk of this steroid cell group. Unilateral salpingo-oophorectomy appears adequate management for small ovarian tumors apparently encapsulated and confined to one ovary at thorough staging laparotomy. Tumors greater than 8 cm in diameter or which show evidence of extraovarian extension should be treated by more extensive surgery. Inadequate experience with adjuvant therapy precludes sensible evaluation of its efficacy.

Macroscopic features

These tumors are almost always well circumscribed, unilateral without predilection for either ovary, and solid. Cystic variants, due to focal degeneration and secondary intracystic hemorrhage, have been observed. They vary greatly in size from 0.5 to 45 cm in diameter. The cut surface, which bulges in the fresh state, is frequently lobulated and ranges in color from bright yellow through reddish-brown to dark green-brown. The smaller tumors tend to occupy the medullary or hilar region of the ovary. Necrosis and hemorrhage may be present in larger tumors.

Microscopic features

The tumors are well demarcated from the surrounding ovarian stroma, which is compressed rather than invaded. They usually have an organoid pattern common to many steroid-producing tumors, consisting of rounded or polygonal vacuolated cells arranged in nests or columns (Fig. 39.1) and separated by a rich network of capillaries and vascular sinusoids. The columns may be arranged centripetally from the capsule, simulating the adrenal cortex. Less commonly, there is a diffuse arrangement of cells (Fig. 39.2). The tumor cell cytoplasm is moderate to abundant in amount and varies correspondingly from granular and eosinophilic (as seen in the adrenal zona reticularis) (Fig. 39.1) to foamy and lipid-rich (as seen in the zona fasciculata) (Fig. 39.2). Stains for neutral lipid are strongly positive in 75% of tumors. Lipochrome pigment granules vary from very sparse to numerous. Cytoplasmic glycogen may be present in some cases. Reticulin fibers invest individual or small groups of cells, but interstitial fibrosis and hyalinization are rarely prominent. Nuclei tend to be small and central with effaced chromatin and, while varying degrees of nuclear pleiomorphism and mitotic activity (usually more than in ovarian Leydig cell tumors) have been observed, a diagnosis of malignancy can only really be made morphologically in the presence of local invasion. Areas of necrosis, hemorrhage, and hyaline fibrosis (which may be calcified) are sometimes present, as are broad areas of myxoid-like connective tissue containing

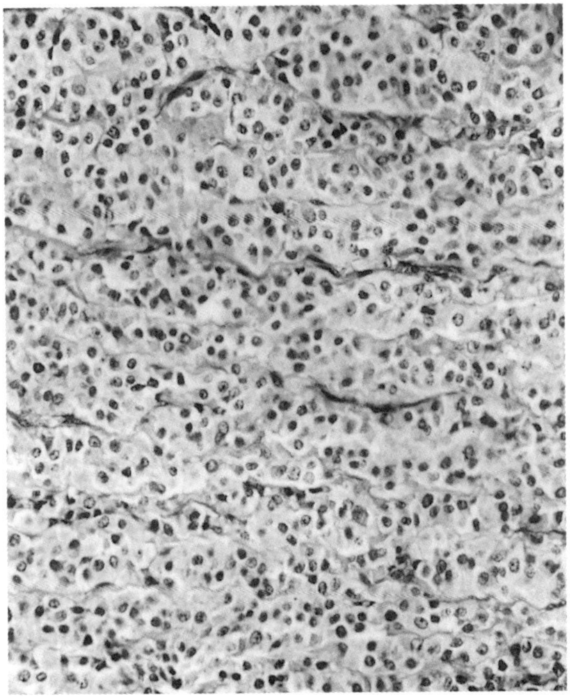

Fig. 39.1 Lipid cell tumor with a fascicular pattern due to the cord-like arrangement of tumor cells and the intervening vascular stroma. H + E ×150

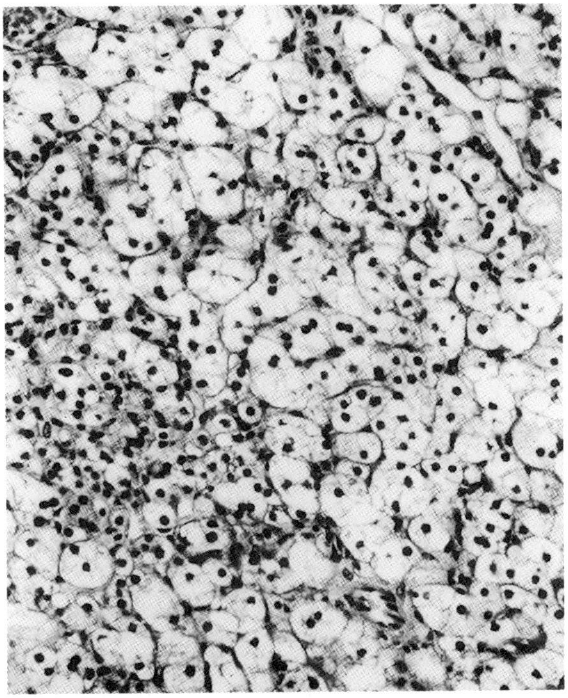

Fig. 39.2 Lipid cell tumor with a solid pattern of growth of large polyhedral cells with vacuolated lipid-rich cytoplasm. H + E ×150

clusters or cords of tumor cells (Osborn et al 1969).

Immunohistochemically, 75% of tumors show staining for vimentin, about 40% focally for various cytokeratins and 30% for smooth muscle actin (Seidman et al 1995). Steroid cell tumors are negative for chromogranin, Leu M1, α-fetoprotein, CEA, and HMB-45.

Differential diagnosis

From the group of solid tumors composed of lipid-rich steroid-producing cells, the diagnosis of steroid cell tumor is basically one of exclusion. The specific histological features that enable identification of Leydig cell tumors are discussed in Chapter 35, and those which clinically distinguish pregnancy luteomas (rare large nodules of lutein cells which develop during pregnancy and regress spontaneously postpartum) from steroid cell tumors are outlined in Table 39.1. Luteinized thecomas (see Ch. 34) exhibit clusters of lutein cells that are very similar to those of steroid cell tumors, but these cells are found in a background of spindled fibroblastic or theca-type cells. Primary clear cell carcinomas of mullerian epithelial type may have a uniform solid pattern of clear cells (see Ch. 27). These latter cells, however, are rich in glycogen and contain scanty lipid, in direct contrast to those of typical steroid cell tumors. They are only occasionally virilizing and are associated with pelvic endometriosis in two-thirds of cases.

REFERENCES

Bonaventura L M, Judd H, Roth L M, Cleary R E 1978 Androgen, estrogen and progestogen production by a lipid cell tumor of the ovary. American Journal of Obstetrics and Gynecology 131: 403–409

Fox H, Langley F A 1976 Tumours of the ovary. Heinemann, London, p 262–277

Harris A C, Wakely P E Jr, Kaplowitz P B, Lovinger R D 1991 Steroid cell tumor of the ovary in a

child. Archives of Pathology and Laboratory Medicine 115: 150–154
Hayes M C, Scully R E 1987 Ovarian steroid cell tumors (not otherwise specified). A clinicopathological analysis of 63 cases. American Journal of Surgical Pathology 11: 835–845
Klaiber H, Genton C, Schreiner W, Keller P J 1987 Extraovariell gelegener virilisierender Lipidzelltumor. Geburtshilfe und Frauenheilkind 47: 817–820
Nirenberg A, Östör A G, Quinn M A 1992 Collision tumor: serous adenocarcinoma and steroid cell tumor of the ovary. Pathology 24: 60–62
Osborn R H, Bradbury J T, Yannone E 1969 Androgen studies in a patient with lipoid-cell tumor of the ovary. Obstetrics and Gynecology 33: 666–672
Scully R E 1964 Stromal luteoma of the ovary. A distinctive type of lipoid-cell tumor. Cancer 17: 769–778
Scully R E 1979 Tumors of the ovary and maldeveloped gonads. AFIP fascicle 16, 2nd series. Armed Forces Institute of Pathology, Washington, DC
Seidman J D, Abbondanzo S L, Bratthauer G L 1995 Lipid cell (steroid cell) tumor of the ovary: immunophenotype with analysis of potential pitfall due to endogenous biotin-like activity. International Journal of Gynecological Pathology 14: 331–338
Sternberg W H, Dhurandhar H M 1977 Functional ovarian tumors of stromal and sex cord origin. Human Pathology 8: 565–582
Sternberg W H, Roth L M 1973 Ovarian stromal tumors containing Leydig cells. I: Stromal–Leydig cell tumor and non-neoplastic transformation of ovarian stroma. Cancer 32: 940–951
Symonds D A, Driscoll S G 1973 An adrenal cortical rest within the fetal ovary. American Journal of Clinical Pathology 60: 562–564

Table 40.1 Percentage histological distribution of germ cell tumors encountered at King George V Hospital (1950–1975)

Tumor type	%
Dysgerminoma	1.0
Endodermal sinus tumor	Rare
Polyvesicular vitelline tumor	
Hepatoid variant	
Embryonal carcinoma	Rare
Polyembryoma	
Choriocarcinoma	Rare
Teratomas (98.5%)	
Immature (embryonal)	1.3
Mature (adult)	95.0
With secondary malignant change	0.5
Monodermal or specialized teratomas:	
–struma ovarii	1.3
–strumal carcinoid	0.4
–primary carcinoid	Rare
–other	Rare
Mixed malignant germ cell tumors	Rare
Total	100.0

Table 40.2 Percentage histological distribution of ovarian tumors occurring in females aged less than 20 years

Tumor type	%
Common epithelial tumors	22
Sex cord–stromal tumors	14
Germ cell tumors	58
Miscellaneous	5
Total	100

1982). Mostly they are encountered in young and fertile women, with a peak incidence in the third decade, and uncommonly over the age of 35 years. It can be seen that almost all are benign adult cystic teratomas and the remainder are infrequently encountered. For females below 20 years of age, however, figures derived from the combined series of Abell et al (1965) and Norris & Jensen (1972) indicate that relative frequencies of germ cell tumors in general (Table 40.2), and the malignant variants in particular, are considerably higher. These two series documented malignancy and potential malignancy rates of 29% and 55%, respectively, for ovarian tumors (these being mostly of germ cell origin) occurring in this age group. The vast majority (about 85%) of germ cell tumors occurring in girls below 10 years of age are malignant.

Malignant germ cell tumors frequently present as an acute condition with abdominal pain and a palpable mass arising from the pelvis. The presentation is commonly mistaken for acute appendicitis. Hemorrhage, cyst rupture and, less commonly, ovarian torsion frequently precipitate patients presenting to hospital emergency rooms outside normal working hours. Appropriate preoperative investigations include serum measurements of β-human chorionic ganadotrophin (β-hCG) and α-fetoprotein (AFP), which form an integral part of postoperative monitoring. The prototypical tumors producing β hCG and AFP are choriocarcinoma and yolk sac tumor, respectively. Dysgerminoma has traditionally been associated with no tumor marker secretion, although small concentrations of β-hCG have been reported (Ueda et al 1972). More recently, elevations of certain isoenzymes of lactic dehydrogenase, a glycolytic enzyme, have been reported in association with dysgerminomas (Friedman et al 1984).

At operation, ovarian germ cell tumors tend to be mostly solid and larger than 10 cm. An accompanying hematoperitoneum or ascites is not uncommon. These tumors are usually unilateral, with the exception of dysgerminomas which are bilateral in 10–15% of cases. Benign cystic teratomas may occur concurrently in either the ipsilateral or contralateral ovary, and rarely in both ovaries.

The dissemination of germ cell tumors is similar to that of epithelial–stromal ovarian tumors. Lymphatic spread is thought to be a more common route, in particular, with dysgerminomas where dissemination demonstrates a predilection for the para-aortic nodes. However, unlike epithelial–stromal tumors, 60% of germ cell tumors are International Federation of Gynecology and Obstetrics FIGO stage 1.

The young age at diagnosis, the desire to preserve fertility, the early stage at presentation, and the sensitivity of these tumors to adjuvant treatment mandate a different surgical approach to that for epithelial ovarian tumors. Unilateral salpingo-oophorectomy is now the standard surgical procedure, with surgical interruption of the contralateral ovary restricted to suspicious enlargement or cysts. A thorough exploration of the abdominal cavity and retroperitoneal nodes is required to stage the disease adequately.

When advanced disease is encountered, cytoreductive surgery is recommended, although there is little evidence to support the efficacy of this approach. Major cytoreductive surgery can be undertaken in this context whilst preserving the contralateral ovary and the uterus. The role of second-look laparotomy for ovarian germ cell tumors remains uncertain. Most patients will demonstrate negative re-explorations and biopsied material is often mature teratoma (Gershenson et al 1986). Postoperative treatment is determined by surgical stage, histology, and tumor grade. Conservative management by surgery alone has been advocated for stage 1a dysgerminomas. Tumor recurrence rates of up to 50% have been reported with expectant postoperative surveillance. This may, in part, be due to suboptimal surgical staging. Other investigators have proposed conservative treatment only where the tumor is confined to one ovary measuring less than 10 cm (Krepart et al 1978). Microscopic prognostic factors that predict recurrence include anaplasia, a medullary tumor pattern, and high mitotic count (Gordon et al 1981). Impressive results following salvage chemotherapy have also added support to conservative postoperative management. Sustained remission following conservative surgery alone for stage 1a disease exceeds 95% (Thomas et al 1987). The current primary chemotherapy treatment for patients with early stage disease considered to be at high risk of recurrence is with combination therapy consisting of bleomycin, etoposide, and cisplatin (BEP) (Gershenson 1993). This regimen has replaced other chemotherapy combinations including VBP (vinblastine, bleomycin, cisplatin) and VAC (vincristine, actinomycin, and cyclophosphamide). For metastatic dysgerminomas, combination chemotherapy has replaced abdominal radiation following cytoreductive surgery, with cure rates approaching 90% (Williams et al 1991).

For all patients with nondysgerminomatous tumors, postoperative chemotherapy is recommended regardless of surgical stage. The exception is a stage 1a, grade 1, immature teratoma, which demonstrates an excellent prognosis with unilateral salpingo-oophorectomy alone. The recommended primary chemotherapy for all nondysgerminomatous tumors is currently bleomycin combination therapy (BEP). The 5-year survival rate for all stages of disease is 70–80% (Mayordomo et al 1994).

Long-term follow-up has demonstrated that 80% of patients resume regular menses and the conception rate is approximately 75%. The risk of birth defects does not appear to be increased (Gershensen 1988).

REFERENCES

Abell M R, Johnson V J, Holtz M 1965 Ovarian neoplasms in childhood and adolescence. Part I. Tumors of germ cell origin. American Journal of Obstetrics and Gynecology 92: 1059–1081

Friedman M, White R G, Nissenbaum M M, Browde S 1984 Serum lactic dehydrogenase – a possible tumor marker for an ovarian dysgerminoma: a literature review and report of a case. Obstetrical and Gynecological Survey 39: 247–251

Gershenson D M 1988 Menstrual and reproductive function after treatment with combination chemotherapy for malignant ovarian germ cell tumors. Journal of Clinical Oncology 6: 270–275

Gershenson D M 1993 Update on malignant ovarian germ cell tumors. Cancer 71 (suppl): 1581–1590

Gershenson D M, Copeland L J, Del Junco G, Edwards C L, Wharton J T, Rutledge F N 1986 Second look laparotomy in the management of malignant germ cell tumors of the ovary. Obstetrics and Gynecology 67: 789–793

Gondos B, Bhiraleus P, Hobel C J 1971 Ultrastructural observations on germ cells in human fetal ovaries. American Journal of Obstetrics and Gynecology 110: 644–652

Gonzales-Crussi F 1982 Extragonadal teratomas. AFIP fascicle 18, 2nd series. Armed Forces Institute of Pathology, Washington, DC, p 1–25

Gordon A, Lipton D, Woodruff J D 1981 Dysgerminoma: a review of 158 cases from the Emil Novak Ovarian Tumor Registry. Obstetrics and Gynecology 58: 497–504

Hecht F, McCaw B K, Patil S 1976 Ovarian teratomas and genetics of germ-cell formation. Lancet ii: 1311

Hou-Jensen K, Kempson R L 1974 The ultrastructure of gonadoblastoma and dysgerminoma. Human Pathology 5: 79–91

Kay S, Silverberg S G, Schatzki P F 1972 Ultrastructure of an ovarian dysgerminoma. Report of a case featuring neurosecretory-type granules in stromal cells. American Journal of Clinical Pathology 58: 458–468

Krepart G, Smith J P, Rutledge F, Delclos L 1978 The treatment of dysgerminoma of the ovary. Cancer 41: 986–990

Linder D, McCaw B K, Hecht F 1975 Parthenogenic origin of benign ovarian teratomas. New England Journal of Medicine 292: 63–66

Mayordomo J I, Paz-Ares L, Rivera F et al 1994 Ovarian and extragonadal malignant germ-cell tumors in females: a single-institution experience with 43 patients. Annals of Oncology 5: 225–231

Norris H J, Jensen R D 1972 Relative frequency of ovarian neoplasms in children and adolescents. Cancer 30: 713–719

Ohama K, Nomura K, Okamoto E, Fukuda Y, Ihara T,

Fujiwara A 1985 Origin of immature teratoma of the ovary. American Journal of Obstetrics and Gynecology 152: 896–900

Parrington J M, West L F, Povey S 1984 The origin of ovarian teratomas. Journal of Medical Genetics 21: 4–12

Russell P, Painter D M 1982 The pathological assessment of ovarian neoplasms. V: The germ cell tumors. Pathology 14: 47–72

Skakkebaek N E 1975 Atypical germ cells in the adjacent 'normal' tissue of testicular tumors. Acta Pathologica et Microbiologica Scandinavica (A) 83: 127–130

Skakkebaek N E 1978 Carcinoma in situ of the testis: frequency and relationship to invasive germ cell tumors in infertile men. Histopathology 2: 157–170

Sobis H, Vandeputte M 1974 Development of teratomas from displaced visceral yolk sac. International Journal of Cancer 13: 444–453

Sobis H, Vandeputte M 1976 Yolk sac-derived rat teratomas are not of germ cell origin. Developmental Biology 51: 320–323

Sobis H, Vandeputte M 1977 Yolk sac-derived teratomas and carcinomas in hamsters. European Journal of Cancer 13: 1175–1181

Teilum G 1976 Special tumors of ovary and testis and related extragonadal lesions, 2nd edn. Munksgaard, Copenhagen, p 68

Thomas G M, Dembo A J, Hacker N F, de Petrillo A D 1987 Current therapy for dysgerminoma of the ovary. Obstetrics and Gynecology 70: 268–275

Ueda G, Hamanaka N, Hayakawa K et al 1972 Clinical, histochemical and biochemical studies of an ovarian dysgerminoma with trophoblasts and Leydig cells. American Journal of Obstetrics and Gynecology 114: 748–754

Williams S D, Blessing J A, Hatch K D, Homesley H D 1991 Chemotherapy of advanced ovarian dysgerminoma: trials of the Gynecologic Oncology Group. Journal of Clinical Oncology 9: 1950–1955

Witschi E 1963 Embryology of the ovary. In Grady H G, Smith D E (eds) The ovary. IAP Monograph Series. Williams & Wilkins, Baltimore, p 1–10

41

Dysgerminomas

P. Russell A. Farnsworth

Dysgerminomas are composed entirely of sheets of large uniform pale cells which show many histological, histochemical, and electron microscopical features (Hou-Jensen & Kempson 1974, Hees et al 1991) in common with primordial germ cells. The tumor cells have abundant pale, slightly granular eosinophilic to clear cytoplasm which is EMA negative and mostly cytokeratin negative (Table 41.1), and exhibit well delineated cell boundaries (Fig. 41.1A) and a large central vesicular nucleus. The cytoplasm contains a variable amount of glycogen demonstrable by the PAS reaction; cytoplasmic lipid can also be demonstrated in frozen sections. Nuclei are oval to round with finely granular chromatin and usually a single prominent eosinophilic nucleolus (Fig. 41.1B).

Dysgerminomas are infrequently encountered neoplasms and, as pure tumors, comprise only about 1% of ovarian germ cell tumors (see Ch. 40) and a similar proportion of all primary ovarian malignant tumors (Kurman & Norris 1977, Scully 1979). They may present at any age from infancy to old age, but are rare below 5 years of age and after the menopause. Most cases occur in the second and third decades; indeed, 80–85% of patients are below the age of 30 years at diagnosis (Scully 1979, Talerman 1982). Therefore, dysgerminomas account for a disproportionately high percentage of malignant ovarian neoplasms of childhood, adolescence, and early adulthood.

Table 41.1 Immunophenotype of dysgerminomas

Antibody against	Expression %
LDH	100
PlAP	100
NSE	75
AE1/AE3	10
β-hCG	5
EMA	–
S-100 protein	–
LCA	–
Vimentin	–
AFP	–

The presenting symptoms of dysgerminomas (a lower abdominal mass or abdominal enlargement, sometimes associated with weight loss and acute pain due to torsion) are similar to those observed in patients with other ovarian neoplasms, although often of shorter duration. Less frequently, they have been found incidentally, such as at a routine antenatal examination (Asadourian & Taylor 1969, Talerman et al 1973, Krepart et al 1978) or during investigation for primary amenorrhea. In the latter 3–5% of cases, one of the various forms of gonadal dysgenesis is usually present in association with a karyotype containing a Y chromosome. In such patients, the resulting dysgerminoma is commonly a small tumor and almost invariably supervenes upon a gonadoblastoma (see Ch. 51) (Scully 1970, Schellhas 1974a,b, Williamson et al 1976). Occasional cases of allegedly pure dysgerminomas have been reported in association with menstrual and endocrine abnormalities in adults, or mildly elevated serum chorionic gonadotrophins (Brettell et al 1984) or signs of isosexual pseudoprecocity in children (Breen & Neubecker 1967, Asadourian & Taylor 1969), these manifestations regressing following removal of the tumor (Burkons & Hart 1978). These symptoms, however, are more typical of dysgerminomas mixed with other malignant germ cell elements, notably choriocarcinoma.

Dysgerminomas are fast growing tumors, but

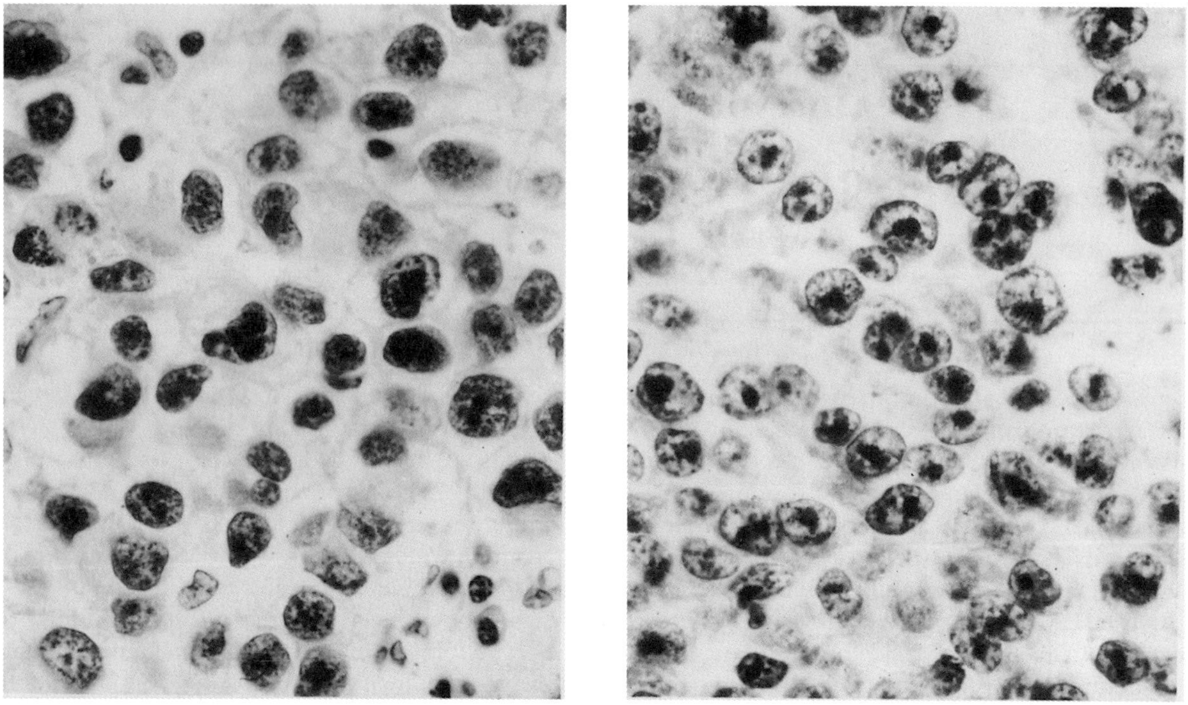

A B

Fig. 41.1 Cellular detail of dysgerminomas. (A) Tumor cells are large (note plasma cell at bottom right for comparison) with round to slightly angular vesicular nuclei, pale cytoplasm and obvious cellular margins. (B) Cytoplasm is more granular and cell borders less distinct here, but nuclear details (with very prominent single nucleolus) are characteristic. H + E ×500

metastases do not commonly occur early in their clinical course. They are confined to one ovary (FIGO stage 1a) in two-thirds of cases at presentation and to both ovaries (stage 1b) in a further 10%, but it should be noted that this figure includes 6% in which contralateral ovarian involvement is only microscopic (Kurman & Norris 1977), thus underpinning the importance of biopsy examination of both ovaries in patients for whom conservative surgery is planned (see below). They are bilateral in about 15% of all cases. A higher proportion of tumors are bilateral when associated with a gonadoblastoma (Scully 1970, Schellhas 1974a,b, Hart & Burkons 1979). Unilateral tumors show a slight tendency to be right-sided (Talerman 1982, La Polla et al 1987). Lymphatic spread affects first the common iliac and lowermost para-aortic groups of nodes, and subsequently the mediastinal and supraclavicular nodes. Blood-borne spread to distant organs typically occurs late, with liver, lungs, kidneys, and bones the most common sites for secondary deposits (Mueller et al 1950, Afridi et al 1976, Burkons & Hart 1978, Freel et al 1979).

FIGO stage at laparotomy and size of tumor are the most important prognostic indicators. Dysgerminomas are associated with an overall 5-year survival rate of 75–90% (Afridi et al 1976, Krepart et al 1978), while survival of patients with 'encapsulated' stage 1a tumors (i.e. the tumor capsules are not invaded by dysgerminoma cells) is over 90% (Afridi et al 1976, Krepart et al 1978, Gallion et al 1988) despite a significant (about 25%) recurrence rate, and 63% for patients with spread beyond the ovaries (Gordon et al 1981, Zaloudek & Kurman 1983, Gallion et al 1988). It is relevant to note here that over 75% of recurrences occur in the first year after diagnosis. Patients aged below 20 years or over 40 years may also be associated with a worse prognosis. Conservative therapy (unilateral salpingo-oophorectomy) is appropriate for the two-thirds of patients who are karyotypically normal young women with an encapsulated unilateral tumor, for whom

cystic spaces are encountered in which the epithelium exhibits more definite intestinal differentiation (Scully 1979). Extremely rarely, entire tumors exhibit the polyvesicular vitelline pattern, and such neoplasms are termed 'polyvesicular vitelline tumors' (Nogales et al 1978).

In addition to these well-defined patterns, further variants termed 'endodermal sinus tumors with hepatoid differentiation' ('hepatoid yolk sac carcinomas') by Prat et al (1982) have a mostly solid pattern typified by sheets and nests of eosinophilic, mitotically active, cells in a cellular fibrous stroma and resembling hepatocellular carcinoma. These authors and others (Ulbright et al 1986, Nakashima et al 1987) have also been able to identify small foci of hepatoid differentiation in 16–48% of otherwise unremarkable yolk sac tumors, thus strengthening this association (Fig. 42.13). How much of this 'somatic' or 'embryonal' differentiation is required to reclassifiy such tumors as mixed malignant germ cell in type (see Ch. 50) has not been determined. No bile is produced in these tumors. Variably sized cystic spaces filled with mucicarmine-positive material may be present, giving a honeycomb appearance, and this tumor pattern occasionally merges with adjacent areas showing the polyvesicular vitelline variant described above. The tumor cells are polygonal with distinct cell borders, eosinophilic cytoplasm, and large rounded central nuclei, each containing a single prominent nucleolus. PAS-positive diastase-resistant hyaline droplets as described above are prominent. AFP and AAT are demonstrable by immunohistochemical techniques in tumor cell cytoplasm and, to a lesser extent, in the hyaline droplets. A related but apparently unique variant reported as showing intestinal differentiation (Cohen et al 1986, 1987, Kim et al 1989) (Figs 42.14, 42.15) is equally interpretable, in our view, as showing true yolk sac differentiation (compare with Fig. 42.1). It is characterized by nests of primitive endodermal glands within loose or hyalinized stroma. These glands contain dense eosinophilic secretion. The glands may also be composed of tall columnar

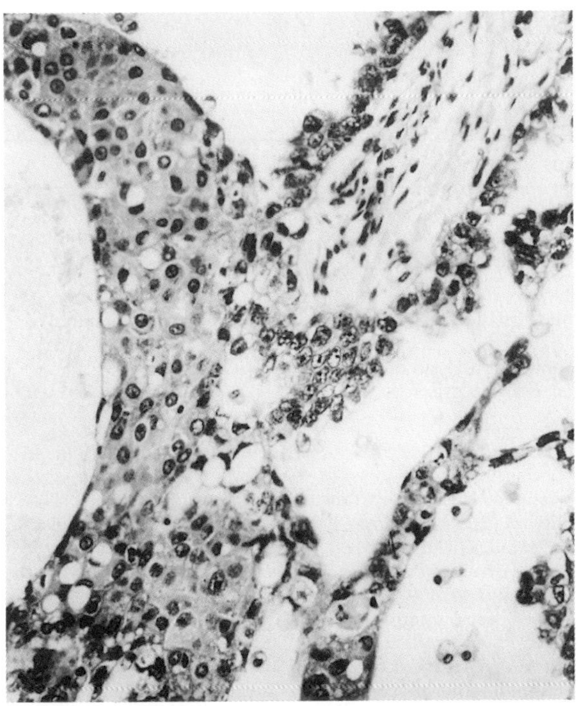

Fig. 42.13 Small focal aggregate of polyhedral eosinophilic hepatoid cells in an otherwise typical yolk sac tumor. H + E ×150

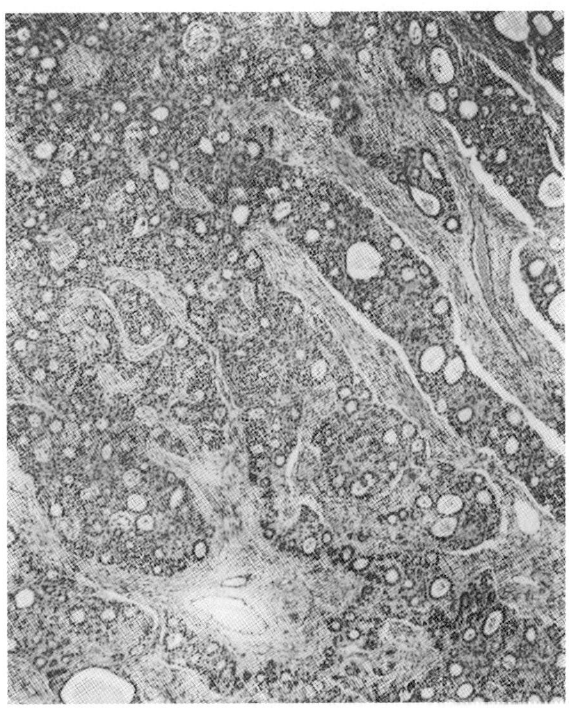

Fig. 42.14 So-called 'endodermal sinus tumor with intestinal differentiation'. Architecturally, this variant resembles normal early human yolk sac (Fig. 42.1). H + E ×30. (Material courtesy of Dr J Molnar, San Francisco)

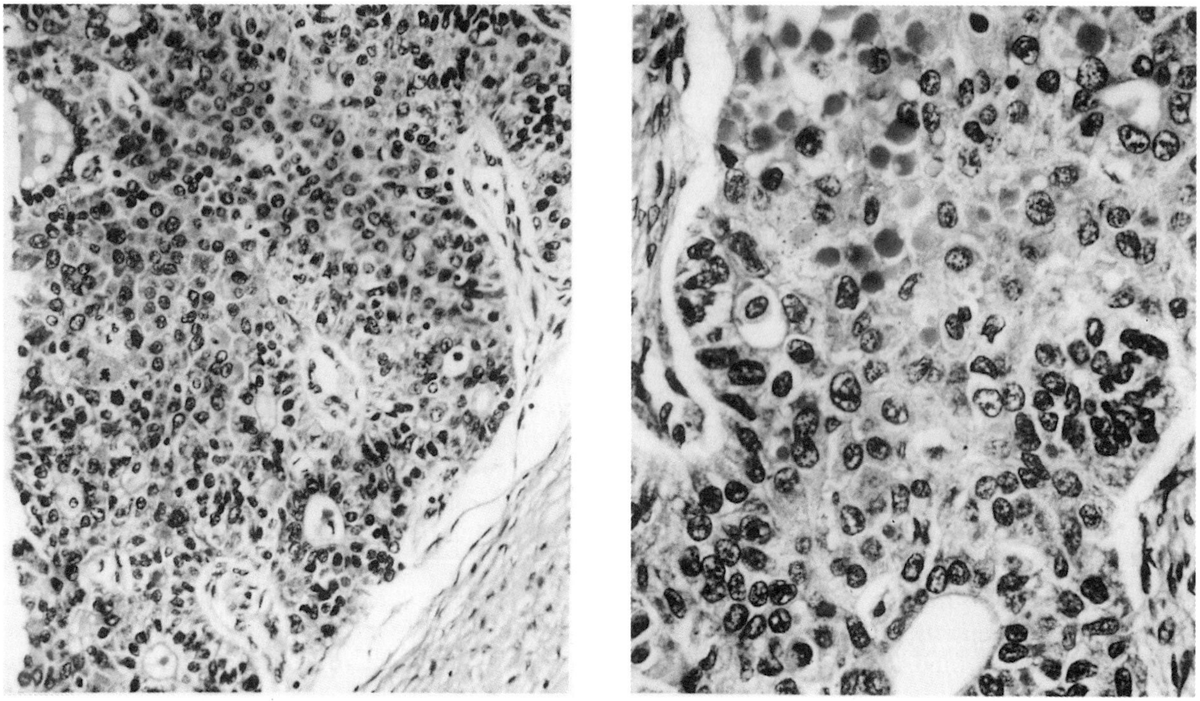

A B

Fig. 42.15 Higher power of same tumor with occasional gland-like spaces. (A) Interspersed amongst polygonal cells with prominent cell borders and eosinophilic cytoplasm. H + E ×150. (B) Polygonal cells in upper portion of figure exhibit many PAS-positive diastase-resistant, eosinophilic hyaline bodies. H + E ×300. (Material courtesy of Dr J Molnar, San Francisco)

or cuboidal cells with vacuolated cytoplasm resembling secretory endometrium (Clement et al 1987).

Differential diagnosis

Mullerian clear cell carcinomas (see Ch. 27) and embryonal carcinomas (see Ch. 43) of the ovaries are the two neoplasms with which yolk sac tumors might be confused histologically. Clear cell carcinomas, which usually occur in the fifth to seventh decades, typically are large thick-walled cystic tumors with numerous yellow-fawn, fleshy nodules projecting into the lumen (Table 42.1). Histologically, they show much more regular tubulopapillary patterns and lack the honeycomb meshwork of cystic spaces and channels of yolk sac tumors. The tubular lining cells either have abundant clear cytoplasm or are hobnailed with nuclei which bulge into the lumen, in contrast to the rather pleiomorphic primitive cells of yolk sac tumors. Hobnail cells are rarely seen in yolk sac tumors. In clear cell carcinomas the papillary processes are finer and more frond like and are

Table 42.1 Differential diagnosis: yolk sac tumor versus mullerian clear cell carcinoma

Yolk sac tumor	Clear cell carcinoma
Clinical	
Almost always occur under 30 years of age	Occur in 5th to 7th decades, peak incidence at 50 years
Macroscopic	
Solid, friable tumors with hemorrhage, necrosis and soft myxoid or gelatinous areas	Thick-walled, unilocular cysts with fleshy, yellow-fawn mural nodules
Histological	
Typical Schiller–Duval bodies in festoon areas	Regular frond-like papillae in tubulopapillary areas
Hobnail cells extremely rare	Hobnail cells common
Solid areas composed mostly of smaller primitive cells	Sheets of pavement-like clear cells with regular nuclei
Hyaline droplets stain for AFP and AAT	Hyaline intracellular bodies do not stain for AFP or AAT
Mitoses very numerous	Mitoses relatively uncommon
Polyvesicular vitelline areas have vesicles lined by cuboidal mucus-secreting cells or mesothelial-like cells	Parvilocular areas show cysts lined by either polyhedral clear cells or hobnail cells

also lined by polyhedral clear cells. Typical Schiller–Duval bodies are absent. Unlike those in yolk sac tumors, the eosinophilic PAS-positive rounded inclusions occasionally seen in clear cell carcinomas do not stain for AFP or AAT. Sheets of large pavement-like cells with clear cytoplasm containing small, dark, uniform, eccentric nuclei, typical of the solid pattern of clear cell carcinoma, are not seen in yolk sac tumors. Parvilocular or benign clear cell tumors are composed entirely of cystic spaces which may resemble superficially the reticular (Fig. 42.4) or polyvesicular vitelline (Fig. 42.12) patterns of yolk sac tumor. However, the epithelial linings in the former are either typical hobnail cells or large clear cells rather than the two types of epithelia (mesothelial-like cells in the broader portion, and columnar mucus-secreting cells in the narrow portion) seen in the different segments of the pear-shaped vesicles characteristic of the polyvesicular vitelline tumors.

Pure embryonal carcinomas are rare in the ovaries (see Ch. 43), are regularly associated with hormonal manifestations and lack any of the specific histological patterns observed in yolk sac tumors, as described above (Table 42.2). Poorly differentiated embryonal carcinomas are composed of masses of cells with more granular amphophilic cytoplasm, greater nuclear pleiomorphism, and even more prominent nucleoli. Syncytiotrophoblastic giant cells are regularly seen and these elaborate immunoreactive chorionic gonadotrophin. Better differentiated embryonal carcinomas exhibit cords, tubules, or cleft spaces lined by primitive epithelial cells, and somewhat more closely resemble poorly differentiated adult type adenocarcinomas rather than particular patterns of yolk sac tumors. Primitive mesenchymal elements such as islands of cartilage may also be present.

Table 42.2 Differential diagnosis: yolk sac tumor versus embryonal carcinoma

Yolk sac tumor	Embryonal carcinoma
Clinical	
No hormonal manifestations	Hormonal manifestations in 60%
Histological	
Spectrum of festoon, solid, reticular and polyvesicular vitelline patterns	Solid sheets of primitive cells with superficial resemblances to adult adenocarcinomas and sarcomas
No trophoblastic giant cells	Syncytiotrophoblastic giant cells which elaborate β-hCG

REFERENCES

Brown J R, Green J D 1976 Yolk sac carcinoma. Southern Medical Journal 69: 728–731

Clement P B, Young R H, Scully R E 1987 Endometrioid-like variant of ovarian yolk sac tumor. A clinicopathologic analysis of eight cases. American Journal of Surgical Pathology 11: 767–778

Clement P B, Young R H, Scully R E 1988 Extraovarian pelvic yolk sac tumors. Cancer 62: 620–626

Cohen M B, Mulchahey K M, Molnar J J 1986 Ovarian endodermal sinus tumor with intestinal differentiation. Cancer 57: 1580–1583

Cohen M B, Friend D S, Molnar J J, Talerman A 1987 Gonadal endodermal sinus (yolk sac) tumor with pure intestinal differentiation: a new histologic type. Pathology Research and Practice 182: 609–616

Gallion H, Van Nagell J R, Powell D F, Donaldson E S, Hanson M 1979 Therapy of endodermal sinus tumor of the ovary. American Journal of Obstetrics and Gynecology 135: 447–451

Gitlin D, Perricelli A 1970 Synthesis of serum albumin, prealbumin, α-fetoprotein, α_1-antitrypsin and transferrin by the human yolk sac. Nature 228: 995–997

Gonzalez-Crussi F, Roth L M 1976 The human yolk sac and yolk sac carcinoma. An ultrastructural study. Human Pathology 7: 675–691

Huntington R W Jr, Bullock W K 1970 Yolk sac tumors of the ovary. Cancer 25: 1357–1376

Jimerson G K, Woodruff J D 1977 Ovarian extra-embryonal teratoma: 1. Endodermal sinus tumor. American Journal of Obstetrics and Gynecology 127: 73–79

Kawai M, Furuhashi Y, Kano T et al 1990 α-Fetoprotein in malignant germ cell tumors of the ovary. Gynecologic Oncology 39: 160–166

Kawai M, Kano T, Furuhashi Y et al 1991 Prognostic factors in yolk sac tumors of the ovary. A clinicopathologic analysis of 29 cases. Cancer 67: 184–192

Kim C R, Hsui J G, Given F T 1989 Intestinal variant of ovarian endodermal sinus tumor. Gynecologic Oncology 33: 379–381

Kinoshita K 1990 A 62-year-old woman with endodermal sinus tumor of the ovary. American Journal of Obstetrics and Gynecology 162: 760–762

Kommoss F, Bibbo M, Talerman A 1990 Nuclear deoxyribonucleic acid content (ploidy) of endodermal sinus (yolk sac) tumor. Laboratory Investigation 62: 223–231

Kurman R J, Norris H J 1976 Endodermal sinus tumor of the ovary. A clinical and pathologic analysis of 71 cases. Cancer 38: 2402–2419

Kurman R J, Norris H J 1977 Malignant germ cell tumors of the ovary. Human Pathology 8: 551–564

Langley F A, Govan A D T, Anderson M C, Gowing N F C, Woodcock A S, Harilal K R 1981 Yolk sac and allied tumors of the ovary. Histopathology 5: 389–401

Mazur M T, Talbot W H Jr, Talerman A 1988 Endodermal sinus tumor and mucinous cystadenofibroma of the ovary. Occurrence in an 82-year-old woman. Cancer 62: 2011–2015

Michael H, Ulbright T M, Brodhecker C A 1989 The pluripotential nature of the mesenchyme-like component of yolk sac tumor. Archives of Pathology and Laboratory Medicine 113: 1115–1119

Morris H H B, La Vecchia C, Draper G J 1985 Endodermal sinus tumor and embryonal carcinoma of the ovary in children. Gynecologic Oncology 21: 7–17

Nakashima N, Fukatsu T, Nagasaki T, Sobue M, Takeuchi J 1987 The frequency and histology of hepatic tissue in germ cell tumors. American Journal of Surgical Pathology 11: 682–692

Nogales F F, Matilla A, Nogales-Ortiz F, Galera-Davidson H L 1978 Yolk sac tumors with pure and mixed polyvesicular vitelline patterns. Human Pathology 9: 553–566

Nogales F F, Beltran E, Pavcovich M, Bustos M 1992 Ectopic somatic endoderm in secondary human yolk sac. Human Pathology 23: 921–924

Okamoto T 1983 Comparative morphology of endodermal sinus tumor (Teilum) to human yolk sac and a proposal of endodermal cell tumor. Acta Pathologica Japonica 33: 1–14

Palmer P E, Safaii H, Wolfe H J 1976 α_1-Antitrypsin and α-fetoprotein, protein markers in endodermal sinus (yolk sac) tumors. American Journal of Clinical Pathology 65: 575–582

Penkar S J, Irani S, Prabhu V L, Candes F P, Nimbkar S A 1992 Endodermal sinus tumor of vulva (a case report). Journal of Postgraduate Medicine 38: 44–45

Prat J, Bhan A K, Dickersin G R, Robboy S J, Scully R E 1982 Hepatoid yolk sac tumor of the ovary (endodermal sinus tumor with hepatoid differentiation). A light microscopic, ultrastructural and immunohistochemical study of seven cases. Cancer 50: 2355–2368

Raghavan D, Friedlander M, Russell P 1985 Tumour markers: applications in the management of cancer of the female genital tract. In: Williams C J, Whitehouse J M A (eds) Cancer of the female reproductive system, Chichester, Wiley, p 61–78

Rutgers J L, Scully R E 1986 Functioning ovarian tumors with peripheral steroid cell proliferation. A report of 24 cases. International Journal of Gynecological Pathology 5: 3190.–337

Salazar H, Kanbour A, Tobon H, Gonzalez-Angulo A 1974 Endoderm cell derivatives in embryonal carcinoma. An electron microscopic study of two cases. American Journal of Pathology 74: 108a

Sawada M, Okudaira Y, Matsui Y, Nishiura H, Iwasaki T, Kasamatsu H 1985 Cisplatin, vinblastine, and bleomycin therapy of yolk sac (endodermal sinus) tumor of the ovary. Gynecologic Oncology 20: 162–169

Scully R E 1979 Tumors of the ovary and maldeveloped gonads. AFIP fascicle 16, 2nd series. Armed Forces Institute of Pathology, Washington, DC

Speleman F, de Potter C, Dal-Cin P et al 1990 i(12p) in a malignant ovarian tumor. Cancer Genetics and Cytogenetics 45: 49–53

Stage A H, Cox E, Rhea W G 1983 Endodermal sinus tumors of gonadal and extragonadal origin. Journal of the Southern California Medical Association 79: 445–448

Stewart K R, Casey M J, Gondos B 1981 Endodermal sinus tumor of the ovary with virilization. Light- and electron-microscopic study. American Journal of Surgical Pathology 5: 385–391

Talerman A, Haije W G, Baggerman L 1978 Serum α-fetoprotein (AFP) in diagnosis and management of endodermal sinus (yolk sac) tumor and mixed germ cell tumor of the ovary. Cancer 41: 272–278

Teilum G 1976 Special tumors of ovary and testis and related extragonadal lesions, 2nd edn. Munksgaard, Copenhagen, p 33–115

Ulbright T M, Roth L M, Brodhecker C A 1986 Yolk sac differentiation in germ cell tumors. A morphologic study of 50 cases with emphasis on hepatic, enteric, and parietal yolk sac features. American Journal of Surgical Pathology 10: 151–164

43

Embryonal carcinomas

P. Russell   A. Farnsworth

Embryonal carcinomas (Kurman & Norris 1976b, Flamant et al 1978) are the least differentiated of the ovarian germ cell tumors and are considered to be homologous to embryonal carcinomas of adult testes. Individual examples show the capacity to differentiate towards either embryonic (teratoid elements) or extraembryonic structures (yolk sac or trophoblast), although, by definition, this is minimal. Tumors exhibiting obvious differentiation in either direction are termed 'mixed malignant germ cell tumors' and are discussed in Chapter 50, and this is the more usual setting in which embryonal carcinoma as a distinct histological pattern in the ovaries is identified.

Pure ovarian embryonal carcinomas are thus extremely rare; the largest reported series of Kurman & Norris (1976b) comprises 15 cases, contrasted with a contemporaneous series of 71 endodermal sinus tumors (yolk sac tumors) from the same source (Kurman & Norris 1976a). The reason for their apparent rarity in the ovaries, while their histological homologs in the testes are relatively more common, is unknown. Embryonal carcinomas have also been observed to arise from pre-existing gonadoblastomas (Scully 1970, Talerman 1974).

As with other malignant germ cell tumors, the majority present in patients in their second and third decades, with a median age of 15 years in the series of Kurman & Norris (1976b), but with exceptional cases occurring in women as old as 50 years (Miyazaki et al 1992). Most patients present with an abdominal or pelvic mass and, unlike yolk sac tumors and dysgerminomas, about two-thirds have hormonal manifestations (precocious pseudopuberty or abnormal uterine bleeding). Serum β-human chorionic gonadotrophin (β-hCG) levels are usually elevated. Familial clustering of cases may occur (Mandel et al 1994).

They are highly malignant neoplasms, are locally aggressive, and spread widely throughout the peritoneal cavity, although extra-abdominal metastases tend to occur somewhat later than with yolk sac tumors. Lungs, liver, and retroperitoneal lymph nodes are documented sites for metastases. stage 1a tumors are found in 60% of patients at laparotomy. There were no stage 1b cases in the series of Kurman & Norris (1976b). One-half of stage 1a cases treated by simple surgical excision alone have a fatal outcome, indicating the high rate of occult metastases at the time of diagnosis and the need for postoperative adjuvant chemotherapy in all cases. Patients with residual extraovarian disease at the time of surgery rarely survive (Ueda et al 1990). The primary treatment of embryonal carcinomas is surgery (unilateral salpingo-oophorectomy is adequate for stage 1a cases) followed by chemotherapy (usually a combination of cisplatinum, vinblastine and bleomycin). Embryonal carcinomas are not radiosensitive. Monitoring the progress of these tumors is facilitated by the serial assessment of both serum β-hCG and α-fetoprotein (AFP).

Macroscopic features

Pure embryonal carcinomas are large, soft, solid unilateral masses with smooth external surfaces. The cut surfaces show yellow-gray tissue with widespread hemorrhage and necrosis, and usually a minor cystic component.

Microscopic features

The least well-differentiated variants are com-

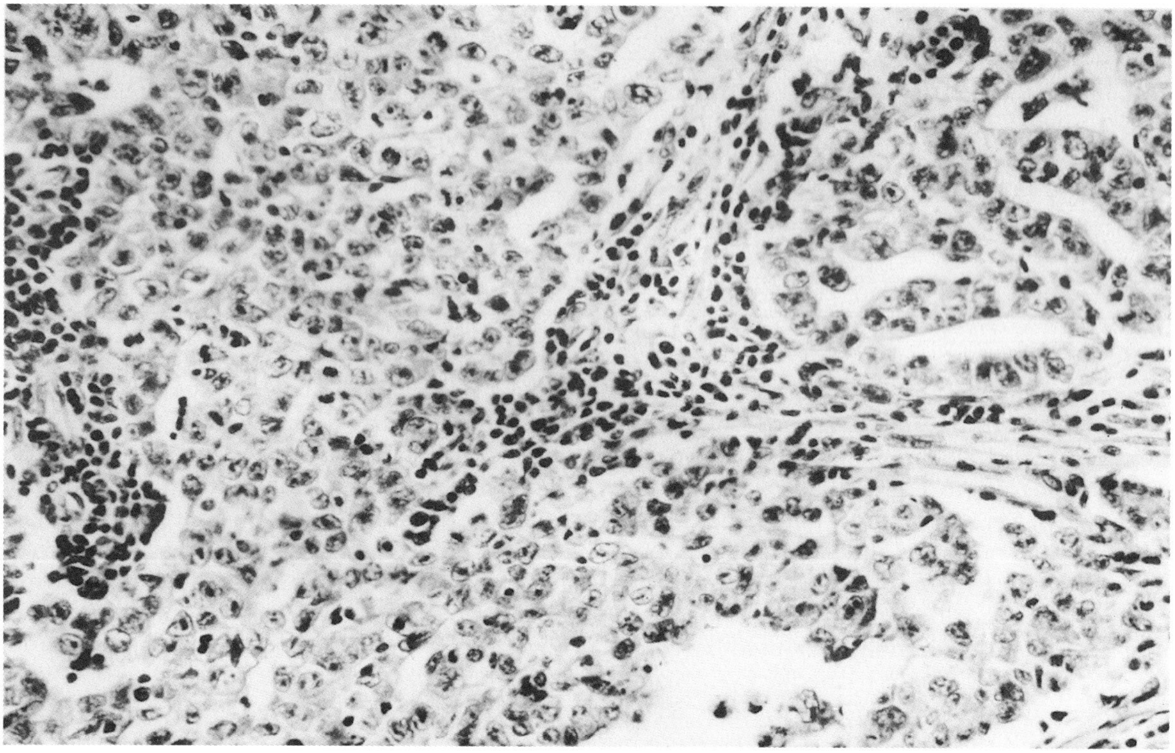

Fig. 43.1 Solid sheets of primitive cells with large vesicular nuclei and prominent nucleoli, characteristic of embryonal carcinomas. Lymphocytes are present in the interstitial tissue, but this is uncommonly a prominent feature. H + E ×150

posed of sheets and masses of pleiomorphic primitive cells, superficially resembling cytotrophoblastic cells, and showing little or no architectural organisation (Fig. 43.1). Tumor cells are medium to large in size, polyhedral in shape, and have obvious pale amphophilic granular cytoplasm but ill-defined cell borders. They often appear to form syncytial cell masses with central necrosis. Nuclei are central and pleiomorphic, with vesicular chromatin, and may contain one or more large nucleoli. Mitoses are frequent and abnormal mitotic figures are regularly seen. Giant multinucleated syncytiotrophoblastic cells, elaborating β-hCG as demonstrated immunohistochemically, are common (see Fig. 43.3). These cells may be clustered at the periphery of tumor nodules or scattered randomly throughout the tumor. Intervening mononuclear tumor cells, however, do not contain β-hCG but stain irregularly for AFP in 85% of cases. Hyaline droplets similar to those described in yolk sac tumors (also staining for AFP) are seen within and between the mononuclear tumor cells. Stromal and epithelial elements consistent with truncated somatic differentiation (minute foci of cartilage and islands of squamous epithelium) are rarely found (Kurman & Norris 1976b). More obvious differentiation is absent (particularly neuroepithelium), thus distinguishing these tumors from immature teratomas.

In the somewhat better differentiated examples, tumor cells tend to line cleft-like glandular spaces (Fig. 43.2) and appear a little more epithelial and less pleiomorphic, thus superficially resembling poorly differentiated adult type carcinomas. True glands are uncommon but, when present, they may be lined by cells elaborating cytoplasmic mucin (Kurman & Norris 1976b). Papillary structures, if present, are composed of solid aggregates of cells and must be differentiated from the typical Schiller–Duval bodies of yolk sac tumors. Occasional abortive embryoid bodies may be seen (Fig. 43.3). Mesenchymal differentiation is recog-

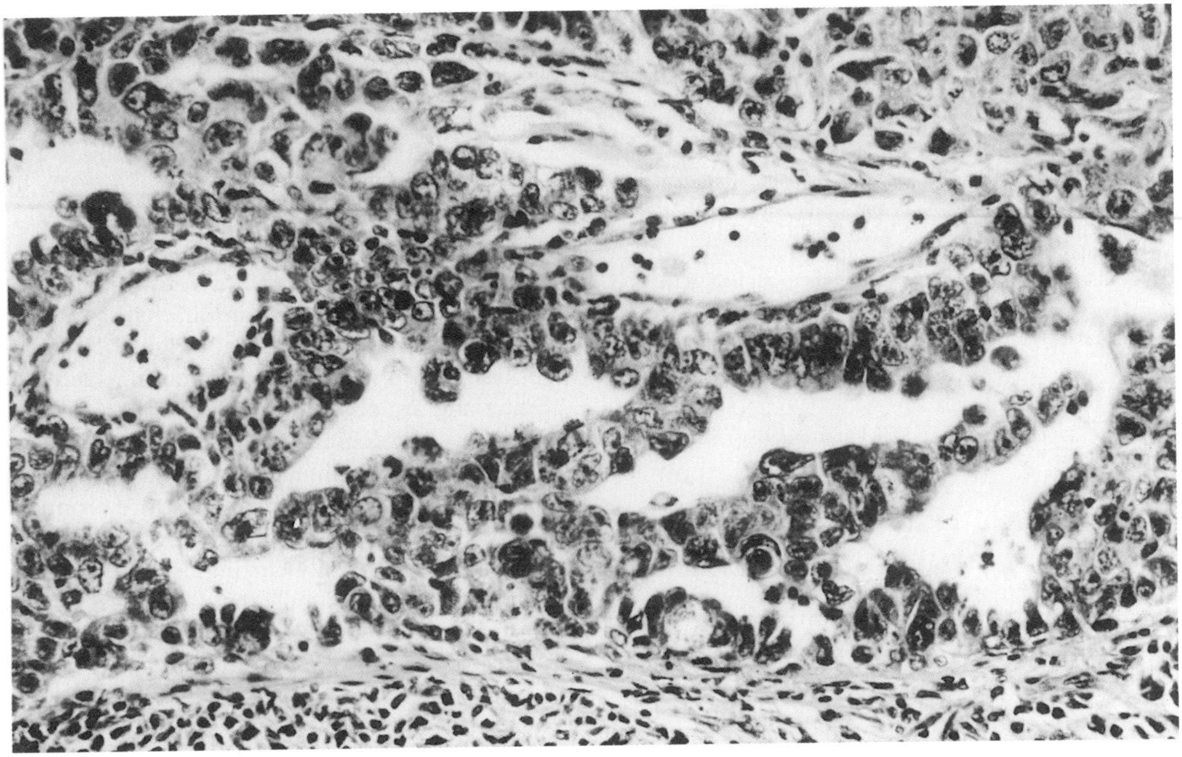

Fig. 43.2 Embryonal carcinoma showing more obvious 'epithelial' differentiation with irregular slit-like spaces lined by primitive cells. H + E ×150

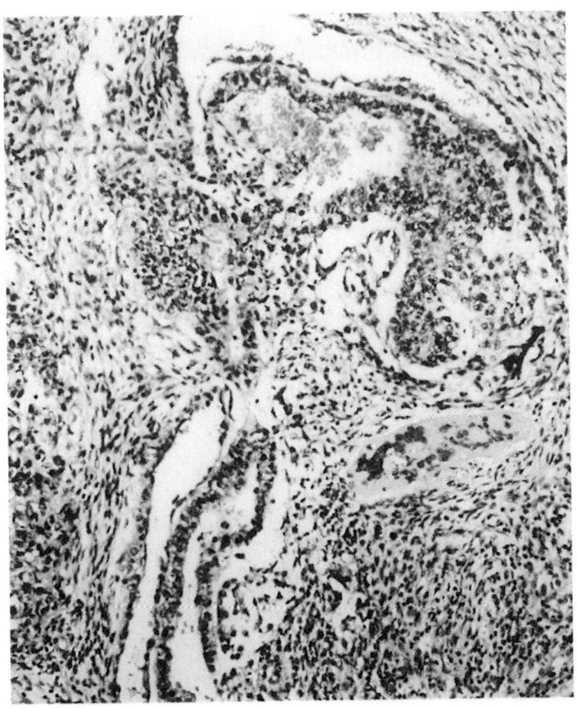

Fig. 43.3 A rare focus in an embryonal carcinoma showing two poorly formed embryoid bodies and a giant multinucleated syncytiotrophoblastic cell. H + E ×75

nizable and manifests as zones of either loose and edematous or dense fibrosarcoma-like tissue containing spindle cells. Focal necrosis and hemorrhage are common. Vascular invasion is more obvious than in other malignant germ cells tumors (with the exception of choriocarcinoma).

The contralateral ovary in many instances show the changes of hyperreactio luteinalis (see Ch. 10) due to the raised β-hCG levels in these patients.

Differential diagnosis

The solid undifferentiated forms of embryonal carcinoma may be occasionally confused with anaplastic dysgerminomas (see Table 41.1), an important discrimination to make because of the markedly

Table 43.1 Differential diagnosis: embryonal carcinoma versus undifferentiated epithelial carcinoma

Embryonal carcinoma	Undifferentiated epithelial carcinoma
Clinical	
Most cases occur before 30 years of age	Occur mostly over 50 years of age
Serum β-hCG and AFP usually raised	Serum β-hCG and AFP almost always normal
Always unilateral	Bilateral in about half of cases
Histological	
Large vesicular 'primitive' nuclei	Irregular hyperchromatic nuclei
Epithelial and mesenchymal components	Carcinomatous elements only
Syncytiotrophoblast-like giant cells in all cases	Syncytiotrophoblast-like giant cells absent
Immunohistochemical	
β-hCG positive, AFP positive, EMA negative,	β-hCG negative, AFP negative, EMA positive
Placental alkaline phosphatase positive	Placental alkaline phosphatase negative

different prognoses of and therapies for these tumors. The presence of clefts, alveoli, or any cell-lined spaces precludes the diagnosis of dysgerminoma. Embryonal carcinoma cells are usually larger and more pleiomorphic and, in contrast to dysgerminoma cells, stain strongly for cytokeratins immunohistochemically. AFP can be readily demonstrated in the mononuclear tumor cells, and syncytiotrophoblastic cells are much more numerous and more frequently seen in embryonal carcinomas than in dysgerminomas.

A more difficult differentiation may be between embryonal carcinomas and undifferentiated carcinomas of common epithelial origin. The latter neoplasms, as a general rule, occur in much older women and are commonly bilateral (Table 43.1). Although, histologically, both may show large sheets of pleiomorphic cells, the large primitive vesicular nuclei, each with one or more prominent central nucleoli, of the embryonal carcinoma cells should be readily distinguishable from the variable hyperchromatic, angular nuclei seen in undifferentiated epithelial malignant tumors. An absence of primitive mesenchyme (except in carcinosarcomas) and syncytiotrophoblast-like giant cells in the latter are also important discriminatory elements, as are the relevant immunophenotypes (Table 43.1).

REFERENCES

Flamant F, Caillou B, Pejovic M H et al 1978 Prognostic factors in germ cell tumors of the ovary in children excluding pure dysgerminoma. European Journal of Cancer 14: 901–906

Kurman R J, Norris H J 1976a Endodermal sinus tumor of the ovary. A clinical and pathologic analysis of 71 cases. Cancer 38: 2402–2419

Kurman R J, Norris H J 1976b Embryonal carcinoma of the ovary. A clinicopathologic entity distinct from endodermal sinus tumor resembling embryonal carcinoma of the adult testis. Cancer 38: 2420–2433

Mandel M, Toren A, Kende G, Newman Y, Kenet G, Rechavi G 1994 Familial clustering of malignant germ cell tumors and Langerhans histiocytosis. Cancer 73: 1980–1983

Miyazaki C, Kato R, Nishimura N, Nagamatsu M, Kodama S, Honna S 1992 A case of embryonal carcinoma of the ovary occurred in a 50-year-old woman. Nippon Sanka Fujinka Gakkai Zasshi 44: 483–486

Scully R E 1970 Gonadoblastoma. A review of 74 cases. Cancer 25: 1340–1356

Talerman A 1974 Gonadoblastoma associated with embryonal carcinoma. Obstetrics and Gynecology 43: 138–142

Ueda G, Abe Y, Yoshida M, Fujiwara T 1990 Embryonal carcinoma of the ovary: a six-year survival. International Journal of Gynaecology and Obstetrics 31: 287–292

44

Polyembryomas

P. Russell   A. Farnsworth

Polyembryomas (polyembryonic embryomas) are extraordinarily rare ovarian germ cell tumors containing myriads of variably formed 'embryoid bodies' (Fig. 44.1), which resemble normal presomite human embryos at approximately day 15–16 of development (Beck et al 1969, Teilum 1976). Occasional embryoid bodies are more readily encountered in ovarian malignant mixed germ cell tumors made up predominantly of other neoplastic elements such as immature teratoma or embryonal carcinoma. Only one ovarian polyembryoma reported to date has been 'pure' (Beck et al 1969). Embryoid bodies have been subtyped as complete, imperfect, or amorphous, depending upon the closeness with which they resemble normal presomite embryos, but this morphological subtyping does not appear to have any pathological significance. Although there are conflicting views on the origin of embryoid bodies, their formation after initiation of teratogenesis from multipotential embryonal cells in the tumors rather than directly from germ cells is the most widely accepted (Talerman 1994). Embryoid bodies should not be regarded as intermediate stages in transformation of embryonal cells towards immature teratomatous structures or tissues, but rather as intransitive end-points of differentiation or maturation in themselves. Histological and immunohistochemical evidence suggests that these embryoid bodies are not real or teratomatous embryos, but rather a 'product during a divergent differentiation into intestine and liver from plastic epithelium, which seems to be derived from an embryonic gut' (Nakashima et al 1988). These investigators noted that embryoid bodies usually showed some contiguity between the 'amniotic cavity'-like structure and intestinal epithelium or squamous cell nests, and between the 'yolk sac' and hepatic tissues. These findings contrast with the normal embryo in which immature somatic structures develop from the embryonic disc.

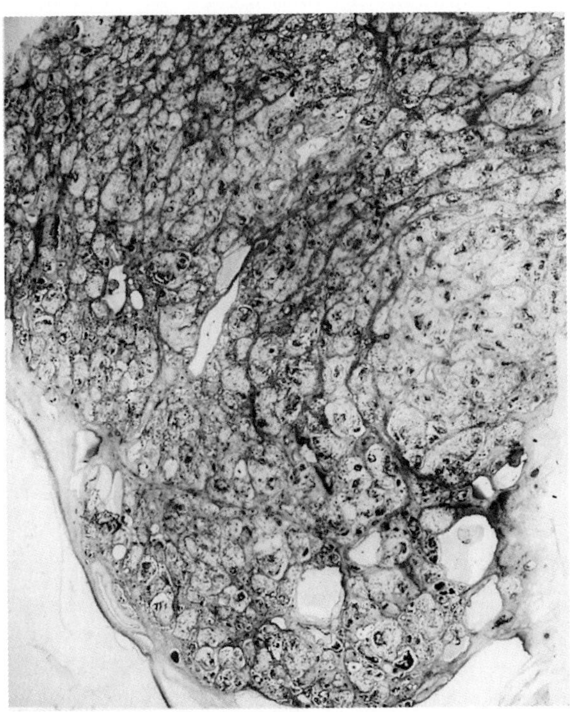

Fig. 44.1 Ovarian polyembryoma. Myriads of discrete islands of loose myxoid tissue representing primitive extraembryonic mesenchyme, separated by hyaline septa, and each containing 'epithelial' structures. H + E ×5. (Material by courtesy of Dr A Takeda, Nagoya)

Fewer than 20 cases of ovarian polyembryoma have been recorded (Simard 1957, Duhig 1959, Marin-Padilla 1965, Beck et al 1969, Gaillard 1972, Takeda et al 1982, Nakashima et al 1987, King et al 1991, Tsukahara et al 1991, Chapman et al 1994), almost all being malignant mixed germ cell tumors with a major component of polyembryoma associated with other germ cell elements, mainly immature teratoma. Most examples occurred in young patients, the oldest being 43 years of age (Chapman et al 1994). Clinical findings are similar to those observed in patients with other ovarian malignant germ cell tumors. In the majority of cases they have been associated with invasion of adjacent structures and organs and intraperitoneal metastases, and have behaved in a highly aggressive fashion. There is little merit in attempting to discriminate at a prognostic or therapeutic level between these and other malignant mixed germ cell tumors on the basis of so few reported cases, although one patient surgically staged and confined to one ovary has been treated successfully by adnexectomy alone (Chapman et al 1994).

Macroscopic features

Polyembryomas are solid, unilateral tumors and grossly resemble other malignant germ cell tumors. They vary in size from about 10 cm in diameter to giant masses filling the whole abdominal cavity (Simard 1957). Hemorrhagic and necrotic areas are prominent.

Microscopic features

The hallmark of polyembryomas is the presence of embryoid bodies, the better differentiated of which include an embryonic disc, amniotic cavity, and yolk sac surrounded by a variable cuff of primitive extraembryonic mesenchyme (Fig. 44.2). In well-formed bodies, the embryonic trilaminar disc is lined on one side by uniform cuboidal epithelial cells, resembling endoderm and continuous with the yolk sac. The epithelium lining the yolk sac stains strongly for α-fetoprotein by immunohistochemical techniques; the primitive 'endodermal' epithelium of the embryonic disc stains weakly (Takeda et al 1982). On the other side of the embryonic disc is tall columnar 'ectodermal' epithelium which merges with the amni-

A 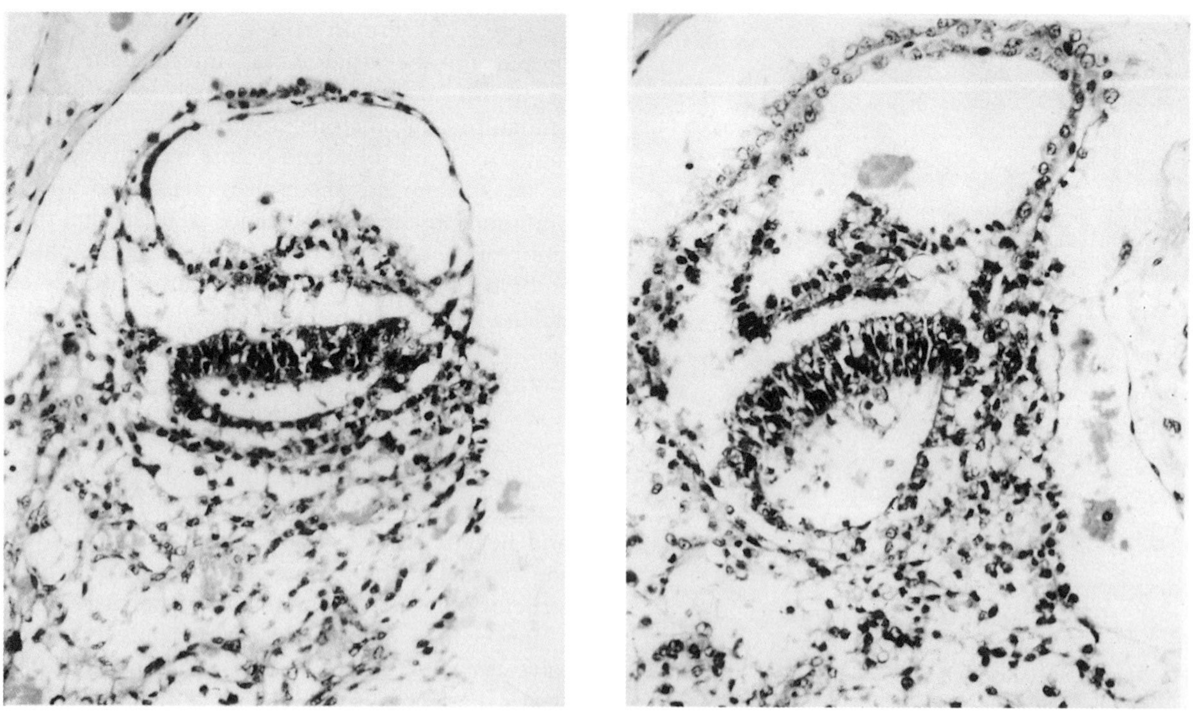 B

Fig. 44.2 Ovarian polyembryoma. (A, B) Two well-formed embryoid bodies each lying in loose myxoid connective tissue. H + E ×150. (Material by courtesy of Dr A Takeda, Nagoya)

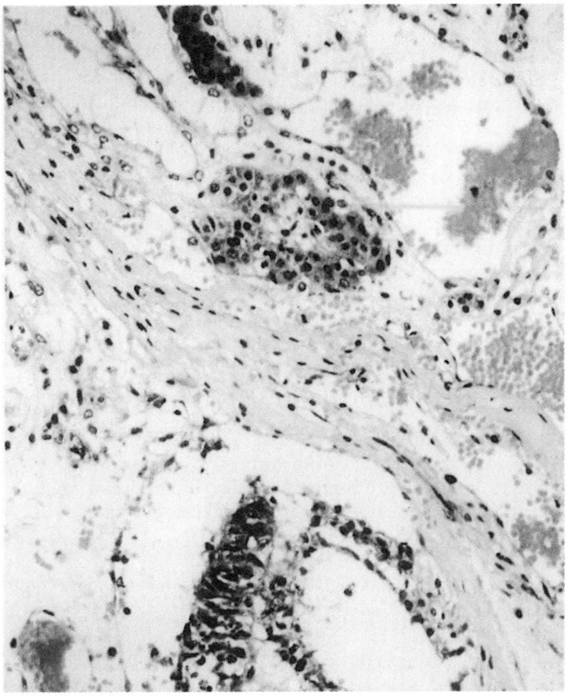

Fig. 44.3 Ovarian polyembryoma. Island of primitive hepatic cells adjacent to an embryoid body. H + E ×150. (Material by courtesy of Dr A Takeda, Nagoya)

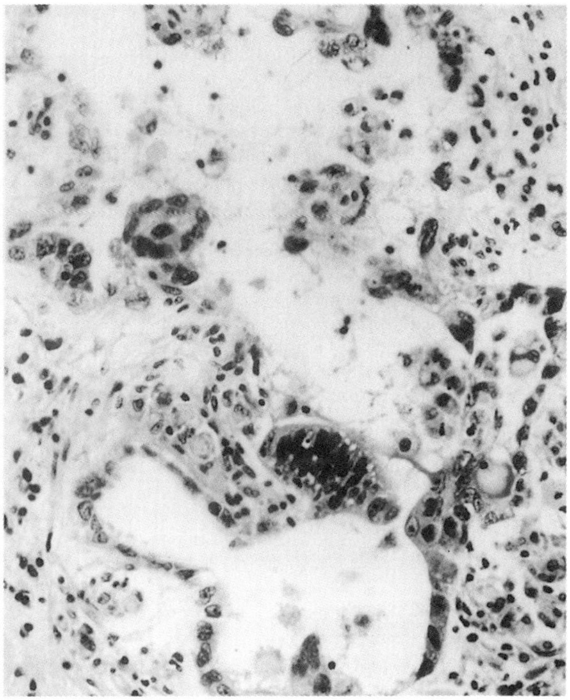

Fig. 44.4 Ovarian polyembryoma. Amorphous embryoid body with bizarre development of amnionic and yolk sac vesicles. H + E ×150

otic epithelium lining the rest of the cavity. The cuff of immature extraembryonic mesenchyme is composed of regular, loosely packed, mitotically active, spindle-shaped cells. Teratomatous structures such as neuroglia, epidermis and skin appendages, cords of liver cells (Fig. 44.3), respiratory and intestinal epithelium, in various stages of differentiation may be seen among the embryoid bodies. Transitions between the 'amniotic cavity' and intestinal or squamous elements, and between the 'yolk sac' and hepatic elements are reported (Nakashima et al 1988), but not between embryoid bodies and other teratomatous elements derived from the embryonic disc. Syncytiotrophoblastic giant cells which stain for β-human chorionic gonadotrophin (β-hCG) and human placental lactogen (hPL) are sometimes present at the periphery of the embryoid bodies. This trophoblastic differentiation, however, is said to be more characteristic of testicular rather than ovarian polyembryomas (Teilum 1976).

When less well-formed, embryoid bodies contain a medullary plate and amnion associated with a blastocystic space or with a cuff of extraembryonic mesenchyme. They may have two or more amniotic cavities and share a single yolk sac cavity, or vice versa (Talerman 1994). There may be disproportion between the two cavities, and the cavities may be malformed. In any one tumor, embryoid bodies may vary in size and their degree of maturation (but not beyond the 18-day stage of embryonic development). Severely malformed and bizarre examples may be encountered (Fig. 44.4).

REFERENCES

Beck J S, Fulmer H F, Lee S T 1969 Solid malignant ovarian teratoma with 'embryoid bodies' and trophoblastic differentiation. Journal of Pathology 99: 67–73

Chapman D C, Grover R, Schwartz P E 1994 Conservative management of an ovarian polyembryoma. Obstetrics and Gynecology 83: 879–882

Duhig J T 1959 An unusual adenocarcinoma of the ovary. A case simulating Schiller's 'Mesonephroma'. American Journal of Obstetrics and Gynecology 77: 201–205

Gaillard J A 1972 Yolk-sac tumor patterns and endoblastic structures in polyembryoma. Acta Pathologica et Microbiologica Scandinavica 80 (suppl 233): 18–25

King M E, Hubbell M J, Talerman A 1991 Mixed germ cell tumor of the ovary with a prominent polyembryoma component. International Journal of Gynecological Pathology 10: 88–95

Marin-Padilla M 1965 Origin, nature and significance of the 'embryoids' of human teratomas. Virchows Archives (A) 340: 105–121

Nakashima N, Fukatsu T, Nagasaki T, Sobue M, Takeuchi J 1987 The frequency and histology of hepatic tissue in germ cell tumors. American Journal of Surgical Pathology 11: 682–689

Nakashima N, Murakami S, Fukatsu T et al 1988 Characteristics of 'embryoid body' in human gonadal germ cell tumors. Human Pathology 19: 1144–1154

Simard L C 1957 Polyembryonic embryoma of the ovary of parthenogenetic origin. Cancer 10: 215–223

Takeda A, Ishizuka T, Goto T et al 1982 Polyembryoma of ovary producing alpha-fetoprotein and HCG. Immunoperoxidase and electron microscopic study. Cancer 49: 1878–1889

Talerman A 1994 Germ cell tumors of the ovary. In: Kurman R J (ed) Blaustein's pathology of the female genital tract, 4th edn. Springer-Verlag, New York, p 849–914

Teilum G 1976 Special tumors of ovary and testis and related extragonadal lesions, 2nd edn. Munksgaard, Copenhagen

Tsukahara Y, Fukuta T, Yamada T, Nakai I 1991 Retroperitoneal giant tumor formed by migrating polyembryoma with numerous embryoid bodies from an ovarian mixed germ cell tumor. Gynecological and Obstetrical Investigation 31: 58–60

ing the rules of normal embryogenesis; skin appendages bear their usual relationship to the epidermis (Fig. 46.3) and intestinal epithelium includes argyrophil (APUD) cells and may be subtended by lymphoid aggregates and smooth muscle (Bosman & Louwerens 1981) (Fig. 46.4). The rare presence of male tissues, e.g. prostatic glands (Fig. 46.5), in cystic teratomas (which always have a 46,XX karyotype) in 46,XX-karyotypic hosts is difficult to explain (Melniker & Slavutin 1980, Russell & Painter 1982, Brumback et al 1985), although induction by locally produced androgens has been suggested (McLachlan & Srigley 1992, Uzoaru et al 1992). The immunophenotype in these areas is identical to that of normal prostate (McLachlan & Srigley 1992, Buzzi et al 1994).

The large and detailed studies of Blackwell et al (1946), Caruso et al (1971), Fox & Langley (1976), Ong & Chan (1977), Abell (1982), and Russell & Painter (1982) are more or less congruent in the proportional representation of various tissues, and a summary is presented below.

- *Tissues very commonly present* (more than two-thirds of cases): epidermis, hair follicles, sebaceous glands, smooth muscle, adipose tissue, cerebrum (children)
- *Tissues commonly present* (one- to two-thirds of cases): sweat glands, cerebrum (adults), peripheral nerve, cartilage, bone, respiratory epithelium (Fig. 46.7)
- *Tissues occasionally present* (less than one-third of cases): teeth (Fig 46.3), gastrointestinal epithelium (Fig. 46.4), thyroid tissue (Fig. 46.8), salivary glands, ependyma
- *Tissues rarely present* (less than 5% of cases): prostate (Fig. 46.5), retina, breast, pituitary, choroid plexus (Fig. 46.6B), ganglia (Fig. 46.9A), lung, kidney, liver, cardiac muscle, adrenal, thymus, cerebellum (Fig 46.9B), striated muscle (Fig. 46.10), erectile tissue (Fig. 46.11).

One characteristic feature of mature cystic ter-

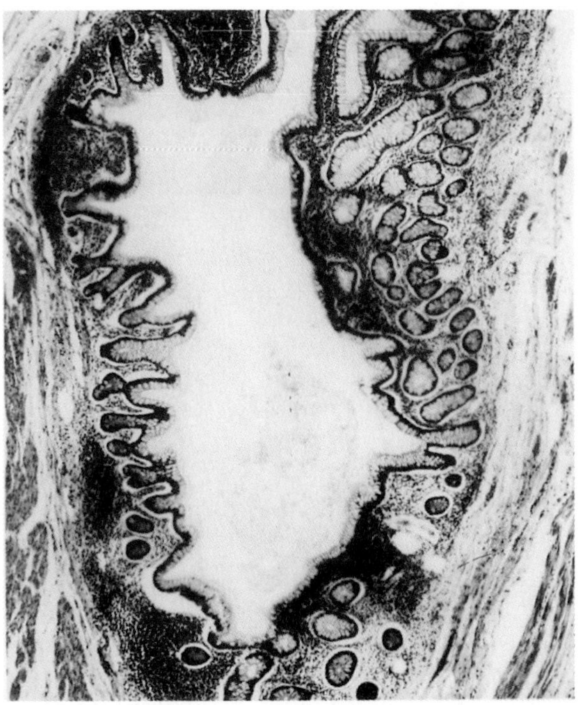

Fig. 46.4 Colonic mucosa with lymphoid aggregates and outer concentric layer of smooth muscle mimicking the appendix. H + E ×35. (Reproduced, with permission, from Painter & Russell 1982)

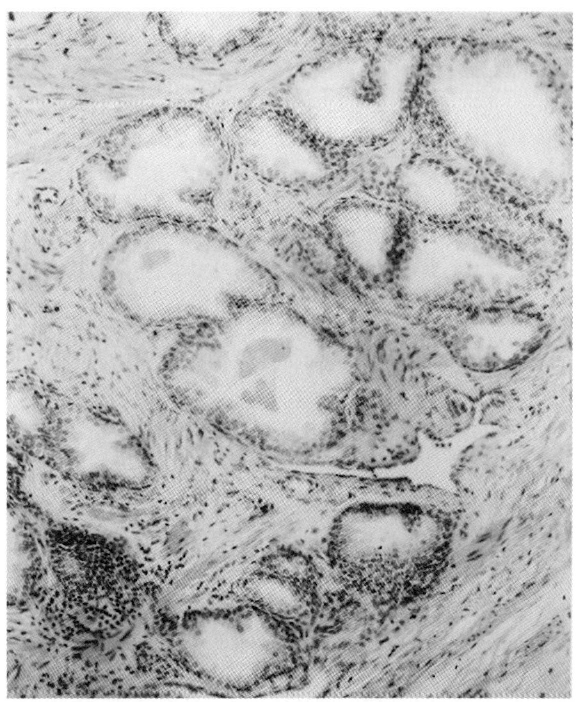

Fig. 46.5 Typical prostatic glands in wall of mature cystic teratoma. H + E ×90

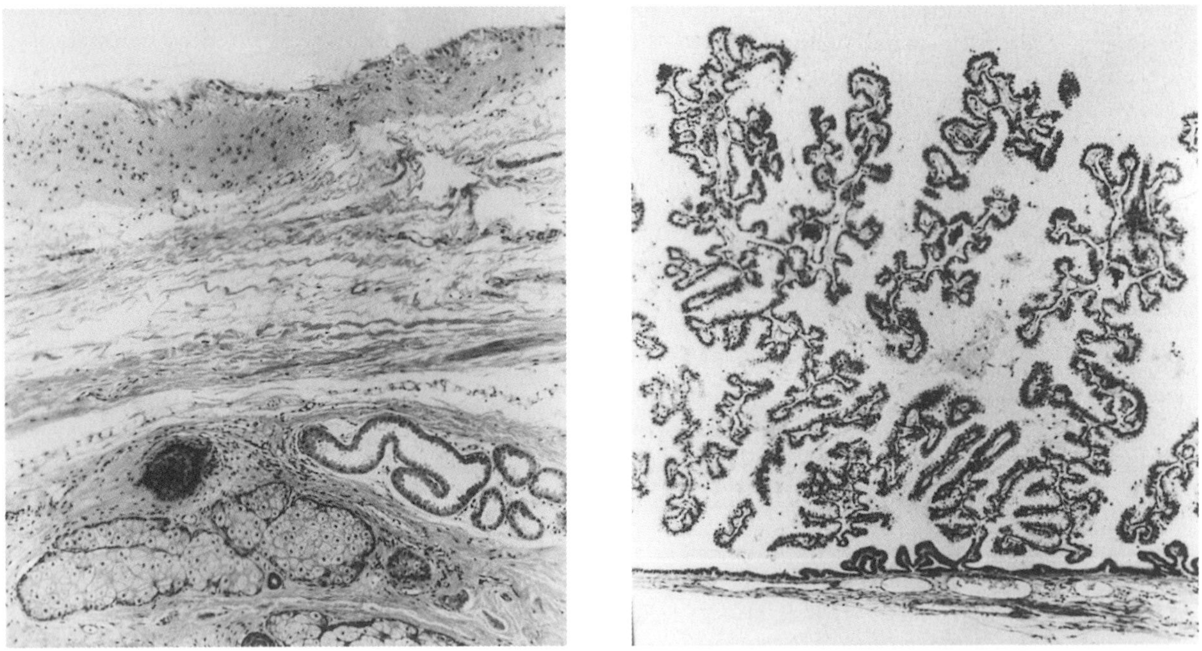

A B

Fig. 46.6 Mature cystic teratomas are occasionally lined by mature neuroglia (A) or ependyma with choroid plexus formation (B). H + E ×50

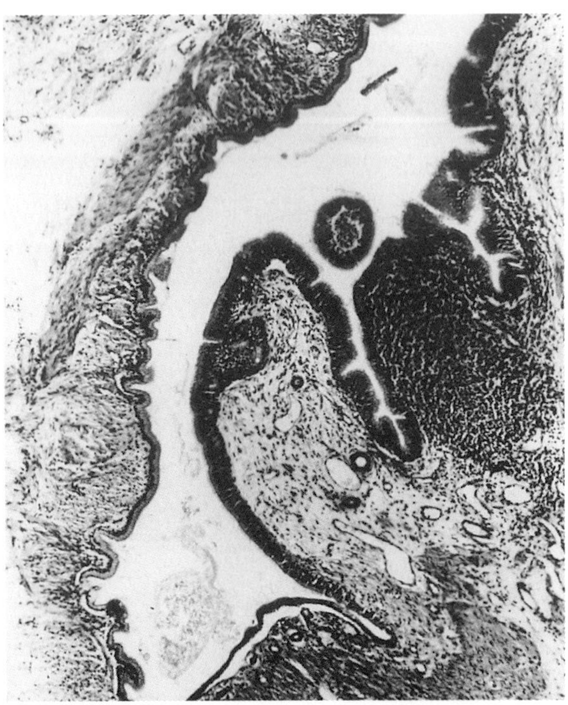

Fig. 46.7 Small cystic space in wall of mature cystic teratoma lined by an endocervical-like simple mucinous epithelium at left and respiratory mucosa at right. H + E ×50

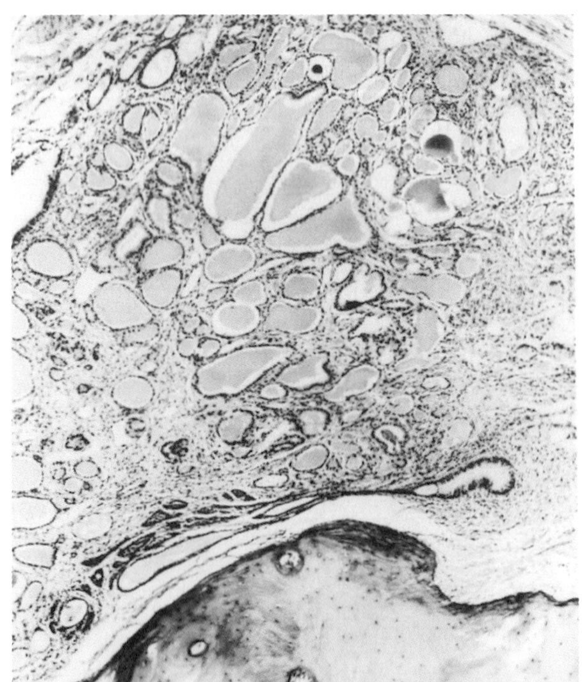

Fig. 46.8 Small focus of thyroid tissue, adjacent to a bony nodule, in cyst wall. H + E ×80

A 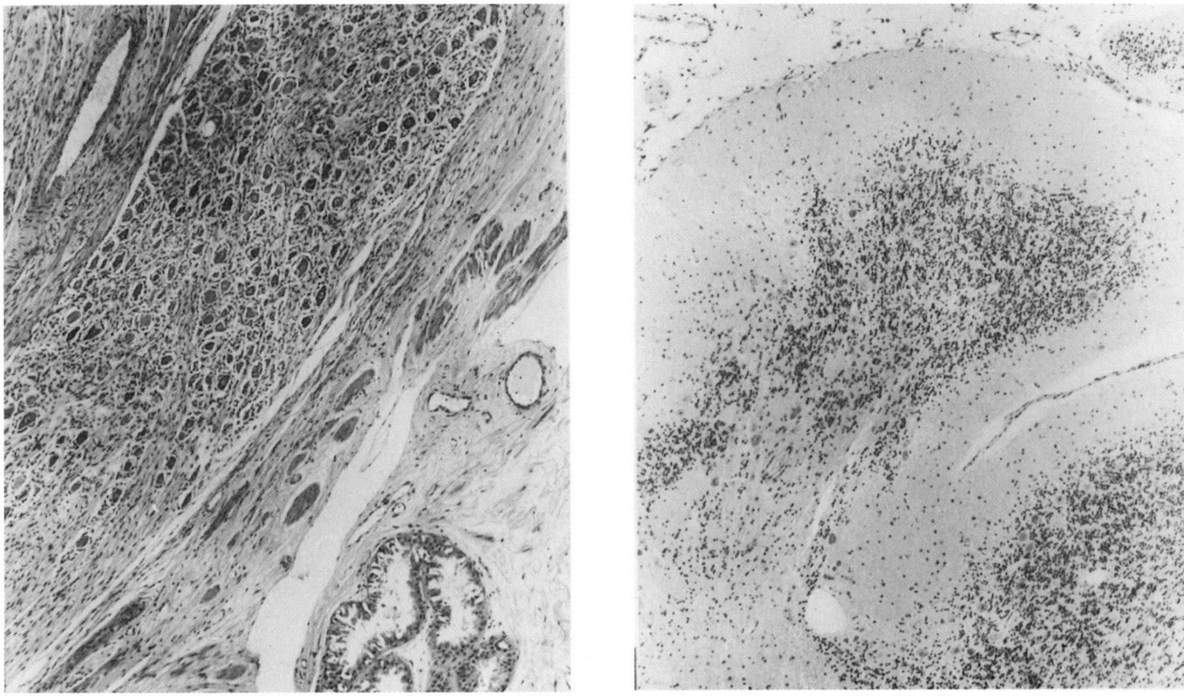 B

Fig. 46.9 Neural tissues in mature cystic teratomas. (A) Ganglion and large nerve bundle, with adjacent bundles of smooth muscle and sweat glands. H + E ×50. (B) Nodule of cerebellar tissue; the cyst was lined by ependyma. H + E ×50

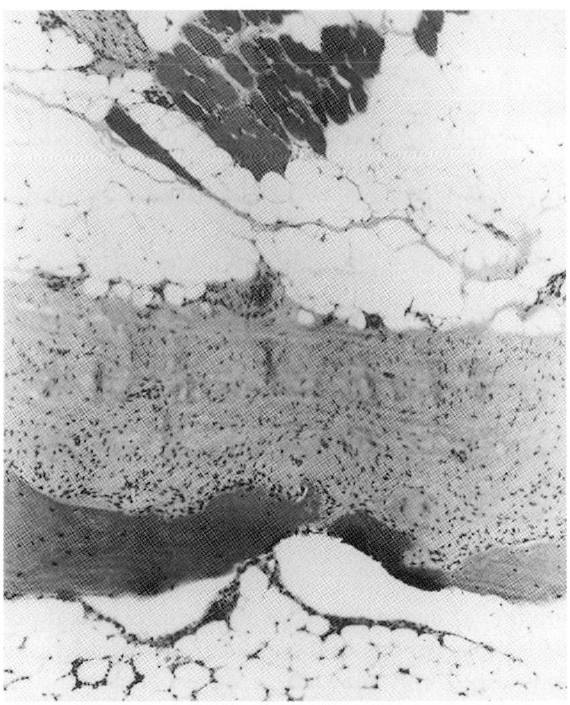

Fig. 46.10 Striated muscle is an unusual finding in mature cystic teratomas. Here it is surrounded by adipose tissue. Bone and marrow below. H + E ×50

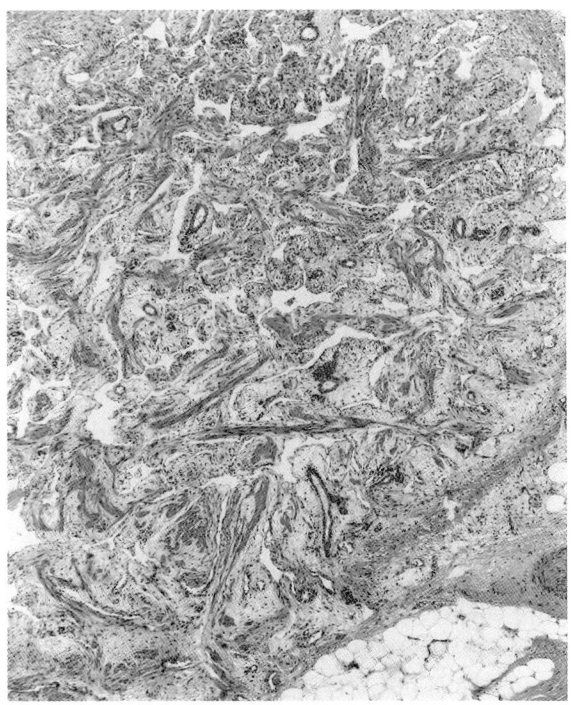

Fig. 46.11 Small discrete and partly organoid focus of vascular erectile tissue. Adipose tissue is seen at bottom. Respiratory epithelium was noted nearby. H + E ×24

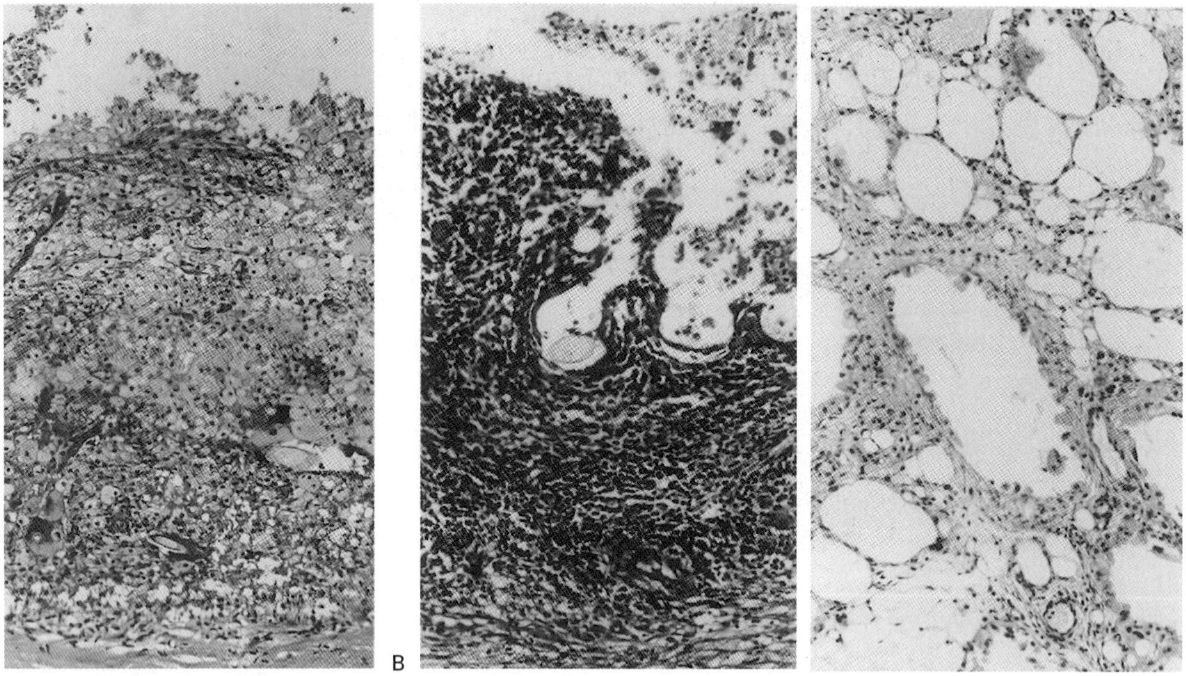
A B C

Fig. 46.12 Reactive changes in walls of cystic teratomas where cyst lining has broken down. (A) Sheets of foamy macrophages, some multinucleated, surround hair fragments. H + E ×80. (B) Heavy lymphoplasmacytic infiltrate. Polymorphs and cellular debris are present in lumen. H + E ×100. (C) Sieve-like pattern in wall of cyst. Some of the fat spaces are lined by large macrophages. H + E ×80

atomas is the focal loss of the squamous epithelial lining, in up to one-quarter of tumors, and consequent florid granulomatous reaction to the exposed hair fragments and keratinous debris (Fig. 46.12). However, the response to exposed lipid, keratinous debris and hair may rarely be extremely florid, even to the extent of simulating a neoplastic process (Fig. 46.13). Another very common finding is a lattice or sieve-like pattern of spaces outlined by attenuated foreign body giant cells (Fig. 46.12C), also referred to as a 'pneumatosis cystoides-like' appearance (Maudsley & Zakhour 1989). This probably represents a granulomatous lipophagic reaction to interstitial oily sebaceous material (Canzonieri et al 1994), but has also been considered to be fat necrosis (Abell 1982).

Individual tissues retain their functional potential and may respond 'appropriately' to an altered hormonal milieu, e.g. secretory activity in mammary tissue of a pregnant host (Nissen 1959, Oi & Dobbs 1978, Russell & Painter 1982). Degenerative and inflammatory changes which occur in normally sited tissues have also been reported in teratomas, e.g. neuronal degeneration, reactive astrocytic changes, and odontogenic structures showing caries or variants of fibrous dysplasia (Fig. 46.14), graying of hair, gastric mucosa showing peptic ulceration (Sahin et al 1990) or ischemic ulceration (Fig. 46.15), and thyroiditis (Pantoja et al 1975, Neilsen 1984, Pesce et al 1985, Farrell et al 1991).

Although melanocytes are not often observed in routine examinations of mature cystic teratomas, their identification can be enhanced by the use of Masson–Fontana silver stains and immunoperoxidase stains for S-100 protein. Epidermal melanocytes have been observed in 40–75% of negroid and 7–12% of caucasian patients (Lewis 1968, Amortegui & Kanbour 1981, Bosman & Louwerens 1981). Intradermal, compound, and blue naevi have been found in association with the epidermal lining of the cysts (Hermann & Humes 1976, Amortegui & Kanbour 1981, Kudo 1985, Tsang et al 1993), and their

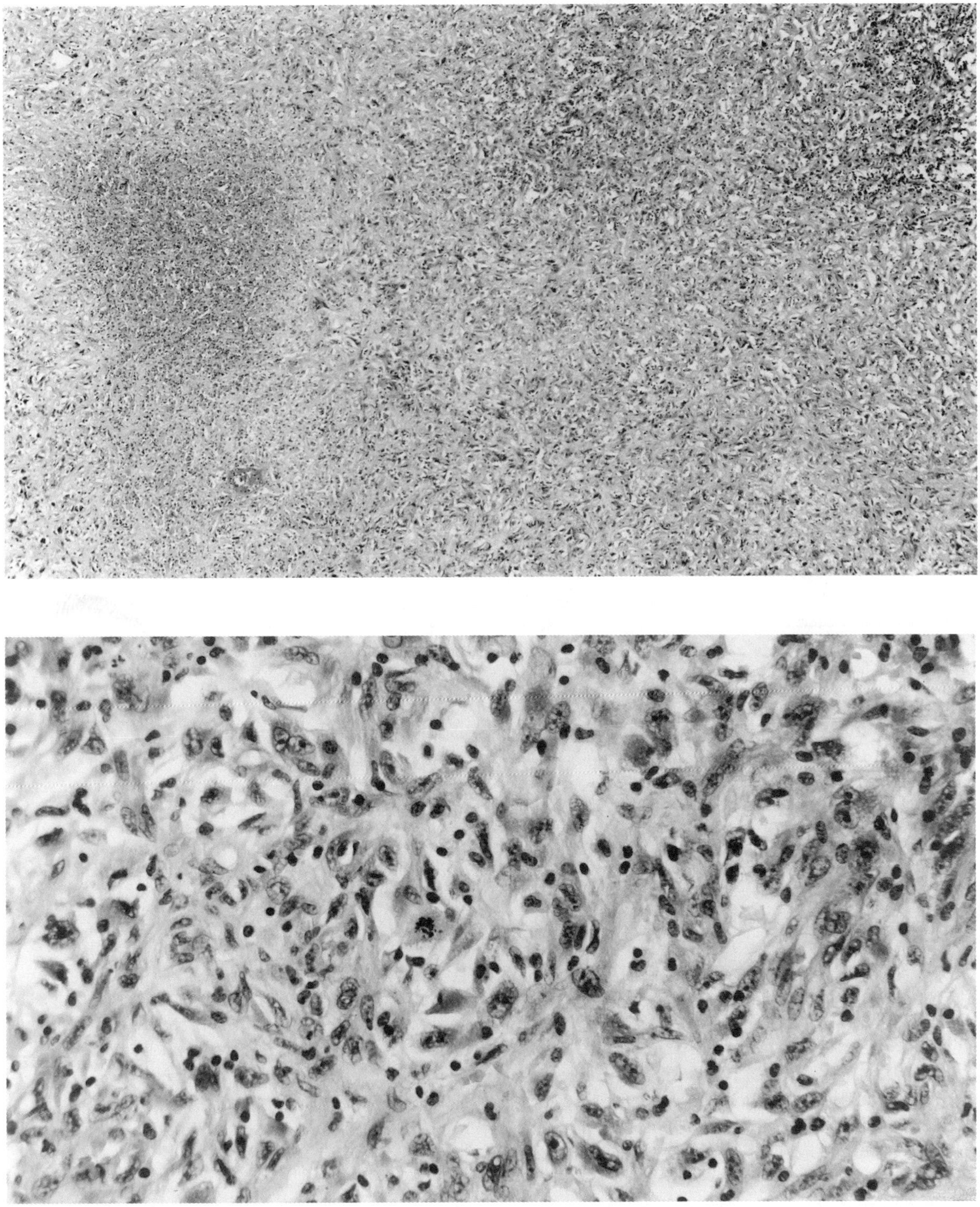

A

B

Fig. 46.13 A 10 cm soft hemorrhagic tumor-like mass occupying much of the lumen of a benign cystic teratoma. (A) An intense fibroxanthomatous response to exposed lipid, keratinous debris and hair fragments with focal necrosis at center left and upper right. H + E ×33. (B) Higher power, demonstrating a vigorous proliferation of atypical fibrohistiocytic cells with a somewhat storiform pattern and a patchy mixed inflammatory infiltrate in the background. H + E ×165

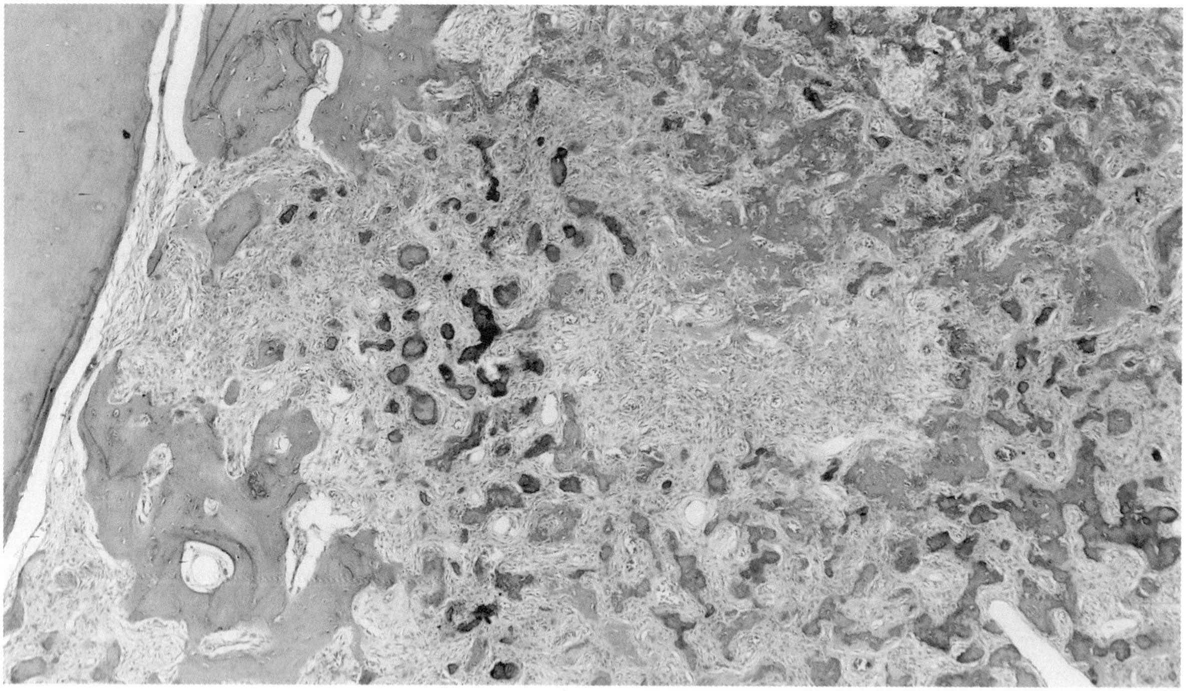

Fig. 46.14 A focus, between an island of cortical bone (left) and a nearby tooth, showing 'cemento-osseous' dysplasia. Florid metaplastic bone formation includes some islands resembling cementum. H + E ×33

existence is of interest when considering the origin of primary ovarian malignant melanomas (see Ch. 48).

Differential diagnosis

The pathological features of mature cystic teratomas are so well known that problems in differential diagnosis rarely arise. Despite the classical macroscopic appearance, the solid portions of the tumor should be well sampled, in accordance with the principles outlined in Chapter 4, to exclude the possibility of immature teratoma, other germ cell tumor elements or secondary malignant transformation, which all carry important prognostic implications. The rarely encountered fetiform teratoma should not be confused with a fetus in fetu, the latter being found in the upper retroperitoneal region and having an axial skeleton with appropriate arrangement of other organs and limbs with respect to it; it probably represents a monozygotic twin of its bearer, included within it during embryonic development (Lord 1956, Chi et al 1984).

Mixed mullerian tumors may include a variety of tissues, both mesenchymal and epithelial, but all are of mesodermal origin and one or more components usually show malignant characteristics (see Ch. 26). When only one, or a very limited number, of benign mature heterologous tissues is present in an ovarian tumor, it may be difficult to feel confident about the diagnosis of teratoma. However, examples such as struma ovarii, and carcinoid are regularly encountered and accepted as teratomatous; by analogy, it seems reasonable to assume teratomatous development for tumors composed of tissues whose presence in the ovary cannot be reasonably explained by other mechanisms (e.g. metaplasia, implantation).

MATURE SOLID TERATOMAS

These are rare compared with the cystic form; they account for only 10% of mature teratomas in the consultation practice of Scully (1979), which is presumably biased towards unusual lesions. The age distribution is comparable to that of

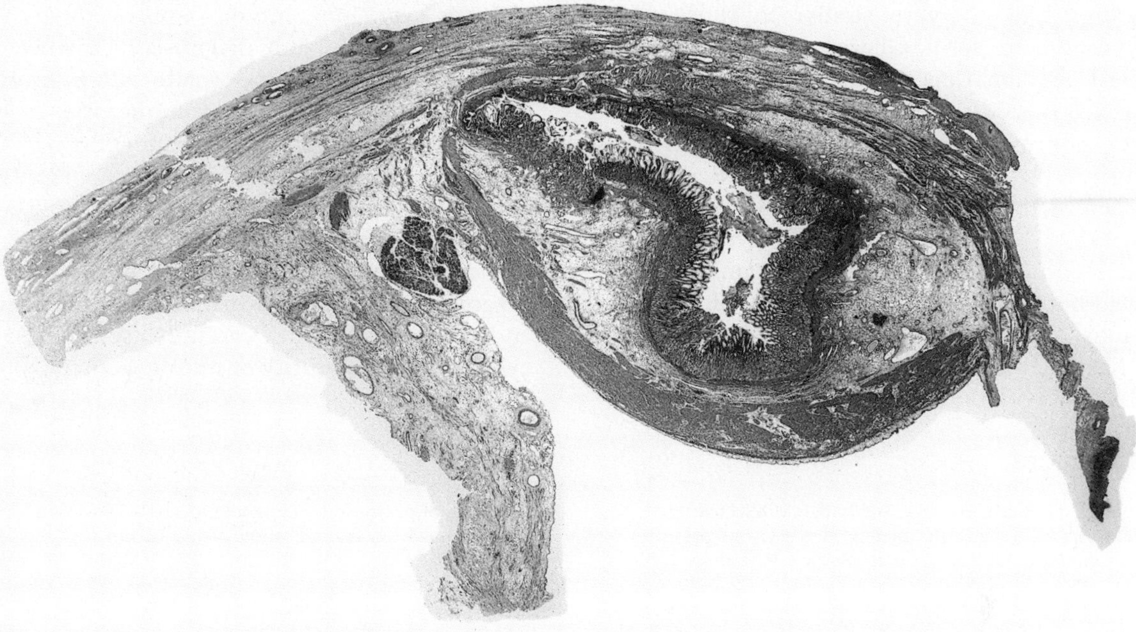

A

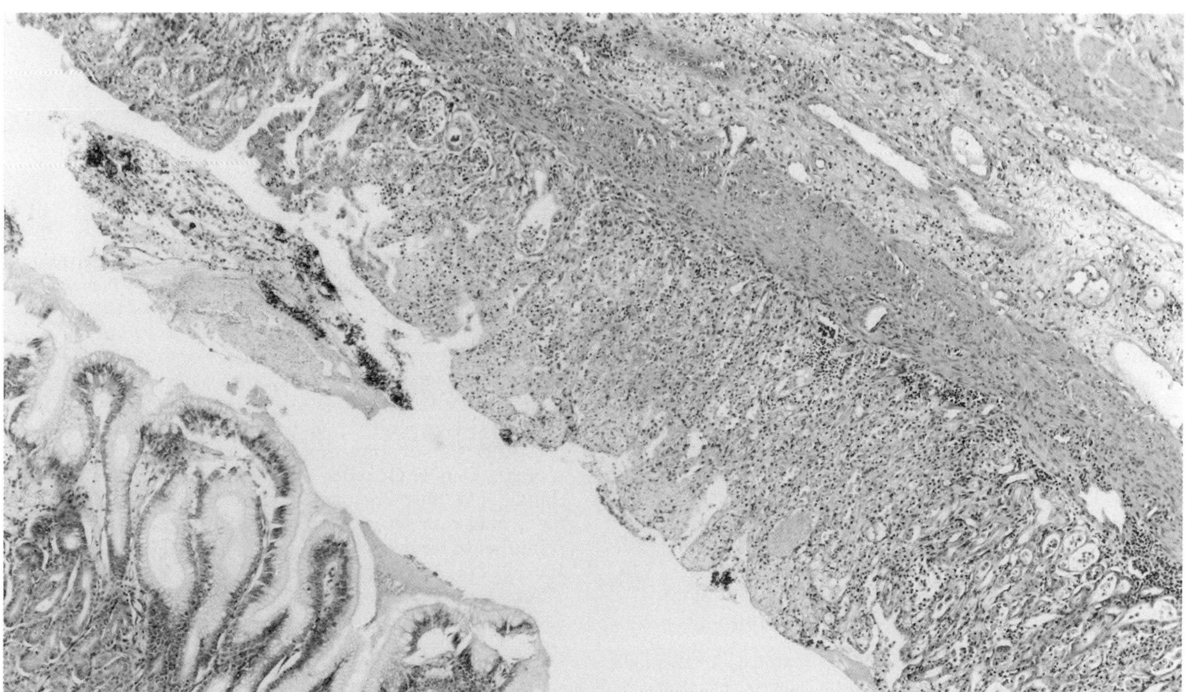

B

Fig. 46.15 Gastric differentiation in mature cystic teratoma. (A) Survey showing transverse section with mixed body type and antral mucosa, and small central, extramural nodule of exocrine pancreas. H + E ×6.6. (B) One of several small punched out ischemic ulcers with mucosal hemorrhage and necrosis and submucosal inflammation. H + E ×33 immature teratomas (see Ch. 47) but the clinical features are otherwise similar to those of the common cystic form. Gliomatosis peritonei – peritoneal implantation of mature glial tissue (see Ch. 47) – occurs in about one-third of cases, but does not indicate malignancy (Peterson 1956, Thurlbeck & Scully 1960, Robboy & Scully 1970, di Zerega et al 1975, El Shafie et al 1984, Vital et al 1985). The clinical course is always benign, and the recommended treatment is unilateral salpingo-oophorectomy with excision of peritoneal lesions, if present, as thoroughly as is practicable.

The macroscopic features are similar to those of immature teratomas, although hemorrhage and necrosis are uncommon unless torsion has occurred. A confident diagnosis of mature solid teratoma can only be made after thorough sampling to exclude areas of immaturity or other malignant germ cell tumor components.

Histological examination reveals a wide variety of mature tissues from all three germ cell layers. These are more finely intermingled than in the cystic variants, but still retain some degree of organization. Neural elements often predominate and these must be carefully scrutinized for evidence of immaturity or mitotic activity.

REFERENCES

Abbott T M, Hermann W J, Scully R E 1984 Ovarian fetiform teratoma (homunculus) in a 9-yr old girl. International Journal of Gynecological Pathology 2: 392–402

Abell M R 1982 Ovarian neoplasms of childhood and adolescence. In: Blaustein A (ed) Pathology of the female genital tract, 2nd edn. Springer-Verlag, New York, p 665–704

Adcock L L 1972 Unusual manifestations of benign cystic teratomas. Obstetrical and Gynecological Survey 27: 471–474

Aiman J, Nalick R H, Jacobs A et al 1977 The origin of androgen and estrogen in a virilized postmenopausal woman with bilateral benign cystic teratomas. Obstetrics and Gynecology 49: 695–704

Amortegui A J, Kanbour A I 1981 Compound nevus in a cystic teratoma of the ovary. Archives of Pathology and Laboratory Medicine 105: 115–116

Anteby E Y, Ron M, Revel A, Shimonovitz S, Ariel I, Hurwitz A 1994 Germ cell tumors of the ovary arising after dermoid cyst resection: a long-term follow-up study. Obstetrics and Gynecology 83: 605–608

Ayhan A, Aksu T, Develioglu O, Tuncer Z S, Ayhan A 1991 Complications and bilaterality of mature ovarian teratomas (clinicopathological evaluation of 286 cases). Australian and New Zealand Journal of Obstetrics and Gynaecology 31: 83–85

Bell D A, Demopoulos R I 1980 Benign cystic teratoma in the omentum. A mechanism of its development. Diagnostic Gynecology and Obstetrics 2: 205–208

Bernstein D, Shimon N, Rikover M, Menahem H 1974 Hemolytic anemia related to ovarian tumor. Obstetrics and Gynecology 43: 276–280

Blackwell W J, Dockerty M B, Masson J C, Mussey T D 1946 Dermoid cysts of the ovary: their clinical and pathologic significance. American Journal of Obstetrics and Gynecology 51: 151–172

Bosman F T, Louwerens J-W K 1981 APUD cells in teratomas. American Journal of Pathology 104: 174–180

Brenner S H, Wallach R C 1983 Familial benign cystic teratomata. International Journal of Gynaecology and Obstetrics 21: 167–169

Brumback R A, Brown B S, di Sant'Agnese P 1985 Unique finding of prostatic tissue in a benign cystic ovarian teratoma. Archives of Pathology and Laboratory Medicine 109: 675–677

Buzzi A, Crescini C, Sonzogni A, Pezzica E 1994 Tessuto prostatico in un teratoma cistico dell'ovaio. Minerva Ginecologica 46: 49–51

Canzonieri V, Volpe R, Gloghini A, Carbone A 1994 Sieve-like areas in mature cystic teratomas of the ovary. A histochemical and immunohistochemical study of 7 cases. Pathologica 86: 43–46

Caruso P A, Marsh M R, Minkowitz S, Karten G 1971 An intense clinicopathologic study of 305 teratomas of the ovary. Cancer 27: 343–348

Chi J G, Lee Y S, Park Y S, Chang K Y 1984 Fetus-in-fetu: report of a case. American Journal of Clinical Pathology 82: 115–119

Comerci J T Jr, Licciardi F, Bergh P A, Gregori C, Breen J L 1994 Mature cystic teratoma: a clinicopathologic evaluation of 517 cases and review of the literature. Obstetrics and Gynecology 84: 22–28

Compton A A, Tandan A, Fleming W P 1985 Coexistent benign teratomas of the omentum and ovary. A case report. Journal of Reproductive Medicine 30: 209–210

Cybulski G R, Von Roenn K A, Bailey O T 1984 Intramedullary cystic teratoid tumor of the cervical spinal cord in association with a teratoma of the ovary. Surgical Neurology 22: 267–272

Dahl N, Gustavson K H, Rune C, Gustavsson I, Pettersson U 1990 Benign ovarian teratomas. An analysis of their cellular origin. Cancer Genetics and Cytogenetics 46: 115–123

Dandia S D 1967 Rectovesical fistula following an ovarian dermoid with recurrent vesical calculus. A case report. Journal of Urology 97: 85–89

di Zerega G, Acosta A, Kaufman R H, Kaplan A L 1975 Solid teratoma of the ovary. Gynecologic Oncology 3: 93–102

Doss N, Forney J P, Vellios F, Nalick R H 1977 Covert bilaterality of mature ovarian teratomas. Obstetrics and Gynecology 50: 651–653

El Shafie M, Furay R W, Chablani L V 1984 Ovarian teratoma with peritoneal and lymph node metastases of mature glial tissue: a benign condition. Journal of Surgical Oncology 27: 18–22

Engel T, Greeley A V, Sweeney W J 1965 Recurrent dermoid cysts of the ovary. Report of two cases. Obstetrics and Gynecology 26: 757–759
Farrell D J, Bloxham C A, Scott D J 1991 Hashimoto's disease in a benign cystic teratoma of the ovary. Histopathology 19: 283–284
Feuerstein I M, Aronson B L, McCarthy E F 1984 Bilateral ovarian cystic teratomata mimicking bilateral pure ovarian hemangiomata: case report. International Journal of Gynecological Pathology 3: 393–397
Forrt R W, Mathie I K 1969 Gliomatosis peritonei caused by ovarian teratoma. Journal of Clinical Pathology 22: 348–353
Fox H, Langley F A 1976 Tumours of the ovary. Heinemann, London, p 210–230
Hermann W J, Humes J J 1976 A compound nevus in a benign cystic teratoma of the ovary. American Journal of Clinical Pathology 66: 54–58
Ireland K, Woodruff J D 1976 Masculinizing ovarian tumors. Obstetrical and Gynecological Survey 31: 83–111
Kommoss F, Emond J, Hast J, Talerman A 1990 Ruptured mature cystic teratoma of the ovary with recurrence in the liver and colon 17 years later. A case report. Journal of Reproductive Medicine 35: 827–831
Kudo M 1985 The nature of 'blue nevus' in cystic teratomas of the ovary. Acta Pathologica Japonica 35: 693–698
Lewis M G 1968 Melanin-pigmented components in ovarian teratomas in Ugandan Africans. Journal of Pathology and Bacteriology 95: 405–409
Livesey S A, Conn P C, Dunn D C 1989 Benign cystic teratoma of the ovary rupturing into the rectum: a rare problem. British Journal of Clinical Practice 43: 77–79
Lord J M 1956 Intra-abdominal foetus in foetu. Journal of Pathology and Bacteriology 72: 627–641
McLachlan C M, Srigley J R 1992 Prostatic tissue in mature cystic teratomas of the ovary. American Journal of Surgical Pathology 16: 780–784
Main D M G 1970 Tooth identity in ovarian teratomas. British Dentistry Journal 129: 328–332
Malkasian G D, Dockerty M B, Symmonds R E 1967 Benign cystic teratomas. Obstetrics and Gynecology 29: 719–725
Maudsley G, Zakhour H D 1989 Pneumatosis cystoides-like appearances in a mature cystic teratoma of the ovary. Histopathology 14: 420–422
Mehra U, O'Connor T, Ostapowicz F, Cavanagh D 1976 Pregnancy with bilateral ruptured benign cystic teratomas. American Journal of Obstetrics and Gynecology 124: 361–366
Melniker L A, Slavutin L J 1980 Prostatic tissue in a benign cystic teratoma of the ovary. Diagnostic Gynecology and Obstetrics 2: 139–145
Mercur L, Farkas T G, Anker P M, Brill R, Mund M L 1976 Developing eye in an ovarian teratoma. Acta Ophthalmologica 94: 597–598
Mulligan R M 1975 Pathogenesis of teratoid tumors of the ovary and testis. Pathology Annual, p 271–298 Appleton-Century Crofts, New York
Neilsen V T 1984 A benign cystic teratoma of the ovary with chronic thyroiditis. American Journal of Obstetrics and Gynecology 148: 1142–1144
Nissen E D 1959 Secretory mammary tissue arising within a benign cystic teratoma of the ovary during pregnancy. American Journal of Obstetrics and Gynecology 77: 663–666
Oi R H, Dobbs M 1978 Lactating breast tissue in benign cystic teratoma of the ovary. American Journal of Obstetrics and Gynecology 130: 729–731
Ong H C, Chan W F 1977 A clinico-pathological review of benign cystic teratoma of the ovary. Singapore Medical Journal 18: 100–104
Palmer P E, Bogojavlensky S, Bhan A K, Scully R E 1990 Prolactinoma in wall of ovarian dermoid cyst with hyperprolactinemia. Obstetrics and Gynecology 75: 540–543
Pantoja E, Noy M A, Axtmayer R W, Colon F E, Pelegrina I 1975 Ovarian dermoids and their complications. Comprehensive historical review. Obstetrical and Gynecological Survey 30: 1–20
Pesce C, Tobia F, Scott T 1985 Microglia in teratomas. Acta Neuropathologica 67: 332–336
Peterson W F 1956 Solid, histologically benign teratomas of the ovary. A report of four cases and review of the literature. American Journal of Obstetrics and Gynecology 72: 1094–1102
Plattner G, Oxorn H 1973 Familial incidence of ovarian dermoid cysts. Canadian Medical Association Journal 108: 892–893
Robboy S J, Scully R E 1970 Ovarian teratoma with glial implants on the peritoneum. An analysis of 12 cases. Human Pathology 1: 643–653
Russell P, Painter D M 1982 The pathological assessment of ovarian neoplasms. V: The germ cell tumors. Pathology 14: 47–72
Rutgers J, Scully R E 1986 An unusual form of ovarian tumor with functioning stroma: a clinicopathological and immunohistological study of 17 cases [abstract]. Laboratory Investigation 54: 55
Sahin A A, Ro J Y, Chen J, Ayala A G 1990 Spindle cell nodule and peptic ulcer arising in a fully developed gastric wall in a mature cystic teratoma. Archives of Pathology and Laboratory Medicine 114: 529–531
Scully R E 1979 Tumors of the ovary and maldeveloped gonads. Atlas of tumor pathology. Fascicle 16, 2nd series. Armed Forces Institute of Pathology, Washington, DC, p 226–286
Serov S F, Scully R E, Sobin L H 1973 Histological typing of ovarian tumors. International histological classification of tumors No. 9. World Health Organization, Geneva, p 48–50
Simon A, Ohel G, Neri A, Schenker J G 1985 Familial occurrence of mature ovarian teratomas. Obstetrics and Gynecology 66: 278–279
Smith R, Deppe G, Selvaggi S, Lall C 1990 Benign teratoma of the omentum and ovary coexistent with an ovarian neoplasm. Gynecologic Oncology 39: 204–207
Stuart G C E, Smith J P 1983 Ruptured benign cystic teratomas mimicking gynecologic malignancy. Gynecologic Oncology 16: 139–143
Thurlbeck W M, Scully R E 1960 Solid teratoma of the ovary. A clinicopathological analysis of 9 cases. Cancer 13: 804–811
Tsang P, Berman L, Kasnica J 1993 Adnexal tumor and a pigmented nevoid lesion in a benign cystic ovarian teratoma. Archives of Pathology and Laboratory Medicine 117: 846–847
Uzoaru I, Akang E E, Aghadiuno P U, Nadimpalli V R 1992 Benign cystic teratomas with prostatic tissue: a report of two cases. Teratology 45: 235–239
Vital A, Rivel J, Verdaguer S, Discamps G, Olivot J, Vital C 1985 Gliomatose péritonéale associée à un tératome mature de l'ovaire. Annales de Pathologie 5: 59–62
Waxman M, Boyce J G 1976 Intraperitoneal rupture of

benign cystic ovarian teratoma. Obstetrics and Gynecology 48: 9s–13s
Weir J H, Janosvski N A 1962 Choroid plexus in benign cystic teratoma of the ovary. American Journal of Obstetrics and Gynecology 84: 682–686
Weldon-Linne C M, Rushovich A M 1983 Benign ovarian cystic teratomas with homunculi. Obstetrics and Gynecology 61: 88s–94s
Woodfield B, Katz D A, Cantrell C J, Bogard P J 1985 A benign cystic teratoma with gastrointestinal development. American Journal of Clinical Pathology 83: 236–240
Zakin D 1976 Radiologic diagnosis of dermoid cysts of the ovary. Obstetrical and Gynecological Survey 31: 165–184

47

Teratomas – immature

P. Russell A. Farnsworth

These teratomas contain immature (embryonal) structures, as well as mature elements in most cases. The additional presence of other malignant germ cell tumor elements (a not uncommon occurrence) places the tumor in the malignant mixed germ cell tumor group (see Ch. 50). Pure immature teratomas comprise 1–2% of ovarian teratomas overall, but 10–20% of those occurring in the first two decades of life (Fox & Langley 1976, Scully 1979, Abell 1982, Russell & Painter 1982, Talerman 1994). Most immature teratomas include elements from all three germ layers, but a small number are predominantly or exclusively monodermal; these rare variants are discussed in Chapter 49.

Immature teratomas occur predominantly in the first two decades of life, with a peak incidence at 14–19 years of age. Tumours have been reported in women up to the age of 47 years, but there are no well-documented postmenopausal cases (Nogales et al 1976, Norris et al 1976, Fox & Langley 1976, Scully 1979, Gallion et al 1983, Gershenson et al 1986, Nielsen et al 1986). Patients usually present with abdominal enlargement, pain, and a readily palpable tumor. The pain is usually dull but may be acute if rupture or torsion supervenes. Ascites is not uncommon at initial presentation and may contribute to the abdominal swelling. Nausea, vomiting, and fever may also occur. A few patients have presented with isosexual pseudoprecocity, but in such cases there was probably histologically undetected choriocarcinoma. Raised serum human chorionic gonadotrophin (hCG) and α-fetoprotein (AFP) levels should alert the clinician and pathologist to the possibility of a mixed malignant germ cell tumor. Elevated serum AFP levels have been found in up to 50% of patients with immature teratomas, including some which have been exhaustively sampled for the presence of other germ cell components (Bahari et al 1980, Gallion et al 1983, Gershenson et al 1986). This apparent conundrum may be explained by the recent detection by Burrus et al (1985) of immunohistochemically positive AFP in a wide variety of both endodermally and ectodermally derived tissues of an immature teratoma, suggesting that endodermal sinus tissue is not the only possible source of this substance.

Two patients with coexisting ovarian and presacral immature teratomas (not evidently metastatic from one site to the other) have been reported (Nielsen et al 1986), but associated pathology is otherwise scarce.

The tumors grow rapidly, and extraovarian spread is present at initial laparotomy in about one-third of cases (Norris et al 1976, Scully 1979, Gallion et al 1983, Gershenson et al 1986, Nielsen et al 1986). As a result of rupture or capsular penetration, the tumor seeds throughout the peritoneal cavity. Direct local spread with formation of adhesions also occurs. In addition, tumors may metastasize to retroperitoneal and para-aortic lymph nodes as well as to liver, lungs and brain, but these distant deposits are rarely found even at autopsy (Fox & Langley 1976, Norris et al 1976, Scully 1979, McLaughlin et al 1989, Talerman 1994).

The prognosis of immature teratomas depends principally on the histological grade of the ovarian tumor (in stage 1 cases) or that of its metastases (in higher stage cases). The grading system for these tumors (see below) is unique in ovarian tumor pathology, being based on the degree of tissue immaturity and the amount of neuroepithelium. The grade of the primary tumor appears to determine the likelihood of extraovarian spread, whereas the grade of the metastases correlates with the likelihood of recurrence and possible death from uncontrolled tumor growth (Norris et al 1976). Large size of tumor (greater than 1500 g), rupture (spontaneous or operative) and increasing age are further adverse factors (Nogales et al 1976, Norris et al 1976, Gallion et al 1983, Harms & Jänig 1985, Talerman 1994). Recurrences, if they occur, usually develop within the first postoperative year, so that the published 2- and 5-year survival rates are similar. Modern combination chemotherapy has seen a marked improvement in long-term clinical outcome, with the largest recent series reporting survival rates of 94% for stage 1 low-grade tumors and 82% for stage 1 high-grade tumors (O'Connor & Norris 1994). These authors noted that only very large grade 1, stage 1 immature teratomas (greater than 1500 g) progressed and warranted consideration of adjuvant chemotherapy. Clinical tumor staging does not correlate with prognosis, as well as might be expected from experience with ovarian tumors in general, since the presence of metastases which are histologically mature may presage maturation of the primary tumor, and therefore confers a paradoxically good prognosis on some high stage tumors.

Peritoneal metastatic deposits of mature teratomatous tissue, sometimes called 'implants', are often composed almost entirely or exclusively of mature glial tissue ('gliomatosis peritonei') (Robboy & Scully 1970, Truong et al 1982, Nielsen et al 1985). This phenomenon occurs in association with approximately 10% of patients with immature teratomas, and is biologically benign. In some instances, gliomatosis peritonei is not evident until 'second-look' laparotomy (Truong et al 1982). It should be noted that gliomatosis peritonei does not develop in association with immature teratoma exclusively; about 10% of all cases are associated with mature solid or cystic teratomas (see Ch. 46) or primary extraovarian immature teratomas (Wheeler 1978, Coulson 1990). At laparotomy the small peritoneal nodules may be mistaken for carcinomatosis or miliary tuberculosis. The lesions are thought to result from release of mature neural tissue through a ruptured capsule (a not uncommon finding in these tumors) or from the maturation of peritoneal deposits of immature neural tissue (a mechanism which we favor as the likely explanation). Lymphatic spread has also been suggested, and this would account for the rare concurrent presence of glial tissue in lymph nodes (Robboy & Scully 1970, El Shafie et al 1984). Follow-up of patients with untreated gliomatosis peritonei shows that the lesions either persist unchanged, undergo fibrous replacement, or disappear entirely.

There is general agreement on management of immature teratomas (Scully 1979, Gallion et al 1983, Gershenson et al 1986, Nielsen et al 1986, Kawai et al 1991, Bonazzi et al 1994). Conservative, fertility-sparing surgery is recommended, with careful follow-up, for patients with stage 1–2, low grade tumors. This is reasonable in view of the rarity of bilateral tumors and the possibility of future fertility which it offers young patients. Patients with high grade, stage 1–2 tumors, or with stage 3 tumors of any grade, or those with tumor recurrence, have benefited from platinum-based chemotherapy. All the excised metastatic tumor tissue should be examined histologically, since the deposits may vary in their degree of maturation. If all are mature (gliomatosis peritonei), no further immediate treatment is required (Harms et al 1989, Gratama et al 1991), although rare malignant transformation of mature peritoneal glial deposits may be encountered (Shefren et al 1991). Radiotherapy has not proved useful in controlling the disease. 'Second-look' laparotomies have demonstrated, in some instances, maturation ('retroconversion') of previously incompletely resected metastases following chemotherapy (Schwartz et al 1979, Dara et al 1982, Caldas et al 1992, Bonazzi et al 1994), but have little else to recommend them (O'Connor & Norris 1994).

Cytogenetic and molecular genetic studies

Chromosomal heteromorphisms identical to those of host cells in a case of a 'grade 3' immature teratoma, suggests a probable premeiotic origin (King et al 1990). Cytogenetic studies have also identified trisomy 12 and translocation (7;9) in an ovarian immature teratoma (Lopez-Gines et al 1989).

Macroscopic features

Immature teratomas are almost always unilateral, but mature cystic teratomas are present in 5–10% of contralateral ovaries (Norris et al 1976, Yanai-Inbar & Scully 1987). Their size is generally in the range 14–18 cm, but may be up to 35 cm. The tumors form round, oval, or lobulated masses which may display capsular adhesions and/or rupture but elsewhere have smooth surfaces. The consistency may be soft or firm, depending on the nature of the teratomatous components. The tumors are predominantly solid, but there are usually multiple small cysts (generally less than 1 cm in diameter) and occasionally one or more large ones are present. Some contain sebaceous

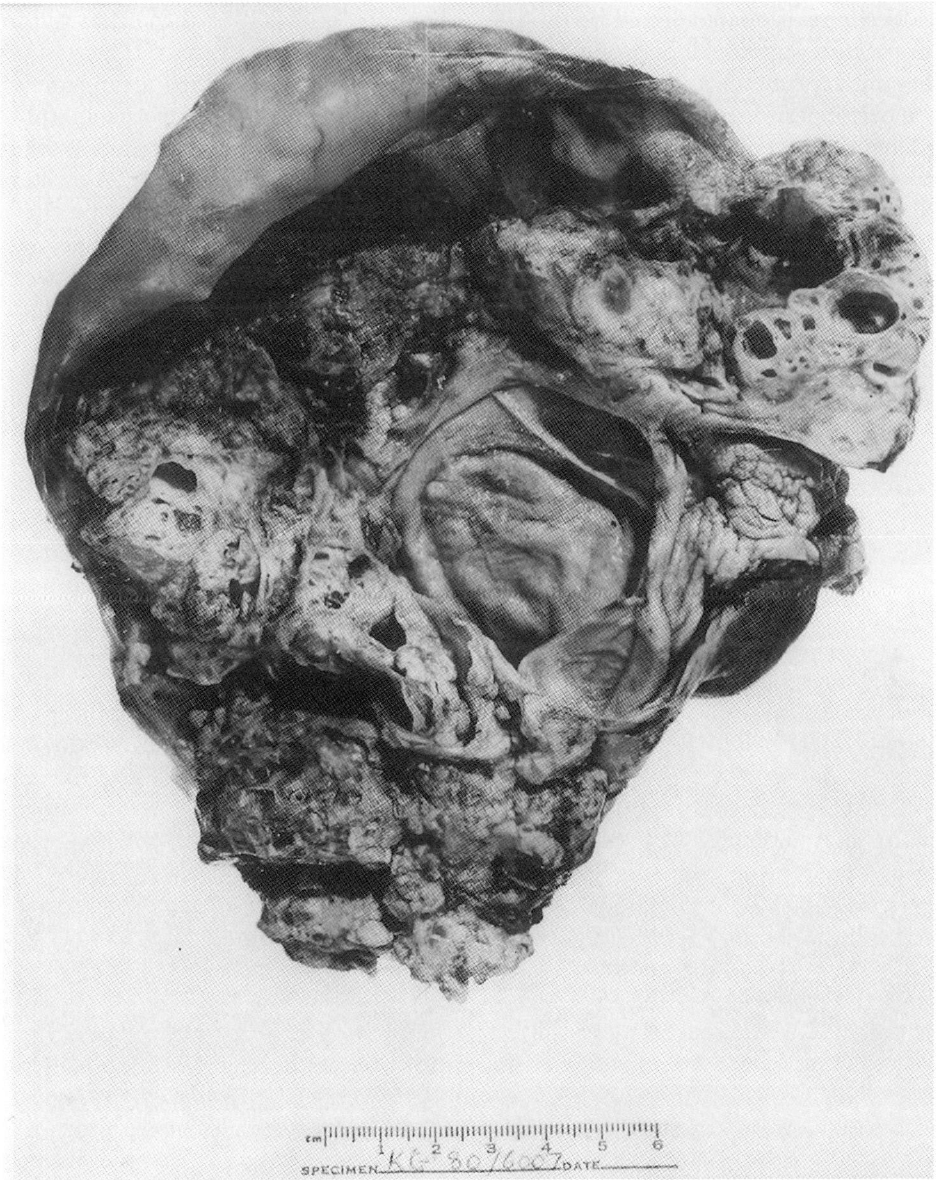

Fig. 47.1 Immature teratoma (grade 2). Large cystic spaces are present at left and center. The 'solid' areas contain multiple tiny cysts. Dark areas are foci of hemorrhage and necrosis.

material or hair, but most are degenerative in type and filled with clear, mucoid, or bloodstained fluid (Fig. 47.1). The solid areas are very variable in appearance; important areas to sample are those with a white or gray soft 'encephaloid' appearance. Hemorrhage and necrosis are relatively common and these foci should also be examined because they are likely to include the less well-differentiated tissues. Bone, cartilage, or gritty calcified areas are often noted.

Gliomatosis peritonei is characterized by multiple tiny firm gray-white superficial peritoneal nodules resembling miliary tubercles. They tend to be localized to the pelvic peritoneum, may be limited to the immediate vicinity of the ovarian tumor, and sometimes appear to be spatially related to the point of tumor rupture. Widespread involvement of both abdominal and pelvic peritoneum may also occur. They are not generally associated with adhesions. The nodules range in size from 0.1 to 1.1 cm, with an average of 0.3 cm (Robboy & Scully 1970, Truong et al 1982). By contrast, immature teratomatous metastatic deposits tend to be fewer in number, larger in size, and associated with adhesions.

Microscopic features

All three germ cell layers are generally evident, and the range of tissues includes all those which may be identified in benign cystic teratomas, as outlined in Chapter 46. There is a marked predominance of ectodermal and mesodermal components, and it is in these that the immaturity is also most clearly evident. The various tissues are admixed in a haphazard arrangement throughout the tumor, and this contrasts sharply with benign cystic teratomas in which there is some semblance of organization (Fig. 47.2). A striking feature on low-power examination may be the proliferation of neural tissues to form nodular masses mimicking some of the familiar intracranial tumors such as glioblastomas, neuroblastomas, medulloblastomas, and ependymomas.

Ectoderm is chiefly represented by neural tissue (Fig. 47.3) in the form of (roughly in decreasing

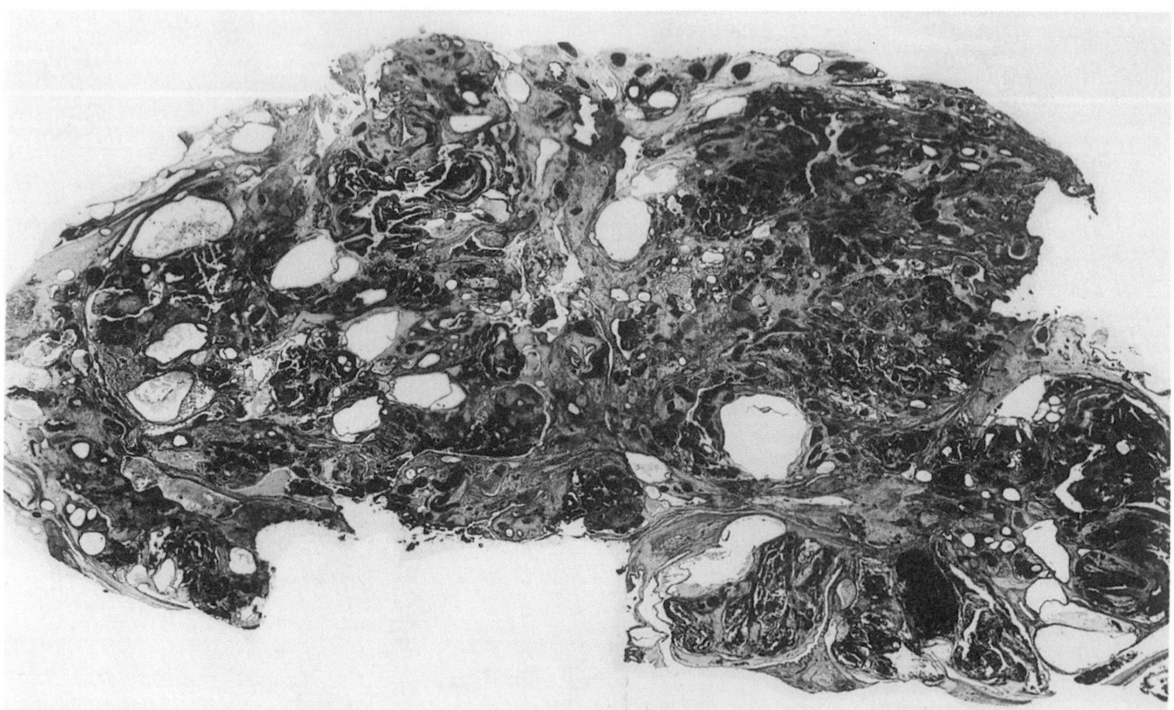

Fig. 47.2 Immature teratoma (grade 3). Tissue components are randomly arranged. Large dark areas are neuroglia. Small dark round areas are cartilage. The cysts are lined by simple columnar epithelium. H + E ×4

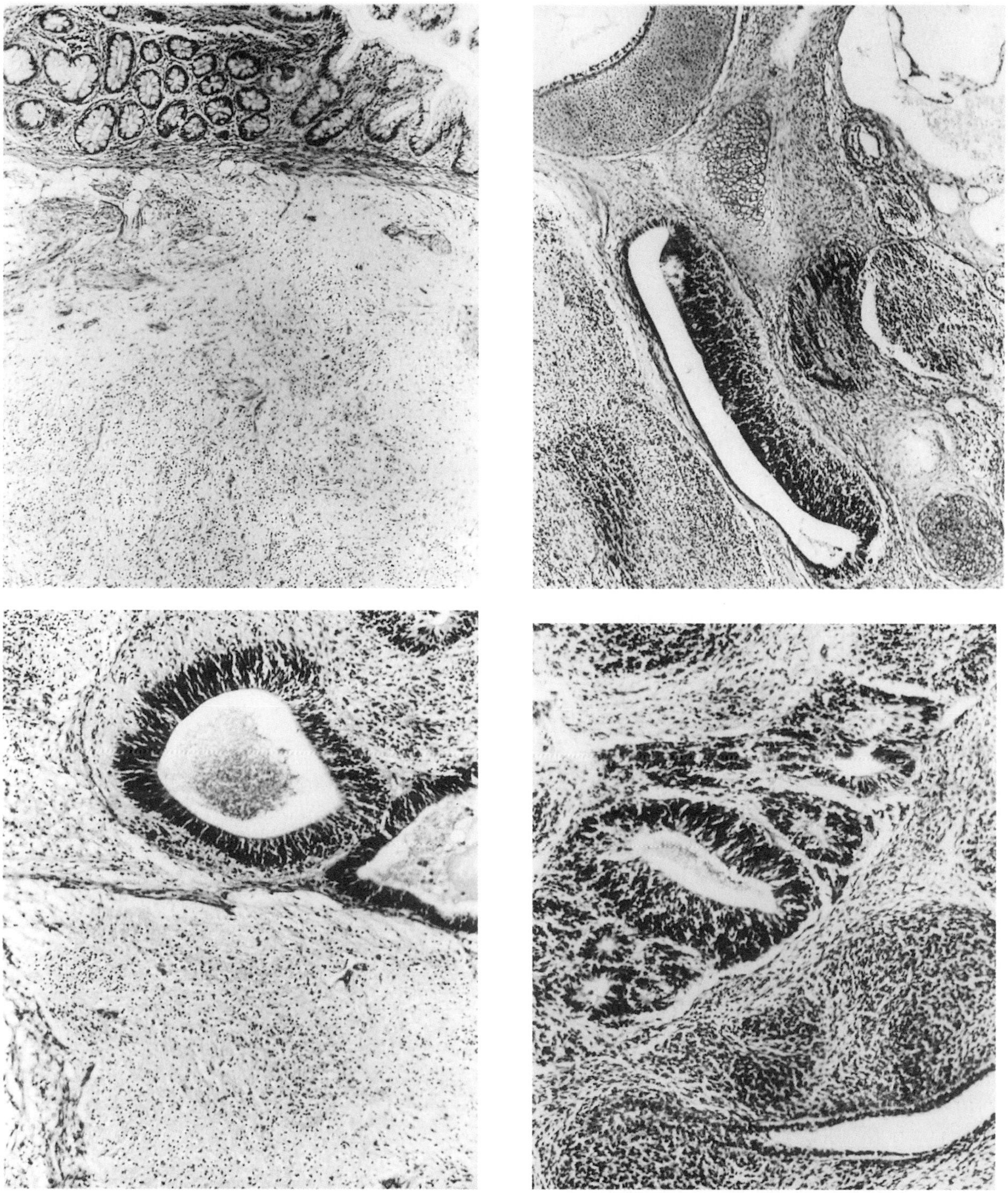

A B C D

Fig. 47.3 Neural elements in grade 3 immature teratomas. (A) Cellular neuroglia resembling glioblastoma. The adjacent gastric epithelium is an unusual finding. H + E ×50. (B) Immature neuroglia (below left) and adjacent pigmented neuroepithelium resembling embryonic optic cup. Note also islands of immature cartilage and degenerative cysts at right. H + E ×64. (C) Neuroglia with neuroepithelial tubules showing well-defined luminal margin and elongate nuclei. H + E ×80. (D) Highly cellular neuroglia forming neuroepithelial tubules. At bottom right, primitive mesenchyme surrounds a space lined by columnar epithelium with subnuclear glycogen vacuoles. H + E ×100 order of frequency): glia, neuroepithelium, neuroblastic tissue, choroid plexus, nerve fibers, microglia, ganglia, cerebellar tissue, and pigmented neuroepithelium (Nogales et al 1976, Scully 1979, Sangruchi & Sobel 1989, Talerman 1994). Gliomatous tissue is present in varying degrees of immaturity and atypicality, and may exhibit the vascular proliferative changes characteristic of astrocytomas. An expected immunoprofile of reactivity to glial fibrillary acid protein (GFAP), neurone specific enolase (NSE) and S-100 protein is seen, with about 50% of tumors also showing expression of vimentin filaments, and infrequently showing staining for neurofilaments (Vance et al 1988). Mitotic activity and atypicality increase in proportion to the degree of immaturity (Figs 47.3A–C). Neuroepithelium is most readily recognizable where it forms tubules, simulating embryonic neural tubes. These have a well-

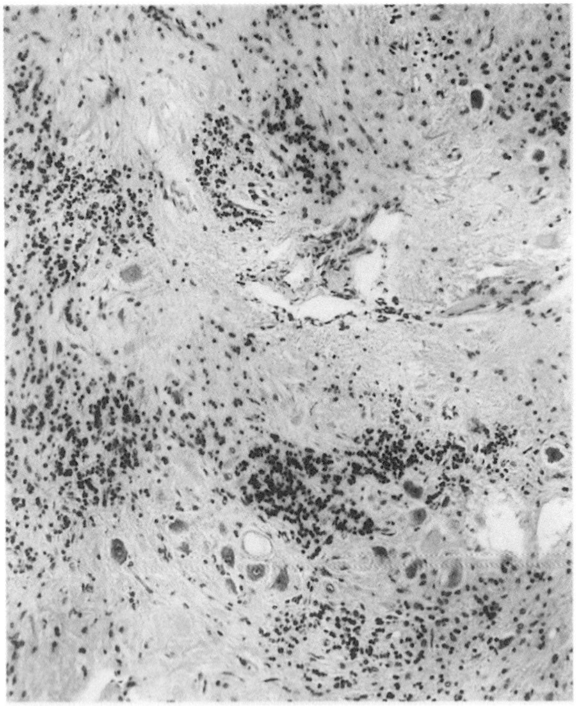

Fig. 47.4 Clusters of neuroblasts admixed with mature neural tissue including neurons (from a grade 1 immature teratoma). H + E ×90 (Reproduced, with permission, from Russell & Painter 1982)

Fig. 47.5 Grade 1 immature teratomas. (A) Cyst lined by mature squamous epithelium and adnexa. Note cellularity of underlying fibroadipose tissue and single focus of neuroglia (arrow). H + E ×25. (B) Three foci of tooth anlage with adjacent mature bony trabeculae and squamous epithelium. This solid tumor displayed immaturity of mesenchyme but not of neuroglia. H + E ×25

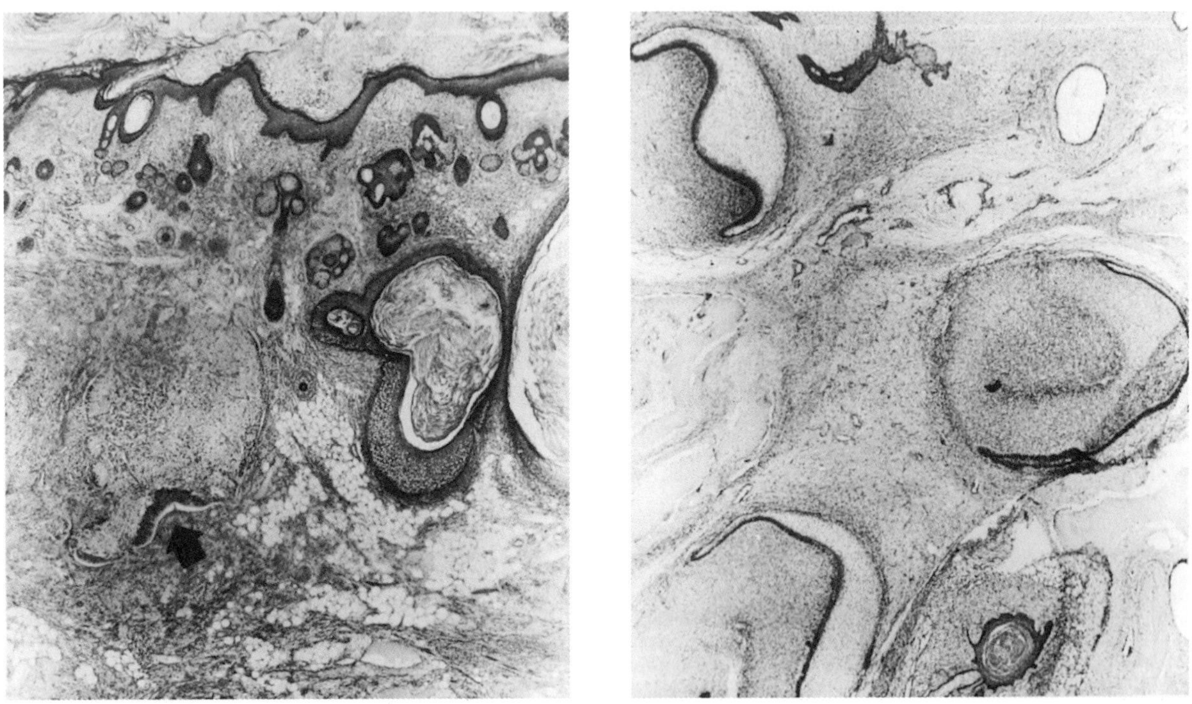

A

B

defined luminal margin lined by tall columnar cells, sometimes ciliated, with elongate hyperchromatic nuclei. Spindle-shaped cells with similar nuclei stream out towards the surrounding tissues. With increasing tumor grade, nuclear atypicality and mitotic activity become more conspicuous (Figs 47.3C,D). Pigmented neuroepithelium is quite common, and foci may resemble embryonic optic discs, pigmented medulloblastoma, or retinal anlage tumor (Fig. 47.3B). Neuroblastomatous areas are recognized by sheets of small cells with hyperchromatic nuclei forming rosettes, as seen in neuroblastomas of the adrenal glands (Fig. 47.4).

Squamous epithelium is usually present, disposed in small islands, and generally does not show cytological malignancy. Skin adnexal structures are also common (Figs 47.5, 47.6). Frank epithelial malignancy, such as adenocarcinoma, is rarely observed (Wisniewski & Deppisch 1973).

Mesoderm is represented by widely distributed loose fibrous connective tissue, which, with increasing tumor immaturity, resembles more closely undifferentiated myxoid embryonic mesenchyme and exhibits increased mitotic activity (Figs 47.3D, 47.5, 47.6). Small islands of cartilage and bone are usually present and these often express immaturity and resemble their embryonic counterparts (Figs 47.2, 47.3B, 47.5B, 47.6A). Immature cartilage characteristically also shows immunoreactivity of chondrocytes for S-100 protein, GFAP, and vimentin (Notohara et al 1990). Tooth anlagen may be prominent in low grade tumors (Fig. 47.5B). Smooth, but not striated, muscle is quite commonly observed.

Endoderm is not as well represented as the above elements in most tumors, and only rarely predominates (Nogales et al 1993). It is usually manifest as tubules lined by nonspecific columnar epithelium, sometimes with subnuclear glycogen vacuoles (Figs 47.3D, 47.5A); gastrointestinal or bronchial epithelium are found less often (Fig. 47.3A), as are

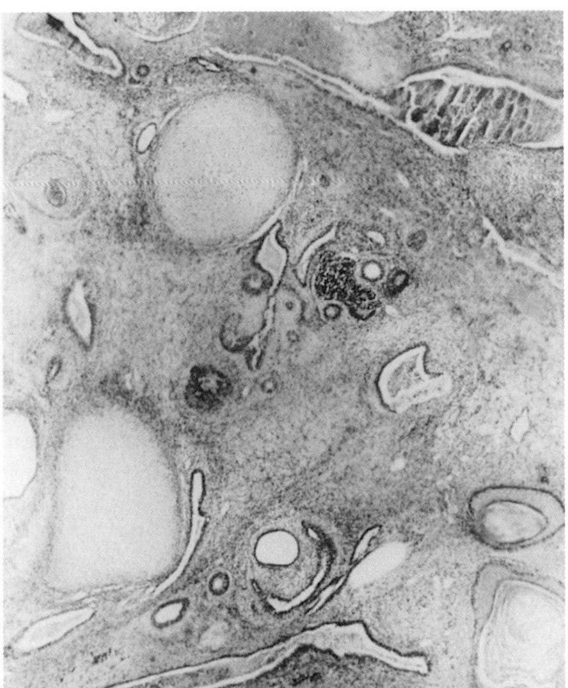

A

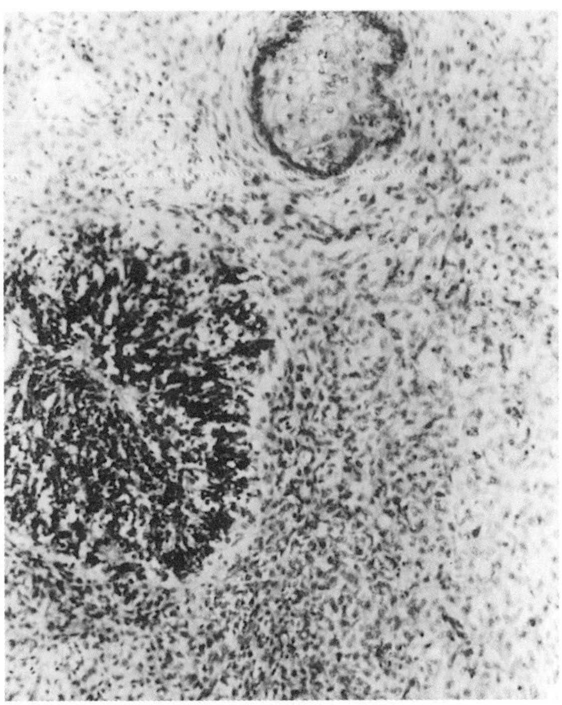

B

Fig. 47.6 Grade 2 immature teratoma. (A) Randomly arranged immature cartilage, squamous epithelial islands and nondescript epithelial structures in a background of immature mesenchyme. Two small foci of immature neuroglia are present at center. Necrosis is seen at top. H + E ×25. (B) Detail of cellular mesenchyme, immature squamous epithelium, and neuroglial focus. H + E ×100

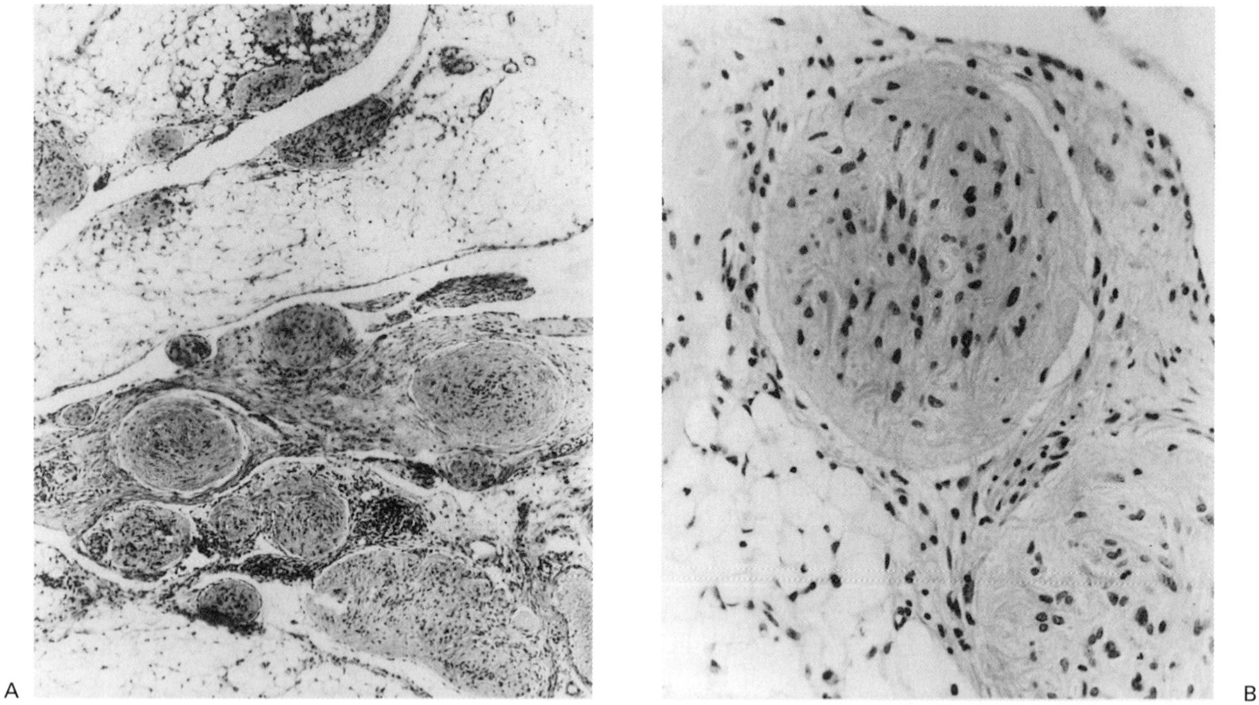

Fig. 47.7 Gliomatosis peritonei. (A) Clustered omental nodules of mature glial tissue. The lesions are well circumscribed and some are surrounded by fibrous tissue or a lymphocytic infiltrate. H + E ×50. (B) Detail of a nodule showing cytologically benign glial nuclei and abundant fibrillary cytoplasm. H + E ×200

isolated groups of hepatic cells (Nakashima et al 1987).

Histological grading of all tumors is recommended and presupposes adequate tumor sampling (see Ch. 4). The semiquantitative system suggested by Steeper & Mukai (1984) based on the overall proportion of neuroepithelium in the tumor, a modification of which has been the preferred grading system in our unit until recently, has been superseded by that of O'Connor & Norris (1994). These authors advocate a two-tiered system for stage 1 tumors with 'low grade' corresponding to grade 1 of the Steeper & Mukai (1984) system and 'high grade' corresponding to combined grades 2 and 3 of the earlier system.

- *Low grade:* neoplasms containing less than one low power field (LPF) of immature neuroepithelium on any one microscope (Fig. 47.6)
- *High grade:* immature neuroepithelium is common and exceeds 1LPF on one or more tumor sections in the tissue available for review (Fig. 47.3).

Gliomatosis peritonei consists of nodules, sometimes agminated, of mature glial tissue with no cytological atypicality and scarce or absent mitotic activity. The individual lesions may be surrounded by loose fibrous connective tissue and a light mixed inflammatory infiltrate in which lymphocytes predominate (Fig. 47.7). A small proportion of lesions include neurons or non-neural teratomatous components such as mature cartilage or squamous elements, the latter sometimes consisting only of some keratinous debris (Robboy & Scully 1970, Nogales et al 1976, Truong et al 1982) (Fig. 47.8). Immunoperoxidase stains for GFAP aid in the localization and identification of gliomatous foci (Truong et al 1982, Steeper & Mukai 1984).

Deposits of metastatic immature teratoma may show a wide variety of tissue components (both neural and other) and degree of immaturity within

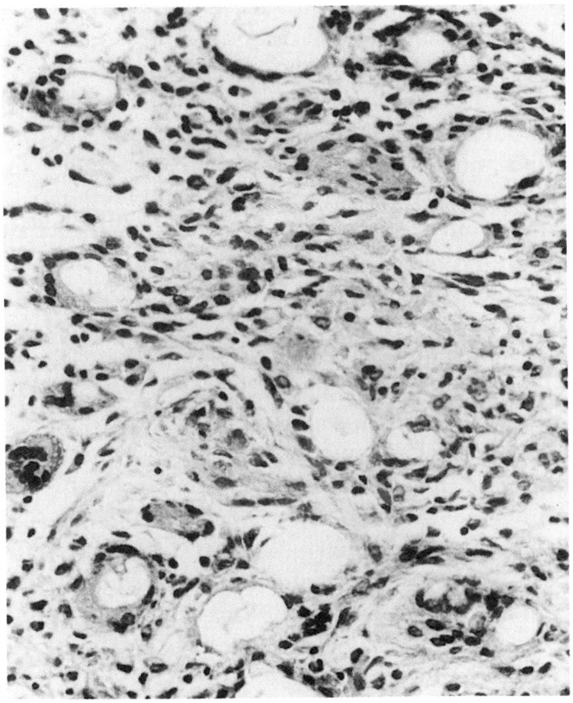

Fig. 47.8 Peritoneal foreign body granulomatous reaction to keratinous debris extruded from an ovarian immature teratoma. H + E ×200

a single patient (Fig. 47.9). There is a tendency for deposits closer to the ovary to be less mature (Nogales et al 1976).

Differential diagnosis

Immature teratomas must be differentiated from benign mature cystic teratomas, since even the low grade lesions have the potential to recur and kill the patient. This diagnostic pitfall can be avoided by adequately sampling all apparently straightforward, predominantly cystic, teratomas – concentrating on solid areas, particularly any which are unusually soft (encephaloid), hemorrhagic, or necrotic. The immunoperoxidase stain for GFAP is useful for identifying mature and immature glial tissue, and, similarly, NSE for other neuroectodermal tissue. In immature teratomas the various tissues are admixed in a haphazard arrangement throughout the tumor,

Fig. 47.9 Peritoneal metastases of immature teratoma. (A) Deposit of slightly immature neuroglia. Note poorly circumscribed margin (arrow) and florid peritoneal inflammatory reaction. H + E ×64. (B) Focus of primitive mesenchyme above, small clusters of mature glial cells below. Note marked peritoneal reaction. H + E ×100

A

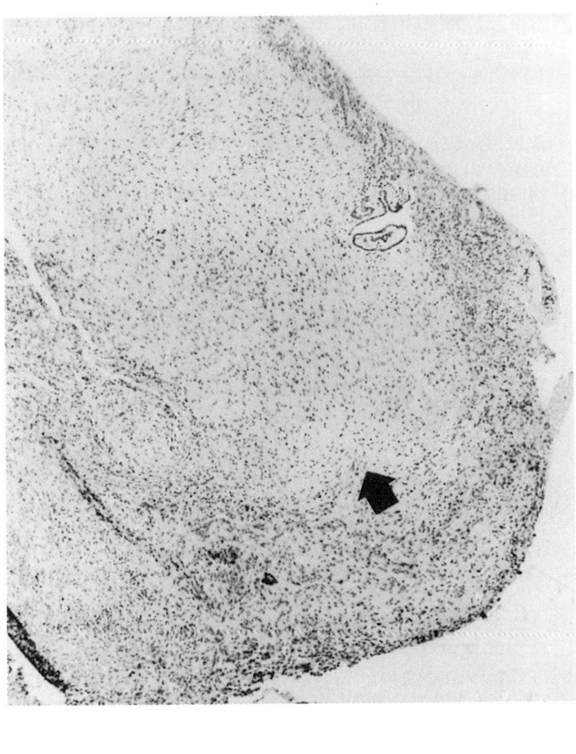

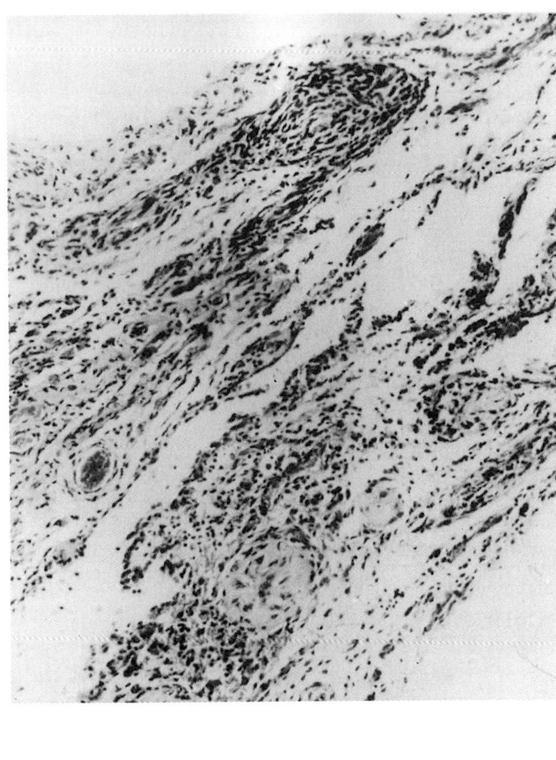

B

contrasting sharply with benign cystic teratomas in which there is some semblance of organization.

Immature teratoma is a common component of malignant mixed germ cell tumors, and the possibility of a mixed tumor should be explored by extensive histological sampling. If more than one LPF of other malignant germ cell tumor elements is found, the tumor must be excluded from the pure immature teratoma category. It is considered that even a small focus of endodermal sinus tumor or choriocarcinoma significantly worsens the prognosis of a germ cell tumor (Norris et al 1976). If preoperative hCG or AFP levels are elevated, it is incumbent on the pathologist to search exhaustively for these components.

Malignant mixed mullerian tumors (see Ch. 26) exhibit a variety of tissue types and may be a source of confusion. However, they are derived from mesoderm only, and therefore neural elements are virtually never present. The adenocarcinomatous components are usually readily distinguishable from the tubular neuroepithelial elements of immature teratoma but, if in doubt, positive cytokeratin and negative GFAP and NSE immunostaining will be confirmatory (Calame & Schaberg 1989). Chondroid elements are frequently present in mullerian tumors, but they are cytologically malignant, contrasting with the common chondroid components of immature teratomas, which have an embryonal rather than a chondrosarcomatous appearance. Rhabdomyoblasts are not uncommon in mullerian tumors, but are rare in immature teratomas (Chan et al 1989). A clinical feature helpful in differential diagnosis is that malignant mixed mullerian tumors occur predominantly in postmenopausal women, whereas immature teratomas have never been reported in this age group (see Table 26.2).

The monodermal variants of immature teratoma, e.g. malignant neuroectodermal tumors, should be clearly identified as such in the final diagnosis, since some of these have a significantly worse prognosis (see Ch. 49).

REFERENCES

Abell M R 1982 Ovarian neoplasms of childhood and adolescence. In: Blaustein A (ed) Pathology of the female genital tract, 2nd edn. Springer-Verlag, New York, p 665–704

Bahari C M, Lurie M, Schoenfeld A, Joel-Cohen S J 1980 Ovarian teratoma with peritoneal gliomatosis and elevated serum alpha-fetoprotein. American Journal of Clinical Pathology 73: 603–607

Bonazzi C, Peccatori F, Colombo N, Lucchini V, Cantu M G, Mangioni C 1994 Pure ovarian immature teratoma, a unique and curable disease: 10 years' experience of 32 prospectively treated patients. Obstetrics and Gynecology 84: 598–604

Burrus D R, Okagaki T, Twiggs L B, Brooker D C 1985 Immunocytochemical evidence of heterogeneous origin of α-fetoprotein in immature teratoma of the ovary. Gynecologic Oncology 21: 73–79

Calame J J, Schaberg A 1989 Solid teratomas and mixed mullerian tumors of the ovary: a clinical, histological, and immunohistochemical comparative study. Gynecologic Oncology 33: 212–221

Caldas C, Sitzmann J, Trimble C L, McGuire W P 3rd 1992 Synchronous mature teratomas of the ovary and liver: a case presenting 11 years following chemotherapy for immature teratoma. Gynecologic Oncology 47: 385–390

Chan Y F, Leung C S, Ma L 1989 Primary embryonal rhabdomyosarcoma of the ovary in a 4-year-old girl. Histopathology 15: 309–311

Coulson W F 1990 Peritoneal gliomatosis from a gastric carcinoma. American Journal of Clinical Pathology 94: 87–89

Dara P, Rich W M, Hodel K, DiSaia P J 1982 Long disease-free survival in immature teratoma of the ovary. Cancer 50: 159–162

El Shafie M, Furay R W, Chablani L V 1984 Ovarian teratoma with peritoneal and lymph node metastases of mature glial tissue: a benign condition. Journal of Surgical Oncology 27: 18–22

Fox H, Langley F A 1976 Tumours of the ovary. Heinemann, London, p 231–248

Gallion H, van Nagell J R, Donaldson E S, Hanson M B, Powell D F 1983 Immature teratoma of the ovary. American Journal of Obstetrics and Gynecology 146: 361–365

Gershenson D M, del Junco G, Silva E G, Copeland L J, Wharton J T, Rutledge F N 1986 Immature teratoma of the ovary. Obstetrics and Gynecology 68: 624–629

Gratama S, Swaak-Saeys A M, van der Weiden R M, Chadra S 1991 Low-grade immature teratomas with peritoneal gliomatosis; a case report. European Journal of Obstetrics and Gynecology and Reproductive Biology 39: 235–241

Harms D, Jänig U 1985 Immature teratomas of childhood. Report of 21 cases. Pathology Research and Practice 179: 388–400

Harms D, Jänig U, Gobel U 1989 Gliomatosis peritonei in childhood and adolescence. Clinicopathological study of 13 cases including immunohistochemical findings. Pathology Research and Practice 184: 422–430

Kawai M, Kano T, Furuhashi Y et al 1991 Immature teratoma of the ovary. Gynecologic Oncology 40: 133–137

King M E, di Giovanni L M, Yung J F, Clarke-Pearson D L

Immature teratoma of the ovary grade 3 with karytype analysis 1990 International Journal of Gynecological Pathology 9: 178–184
Lopez-Gines C, Gil R, Pellin A, Martorelli M, Vilar F, Llombart-Bosch A 1989 Trisomy 12 and translocation (7;9) in an ovarian immature teratoma. International Journal of Gynecological Pathology 8: 277–285
McLaughlin J E, Diebold M D, Rigaud C 1989 Blood-borne metastases from an immature teratoma of the ovary in a 36-year-old woman. Histopathology 15: 546–550
Nakashima N, Fukatsu T, Nagasaki T, Sobue M, Takeuchi J 1987 The frequency and histology of hepatic tissues in germ cell tumors. American Journal of Surgical Pathology 11: 682–692
Nielsen S N J, Scheithauer B W, Gaffey T A 1985 Gliomatosis peritonei. Cancer 56: 2499–2503
Nielsen S N J, Gaffey T A, Malkasian G D 1986 Immature ovarian teratoma: a review of 14 cases. Mayo Clinic Proceedings 61: 110–115
Nogales F F, Favara B E, Major F J, Silverberg S G 1976 Immature teratoma of the ovary with a neural component ('solid' teratoma). A clinicopathologic study of 20 cases. Human Pathology 7: 625–642
Nogales F F, Ruiz-Avila I, Concha A, del Moral E 1993 Immature endodermal teratoma of the ovary: embryologic correlations and immunohistochemistry. Human Pathology 24: 364–370
Norris H J, Zirkin H J, Benson W L 1976 Immature (malignant) teratoma of the ovary. A clinical and pathologic study of 58 cases. Cancer 37: 2359–2372
Notohara K, Hsueh C L, Awai M 1990 Glial fibrillary acidic protein immunoreactivity of chondrocytes in immature and mature teratomas. Acta Pathologica Japonica 40: 335–342
O'Connor D M, Norris H J 1994 The influence of grade on the outcome of stage 1 ovarian immature (malignant) teratomas and the reproducibility of grading. International Journal of Gynecological Pathology 13: 283–289
Robboy S J, Scully R E 1970 Ovarian teratoma with glial implants on the peritoneum. An analysis of 12 cases. Human Pathology 1: 643–653
Russell P, Painter D M 1982 The pathological assessment of ovarian neoplasms. V: The germ cell tumors. Pathology 14: 47–72
Sangruchi T, Sobel R A 1989 Microglial and neural differentiation in human teratomas. Acta Neuropathologica Berlin 78: 258–263
Schwartz P E, Merino M J, LiVolsi V A 1979 Immature ovarian teratomas. Maturation following chemotherapy. American Journal of Diagnostic Gynecology and Obstetrics 1: 361–366
Scully R E 1979 Germ cell tumors. In: Tumors of the ovary and maldeveloped gonads. Atlas of tumor pathology. Fascicle 16, 2nd series. Armed Forces Institute of Pathology, Washington, DC, p 226–286
Shefren G, Collin J, Soriero O 1991 Gliomatosis peritonei with malignant transformation: a case report and review of the literature. American Journal of Obstetrics and Gynecology 164: 1617–1620
Steeper T A, Mukai K 1984 Solid ovarian teratomas: an immunocytochemical study of thirteen cases with clinicopathologic correlation. Pathology Annual (Part 1) 19: 81–92
Talerman A 1994 Germ cell tumors of the ovary. In: Kurman R J (ed) Blaustein's pathology of the female genital tract, 4th edn. Springer-Verlag, New York. Ch 20, p 849–914
Truong L D, Jurco S, McGavran M H 1982 Gliomatosis peritonei. Report of 2 cases and review of literature. The American Journal of Surgical Pathology 6: 443–449
Vance R P, Geisinger K R, Randall M B, Marshall R B 1988 Immature neural elements in immature teratomas. An immunohistochemical and ultrastructural study. American Journal of Clinical Pathology 90: 397–411
Wheeler J E 1978 Extraovarian teratoma with peritoneal gliomatosis. Human Pathology 9: 232–234
Wisniewski M, Deppisch L M 1973 Solid teratomas of the ovary. Cancer 32: 440–446
Yanai-Inbar I, Scully R E 1987 Relation of ovarian dermoid cysts and immature teratomas: an analysis of 350 cases of immature teratoma and 10 cases of dermoid cyst with microscopic foci of immature tissue. International Journal of Gynecological Pathology 6: 203–212

48

Teratomas with secondary malignant transformation

P. Russell   A. Farnsworth

This category does not include all malignant neoplasms arising from, or in association with, benign cystic teratomas. By convention, malignancies associated with monodermal teratomas are excluded; thyroid carcinomas and carcinoids are therefore discussed separately (see Ch. 49). Tumors which include malignant germ cell tumor elements, such as choriocarcinoma, as well as teratomatous elements are also excluded as these form part of the malignant mixed germ cell tumor group (see Ch. 50).

Malignant transformation, as defined above, develops in a little less than 2% of mature cystic teratomas. This complication occurs most often in postmenopausal women, but is also, albeit rarely, seen in younger women (including those who are pregnant) and girls as young as 9 years. There are no distinctive clinical features, although as a group they are more likely than uncomplicated teratomas to be associated with abdominal swelling (sometimes due to ascites), pain, and systemic symptoms (Peterson 1957, Malkasian et al 1965, Caruso et al 1971, Fox & Langley 1976, Scully 1979).

At laparotomy, malignancy can be suspected in more than half the cases because of the presence of capsular tumor penetration and adhesions, infiltration of adjacent structures, or peritoneal metastases. In others the diagnosis is suspected on incising the excised ovarian mass, but in about one-quarter the diagnosis is not made until the tumor is examined histologically.

A wide variety of malignant tumors may arise within previously benign mature cystic teratomas, but by far the most common are squamous cell carcinomas (Hirakawa et al 1989) which account for 75–85% of all cases. The remainder is made up of: adenocarcinomas (about 7%); undifferentiated carcinomas, melanomas (Takubo et al 1991, Borup et al 1992, Carlson & Wheeler 1993, di Vagno et al 1993), and basal cell carcinomas (less than 1%); and various sarcomas (about 7%) (Peterson 1957, Climie & Heath 1968, Pantoja et al 1975, Fox & Langley 1976, Ueda et al 1977, Genadry et al 1979, Stamp & McConnell 1983). Malignant tumors documented to have arisen in mature cystic teratomas of the ovary are listed below:

- Squamous cell carcinoma
- Adenocarcinoma
- Malignant melanoma
- Thyroid carcinoma (see Ch. 49)
- Carcinoid tumor (see Ch. 49)
- Sebaceous carcinoma (Betta & Cosimi 1984, Chumas & Scully 1991, Changchien et al 1994, Papadopoulos et al 1995)
- Apocrine adenocarcinoma (Morimitsu et al 1993)
- Adenosquamous carcinoma (Climie & Heath 1968, Sekiya et al 1984, Manson et al 1993)
- Extramammary Paget's disease (Randall et al 1991, Shimizu et al 1991)
- Clear cell carcinoma (Sekiya et al 1984)
- Undifferentiated carcinoma (Kelly & Scully 1961, Climie & Heath 1968, Stamp & McConnell 1983, Chang et al 1992)
- Basal cell carcinoma (Mathios & McCausland 1973, Talerman 1982, Chumas & Scully 1991)
- Fibrosarcoma (Peterson 1957, Stamp & McConnell 1983)
- Osteogenic sarcoma (Ngwalle et al 1990)
- Chondrosarcoma (Climie & Heath 1968)
- Leiomyosarcoma (Kelly & Scully 1961, Tyagi et al 1993)

- Malignant fibrous histiocytoma (Ueda et al 1977)
- Histiocytoid (epithelioid) angiosarcoma (Madison & Cooper 1989)
- Lymphoma (Seifer et al 1986)
- Neuroblastoma (McCullough & Hardart 1963, Reid et al 1983)
- Glioblastoma (Shirley et al 1971).

In exceptional cases more than one malignant component is identified (Peterson 1957, Kelly & Scully 1961, Tyagi et al 1993). The validity of malignant neural tumors arising in mature cystic teratomas has been questioned (Reid et al 1983), and those reported in young women more probably represent immature teratomas which characteristically contain neural elements (see Ch. 47). Rare lesions will not be described in detail in this text, but references are provided. The pathological features generally represent a composite of mature cystic teratoma and the malignant tumor, as encountered in nonovarian tissues.

Tumor spread is predominantly by local direct infiltration and subsequent intraperitoneal dissemination. Distant lymphatic and blood-borne metastases are distinctly unusual except in sarcomas.

The prognosis for patients with malignant transformation in teratomas is very poor, with most women dying within a year. If extraovarian spread is present at the time of diagnosis the outlook is universally dismal. Outcome is less gloomy for patients with squamous cell carcinomas confined to the ovary at the time of surgical treatment (Chadha & Schaberg 1988, Hirakawa et al 1989). For this group Peterson (1957) found a 5-year survival rate of 63%, compared with 15% for the remainder. Poor prognostic factors are considered to be dissemination, cyst wall invasion, ascites, spontaneous or accidental rupture, adhesions (these may indicate capsular invasion or, at best, represent a risk of rupture during surgical removal), and tumor type other than squamous carcinoma (Peterson 1957, Climie & Heath 1968, Pantoja et al 1975, Krumerman & Chung 1977, Genadry et al 1979, Stamp & McConnell 1983).

The mainstay of treatment is surgery, with pelvic clearance being indicated in most cases. Unilateral oophorectomy may represent sufficient treatment in younger women in whom the ovarian capsule is not breached and the diagnosis is made only on pathological examination (Fox & Langley 1976, Talerman 1982).

Macroscopic features

Malignant transformation is always unilateral, but an uncomplicated mature cystic teratoma may be present in the contralateral ovary. They tend to be larger than their benign counterparts, generally in the range 15–20 cm in diameter. At least one half display tumor-associated adhesions and capsular penetration. In these more advanced cases, malignant tumor is generally obvious on bisecting the ovaries, presenting as necrotic crumbly masses projecting into the cavity and/or infiltrating the cyst wall. Carcinomas often develop in or close to the dermal papilla. Malignant melanomas form pigmented mural nodules (Fig. 48.1). Sarcomas are generally very hemorrhagic. However, in many cases tumor growth is more subtle and may only be represented by a plaque-like focus in the cyst lining or an area of induration in the wall. It is imperative, therefore, that all mature cystic teratomas should be examined histologically with particular attention paid to any unusual areas. Even if there is an overgrowth of malignant tumor

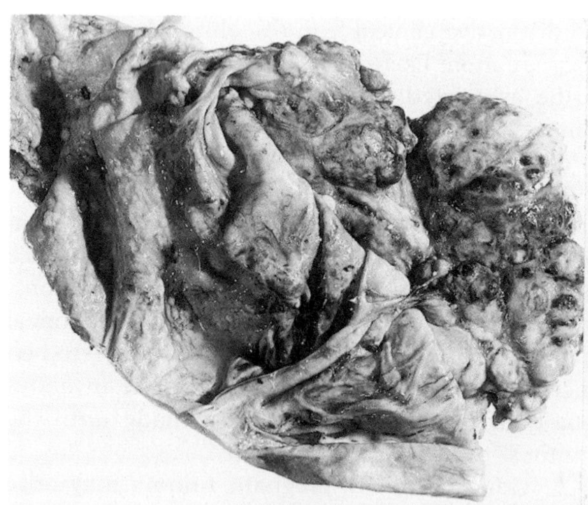

Fig. 48.1 Malignant melanoma arising in a benign cystic teratoma. Fungating, variably pigmented polypoid projections are seen at right, projecting into the lumen of a somewhat crenated, thick-walled cyst. Sebaceous debris has been removed to demonstrate the solid tumor mass

tissue, the presence of an underlying mature cystic teratoma usually declares itself by the presence of hair and/or sebaceous material in the cyst cavity.

Microscopic features

The histological appearances are diverse, reflecting the wide range of malignancies which may arise within teratomas. Squamous cell carcinomas (the most commonly observed tumors) can often be seen to arise from metaplastic squamous epithelium lining the cyst (Fig. 48.2), sometimes within a zone of dysplastic or in situ carcinomatous epithelium (Peterson et al 1956, Klionsky et al 1972, Fox & Langley 1976, Genadry et al 1979, Russell & Painter 1982) or from a focus of ciliated or nonciliated columnar mucosa (Fox & Langley 1976, Krumerman & Chung 1977, Hirakawa et al 1989). A pseudosarcomatous stromal reaction to invading squamous cell carcinoma has been documented (Czernobilsky et al 1972).

Adenocarcinomas may potentially arise from a variety of tissues, but a specific histogenesis is usually difficult to confirm except in tumors of distinctive histology such as sebaceous carcinoma (Betta & Cosimi 1984, Chumas & Scully 1991, Changchien et al 1994, Papadopoulos et al 1995). Tumors suggestive of mammary, sweat gland, or salivary gland, origin have been described (Peterson 1957, Curling et al 1979). Mucinous carcinoma of colonic type may occasionally develop (Ueda et al 1993), but it should be remembered that pure primary mucinous tumors of the ovary (part of the epithelial–stromal tumor group) quite commonly accompany mature cystic teratomas, and no clear policy exists as to whether malignancy of this type should be attributed to a pre-existing benign mucinous tumor or a teratoma if evidence of both is present.

Ovarian malignant melanomas are usually pig-

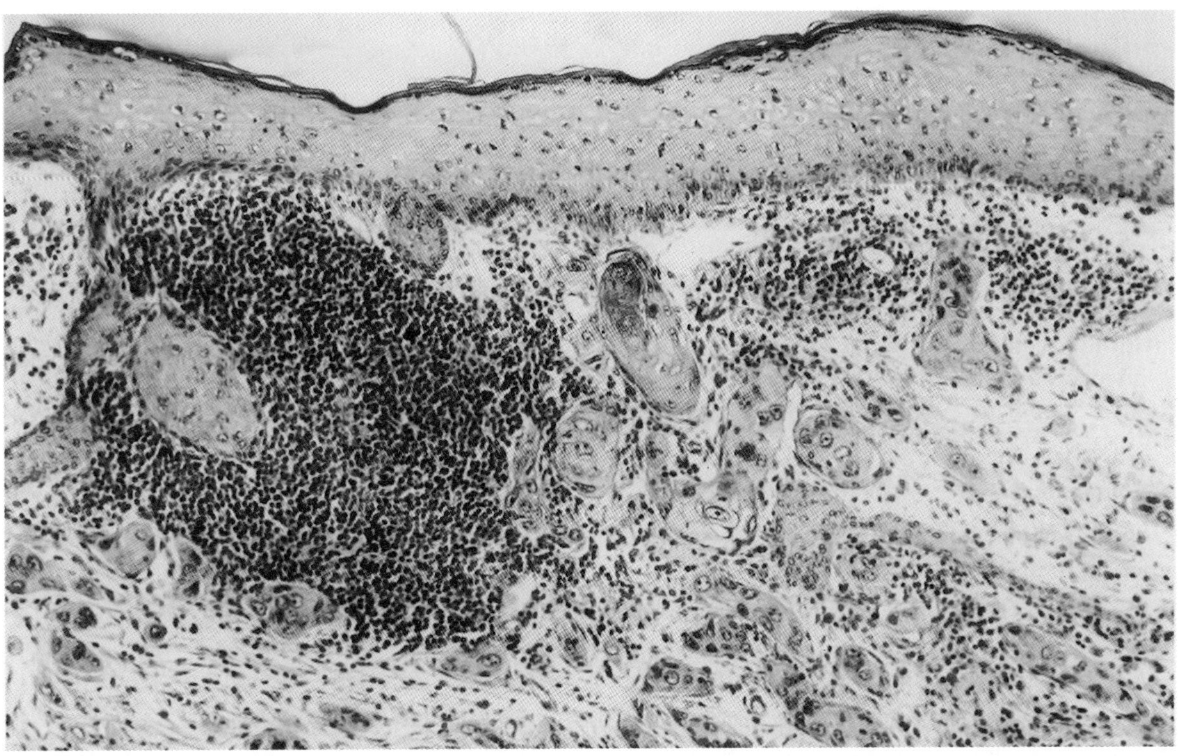

Fig. 48.2 Squamous cell carcinoma arising in the mature cystic teratoma of a 61-year-old woman. The carcinoma formed an 11 cm nodule in the cyst wall. Clusters of carcinoma cells invade the cyst wall from the squamous epithelial lining. H + E ×125

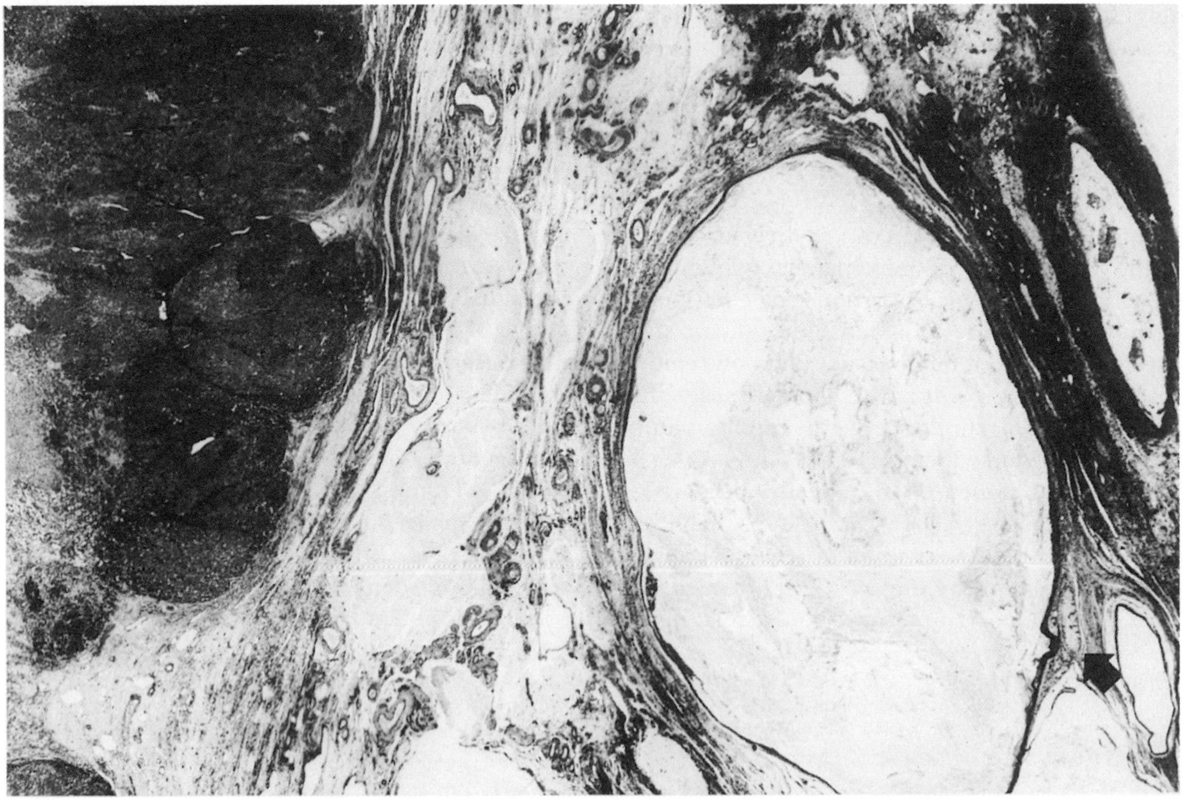

Fig. 48.3 Malignant melanoma (left) formed a 13 cm ovarian mass in a 37-year-old woman. There was an adjacent 1 cm squamous epithelium-lined cyst (right) and sebaceous gland (arrow), indicative of a mature teratoma. The subsequent clinical course of the patient (alive with disease at 4 years) supported a primary (teratomatous) origin rather than a metastasis. H + E ×10

mented and show any of the histological patterns seen at other sites (Fig. 48.3). Some are associated with junctional activity in the adjacent epidermis-lined cyst (Park et al 1970, Leo et al 1973, Cronje & Woodruff 1981, Ueda et al 1991).

Differential diagnosis

The teratomatous origin of these tumors may be overlooked if histological sampling is not adequate; the lesion is then likely to be misdiagnosed as a metastasis. However, there is the possibility that growth of the malignant component may have obliterated the pre-existing teratoma. The clinical presentation should always be taken into account and the pattern of extraovarian spread, if present, should be consistent with a primary ovarian neoplasm.

The most frequent misdiagnosis is immature teratoma (see Ch. 47), a clinically malignant neoplasm which is found in girls and young women. This tumor, almost always a predominantly solid lesion, is characterized by an abundance of immature neural components. In addition, other tissue components often show immaturity and malignant cytological features, unlike mature cystic teratomas with malignant transformation in which only one cancerous component (which is very rarely neural) is demonstrable.

The identification of germ cell tumor components other than mature cystic teratoma, such as choriocarcinoma, places the tumor in the category of malignant mixed germ cell tumor (see Ch. 50).

Malignant mixed mullerian tumors (see Ch. 26) occur in the same age group as the tumors under discussion and exhibit a variety of tissue components. However, they are generally solid tumors and lack the characteristic squamous epithelium-lined cyst and associated adnexal structures. Malignancy is commonly expressed in both the epithelial component (generally resembling serous carcinoma) and the mesenchymal component (usually resembling endometrial stromal sarcoma, at least in part). Endodermally and ectodermally derived structures are absent, but islands of malignant squamous epithelium (of mullerian mesodermal origin) are occasionally present (see Ch. 26).

Some Sertoli–Leydig cell tumors include heterologous elements and these variants (see Ch. 35) may mimic adenocarcinomas or sarcomas arising in mature cystic teratomas. Mucinous epithelium of colonic type is the most common heterologous element, but squamous epithelium, which is almost universal in mature cystic teratomas, is not seen. Sertoli cell tubules tend to be admixed with other heterologous tissues rather than forming a discrete mass, as would carcinoma arising in a mature cystic teratoma. When the heterologous elements are malignant and form the major element of the tumor, exhaustive sampling may be the only means of establishing the androblastomatous, as opposed to teratomatous, origin of the malignancy. Leydig cells may be scattered in groups throughout the stroma; they are only rarely present in teratomas (at the margins). A clinical point of distinction is the occurrence of androblastomas predominantly in young women, whereas teratomas with secondary malignant transformation tend to develop in postmenopausal women.

The difficulties in distinguishing primary ovarian malignant melanomas from the more common metastatic lesions are discussed in Chapter 54.

REFERENCES

Betta P G, Cosimi M F 1984 Sebaceous carcinoma arising in benign cystic teratoma of the ovary. Case report. European Journal of Gynaecological Oncology 5: 146–149

Borup K, Leisgard-Rasmussen K, Scheirup L, Moller J C 1992 Amelanotic malignant melanoma arising in an ovarian dermoid cyst. Acta Obstetricia et Gynecologica Scandinavica 71: 242–244

Carlson J A Jr, Wheeler J E 1993 Primary ovarian melanoma arising in a dermoid stage. IIIc: Long-term disease-free survival with aggressive surgery and platinum therapy. Gynecologic Oncology 48: 397–401

Caruso P A, Marsh M R, Minkowitz S, Karten G 1971 An intense clinicopathologic study of 305 teratomas of the ovary. Cancer 27: 343–348

Chadha S, Schaberg A 1988 Malignant transformation in benign cystic teratomas: dermoids of the ovary. European Journal of Obstetrics Gynecology and Reproductive Biology 29: 329–338

Chang D H, Hsueh S, Soong Y K 1992 Small cell carcinoma with neurosecretory granules arising in an ovarian dermoid cyst. Gynecologic Oncology 46: 246–250

Changchien C C, Chen L, Eng H L 1994 Sebaceous carcinoma arising in a benign dermoid cyst of the ovary. Acta Obstetricia et Gynecologica Scandinavica 73: 355–358

Chumas J C, Scully R E 1991 Sebaceous tumors arising in ovarian dermoid cysts. International Journal of Gynecological Pathology 10: 356–363

Climie A R W, Heath L P 1968 Malignant degeneration of benign cystic teratomas of the ovary. Review of the literature and report of a chondrosarcoma and carcinoid tumor. Cancer 22: 824–832

Cronje H S, Woodruff J D 1981 Primary ovarian malignant melanoma arising in cystic teratoma. Gynecologic Oncology 12: 379–383

Curling O M, Potsides, Hudson C N 1979 Malignant change in benign cystic teratoma of the ovary. British Journal of Obstetrics and Gynaecology 86: 399–402

Czernobilsky B, Rotenstreich L, Lancet M 1972 Ovarian dermoid with squamous carcinoma-pseudosarcoma. Archives of Pathology 93: 141–144

di Vagno G, Mele M, Resta L et al 1993 Primary malignant melanoma arising in an ovarian dermoid cyst: proposed use of radioimmunoscintigraphy with 99mTc-F(ab')2 antimelanoma antibody for staging and follow-up. Case report. European Journal of Gynaecological Oncology 14: 237–245

Fox H, Langley F A 1976 Tumours of the ovary. Heinemann, London, p 210–230

Genadry R, Parmley T, Woodruff J D 1979 Secondary malignancies in benign cystic teratomas. Gynecologic Oncology 8: 246–251

Hirakawa T, Tsuneyoshi M, Enjoji M 1989 Squamous cell carcinoma arising in mature cystic teratoma of the ovary. Clinicopathologic and topographic analysis. American Journal of Surgical Pathology 13: 397–405

Kelly R R, Scully R E 1961 Cancer developing in dermoid cysts of the ovary: a report of 8 cases including a carcinoid and a leiomyosarcoma. Cancer 14: 989–1000

Klionsky B L, Nickens O J, Amortegui A J 1972 Squamous cell carcinoma in situ arising in adult cystic teratoma of the ovary. Archives of Pathology 93: 161–163

Krumerman M S, Chung A 1977 Squamous carcinoma arising in benign cystic teratoma of the ovary. A report of four cases and review of the literature. Cancer 39: 1237–1242

Leo S, Rorat E, Parekh M 1973 Primary malignant melanoma in a dermoid cyst of the ovary. Obstetrics and Gynecology 41: 205–210

McCullough C D, Hardart F 1963 Neuroblastomatous transformation in a benign cystic teratoma. Obstetrics and Gynecology 21: 259–261

Madison J F, Cooper P H 1989 A histiocytoid (epithelioid) vascular tumor of the ovary: occurrence within a benign cystic teratoma. Modern Pathology 2: 55–58

Malkasian G D, Symmonds R E, Dockerty M B 1965 Malignant ovarian teratomas. Report of 31 cases. Obstetrics and Gynecology 25: 810–814

Manson C M, Cross P A, Herd M E, Wake C R 1993 Mixed adeno- and squamous carcinoma in a mature cystic teratoma in a young woman. Histopathology 23: 481–482

Mathios A J, McCausland A M 1973 Basal cell carcinoma originating in a benign cystic teratoma of the ovary. Obstetrics and Gynecology 42: 892–896

Morimitsu Y, Nakashima O, Nakashima Y, Kojiro M, Shimokobe T 1993 Apocrine adenocarcinoma arising in cystic teratoma of the ovary. Archives of Pathology and Laboratory Medicine 117: 647–649

Ngwalle K E, Hirakawa T, Tsuneyoshi M, Enjoji M 1990 Osteosarcoma arising in a benign dermoid cyst of the ovary. Gynecologic Oncology 37: 143–147

Pantoja E, Rodriguez-Ibanez I, Axtmayer R W, Noy M A, Pelegrina I 1975 Complications of dermoid tumors of the ovary. Obstetrics and Gynecology 45: 89–94

Papadopoulos A J, Ahmed H, Pakarian F B, Caldwell C J, McNicholas J, Raju K S 1995 Sebaceous carcinoma arising within an ovarian cystic mature teratoma. International Journal of Gynecological Cancer 5: 76–79

Park H, Kramer E E, Gray G F 1970 Primary malignant melanoma in an ovarian dermoid cyst. American Journal of Obstetrics and Gynecology 106: 942–943

Peterson W F 1957 Malignant degeneration of benign cystic teratomas of the ovary. A collective review of the literature. Obstetrical and Gynecological Survey 12: 793–830

Peterson W F, Prevost E C, Edmunds F T, Hundley J M, Morris F K 1956 Epidermoid carcinoma arising in a benign cystic teratoma. A report of 15 cases. American Journal of Obstetrics and Gynecology 71: 173–189

Randall B J, Ritchie C, Hutchison R S 1991 Paget's disease and invasive undifferentiated carcinoma occurring in a mature cystic teratoma of the ovary. Histopathology 18: 469–470

Reid H A S, Van der Walt J D, Fox H 1983 Neuroblastoma arising in a mature cystic teratoma of the ovary. Journal of Clinical Pathology 36: 68–73

Russell P, Painter D M 1982 The pathological assessment of ovarian neoplasms. V: The germ cell tumors. Pathology 14: 47–72

Scully R E 1979 Tumors of the ovary and maldeveloped gonads. Atlas of tumor pathology. Fascicle 16, 2nd series. Armed Forces Institute of Pathology, Washington, DC, p 226–286

Seifer D B, Weiss L M, Kempson R L 1986 Malignant lymphoma arising within thyroid tissue in a mature cystic teratoma. Cancer 58: 2459–2461

Sekiya S, Iwasawa H, Morikawa S, Takamizawa H 1984 Malignant change of dermoid cysts of the ovary. Report on an adenosquamous cell carcinoma and a clear cell carcinoma. European Journal of Gynaecological Oncology 5: 16–20

Shimizu S, Kobayashi H, Suchi T, Torii Y, Narita K, Aoki S 1991 Extramammary Paget's disease arising in mature cystic teratoma of the ovary. American Journal of Surgical Pathology 15: 1002–1006

Shirley R L, Piro A J, Crocker D W 1971 Malignant neural elements in a benign cystic teratoma. A case report. Obstetrics and Gynecology 37: 402–407

Stamp G W H, McConnell E M 1983 Malignancy arising in cystic ovarian teratomas. A report of 24 cases. British Journal of Obstetrics and Gynaecology 90: 671–675

Takubo K, Kimura T, Suzuki K et al 1991 Malignant melanoma arising in ovarian cystic teratoma. Gynecologic Oncology 43: 77–80

Talerman A 1982 Germ cell tumors of the ovary. In: Blaustein A (ed) Pathology of the female genital tract, 2nd edn. Springer-Verlag, New York, p 602–664

Tyagi S P, Maheshwari V, Tyagi N, Tewari K 1993 Double malignancy in a benign cystic teratoma of the ovary (a case report). Indian Journal of Cancer 30: 140–142

Ueda G, Sato Y, Yamasaki M et al 1977 Malignant fibrous histiocytoma arising in a benign cystic teratoma of the ovary. Gynecologic Oncology 5: 313–322

Ueda G, Fujita M, Ogawa H, Sawada M, Inoue M, Tanizawa O 1993 Adenocarcinoma in a benign cystic teratoma of the ovary: report of a case with a long survival period. Gynecologic Oncology 48: 259–263

Ueda Y, Kimura A, Kawahara E, Kitagawa H, Nakanishi I 1991 Malignant melanoma arising in a dermoid cyst of the ovary. Cancer 67: 3141–3145

49

Monodermal and highly specialized teratomas

P. Russell   A. Farnsworth

These are teratomas which consist predominantly or exclusively of one adult tissue and are presumed to result either from teratomatous development involving only one germ cell layer or overgrowth of one tissue at the expense of others originally present. Examples include struma ovarii, carcinoid tumors, epidermoid cysts, and neuroectodermal tumors. There is clearly some conceptual overlap between this and the preceding chapter with regard to those monodermal teratomas which are clinically malignant, a difficulty which is not overcome by rational argument.

STRUMA OVARII

The World Health Organization (WHO) definition of struma ovarii is 'a teratoma in which thyroid tissue is exclusively present or constitutes a grossly recognizable component of a more complex teratoma' (Serov et al 1973). Since 5–13% of mature cystic teratomas of the ovary contain some thyroid tissue, it is useful to have a semiquantitative definition. Caruso et al (1971) used the criterion of at least 50% thyroid tissue content, an example we followed in analyzing our series of teratomas. Kempers et al (1970) recommended that a 'significant thyroid component', i.e. struma, should represent at least 50% of the ovarian tumor or show evidence of function as indicated by hyperthyroidism. Strumas are generally considered to account for less than 5% of mature teratomas (Scully 1979, Talerman 1994); using the 50% thyroid tissue criterion, Caruso et al (1971) and ourselves (Russell & Painter 1982) both arrived at a figure of 1.4%. Conversely, while 50–60% of strumas are associated with, or part of, mature cystic teratomas, most of the remainder are pure, and a very small percentage is associated with carcinoid tumors (strumal carcinoids) or mucinous cystadenomas in the same ovary (Kempers et al 1970, Fox & Langley 1976, Scully 1979).

The age range for struma ovarii is a little narrower than for mature cystic teratomas in general, most cases occurring in the reproductive years with a peak in the early forties. Like mature cystic teratomas of the ovary, they usually present with nonspecific abdominal symptoms or are incidental findings. Rarely, patients develop symptoms or signs indicating estrogen excess, considered to be due to the activity of luteinized stromal cells surrounding the tumor (Ober 1960, Rutgers & Scully 1986). Up to one-third develop ascites, which can be quite marked but does not signify malignancy and settles rapidly after tumor removal. Some of these patients also develop a hydrothorax (Meigs' syndrome) (Kempers et al 1970, Fox & Langley 1976, Scully 1979).

Hyperthyroidism is a much discussed complication of struma ovarii but, using biochemical criteria to confirm the clinical impression (not available in most early studies), less than 5% of strumas have this association. A causal relationship is often very difficult to establish, since about one-sixth of all struma ovarii patients and one-half of those with hyperthyroidism have an enlarged cervical thyroid gland; some also have a history of partial thyroidectomy (Marcus & Marcus 1961, Kempers et al 1970, Brown et al 1973, Fox & Langley 1976). In order to attribute biochemically established hyperthyroidism to struma ovarii, thyroid activity should be demonstrated in the ovary by means of an iodine-131 scan and, preferably, a radionucleotide angiogram. Fox & Langley

(1976) found 17 acceptable cases in the literature; symptoms and signs of hyperthyroidism resolved after oophorectomy (Dalgaard & Wetteland 1956, Judd & Buie 1962, Kempers et al 1970, Brown et al 1973). The pathogenesis of hyperthyroidism associated with struma ovarii is of interest. The ectopic thyroid tissue appears to act autonomously in a manner analogous to toxic nodular goitre, and the thyroid gland itself may be suppressed. Long-acting thyroid stimulator has not been identified in these patients (Marcus & Marcus 1961, Kempers et al 1970, Brown et al 1973, Fox & Langley 1976). In patients without hyperthyroidism, excision of the struma ovarii may result in transient compensatory enlargement of the thyroid gland and, rarely, mild hyperthyroidism (Fox & Langley 1976).

Approximately 5% of strumas are clinically malignant, i.e. associated with metastatic disease (Fox & Langley 1976, Scully 1979). The well-known difficulties in diagnosing malignancy in the thyroid gland are exaggerated in ectopically sited tissue, where criteria such as capsular invasion cannot be readily applied. Extraovarian spread appears to be the only valid criterion, so that many cases from the older literature have been discredited by modern reviewers; the original diagnoses were sometimes based on morphology alone (anaplasia and mitotic activity) or on a misinterpretation of what we now know to be strumal carcinoid tumors. Metastases, occurring up to 26 years after oophorectomy, to peritoneum, mesentery, contralateral ovary, liver, bones, mediastinum, lung, and brain have been reported (Kempers et al 1970, Fox & Langley 1976, Hasleton et al 1978, Pardo-Mindan & Vazquez 1983, Willemse et al 1987, Rosenblum et al 1989). The assessment of the malignant potential of struma ovarii has been further confounded by the half-hearted acceptance of the concept of 'benign strumosis'. This term was applied by Emge (1940) to histologically benign peritoneal deposits of thyroid tissue which he identified in a few patients with apparently benign struma ovarii; although untreated, the peritoneal lesions did not progress over many years of observation. Endorsement of 'strumosis' may be unwise, considering the notorious histological fickleness of thyroid carcinoma and its ability to follow a very protracted course. At best it can be said that well-differentiated peritoneal metastases are compatible with long survival (Gonzalez-Angulo et al 1963, Woodruff et al 1966, Caruso et al 1971, Fox & Langley 1976, Scully 1979). Strumosis, as a bona fide process, is a possible alternative explanation to multifocal germ cell neoplasia, to account for occasional concurrence of thyroid-like tissue in ovary and adjacent fallopian tube (Hoda & Huvos 1993).

Oophorectomy is adequate treatment for straightforward struma ovarii. Pelvic clearance is recommended for malignant tumors, with additional thyroidectomy and adjunctive therapy, e.g. iodine-131 for those with extraovarian spread (Kempers et al 1970, Willemse et al 1987).

Macroscopic features

Struma ovarii are almost always unilateral. The contralateral ovary has rarely been reported to harbor an additional struma, but is more likely to contain an uncomplicated mature cystic teratoma. The tumors vary greatly in size, but typical lesions are about 10 cm in diameter (but somewhat larger if cystic in nature or if associated with mature cystic teratomas). Strumas associated with hyperthyroidism are generally more than 6 cm in diameter (Kempers et al 1970). They are most often found as circumscribed nodules in the walls of mature cystic teratomas but, if pure, form encapsulated lobulated masses with smooth surfaces, often displaying prominent blood vessels. Sectioning of the tumors reveals soft or firm red-brown or yellowish tissue with a glistening surface. Tumors are mostly solid, but usually include multiple small cystic spaces containing colloid or mucoid material. Cystic variants contain clear to green-brown fluid. Hemorrhage, necrosis, and fibrosis may be apparent and, in fact, the gross appearance may closely resemble that of nodular colloid or adenomatous goitres (Fig. 49.1).

Microscopic features

The thyroid tissue of struma ovarii exhibits morphological and biochemical identity with cervical thyroid tissue (Marcus & Marcus 1961, Fox & Langley 1976). It may appear histologically 'normal', but more commonly shows a range of minor

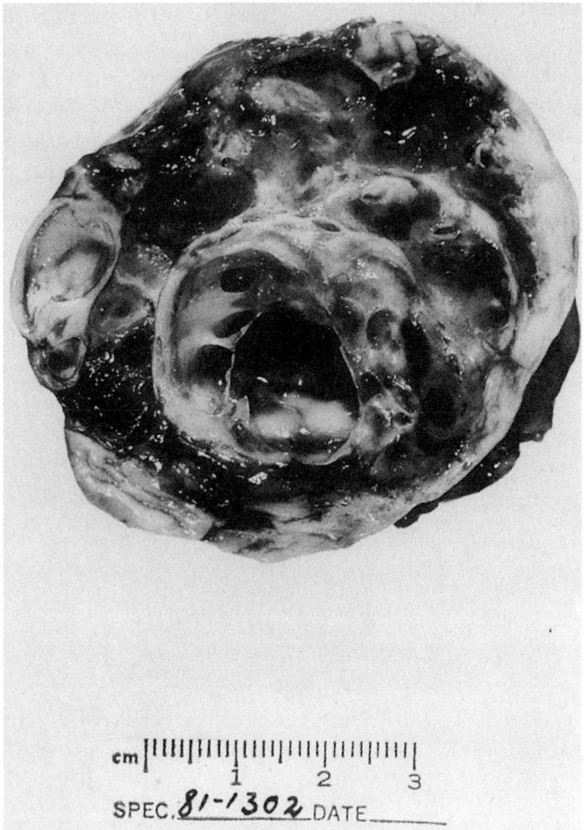

Fig. 49.1 Struma ovarii. Encapsulated mass of glistening thyroid tissue with foci of cystic degeneration and fibrosis. No other heterologous elements were present in this tumor, but there was a contralateral mature cystic teratoma

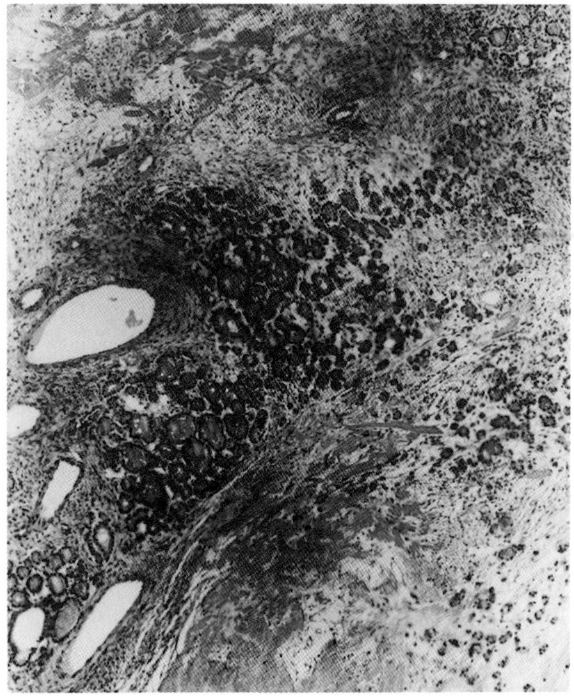

Fig. 49.2 Struma ovarii. Small thyroid follicles in an area of 'fibrinoid' degeneration and fibrosis. H + E ×50

abnormalities. There is generally a great variability in follicular size and maturity, with macrofollicular, microfollicular, and solid (embryonal) patterns being commonly observed. Small numbers of oxyphil cells may also be encountered (Scully 1979). The colloid is PAS positive and contains birefringent oxalate crystals. The identity of the tissue can be readily confirmed with an immunohistochemical stain for thyroglobulin. All the microscopic features associated with nodular colloid or adenomatous goitres (e.g. fibrosis, hemorrhage, and cystic degeneration) may be encountered (Fig. 49.2). Cystic degeneration may lead to a paucity of thyroid follicles in the cyst wall, with an accompanying danger of the diagnosis being overlooked (Szyfelbein et al 1994). Follicular adenoma-like areas are not infrequently seen, but their significance is unknown. Devaney et al (1993) have subcategorized the largest series of such cases as 'proliferative struma' to indicate tumor-like architectural and cellular features, but separable from 'malignant struma' by the lack of 'ground glass', overlapping nuclei, vascular space invasion, or mitotic activity. All their 'proliferative struma' cases pursued a benign clinical course. No capsule normally separates thyroid tissue from adjacent teratomatous elements, if present, or residual ovarian parenchyma, and capsular invasion, an important parameter in the assessment of follicular tumors in the cervical thyroid, is not available in equivalent ovarian thyroid masses. Stromal luteinization or, rarely, Leydig cell hyperplasia, may be seen at the margins of the tumor (Fig. 49.3). In patients with hyperthyroidism, and some without, histological features of hyperplasia may be evident, i.e. diminution in colloid with scalloping of its margin and tall columnar epithelium with focal intraluminal tufting. Florid diffuse hyperplasia is rarely seen and the overall impression is that the morphology correlates poorly with

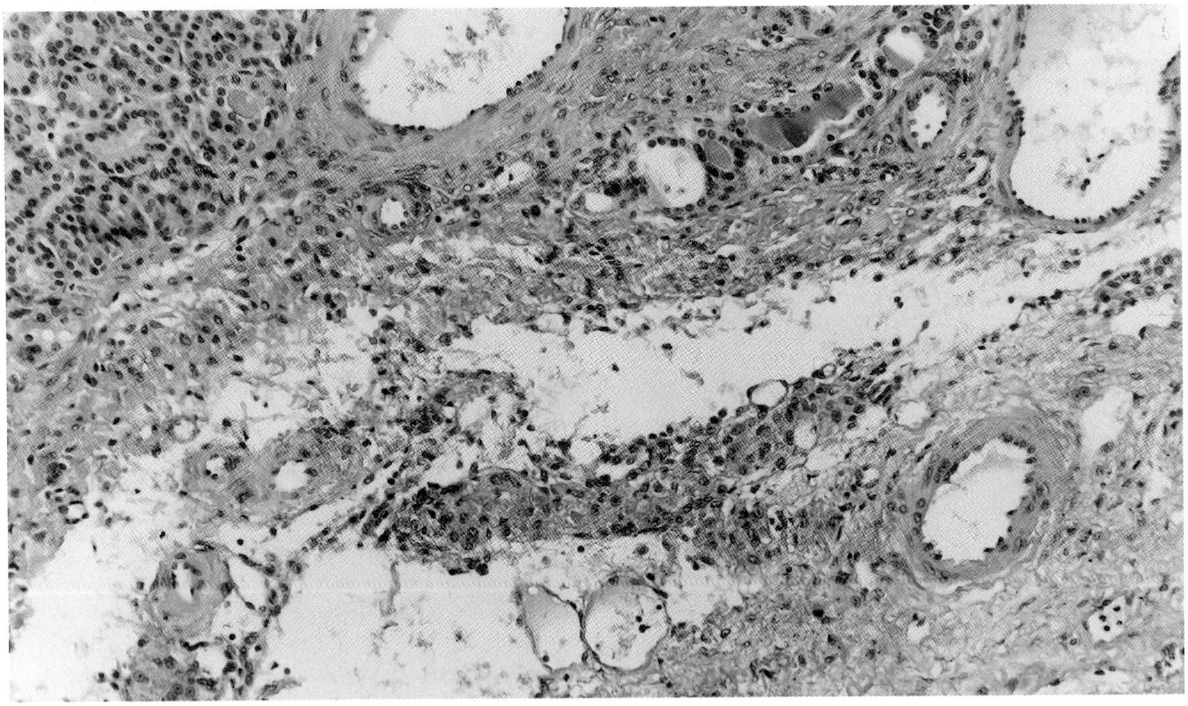

Fig. 49.3 Margin of a struma ovarii showing a focus of Leydig cell hyperplasia (center). Such Leydig cell clusters were prominently situated around much of the perimeter of the struma. H + E ×82.5

the degree of toxicity (Kempers et al 1970). As in the thyroid gland, mild nuclear atypia and mitotic activity can be present without generating suspicions of malignancy. Gross anaplasia and vascular invasion should be regarded as indicating a tumor of uncertain malignant potential. Indisputable malignant strumas, i.e. with documented extra-ovarian spread, have manifested both follicular and papillary patterns, but with a predominance of the former (Kempers et al 1970, Yannopoulos et al 1976, Scully 1979, Pardo-Mindan & Vazquez 1983, Brunskill et al 1990, Ro et al 1991, Talerman 1994).

Differential diagnosis

Colloid-like follicles or microfollicular foci may be encountered in some clear cell carcinomas, androblastomas, endometrioid carcinomas, granulosa cell tumors, and pregnancy luteomas. These areas, however, constitute only minor components of these tumors, and other characteristic patterns will be seen elsewhere. Teratomatous elements are very unlikely to be present. If still in doubt, the demonstration of birefringent oxalate crystals in the acini or immunohistochemical positivity for thyroglobulin in the lining epithelium will be conclusive.

Metastatic thyroid carcinoma should not be seriously considered except in a patient with a known primary, since, even in this situation, ovarian metastases are exceedingly rare (see Ch. 53).

Care must be taken not to overlook a strumal carcinoid (see below). The carcinoid component of these tumors is usually trabecular in type and is either intimately admixed with the thyroid follicles or occurs as a discrete focus. The cellular characteristics are the same as in pure carcinoid tumors and most are argyrophilic (see below). Mitotic activity is minimal.

The difficulties in identifying malignancy in struma ovarii have been discussed above.

CARCINOID TUMORS

Primary carcinoid tumors constitute less than 5%

of ovarian teratomas and are rarer than struma ovarii (Climie & Heath 1968, Robboy et al 1975), yet they outnumber metastatic carcinoids by a factor of four (Talerman 1984). Approximately one-half are insular, one-third trabecular, and one-sixth strumal in type (Scully 1979). A few cases of mucinous carcinoid (goblet cell or adenocarcinoid) have been reported (Talerman 1982, 1984, Alenghat et al 1986, Wolpert et al 1989, Ammaturo et al 1990). A case of strumal carcinoid has been encountered in a patient with multiple endocrine neoplasia syndrome type IIA (Sipple's syndrome) (Tamsen & Mazur 1992).

The origin of carcinoid tumors in organs in which there is no normal population of APUD cells has caused great controversy, the details of which are not germane to this text. However, the majority of primary ovarian carcinoids are associated with teratomatous elements, and some have been noted to arise in close proximity to gastrointestinal or respiratory epithelium which includes APUD cells, a possible source of the neoplastic proliferation (Robboy et al 1975, Fox & Langley 1976, Scully 1979, Bosman & Louwerens 1981). Alternatively, the tumors could arise directly from teratomatous primitive neuroectodermal cells or uncommitted endodermal epithelial cells which have the potential for APUD cell differentiation. Rarely, they are found in association with Sertoli–Leydig cell tumors (Young et al 1982). Hidvegi et al (1982) have identified neuroendocrine cells in 6% of non-neoplastic ovaries, and have suggested that these may be the origin of carcinoids not associated with teratomas.

Biochemical, histochemical, and morphological (including ultrastructural) studies indicate that ovarian insular carcinoids are analogous to midgut carcinoids, whereas trabecular carcinoids are analogous to foregut or hindgut carcinoids (Scully 1979, Sporrong et al 1982, Talerman & Evans 1982, Talerman 1984). Strumal carcinoids are composed of carcinoid (mostly trabecular and analogous to hindgut carcinoid) and thyroid elements, both considered to be of endodermal teratomatous origin (Robboy & Scully 1980, Senterman et al 1984, Morgan et al 1985, Stagno et al 1987). Mucinous carcinoids are analogous to the more familiar appendiceal tumors (Warkel et al 1978), and are considered to represent biphasic differentiation along mucinous and argentaffin cell lines.

The age range of patients with ovarian carcinoids is wide, but most tumors are seen in peri- or postmenopausal women. Mucinous carcinoids tend to occur in somewhat younger women. Exceptional cases have been reported in teenage girls (Talerman 1984, Harling et al 1986). Most patients present with symptoms relating to an enlarging ovarian mass, or the lesion is an incidental finding. A small percentage of patients present with manifestations of estrogen or androgen excess (abnormal uterine bleeding or virilization) (Dikman & Toker 1971, Robboy et al 1977) or features of hyperthyroidism (Robboy & Scully 1980). One-third of patients with insular carcinoids present with symptoms or signs of the carcinoid syndrome. In decreasing order of frequency these are: flushing, diarrhea/constipation, cardiac murmurs, and pedal edema. The flushing attacks must be carefully distinguished from menopausal symptoms, which are likely to be quite common in the age group in which these tumors most commonly occur (Robboy et al 1975, Fox & Langley 1976). The syndrome is generally seen only in women more than 50 years of age and in whom the tumor is greater than 4 cm in diameter (Robboy et al 1975). It is a more common complication of ovarian, contrasted with gastrointestinal, carcinoids since the secretory products of the tumor (particularly 5-hydroxytryptamine (serotonin)) can reach the systemic circulation without passing through the liver where they would be detoxified. If the syndrome is suspected preoperatively, it may be confirmed by measuring serum serotonin or urinary 5-hydroxyindoleacetic acid (5-HIAA) levels, which are always raised in these patients.

Insular and 'mixed' carcinoids are best considered as tumors of low malignant potential. The tumors grow slowly and recurrences or metastases are rare. Trabecular carcinoids are not associated with metastases (Talerman 1994). The metastases of strumal carcinoids may be either thyroidal or carcinoid in type (Armes & Östör 1993). Approximately 5% of cases have proved fatal, with extensive peritoneal, liver, and abdominal lymph node deposits and, rarely, widespread systemic dissemination (Haines 1971, Fox & Langley 1976, Robboy et al 1975, 1977, Robboy & Scully

1980, Russell & Painter 1982, Sens et al 1982, Harling et al 1986). Some patients have succumbed to carcinoid heart disease which has progressed even after successful tumor excision (Robboy et al 1975).

Treatment of uncomplicated carcinoid tumors is bilateral salpingo-oophorectomy and hysterectomy. In the rare young patient desirous of retaining her fertility, or in cases with trabecular carcinoid tumors, unilateral salpingo-oophorectomy is acceptable. Close clinical follow-up is mandatory in all patients. In cases of extraovarian spread, excision of metastases, insofar as is practicable, is recommended, followed by chemotherapy (Robboy et al 1975, Talerman 1984). Serum serotonin or urinary 5-HIAA levels can be used to monitor the progress of the disease. Most symptoms and signs of the carcinoid syndrome regress quickly postoperatively. However, carcinoid heart disease (pulmonary stenosis, tricuspid stenosis/incompetence, and right-sided heart failure) can continue to progress without obvious recurrence of tumor (Trell et al 1973).

The clinical course of mucinous carcinoids is more aggressive, and in this respect they are comparable with their homologs in the appendix. Metastases may be present at the time of laparotomy. Treatment therefore needs to be radical, more in keeping with that employed in patients with ovarian mullerian carcinomas (Talerman 1984, Alenghat et al 1986).

Macroscopic features

Primary ovarian carcinoids are virtually always unilateral, but in up to 15% of cases there is a mature cystic teratoma or mucinous tumor in the contralateral ovary. Most (60–80%) are components of mature cystic teratomas or, less commonly, mucinous cystadenomas; mucinous carcinoids tend to be pure (Robboy et al 1975, Robboy et al 1977, Robboy & Scully 1980, Talerman 1984, Wolpert et al 1989). Carcinoid tumors most commonly appear as firm circumscribed nodules in the walls of mature cystic teratomas (or mucinous cystadenomas). The size of the carcinoid component ranges from small to massive, but the maximum dimension is generally about 10 cm. Unlike struma ovarii there is, as yet, no minimum size criterion for the diagnosis of carcinoid tumors, but a 1 cm nodular proliferation would seem to be a reasonable lower limit. On sectioning, the tumor tissue is gray-yellow or tan colored. Hemorrhage and necrosis are generally not apparent, but may occasionally be seen in strumal and mucinous carcinoids. Cystic spaces containing clear or mucoid fluid are usually present in addition to the cystic teratomatous components. The thyroid component of strumal carcinoids may sometimes be recognized macroscopically, especially if it forms a discrete mass. These areas are soft to very firm and the cut surface is red-brown and glistening, contrasted with the yellow-gray of carcinoid tissue. Pure tumors form firm nodular masses with smooth bosselated surfaces.

Microscopic features

Ovarian insular carcinoids resemble midgut carcinoids of appendix or ileum. Tumor cells are arranged in round, oval, or angular islands with some peripheral palisading. Small acini are present, typically at the margins of the islands, but sometimes diffusely. They contain eosinophilic secretions which stain positively for mucin and may become inspissated and calcified resembling psammoma bodies. The tumor cells are quite uniform in appearance. Cytoplasm is abundant and may exhibit eosinophilic granules, particularly at the periphery of the islands. The nuclei are central and round, with evenly distributed clumped chromatin. Mitotic activity is rarely observed. The proportion of stroma is very variable; it is dense and fibroma like and is occasionally focally luteinized. Minor trabecular areas are seen in less than 5% of cases (Robboy et al 1975) (Fig. 49.4). All tumors are argentaffinic (as demonstrated by Fontana–Masson silver stain, ferric ferricyanide, or diazo methods) and this is most readily appreciated in the granular cells described above. The argyrophilic reaction (Grimelius and Bodian protargol stain) is usually weakly positive. An immunoprofile of positivity for neuron-specific enolase (NSE), serotonin, chromogranin, and various neuronal peptides, including calcitonin, can be demonstrated (Sporrong et al 1982, Talerman 1984), as well as prostatic acid phosphatase (Sidhu & Sanchez 1993), this latter interpreted as

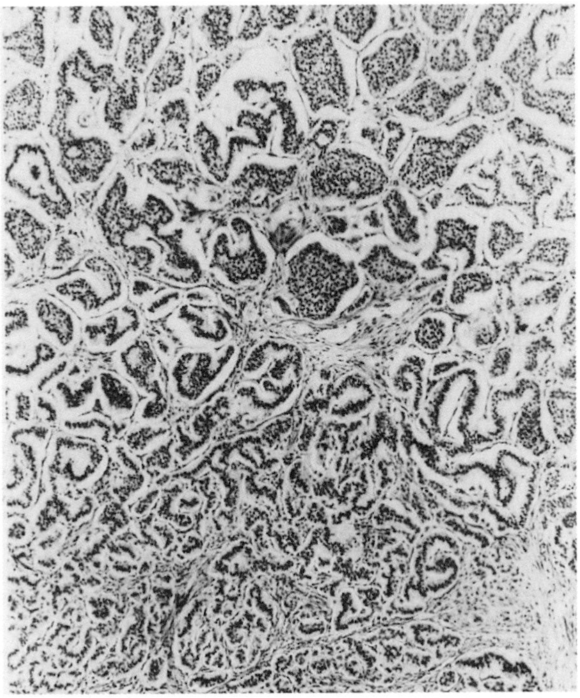

Fig. 49.4 Ovarian carcinoid tumor with insular pattern above and trabecular area below. H + E ×50

a further similarity between such tumors in the ovaries and rectal carcinoids. Microscopic features which best correlate with the presence of the carcinoid syndrome are abundance of acini and prominence of argentaffin granules (Robboy et al 1975). Electron microscopy confirms the neuroendocrine nature of the cells and their similarity to those of midgut carcinoids. The diagnostic neurosecretory granules are pleiomorphic (typically dumb-bell shaped or reniform) within the size range 90–410 nm (average 210–260 nm) (Serratoni & Robboy 1975, Sens et al 1982). The associated teratomatous components are chiefly of endodermal derivation (Robboy et al 1975).

The histological features of ovarian trabecular carcinoids resemble those of hindgut, e.g. rectal carcinoids. The most characteristic pattern is that of orderly long wavy ribbons, one to two cells thick, interspersed with a small amount of loose fibrous connective tissue. Where the ribbons

Fig. 49.5 Detail of trabecular carcinoid tumor. (A) Neat sinuous ribbons of elongate cells are orientated at right angles to the long axes of the ribbons. The small nuclei are round or ovoid with dense but regular chromatin. H + E ×100. (B) One of a myriad of small scattered cell nests around the perimeter of the main tumor mass, this one beneath the squamous lining of the teratomatous cyst. H + E ×99

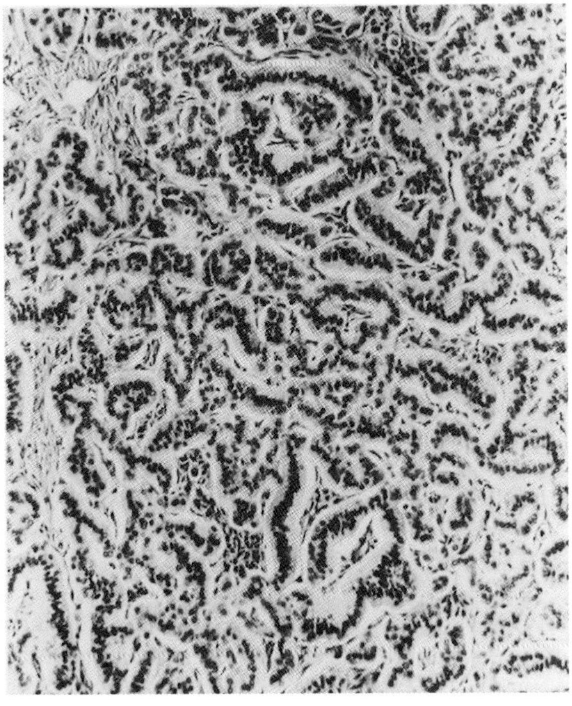

A

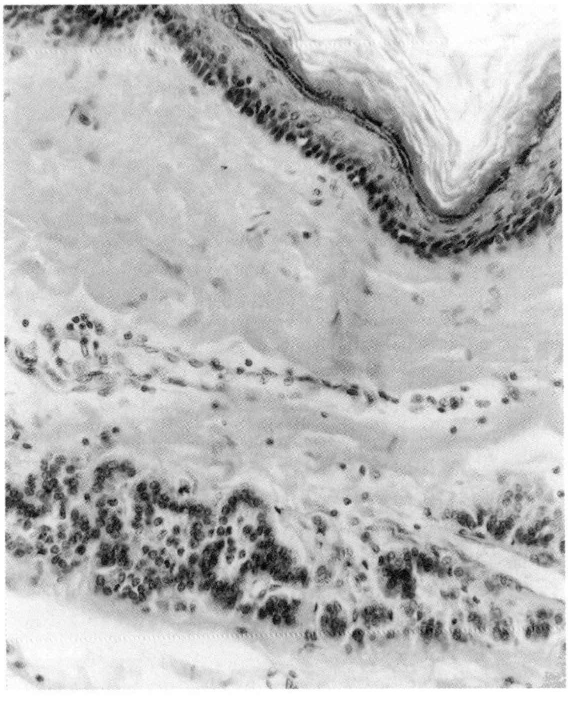

B

appear shorter, the stroma tends to be denser. The elongate cells are orientated perpendicularly to the long axes of the ribbons (Fig. 49.5A). Wide bands and trabeculae are also present, as are scattered small cell nests (Fig. 49.5B). This latter feature should not be misinterpreted as vascular permeation or evidence of aggressive local invasion. A minor but definite insular component is seen in 20% of cases (Robboy et al 1977). The tumor often includes multiple small cystic spaces, lined by mucinous epithelium, which appear to form an intrinsic part of the tumor. The cytological characteristics are similar to insular carcinoids as described above. The tumor cells are argyrophilic, but argentaffinicity is present in only two-thirds. Neuronal peptides, including calcitonin, have been identified immunohistochemically (Robboy et al 1977, Sporrong et al 1982). Stromal luteinization is quite common (Robboy et al 1977, Talerman 1984). Electron microscopy reveals uniform round or oval granules 150–500 nm in diameter (Serratoni & Robboy 1975, Talerman & Okagaki 1985).

The diagnostic feature of strumal carcinoids is the admixture of carcinoid and thyroid elements. These vary in their relative proportions and may be intimately admixed throughout the mass or merge only at the interface between separate masses of thyroid and carcinoid tissue (Fig. 49.6A). The carcinoid component is purely trabecular in half the cases and, in most of the remainder, is a mixture of trabecular and insular patterns. Rarely it is entirely insular in type. The thyroid component is both macro- and microfollicular and includes typical colloid. Where the tissues are admixed, follicular epithelium appears to stream into the ribbons of carcinoid cells, or carcinoid cells seem to replace part of the follicular lining (Fig. 49.6B). The individual components retain their innate cytological and immunohistochemical characteristics; the follicular epithelium is thyroglobulin positive, while the carcinoid component contains various neuropeptides, including calcitonin in a small number of cases (Stagno et al 1987). Some workers have identified, in the transitional zones, an intermediate cell population (resembling thy-

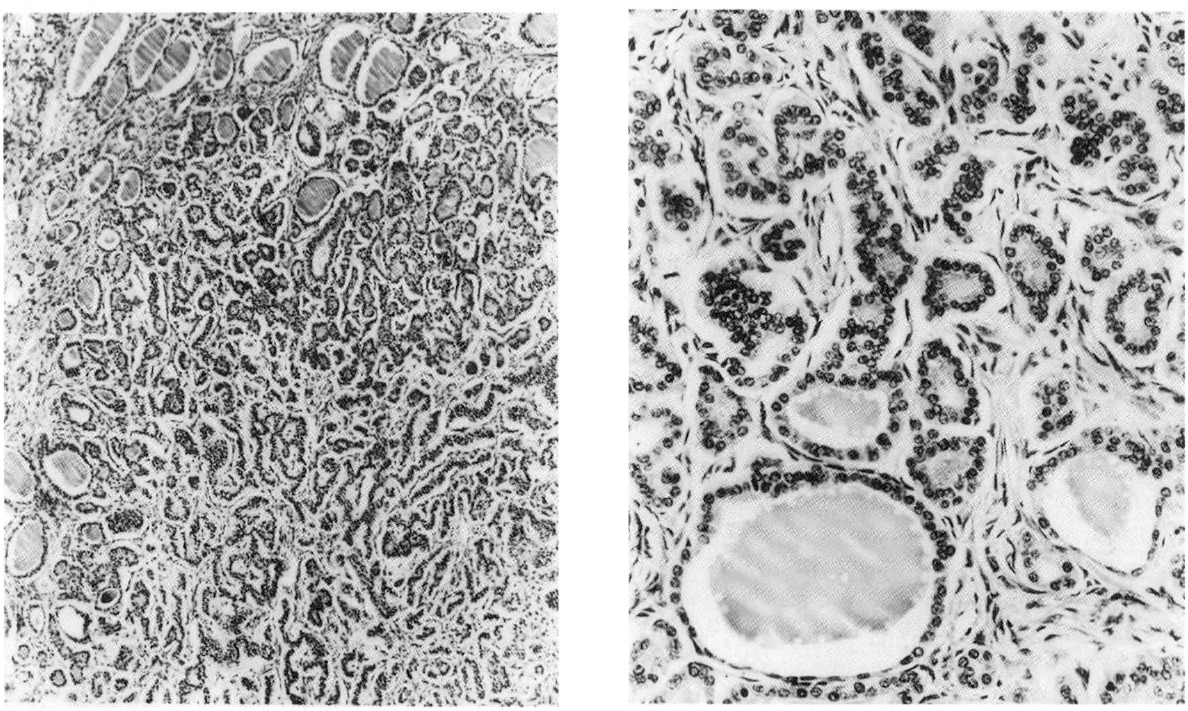
A B

Fig. 49.6 Strumal carcinoid tumor. (A) Low-power view of a transitional area between the two components. H + E ×50. (B) Detail of this area showing subtle transitions between thyroid follicles and carcinoid ribbons. H + E ×200 roid 'C' cells), showing both follicular thyroid and neuroendocrine differentiation (Greco et al 1979, Ulbright et al 1982, Snyder & Tavassoli 1986). Mucinous epithelium may be evident as a few or many cysts or as individual cells within the carcinoid component. The stroma is very variable in quantity and character and may contain amyloid, a property which enhances the morphological similarity of some of these lesions to medullary carcinomas of the thyroid gland (Blaustein 1979, Dayal et al 1979, Robboy & Scully 1980, Morgan et al 1985). Stromal luteinization has been observed in one-third of cases (Robboy & Scully 1980).

No histological features which are reliably predictive of a malignant clinical course in nonmucinous carcinoids can be gleaned from the few cases reported (Fox & Langley 1976). However, unusual features observed in metastasizing tumors have included prominent mitotic activity (more than 3 per HPF), conspicuous nucleoli, necrosis, paucity of acini and 'anaplasia'. The histological descriptions of these tumors (often limited) suggest that some of them are more in keeping with 'atypical' or malignant carcinoid tumors as documented in extraovarian sites (Haines 1971, Robboy et al 1975, Sens et al 1982, Harling et al 1986).

An unusual tumor associated with the carcinoid syndrome has been described (Czernobilsky et al 1984). As well as some typical insular and trabecular foci, atypical solid and papillary growth patterns composed of pleiomorphic and clear cells were present. Moderate mitotic activity and anaplasia were noted. All the diverse areas fulfilled the ultrastructural and immunohistochemical criteria of carcinoid tumor. It was suggested that such a tumor might behave more like a carcinoma than a typical carcinoid.

Mucinous carcinoids are composed of small and large acini containing mucin surrounded by cuboidal or columnar cells. Interstitial mucin and signet-ring cells may be observed occasionally to the point of resembling Krukenberg tumors. The small round or oval nuclei resemble more closely those of carcinoid tumors rather than colonic adenocarcinomas, but show more nuclear atypia and mitotic activity than other varieties of primary ovarian carcinoids. The cytoplasm of some cells is argyrophilic and sometimes argentaffinic as well, corresponding to the presence of immunoreactive neuropeptides (e.g. serotonin, chromogranin A). Electron microscopy demonstrates neurosecretory granules in the non-mucin-secreting cells. The stroma is not abundant and may be loose or dense (Talerman 1984, Alenghat et al 1986).

Differential diagnosis

Metastatic carcinoids (see Ch. 54), which are usually insular in type, are histologically indistinguishable from primary ovarian lesions, but there are usually discriminating clinical and surgical features. Metastatic tumors are almost always bilateral, and extraovarian metastases may be evident. The tumors are multinodular and not associated with teratomatous elements. Identification of a primary tumor, usually in the ileum, clinches the diagnosis (see Table 54.2).

Granulosa cell tumors (see Ch. 33) are the neoplasms which are most likely to be confused with insular carcinoids. Call–Exner bodies may resemble carcinoid acini, but their margins are less regular and the lumens may contain nuclear debris as well as eosinophilic material. The cells have grooved nuclei, and the scanty cytoplasm is not argyrophilic or argentaffinic. Teratomatous elements are not present (see Table 33.3).

Poorly differentiated primary or metastatic adenocarcinomas may superficially resemble insular carcinoid tumors, but the nuclei are never as uniform and there is always obvious mitotic activity. Argentaffin and argyrophil reactions are usually negative, as are immunohistochemical stains for neurosecretory granules.

Brenner tumors (see Ch. 28) display epithelial islands, but these are broken up by large amounts of fibromatous stroma. The epithelial component is composed of transitional cells without acini formation. The nuclei are often grooved and the cytoplasm is not argyrophilic or argentaffinic.

Androblastomas (see Ch. 35) may be confused with trabecular carcinoids, particularly those with luteinized stroma. The Sertoli cell ribbons are, however, thinner and shorter, and the constituent cells have sparser cytoplasm which is sometimes vacuolated and lacks granularity or argyrophilia. Examination of further sections will usually reveal other typical growth patterns and clumps of

Table 49.1 Differential diagnosis: trabecular carcinoid versus androblastoma

Trabecular carcinoid	Androblastoma
Clinical	
Virilization very rare	Virilization common
Histological	
Ribbons of uniform width throughout tumor	Narrower ribbons, other patterns present
Stroma fibromatous	Stroma often contains Leydig cells
Cytoplasm copious, often granular	Less cytoplasm, sometimes vacuolated
Argyrophilic, usually argentaffinic	Both reactions negative
Teratomatous elements almost always present	Mucinous cysts may be present

Leydig cells. Teratomatous elements are absent, but cysts lined by mucinous epithelium including occasional argentaffin cells may be present in both (Table 49.1).

Malignant strumas need to be distinguished from strumal carcinoids, with which they have often been confused in the past. Thyroid carcinomas generally show a fair degree of anaplasia and mitotic activity. Ribbon-like growth is not apparent and the cells are not argyrophilic or argentaffinic.

Primary mucinous adenocarcinomas of the ovary may be confused with mucinous carcinoids. Carcinomas are distinguished by more marked cytological atypia and relative paucity of argyrophilic or argentaffinic cells. The glandular spaces in adenocarcinomas tend to be larger, and substantial cysts are usually evident macroscopically.

OTHER (RARE) MONODERMAL AND HIGHLY SPECIALIZED TERATOMAS

Pituitary adenomas

A corticotrophin adenoma, arising in a mature cystic teratoma, has been reported in a 24-year-old woman with Cushing's syndrome. The tumor formed a discrete 2 cm nodule in the wall of a 3 cm cyst (Axiotis et al 1987).

Epidermoid cysts

These cysts are most often considered to be of teratomatous origin, but there are other histogenetic possibilities and the lesions are therefore discussed with other miscellaneous epithelial lesions in Chapter 31.

Endodermal variants of mature cystic teratomas

A mature monodermal teratoma, consisting of a cyst lined by respiratory epithelium (with focal squamous metaplasia), has been reported; the 9 cm lesion developed in a 5-year-old girl (Clement & Dimmick 1979).

Giant sebaceous tumors

A very large (3345 g) ovarian tumor consisting almost exclusively of sebaceous glandular tissue has been reported (Strauss & Gates 1964). Teratomatous development was suggested by the presence of a small amount of adipose tissue, keratin, and hair shafts. Although the tumor displayed focally brisk mitotic activity, the clinical course was benign. Four similar, but cystic, lesions have since been described (Kaku et al 1987, Chumas & Scully 1991), which included nodules of benign sebaceous glandular tissue protruding into the lumen. Three of five patients had mature cystic teratomas in the contralateral ovaries.

Salivary tumors

We have encountered a benign monomorphic (basal cell) salivary adenoma in a 26-year-old patient (Fig. 49.7), characterized by mixed adenoid cystic and cribriform patterns of growth (Russell et al 1995). Small discrete cribriform nests of basaloid cells showed peripheral palisading and cuffing with hyalinized basal lamina material (Fig. 49.8). Centrally, epithelial islands showed a sponge-like arrangement with deposits of sialomucins. Cells immunostained for cytokeratins, S-100 protein, and salivary amylase. Ultrastructural features were similar to those reported for basal cell adenomas of the major salivary glands.

Neuroectodermal tumors

Although rare, there is a wide variety of reported

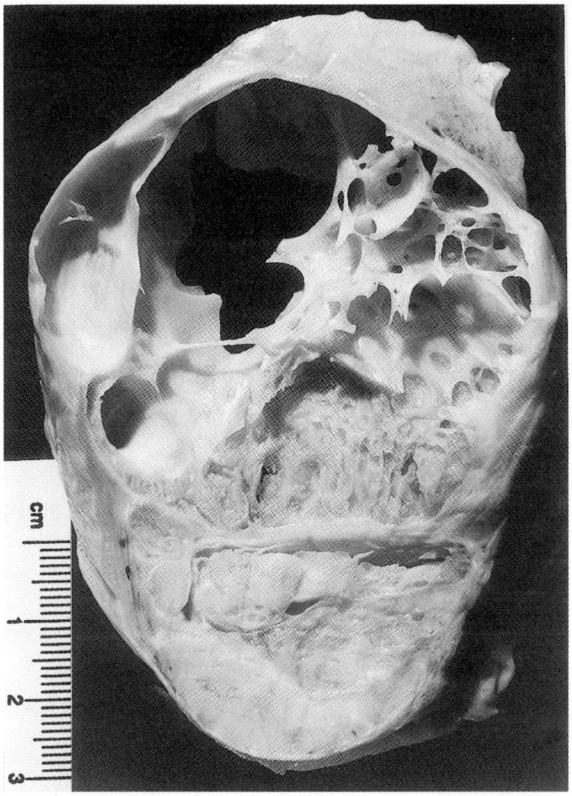

Fig. 49.7 Monomorphic (basal cell) salivary adenoma. Slice through tumor to reveal various sized cystic spaces, fine 'honeycomb' areas and solid nodules

cases of ovarian tumors of neuroectodermal origin. Some are dominant components of otherwise typical mature or immature teratomas, while others are apparently pure and may, indeed, produce cystic lesions composed exclusively of mature brain tissue (Spaun & Rix 1990, Fogt et al 1994). It is possible that some may arise as a result of secondary malignant transformation in pre-existing mature cystic teratomas, but the majority probably represent monodermal teratomatous development. The tumors are difficult to classify, but an important and perhaps definitional feature is that they resemble well-characterized tumors of the central nervous system, such as neuroblastomas, glioblastomas, and ependymomas. Some investigators attempt to distinguish between immaturity and 'intrinsic malignancy' in this group of tumors, but both qualities have similar clinical implications. Most of the tumors occur in young women (rarely in postmenopausal women) and many of the poorly differentiated examples are clinically aggressive (Theppisai et al 1977, Aguirre & Scully 1982, Reid et al 1983, Block et al 1984, Burke & Beilby 1984, Kleinman et al 1993).

Primitive neuroectodermal tumors (PNETs) in the ovary resemble the lesions of the same name occurring in the brains of children (Becker & Hinton 1983). The average age of patients is about 19 years and there is a high mortality rate. The tumors are unilateral, large, and partly solid and partly cystic. They consist chiefly of patternless sheets of undifferentiated small pleiomorphic cells (Fig. 49.9) resembling neuroblasts. There are also foci of glial differentiation, and some tumors include ependymal rosettes, medulloepitheliomatous, or medulloblastomatous patterns (Fig. 49.10), and primitive neural tube-like structures. Some show foci of mature teratoma, including typical dermoid cysts. Those which lack these components may be confused with other types of ovarian neoplasm such as granulosa cell tumors, undifferentiated small cell carcinomas of hypercalcaemic type, or desmoplastic small cell tumors (see Ch. 31). The background of small undifferentiated pleiomorphic cells distinguishes these tumors from the other ovarian neuroectodermal tumors mentioned above (Aguirre & Scully 1982, Harms & Jänig 1985). The immunophenotype of the cells generally includes focal staining for GFAP, synaptophysin, and neurofilaments, and negative staining for cytokeratins (Kleinman et al 1993, Kanbour-Shakir et al 1993).

Anaplastic neuroectodermal tumors, resembling high grade gliomas (glioblastoma) have also been described. Focal squamous differentiation is an indication of their teratomatous origin. Anaplastic tumor cells are arranged in sheets and contain variable amounts of cytoplasm with eosinophilic processes. Bizarre nuclei and mitoses are common. Cells immunostain for GFAP (Bjersing et al 1989).

Melanotic neuroectodermal tumors of the ovary are similar to the retinal anlage tumors or pigmented progonomas of infancy (Dehner et al 1979). They are generally cystic and are characterized by sheets of small dark cells with scant cytoplasm, among which are tubules lined by larger cells containing abundant melanin. Structures resembling primitive optic vesicles may be found. Two cases, one including immature teratomatous components,

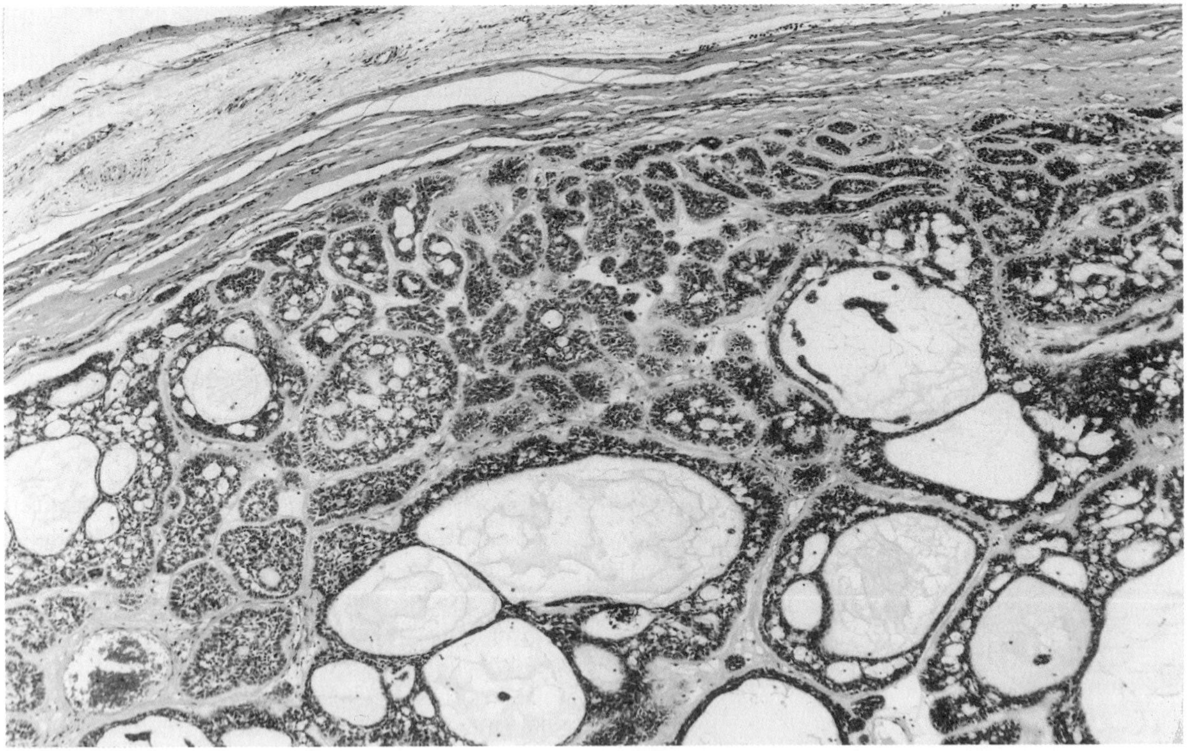

A

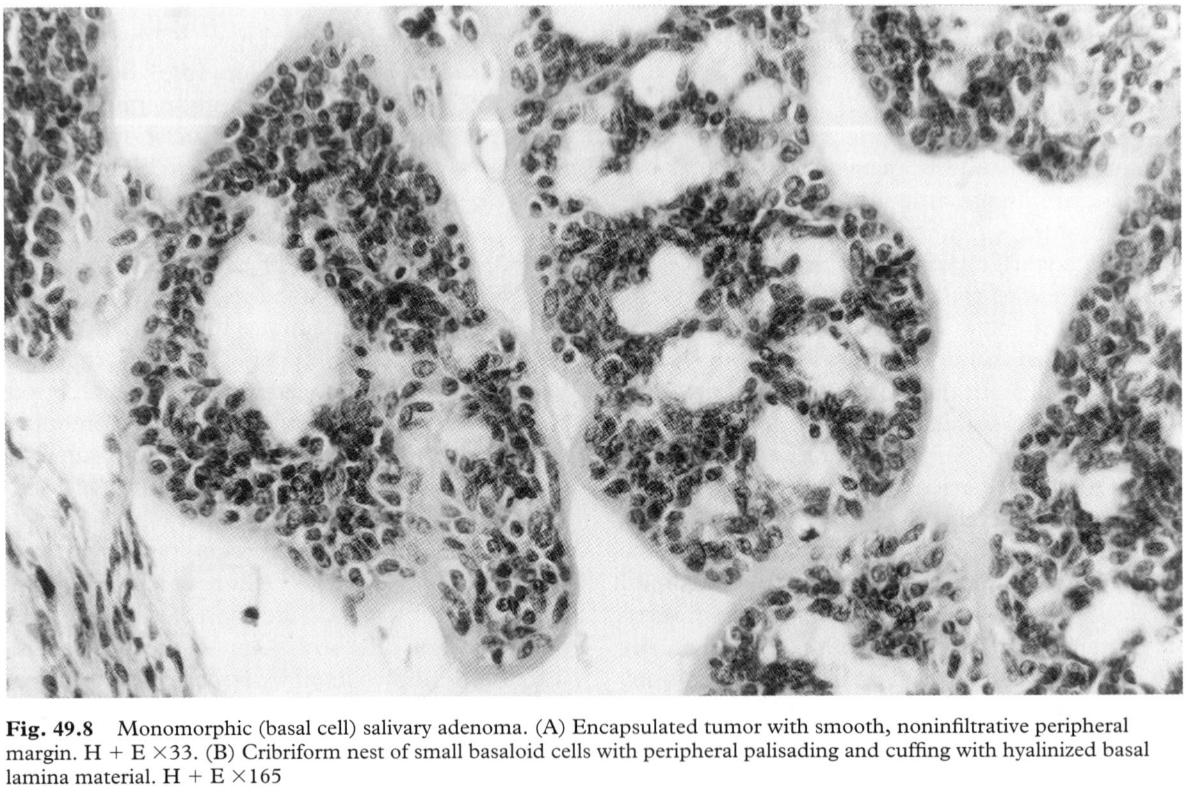

B

Fig. 49.8 Monomorphic (basal cell) salivary adenoma. (A) Encapsulated tumor with smooth, noninfiltrative peripheral margin. H + E ×33. (B) Cribriform nest of small basaloid cells with peripheral palisading and cuffing with hyalinized basal lamina material. H + E ×165

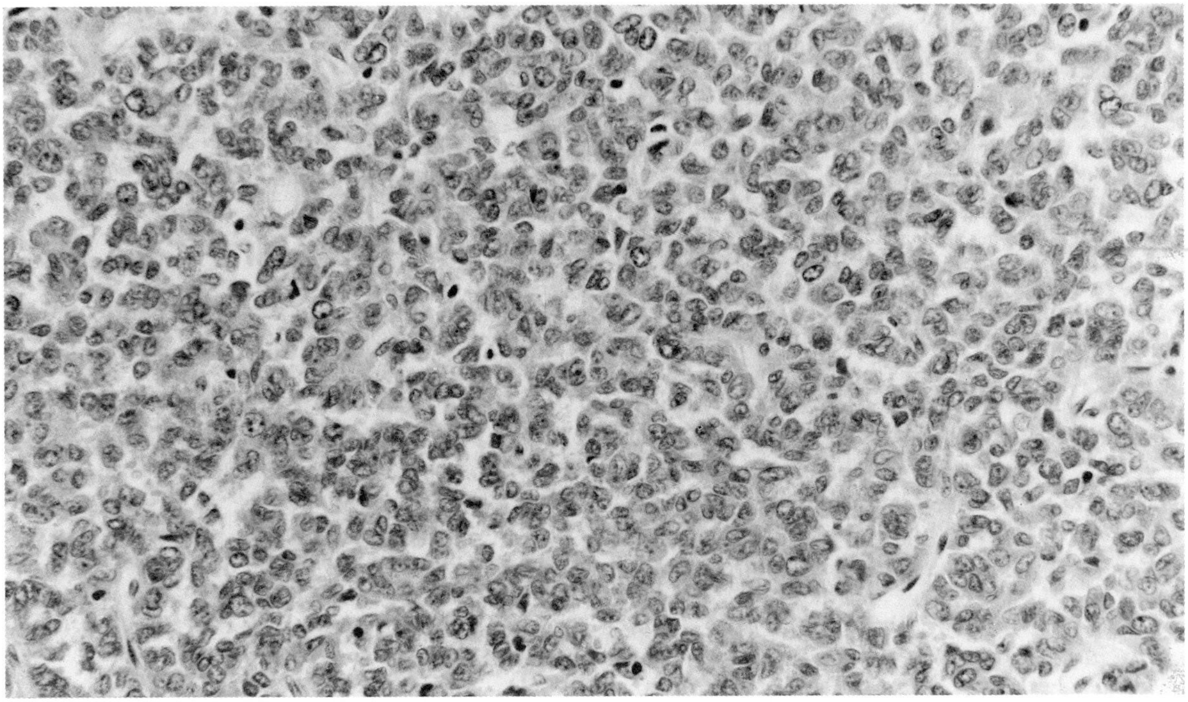

Fig. 49.9 Apparently pure primitive neuroectodermal tumor from an 18-year-old girl. Patternless sheets of small pleiomorphic cells. In a patient of this age, differentiation is required from undifferentiated small cell tumor of hypercalcemic type and from desmoplastic small cell tumor of peritoneum. H + E ×165

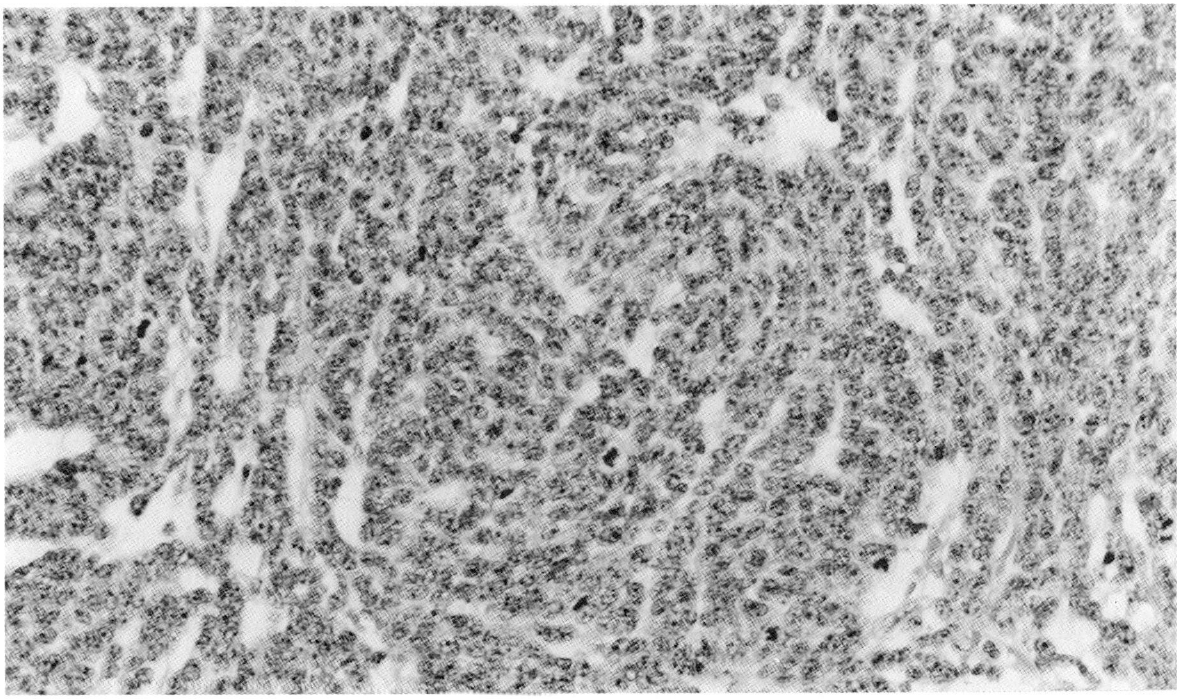

Fig. 49.10 Primitive neuroectodermal tumor with some focal suggestion of medulloblastomatous differentiation. H + E ×165

were clinically malignant (Hameed & Burslem 1970, King et al 1985), while three further cases, one associated with typical mature cystic teratomatous components, were clinically benign (Anderson & McDicken 1971, Sinniah & O'Brien 1973, Fox & Langley 1976).

Ependymomas occurring in women aged 16–68 years (Kleinman et al 1984, 1993, Carlsson et al 1989, Guerrieri & Jarlsfelt 1993) have been reported, with over one-half of cases being confined to one ovary and the remainder with intraperitoneal metastases. Similar tumors have been identified in the broad ligament (Bell et al 1984) and mesovarium (Grody et al 1985). As noted above, the ovarian tumors are unilateral and at least partly cystic. Microscopically, ependymomas are indistinguishable from those of the central nervous system (contrasting with those of the sacrococcygeal region) and show predominantly a diffuse or lobular pattern of cells separated by relatively acellular stroma. Perivascular pseudorosettes are prominent, as are fibrillary cytoplasmic processes. Occasional true rosettes are noted. The nature of the cells is confirmed by immunostaining for GFAP, cytokeratins, S-100 protein, and vimentin. The tumors may superficially resemble endometrioid (with large gland-like spaces) or serous carcinomas (with complex papillary patterns and psammoma bodies). Although other obvious heterologous tissues are absent, the teratomatous origin of these tumors is supported by the known occurrence of ependymal tissue in ovarian mature cystic teratomas (sometimes forming the dominant component) (Tiltman 1985), and of focal ependymal differentiation in immature teratomas. A suggested alternative histogenesis is neometaplasia of mullerian-duct-derived tissue (Guerrieri & Jarlsfelt 1993). The identification of progesterone receptors in a bilateral ovarian ependymoma (Carr et al 1992) suggests the possibility of hormone responsiveness, which may be of value in management.

Other differentiated neuroectodermal tumors such as *nonchromaffin paragangliomas* are occasionally encountered, and some are presumably of

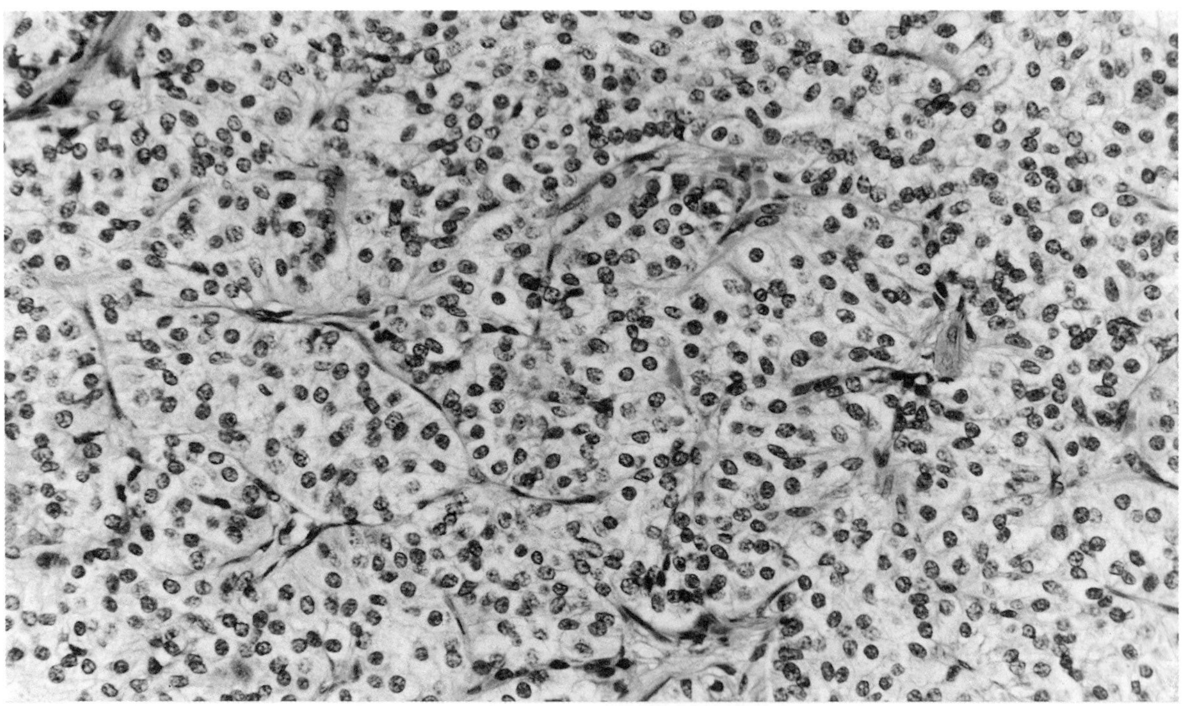

Fig. 49.11 A 13 cm nonchromaffin paraganglioma. Other teratomatous elements were sought and not found and the origin of the tumor is unclear (see Fig. 52.2). Organoid pattern of small cells with rounded central nuclei and pale, slightly granular cytoplasm. H + E ×165

teratomatous origin (Fig. 49.11). Morphologically, they exhibit the typical organoid pattern of 'zellballen', or nests of uniform rounded cells with small central nuclei, showing delicate stippled chromatin, and pale or granular cytoplasm. Reticulin fibers separate cell nests from the vascular network of the stroma. Immunostaining of the main tumor cells ('chief cells') for NSE and chromogranin A is the rule. Peripheral sustentacular cells are highlighted by strong immunostaining for S-100 protein. Other possible origins are from hilar neural elements (see Ch. 52).

REFERENCES

Aguirre P, Scully R E 1982 Malignant neuroectodermal tumor of the ovary, a distinctive form of monodermal teratoma. Report of five cases. American Journal of Surgical Pathology 6: 283–292

Alenghat E, Okagaki T, Talerman A 1986 Primary mucinous carcinoid of the ovary. Cancer 58: 777–783

Ammaturo C, Gerardi G, Giardello C, Tufano G, Romano C, de Angelis P 1990 Il carcinoide mucinoso primitivo dell'ovaio. Minerva Chirurgia 45: 535–537

Anderson M C, McDicken I W 1971 Melanotic cyst of the ovary. Journal of Obstetrics and Gynaecology of the British Commonwealth 78: 1047–1049

Armes J E, Östör A G 1993 A case of malignant strumal carcinoid. Gynecologic Oncology 51: 419–423

Axiotis C A, Lippes H A, Merino M J, de Lanerolle N C, Stewart A F, Kinder B 1987 Corticotroph cell pituitary adenoma within an ovarian teratoma. A new cause of Cushing's syndrome. American Journal of Surgical Pathology 11: 218–224

Becker L E, Hinton D 1983 Primitive neuroectodermal tumors of the central nervous system. Human Pathology 14: 538–550

Bell D A, Woodruff J M, Scully R E 1984 Ependymoma of the broad ligament. Report of two cases. American Journal of Surgical Pathology 8: 203–209

Bjersing L, Cajander S, Rogo K, Ottosson U B, Stendahl U 1989 Glioblastoma multiforme in a dermoid cyst of the ovary. European Journal of Gynaecological Oncology 10: 389–392

Blaustein A 1979 Calcitonin secreting struma – carcinoid tumor of the ovary. Human Pathology 10: 222–228

Block M, Gilbert E, Davis C 1984 Metastatic neuroblastoma arising in an ovarian teratoma with long-term survival. Cancer 54: 590–595

Bosman F T, Louwerens J-W K 1981 APUD cells in teratomas. American Journal of Pathology 104: 174–180

Brown W W, Shetty K R, Rosenfeld P S 1973 Hyperthyroidism due to struma ovarii: Demonstration by radioiodine scan. Acta Endocrinologica 73: 266–272

Brunskill P J, Rollason T P, Nicholson H O 1990 Malignant follicular variant of papillary struma ovarii. Histopathology 17: 574–576

Burke M, Beilby J O W 1984 Unusual malignant neuroectodermal tumors of the ovary – case report and literature review. Histopathology 8: 1059–1067

Carlsson B, Havel G, Kindblom L G, Knutson F, Mark J 1989 Ependymoma of the ovary. A clinicopathologic, ultrastructural and immunohistochemical investigation. A case report. Acta Pathologica Microbiologica et Immunologica Scandinavica 97: 1007–1012

Carr K A, Roberts J A, Frank T S 1992 Progesterone receptors in bilateral ovarian ependymoma presenting in pregnancy. Human Pathology 23: 962–965

Caruso P A, Marsh M R, Minkowitz S, Karten G 1971 An intense clinicopathologic study of 305 teratomas of the ovary. Cancer 27: 343–348

Chumas J C, Scully R E 1991 Sebaceous tumors arising in ovarian dermoid cysts. International Journal of Gynecological Pathology 10: 356–363

Clement P B, Dimmick J E 1979 Endodermal variant of mature cystic teratoma of the ovary. Report of a case. Cancer 43: 383–385

Climie A R W, Heath L P 1968 Malignant degeneration of benign cystic teratomas of the ovary. Review of the literature and report of a chondrosarcoma and carcinoid tumor. Cancer 22: 824–832

Czernobilsky B, Segal M, Dgani R 1984 Primary ovarian carcinoid with marked heterogeneity of microscopic features. Cancer 54: 585–589

Dalgaard J B, Wetteland P 1956 Struma ovarii. A follow up of 20 cases. Acta Chirurgica Scandinavica 112: 1–17

Dayal Y, Tashjian A H, Wolfe H J 1979 Immunocytochemical localization of calcitonin-producing cells in a strumal carcinoid with amyloid stroma. Cancer 43: 1331–1338

Dehner L P, Sibley R K, Sauk J J et al 1979 Malignant neuroectodermal tumor of infancy. A clinical, pathologic, ultrastructural and tissue culture study. Cancer 43: 1389–1410

Devaney K, Snyder R, Norris H J, Tavassoli F A 1993 Proliferative and histologically malignant struma ovarii: a clinicopathologic study of 54 cases. International Journal of Gynecological Pathology 12: 333–343

Dikman S H, Toker C 1971 Strumal carcinoid of the ovary with masculinization. Cancer 27: 925–930

Emge L A 1940 Functional and growth characteristics of struma ovarii. American Journal of Obstetrics and Gynecology 40: 738–750

Fogt F, Vortmeyer A O, Ahn G et al 1994 Neural cyst of the ovary with central nervous system microvasculature. Histopathology 24: 477–480

Fox H, Langley F A 1976 Tumours of the ovary. Heinemann, London, p 231–248

Gonzalez-Angulo A, Kaufman R H, Braungardt C D, Chapman F C, Hinshaw A J 1963 Adenocarcinoma of thyroid arising in struma ovarii (malignant struma ovarii). Report of two cases and review of the literature. Obstetrics and Gynecology 21: 567–576

Greco M A, Li Volsi V A, Pertschuk L P, Bigelow B 1979 Strumal carcinoid of the ovary. An analysis of its components. Cancer 43: 1380–1388

Grody W W, Nieberg R K, Bhuta S 1985 Ependymoma-like tumor of the mesovarium. Archives of Pathology and Laboratory Medicine 109: 291–293

Guerrieri C, Jarlsfelt I 1993 Ependymoma of the ovary. A case report with immunohistochemical, ultrastructural, and

DNA cytometric findings, as well as histogenetic considerations. American Journal of Surgical Pathology 17: 623–632

Haines M 1971 Carcinoid tumors of the ovary. Journal of Obstetrics and Gynaecology of the British Commonwealth 78: 1123–1127

Hameed K, Burslem M R G 1970 A melanotic ovarian neoplasm resembling the 'retinal anlage' tumor. Cancer 25: 564–567

Harling H, Paulsen S M, Sørenson J 1986 Primary malignant ovarian carcinoid. Gynecologic Oncology 24: 265–267

Harms D, Jänig U 1985 Immature teratomas of childhood. Report of 21 cases. Pathology Research and Practice 179: 388–400

Hasleton P S, Kelehan P, Whittaker J S, Burslem R W, Turner L 1978 Benign and malignant struma ovarii. Archives of Pathology and Laboratory Medicine 102: 180–184

Hidvegi D, Cibils L A, Sorensen K, Hidvegi I 1982 Ultrastructural and histochemical observations of neuroendocrine granules in nonneoplastic ovaries. American Journal of Obstetrics and Gynecology 143: 590–594

Hoda S A, Huvos A G 1993 Struma salpingis associated with struma ovarii. American Journal of Surgical Pathology 17: 1187–1189

Judd E S, Buie L A 1962 Hyperthyroidism associated with struma ovarii. A rare surgical challenge. Archives of Surgery 84: 692–697

Kaku T, Toyoshima S, Hachisuga T, Enjoji M, Tanaka M 1987 Sebaceous gland tumor of the ovary. Gynecologic Oncology 26: 398–402

Kanbour-Shakir A, Sawaday J, Kanbour A I, Kunschner A, Stock R J 1993 Primitive neuroectodermal tumor arising in an ovarian mature cystic teratoma: immunohistochemical and electron microscopic studies. International Journal of Gynecological Pathology 12: 270–275

Kempers R D, Dockerty M B, Hoffman D L, Bartholomew L G 1970 Struma ovarii – ascitic, hyperthyroid and asymptomatic syndromes. Annals of Internal Medicine 72: 883–893

King M E, Mouradian J A, Micha J P, Chaganti R S K, Allen S L 1985 Immature teratoma of the ovary with predominant malignant retinal anlage component. A parthenogenically derived tumor. American Journal of Surgical Pathology 9: 221–231

Kleinman G M, Young R H, Scully R E 1984 Ependymoma of the ovary: Report of three cases. Human Pathology 15: 632–638

Kleinman G M, Young R H, Scully R E 1993 Primary neuroectodermal tumors of the ovary. A report of 25 cases. American Journal of Surgical Pathology 17: 764–778

Marcus C C, Marcus S L 1961 Struma ovarii. A report of seven cases and a review of the subject. American Journal of Obstetrics and Gynecology 81: 752–762

Morgan K, Wells M, Scott J S 1985 Ovarian strumal carcinoid tumor with amyloid stroma – report of a case with 20-year follow-up. Gynecologic Oncology 22: 121–128

Ober W B 1960 Solid ovarian teratoma with struma ovarii, theca lutein reaction, and endometrial hyperplasia. Journal of Obstetrics and Gynaecology of the British Empire 67: 451–454

Pardo-Mindan F J, Vazquez J J 1983 Malignant struma ovarii. Light and electron microscopic study. Cancer 51: 337–443

Reid H A S, van der Walt J D, Fox H 1983 Neuroblastoma arising in a mature cystic teratoma of the ovary. Journal of Clinical Pathology 36: 68–73

Ro J Y, Sahin A A, el Naggar A K et al 1991 Intraluminal crystalloids in struma ovarii. Immunohistochemical. DNA flow cytometric, and ultrastructural study. Archives of Pathology and Laboratory Medicine 115: 145–149

Robboy S J, Scully R E 1980 Strumal carcinoid of the ovary: an analysis of 50 cases of a distinctive tumor composed of thyroid tissue and carcinoid. Cancer 46: 2019–2034

Robboy S J, Norris H J, Scully R E 1975 Insular carcinoid primary in the ovary. A clinicopathologic analysis of 48 cases. Cancer 36: 404–418

Robboy S J, Scully R E, Norris H J 1977 Primary trabecular carcinoid of the ovary. Obstetrics and Gynecology 49: 202–207

Rosenblum N G, Li Volsi V A, Edmonds P R, Mikuta J J 1989 Malignant struma ovarii. Gynecologic Oncology 32: 224–227

Russell P, Painter D M 1982 The pathological assessment of ovarian neoplasms. V: The germ cell tumors. Pathology 14: 47–72

Russell P, Wills E J, Watson G, Lee J, Geraghty T 1995 Monomorphic (basal cell) adenoma of ovary: report of a case. Ultrastructural Pathology 19: 431–438

Rutgers J L, Scully R E 1986 Functioning ovarian tumors with peripheral steroid cell proliferation. International Journal of Gynecological Pathology 5: 319–337

Scully R E 1979 Tumors of the ovary and maldeveloped gonads. Atlas of tumor pathology. Fascicle 16, 2nd series. Armed Forces Institute of Pathology, Washington, DC, p 269–285

Sens M A, Levenson T B, Metcalf J S 1982 A case of metastatic carcinoid arising in an ovarian teratoma. Case report with autopsy findings and review of the literature. Cancer 49: 2541–2546

Senterman M K, Cassidy P N, Fenoglio C M, Ferenczy A 1984 Histology, ultrastructure, and immunohistochemistry of strumal carcinoid: a case report. International Journal of Gynecological Pathology 3: 232–240

Serov S F, Scully R E, Sobin L H 1973 Histological typing of ovarian tumors. International histological classification of tumors No. 9. World Health Organization, Geneva, p 48–50

Serratoni F T, Robboy S J 1975 Ultrastructure of primary and metastatic ovarian carcinoids: analysis of 11 cases. Cancer 36: 157–160

Sidhu J, Sanchez 1993 Prostatic acid phosphatase in strumal carcinoids of the ovary. An immunohistochemical study. Cancer 72: 1673–1678

Sinniah R, O'Brien F V 1973 Pigmented progonoma in a dermoid cyst of the ovary. Journal of Pathology 109: 357–359

Snyder R R, Tavassoli F A 1986 Ovarian strumal carcinoid: immunohistochemical, ultrastructural, and clinicopathologic observations. International Journal of Gynecological Pathology 5: 187–201

Spaun E, Rix P 1990 Benign cystic monodermal teratoma of neurogenic type. International Journal of Gynecological Pathology 9: 283–290

Sporrong B, Falkmer S, Robboy S J et al 1982 Neurohormonal peptides in ovarian carcinoids: an immunohistochemical study of 81 primary carcinoids and of intraovarian metastases from six mid-gut carcinoids. Cancer 49: 68–74

Stagno P A, Petras R E, Hart W R 1987 Strumal carcinoids of the ovary. An immunohistologic and ultrastructural study.

Archives of Pathology and Laboratory Medicine 111: 440–446

Strauss A F, Gates H S 1964 Giant sebaceous tumor of the ovary. American Journal of Clinical Pathology 41: 78–83

Szyfelbein W M, Young R H, Scully R E 1994 Cystic struma ovarii: a frequently unrecognised tumor. A report of 20 cases. American Journal of Surgical Pathology 18: 785–788

Talerman A 1982 Mucinous carcinoid tumor of the ovary. In: Dallenbach-Hellweg G (ed) Ovarial tumoren. Springer-Verlag, Heidelberg, p 73–75

Talerman A 1984 Carcinoid tumors of the ovary. Journal of Cancer Research and Clinical Oncology 107: 125–135

Talerman A 1994 Germ cell tumors of the ovary. In: Kurman R J (ed) Blaustein's pathology of the female genital tract, 4th edn. Springer-Verlag, New York, p 849–914

Talerman A, Evans M I 1982 Primary trabecular carcinoid tumor of the ovary. Cancer 50: 1403–1407

Talerman A, Okagaki T 1985 Ultrastructural features of primary trabecular carcinoid tumor of the ovary. International Journal of Gynecological Pathology 4: 153–160

Tamsen A, Mazur M T 1992 Ovarian strumal carcinoid in association with multiple endocrine neoplasia type IIA. Archives of Pathology and Laboratory Medicine 116: 200–203

Theppisai H, Shuangshoti S, Amatyakul A 1977 Neuroblastoma arising in metastasizing ovarian teratoma. Journal of the Medical Association of Thailand 60: 396–404

Tiltman A J 1985 Ependymal cyst of the ovary. A case report. South African Medical Journal 68: 424–425

Trell E, Rausing A, Ripa J, Torp A, Waldenström J 1973 Carcinoid heart disease. Clinicopathologic findings and follow-up in 11 cases. American Journal of Medicine 54: 433–444

Ulbright T M, Roth L M, Ehrlich C E 1982 Ovarian strumal carcinoid. An immunocytochemical and ultrastructural study of two cases. American Journal of Clinical Pathology 77: 622–631

Warkel R L, Cooper P H, Helwig E B 1978 Adenocarcinoid, a mucin-producing carcinoid tumor of the appendix. Cancer 42: 2781–2793

Willemse P H B, Oosterhuis J W, Aalders J G et al 1987 Malignant struma ovarii treated by ovariectomy, thyroidectomy, and ^{131}I administration. Cancer 60: 178–182

Wolpert H R, Fuller A F, Bell D A 1989 Primary mucinous tumor of the ovary. A case report. International Journal of Gynecological Pathology 8: 156–162

Woodruff J D, Rauh J T, Markley R L 1966 Ovarian struma. Obstetrics and Gynecology 27: 194–201

Yannopoulos D, Yannopoulos K, Ossowski R 1976 Malignant struma ovarii. Pathology Annual 11: 403–413

Young R H, Prat J, Scully R E 1982 Ovarian Sertoli–Leydig cell tumors with heterologous elements. (1) Gastrointestinal epithelium and carcinoid: a clinicopathologic analysis of thirty-six cases. Cancer 50: 2448–2456

50

Malignant mixed germ cell tumors

P. Russell   A. Farnsworth

Malignant mixed germ cell tumors are composed of two or more of the neoplastic germ cell elements described in the previous chapters. By convention, benign mature cystic teratomas with secondary malignant change (most commonly squamous carcinoma and occurring in much older women – see Ch. 48) are excluded from this category. Gonadoblastomas and other mixed germ cell–sex cord–stromal tumors are also excluded (these tumors containing sex cord–stromal derivatives as well as germ cells or germ cell tumors – see Ch. 51). Although mixed germ cell tumors have,

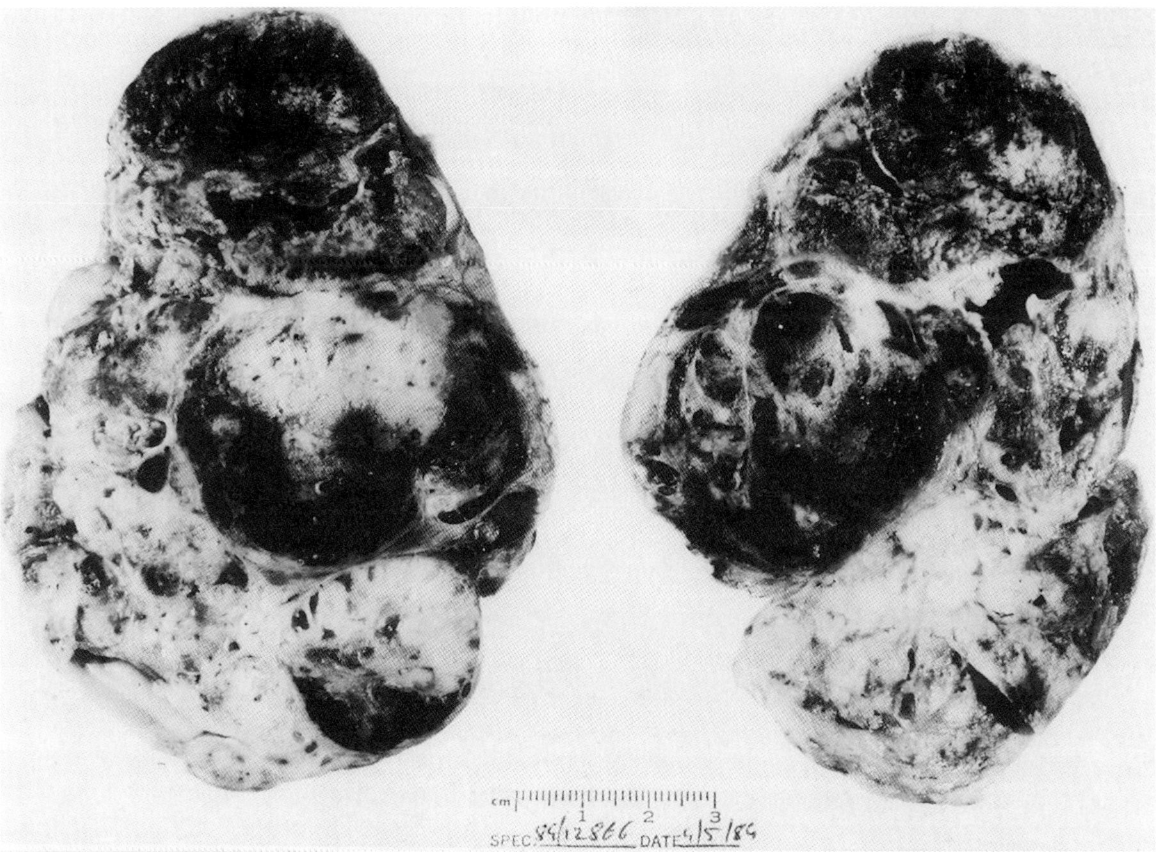

Fig. 50.1 The cut surface of a solid malignant mixed germ cell tumor showing variation from area to area characteristic of such neoplasms

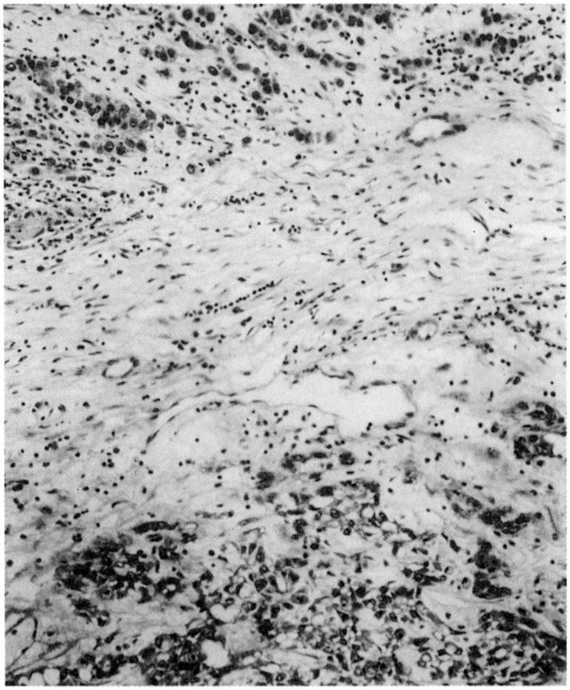

Fig. 50.2 Malignant mixed germ cell tumor – dysgerminoma (top) and reticular pattern of yolk sac tumor (lower). H + E ×75

in the past, been considered uncommon (many such tumors were classified according to their dominant component), a better appreciation of the various 'pure' patterns of malignant germ cell tumors, as well as more detailed histological examination of such neoplasms, has led to an increased awareness of their true frequency (Huntington & Bullock 1970, Talerman et al 1973, Norgaard-Pedersen et al 1975, Fox & Langley 1976, Kurman & Norris 1976, Jimerson & Woodruff 1977, Flamant et al 1978, Talerman et al 1978, Martinazzi et al 1989, Vos et al 1990). For example, they comprised about 8% of all malignant ovarian germ cell tumors in a large series published from the Armed Forces Institute of Pathology (Kurman & Norris 1977).

These tumors occur in young women, almost all below 30 years of age, and with a mean age of 16 years at presentation. About one-third of all malignant mixed germ cell tumors occurring in prepubertal girls are associated with isosexual pseudoprecocity (Kurman & Norris 1976).

Fig. 50.3 Malignant mixed germ cell tumor – dysgerminoma (left) and embryonal carcinoma (right). H + E ×125

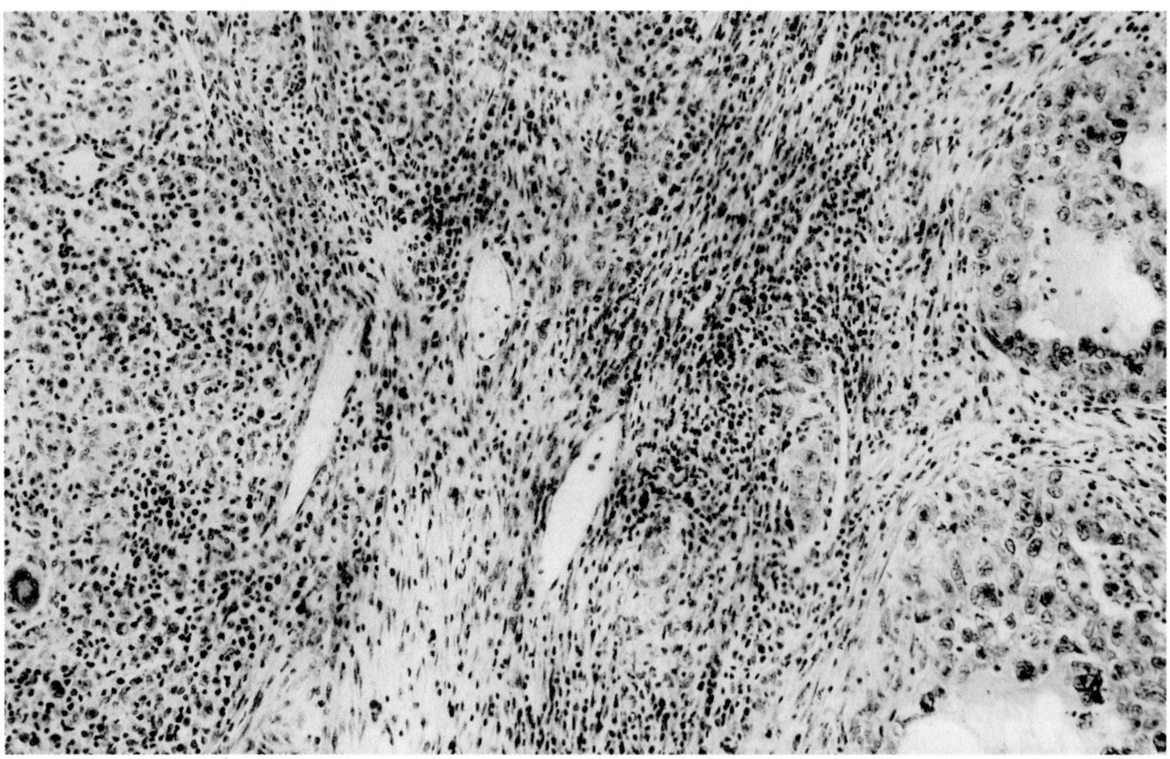

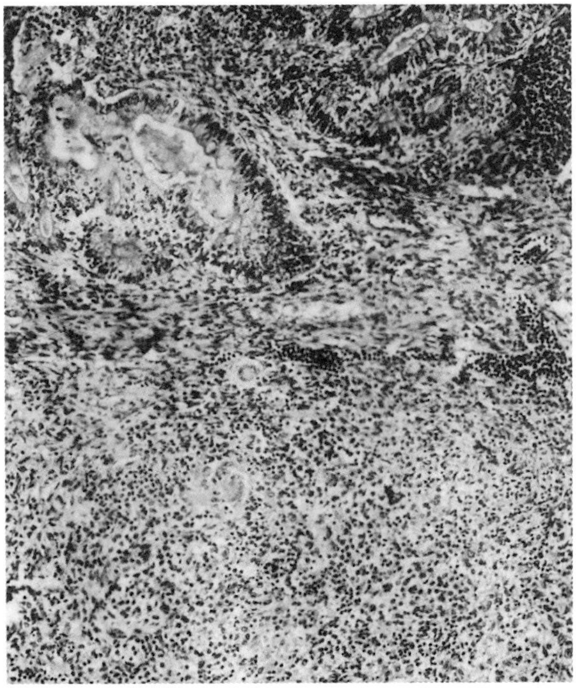

Fig. 50.4 Malignant mixed germ cell tumor – high grade immature teratoma (top) and dysgerminoma (lower). H + E ×75

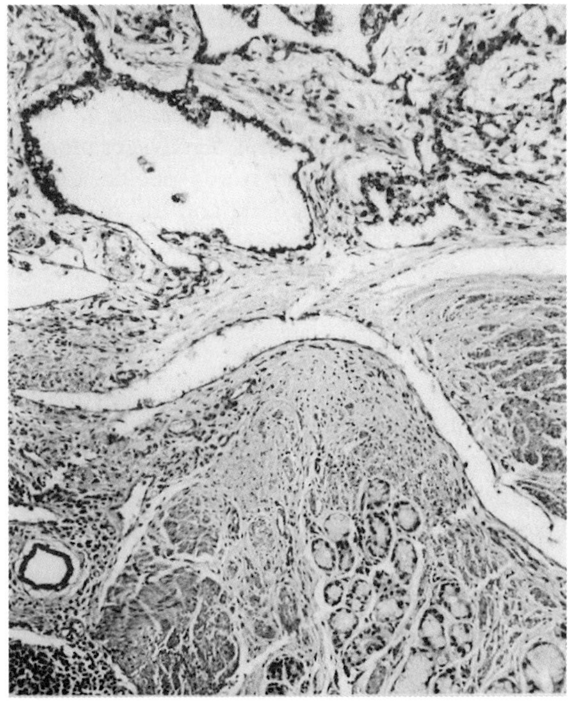

Fig. 50.5 Malignant mixed germ cell tumor – yolk sac tumor with reticular pattern (top) and adjacent mature teratoma (immature elsewhere). H + E ×75

Serum levels of β-human chorionic gonadotrophin (β-hCG), α-fetoprotein (AFP), or both may be raised, depending on the composition of the individual tumor, although it should be noted that a raised serum β-hCG does not necessarily indicate choriocarcinoma, since isolated syncytiotrophoblastic cells as part of embryonal carcinoma, polyembryoma, or dysgerminoma (and, rarely, non-germ-cell tumors) may be associated with the elaboration of this hormone.

Of the malignant mixed germ cell tumors 60% are apparently confined to one ovary (stage 1a) at presentation but, prior to the advent of modern chemotherapy, 50% of these patients died from tumor, indicating a considerable proclivity for occult metastases. They are unilateral, unless dysgerminoma is a component of the tumor, in which case there is about a 5–10% likelihood of neoplastic involvement of the other ovary. Biopsy of the second ovary, and exclusion of bilaterality in such instances, should thus precede any decision to employ conservative surgery (Kurman & Norris 1976). These authors have suggested that tumor size (greater than 10 cm in diameter) and histological composition (more than one-third of choriocarcinoma, yolk sac tumor, and/or high grade teratoma) are the two major pathological correlates of poor clinical outcome for stage 1 malignant mixed germ cell tumors, but a subsequent study (Gershenson et al 1984) suggested that FIGO stage alone may be the most important prognostic factor. Postoperative multiple-agent chemotherapy, an integral component of management based partly on the microscopic composition of the individual tumor, has dramatically improved the prognosis for these patients (Gershenson et al 1984, Micha et al 1985), yielding survival rates of about 80% for patients with stage 1 lesions and 50% for more advanced cases.

Macroscopic features

They tend to be large tumors, averaging about 15 cm in diameter, with smooth or bosselated external surfaces and cut surfaces which vary markedly, depending on the histological components present (Fig. 50 1). Microcystic or 'honeycomb' areas suggest immature teratoma. Solid, soft fleshy areas usually indicate dysgerminoma. Hemorrhage, although often nonspecific, may be a pointer to choriocarcinoma, and the margins of such areas must be adequately sampled. Necrosis is almost always obvious.

Microscopic features

The various elements in these tumors may be extensively admixed or may form separate areas in juxtaposition or separated by fibrous tissue septa. Malignant neoplasms in this group are classified according to component elements listed in decreasing order of prominence, but this depends on all areas of varying appearance being thoroughly sampled and examined histologically (a minimum of one block per centimeter of tumor diameter is suggested). Dysgerminoma is the commonest component of malignant mixed germ cell tumors, being present in over 75% of published cases (Figs 50.2–50.4). Only slightly less frequently encountered are the various patterns of yolk sac tumor (Figs 50.2, 50.5). Immature teratoma is seen in about 50% of these tumors (Figs 50.4, 50.5), while embryonal carcinoma (Fig. 50.3) and choriocarcinoma are relatively uncommonly seen (about 20% of cases). Rare examples of soft tissue sarcomas (rhabdomyosarcomas) mixed with dysgerminoma are reported in the testes and ovaries (Akhtar et al 1989).

REFERENCES

Akhtar M, Bakri Y, Rank F 1989 Dysgerminoma of the ovary with rhabdomyosarcoma. Report of a case. Cancer 64: 2309–2312

Flamant F, Caillou B, Pejovic M H et al 1978 Prognostic factors in malignant germ cell tumors of the ovary in children excluding pure dysgerminoma. European Journal of Cancer 14: 901–906

Fox H, Langley F A 1976 Tumors of the ovary. Heinemann, London, p 74–137

Gershenson D M, del Junco G, Copeland L J, Rutledge F N 1984 Mixed germ cell tumors of the ovary. Obstetrics and Gynecology 64: 200–206

Huntington R W Jr, Bullock W K 1970 Yolk sac tumors of the ovary. Cancer 25: 1357–1367

Jimerson G K, Woodruff J D 1977 Ovarian extra-embryonal teratoma: 2. Endodermal sinus tumor mixed with other germ cell tumors. American Journal of Obstetrics and Gynecology 127: 302–305

Kurman R J, Norris H J 1976 Malignant mixed germ cell tumors of the ovary. A clinical and pathologic analysis of 30 cases. Obstetrics and Gynecology 48: 579–589

Kurman R J, Norris H J 1977 Malignant germ cell tumors of the ovary. Human Pathology 8: 551–564

Martinazzi M, Bertoli G, Crivelli F, Zampatti C, Bersiga A 1989 Neoplasia germinale ovarica complessa: carcinoma embrionala adulto e disgerminoma con trofoblasto. Pathologica 81: 537–542

Micha J P, Kucera P R, Berman M L et al 1985 Malignant ovarian germ cell tumors: a review of thirty-six cases. American Journal of Obstetrics and Gynecology 152: 842–846

Norgaard-Pedersen B, Albrechtsen R, Teilum G 1975 Serum α-fetoprotein as a marker for endodermal sinus tumor (yolk sac tumor), or a vitelline component of teratocarcinoma. Acta Pathologica et Microbiologica Scandinavica (A) 83: 573–589

Talerman A, Haije W G, Baggerman L 1978 Serum alpha-fetoprotein in diagnosis and management of endodermal sinus (yolk sac) tumor and mixed germ cell tumor of the ovary. Cancer 41: 272–278

Talerman A, Huyzinga W T, Kuipers T 1973 Dysgerminoma. Clinicopathologic study of 22 cases. Obstetrics and Gynecology 41: 137–147

Vos A, Oosterhuis J W, de Jong B et al 1990 Karyotyping and DNA flow cytometry of metastatic ovarian yolk sac tumor. Cancer Genetics and Cytogenetics 44: 223–228

51

Germ cell–sex cord–stromal tumors ('gonadal anlage tumors')

P. Russell A. Farnsworth

The descriptive term 'mixed germ cell–sex cord–stromal tumor' was originally intended to embrace all the tumors composed of these cell types, including gonadoblastomas (Talerman 1972a,b). The latter entity is now so well established, however, that by general usage the term mixed germ cell–sex cord–stromal tumor is reserved for those few otherwise unclassified neoplasms composed of these cell types but which exhibit distinctive histological appearances and clinicopathological features differing from those of gonadoblastomas (Table 51.1). An alternative terminology, 'gonadal anlage tumor with male differentiation' (gonadoblastoma) and 'gonadal anlage tumor with female differentiation' (pflugeroma or mixed germ cell–sex cord–stromal tumor), has been proposed (Minh et al 1990).

Table 51.1 Differential diagnosis: gonadoblastoma versus unclassified mixed germ cell–sex cord–stromal tumor

Gonadoblastoma	Unclassified
Clinical	
Most common in second and third decades	Almost all under the age of 10 years
Most have abnormal karyotype (including Y chromosome)	All have 46XX karyotype
Tumors hormonally inert or associated with masculinization and primary amenorrhea	Phenotypically normal females, isosexual pseudoprecocity in occasional cases
Macroscopic	
Small tumors, bilateral in 38%, grossly calcified in 45%	Large tumors, always unilateral, not calcified
Histological	
Typical nest-like pattern	Multiplicity of patterns
Hyaline bodies and microcalcification common	Hyaline bodies and microcalcification absent
Stromal lutein cells common	Stromal lutein cells rare
Supervention of dysgerminoma or other germ cell tumor in 60%	Supervention of other germ cell tumor types very rare

As a group, these mixed tumors are composed of two and commonly three cell types. The two cellular elements common to all are germ cells and cells of sex cord origin resembling immature granulosa or Sertoli cells. Theca-lutein or Leydig-like cells are also present in most examples of gonadoblastoma type.

Over 80% of acceptable examples of gonadoblastoma have occurred in phenotypic females. However, over 95% of 'females' with gonadal tumors of this type have been shown to have abnormal karyotypes, which include a Y chromosome. The additional evidence of electron microscopic similarities between the sex cord elements of gonadoblastomas and those of normal testes supports the hypothesis that they represent disordered or abortive attempts at testicular differentiation (Scully 1979, Roth & Eglen 1989). Justification for inclusion of such tumors in a text of ovarian pathology is principally one of tradition and pragmatism. These lesions are mostly presented to the surgical pathologist as 'ovarian tumors'. Also, rare cases genuinely arise in essentially normal ovaries (Fig. 51.1).

GONADOBLASTOMAS

Gonadoblastomas are the best characterized of the mixed germ cell–sex cord–stromal tumors. The component germ cells closely resemble dysgerminoma cells, while the intermixed cells are similar to immature granulosa- or Sertoli-type cells. This basic cellular composition has been

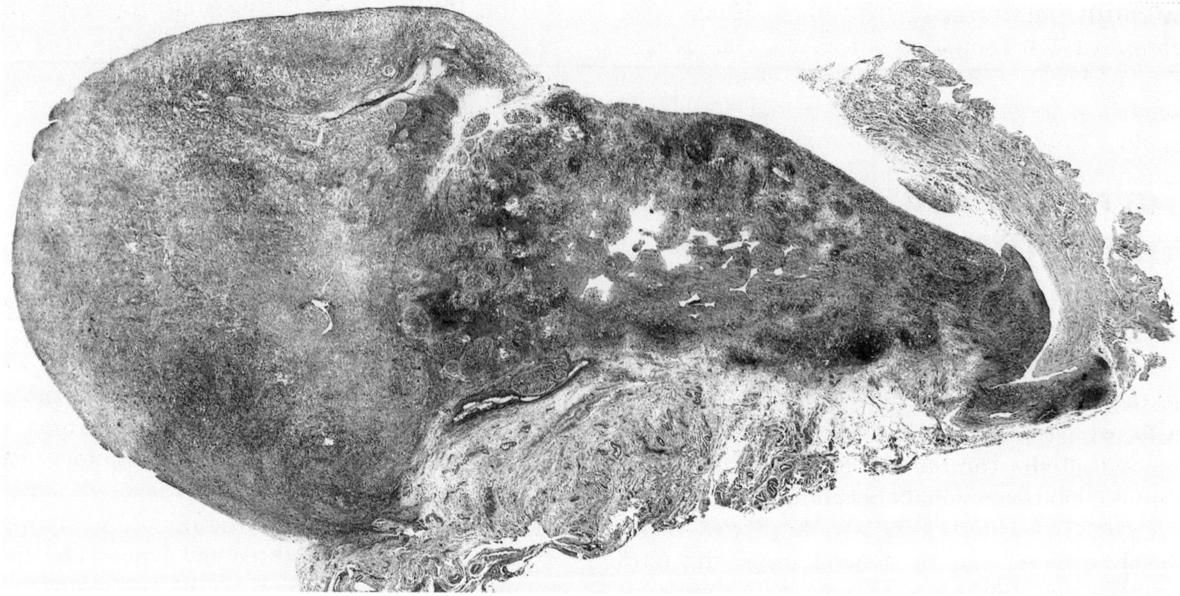

A

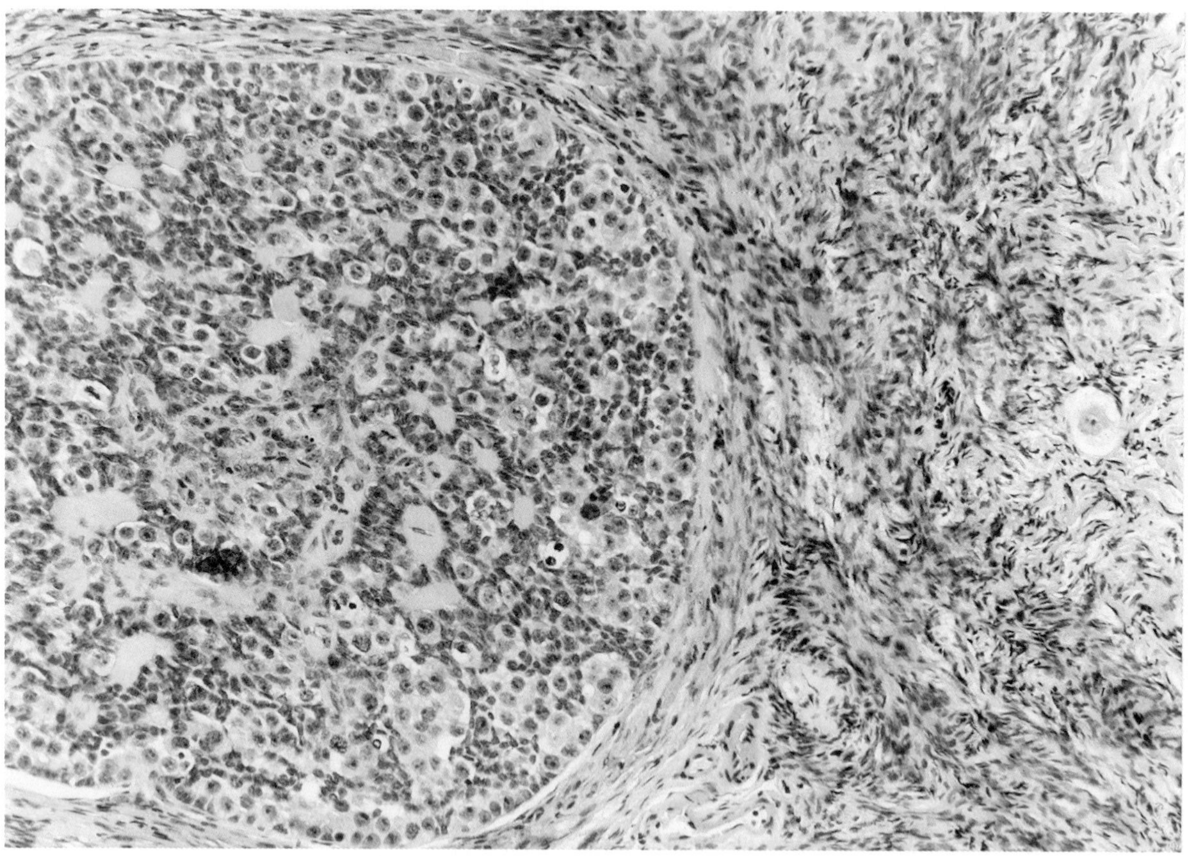

B

Fig. 51.1 Rare gonadoblastoma arising in normal ovary of a 13-year-old prepubertal girl with a 46,XX karyotype. (A) Survey of ovary. Note primordial follicles in adjacent cortex. H + E ×6.6. (B) Gonadoblastoma nests with germ cell and granulosa cell populations. Primordial follicle at center right. H + E ×82.5. (Material courtesy of Dr R. Osborn, Westmead) confirmed ultrastructurally (Hou-Jensen & Kempson 1974, Damjanov et al 1975, Garvin et al 1976, Ishida et al 1976). Isolated nests of cells resembling those of gonadoblastoma are occasionally seen in abnormal gonads and malformed seminiferous tubules, and have been variously termed 'gonadoblastosis', 'intersexual formations', and 'ring tubules'. While it is generally held that these differ from the grossly visible tumors only in size (Scully 1979), this continuous morphological spectrum has also been interpreted as suggesting a hamartomatous nature for gonadoblastomas (Fox & Langley 1976), a concept with which we are in agreement. No case of pure gonadoblastoma has been associated with documented metastases. Where a superimposed malignant germ cell tumor has led to metastases, the secondary deposits have not recapitulated the patterns of gonadoblastoma. This suggests that these tumors should be regarded, at most, as in situ malignant germ cell neoplasms (Muller et al 1992).

Over 80% of patients with gonadoblastomas are phenotypically female, while the remainder are cryptorchid males. Of the 'females', 60% are virilized (Scully 1970a), and over 95% of them have an abnormal karyotype which includes a Y chromosome (46,XY in 50%, 45,X/46,XY in 25%) and underlying anomalies of gonadal development. Rare patients have stigmata of Turner's syndrome, one with a 45,X karyotype (Schellhas 1974a). Gonadoblastomas have also been seen in true hermaphrodites, with a 46,XX karyotype (McDonough et al 1976, Talerman et al 1990, Talerman 1994) or a 46,XY karyotype (Park et al 1972, Szokol et al 1977). Rarely, these tumors have occurred in siblings (Frazier et al 1964, Talerman 1971, Anderson & Carlson 1975).

Patient age at diagnosis is 6–38 years, with most presenting in the second and third decades. The majority of somatosexual females with gonadoblastomas present with primary amenorrhea or early-onset secondary amenorrhea, during the investigation of which the lesions are identified. Much less commonly, they may present as unilateral or bilateral gonadal masses (radiographic examination frequently shows fine stippled calcification in such pelvic masses), presumptive evidence of gonadoblastoma. Occasional patients have exhibited isosexual pseudoprecocity, while very rare women have cycled spontaneously and become pregnant (Pratt-Thomas & Cooper 1976, Nakashima et al 1989, Elemenoglou et al 1990, Erhan et al 1992).

The germ cell component penetrates the boundaries of the nests in about one-half of cases to become typical dysgerminoma (Scully 1970a, Hart & Burkons 1979). Other categories of malignant germ cell tumors may be seen in an additional 10% of gonadoblastomas (Talerman 1974). It is important to note that superimposed malignancy manifests exclusively as a germ cell neoplasm in spite of gonadoblastomas being composed of at least two and usually three different cell types. In the case of dysgerminoma, the clinical outcome is still very good (Schellhas et al 1971, Hart & Burkons 1979). Metastases appear to occur later and less frequently than in dysgerminomas unassociated with gonadoblastoma, and are rarely fatal (Hart & Burkons 1979, Gadducci et al 1994). By contrast, the more malignant forms of germ cell tumor can be expected to behave in a fashion similar to those unassociated with gonadoblastoma (Gallager & Lewis 1973, la Polla et al 1990). We have seen personally a case of bilateral oophorectomy (?incomplete) in a phenotypically normal female for gonadoblastoma being followed 20 years later by the development of a typical adnexal granulosa cell tumor, at which time cytogenetic studies revealed a normal 46,XX karyotype. The relationship between these two entities is uncertain, especially as the completeness of the original oophorectomy cannot be confirmed.

Female patients with dysgenetic gonads whose genotype includes a Y chromosome have an approximately 25% likelihood of harboring a gonadoblastoma or malignant germ cell tumor, a risk which argues strongly in favour of prophylactic bilateral adnexectomy (Schellhas 1974b, Talerman 1974, Garvin et al 1976, Williamson et al 1976, Hart & Burkons 1979, Wilson et al 1992), especially as these dysgenetic gonads are incapable of normal function and retention of reproductive capability is not at issue. Furthermore, the dysgenetic gonads may be virilizing influences, even if a malignant tumor does not supervene.

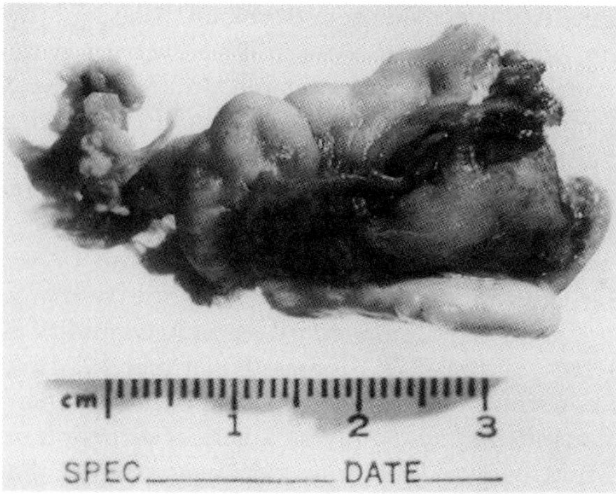

Fig. 51.2 Below the fallopian tube is a small 20 mm streak gonad which, histologically, showed 'burnt-out' gonadoblastoma

Macroscopic features

These tumors are bilateral in over one-third of cases. Unilateral cases show a slight right-sided predominance. About one-quarter are diagnosed only after microscopic examination (Fig. 51.2). The macroscopic appearances of the obvious gonadoblastomas vary with size (usually 2–3 cm across, but up to 10 cm in diameter), the presence or absence of a supervening malignant germ cell tumor, and whether or not calcification is prominent (in 45% of cases). Pure gonadoblastomas are almost always solid tumors (although cystic variants have been encountered) with smooth or slightly lobulated external surfaces. They vary in consistency from soft and fleshy to firm and densely calcified. The cut surface is gray-yellow or white and granular, if calcified (Fig. 51.3).

A

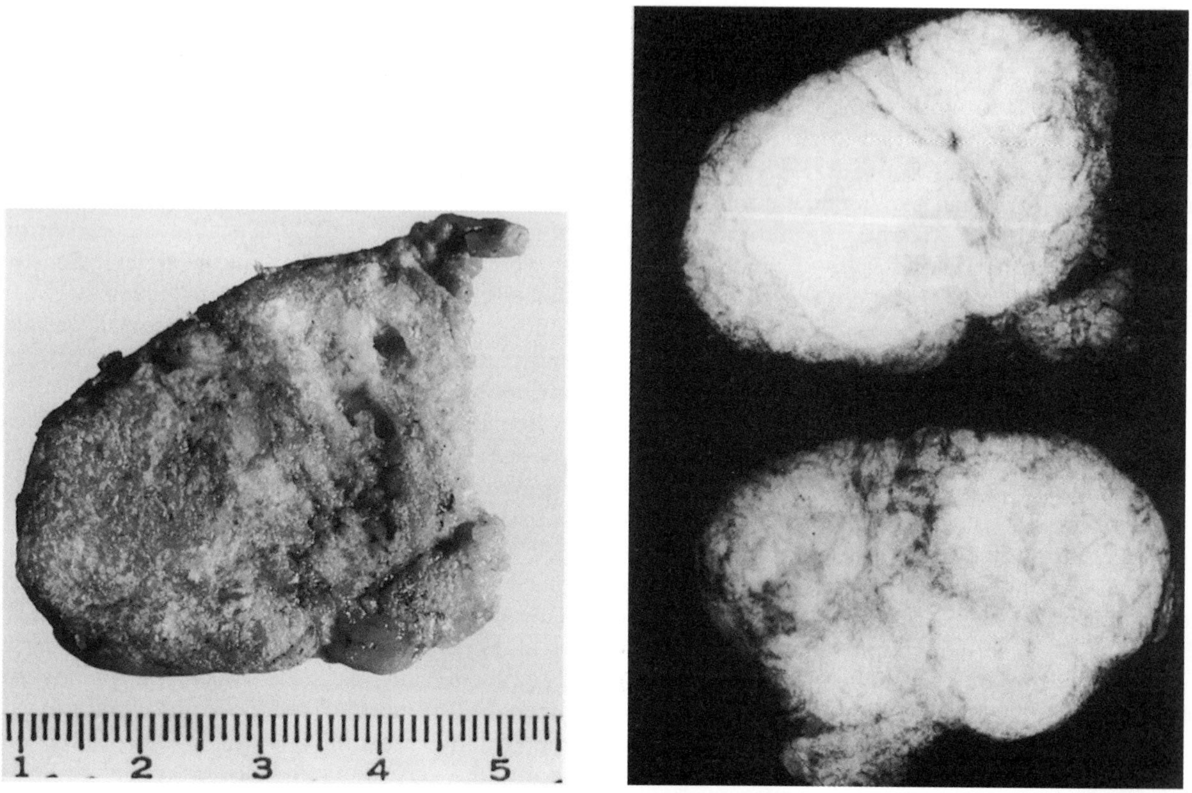

B

Fig. 51.3 Heavily calcified gonadoblastoma. (A) Pale, gritty cut surface with a small soft tissue nodule in the lower right corner which was histologically dysgerminoma. (B) Specimen radiograph of the same tumor

Microscopic features

The basic architecture of gonadoblastomas depends on the presence of numerous well-circumscribed cell nests, each invested by a very thick basal lamina and embedded in fibrous connective tissue stroma (Fig. 51.4). The nests are small, oval to round, and solid (only rarely cystic) (Fig. 51.5); they contain an intimate mixture of germ cells and other cells of sex cord type resembling immature granulosa or Sertoli cells. Lymphocytes and even granulomas (Fig. 51.6) are occasionally seen within the discrete nests (Scully 1979).

The germ cells show histological, histochemical, and electron microscopic similarities to dysgerminoma cells. They are large and polyhedral, with pale, slightly granular cytoplasm and large round vesicular nuclei, often with a prominent nucleolus, sometimes exhibit appreciable mitotic activity, and immunostain for placental alkaline phosphatase. The small ovoid sex cord cells have dark, slightly elongated nuclei (Fig. 51.7). Mitoses are not seen in these cells. They are considered by some to be Sertoli cells or their precursors (Roth & Eglen 1989), while others regard them as primitive sex cord stromal cells defying further categorization (Scully 1970a, Hou-Jensen & Kempson 1974, Damjanov et al 1975, Talerman 1980). They are organized within the cell nests in three different patterns:

- to form a peripheral palisade around aggregates of germ cells (Figs 51.3, 51.5)
- to form a corona around individual or groups of germ cells in a microfollicular pattern similar to the granulosa of primary follicles
- to radially surround small deposits of hyaline, eosinophilic PAS-positive material similar to Call–Exner bodies (Fig. 51.7).

These rounded, hyaline deposits, composed

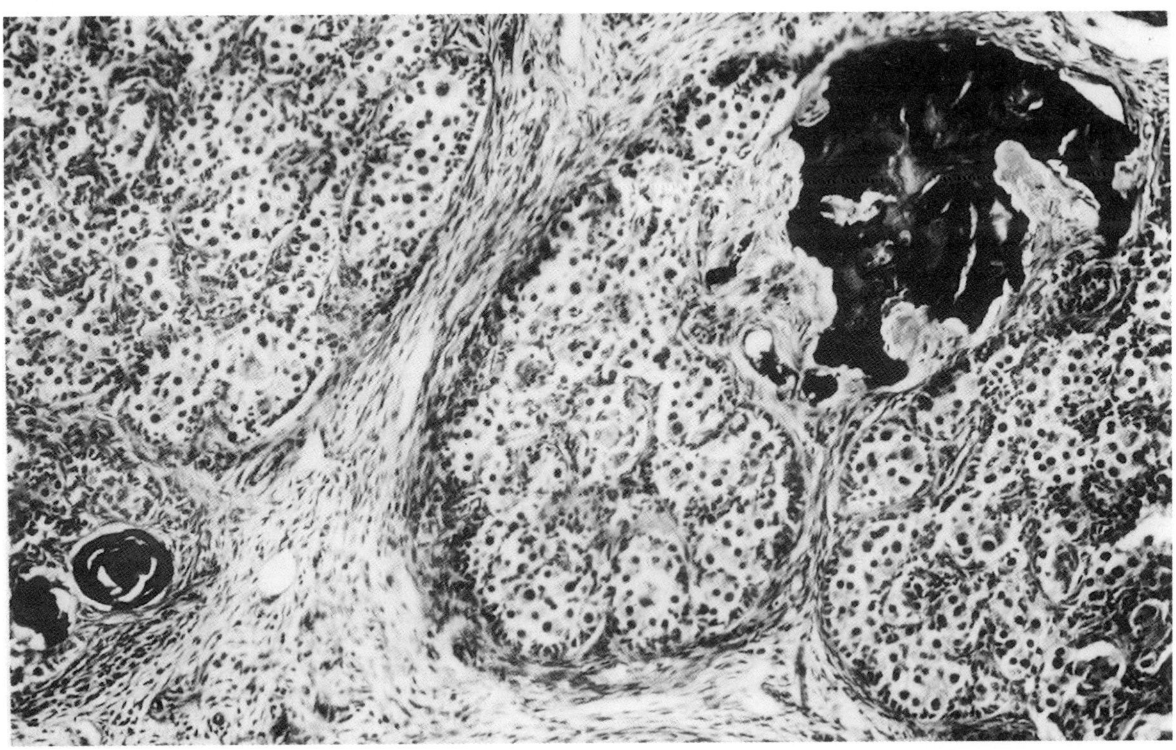

Fig. 51.4 Well-circumscribed nests of a gonadoblastoma with dystrophic calcification. Small rounded calcified bodies resembling psammoma bodies (lower left) coalesce to form larger irregular masses (upper right). H + E ×125

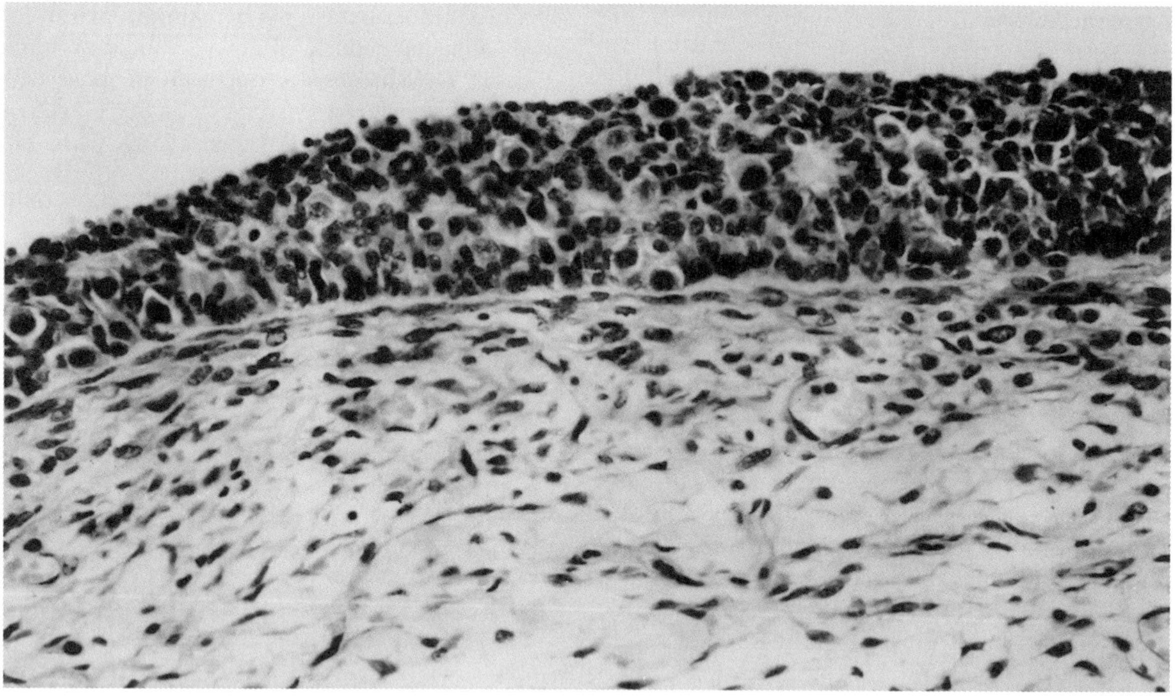

Fig. 51.5 Rare cystic gonadoblastoma showing the same intimate mixture of large germ cells and smaller 'supportive' or sex cord stromal cells. H + E ×250

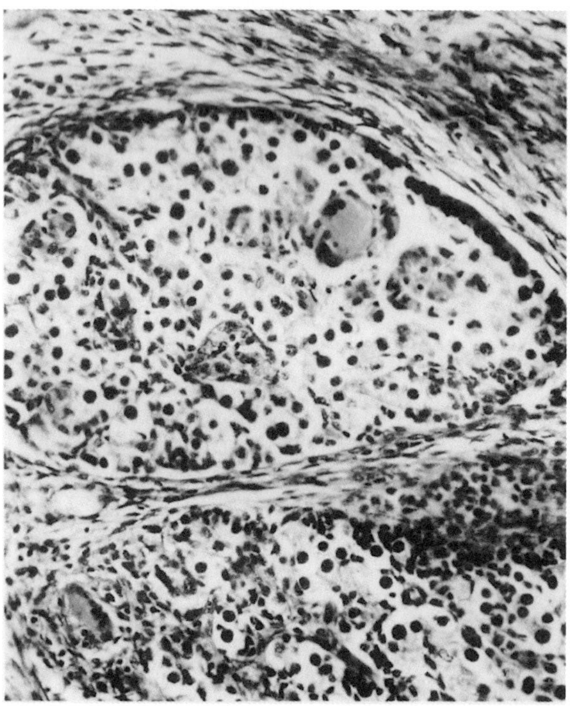

Fig. 51.6 Gonadoblastoma. Two histiocytic giant cells included within the cell nests. H + E ×150

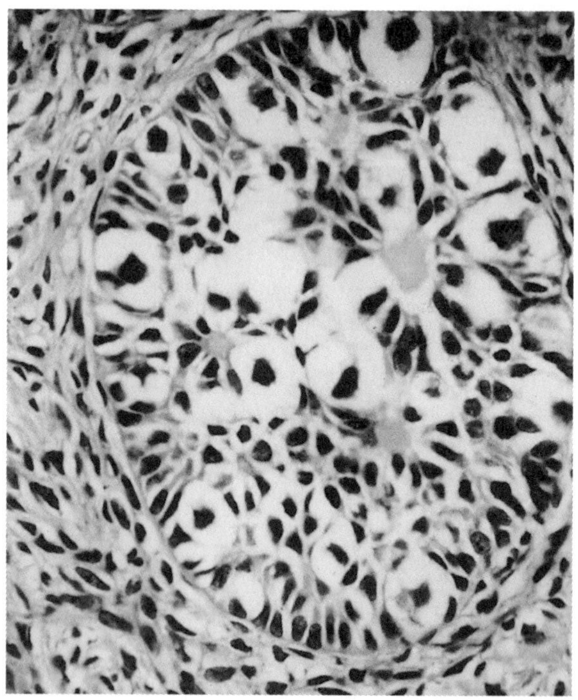

Fig. 51.7 Gonadoblastoma. A typical cell nest showing Sertoli-like cells arranged radially around individual germ cells and around hyaline deposits. H + E ×300

of aggregated basal lamina material (laminin) Damjanov et al 1975, Ishida et al 1976, Roth & Eglen 1989), are sometimes continuous with linear hyaline deposits around the periphery of the cell nests. Similarities with the hyaline bodies of the sex cord tumor with annular tubules (see Ch. 37), and differences from typical Call–Exner bodies, have been noted ultrastructurally.

The fibrous connective tissue stroma which separates the cellular nests contains lutein or Leydig-like cells in 66–75% of cases overall, but significantly more commonly in patients over 15 years of age (postpubertal) than in those below this age, possibly in response to gonadotrophin stimulation. They vary considerably in their numbers from case to case and, although they usually contain lipochrome pigment, Reinke crystals have been observed in only one case (Fox & Langley 1976). This intervening fibrous stroma also varies greatly in amount and in cellularity, from dense and hyalinized to tissue more closely resembling ovarian cortex, the latter particularly so in tumors that have arisen in a gonadal streak (Scully 1970a). In some gonadoblastomas, the stroma is loose and edematous.

Gonadoblastomas usually obliterate most or all of the gonads in which they arise; these, in turn, in the case of smaller tumors, can be shown to be gonadal streaks (Fig. 51.2) or abnormal abdominal testes of pure gonadal dysgenesis or mixed gonadal dysgenesis types.

The appearances of gonadoblastomas may be considerably modified by hyalinization, calcification, and the supervention of dysgerminoma or other malignant germ cell tumor (Scully 1970a, Garvin et al 1976). Hyalinization occurs by coalescence and extension of the amorphous, hyaline bodies and the peripheral basal lamina-like band. The hyaline material replaces tumor cells, sometimes entirely. Calcification, seen microscopically in 80% of lesions, usually begins in the hyaline bodies with formation of small laminated calcispherules resembling psammoma bodies (Fig. 51.4). The process continues with enlargement and fusion of the calcified bodies and spiculate dystrophic calcification of the hyaline material, finally forming a calcified mass around the whole nest. The process may extend to the stroma between the cellular nests. In such cases, the tumor cells are sparse or even absent, and the pattern of calcification (Fig. 51.8) and the presence of lutein or Leydig-like cells may be the only indication of gonadoblastoma (Garvin et al 1976). Although this appearance is not considered pathognomonic of gonadoblastoma (it has been graced with the term 'burnt-out' gonadoblastoma (Scully 1970a, Talerman 1971)) it is highly suggestive and, in such circumstances, a careful search for more typical areas of tumor should be undertaken.

Gonadoblastomas are overgrown by otherwise typical dysgerminoma in 50% of cases (Scully 1970a). This overgrowth may vary from a small focus of germ cells in the stroma outside the gonadoblastomatous nests to gross tumor growth with obliteration of the antecedent tumor (Fig. 51.9). The only clue to the presence of the original lesion may be tiny foci of calcification (the detection of which is facilitated by radiographic examination of the specimen) and the genotype of the patient. Gonadoblastomas may be associated with other more malignant germ cell tumor types, such as immature teratoma, yolk sac tumor,

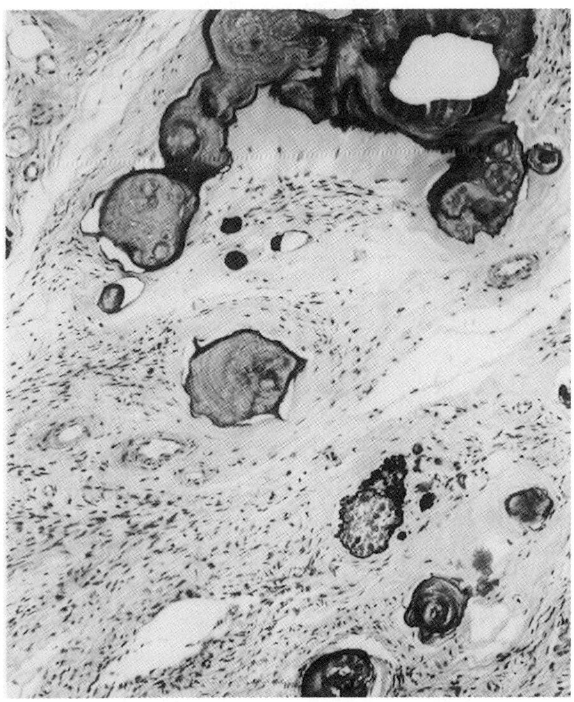

Fig. 51.8 So-called 'burnt-out' gonadoblastoma. A streak gonad (Fig. 51.2) characterized by the pattern of calcification set in fibrous gonadal stroma. H + E ×75

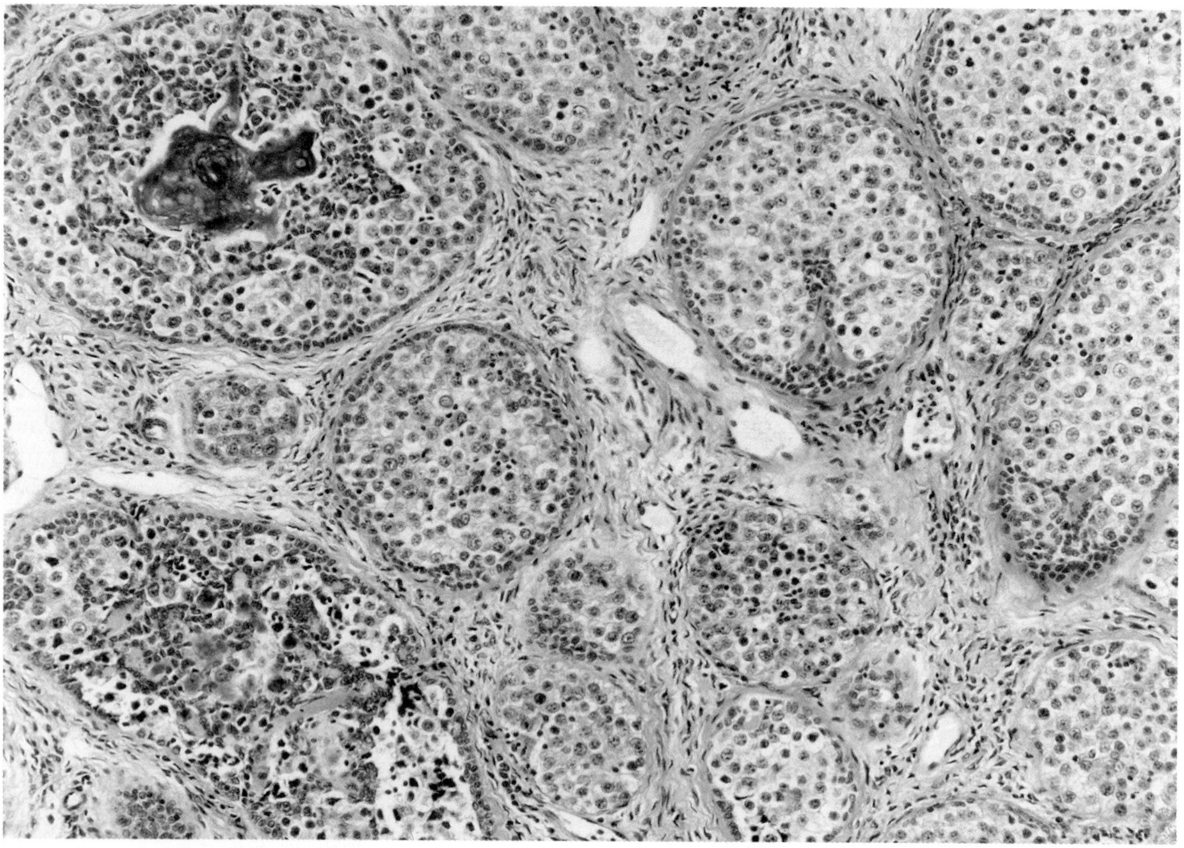

A

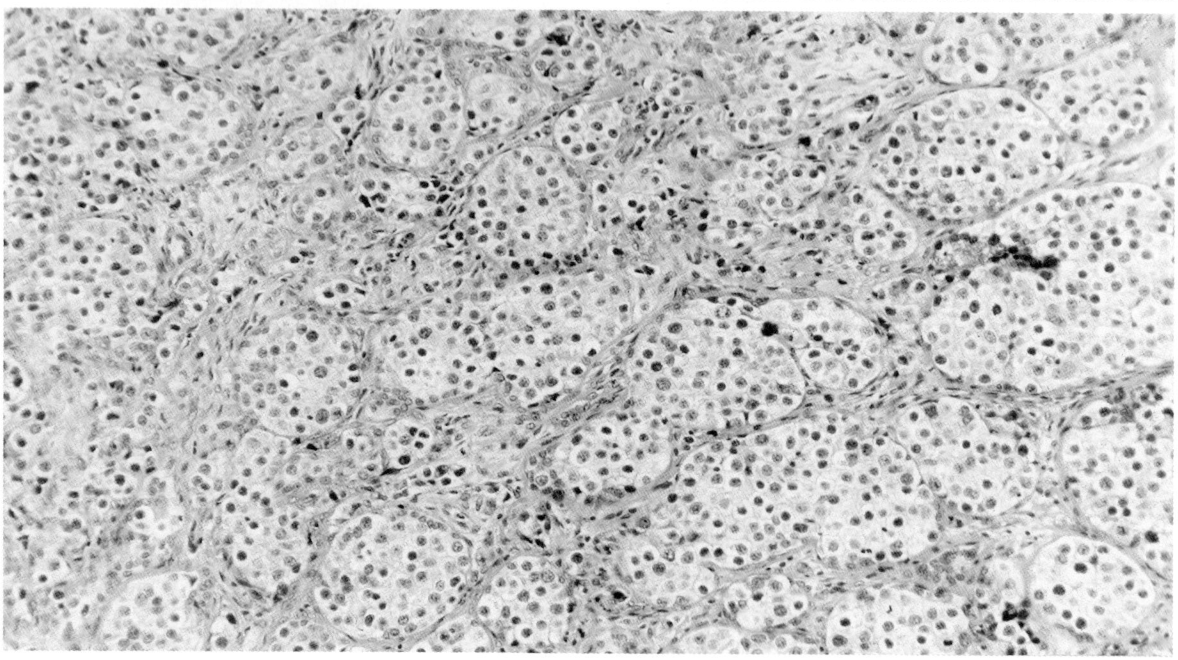

B

Fig. 51.9 Gonadoblastoma exhibiting progressive supervention by dysgerminoma. (A) Typical gonadoblastoma nests are seen in which germ cell proliferation is still confined to the cell nests ('dysgerminoma in situ'). H + E ×82.5. (B) Stromal invasion by malignant germ cells takes place, destroying the architectural pattern. H + E ×82.5

embryonal carcinoma, or choriocarcinoma, in a further 10% of cases (Talerman 1974).

Differential diagnosis

Gonadoblastomas, because of their distinctive histological appearances and cellular composition, are readily distinguished from the more frequently encountered gonadal neoplasms. Those from which differentiation may be problematical are the mixed germ cell–sex cord–stromal tumors (see below), and the ovarian sex cord tumors with annular tubules (Scully 1970b, 1979), which are usually found in patients with Peutz–Jeghers syndrome (see Ch. 37). These latter lesions are composed of tubules lined by Sertoli and granulosa-like cells arranged in nests, contain similar round, eosinophilic, hyaline deposits, and tend to calcify in the same manner as gonadoblastomas. They are, however, completely devoid of germ cells.

UNCLASSIFIED GERM CELL–SEX CORD–STROMAL TUMORS

Only rare examples have been adequately documented of this category of tumors, which includes all neoplasms containing variable mixtures of germ cells and sex cord elements (Talerman 1972a,b, 1980, Talerman & van der Harten 1977, Tokuoka et al 1985, Lacson et al 1988, Minh et al 1990, Jacobsen et al 1991, Zuntova et al 1992), but lacking the characteristic cellular arrangements of gonadoblastomas. Occasionally theca-lutein and Leydig-like cells are encountered. They arise from normally developed ovaries. All but one have occurred in karyotypically and somatosexually normal children under 10 years of age, and 6 of these below 1 year of age (Talerman 1972b, 1980, Tavassoli 1983). The exceptional case occurred in a 31-year-old parous woman. A solitary case has been reported arising in a normal adult testis (Bolen 1981).

The most frequent presenting symptoms have been an abdominal mass and acute abdominal pain due to torsion. Four children have exhibited signs of isosexual pseudoprecocity (Talerman & van der Harten 1977, Lacson et al 1988).

The true malignant potential of these tumors has not been firmly determined but, to date, recurrences and/or metastases after unilateral salpingo-oophorectomy have been recorded only once (Lacson et al 1988), and this therefore remains the recommended therapy. Furthermore, in the case of the 31-year-old woman, a dysgerminoma had supervened upon the mixed germ cell–sex cord–stromal tumor, yet the patient was free of disease 4 years after local excision and radiotherapy. It is axiomatic that careful examination of the abdomen and a biopsy of the contralateral ovary be performed at the time of surgery.

Cytogenetic and molecular genetic studies

All females who have been studied cytogenetically have demonstrated a 46,XX karyotype with normal somatosexual development (Talerman 1994).

Macroscopic features

These tumors are almost always unilateral and vary in size up to 18 cm in diameter and 1 kg in weight. They are usually round to oval and of firm consistency, with a smooth, glistening capsule and a gray-pink to pale fawn solid cut surface. Cysts are occasionally present (Talerman & van der Harten 1977). Necrosis and macroscopic calcification have not been observed.

Microscopic features

The germ cells are similar to those in dysgerminomas and seminomas (Fig. 51.10). They show brisk mitotic activity. Some of the germ cells occasionally appear to be more mature than those seen in gonadoblastomas or dysgerminomas, with large round nuclei lacking a prominent nucleolus, and tend to resemble 'primordial cells' (Talerman 1994) or 'clear cells of another type' (Scully 1979). The cells of sex cord origin resemble Sertoli cells rather more closely than granulosa cells (Fig. 51.10), but may be very immature, and also show variable mitotic activity. While the relative proportions of germ cells and sex cord cells varies from area to area within individual tumors, their intimate admixture is universal. Tumors are predominantly solid in pattern (Fig. 51.11), but with occasional small cleft-like or cystic spaces, the latter resembling the follicle-like spaces of granulosa cell tumors or the retiform pattern of moderately

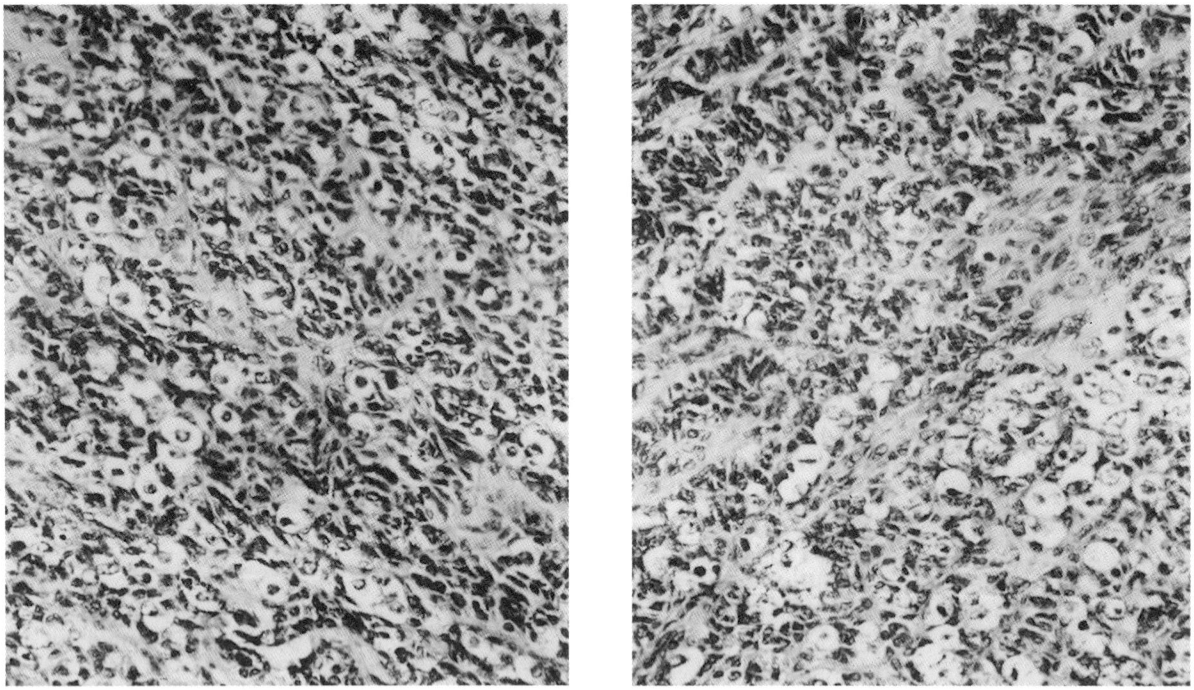

A B

Fig. 51.10 A mixed germ cell–sex cord–stromal tumor. In (A) and (B) the presence of large germ cells and smaller 'supportive' or sex cord–stromal cells is universal, although their proportions vary from field to field. H + E ×150. (Material courtesy of Dr A. Talerman, Chicago)

or poorly differentiated Sertoli–Leydig cell tumors (Tokuoka et al 1985). The apparently unique and controversial case of Tavassoli (1983) was characterized by the additional presence of slit-like spaces and tubules lined by 'epithelial cells'. These structures were focally continuous with the surface epithelium of the ovary, yet, in the deeper portions of the tumor, the 'epithelial cells' merged imperceptibly with the cells of sex cord type at both light and electron microscopic levels. No mullerian differentiation was noted, and an alternative interpretation of this third structural element is that it also represents a retiform Sertoli cell component (Talerman 1984). Another apparently unique variation is the presence of heterologous elements, comprised of intestinal type glands or cysts containing goblet and neuroendocrine cells, analogous to those seen in Sertoli–Leydig cell tumors (Zuntova et al 1992).

Three discernible architectural arrangements of the component cells may be seen. The first is represented by long, branching cords of variable thickness surrounded by moderate amounts of loose, edematous, or dense, fibrous connective tissue. There is some similarity between these trabeculae and the primitive sex cords of the developing ovary. The second pattern shows pseudotubular structures surrounded by a fine network of similar fibrous connective tissue, and resembling the gonadal Sertoli cell congeries of the androgen insensitivity syndrome (testicular feminization syndrome). There may be merging of this pseudotubular pattern, via small clusters of larger round or oval cellular masses, with the third pattern, which exhibits germ cell aggregates surrounded by variable, but usually prominent, sex cord elements. The nest-like pattern of gonadoblastomas is not observed in these tumors. Hyaline bodies and focal stromal dystrophic calcification are very rare or absent. In one case, rare small collections of luteinized stromal cells (Leydig or theca-lutein cells) were observed (Talerman 1972a), but these cells were conspicuously absent in all other cases.

Normal ovarian stroma with primordial or

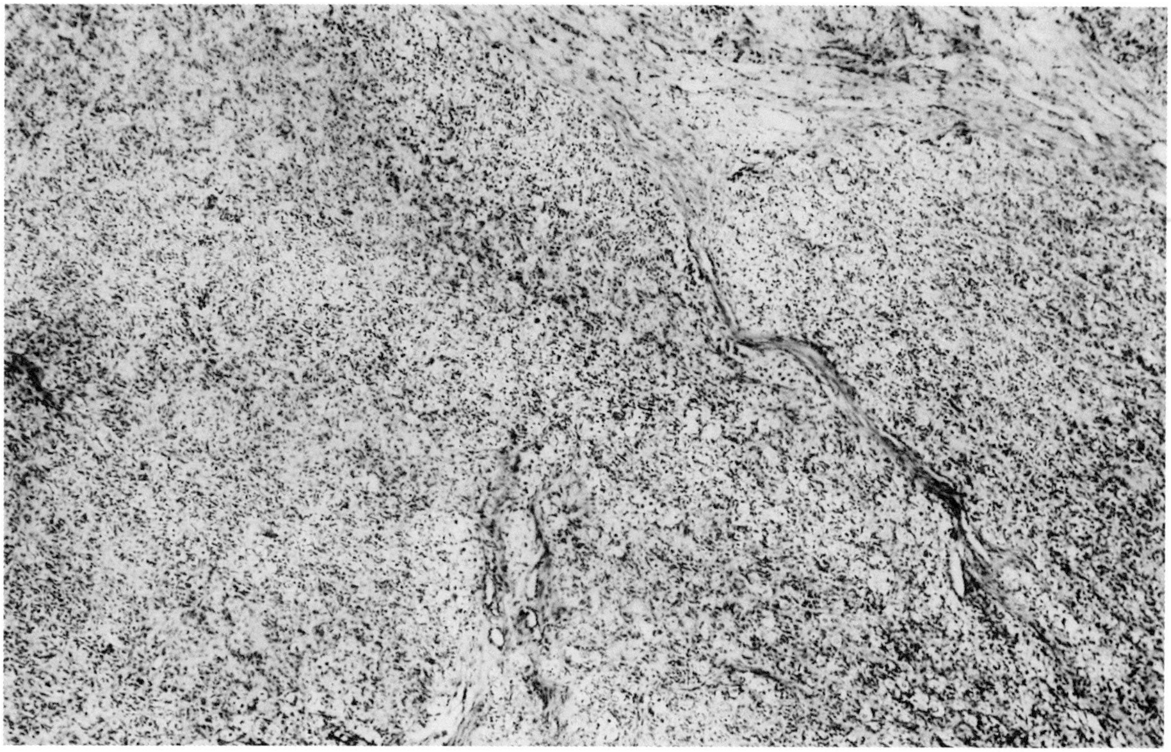

Fig. 51.11 A mixed germ cell–sex cord–stromal tumor. Low power demonstrating the diffuse pattern of growth, to be contrasted with the circumscribed cell nests of gonadoblastoma. H + E ×50. (Material courtesy of Dr A. Talerman, Chicago)

developing follicles is present at the periphery in all cases (Talerman 1972a, Talerman & van der Harten 1977). A pure dysgerminoma has been reported as supervening upon the germ cell element in this type of tumor (Talerman 1994), and Scully (1979) has observed one case in which a mixed germ cell–sex cord–stromal tumor was partly surrounded by choriocarcinoma. Intermediate patterns between typical gonadoblastomas and tumors in this category have also been encountered (Bhathena et al 1985).

Differential diagnosis

The neoplasms with which mixed germ cell–sex cord–stromal tumors may be most easily confused are, of course, gonadoblastomas (Table 51.1). These girls have a normal female 46,XX karyotype, while those patients with gonadoblastomas are mostly chromosomally abnormal, the karyotype containing a Y chromosome. There is no evidence of virilization, and if signs of hormonal activity are present, these are usually estrogenic (isosexual pseudoprecocity). Macroscopically these tumors are generally larger than uncomplicated gonadoblastomas and they arise in normal ovaries, without evidence of gonadal dysgenesis or somatosexual abnormality. They can be distinguished microscopically from gonadoblastomas by the presence of multiple histological patterns (described above) and greater proliferative activity, particularly in the sex cord elements. Calcification and stromal hyalinization are absent in these tumors, and in the vast majority of cases no theca-lutein or Leydig cells are seen either.

Confusion between mixed germ cell–sex cord–stromal tumors and pure sex cord–stromal tumors should be countered by sampling sufficiently to find the germ cell element and, conversely, they can be differentiated from dysgerminomas by correctly identifying the sex cord component, which may be scanty but is always present.

REFERENCES

Anderson C T Jr, Carlson I H 1975 Elevated plasma testosterone and gonadal tumors in two 46XY 'sisters'. Archives of Pathology 99: 360–363

Bhathena D, Haning R V Jr, Shapiro S, Hafez G R 1985 Coexistence of a gonadoblastoma and mixed germ cell–sex cord stromal tumor. Pathology Research and Practice 180: 203–206

Bolen J W 1981 Mixed germ cell–sex cord stromal tumor. A gonadal tumor distinct from gonadoblastoma. American Journal of Clinical Pathology 75: 565–573

Damjanov I, Drobnjak P, Grizelj V 1975 Ultrastructure of gonadoblastoma. Archives of Pathology 99: 25–31

Elemenoglou J, Korkolopoulou P, Zizi A, Delides G S 1990 A case of gonadoblastoma in a normal woman with tubal pregnancy. Archiv für Geschwulstforschrift 60: 223–226

Erhan Y, Toprak A S, Ozdemir N, Tiras B 1992 Gonadoblastoma and fertility. Journal of Clinical Pathology 45: 828–829

Fox H, Langley F A 1976 Tumours of the ovary. Heinemann, London, p 249–261

Frazier S D, Bashore R A, Mosier H D 1964 Gonadoblastoma associated with pure gonadal dysgenesis in monozygous twins. Journal of Pediatrics 64: 740–745

Gadducci A, Madrigali A, Simeone T, Facchini V, Singer M T, Marchetti G 1994 The association of ovarian dysgerminoma and gonadoblastoma in a phenotypic female with 46XY karyotype. European Journal of Gynaecological Oncology 15: 125–131

Gallager H S, Lewis R P 1973 Sequential gonadoblastoma and choriocarcinoma. Obstetrics and Gynecology 41: 123–128

Garvin A J, Pratt-Thomas H R, Spector M, Spicer S S, Williamson H O 1976 Gonadoblastoma: histologic, ultrastructural and histochemical observations in five cases. American Journal of Obstetrics and Gynecology 125: 459–471

Hart W R, Burkons D M 1979 Germ cell neoplasms arising in gonadoblastoma. Cancer 43: 669–678

Hou-Jensen K, Kempson R L 1974 The ultrastructure of gonadoblastoma and dysgerminoma. Human Pathology 5: 79–91

Ishida T, Tagatz G E, Okagaki T 1976 Gonadoblastoma. Ultrastructural evidence of testicular origin. Cancer 37: 1770–1781

Jacobsen G K, Braendstrup O, Talerman A 1991 Bilateral mixed germ cell sex–cord stroma tumor in a young adult woman. Case report. Acta Pathologica Microbiologica et Immunologica Scandinavica 23: 132–137

Lacson A G, Gillis D A, Shawwa A 1988 Malignant mixed germ cell–sex cord–stromal tumors of the ovary associated with isosexual precocious puberty. Cancer 61: 2122–2133

la Polla J P, Fiorica J V, Turnquist D, Nicosia S, Wilson J, Cavanagh D 1990 Successful therapy of metastatic embryonal carcinoma coexisting with gonadoblastoma in a patient with 46,XY pure gonadal dysgenesis (Swyer's syndrome). Gynecologic Oncology 37: 417–421

McDonough P G, Byrd J R, Tho P T, Otken L 1976 Gonadoblastoma in a true hermaphrodite with 46XX karyotype. Obstetrics and Gynecology 47: 355–358

Minh H N, Smadja A, Delteil C, Sevestre C 1990 A propos d'un cas de pflugerome ou 'tumeur mixte germinale des cordons sexuels et du stroma'. Archives d'Anatomie Cytologie et Pathologie 38: 11–17

Muller J, Visfeldt J, Philip J, Skakkebaek N E 1992 Carcinoma in situ, gonadoblastoma, and early invasive neoplasia in a nine-year-old girl with 46,XY gonadal dysgenesis. Acta Pathologica Microbiologica et Immunologica Scandinavica 100: 170–174

Nakashima N, Nagasaka T, Fukata S et al 1989 Ovarian gonadoblastoma with dysgerminoma in a woman with two normal children. Human Pathology 20: 814–816

Park I J, Pyeatte J C, Jones H W, Woodruff J D 1972 Gonadoblastoma in a true hermaphrodite with 46XY genotype. Obstetrics and Gynecology 40: 466–472

Pratt-Thomas H R, Cooper J M 1976 Gonadoblastoma with tubal pregnancy. American Journal of Clinical Pathology 65: 121–125

Roth L M, Eglen D E 1989 Gonadoblastoma. Immunohistochemical and ultrastructural observations. International Journal of Gynecological Pathology 8: 72–81

Schellhas H F 1974a Malignant potential of the dysgenetic gonad. Part I. Obstetrics and Gynecology 44: 298–309

Schellhas H F 1974b Malignant potential of the dysgenetic gonad. Part II. Obstetrics and Gynecology 44: 455–462

Schellhas H F, Trujillo J M, Rutledge F N, Cork A 1971 Germ cell tumors associated with XY gonadal dysgenesis. American Journal of Obstetrics and Gynecology 109: 1197–1204

Scully R E 1970a Gonadoblastoma. A review of 74 cases. Cancer 25: 1340–1356

Scully R E 1970b Sex cord tumor with annular tubules. A distinctive ovarian tumor of the Peutz–Jeghers syndrome. Cancer 25: 1107–1121

Scully R E 1979 Tumors of the ovary and maldeveloped gonads. AFIP fascicle 16, 2nd series. Armed Forces Institute of Pathology, Washington, DC

Szokol M, Kondrai G, Papp Z 1977 Gonadal malignancy and 46XY karyotype in a true hermaphrodite. Obstetrics and Gynecology 49: 358–360

Talerman A 1971 Gonadoblastoma and dysgerminoma in two siblings with dysgenetic gonads. Obstetrics and Gynecology 38: 416–426

Talerman A 1972a A distinctive gonadal neoplasm related to gonadoblastoma. Cancer 36: 1219–1224

Talerman A 1972b A mixed germ cell-sex cord stroma tumor in a normal female infant. Obstetrics and Gynecology 40: 473–478

Talerman A 1974 Gonadoblastoma associated with embryonal carcinoma. Obstetrics and Gynecology 43: 138–142

Talerman A 1980 The pathology of gonadal neoplasms composed of germ cells and sex cord stroma derivatives. Pathology Research and Practice 170: 24–38

Talerman A 1984 A combined germ cell–sex cord–stromal–epithelial tumor of the ovary or a hamartoma (letter). American Journal of Surgical Pathology 8: 638–639

Talerman A 1994 Germ cell tumors of the ovary. In: Kurman R J A (ed) Blaustein's pathology of the female genital tract, 4th edn. Springer-Verlag, New York, p 849–914

Talerman A, van der Harten J J 1977 A mixed germ cell–sex cord stroma tumor of the ovary associated with iso-sexual precocious puberty in a normal female child. Cancer 40: 889–894

Talerman A, Verp M, Senekjian E, Gilewski T, Vogelkanz N

1990 True hermaphrodite with normal female 46, XX karyotype, bilateral gonadoblastomas and dysgerminomas and normal pregnancy. Cancer 66: 2668

Tavassoli F A 1983 A combined germ cell–gonadal stromal–epithelial tumor of the ovary. American Journal of Surgical Pathology 7: 73–84

Tokuoka S, Aoki Y, Hayashi Y, Yokoyama T, Ishii T 1985 A mixed germ cell–sex cord–stromal tumor of the ovary with retiform tubular structure: a case report. International Journal of Gynecological Pathology 4: 161–170

Williamson H O, Underwood P B Jr, Kreutner A Jr, Rogers J F, Mathur R S, Pratt-Thomas H R 1976 Gonadoblastoma: clinicopathologic correlation in six patients. American Journal of Obstetrics and Gynecology 126: 579–584

Wilson E E, Vuitch F, Carr B R 1992 Laparoscopic removal of dysgenetic gonads containing a gonadoblastoma in a patient with Swyer syndrome. Obstetrics and Gynecology 79: 842–844

Zuntova A, Motlik K, Horejsi J, Eckschlager T 1992 Mixed germ cell–sex cord–stromal tumor with heterologous structures. International Journal of Gynecological Pathology 11: 227–233

SECTION 8

Miscellaneous and metastatic tumors

52

Miscellaneous mesenchymal tumors

P. Russell   A. Farnsworth

Ovarian mesenchymal tumors are of diverse origin. Tumors of fibrous tissue are considered to be part of the spectrum of fibrothecomas and, as such, to be of specific gonadal stromal origin (see Ch. 34). Smooth muscle tumors, on the basis of their homology with tumors occurring more commonly in the uterus, are included in the group of mullerian mesenchymal tumors (see Ch. 26). The remaining mesenchymal tumors discussed below are considered to arise directly from those elements of the ovary not committed to its specific gonadal function, e.g. connective tissue, vessels, and nerves (Fox & Langley 1976). They may also arise from monophyletic teratomas (as proposed for struma ovarii and ovarian carcinoids), secondary malignant transformation in mature cystic teratomas, or be the predominant sarcomatous component in mixed mullerian tumors or Sertoli–Leydig cell tumors (Fox & Langley 1976, Talerman 1982, Prat & Scully 1986).

In view of the diverse nature of these mesenchymal tumors, the ovaries should be sampled extensively for evidence of a specific origin, since this may have a bearing on prognosis. In general, pure sarcomas have a better outlook than those which are components of teratomas or malignant mixed mullerian tumors. Primary pure ovarian sarcomas also seem, from the limited reports available for analysis, to have a better prognosis than the same tumors occurring in extraovarian sites; this may relate to their greater ease of local excision (oophorectomy) compared with similar tumors occurring in the deep soft tissues.

In addition, it is important that the possibility, although rare, that a sarcoma occurring in the ovary is metastatic (see Ch. 53) should be investigated clinically.

VASCULAR AND RELATED TUMORS

Hemangiomas

These are the most common of the miscellaneous mesenchymal ovarian tumors, although some controversy exists to whether they represent malformations, hamartomas, or true tumors. About 40 cases have been reported (Gunes et al 1990). They occur at any age, but most are found in children or young adults (Ebrahimi et al 1971, Janovski & Paramanandhan 1973). They are usually incidental findings at surgery or autopsy, but some patients present with abdominal masses or pain due to torsion. Ascites (Fox & Langley 1976), thrombocytopenia (Lawhead et al 1985) or hemoperitoneum (di Orio & Lowe 1980) occur rarely. In some cases there is an association with generalized or abdominopelvic hemangiomatosis, or with hemangioma elsewhere in the genital tract (Talerman 1967, 1982).

Hemangiomas are usually unilateral, bilaterality being associated with some cases of generalized or abdominopelvic hemangiomatosis (Fox & Langley 1976, Lawhead et al 1985). Most lesions are small, less than 1.5 cm in diameter, and located in the hilus or medulla. They are clearly demarcated from the surrounding tissues, a feature which distinguishes them from the prominent coils of blood vessels normally present in this region (see Fig. 3.4). Hemangiomas up to 24 cm in diameter have been described, but such large tumors are rare (Ebrahimi et al 1971, Alvarez & Cerezo 1986). The capsule is smooth and the cut surface shows spongy red or purplish tissue. Most tumors are of the cavernous or mixed cavernous–capillary type. The vascular channels are lined by a single layer of endothelial cells and focal thrombosis may be present. The intervening scanty fibrous tissue may show some hyalinization or calcification.

The differential diagnosis includes normal medullary vasculature, lymphangiomas (see below), and cystic teratomas with prominent vascular components (Feuerstein et al 1984).

Hemangioendotheliomas (angiosarcomas)

These rare tumors have been reported only in adults and have presented as abdominal masses. Torsion and rupture are not uncommon complications. They pursue a malignant course with local infiltration, peritoneal seeding and vascular dissemination (Fox & Langley 1976, Talerman 1982). There is a recent report of an epithelioid angiosarcoma arising in a leiomyoma (Drachenberg et al 1994). The tumors are large soft friable spongy masses with areas of hemorrhage and necrosis. The vascular spaces are lined by endothelial cells showing nuclear pleiomorphism and mitotic activity which, although sometimes only focal, may be the only features that distinguish them from hemangiomas. The presence of solid cores of endothelial cells helps to confirm the diagnosis. The differential diagnosis also includes teratomas with prominent vascular components, lymphangiosarcomas, hemangiopericytomas, and metastatic angiosarcomas.

Lymphangiomas

These are rarer than hemangiomas (Janovski & Paramanandhan 1973, Fox & Langley 1976). The tumors are unilateral, up to 6 cm in diameter, with smooth gray capsules. The cut surfaces show cystic spaces containing clear yellowish fluid. The microscopic features are typical of extraovarian lymphangiomas and differ from hemangiomas by the absence of red cells in the anastomosing channels and the frequent presence of lymphocytes in their walls. The differential diagnoses also include adenomatoid tumors, cystic mesotheliomas (see Ch. 31), and cystic teratomas with sieve-like foci (see Ch. 46).

Lymphangiosarcomas

The only reported case of which we are aware occurred in a 31-year-old woman who died within a year from widespread metastases. The 15 cm tumor was distinguished from a lymphangioma by the presence of focal endothelial proliferation with some pleiomorphism and nuclear hyperchromatism (Rice et al 1943).

Hemangiopericytomas

Ovarian hemangiopericytomas have only been reported in the last decade. Nørgaard et al (1985) described a 48-year-old woman who developed bilateral 10 cm ovarian tumors with a small subperitoneal metastasis in the terminal ileum. Histological features were typical of hemangiopericytoma and mitotic activity was present (not quantitated). The patient was given postoperative chemotherapy, but died from surgical complications and inanition 2 years later with residual (but nonprogressive) disease. Shakfeh & Woodruff (1987) reported a 63-year-old woman with a 28 cm tumor, associated with adhesions and ascites, who was alive with disease 5 years postoperatively.

Tumors which may, wholly or in part, resemble hemangiopericytomas are endometrial stromal tumors, sclerosing stromal tumors, granulosa cell tumors, and leiomyomas, and these probably account for most of the tumors previously designated as hemangiopericytomas (Fox & Langley 1976). Hemangiopericytomas have a complex vascular network composed of gaping thin-walled channels which often show a staghorn pattern of branching. The tumor cells which surround the vessels are regular ovoid fibroblast-like cells, each surrounded by abundant reticulin fibres. Fibrosis and myxoid change may be present (Enzinger &

Smith 1976). Electron microscopy confirms the pericytic origin of hemangiopericytomas – abundant cytoplasmic fibrils, basal lamina, and micropinocytotic vesicles (Battifora 1973). In endometrial stromal tumors, abundant, regularly distributed, small blood vessels are present, but they do not form the branching pattern characteristic of hemangiopericytomas. Collagenization and myxoid change are rarely present. Ultrastructural features of pericytic differentiation are absent.

TUMORS OF STRIATED MUSCLE ORIGIN

No case of ovarian rhabdomyoma has been reported. By contrast, rhabdomyosarcomas are the most common of the pure heterologous ovarian sarcomas (Prat & Scully 1986, Shakfeh & Woodruff 1987). Although they possibly arise from undifferentiated ovarian mesenchyme, they may also represent one-sided development of mixed mullerian tumors (in which rhabdomyosarcoma is a relatively frequent component – see Ch. 26) or Sertoli–Leydig cell tumors (see Ch. 35). Diagnosis of pure primary rhabdomyosarcoma requires the examination of multiple blocks in order to exclude other diagnostic possibilities, as indicated at the beginning of this chapter. The age at presentation ranges from early childhood to old age, usually with an initial complaint of a rapidly enlarging abdominal mass. The tumors are unilateral and usually greater than 10 cm in diameter. The cut surfaces show soft gray-white tissue, with areas of hemorrhage, necrosis, and cystic degeneration. The histological subtypes are comparable with extraovarian rhabdomyosarcomas; embryonal and alveolar types are most common in young patients and the pleiomorphic type is most common in the elderly. Although metastases are often apparent at initial presentation and death usually occurs within a year (Fox & Langley 1976, Shakfeh & Woodruff 1987), there have been some good responses to surgery, chemotherapy, and radiotherapy (Talerman 1982), as well as a report of a disease-free period of 2 years following surgical removal alone (Sandison 1955).

CHONDROGENIC TUMORS

Only one case of an ovarian chondroma has been reported (Ramos-Martinez et al 1983). Ovarian tumors with conspicuous benign cartilaginous components are most likely to be fibromas with cartilaginous metaplasia, or teratomas with prominent cartilage formation (Fox & Langley 1976).

Talerman et al (1981) have reported a pure primary ovarian chondrosarcoma. The large tumor occurred in a 61-year-old woman who was free of tumor 4.5 years after total hysterectomy and bilateral salpingo-oophorectomy. Extensive sampling of the tumor revealed no other histological elements, but the authors nonetheless suggested that the tumor probably resulted from malignant transformation of cartilage in a mature cystic teratoma (an example of which has been documented previously (Climie & Heath 1968). A subsequent case, briefly described by Shakfeh & Woodruff (1987), died of disease 8 years postoperatively.

BONE TUMORS

The rare reports of ovarian osteomas probably represent examples of osseous metaplasia in fibromas, leiomyomas or non-neoplastic lesions (Shipton & Meares 1965, Janovski & Paramanandhan 1973, Fox & Langley 1976, Talerman 1982).

Osteogenic sarcomas

Pure osteogenic sarcomas, i.e. with no evidence of associated teratoma or malignant mixed mullerian tumor, have been described rarely (Azoury & Woodruff 1971, Shakfeh & Woodruff 1987, Hirakawa et al 1988, Hines et al 1990). Patient age ranged from 24 to 75 years, and prognosis was poor, with many dying within months of diagnosis. The large tumors had histological features similar to those of skeletal osteogenic sarcomas. Some cases (Stowe & Watt 1952, Sakata et al 1991) have been described which are associated with a cyst lined by ciliated epithelium.

Giant cell tumors

A benign giant cell tumor, histologically similar to the familiar skeletal lesion, has been reported in the form of a 3 cm mural nodule in an ovarian

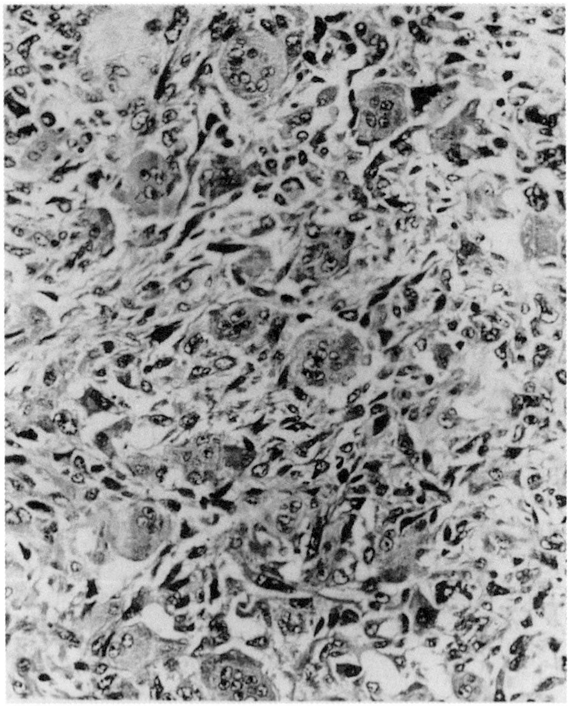

Fig. 52.1 Malignant giant cell tumor of ovary, composed of multinucleated giant cells and background of mononuclear cells which show more marked nuclear pleiomorphism. H + E ×200. (Courtesy of Dr D Buntine, Brisbane)

cyst (uncertain type) from a 31-year-old woman with infertility and endometriosis (Lorentzen 1980). Ovarian lesions of this type have more commonly been associated with mucinous tumors (see Ch. 24). We have seen, in consultation, an apparently pure giant cell tumor which presented as a 10 cm solid ovarian mass in a 78-year-old woman; no epithelial components could be demonstrated. Although confined to the ovary, it was cytologically malignant (Fig. 52.1).

MYXOMAS

Eichhorn & Scully (1991) have recently described five ovarian myxomas and reviewed the few similar tumors previously described in the literature (Dutz & Stout 1961, Masubuchi et al 1970, Majmudar et al 1978, Brady et al 1987). A further two cases have also been reported (Tetu & Bonefat 1991). The age of the patients ranged from 13 to 65 years. Presentation was usually with an asymptomatic unilateral adnexal mass.

Macroscopic features

Published examples measure 5–22 cm in diameter. The tumors are well-encapsulated, gray-white tumors which are partly solid and partly cystic, both areas containing viscid gelatinous material (the cysts are occasionally blood filled).

Microscopic features

Tumors show stellate and spindle cells in a myxoid stroma containing mucopolysaccharides stainable by alcian blue. Hyaluronic acid is present. Tumors are well vascularized and the vessels are capillary like. The overall picture is typically uniform, and fibrosis, if present, is limited and focal. Immunohistochemically, tumor cells stain for vimentin and smooth muscle actin, but not desmin, features shared with some tumors of the thecoma–fibroma group and raised as evidence by Costa et al (1993) for myxomas being part of this neoplastic spectrum.

Differential diagnosis

The tumors most frequently encountered that are likely to cause difficulties are edematous fibromas. However, these are composed predominantly of fibrous tissue, with only focal edematous or myxoid areas, similar to the patterns seen in uterine leiomyomas.

More important distinctions are from myxoid liposarcomas (distinguished by their characteristic plexiform vascular patterns and lipoblasts), pseudomyxoma ovarii (strips and clusters of mucin-secreting epithelial cells in pools of extracellular mucin), and sarcoma botryoides (pleiomorphic cells, including rhabdomyoblasts). They also should not be confused with massive edema. In the series of Eichhorn & Scully (1991), each was treated by conservative surgery, and none of the five tumors recurred after 5 years follow-up. One of two cases reported by Tetu & Bonefat (1991) recurred. In this latter study, DNA flow cytometry showed an aneuploid cell population; tumor cells were immunoreactive for vimentin and usually actin, but only focally for desmin, and stains for S100-protein, neuron-specific enolase, neurofilament, Leu-M7, EMA, cytokeratins, and factor VIII-related antigen were all negative.

LIPOGENIC TUMORS

There are no well-documented cases of pure ovarian lipomas. Lesions which simulate lipomas are: benign cystic teratomas with prominent adipose tissue; adherent adipose tissue or autoamputated infarcted appendices epiploicae; and adipocytic prosoplasia (Kanter & Zummo 1956, Janovski & Paramanandhan 1973, Fox & Langley 1976). In the latter condition, most often observed in perimenopausal obese women, small accumulations of fat cells are found in the ovarian cortex (see Fig. 3.23). No pure primary ovarian liposarcoma has been reported, but liposarcoma may be identified in the ovary as a component of a malignant mixed mullerian tumor or as a metastasis (Talerman 1982).

NEURAL AND RELATED TUMORS

These are very rare and their histogenesis is similar to that proposed for other mesenchymal ovarian tumors. Some are associated with von Recklinghausen's disease. Neuroectodermal tumors (ependymomas, neuroblastomas, glioblastomas), even if apparently pure, are considered to be of teratomatous origin, and are discussed with immature and monodermal teratomas (see Chs 47, 49).

Neurofibromas, neurofibrosarcomas

Each of these has been described in association with von Recklinghausen's disease (Smith 1931, Dover 1950, Hegg & Flint 1990). These neoplasms may cause ovarian enlargement, simulating a malignant tumor in such patients.

Neurilemmomas (schwannomas)

Three cases have been reported, all with symptoms of a pelvic mass and an uneventful postoperative course. The tumors were solid and histologically similar to nonovarian neurilemmomas (Talerman 1982). Two malignant schwannomas have been reported in old women who died with metastatic disease 5–18 months after initial surgery (Shetty et al 1982, Stone et al 1986). One presented with episodic hypoglycemia; insulin was extracted from the 12 cm tumor (Shetty et al 1982).

Ganglioneuromas

Meyer (1943) described small ganglioneuromas in the ovarian hilus, but such diminutive lesions would have to be distinguished from the non-neoplastic proliferations of ganglion cells sometimes seen in this region (Talerman 1982). Schmeisser & Anderson (1938) reported a 200 g ganglioneuroma in a 4-year-old child, and Stout (1947) included six ovarian examples in his series of 243 ganglioneuromas.

Phaeochromocytomas

One ovarian phaeochromocytoma has been reported (Fawcett & Kimbell 1971). A 15-year-

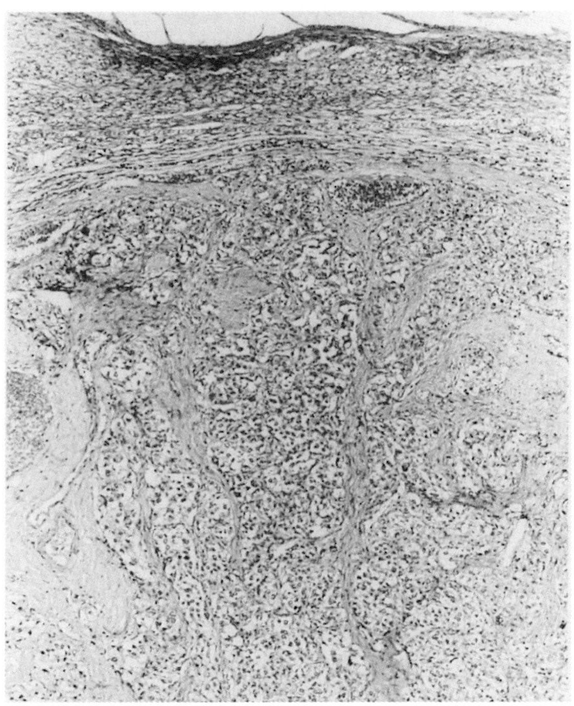

Fig. 52.2 Ovarian paraganglioma; the tumor has an alveolar pattern broken up by vascular fibrous septa. H + E ×64

old girl presented with hypertension, fits and a left-sided abdominal mass. The 970 g tumor showed the typical histological features of phaeochromocytoma, and catecholamines were extracted from it. The symptoms disappeared rapidly postoperatively and the patient was well 15 months later. We have encountered a 1.5 cm ovarian paraganglioma as an incidental finding at hysterectomy in a 59-year-old woman (Fig. 52.2).

SARCOMAS NOT OTHERWISE DIFFERENTIATED

Rarely, one may encounter malignant mesenchymal tumors with no apparent specific differentiation or evidence of underlying lesions known to be associated with, or complicated by, sarcomas. Multiple blocks should be examined closely for evidence of mullerian epithelial components or teratomatous elements. It is also worth performing immunohistochemical stains for epithelial markers to exclude undifferentiated carcinoma. The possibility of a metastasis should also be considered; the clinical history and operative findings should be reviewed. If the patient is a young woman with hypercalcemia, primary small cell 'carcinoma' enters the differential diagnosis (see Ch. 31).

REFERENCES

Alvarez M, Cerezo L 1986 Ovarian cavernous hemangioma. Archives of Pathology and Laboratory Medicine 110: 77–78

Azoury R S, Woodruff J D 1971 Primary ovarian sarcomas. Report of 43 cases from the Emil Novak Tumor Registry. Obstetrics and Gynecology 37: 920–941

Battifora H 1973 Hemangiopericytoma: ultrastructural study of five cases. Cancer 31: 1418–1432

Brady K, Page D V, Benn L E, de las Morenas A, O'Brien M 1987 Ovarian myxoma. American Journal of Obstetrics and Gynecology 156: 1240–1242

Climie A R W, Heath L P 1968 Malignant degeneration of benign cystic teratomas of the ovary; review of the literature and report of a chondrosarcoma and carcinoid tumor. Cancer 22: 824–832

Costa M J, Morris R, de Rose P B, Cohen C 1993 Histologic and immunohistochemical evidence for considering myxoma as a variant of the thecoma–fibroma group of ovarian stromal tumors. Archives of Pathology and Laboratory Medicine 117: 802–808

di Orio J, Lowe L C 1980 Hemangioma of the ovary in pregnancy. A case report. Journal of Reproductive Medicine 24: 232–234

Dover H 1950 Neurofibrosarcoma of the ovary, associated with neurofibromatosis. Canadian Medical Association Journal 63: 488–490

Drachenberg C B, Faust F J, Borkowski A, Papadimitriou J C 1994 Epithelioid angiosarcoma of the uterus arising in a leiomyoma with associated ovarian and tubal angiomatosis. American Journal of Clinical Pathology 102: 388–389

Dutz W, Stout A P 1961 The myxoma in childhood. Cancer 14: 629–635

Ebrahimi T, Goldsmith J W, Okagaki T 1971 Hemangioma of the ovary. A case report. Obstetrics and Gynecology 38: 677–679

Eichhorn J H, Scully R E 1991 Ovarian myxoma: clinicopathologic and immunocytologic analysis of five cases and a review of the literature. International Journal of Gynecological Pathology 10: 156–169

Enzinger F, Smith B H 1976 Hemangiopericytoma: an analysis of 106 cases. Human Pathology 7: 61–82

Fawcett F J, Kimbell N K B 1971 Phaeochromocytoma of the ovary. British Journal of Obstetrics and Gynaecology 78: 458–459

Feuerstein I M, Aronson B L, McCarthy E F 1984 Bilateral ovarian cystic teratomata mimicking bilateral pure ovarian hemangiomata: case report. International Journal of Gynecological Pathology 3: 393–397

Fox H, Langley F A 1976 Tumors of the ovary. Heinemann, London, p 278–292

Gunes H A, Egilimez R, Dulger M 1990 Ovarian haemangioma. British Journal of Clinical Practice 44: 734–735

Hegg C A, Flint A 1990 Neurofibroma of the ovary. Gynecologic Oncology 37: 437–438

Henes J F, Compton D M, Stacy C C, Potter M E 1990 Pure primary osteosarcoma of the ovary presenting as an extensively calcified adnexal mass: a case report and review of the literature. Gynecologic Oncology 39: 259–263

Hirakawa T, Tsuneyoshi M, Enjojil M, Shigyo R 1988 Ovarian sarcoma with histologic features of telangiectatic osteosarcoma of the bone. American Journal of Surgical Pathology 12: 567–572

Janovski N A, Paramanandhan T L 1973 Ovarian tumors. Tumors and tumor-like conditions of the ovaries, fallopian tubes and ligaments of the uterus. Saunders, Philadelphia, p 46–60

Kanter A E, Zummo B P 1956 Lipomas of gynecologic interest. American Journal of Obstetrics and Gynecology 71: 376–385

Lawhead R A, Copeland L J, Edwards C L 1985 Bilateral ovarian hemangiomas associated with diffuse abdomino-pelvic hemangiomatosis. Obstetrics and Gynecology 65: 597–599

Lorentzen M 1980 Giant cell tumor of the ovary. Virchows Archiv A 388: 113–122

Majmudar B, Kapernick P S, Phillips R S 1978 Ovarian myxoma. Human Pathology 9: 723–725

Masubuchi K, Kimura M, Suzuki H, Suzuki P, Aoki M 1970 Case of ovarian myxoma. Japanese Journal of Cancer Clinics 16: 156–159

Meyer R 1943 Nerve tumors of the female genitals and pelvis. Archives of Pathology 36: 437–464

Nørgaard M, Hansborg N, Fischer-Rasmussen W 1985

Malignant hemangiopericytoma of the ovary. Acta Obstetricia et Gynecologica Scandinavica 64: 87–89
Prat J, Scully R E 1986 Ovarian sarcomas and related tumors. A clinicopathologic analysis of 98 cases [abstract]. Laboratory Investigation 54: 50A
Ramos-Martinez E, Rodriguez Moguel L, Quijano Narezo M, Santiago Payan H 1983 Condroma primario del ovario. Informe de un caso. Ginecologia y Obstetricia de México 51: 95–98
Rice M, Pearson B, Treadwell W B 1943 Malignant lymphangioma of the ovary. American Journal of Obstetrics and Gynecology 45: 884–889
Sakata H, Hirahara T, Ryu A, Sawada T, Yamamoto M, Sakuram I 1991 Primary osteosarcoma of the ovary. A case report. Acta Pathologica Japonica 41: 311–317
Sandison A T 1955 Rhabdomyosarcoma of the ovary. Journal of Pathology and Bacteriology 70: 433–438
Schmeisser H C, Anderson W A D 1938 Ganglioneuroma of the ovary. Journal of the American Medical Association 111: 2005–2007
Shakfeh S M, Woodruff J D 1987 Primary ovarian sarcomas: report of 46 cases and review of the literature. Obstetrical and Gynecological Survey 42: 331–349
Shetty M R, Boghossian H M, Duffell D, Freel R, Gonzales J C 1982 Tumor-induced hypoglycemia. A result of ectopic insulin production. Cancer 49: 1920–1923
Shipton E A, Meares S D 1965 Heterotopic bone formation in the ovary. Australian and New Zealand Journal of Obstetrics and Gynaecology 5: 100–102
Smith F R 1931 Neurofibroma of the ovary associated with Recklinghausen's disease. American Journal of Cancer 15: 859–862
Stone G C, Bell D A, Fuller A, Dickersin G R, Scully R E 1986 Malignant schwannoma of the ovary. Report of a case. Cancer 58: 1575–1582
Stout A P 1947 Ganglioneuroma of the sympathetic nervous system. Surgery, Gynecology and Obstetrics 84: 101–110
Stowe L M, Watt J Y 1952 Osteogenic sarcoma of the ovary. American Journal of Obstetrics and Gynecology 64: 422–426
Talerman A 1967 Hemangiomas of the ovary and the uterine cervix. Obstetrics and Gynecology 30: 108–113
Talerman A 1982 Mesenchymal tumors and malignant lymphoma of the ovary. In: Blaustein A (ed) Pathology of the female genital tract, 2nd edn. Springer-Verlag, New York, p 561–580
Talerman A, Auerbach W M, van Meurs A J 1981 Primary chondrosarcoma of the ovary. Histopathology 5: 319–324
Tetu B, Bonefat J L 1991 Ovarian myxoma. A study of two cases with long-term follow up. American Journal of Clinical Pathology 95: 340–346

53

Tumors metastatic to the ovaries – introduction, metastases from the female genital tract and breasts

P. Russell A. Farnsworth

The ovaries provide fertile soil for metastases and are the most commonly involved organs in the female genital tract, regardless of the location of the primary tumor (Mazur et al 1984). The frequency with which the ovaries are involved in metastatic malignancy is difficult to assess from the literature because of the differing methods of pathological examination and analysis as well as the variable inclusion of lymphomas, subclinical metastases in patients undergoing prophylactic or therapeutic oophorectomy for breast carcinoma, and ovarian tumors which are associated with uterine carcinomas but are not necessarily metastatic. There is also a wide geographical variation in the incidence of the common gastric, mammary, and colonic carcinomas as well as a changing incidence in many population groups over recent decades, gastric carcinoma becoming less common and the others more common. Overall, in cancer-associated deaths, ovarian metastases are likely to be macroscopically evident in approximately 6% and histologically identifiable in an additional 6% (Fox & Langley 1976). For individual tumors this figure rises to a peak of 50% for gastric carcinoma (Virieux 1962). Since primary ovarian carcinomas account for only 6% of cancer deaths, malignant ovarian tumors identified at autopsy are more likely to be secondary than primary lesions. By contrast, the probability that a malignant ovarian tumor encountered at laparotomy is metastatic is approximately 6–7% (Fox & Langley 1976, Blaustein 1982, Ulbright et al 1984, Demopoulos et al 1987).

MECHANISMS OF SPREAD

There are several routes of tumor spread to the ovaries, one or more of which can often be inferred from careful histological examination in a given case. The lymphatic route is probably the most important and accounts for many metastases from the genitourinary tract as well as from the colon, stomach, and breast. With these latter tumors, blockage of lymphatics and retrograde spread may be responsible for the appearance of a symptomatic ovarian mass before the primary tumor declares itself. Lymphatic permeation is most readily recognized in the ovarian hilus (Fig. 53.1) and may also

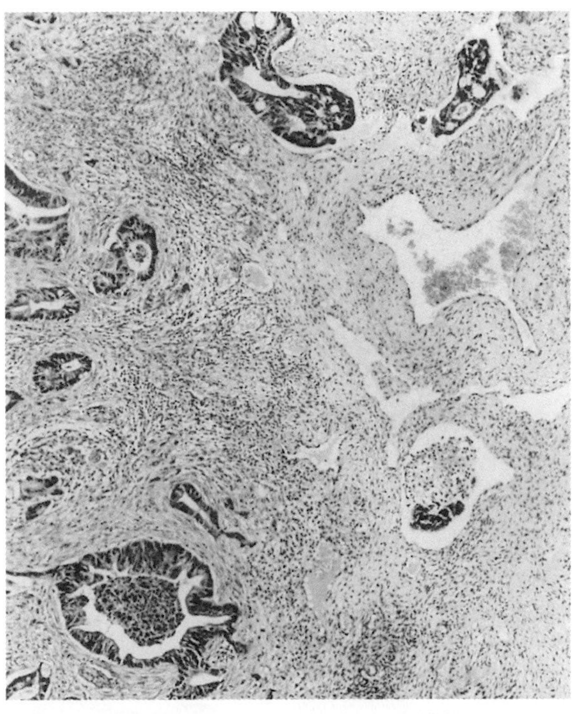

Fig. 53.1 Metastatic colonic adenocarcinoma in lymphatics of ovarian hilus/medulla. H + E ×50

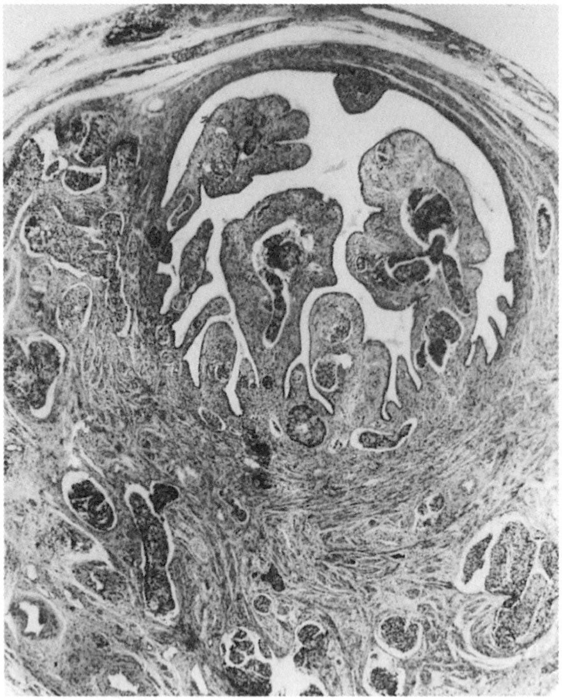

Fig. 53.2 Extensive infiltration of mucosal and mural lymphatics of fallopian tube by metastatic colonic adenocarcinoma. H + E ×20

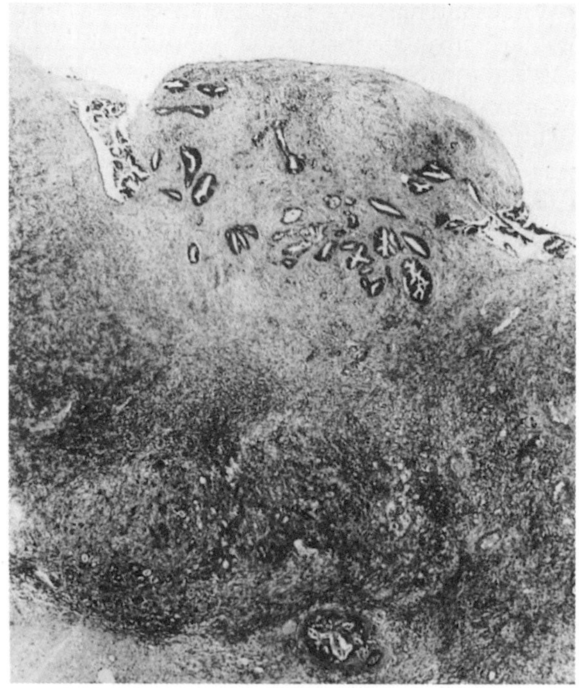

Fig. 53.3 Metastatic colonic adenocarcinoma. Capsular nodule of carcinoma with adjacent loosely adherent clusters of tumor cells. Carcinoma also infiltrates cortical stroma below. H + E ×20

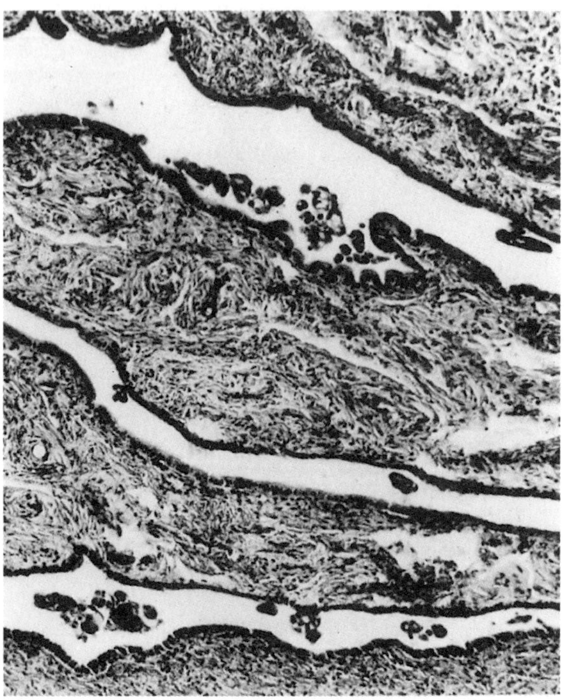

be conspicuous in the submucosal lymphatics of the fallopian tube (Fig. 53.2).

Evidence of hematogenous dissemination is most often seen in patients with advanced disease, and other blood-borne metastases are usually apparent. The well-vascularized ovaries of premenopausal women are said to be particularly receptive to seeding in this way (MacKeigan & Ferguson 1979, Scully 1979, Parker & Currie 1981).

Transcoelomic spread is associated principally with primary tumors of the abdominal viscera. Viable malignant cells are exfoliated into the peritoneal cavity and may establish themselves on the surface of the ovaries, as well as other pelvic and abdominal organs (Fig. 53.3). It has been suggested that ovulation stigmas may allow ingress of these free-floating malignant cells into the ovarian parenchyma (Scully 1979, Parker & Currie 1981).

Fig. 53.4 Clusters of carcinoma cells in the lumen of the fallopian tube. H + E ×50

A transluminal route may be utilized by endometrial and tubal carcinomas. Clusters of carcinoma cells can regularly be identified in the tubal lumen in these cases (Fig. 53.4) and it is feasible that cells shed from the ostia could implant on the ovary. This route is said to be especially common with adenosquamous carcinomas of endometrium (Scully 1979).

Direct infiltration by tumors arising in pelvic organs is also an important mechanism, especially in advanced disease. Uterine, tubal, colonic, bladder, mesothelial, and retroperitoneal tumors may involve the ovaries in this way.

As well as metastasizing to the ovarian parenchyma, spread to pre-existing primary ovarian neoplasms has also been reported; for example, breast tumors to Brenner tumors (Hines et al 1976, Smale 1980), and melanoma (see Ch. 54) and colonic adenocarcinoma to mature cystic teratomas (Fig. 53.5).

CLINICAL FEATURES

Ovarian metastases are usually a manifestation of advanced disease, developing within a few years of the diagnosis of the primary neoplasm. Sometimes they simulate primary ovarian carcinomas clinically, and the source of the metastases may remain obscure for some months or even years after oophorectomy (Johansson 1960). Diagnosis may be incidental at the time of laparotomy for gastrointestinal carcinoma, or follow histological examination of ovaries removed for control of breast cancer.

Patients with metastases to the ovaries tend to be younger than those with primary ovarian neoplasms. This is partly a reflection of the propensity

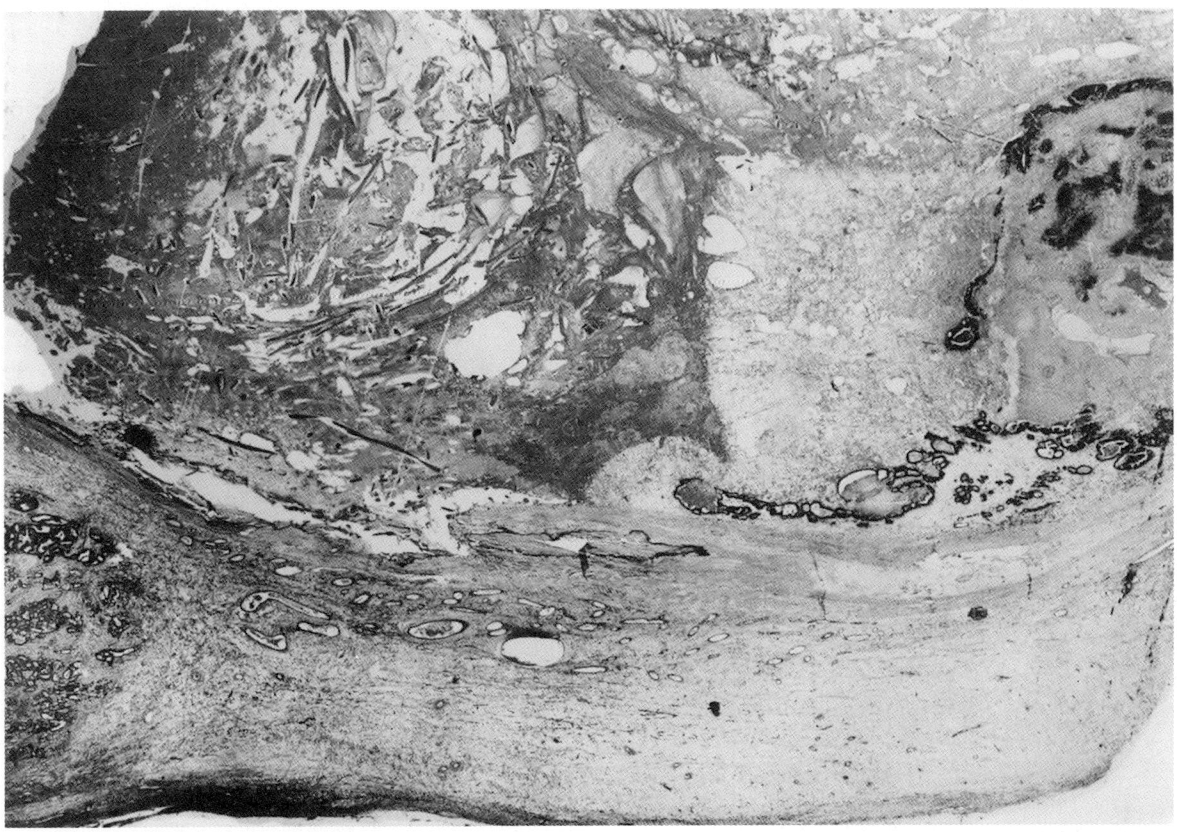

Fig. 53.5 Colonic adenocarcinoma (Dukes stage C) metastatic to a mature cystic teratoma. The 15 cm cyst was filled with necrotic tumor tissue (right), sebaceous material and hair fragments (left). The thick fibrous wall was also infiltrated by carcinoma (below left). H + E ×7

of tumors to seed to the well-vascularized premenopausal ovaries and partly a reflection of the fact that tumors which commonly metastasize to the ovaries, especially gastric and mammary carcinomas, tend to occur in a younger age group. For example, most women with Krukenberg tumors are premenopausal. The prognosis for the majority of patients with ovarian metastases is very poor, with an overall 5-year survival rate of 12% (Webb et al 1975).

A small percentage of women with metastatic ovarian neoplasms may suffer from menstrual abnormalities, postmenopausal bleeding, virilization, or the delivery of a masculinized female fetus (Fox & Langley 1976, Bell 1977, Scully 1979, Vicens et al 1980, Rome et al 1981). These manifestations are considered to be the result of the endocrine activity of luteinized stromal cells (Figs 53.6, 54.11) which have been identified in approximately one-third of metastatic neoplasms, especially those of colorectal origin (Scully & Richardson 1961, Scully 1979, Ulbright et al 1984; see Ch. 54). Estrogen and progesterone production has been demonstrated in tumors from postmenopausal patients (Rome et al 1981, Jolles et al 1985). Correlation between the amount of stromal luteinization, histological type of tumor, and endocrine manifestation (estrogenic versus androgenic) is not established. MacDonald et al (1976) have postulated that the tumor stroma produces the prehormone androstenedione which is converted to either testosterone or estrone peripherally. The final balance depends on the rate of production of the prehormone and the patient's capacity for peripheral aromatization. This hypothesis is supported by Brennecke et al (1986). There is some evidence that the stromal luteinization is human chorionic gonadotrophin (hCG) and leutenizing hormone (LH) responsive, thus explaining its relative frequency in pregnancy and in the postmenopausal period when these hormone levels are elevated (Scully 1979). The

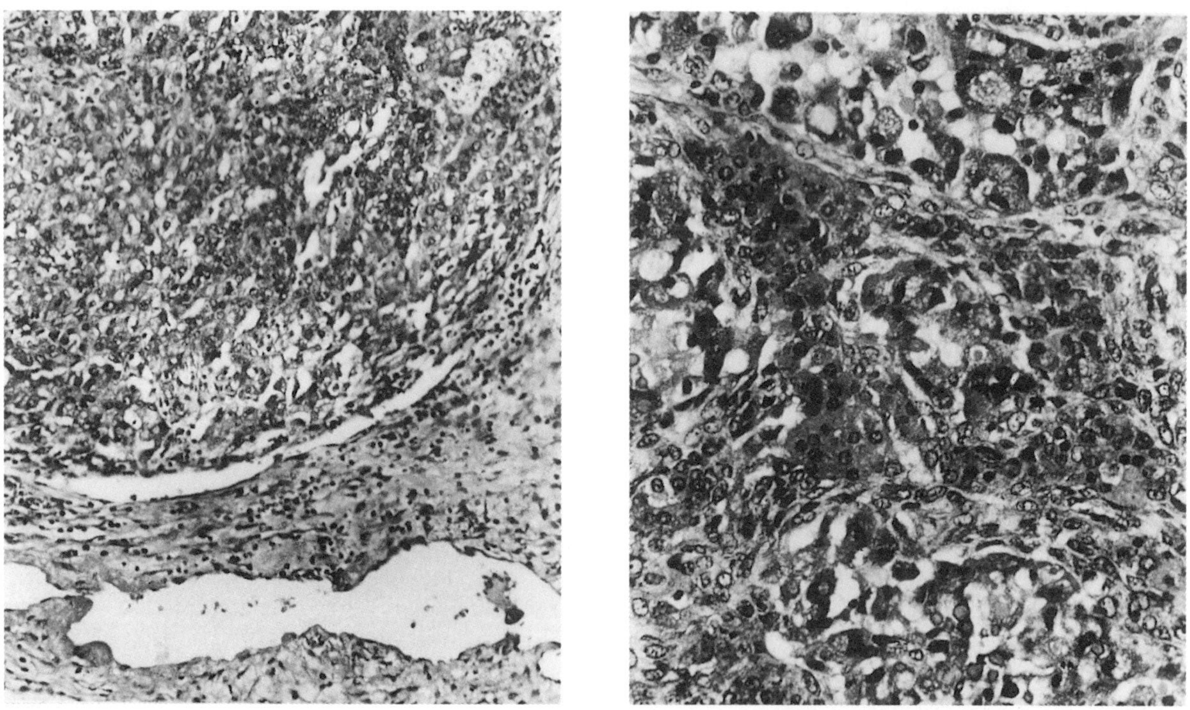

A B

Fig. 53.6 Metastatic hepatocellular carcinoma. Large ovarian mass from a woman with a history of a primary hepatic tumor resected a few months previously. (A) Solid tumor mass abutting medulla. Note cluster of tumor cells in lymphatic below. H + E ×100. (B) Trabeculae of tumor cells, some vacuolated and some containing hyaline globules (most conspicuous below) which are a-fetoprotein positive. There is marked stromal luteinization, manifest as compact groups of smaller cells with dense cytoplasm. H + E ×250

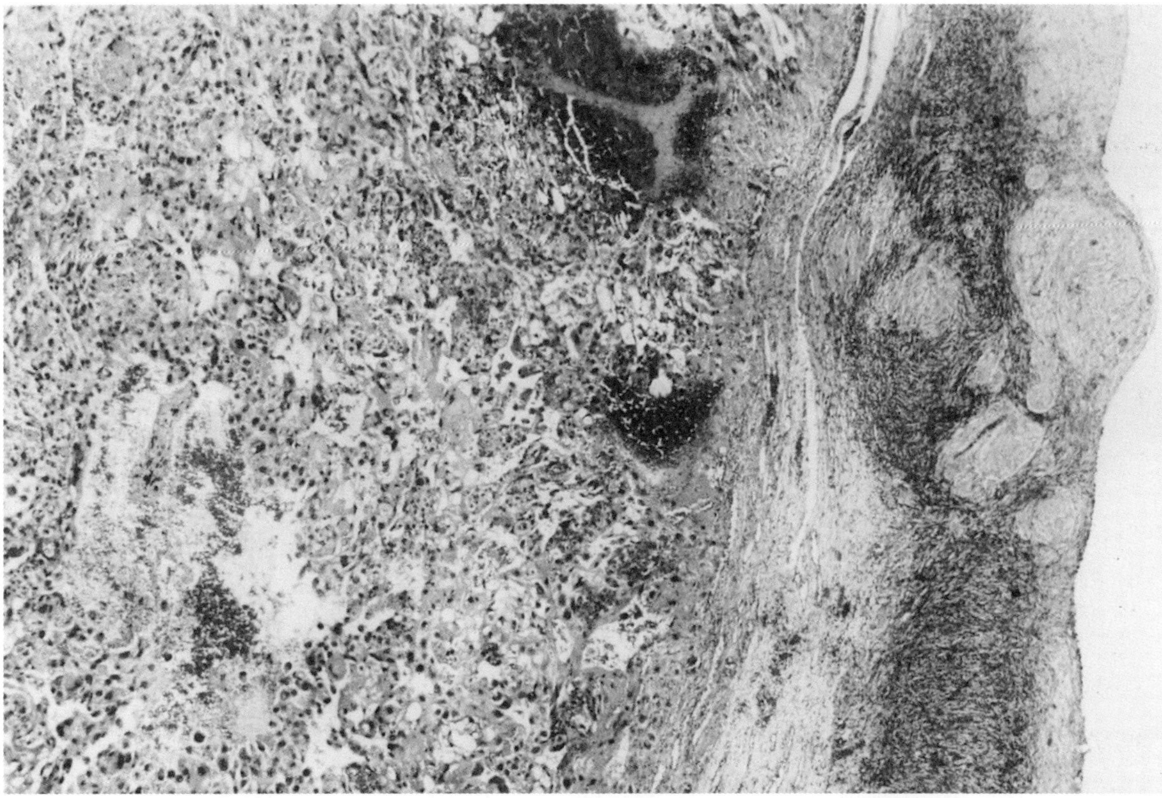

Fig. 53.7 Metastatic choriocarcinoma. The hemorrhagic tumor displays both syncytio- and cytotrophoblastic proliferation. The adjacent cortical stroma shows conspicuous deciduosis, secondary to the high circulating levels of hCG. From a 53-year-old woman with irregular vaginal bleeding; no history of gestational trophoblastic disease or germ cell tumor. H + E ×40

metastatic tumor cells may, in some cases, produce hCG (Fig. 53.7) and possibly also a mitogenic agent which stimulates stromal proliferation and facilitates the response to hCG or LH (MacDonald et al 1976, Rome et al 1981, Quinn et al 1983). It has also been suggested that the expanding tumor mass physically stimulates the surrounding stroma in a manner similar to that which occurs during physiological follicular growth (Scott et al 1967, Woodruff et al 1968) and massive ovarian edema and fibromatosis (see Ch. 16).

DIAGNOSIS

The recognition of an ovarian tumor as metastatic is of vital clinical importance, determining appropriate management and likely outcome of the patient. Such recognition will depend on: (a) an awareness of the frequency of metastases to the ovary which may stimulate primary tumor; (b) a detailed clinical history; (c) a clinical search by the gynecologist for a primary tumor outside the ovary and for other sites of spread; and (d) a careful evaluation of the tumor by the pathologist.

Obviously, if it is known that a primary malignant tumor outside the ovary exists, in the presence of an ovarian mass or masses, appropriate assessment can take place. Unusual patterns of spread for a primary ovarian tumor and even the presence of any extraovarian tumor (e.g. lung, liver, peritoneum) should alert the pathologist that ovarian metastasis rather than primary neoplasm must be considered and confirmed or excluded. It may be necessary to instigate a search for an extraovarian primary neoplasm if the pathological features of the ovarian mass indicate this likelihood. The following general features may be helpful in making such a decision.

PATHOLOGICAL FEATURES

Macroscopic features

Appearances of ovaries containing metastases will vary greatly and may resemble a primary ovarian tumor. Macroscopic features that are the most helpful are bilaterality and the presence of multiple large nodules either within the substance of the ovary or on the surface (Figs 53.8, 53.9). The tumors may be solid or cystic. It is important to note that the presence of a cyst, while favoring primary neoplasia, does not exclude a metastasis.

Metastases are bilateral in 65–75% of all cases. Primary ovarian serous and undifferentiated carcinomas are also commonly bilateral, but tumors showing mucinous or endometrioid features are bilateral in less than 15% of cases. When bilateral

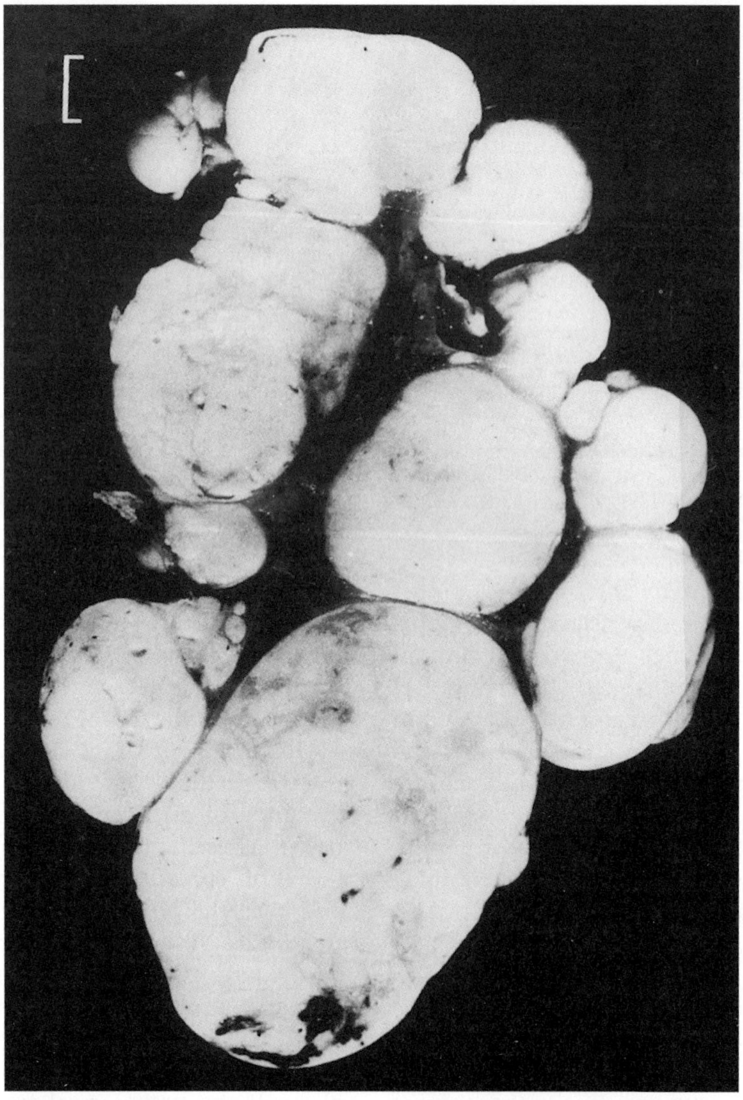

Fig. 53.8 Metastatic adenocarcinoma, probably colonic in origin. Such a multinodular mass would be quite uncharacteristic of a primary ovarian carcinoma. Scale bar equals 1 cm.

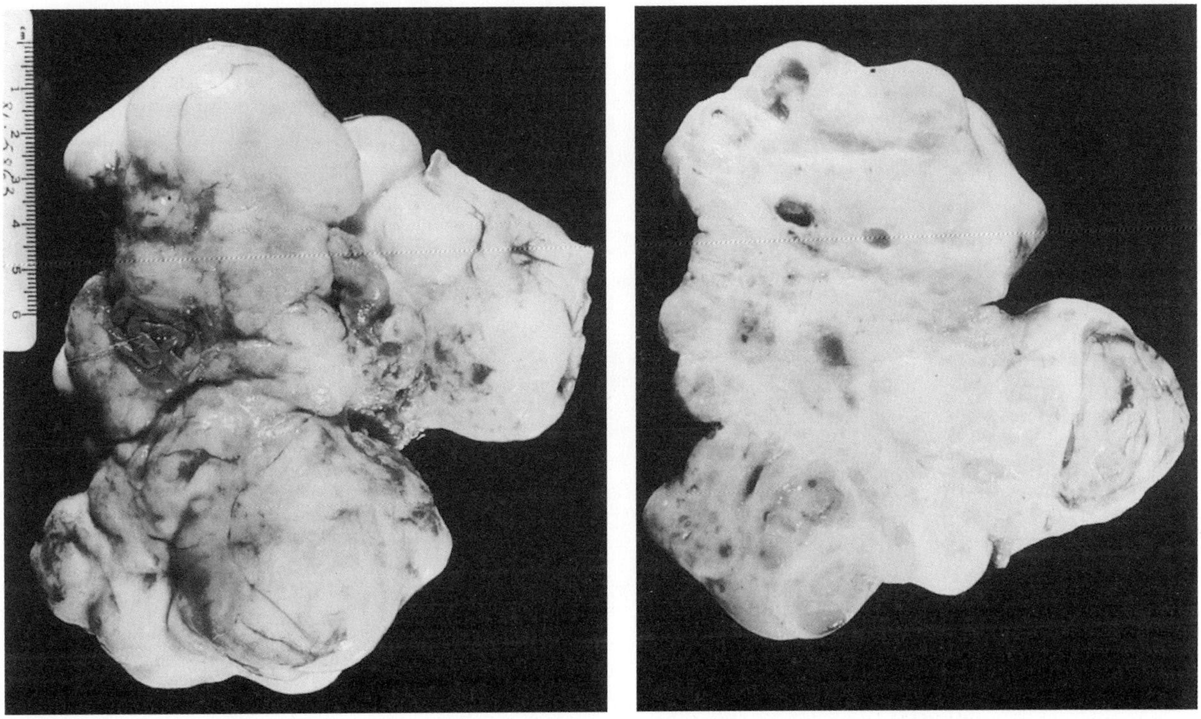

Fig. 53.9 Breast carcinoma metastatic to the ovary. External surface (left) is smooth and bosselated. Cut surface (right) shows uniform firm tumor tissue with a few small foci of cystic degeneration. Scale is in centimeters.

tumors are shown to be mucinous or endometrioid they are likely to be metastatic.

Microscopic features

Metastatic tumors will have a variety of appearances, largely depending on their site of origin. Features that are more commonly observed in metastatic lesions include lymphatic or blood vessel invasion (indeed, lymphatic permeation is only extremely infrequently seen at the periphery of primary ovarian carcinomas), growth in multiple nodules, and the presence of implants on the surface (which may have been visible macroscopically). The tumors may form both small and large cysts.

Other features to consider are small tumors confined to the medulla, relative sparing or infiltration (rather than obliteration) of follicular structures (Figs 53.10, 53.12, 53.13) and lack of transition from benign through proliferating to malignant. If stromal luteinization is prominent around the tumor nodules, metastases should be strongly considered (Figs 53.6, 54.11).

SOURCE OF PRIMARY TUMOR

Despite interseries variation based on geographical, temporal, and case selection (factors alluded to above), there is general agreement that the bulk of ovarian metastases are from the *breast, gastrointestinal tract,* and *female genital tract,* these three together constituting up to 90% of all cases (Johansson 1960, Woodruff et al 1970, Fox & Langley 1976, Scully 1979, Parker & Currie 1981, Mazur et al 1984, Ulbright et al 1984, Demopoulos et al 1987). Gastrointestinal metastasis are discussed in Chapter 54, and the rarer primary sites are discussed in Chapter 55.

METASTASES FROM THE FEMALE GENITAL TRACT

Carcinoma of the cervix

Ovarian metastases from carcinoma of the cervix are considered rare. Examples occur, however, of coexistent cervical and ovarian cancers, frequently of similar histological type, and analogous to the

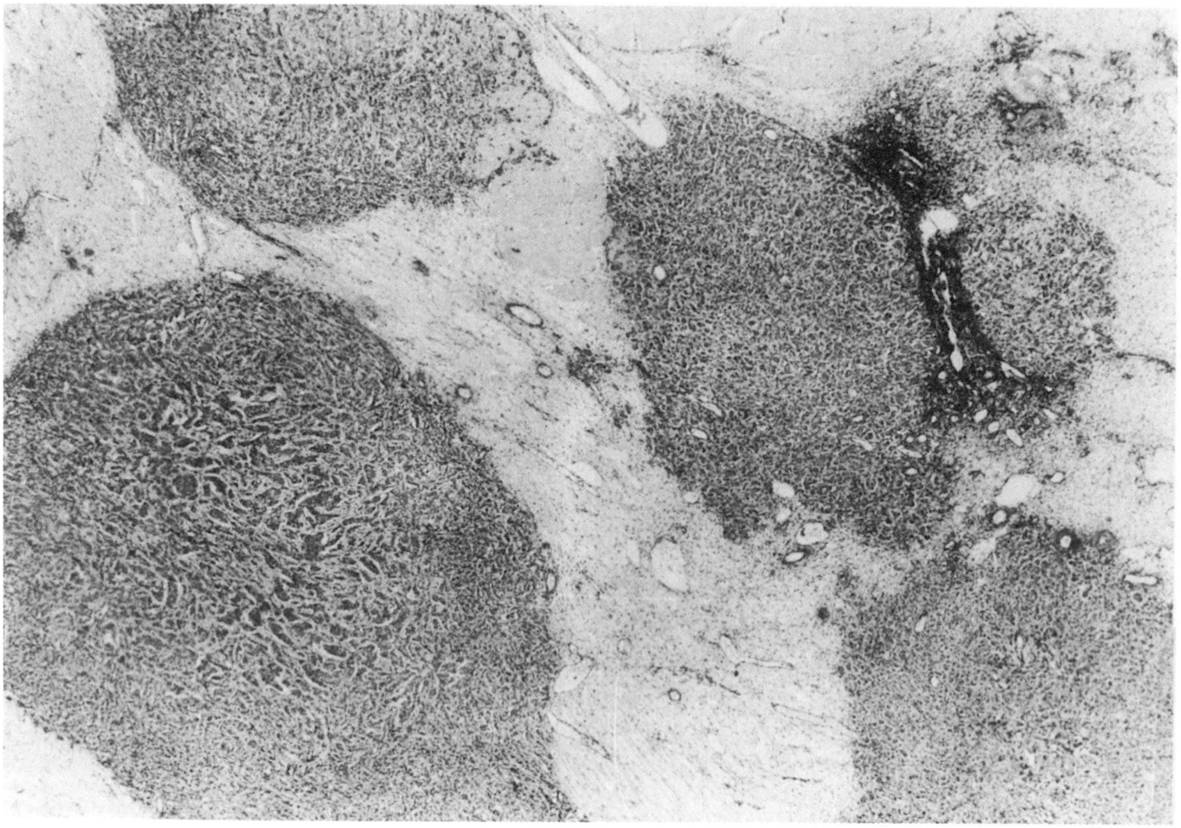

Fig. 53.10 Metastatic breast carcinoma. Multiple discrete nodules are present in the ovarian stroma and there is invasion of a corpus albicans (top). H + E ×40

more commonly encountered synchronous or metachronous carcinomas in ovaries. In a study of such patients reported by Young et al (1993), the ovarian tumors were diagnosed as metastatic on the basis of their bilaterality, pathological features unusual for primary ovarian carcinomas (i.e. squamous, small cell, adenocarcinoma, adenosquamous, transitional cell carcinomas) and the presence of extensive extracervical disease. The importance of this distinction relates to treatment protocols for removal of the ovaries in premenopausal women undergoing radical hysterectomy for cervical carcinoma; the overall incidence of ovarian metastases from cervical squamous carcinoma is relevant in deciding this issue.

A number of studies have addressed at this issue, particularly the incidence of ovarian involvement in cervical adenocarcinoma versus squamous carcinoma (Mann et al 1987). A large series reported by Tabata et al (1987) showed no ovarian metastases in 278 patients with stages Ib–III squamous cell carcinoma, but six metastases in 48 patients with equivalent stages of cervical adenocarcinoma. In the same study, but looking at cases diagnosed at autopsy (Tabata et al 1987), 17.4% of cases of squamous cell carcinoma and 28.6% of cases of adenocarcinoma had ovarian metastases. A Gynaecological Oncology Group (GOG) study (Sutton et al 1992) and a smaller series by Brown et al (1990) both showed the incidence in stage I cervical cancers to be small. Brown et al looked exclusively at adenocarcinomas and, including a review of the literature, estimated a rate of 1.8%. The GOG study showed a rate of ovarian spread of 0.5% for squamous carcinomas and 1.7% for adenocarcinomas. In both studies ovarian metastases were only present when there was

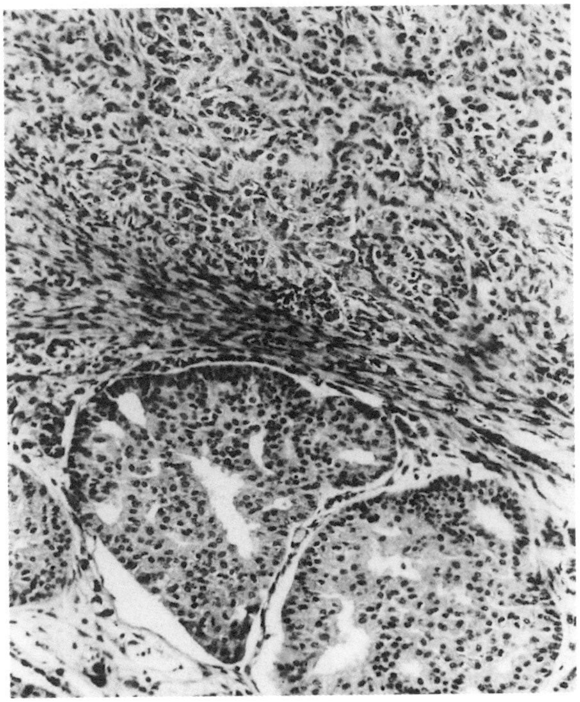

Fig. 53.11 Patterns of breast carcinoma metastatic to the ovary – trabecular (above) and cribriform (below). H + E ×100

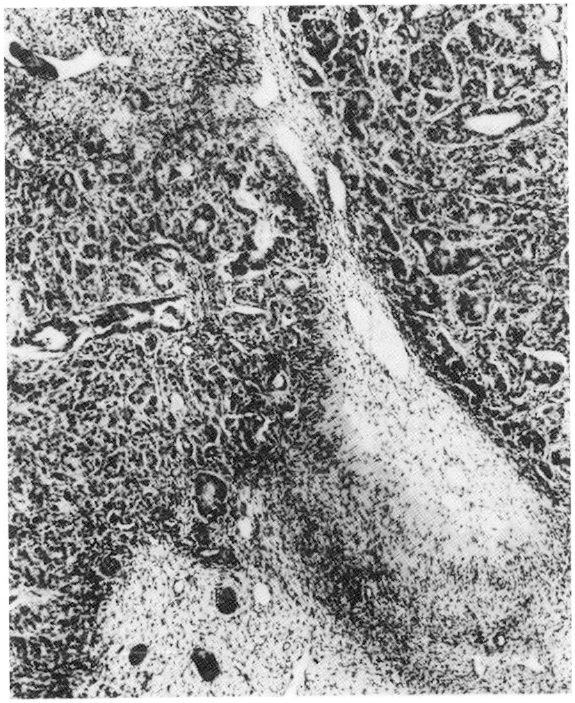

Fig. 53.12 Metastatic breast carcinoma invading the wall of an atretic follicle. Lymphatic permeation is seen at top left and bottom center. H + E ×50

evidence of extracervical disease elsewhere or the patient was postmenopausal.

Carcinoma of fallopian tubes

Metastases from fallopian tube carcinomas are rarely reported (Woodruff et al 1970, Webb et al 1975). This is partly a reflection of the rarity of these tumors and partly a result of the difficulty in establishing the anatomical and pathogenetic relationships between coexisting tubal and ovarian lesions.

Given that most tubal carcinomas show similar microscopic features to serous or undifferentiated tumors of the ovary, where both organs are involved it is often not possible to say where the tumor originated. In cases of mucinous, endometrioid, or clear cell carcinoma, as these are so rare in the tube, they are usually ascribed an ovarian primary. Surface growth of tumor with the tube may occur as spread from an ovarian primary and does not indicate origin in the tube (Blaustein 1982).

Carcinoma of endometrium

When carcinomas are found in one or both ovaries and the endometrial cavity, they are usually of similar histological type, raising the question as to whether they are synchronous primary or metastatic lesions. The principles used in distinguishing primary independent ovarian carcinomas from metastatic endometrial carcinoma are discussed in Chapter 25.

Sarcoma of the uterus

In a large series of 21 sarcomas metastatic to the ovaries, 11 were from uterine primaries (three leiomyosarcomas and eight endometrial stromal sarcomas) (Young & Scully 1990). Leiomyosarcomas usually involve the ovaries when there is evidence of widespread disease. The ovaries may be enlarged, but microscopic metastases can occur. Secondary stromal sarcoma also needs to be distinguished from a primary ovarian endometrioid

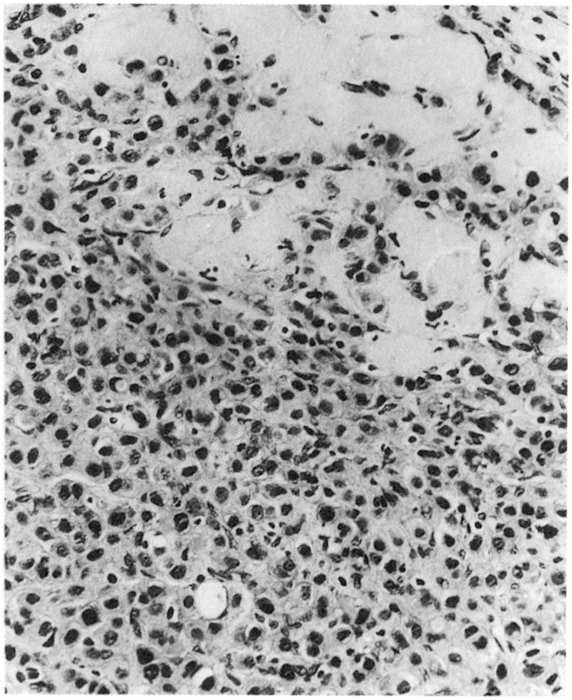

Fig. 53.13 Metastatic breast carcinoma infiltrating a corpus albicans. Tumor cells have a moderate amount of cytoplasm. Nuclei are pleiomorphic and hyperchromatic. H + E ×200

stromal sarcoma. The latter is usually associated with endometriosis. Stromal sarcoma may also mimic thecoma (Yu et al 1986) or other sex cord–stromal tumors, including granulosa cell tumors. The metastatic lesions are usually bilateral and extraovarian disease is regularly present.

Trophoblastic tumors

It may be impossible to distinguish primary choriocarcinoma of the ovary of either gestational or germ cell origin from metastasis from a uterine tumor which has regressed (Fig. 53.7). The age of the patient will only help in prepubertal girls, and thorough sampling of the ovarian tumor to identify other germ cell elements will be necessary.

Placental site trophoblast tumors metastatic to the ovaries have been described (Abdul Hafeez et al 1987), as has an invasive hydatidiform mole with ovarian involvement (Wei & Ouyang 1963).

METASTATIC BREAST CARCINOMAS

Breast carcinomas account for a considerable percentage of lesions metastatic to the ovaries. Ovarian secondaries have been identified at autopsy in up to 40% of women dying with widespread breast cancer (Abrams et al 1950, Saphir 1951, Luisi 1968). The incidence of ovarian involvement in patients undergoing therapeutic oophorectomy for advanced disease is 20–30% and for prophylactic oophorectomy 2–11% (Kasilag & Rutledge 1957, Turksoy 1960, Lee & Hori 1971, Scully 1979). Ovarian metastases are usually clinically silent (Scully 1979, Mazur et al 1984), only rarely producing endocrine symptoms; they do occasionally present as primary ovarian neoplasms, sometimes prior to the discovery of the breast tumor (Johansson 1960, Young et al 1981).

Macroscopic features

Bilateral involvement occurs in at least 75% of cases, but is frequently microscopic only (Saphir 1951, Lumb & MacKenzie 1959, Woodruff et al 1970, Scully 1979). The tumors are usually small; lesions larger than 5 cm are very uncommon (Gagnon & Tetu 1989). If enlarged, ovaries display large smooth bosselated masses or multiple small firm white nodules (Fig. 53.9). Rarely, the involved ovaries may contain cysts or be entirely cystic.

Microscopic features

Multiple small nodules or a confluent mass may be evident (Fig. 53.10). Any of the various histological patterns of primary breast carcinomas may be recapitulated in ovarian metastases, such as trabeculae, acini, sheets, and indian files; several different patterns may be evident in a single tumor (Fig. 53.11). Infiltration of follicular structures is frequently observed, and lymphatic permeation is usually readily apparent (Figs 53.10, 53.12, 53.13). In one large series, 75% showed either an indian file or ductal pattern (Gagnon & Tetu 1989). Small lesions may merge imperceptibly with the adjacent stroma and simulate foci of nodular stromal hyperplasia, especially if the interspersed stromal cells show luteinization (Fig. 53.14).

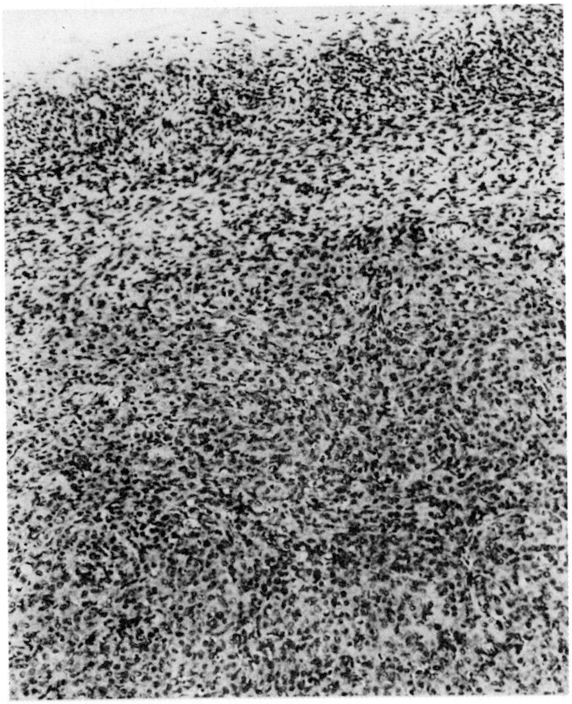

Fig. 53.14 Nodule of metastatic breast carcinoma which merges imperceptibly with adjacent stroma, simulating a focus of stromal hyperplasia. H + E ×80

However, the malignant cytological characteristics of the infiltrate are readily apparent on closer inspection. Krukenberg-type metastases from the breast have also been reported (see Ch. 54).

Differential diagnosis

Diffuse and indian file patterns are often found in lymphomas and leukemias, and these differential diagnoses are discussed in Chapter 56. In the study by Gagnon & Tetu (1989), the ovarian lesions most commonly mimicked by the metastatic breast carcinomas were sex cord–stromal tumors, dysgerminomas, granulosa cell tumors, and carcinoid tumors.

Carcinoid and sex cord–stromal tumors, especially Sertoli-cell tumors, may simulate the cord-like and trabecular patterns of metastatic breast carcinomas. However, these tumors have regular round to elongate nuclei and lack the obvious malignant cytological features of metastatic breast carcinomas. Breast carcinoma cells are EMA positive, nonargyrophilic, and NSE and chromogranin negative, and the cells often exhibit luminal or cytoplasmic mucin.

Metastases from intestinal carcinomas, while tending to form pseudocystic necrotic masses with obvious mucinous glandular differentiation, may occasionally form small acini and cords with only scanty mucin production and thus resemble metastases from breast. The clinical history and surgical findings should provide the necessary information to establish the site of the primary tumor.

Metastatic breast carcinomas may need to be distinguished from poorly differentiated primary ovarian adenocarcinomas, especially serous. Patients with breast carcinoma have an increased risk of ovarian carcinoma and as there is, unfortunately, considerable morphological and immunohistochemical overlap between these lesions, which can pose a difficult diagnostic problem (see Ch. 23). A recent study has shown that immunostaining for gross cystic disease fluid protein 15 (GCDFP-15) may be helpful in distinguishing between the two lesions (Monteagudo et al 1991).

REFERENCES

Abdul Hafeez M, Akhtar M, Ageel H S Ba, Kidess E A 1987 Placental site trophoblast tumor: report of a case with review of literature. Annals of Saudi Medicine 7: 340–344

Abrams H L, Spiro R, Goldstein N 1950 Metastases in carcinoma; analysis of 1000 autopsied cases. Cancer 3: 74–85

Bell R J M 1977 Fetal virilisation due to maternal Krukenberg tumor. Lancet i: 1162–1163

Blaustein A 1982 Pathology of the female genital tract, 2nd edn. Springer-Verlag, New York, p 705–715

Brennecke S P, McEvoy M I, Seymour A E, Bessell C K, Munday R N 1986 Caecal adenocarcinoma metastatic to ovary inducing increased oestrogen production and postmenopausal bleeding. Australian and New Zealand Journal of Obstetrics and Gynaecology 26: 158–161

Brown J V, Fu Y S, Berek J S 1990 Ovarian metastases are rare in stage I adenocarcinoma of the cervix. Obstetrics and Gynecology 76: 623–626

Demopoulos R I, Touger L, Dubin N 1987 Secondary ovarian carcinoma: a clinical and pathological evaluation. International Journal of Gynecological Pathology 6: 166–175

Fox H, Langley F A 1976 Tumors of the ovary. Heinemann, London, p 300–306

Gagnon Y, Tetu B 1989 Ovarian metastases of breast carcinoma. A clinicopathological study of 59 cases. Cancer 64: 892–898

Hines J R, Gordon R T, Widger C, Kolb T 1976 Cystosarcoma phyllodes metastatic to a Brenner tumor of the ovary. Archives of Surgery 111: 299–300

Johansson H 1960 Clinical aspects of metastatic ovarian cancer of extragenital origin. Acta Obstetricia et Gynecologica Scandinavica 39: 681–697

Jolles C J, Beeson J H, Abbott T 1985 Progesterone production in adenocarcinoma of the colon metastatic to the ovaries. Obstetrics and Gynecology 65: 853–857

Kasilag F B, Rutledge F N 1957 Metastatic breast carcinoma in the ovary. American Journal of Obstetrics and Gynecology 74: 989–992

Lee Y T N, Hori J M 1971 Significance of ovarian metastasis in therapeutic oophorectomy for advanced breast cancer. Cancer 27: 1374–1378

Luisi 1968 Metastatic ovarian tumors. In: Gentil F, Junqueira A C (eds) Ovarian cancer. UICC monograph series, Vol II. Springer-Verlag, Berlin, p 87–104

Lumb G, MacKenzie D H 1959 The incidence of metastases in adrenal glands and ovaries removed for carcinoma of the breast. Cancer 12: 521–526

MacDonald P C, Grodin J M, Edman C D, Vellios F, Siiteri P K 1976 Origin of estrogen in a postmenopausal woman with a nonendocrine tumor of the ovary and endometrial hyperplasia. Obstetrics and Gynecology 47: 644–650

MacKeigan J M, Ferguson J A 1979 Prophylactic oophorectomy and colorectal cancer in premenopausal patients. Diseases of the Colon and Rectum 22: 401–405

Mann W J, Chumas J, Amalfitano T, Westermann C, Patsner B 1987 Ovarian metastases from stage 1B adenocarcinoma of the cervix. Cancer 60: 1123–1126

Mazur M T, Hsueh S, Gersell D J 1984 Metastases to the female genital tract; analysis of 325 cases. Cancer 53: 1978–1984

Monteagudo C, Merino M J, Laporte N, Neumann R D 1991 Value of gross cystic disease fluid protein 15 in distinguishing metastatic breast carcinoma among poorly differentiated neoplasms involving the ovary. Human Pathology 22: 368–372

Parker R T, Currie J L 1981 Metastatic tumors of ovary. In: Coppleson M (ed) Gynecologic oncology. Churchill Livingstone, Edinburgh, p 731–742

Quinn M A, Baker H W G, Rome R, Fortune D, Brown J B 1983 Response of a mucinous ovarian tumor of borderline malignancy to human chorionic gonadotropin. Obstetrics and Gynecology 61: 121–126

Rome R M, Fortune D W, Quinn M A, Brown J B 1981 Functioning ovarian tumors in postmenopausal women. Obstetrics and Gynecology 57: 705–710

Saphir O 1951 Signet-ring carcinoma. Military Surgeon 109: 360–369

Scott J S, Lumsden C E, Levell M J 1967 Ovarian endocrine activity in association with hormonally inactive neoplasia. American Journal of Obstetrics and Gynecology 97: 161–170

Scully R E 1979 Tumors of the ovary and maldeveloped gonads. Atlas of tumor pathology. Fascicle 16, 2nd series. Armed Forces Institute of Pathology, Washington, DC, p 323–363

Scully R E, Richardson G S 1961 Luteinization of the stroma of metastatic cancer involving the ovary and its endocrine significance. Cancer 14: 827–840

Smale L E 1980 Metastatic breast adenocarcinoma to Brenner tumors. Gynecologic Oncology 9: 251–253

Sutton G P, Bundy B N, Delgado G et al 1992 Ovarian metastases in Stage Ib carcinoma of the cervix: a Gynecologic Oncology Group study. American Journal of Obstetrics and Gynecology 166: 50–53

Tabata M, Ichinoe K, Sakaragi N, Shena Y, Yamaguchi T, Mabuchi Y 1987 Incidence of ovarian metastases in patients with cancer of the uterine cervix. Gynecolic Oncology 28: 255–261

Turksoy N 1960 Ovarian metastasis of breast carcinoma: a surgical surprise. Obstetrics and Gynecology 15: 573–578

Ulbright T M, Roth L M, Stehman F B 1984 Secondary ovarian neoplasia; a clinicopathologic study of 35 cases. Cancer 53: 1164–1174

Vicens E, Martinez-Mora J, Potau N, Sans M, Boix-Ochoa J 1980 Masculinization of a female fetus by Krukenberg tumor during pregnancy. Journal of Pediatric Surgery 15: 188–190

Virieux C 1962 Untersuchungen über Häufigkeit und Entstehungweise von Krebsmetastasen in den Eierstöcken. Gynaecologia 153: 209–224

Webb M J, Decker D G, Mussey E 1975 Cancer metastatic to the ovary; factors influencing survival. Obstetrics and Gynecology 45: 391–396

Wei P-Y, Ouyang P-C 1963 Trophoblastic disease in Taiwan. A review of 157 cases in a 10 year period. American Journal of Obstetrics and Gynecology 85: 844–849

Woodruff J D, Goldberg B, Jones G S 1968 Enzymic histochemical reactions in two Krukenberg tumors associated with clinically different endocrine patterns. American Journal of Obstetrics and Gynecology 100: 405–417

Woodruff J D, Murthy Y S, Bhaskar T N, Bordbar F, Tseng S S 1970 Metastatic ovarian tumors. American Journal of Obstetrics and Gynecology 107: 202–209

Young R H, Scully R E 1990 Sarcomas metastatic to the ovary: a report of 21 cases. International Journal of Gynecological Pathology 9: 231–252

Young R H, Carey R W, Robboy S J 1981 Breast carcinoma masquerading as primary ovarian neoplasm. Cancer 48: 210–212

Young R H, Gersell D J, Roth L M, Scully R E 1993 Ovarian metastases from cervical carcinomas other than pure adenocarcinomas. Cancer 71: 407–418

Yu T J, Iwasaki I, Horie H, Tamaru J, Takahashi A 1986 Endolymphatic stromal myosis of the uterus with metastasis to ovary and recurrence in vagina. Acta Pathologica Japonica 36: 301–308

54

Metastatic gastrointestinal carcinomas and carcinoids

P. Russell A. Farnsworth

In recent decades the incidence of gastric carcinoma has fallen, and in most western countries colonic carcinomas are now encountered more frequently by a factor of three or four (Johansson 1960, Scully & Richardson 1961, Webb et al 1975, Parker & Currie 1981, Mazur et al 1984, Ulbright et al 1984). Both carcinomas spread readily to the ovaries, and together they form the bulk of tumors metastatic to these organs (see Ch. 53). Ovarian secondaries are identified at autopsy in 15–50% of women with gastric carcinoma (Abrams et al 1950, Saphir 1951, Virieux 1962, Duarte & Llanos 1981) and in 15–30% of those with colorectal carcinoma (Abrams et al 1950, Virieux 1962). However, in clinical series of colorectal carcinomas they are diagnosed in only 3–8% of cases (Harcourt & Dennis 1968, Antoniades et al 1977, MacKeigan & Ferguson 1979, O'Brien et al 1981, Morrow & Enker 1984).

A very small percentage of gastrointestinal tumors metastatic to the ovaries originate in the appendix (mostly adenocarcinoids) (Merino et al 1985, Thomas et al 1985, Hood et al 1986), pancreas (Johansson 1960, Scully & Richardson 1961, Mazur et al 1984, Ulbright et al 1984), gallbladder (Woodruff & Novak 1960, Mazur et al 1984), small intestine (Mazur et al 1984, Gallup et al 1985), or esophagus (squamous cell carcinoma) (Takita et al 1977).

Krukenberg tumors

We reserve the term 'Krukenberg tumor', in accordance with the recommendations of Woodruff & Novak (1960) and endorsed by the World Health Organization (Serov et al 1973), for ovarian adenocarcinomas with a distinctive histological pattern characterized by pleiomorphic mucin-filled signet-ring cells accompanied by a sarcomatoid proliferation of the ovarian stroma. Krukenberg tumors account for 3–8% of all carcinomas metastatic to the ovaries (Metz et al 1980), and most commonly originate in the gastrointestinal tract. Gastric carcinomas are identified in 40–95% of all cases (depending on the characteristics of the population studied) and colorectal carcinomas in less than 20%. Indeed most, if not all, metastases to the ovaries from the stomach are of the Krukenberg type (Scully & Richardson 1961, Holtz & Hart 1982, Mazur et al 1984, Ulbright et al 1984). It appears that the signet-ring type of gastric carcinoma has a greater propensity to metastasize to the ovaries than does the intestinal type (Saphir 1951, Duarte & Llanos 1981). Its predilection for young Japanese women can be seen in Hale's series from Hawaii (1968).

Breast carcinomas uncommonly produce metastases of Krukenberg type (Woodruff & Novak 1960, Hale 1968, Scully 1979, Holtz & Hart 1982, Mazur et al 1984). Rare sources are the gallbladder (Woodruff & Novak 1960), ampulla of Vater (Wong et al 1986), appendix (de Graaf et al 1984, Mazur et al 1984, Hirschfield et al 1985, Thomas et al 1985), cervix, and bladder (Scully 1979, Bowlby & Smith 1986). In up to 40% of reported cases no primary lesions were found. Although many of these cases did not have the benefit of a thorough autopsy examination, some may have been examples of so-called primary ovarian Krukenberg tumors (Joshi 1968; see Ch. 24). The clinical criteria for this diagnosis include survival for at least 5 years after surgical treatment, or, if death occurs at an earlier stage, exclusion of any other possible primary tumor by detailed autopsy examination.

The average age of patients with Krukenberg tumors is approximately 45 years (Hale 1968, Scully 1979, Holtz & Hart 1982). Common presenting symptoms are abdominal pain and swelling, which relate to the ovarian masses; the latter are usually bilateral and often large. Gastrointestinal disturbances are less common, and endocrine symptoms are rare and generally restricted to pregnant patients who may become virilized or deliver a masculinized female fetus (Bell 1977, Vicens et al 1980, Fung et al 1991). Ascites is present in more than 50% of the cases. Only 25% of patients have a history of prior tumor, with an average elapsed interval before the appearance of ovarian lesions of less than 6 months (Hale 1968, Holtz & Hart 1982). The primary carcinoma is sometimes occult, even at laparotomy, and may not be detected until the postoperative period (and rarely not at all). Peritoneal involvement is usually inconspicuous, an observation which supports the theory of retrograde lymphatic spread as the pathogenesis of these tumors. The prognosis is very poor, with death usually occurring within a year. However, surgical treatment of the primary and secondary tumors is often still worthwhile (Scully 1979).

Macroscopic features

The tumors are bilateral in over 80% of cases (Woodruff & Novak 1960, Hale 1968, Scully 1979, Holtz & Hart 1982). The ovaries are asymmetrically enlarged, with one usually greater than 10 cm in maximum diameter and sometimes as large as 25 cm. The ovaries are transformed into rounded or lobulated masses of firm white or yellowish tissue with brown or purple foci of degeneration. In smaller tumors the overall ovarian contours may be preserved. The capsular surface is typically free of adhesions or peritoneal deposits. Parts of the tumors may be gelatinous, spongy or edematous; cystic degeneration is quite common in larger masses. Frank necrosis is generally not conspicuous (Fig. 54.1).

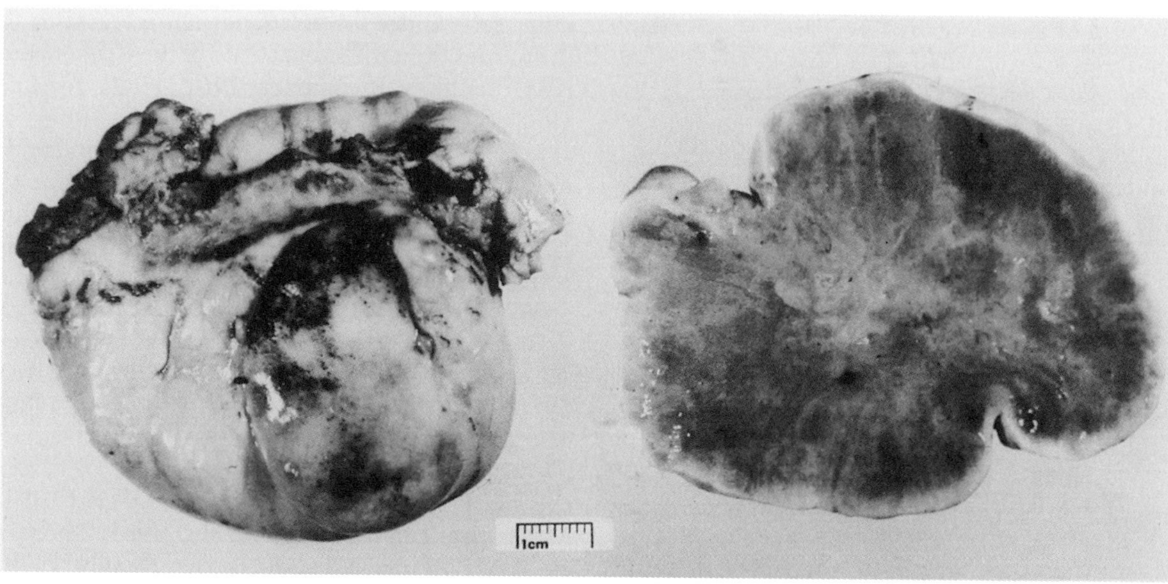

Fig. 54.1 Krukenberg tumor from 61-year-old woman with primary gastric carcinoma. Capsular surface (left) is bosselated. Cut surface (right) shows uniform oedematous gelatinous tumor tissue. No normal ovarian structures are evident. The other ovary was only slightly enlarged, but was also infiltrated by metastatic carcinoma.

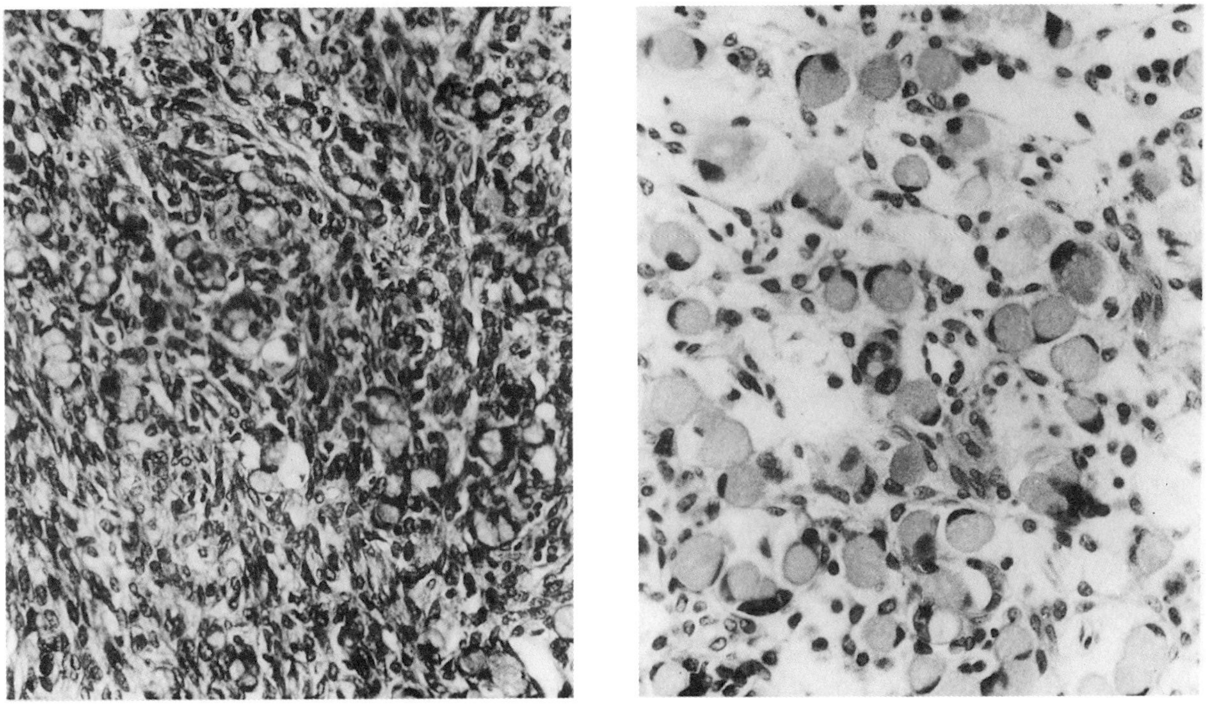

A B

Fig. 54.2 Krukenberg tumors. (A) Single and clustered vacuolated carcinoma cells, including signet-ring forms, infiltrate between hyperplastic stromal cells. H + E ×160. (B) Signet-ring cells, with abundant granular eosinophilic cytoplasm and pleiomorphic nuclei, lying in edematous stroma. H + E ×200

Microscopic features

By definition, the tumors exhibit an intimate admixture of pleiomorphic signet-ring cells and plump spindled stromal cells, the latter presenting a sarcomatoid appearance (Figs 54.2A, 54.3A). The epithelial component is composed chiefly of single or clustered signet-ring cells, but trabeculae, tubules, acini, and small cysts may also be present. The signet-ring cells are identical to those seen in gastric carcinomas, with vacuolated cytoplasm and eccentric hyperchromatic nuclei. Mitotic activity is sparse. The carcinoma cells may also display granular eosinophilic cytoplasm, particularly when located within tubules (Fig. 54.2). Neutral mucin is the predominant secretion and the diastase–PAS stain best demonstrates the nature and arrangement of the cells (Fig. 54.3B). Immunohistochemical stains for epithelial markers, such as cytokeratins (AE1/AE3, CAM 5.2) and EMA, also successfully highlight the carcinoma cells.

The mesenchymal component varies considerably in amount. It is of ovarian stromal origin and is composed of bundles of spindle cells resembling those seen in stromal hyperplasia (Figs 54.2A, 54.3A). There is minimal cytological atypia or mitotic activity. The stroma may become collagenized and may also show a storiform pattern, resembling a fibroma, particularly in the superficial portions of the tumors. The deeper portions of the tumors are generally more cellular and the stromal cells plumper. Edema is present focally (Fig. 54.2B), especially in the medulla, but is sometimes diffuse and marked, to the extent of simulating 'massive edema' (see Ch. 16) and forming pseudocysts. Rarely, pools of interstitial mucin are present.

Luteinized stromal cells are only rarely identified and are certainly not as common as in metastatic colorectal carcinomas (Scully & Richardson 1961, Holtz & Hart 1982). Electron microscopic studies of the hypercellular stroma of Krukenberg tumors shows hypertrophic fibroblasts and myofibroblasts, as well as sparse luteinized stromal cells with ultra-

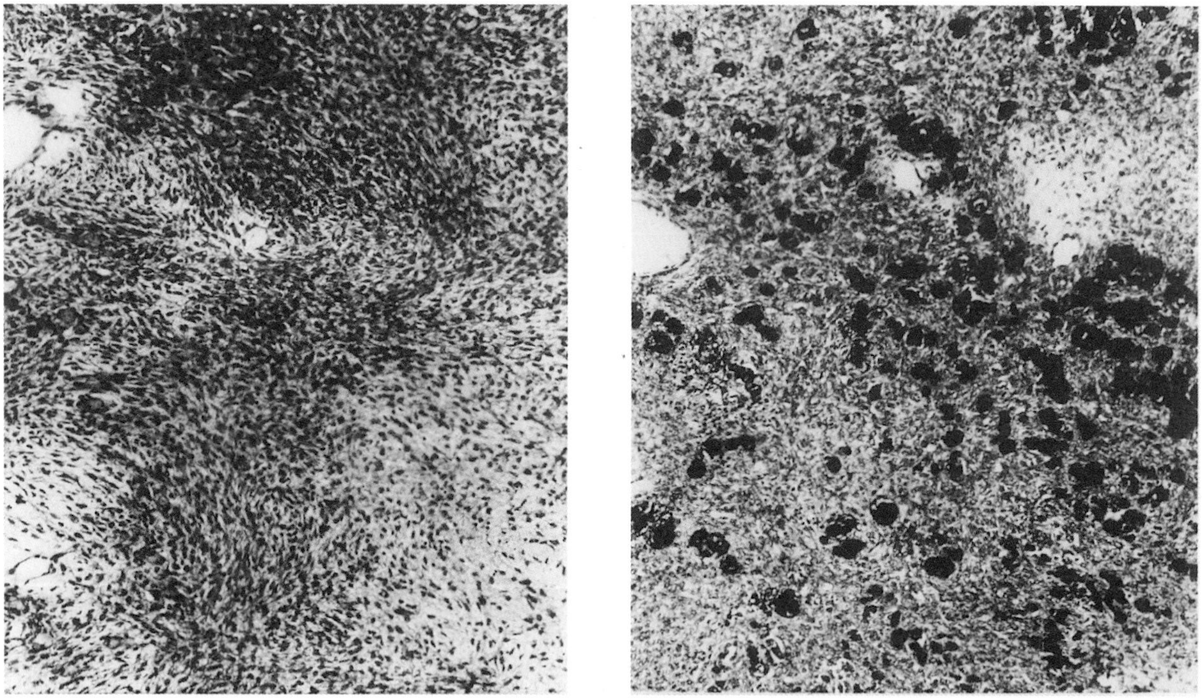

A B

Fig. 54.3 Krukenberg tumor. The ovarian stroma is hyperplastic and focally edematous. (A) The infiltrate of carcinoma cells is difficult to appreciate in this H + E section. ×80. (B) Same area with carcinoma cells highlighted by PAS stain. ×80

structural features typical of endocrinologically active cells (Wong et al 1986).

Lymphatic invasion is generally conspicuous and is best observed in the hilus, but can also readily be demonstrated in the mesosalpinx and mesovarium if these tissues are available for review.

Some Krukenberg tumors display a predominant tubular pattern and have been subclassified as 'tubular Krukenberg tumors', as distinct from the classical type (Bullon et al 1981). They constitute approximately 20% of all Krukenberg tumors and may represent a better differentiated group. Signet-ring cells are present both in tubules and intermingled with stromal cells (Fig. 54.4). Scattered argentaffinic and argyrophilic cells may be identified (Bullon et al 1981, Wong et al 1986). Luteinized stromal cells are relatively more frequent than in the classic variant (Bullon et al 1981, Ulbright et al 1984, Wong et al 1986).

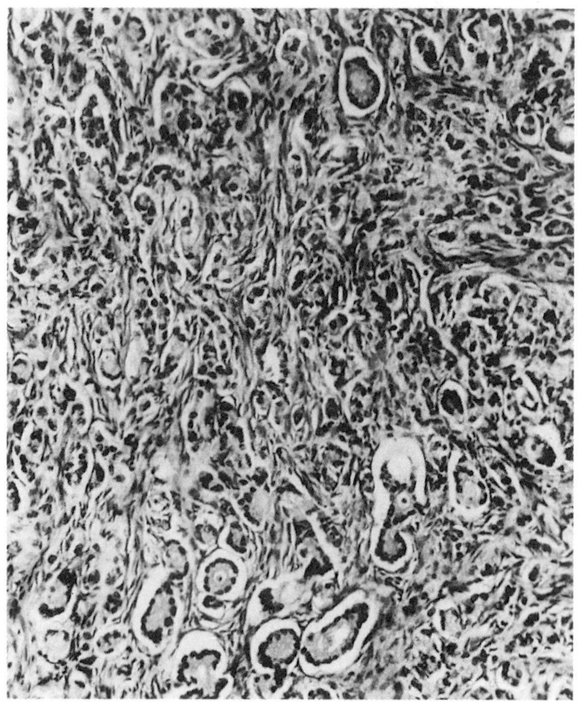

Fig. 54.4 Tubular Krukenberg tumor. Small glandular structures infiltrate the ovarian stroma. H + E ×100

Differential diagnosis

Fibromas may resemble Krukenberg tumors

macroscopically, although the former are usually unilateral. The erroneous impression may be reinforced microscopically if the Krukenberg tumor has abundant fibromatous stroma with only sparse carcinoma cells. The correct diagnosis will not be missed if tumors are well sampled and sections showing vacuolated cells are stained for mucin.

Sertoli–Leydig cell tumors may simulate tubular Krukenberg tumors. Although vacuolated cells are sometimes present in Sertoli cell tubules, they do not contain mucin and the cells lack significant cytological atypia. The stromal components of Sertoli–Leydig cell tumors lack signet-ring cells but contain Leydig cells which may be difficult to distinguish from the luteinized stromal cells of Krukenberg tumors.

Vacuolated cells are present in sclerosing stromal tumors and in its apparently unique variant 'signet-ring stromal tumor of ovary' (Ramzy 1976), but neither of these contain mucin.

Note that metastatic carcinomas in the ovary typically show a range of histological patterns within individual tumors, and some (of diverse origin) may include focal areas which resemble Krukenberg tumors.

Metastases from colorectal carcinoma

The most commonly occurring metastatic carcinoma to mimic primary ovarian carcinoma is that of large bowel origin (Daya et al 1992). Patients with ovarian metastases of colorectal origin tend to be older than those with gastric carcinoma, and

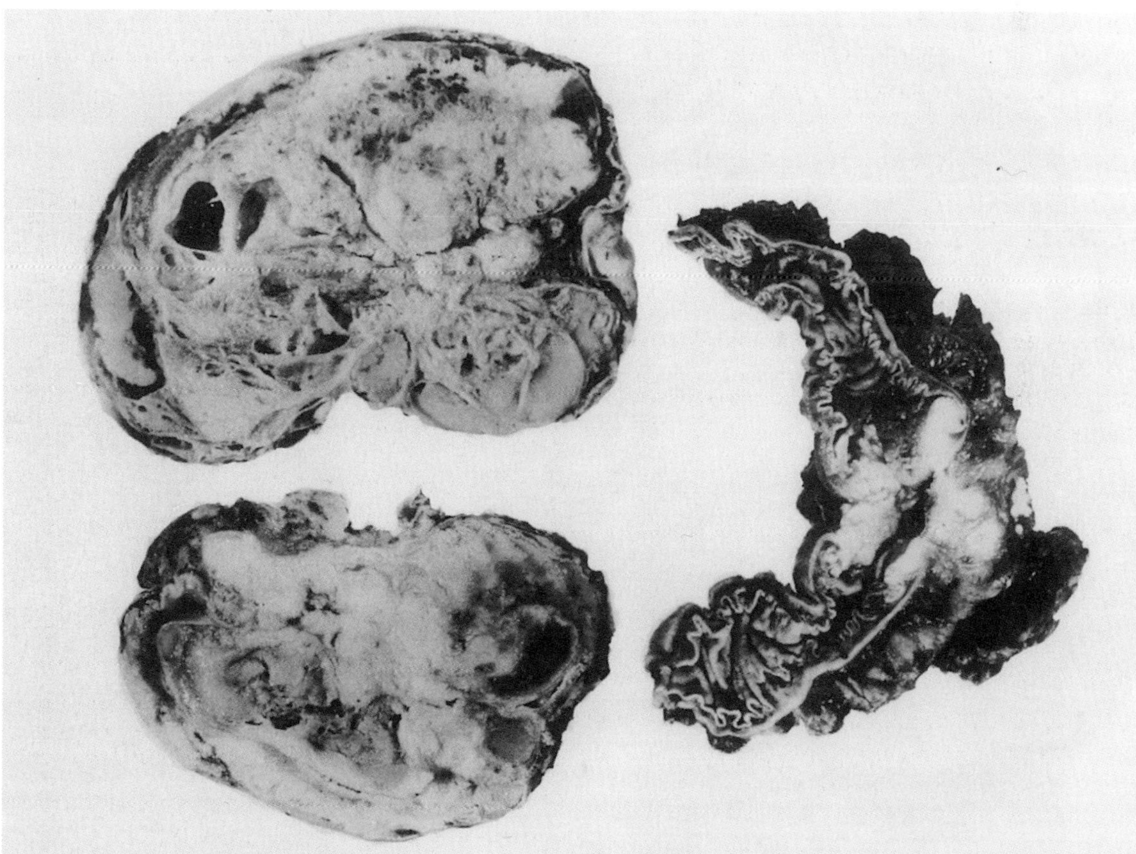

Fig. 54.5 Bilateral large solid/cystic ovarian metastases from adenocarcinoma of transverse colon. Multiple peritoneal deposits were also present

are generally peri- or postmenopausal. In over 50% of patients the ovarian metastases are part of diffuse intraperitoneal disease (MacKeigan & Ferguson 1979, Morrow & Enker 1984). A few have abnormal uterine bleeding or virilization as a result of the endocrine activity of luteinized ovarian stromal cells (Scully & Richardson 1961; see Ch. 53). About 75% have had an intestinal carcinoma removed, in most cases less than 3 years previously. In the remainder the presentation is that of an apparent primary ovarian neoplasm (Johansson 1960, Scully 1979, Herrera-Ornelas et al 1983, Mazur et al 1984, Ulbright et al 1984, Lash & Hart 1987), and such patients present with approximately the same order of frequency as those with true primary mucinous ovarian carcinomas. It should be noted that women with colorectal carcinomas have an increased risk of developing primary ovarian carcinomas, and for this reason, as well as to avoid the possibility of subsequent bulky ovarian metastases and the need for further surgery, it has been recommended that peri- or postmenopausal women should have prophylactic bilateral oophorectomies at the time of initial colorectal surgery (Antoniades et al 1977, MacKeigan & Ferguson 1979, O'Brien et al 1981, Morrow & Enker 1984).

Macroscopic features

Approximately 70% of colorectal metastases are bilateral and, like those of gastric origin, may be very large (Fig. 54.5). Capsular adhesions, associated with peritoneal metastases or direct tumor

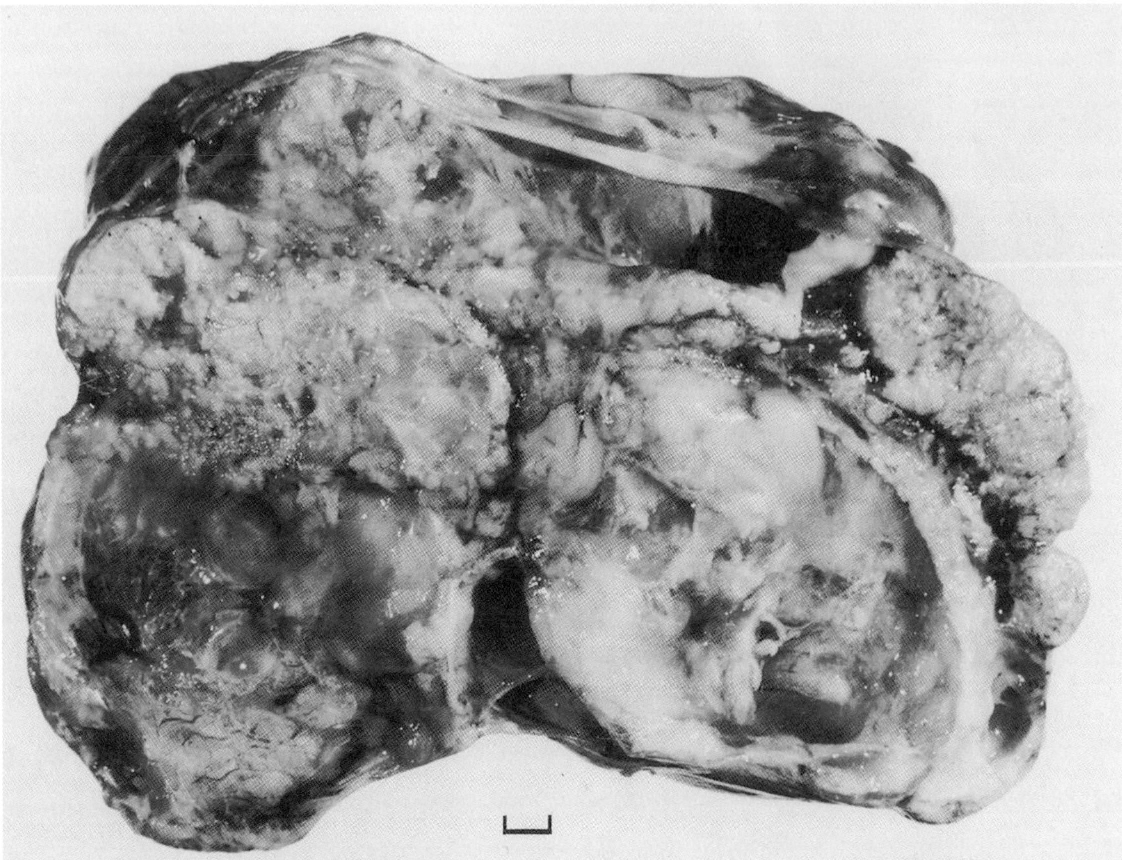

Fig. 54.6 Large unilateral ovarian metastasis from adenocarcinoma of ascending colon. Note degenerative cystic change (best seen top center), necrosis and mucoid areas. Scale bar equals 1 cm

infiltration, are sometimes present. The lobulated or multinodular masses frequently have a cystic component with spaces filled with necrotic debris or, less often, clear or mucinous fluid (Fig. 54.6), and they may thus simulate primary ovarian mucinous carcinomas. Other intra-abdominal metastases are commonly present; lymph nodes and liver parenchyma are often involved.

Microscopic features

Metastases typically resemble the corresponding primary colorectal carcinomas, which are most often moderately differentiated. A characteristic feature is pseudocystic change which results from central necrosis of tumor nodules, leaving a rim of viable epithelium (Fig. 54.7). The presence of a prominent neutrophil infiltrate in the necrotic debris has led to the term 'dirty necrosis' for this appearance. Individual glands may also show segmental necrosis of their epithelial lining (Fig. 54.8). Glandular spaces of various sizes are present and cribriform foci are common (Figs 54.8, 54.9). Mucin production is almost always demonstrable, but is generally limited to the apical cytoplasm and gland lumens. The overall appearances may closely mimic endometrioid adenocarcinoma (Lash & Hart 1987). Frankly mucinous glands are uncommon, but when present are sometimes lined by relatively bland epithelium, thus simulating primary ovarian mucinous neoplasms (Fig. 54.10). Trabecular patterns and foci of Krukenberg-type infiltration are occasionally encountered.

The stroma is very variable in amount and may show collagenization, edema, or myxoid change. In up to 50% of tumors the stroma is thecoma like, being composed of plump spindle cells. In

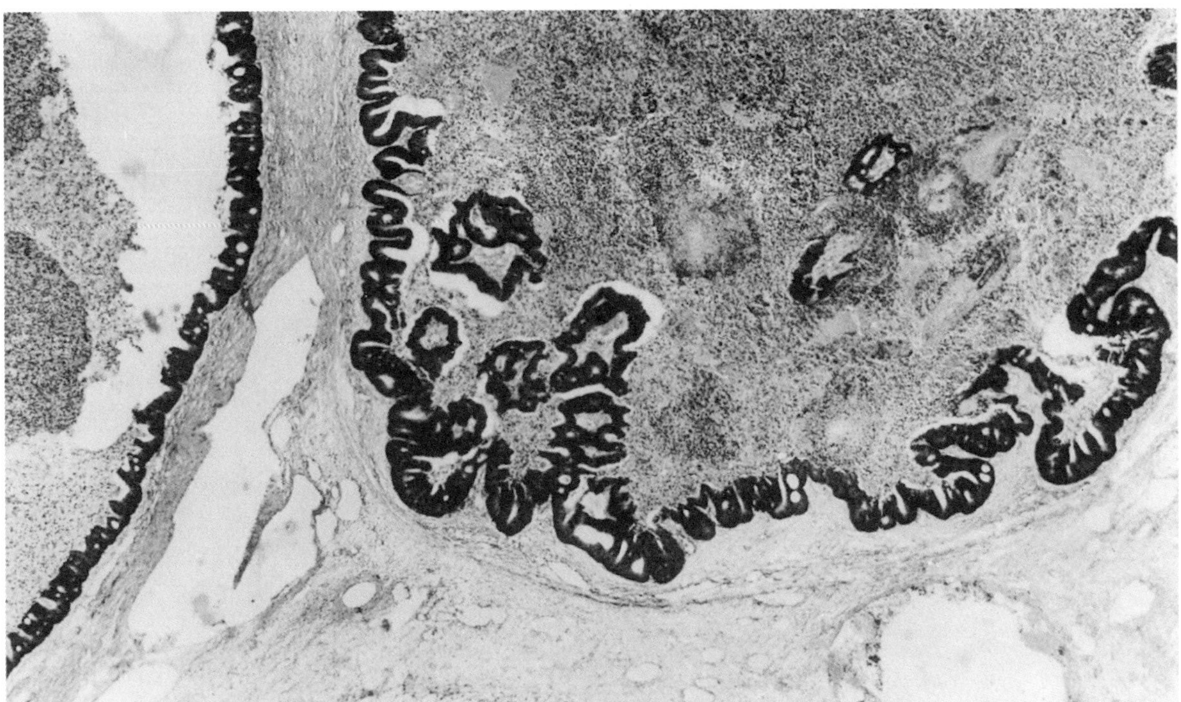

Fig. 54.7 Pseudocystic change in metastatic colonic carcinoma. Necrosis in center of tumor nodules leaves a rim of viable epithelium (the so-called 'garland' pattern) and is responsible for specific cytological features (see Ch. 57). Note lymphatic permeation (lower right). H + E ×32.

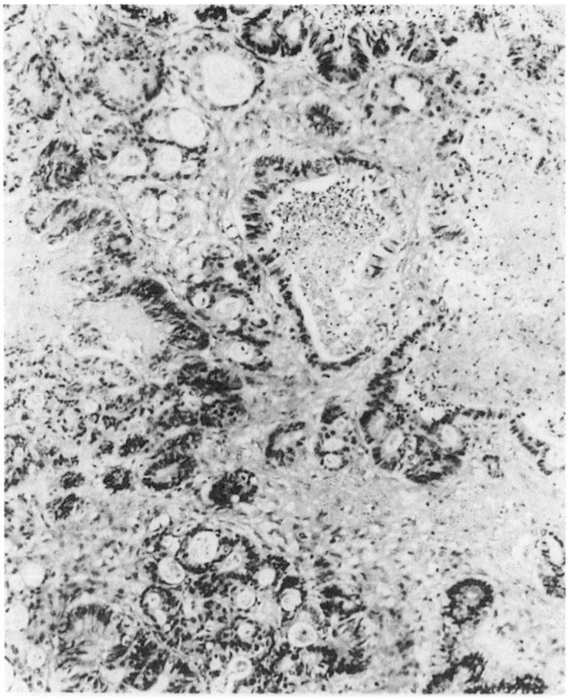

Fig. 54.8 Metastatic colonic adenocarcinoma showing a cribriform pattern resembling endometrioid carcinoma. The glandular epithelium is focally necrotic (center and right). Compare with Fig. 54.10 (mucinous type). H + E ×80

many of these (about 35% of all colorectal metastases) there are foci of frank stromal cell luteinization (Scully & Richardson 1961, Ulbright et al 1984, Lash & Hart 1987). Luteinized cells have abundant vacuolated or granular eosinophilic cytoplasm; they are arranged in small clusters or appear to unsheathe groups of carcinoma cells, and are often most conspicuous at the margins of the tumor (Figs 53.6, 54.11). In pregnancy, luteinized cells may become confluent and fill the spaces between the epithelial components (Scully 1979).

Less than 10% of colorectal metastases have the pathological characteristics of Krukenberg tumors (see above).

Sections of capsular adhesions may reveal direct tumor infiltration or small discrete peritoneal metastases (see Fig. 53.3). Lymphatic permeation is often present in the ovarian hilus and accompanying fallopian tube (see Figs 53.1, 53.2).

Fig. 54.9 Multinodular ovarian metastasis from colonic adenocarcinoma. Nodules at top left and center right are cribriform (pseudoendometrioid), while remainder are mucinous. H + E ×10

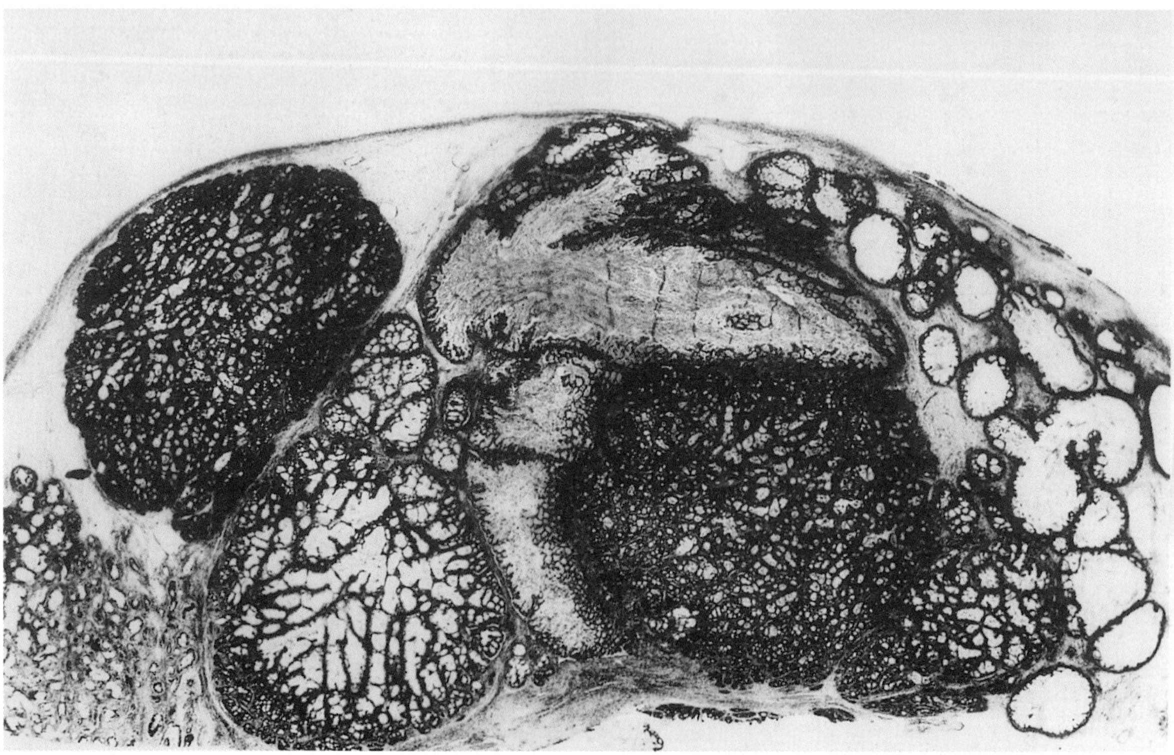

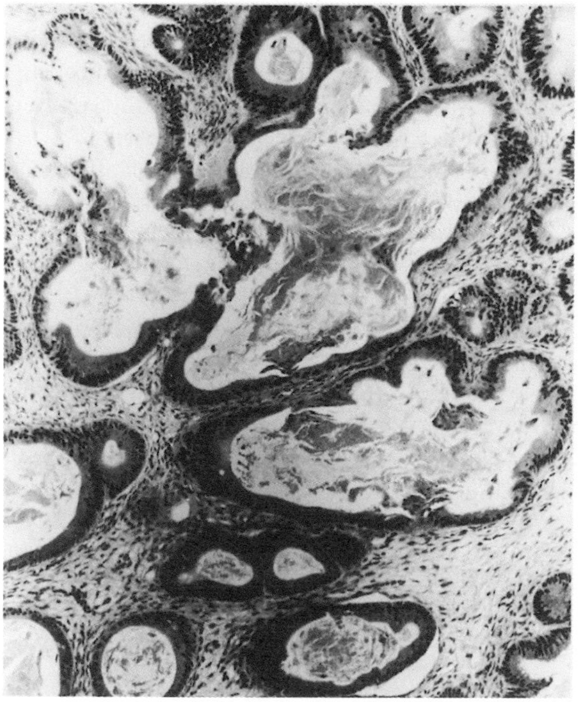

Fig. 54.10 Metastatic colonic carcinoma of mucinous type. Epithelium lining glands appears deceptively bland at this magnification. Compare with Fig. 54.8 (pseudoendometrioid pattern). H + E $\times$80

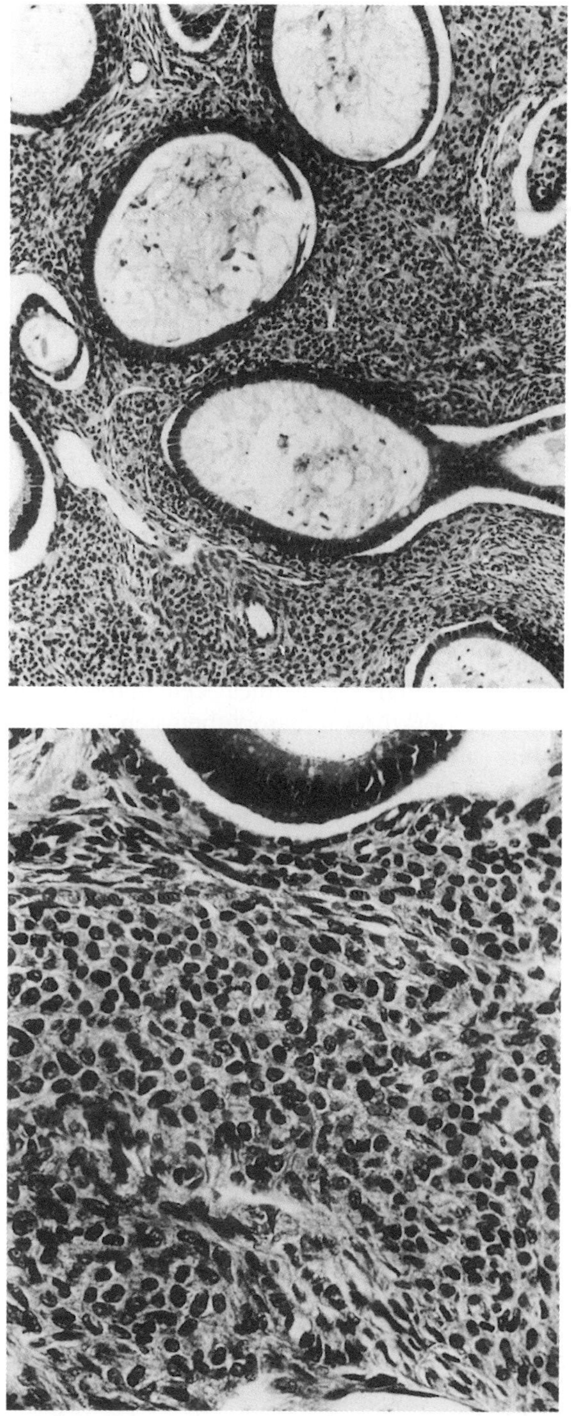

A

B

Fig. 54.11 Stromal luteinization associated with metastatic colonic carcinoma. (A) Hyperplastic stroma separates the malignant glands. H + E $\times$80. (B) Detail of stromal cells showing abundant eosinophilic cytoplasm. The nuclei are round to oval and cytologically benign. H + E $\times$250

Differential diagnosis

In women without a history of prior intestinal carcinoma and in whom no other abdominal neoplasm is readily apparent at the time of oophorectomy, the often difficult problem arises of distinguishing a primary ovarian adenocarcinoma (mucinous or endometrioid) from a colorectal metastasis. Features favoring metastatic carcinoma are bilaterality, multinodular pattern, extensive necrosis, lack of a fibrous capsule or of a true cystic component, prominent stromal luteinization, and only rare transitions from bland through atypical to frankly malignant epithelium (Table 54.1). Daya et al (1992) found a 'garland' pattern with cribriform areas and 'dirty' necrosis to be the most useful microscopic features that allowed differentiation from primary endometrioid carcinoma. The presence of squamous differentiation virtually excludes metastatic colonic carcinoma and indicates primary or metastatic endometrioid adenocarcinoma. Unfortunately, currently

Table 54.1 Differential diagnosis: primary mucinous adenocarcinoma of ovary versus metastatic colonic carcinoma

Primary mucinous carcinoma	Metastatic colonic carcinoma
Clinical	
Bilateral in 20%	Bilateral in 70%
Metastases, if present, are peritoneal and superficial	Other metastases common, in lymph nodes and liver parenchyma
Macroscopic	
Cystic component prominent	Multinodular solid tumors
Necrosis mild to moderate	Necrosis usually marked, producing pseudocysts
Microscopic	
Thick acellular fibrous capsule around periphery in many	No peripheral capsule
Epithelial transitions common	Epithelial transitions uncommon
Stromal luteinization uncommon	Stromal luteinisation common
Immunohistochemical	
Cytokeratin 7 positive	Cytokeratin 7 negative

available immunohistochemical cell markers are generally poor discriminators between primary ovarian and metastatic mucinous carcinoma because of the histogenetic analogy of the tumors in question. For example, CEA is typically positive in colonic carcinomas, but is also positive in at least 80% of primary mucinous carcinomas (Heald et al 1979, Casper et al 1984, Lash & Hart 1987). By contrast, Daya et al (1992) showed strong *intracytoplasmic* positive staining for CEA in all cases of metastatic intestinal adenocarcinoma, while CEA was either negative or showed intraluminal or apical positivity in primary ovarian endometrioid adenocarcinoma. Ueda et al (1993) have suggested that cytokeratin 7 is a useful discriminator between mucinous ovarian masses of mullerian type (positive) and intestinal type or derivation (negative). Mucin and argyrophil stains are noncontributory. Electron microscopy may be helpful if the very prominent microvilli and glycocalyceal bodies said to be typical of colorectal carcinomas are identified (Hickey & Seiler 1981, Lash & Hart 1987).

Metastatic carcinoid tumors

Carcinoid tumors account for less than 2% of metastatic ovarian tumors (Scully 1979), but it is important to distinguish them from primary ovarian carcinoid tumors and other ovarian tumors with which they share some histological characteristics but carry quite disparate prognoses.

The age range of patients with metastatic carcinoids is wide, but most patients are over 40 years of age. Symptoms of a pelvic or abdominal mass are commonly present, and the carcinoid syndrome is present preoperatively in 40% of surgical cases (Robboy et al 1974). The ileum is the most common site of the primary tumor; caecum, appendix, jejunum, and pancreas are less common sources. Metastasis from a bronchial carcinoid has also been reported (Brown et al 1980, Ulbright et al 1984). In the series of Robboy et al (1974), a primary lesion was identified in 20 of 25 surgical cases, although in 8 of these it was only detected postoperatively.

At operation both ovaries are found to be involved almost invariably. Abdominal metastases (mesenteric, omental, and peritoneal) are usually also evident, but liver involvement is often only minimal or absent (except in patients with the carcinoid syndrome).

The prognosis for patients with ovarian metastases from a carcinoid tumor is poor. One-third die within 1 year and two-thirds within 4 years. At autopsy there is usually extensive peritoneal and nodal disease, as well as hepatic and other visceral metastases. Morphological evidence of carcinoid heart disease is present in 70% (Robboy et al 1974).

Macroscopic features

Almost all metastatic carcinoid tumors in the ovaries are bilateral but of unequal size (range 1–20 cm; mean 8 cm) (Robboy et al 1974). The external surfaces are smooth but bosselated, and there may be adhesions to adjacent organs. The cut surfaces display firm confluent tan, gray, or yellowish nodules. Degenerative cysts containing clear fluid and foci of necrosis are occasionally present.

Microscopic features

Any or all of the typical histological patterns of

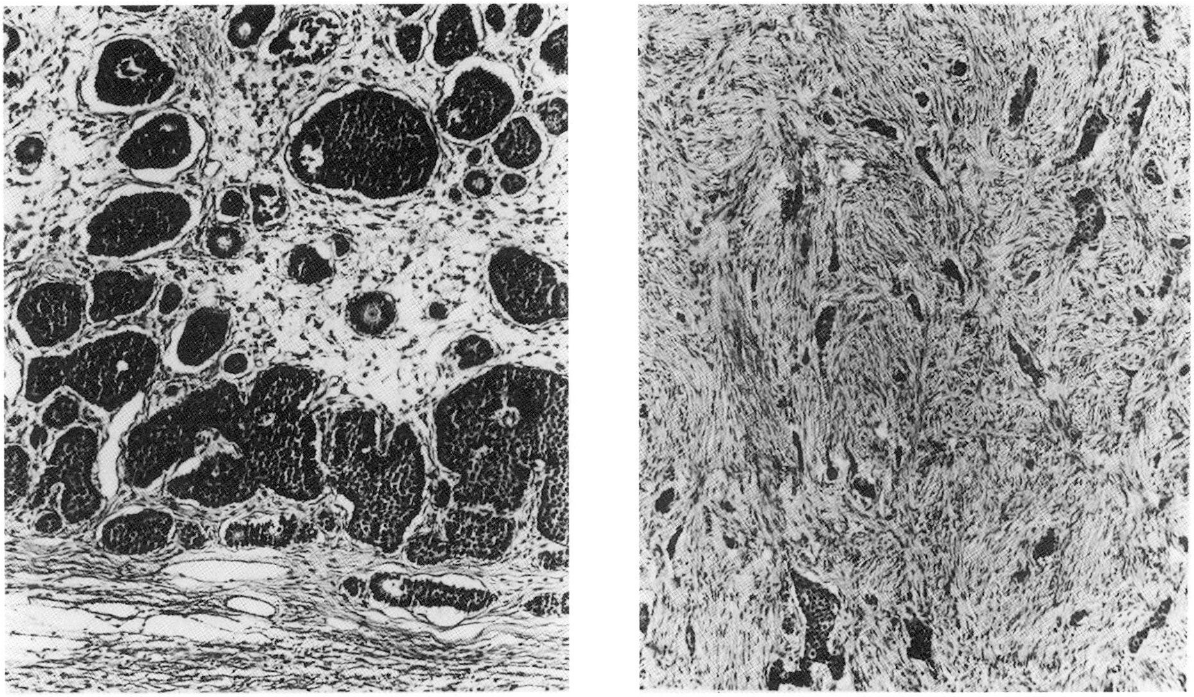

Fig. 54.12 Metastatic carcinoid tumor – insular type. (A) Uniform, closely packed groups of cells with peripheral palisading. A few acini are present. From a 58-year-old woman with widespread intraperitoneal disease; a primary ileal tumor had been resected 2 years previously. H + E ×80. (B) In this example, the cell groups are separated by abundant sclerotic stroma. The low-power pattern mimics a transitional cell tumor. H + E ×80

carcinoid tumors may be present, but the most common is the insular pattern typical of midgut carcinoids, reflecting the most frequent source of these tumors. The cell groups often show peripheral palisading of nuclei, and small acini may be present at the margins of the islands (Figs 54.12A, 54.13). An unusual variant has shown central spindling within the islands of metastatic carcinoid cells (Fig. 54.14). The nuclei are central with coarse but evenly clumped chromatin; mitoses are sparse. The eosinophilic, sometimes granular, cytoplasm is argyrophilic, and may be argentaffinic as well. The neuroendocrine nature of the cells can be confirmed simply by demonstrating immunohistochemically the presence of NSE, chromogranin, synaptophysin, or specific secretory products such as serotonin. The fibromatous stroma may become hypocellular and hyalinized (Fig. 54.12B) or, less commonly, luteinized. Calcification of the stroma or intraluminal secretions may be present. Vascular invasion is sometimes observed. The microscopic pattern of

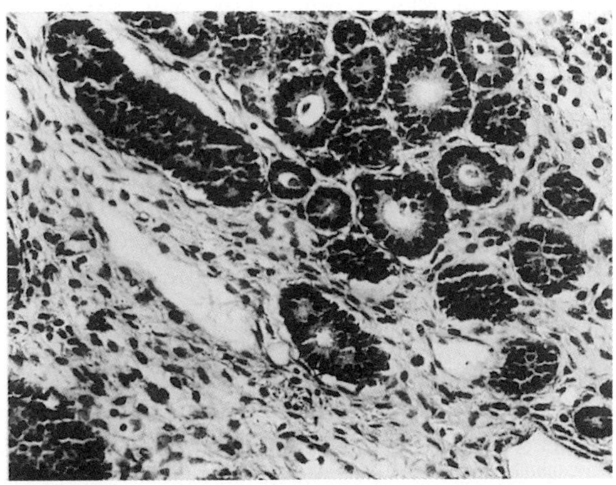

Fig. 54.13 Metastatic carcinoid tumor. Some cell groups form acini; central lumens are surrounded by radially orientated low columnar cells compared with Call–Exner bodies (same case as in Fig. 54.12A). H + E ×150

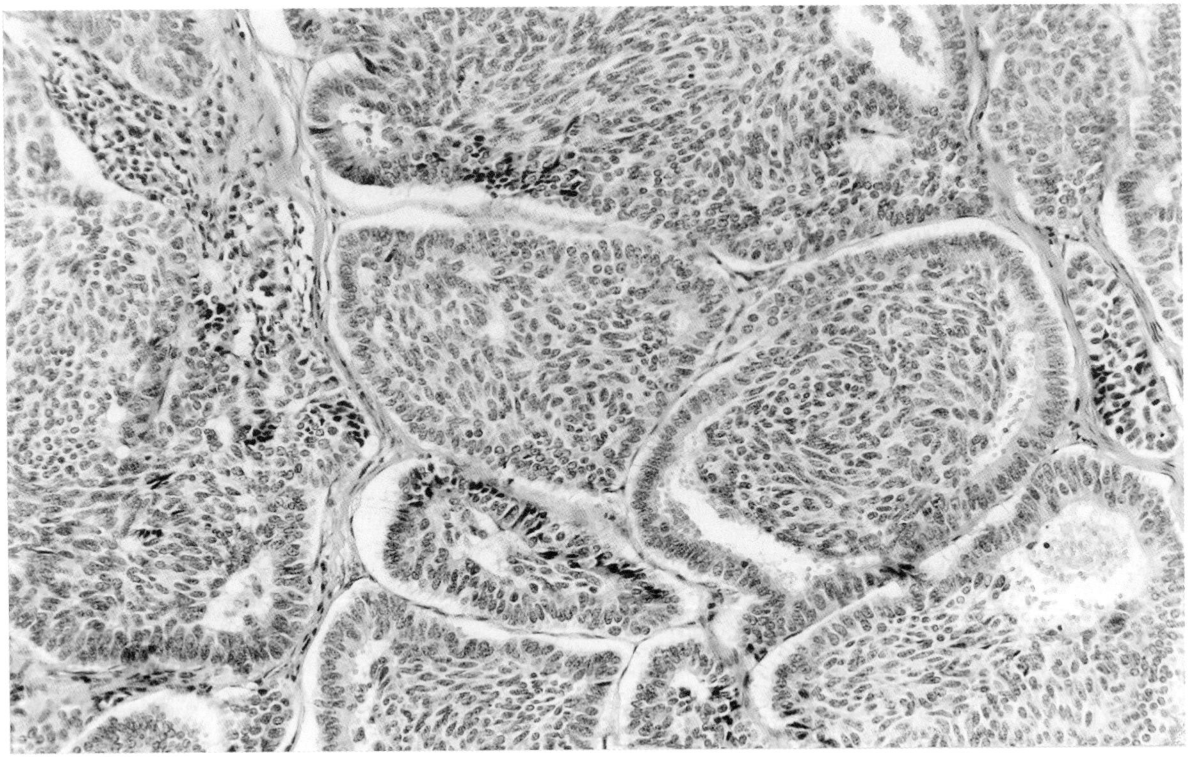

Fig. 54.14 Metastatic carcinoid tumor in an 89-year-old woman. The large solid right ovarian mass was characterized by islands of small central spindle cells with distinct peripheral palisading by tall columnar cells with eosinophilic cytoplasm. Immunostains were strongly positive for chromogranin and synaptophysin. H + E ×165. (Material courtesy of Dr J Ferguson, Canberra)

mucinous or goblet cell carcinoid should also be recognized. These are almost always of appendiceal origin (see below). They contain goblet cells as well as argentaffin or argyrophil cells.

Differential diagnosis

Distinction from a primary ovarian carcinoid tumor may be very difficult except when there is evidence of coexisting cystic teratoma, on the one hand, or an intestinal tumor on the other. In the absence of these strong clues, the most useful discriminator is bilaterality (Table 54.2); bilateral tumors should be considered metastatic until proved otherwise (Robboy et al 1974, Talerman 1984). Primary tumors are unlikely to be associated with peritoneal deposits at initial presentation. The above observations mandate that if an ovarian carcinoid tumor is diagnosed at frozen section, the contralateral ovary and abdominal contents should be carefully examined for evidence of further tumor. If the contralateral ovary is excised, it must be examined microscopically, even if not enlarged

Table 54.2 Differential diagnosis: primary versus secondary carcinoid tumor

Metastatic carcinoid	Primary carcinoid
Clinical	
Primary site apparent in 80%	No intestinal tumor
Peritoneal seeding and abdominal metastases frequent	Extra–ovarian spread uncommon
Early recurrence and progression	Low rate of recurrence
Macroscopic	
Bilateral almost always	Unilateral always
Cut surface nodular and variegated	Cut surface homogeneous
Microscopic	
Teratomatous elements absent	Teratomatous elements present usually

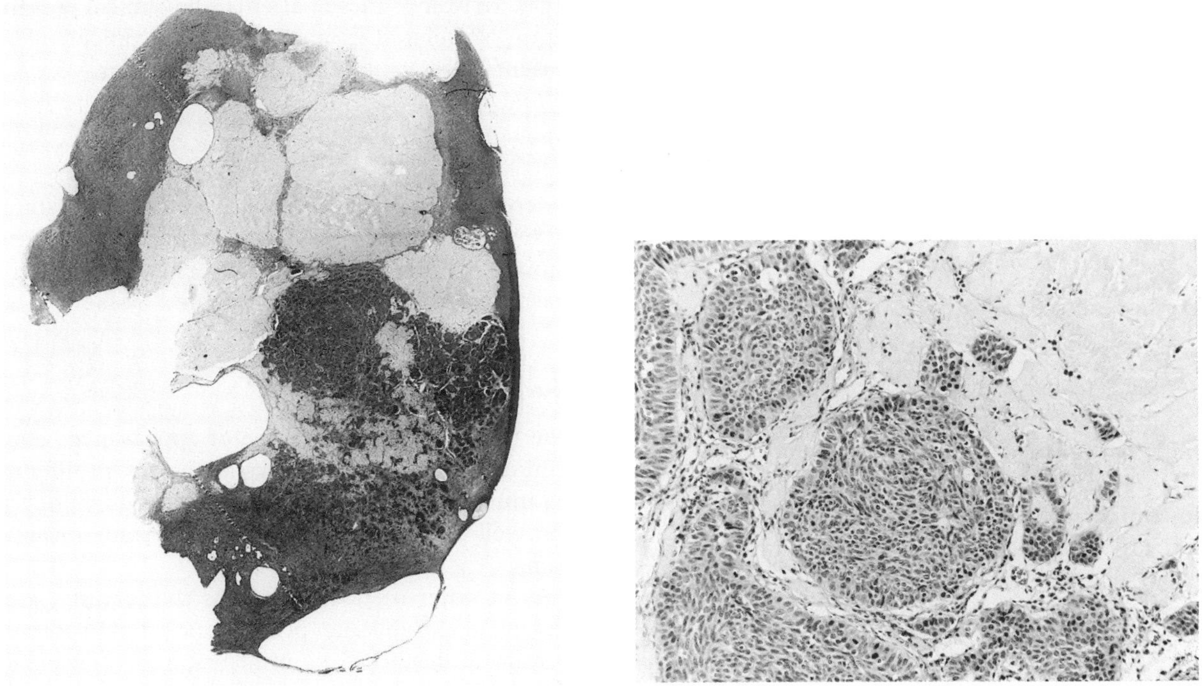

Fig. 54.15 Metastatic carcinoid tumor. Small atrophic contralateral ovary from same patient as in Fig. 54.14. (A) Survey of ovary. H + E ×6.6. (B) Carcinoid tumor infiltrating the margin of an old corpus albicans. H + E ×99. (Material courtesy of Dr J Ferguson, Canberra)

(Fig. 54.15). On macroscopic examination, primary tumors present a more homogeneous and less nodular appearance than that of secondary tumors; there are no useful microscopic discriminatory features. Postoperative radiological examination of the abdomen and urinary 5-hydroxyindole acetic acid estimations may be helpful. If the ovarian tumors are metastatic, abdominal recurrences usually become apparent within a few months.

Other ovarian neoplasms which may be confused with metastatic carcinoids are granulosa cell tumors, transitional cell tumors, adenofibromas, and adenocarcinomas.

Granulosa cell tumors display insular and trabecular patterns, but other patterns (e.g. diffuse and follicular) not found in carcinoids are also present. Call–Exner bodies are distinguished from the acinar spaces of carcinoid tumors by the haphazard rather than radial arrangement of cells which border them (Fig. 54.13). Granulosa cells have grooved oval rather than round nuclei. The scanty cytoplasm is nonargyrophilic and negative for cytokeratins and neuroendocrine markers.

Transitional cell tumors have abundant fibromatous stroma surrounding islands of multilayered cells with elongate grooved nuclei. The cytoplasm is only focally argyrophilic. The islands often include central mucinous epithelial cells, and there may also be separate simple mucinous cysts.

Adenofibromas may resemble carcinoid tumors macroscopically and on low power microscopic examination. However, higher magnification will reveal that the cystic spaces are lined by typical mullerian epithelia.

Poorly differentiated primary or metastatic adenocarcinomas may superficially resemble metastatic carcinoid tumors, but closer inspection will reveal foci of necrosis, obvious nuclear pleiomorphism, and numerous mitoses. The neat organoid patterns of carcinoids are absent.

Metastatic mucinous carcinoids need to be distinguished from metastatic adenocarcinomas. Mucinous carcinoids may contain foci of pure adenocarcinoma and, conversely, metastatic gastric carcinoma may contain scattered argentaffin or argyrophil cells. The diagnosis of a mucinous carcinoid (apart from finding the appendiceal primary tumor) should be made in the presence of the typical pattern of nests containing an admixture of signet ring cells and cells containing argentaffin granules. Distinction from the extremely rare ovarian mucinous carcinoid is difficult, and is discussed in Chapter 49.

Metastases from appendix

Appendiceal metastases are of three main types: frankly invasive adenocarcinoma; carcinoid, usually mucinous; and low grade mucinous epithelial tumors.

It is estimated that adenocarcinoma of the appendix spreads to the ovary in 8% of cases (Fichera et al 1976). They can present, however, as an ovarian mass. A similar approach as for metastatic large bowel tumors should be taken (see above).

Metastatic carcinoids also occur (Robboy et al 1974). The most common types of carcinoma to metastasize from the appendix are adenocarcinoids or goblet cell carcinoids, these metastases either presenting as a Krukenberg tumor (Miller et al 1988) or mimicking a mucinous cystadenocarcinoma (Chen 1990, Ikeda et al 1991). Metastases of these rare tumors occur at a rate that warrants bilateral oophorectomy at the time of resection of primary tumor (Young & Scully 1994). Conversely, close inspection of the appendix at the time of removal of any mucinous tumor of the ovary is advisable. Microscopically they show rounded nests containing goblet cells and argentaffin or argyrophil cells. They may also have foci resembling Krukenberg tumor or cystic glands filled with mucin.

The incidence of patients with low grade tumors of the appendix who also have similar tumors in one or both ovaries and pseudomyxoma peritonei is quite high. The origin of these tumors is controversial and is discussed in Chapter 23.

Metastases from pancreas

Young & Hart (1989) have reported a series of seven patients with mucinous tumors of the ovary interpreted as metastatic from the exocrine pancreas. In four of these patients, the clinical presentation simulated primary ovarian cancer. The patients' ages ranged from 29 to 87 years.

Macroscopic features

Macroscopically the ovarian tumors were bilateral in six, with the status of the opposite ovary not known in the remaining case. The ovarian neoplasms were all large multiloculated cysts.

Microscopic features

The tumors showed a range of appearances containing foci of mucinous cystadenoma, proliferating mucinous tumor ('of borderline malignancy'), and well-differentiated mucinous cystadenocarcinoma.

As in other metastatic lesions the features suggesting an extraovarian primary included bilaterality, surface desmoplastic implants, and widespread intra-abdominal spread.

There is a solitary reported case of possible metastatic islet cell carcinoma (Wertberg & Wertzman 1983). Young and Scully (1994) also describe two cases of metastatic microadenocarcinomas to the ovary. These may mimic carcinoid tumors, but are negative with silver stains.

Metastases from gallbladder and bile ducts

Six cases of ovarian metastases from carcinoma of the gallbladder or bile ducts have been described by Young & Scully (1990). The patients' ages ranged from 33 to 72 years (mean 57 years). In one case of gallbladder adenocarcinoma, the presentation was that of an ovarian mass. A further case of carcinoma of the cystic duct presenting with an ovarian mass is also reported Nashgari et al (1992). In other cases the two sites were discovered synchronously or the ovarian metastasis appeared up to 2 years after the biliary primary.

Macroscopic features

The ovarian tumors were usually bilateral. One metastatic mass was cystic; the others were solid, ranging up to 6.5 cm in diameter. They had a lobulated external surface and were usually multinodular on cut surface.

Microscopic features

The tumors described by Young & Scully (1990) had varying appearances. One resembled endometrioid carcinoma, one simulated mucinous cystadenocarcinoma, and a third had the appearance of a Sertoli–Leydig cell tumor. As with other metastases, the diagnosis depended on awareness of the possibility of an extraovarian origin as well as the usual features of bilaterality, multinodularity (macroscopically and/or microscopically), and surface implants.

Metastases from liver

Hepatocellular carcinoma metastasizing to the ovary is extremely rare (Fig. 53.6), but must be included in the differential diagnosis of oxyphil cell tumors of the ovary. Only a handful of cases of metastatic hepatocellular carcinoma have been described (Oortman & Elliott 1983, Young et al 1992). The patients' ages ranged from 31 to 67 years. The ovarian masses may be identified synchronously with the liver tumor or occur at some later time.

Macroscopically the tumors are usually bilateral, range from 4 to 11 cm in diameter, and may be solid or cystic. Microscopically they are composed of cells with moderate to abundant eosinophilic cytoplasm (either diffuse or in nodules), nests, and trabeculae. Cysts or glands and bile may be present.

A *hepatoblastoma* in a 19-year-old woman and associated with bilateral ovarian metastases has been described (Green & Silva 1989).

The main differential diagnosis is hepatoid yolk sac tumor (especially in a young patient) and hepatoid carcinoma (see Ch. 31), either primary or metastatic in the ovary.

REFERENCES

Abrams H L, Spiro R, Goldstein N 1950 Metastases in carcinoma; analysis of 1000 autopsied cases. Cancer 3: 74–85

Antoniades K, Spector H B, Hecksher R H 1977 Prophylactic oophorectomy in conjunction with large-bowel resection for cancer: report of two cases. Diseases of the Colon and Rectum 20: 506–510

Bell R J M 1977 Fetal virilisation due to maternal Krukenberg tumor. Lancet i: 1162–1163

Bowlby L S, Smith McC L 1986 Signet-ring cell carcinoma of the urinary bladder primary presentation as a Krukenberg tumor. Gynecologic Oncology 25: 376–381

Brown B L, Scharifker D A, Gordon R, Deppe G G, Cohen C J 1980 Bronchial carcinoid tumor with ovarian metastasis. A light microscopic and ultrastructural study. Cancer 46: 543–546

Bullon A, Arsenau J, Prat J, Young R H, Scully R E 1981 Tubular Krukenberg tumor. A problem in histopathologic diagnosis. American Journal of Surgical Pathology 5: 225–232

Casper S, van Nagell J R, Powell D F et al 1984 Immunohistochemical localisation of tumor markers in epithelial ovarian cancer. American Journal of Obstetrics and Gynecology 149: 154–158

Chen K T K 1990 Appendiceal adenocarcinoid with ovarian metastasis. Gynecological Oncology 38: 286–288

Daya D, Nazerali L, Frank G L 1992 Metastatic ovarian carcinoma of large intestinal origin simulating primary ovarian carcinoma. American Journal of Clinical Pathology 97: 751–758

de Graaf J, Puyenbroek J I, van der Harten J J 1984 Primary mucinous adenocarcinoma of the appendix with bilateral Krukenberg tumors of the ovary and primary adenocarcinoma of the endometrium. Gynecologic Oncology 19: 358–364

Duarte I, Llanos O 1981 Patterns of metastases in intestinal and diffuse types of carcinoma of the stomach. Human Pathology 12: 237–242

Fichera A, Petty N M, Park R C, Muir P W 1976 Primary adenocarcinoma of the vermiform appendix in gynecologic patient. American Journal of Obstetrics and Gynecology 124: 663–664

Fung M F, Vadas G, Lotocki R, Heywood M, Krepart G 1991 Tubular Krukenberg tumor in pregnancy with virilization. Gynecologic Oncology 41: 81–84

Gallup D G, Stock R J, Sammons J J, Paulk W E 1985 Primary small bowel adenocarcinoma presenting as a malignant ovarian neoplasm. Military Medicine 150: 105–106

Green L K, Silva E G 1989 Hepatoblastoma in an adult with metastases to the ovaries. American Journal of Clinical Pathology 92: 110–115

Hale R W 1968 Krukenberg tumor of the ovaries. A review of 81 records. Obstetrics and Gynecology 32: 221–225

Harcourt K F, Dennis D L 1968 Laparotomy for 'ovarian tumors' in unsuspected carcinoma of the colon. Cancer 21: 1244–1246

Heald J, Buckley C H, Fox H 1979 An immunohistochemical study of the distribution of carcinoembryonic antigen in epithelial tumors of the ovary. Journal of Clinical Pathology 32: 918–926

Herrera-Ornelas L, Natarajan N, Tsukada Y et al 1983 Adenocarcinoma of the colon masquerading as primary ovarian neoplasia. An analysis of ten cases. Diseases of the Colon and Rectum 26: 377–380

Hickey W F, Seiler M W 1981 Ultrastructural markers of colonic adenocarcinoma. Cancer 47: 140–145

Hirschfield L S, Kahn L B, Winkler B, Bochner R Z, Gibstein A A 1985 Adenocarcinoid of the appendix presenting as bilateral Krukenberg's tumor of the ovaries. Archives of Pathology and Laboratory Medicine 109: 930–933

Holtz F, Hart W R 1982 Krukenberg tumors of the ovary. A clinicopathologic analysis of 27 cases. Cancer 50: 2438–2447

Hood I C, Jones B A, Watts J C 1986 Mucinous carcinoid tumor of the appendix presenting as bilateral ovarian tumors. Archives of Pathology and Laboratory Medicine 110: 336–340

Ikeda E, Tsutsumi Y, Yoshida H, Yahagi K 1991 Goblet cell carcinoid of the vermiform appendix with ovarian metastasis mimicking mucinous cystadenocarcinoma. Acta Pathologica Japonica 41: 455–460

Johansson H 1960 Clinical aspects of metastatic ovarian cancer of extragenital origin. Acta Obstetricia et Gynecologica Scandinavica 39: 681–697

Joshi V V 1968 Primary Krukenberg tumor of ovary. Review of literature and case report. Cancer 22: 1199–1207

Lash R H, Hart W R 1987 Intestinal adenocarcinomas metastatic to the ovaries. A clinicopathologic evaluation of 22 cases. American Journal of Surgical Pathology 11: 114–121

MacKeigan J M, Ferguson J A 1979 Prophylactic oophorectomy and colorectal cancer in premenopausal patients. Diseases of the Colon and Rectum 22: 401–405

Mazur M T, Hsueh S, Gersell D J 1984 Metastases to the female genital tract; analysis of 325 cases. Cancer 53: 1978–1984

Merino M J, Edmonds P, LiVolsi V 1985 Appendiceal carcinoma metastatic to the ovaries and mimicking primary ovarian tumors. International Journal of Gynecological Pathology 4: 110–120

Metz S A, Karnei R F, Veach S R, Hoskins W J 1980 Krukenberg carcinoma of the ovary with bone marrow involvement; report of two cases and review of the literature. Obstetrics and Gynecology 55: 99–104

Miller R T, Sarikaya H, Jenison E L 1988 Adenocarcinoid tumor of appendix presenting as unilateral Krukenberg tumor. Journal of Surgical Oncology 37: 65–71

Morrow M, Enker W E 1984 Late ovarian metastases in carcinoma of the colon and rectum. Archives of Surgery 119: 1385–1388

Nashgari M, Behmaram B, Hoffman J S, Carcia J 1992 Primary biliary carcinoma with metastases to the ovary. Gynecologic Oncology 47: 272–274

O'Brien P H, Newton B B, Metcalf J S, Rittenbury M S 1981 Oophorectomy in women with carcinoma of the colon and rectum. Surgery, Gynecology and Obstetrics 153: 827–830

Oortman E H, Elliott J P 1983 Hepatocellular carcinoma metastatic to the ovary: a case report. American Journal of Obstetrics & Gynecology 146: 715–718

Parker R T, Currie J L 1981 Metastatic tumors of ovary. In: Coppleson M (ed) Gynecologic oncology. Churchill Livingstone, Edinburgh, p 731–742

Ramzy I 1976 Signet-ring stromal tumor of ovary: histochemical, light and electronmicroscopic study. Cancer 38: 166–172

Robboy S J, Scully R E, Norris H J 1974 Carcinoid metastatic to the ovary. A clinicopathologic analysis of 35 cases. Cancer 33: 798–811

Saphir O 1951 Signet-ring carcinoma. Military Surgeon 109: 360–369

Scully R E 1979 Tumors of the ovary and maldeveloped gonads. Atlas of tumor pathology. Fascicle 16, 2nd series. Armed Forces Institute of Pathology, Washington, DC, p 323–363

Scully R E, Richardson G S 1961 Luteinization of the stroma of metastatic cancer involving the ovary and its endocrine significance. Cancer 14: 827–840

Serov S F, Scully R E, Sobin L H 1973 Histological typing of ovarian tumors. International histological classification of tumors No. 9. World Health Organization, Geneva, p 51

Takita H, Vincent R G, Caicedo V, Gutierrez A C 1977 Squamous cell carcinoma of the esophagus: a study of 153 cases. Journal of Surgical Oncology 9: 547–554

Talerman A 1984 Carcinoid tumors of the ovary. Journal of Cancer Research and Clinical Oncology 107: 125–135

Thomas R, Barnhill D, Worsham F, Hoskins W 1985 Krukenberg tumor of the ovary from an occult appendiceal primary: case report and literature review. Obstetrics and Gynecology 65: 95s–98s

Ueda G, Sawada M, Ogawa H, Tanizawa O, Tsujimoto M 1993 Immunohistochemical study of cytokeratin 7 for the differential diagnosis of adenocarcinomas in the ovary. Gynecologic Oncology 51: 219–223

Ulbright T M, Roth L M, Stehman F B 1984 Secondary ovarian neoplasia. A clinicopathologic study of 35 cases. Cancer 53: 1164–1174

Vicens E, Martinez-Mora J, Potau N, Sans M, Boix-Ochoa J 1980 Masculinization of a female fetus by Krukenberg tumor during pregnancy. Journal of Pediatric Surgery 15: 188–190

Virieux C 1962 Untersuchungen über Häufigkeit und Entstehungweise von Krebsmetastasen in den Eierstöcken. Gynaecologia 153: 209–224

Webb M J, Decker D G, Mussey E 1975 Cancer metastatic to the ovary; factors influencing survival. Obstetrics and Gynecology 45: 391–396

Wertberg A B, Wertzman S A 1983 Metastatic islet cell carcinoma. A potentially treatable cause of carcinoma of unknown origin. Cancer a Journal for Clinicians 33: 167–171

Wong P C, Ferenczy A, Fan L D, McCaughey E 1986 Krukenberg tumors of the ovary. Ultrastructural, histochemical, and immunohistochemical studies of 15 cases. Cancer 57: 751–760

Woodruff J D, Novak E R 1960 The Krukenberg tumor. Study of 48 cases from the Ovarian Tumor Registry. Obstetrics and Gynecology 15: 351–360

Young R H, Hart W R 1989 Metastases from carcinomas of the pancreas simulating primary mucinous tumors of the ovary. A report of seven cases. American Journal of Surgical Pathology 13: 748–756

Young R H, Scully R E 1990 Ovarian metastases from carcinoma of the gallbladder and extrahepatic bile ducts simulating primary tumors of the ovary. A report of 6 cases. International Journal of Gynecological Pathology 9: 60–72

Young R H, Scully R E 1994 Metastatic tumors of the ovary. In: Kurman RJ (ed) Blaustein's pathology of the female genital tract, 4th edn. Springer-Verlag, New York, p 958

Young R H, Gersell D J, Clement P B, Scully R E 1992 Hepatocellular carcinoma metastatic to the ovary: a report of three cases discovered during life with discussion of the differential diagnosis of hepatoid tumors of the ovary. Human Pathology 23: 574–580

55

Metastatic melanomas, nongenital carcinomas and sarcomas

P. Russell   A. Farnsworth

Metastatic melanoma

Ovarian metastases are present in 16% of women dying with malignant melanoma (das Gupta & Brasfield 1964). They are usually the result of hematogenous spread and occur in a setting of disseminated disease. The ovarian lesions are generally not clinically manifest, but may occasionally present as apparent primary neoplasms (Morrow & di Saia 1976, Silveira et al 1977, Ulbright et al 1984, Fitzgibbons et al 1987, Young & Scully 1991). In countries with a high incidence of cutaneous melanomas, such as Australia, these tumors may constitute up to 10% of surgically resected ovarian metastases. They may present up to 25 years after the primary lesion has been excised (Thiery & Willighagen 1966, Ben David et al 1984). Sometimes the primary lesion undergoes regression or is clinically occult (adrenal gland, eye) and is not identified during life or even by thorough autopsy examination. Rare ovarian melanomas are true primary neoplasms, generally considered to be of teratomatous origin (see Ch. 48).

Macroscopic features

Ovarian metastases of malignant melanoma usually form bilateral, soft, multinodular masses. The involved ovaries are enlarged, averaging 11 cm in diameter. Hemorrhage, cystic degeneration, and necrosis are usually conspicuous, but pigmentation is variable (Fig. 55.1).

Microscopic features

The microscopic features are those of metastatic melanoma elsewhere, but can be extremely variable and can simulate a variety of primary ovarian neoplasms (Fig. 55.2).

Differential diagnosis

Pigmented metastases generally cause no problem in differential diagnosis, particularly if there is a known extraovarian primary lesion. Amelanotic melanomas can be confused with primary or metastatic undifferentiated carcinomas, endometrial stromal sarcomas, primary ovarian undifferentiated small cell carcinomas (see Ch. 31), and dysgerminomas (see Ch. 41). An immunoprofile of S-100 protein, NKI/C3 positivity and cytokeratin negativity, and electron microscopy are the most useful tools for confirming the diagnosis.

A difficult differential diagnosis is between primary and metastatic ovarian melanomas, a distinction of importance since the former are associated with a better prognosis (Fox & Langley 1976, Morrow & Di Saia 1976). Bilaterality is a strong point in favor of metastases. Unilateral tumors associated with teratomatous elements suggest primary ovarian origin. The presence of teratomatous elements in the same ovary is not conclusive evidence, however, that the tumor is primary, since melanomas have been reported to metastasize to mature cystic teratomas (el Minawi & Hori 1973). Conversely, lack of teratomatous elements does not exclude primary ovarian origin, since such evidence may have been obliterated by tumor growth or missed as a result of inadequate sampling. Evidence of primary origin is most convincing if lesions can be demonstrated to arise from a focus of preinvasive melanocytic proliferation such as junctional activity in the cyst lining of a teratoma (see Chs 46, 48). However, this is not

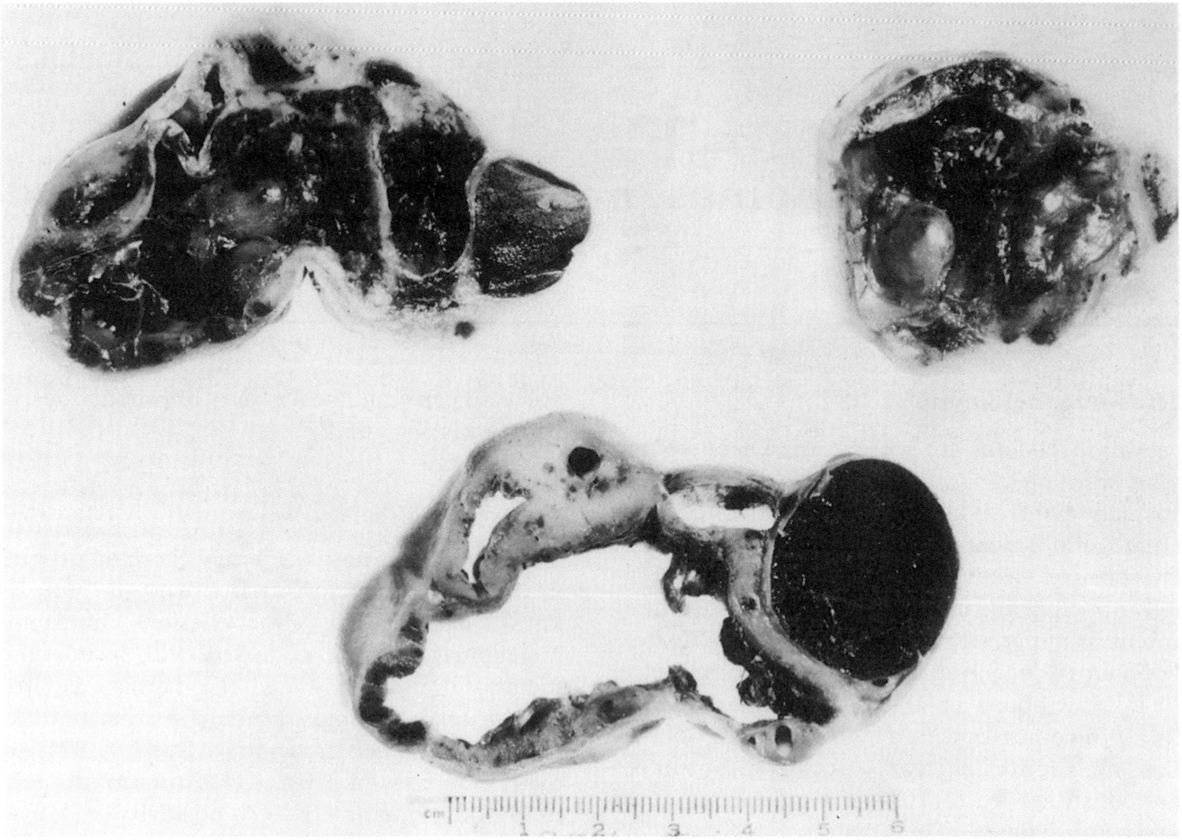

Fig. 55.1 Malignant melanoma metastatic to the ovary of an 18-year-old girl. A skin lesion had been excised a few weeks previously. The large mass is hemorrhagic, cystic, and focally pigmented

necessary for confident diagnosis if other features, including the clinical findings, are consistent with a primary ovarian neoplasm (Tham et al 1981, Gregg 1982, Tsukamoto et al 1986).

Renal tumors

Metastases are found at autopsy in less than 1% of women with renal adenocarcinomas. They rarely present clinical problems, but they can be the initial manifestation of the disease (Martzloff & Manlove 1949, Webb et al 1975, Mazur et al 1984, Spencer et al 1993) or present as isolated secondary lesions many years after nephrectomy (Vorder-Bruegge et al 1957, Adachi et al 1994).

On the rare occasion that clear cell adenocarcinoma of the kidney metastasises to the ovary it must be distinguished from primary ovarian clear cell carcinoma (Young & Hart 1992). Many of the features which usually suggest metastasis to the ovary (e.g. bilaterality, macroscopic appearance of multiple nodules) are not present in these cases. The microscopic features that suggest metastatic renal cell tumor are a characteristic sinusoidal vascular pattern, the absence of hobnail cells lining the tubules and glands, the absence of intraluminal mucin, and hyaline basement-membrane-like material. The only other tumor that could enter the differential diagnosis is a steroid cell tumor, but such neoplasms do not usually have a tubular pattern. Immunohistochemistry is of little help (Young & Hart 1992).

Other urinary tract tumors

There is a solitary report of metastasis from a

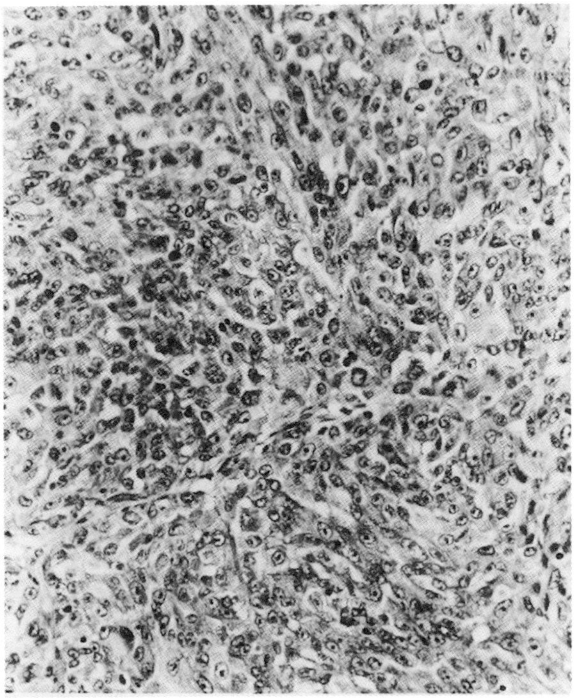

Fig. 55.2 Typical microscopic appearance of metastatic malignant melanoma. Diffuse pattern, large elongate cells, with oval nuclei and single prominent nucleolus. H + E ×200

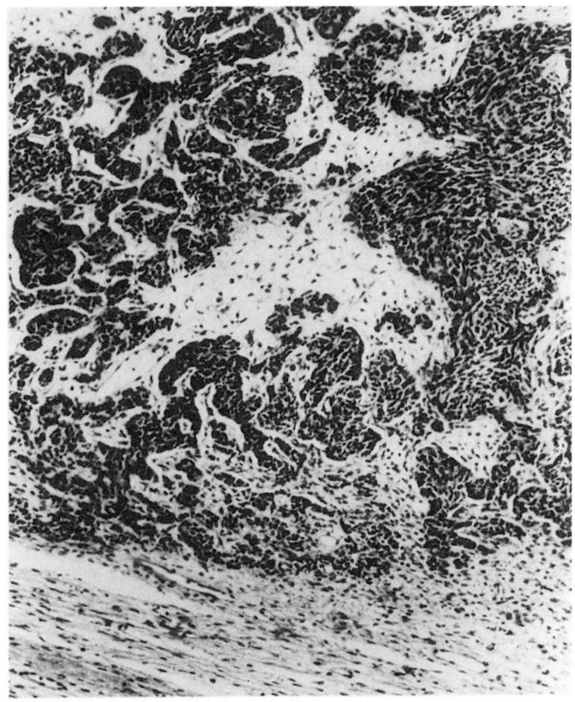

Fig. 55.3 Metastatic small cell undifferentiated carcinoma of the lung, previously treated. The cell groups show central necrosis. Nuclei are hyperchromatic and cytoplasm is scanty. H + E ×80

transitional cell carcinoma of the renal pelvis presenting as a primary ovarian carcinoma (Hsui et al 1991). A Wilm's tumor and a rhabdoid tumor have also been described metastasizing to the ovary where they were confused with ovarian primaries. An adenocarcinoma of the bladder has been reported to present initially as a Krukenberg tumor (Bowlby & Smith 1986).

Lung and mediastinal tumors

Metastases from lung carcinomas have rarely been reported, and have been identified in less than 5% of women with the disease (Abrams et al 1950, Woodruff et al 1970, Webb et al 1975, Mazur et al 1984, Young & Scully 1985), but their frequency may increase as the disease becomes more common in women (Figs 55.3, 55.4). They present considerable diagnostic difficulty if the ovarian lesions become manifest before the lung tumors declare themselves (Young & Scully 1985). Metastatic small cell undifferentiated (oat cell) carcinomas of the lung, the most common type of tumor to metastasize, should not be confused with primary small cell carcinomas of ovary of either 'hypercalcemic type' (see Ch. 31) or 'pulmonary type' (see Chs 24, 25, 28), although the prognosis of all of these tumor types is very poor.

Small cell carcinomas arising in sites other than lung, such as mediastinum, may also metastasize to the ovary (Eichhorn et al 1993). A case of posterior mediastinal neuroblastoma, metastatic to the ovary has also been described (Young et al 1993), as has an example of mediastinal thymoma (Briese & Rohde 1984).

Metastases from endocrine tumors

Carcinomas of the endocrine glands rarely feature in series of metastatic ovarian tumors. Two cases of metastatic thyroid carcinoma are included in the series of Woodruff et al (1970). A case of ovarian metastasis from thyroid carcinoma mimicking struma ovarii has also been reported (Young et al 1994).

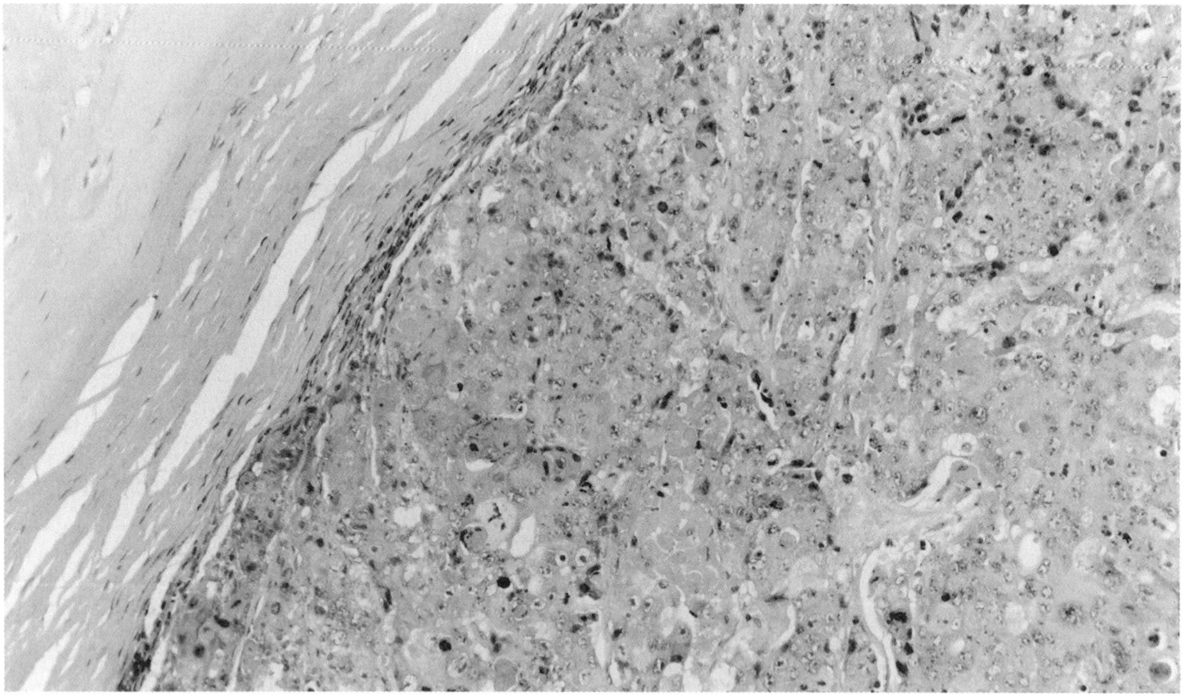

A

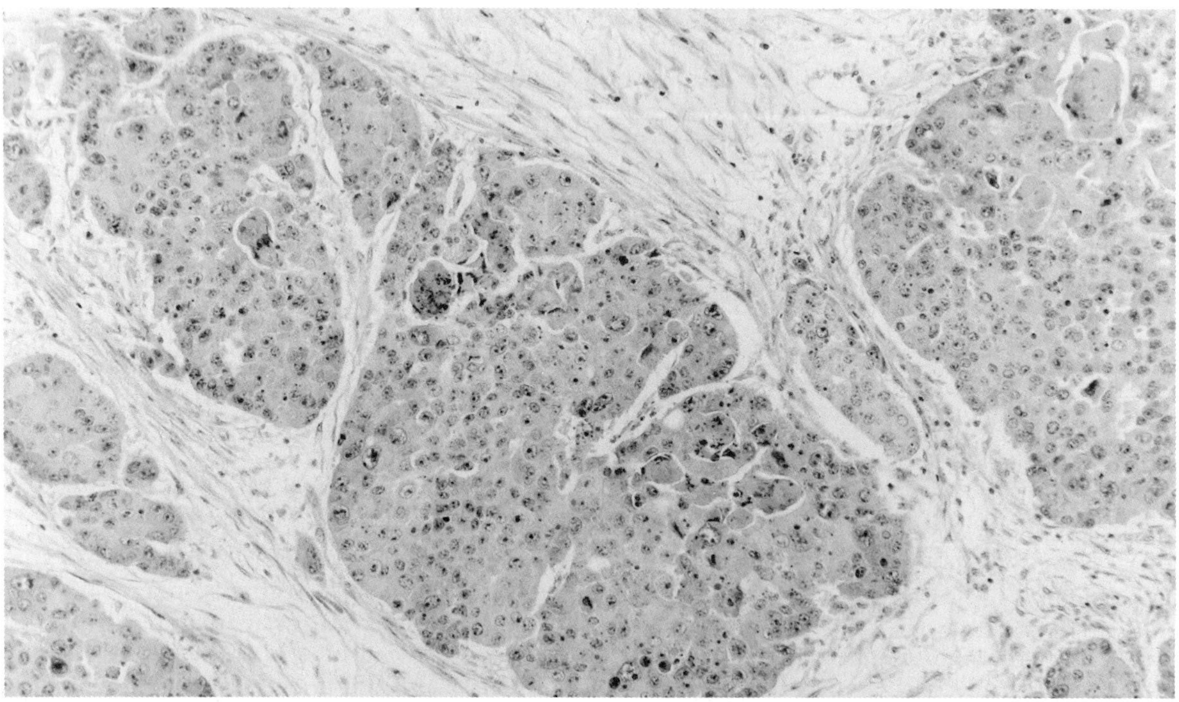

B

Fig. 55.4 Keratinizing squamous carcinoma of lung metastatic to the ovaries in a 44-year-old woman. (A) Primary tumor, adjacent to bronchial cartilage. H + E ×165. (B) Metastatic deposit within right ovary. H + E ×165

Neuroblastoma of the adrenal gland does metastasize to the ovary, but this is usually an autopsy finding (Meyer et al 1979). Rarely, the metastasis can present clinically (Young et al 1993). The typical histological features of neuroblastoma are present. The clinical context is a reliable discriminator between such lesions and the even rarer neuroblastomas primary in the ovary (Kleinman et al 1993).

Extragenital sarcomas

Sarcomas rarely metastasize to the ovaries and are more likely to be primary tumors at that site (see Ch. 52). Reported cases include angiosarcoma (Chen et al 1980, Sedgely et al 1985, Patel et al 1991) (Fig. 55.5), Ewing's sarcoma (Woodruff et al 1970), alveolar rhabdomyosarcoma (Young & Scully 1989), and chordoma (Zukerberg & Young 1990).

In the largest series of sarcomas metastatic to the ovaries, Young & Scully (1990) describe 10 extragenital sarcomas: four leiomyosarcomas (one from stomach, two from small bowel, one from retrovesical tissue); and a single example each of fibrosarcoma of the anterior abdominal wall, sarcoma of the mesentery of smooth muscle or neural type, a hemangiosarcoma of the heart, an osteosarcoma of the maxilla, a chondrosarcoma of the rib, and a Ewing's sarcoma of a pubic bone.

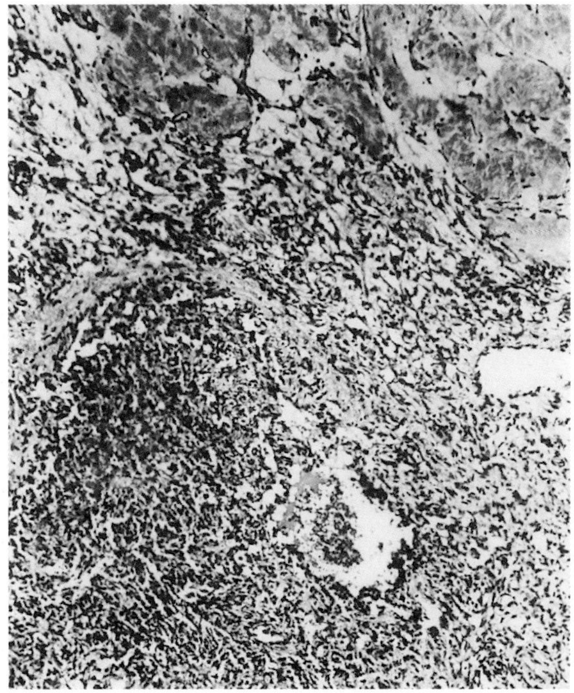

Fig. 55.5 Metastatic angiosarcoma from the breast in a 42-year-old woman. The tumor, which impinges on a corpus albicans (above), consists of a network of small vascular spaces. A larger space (center below) contains numerous red blood cells. H + E ×80

REFERENCES

Abrams H L, Spiro R, Goldstein N 1950 Metastases in carcinoma; analysis of 1000 autopsied cases. Cancer 3: 74–85

Adachi Y, Sasagawa I, Nakada T et al 1994 Bilateral ovarian metastasis from left renal cell carcinoma. Urology International 52: 169–171

Ben David M, Feldberg D, Dicker D, Kessler H, Goldman J A 1984 Ovarian melanoma. An interesting case. International Journal of Gynaecology and Obstetrics 22: 77–79

Bowlby L S, Smith McC L 1986 Signet-ring cell carcinoma of the urinary bladder primary presentation as a Krukenberg tumor. Gynecologic Oncology 25: 376–381

Briese V, Rohde E 1984 Ovarielle Metastasierung eines Thymoms. Zentralblatt für Gynäkologie 106: 472–476

Chen K T K, Kirkegaard D D, Bocian J J 1980 Angiosarcoma of the breast. Cancer 46: 368–371

das Gupta T, Brasfield R 1964 Metastatic melanoma: a clinicopathological study. Cancer 17: 1323–1339

Eichhorn J H, Young R H, Scully R E 1993 Non-pulmonary small cell carcinomas of extragenital origin metastatic to ovary: a report of 7 cases. Cancer 71: 177–186

el Minawi M F, Hori J M 1973 Malignant melanoma in bilateral dermoid cysts of the ovary. International Journal of Gynaecology and Obstetrics 11: 218–222

Fitzgibbons P L, Martin S E, Simmons T J 1987 Malignant melanoma metastatic to the ovary. American Journal of Surgical Pathology 11: 959–964

Fox H, Langley F A 1976 Tumours of the ovary. Heinemann, London, p 300–306

Gregg R H 1982 Primary malignant melanoma arising in an ovarian dermoid cyst. American Journal of Obstetrics and Gynecology 143: 25–26

Hsui J G, Kemp G M, Singer G A, Rawls W H, Siddiky M A 1991 Transitional cell carcinoma of the renal pelvis with ovarian metastasis. Gynecologic Oncology 41: 178–181

Kleinman G M, Young R H, Scully R E 1993 Primary neuroectodermal tumors of the ovary. A report of 25 cases. American Journal of Surgical Pathology 17: 764–778

Martzloff K H, Manlove C H 1949 Vaginal and ovarian metastases from hypernephroma: report of case and review of literature. Surgery, Gynecology, and Obstetrics 88: 145–154

Mazur M T, Hsueh S, Gersell D J 1984 Metastases to the female genital tract; analysis of 325 cases. Cancer 53: 1978–1984

Meyer W H, Yu G W, Milvenan E S, Jeffs R D, Kaizer H, Leventhal B G 1979 Ovarian involvement in neuroblastoma. Medical and Pediatric Oncology 7: 49–54

Morrow C P, di Saia P J 1976 Malignant melanoma of the female genitalia; a clinical analysis. Obstetrical and Gynecological Survey 31: 233–271

Patel T, Ohri S K, Sundaresan M et al 1991 Metastatic angiosarcoma of the ovary. European Journal of Surgical Oncology 17: 295–299

Sedgely M G, Östör A G, Fortune D W 1985 Angiosarcoma of breast metastatic to the ovary and placenta. Australian and New Zealand Journal of Obstetrics and Gynaecology 25: 299–302

Silveira E, Palhares F A B, de Oliveira Filho J A, Alberti O, Alberti V N, Silveira M I G S 1977 Peritonitis following rupture of metastatic malignant melanoma of the ovary. Gynecologic Oncology 5: 305

Spencer J R, Eriksen B, Garnett J E 1993 Metastatic renal tumor presenting as ovarian clear cell carcinoma. Urology 49: 582–584

Tham K T, Ma P H, Kung T M 1981 Malignant melanoma in an ovarian teratoma. Human Pathology 12: 577–579

Thiery M, Willighagen R 1966 Melanoma of the female genital tract. Gynaecologia 161: 466–480

Tsukamoto N, Matsukuma K, Matsumura M, Kamura T, Matsuyama T, Kinjo M 1986 Malignant melanoma arising in a cystic teratoma of the ovary. Gynecologic Oncology 23: 395–400

Ulbright T M, Roth L M, Stehman F B 1984 Secondary ovarian neoplasia. A clinicopathologic study of 35 cases. Cancer 53: 1164–1174

Vorder-Bruegge C F, Hobbs J E, Wegner C R, Winter Mutte R W 1957 Bilateral ovarian metastases from renal adenocarcinoma: report of a case and discussion of pathogenesis. Obstetrics and Gynecology 9: 198–205

Webb M J, Decker D G, Mussey E 1975 Cancer metastatic to the ovary; factors influencing survival. Obstetrics and Gynecology 45: 391–396

Woodruff J D, Murthy Y S, Shaskar T N, Bordbar F, Tseng S S 1970 Metastatic ovarian tumors. American Journal of Obstetrics and Gynecology 107: 202–209

Young R H, Hart W R 1992 Renal cell carcinoma metastatic to the ovary. A report of 3 cases emphasising possible confusion with ovarian clear cell carcinoma. International Journal of Gynecological Pathology 11: 96–104

Young R H Scully R E 1985 Ovarian metastases from cancer of the lung. Problems in interpretation: a report of seven cases. Gynecologic Oncology 21: 337–350

Young R H, Scully R E 1989 Alveolar rhabdomyosarcoma metastatic to the ovary. A report of two cases and a discussion of the differential diagnosis of small cell malignant tumors of the ovary. Cancer 64: 899–904

Young R H, Scully R E 1990 Sarcomas metastatic to the ovary: a report of 21 cases. International Journal of Gynecological Pathology 9: 231–252

Young R H, Scully R E 1991 Malignant melanoma metastatic to the ovary. A clinicopathologic analysis of 20 cases. American Journal of Surgical Pathology 15: 849–860

Young R H, Kozakewich H P W, Scully R E 1993 Metastatic ovarian tumors in children: a report of 14 cases and review of the literature. International Journal of Gynecological Pathology 12: 8–19

Young R H, Jackson A, Wells M 1994 Ovarian metastasis from thyroid carcinoma 12 years after partial thyroidectomy mimicking stroma ovarii: a report of a case. International Journal of Gynecological Pathology 13: 181–185

Zukerberg L R, Young R H 1990 Chordoma metastatic to the ovary. Archives of Pathology and Laboratory Medicine 114: 208–210

56

Lymphomas and leukemias

P. Russell A. Farnsworth

Lymphomas

Ovarian involvement by malignant lymphomas can take three forms.

The first and most common is ovarian involvement in patients with disseminated lymphoma where the ovaries are found to be involved as a secondary phenomenon. Autopsy studies of patients dying of lymphoma have shown such ovarian disease in approximately 25% of cases (Chorlton et al 1974, Scully 1979).

Secondly, the initial presentation of a malignant lymphoma may be as an ovarian mass. Approximately 0.3% of lymphomas present as gonadal disease (Freeman et al 1972). Most of these patients probably have occult nodal involvement (Osborne & Robboy 1983, Ulbright et al 1984), and overt generalized disease usually develops within a short time (Paladugu et al 1980, Talerman 1982).

Thirdly, malignant lymphoma may arise in the ovaries as a primary extranodal lymphoma. This diagnosis is only made where staging and follow-up studies show no evidence of any systemic disease. Although there has been skepticism about the occurrence of such an entity, given the lack of a normal lymphocyte population in the ovaries (Halpin 1975, Osborne & Robboy 1983), rare but well-documented reports in the literature support the existence of primary ovarian lymphoma (Monterosso et al 1993, Boyle et al 1991, Imaizumi et al 1993). A solitary case has been reported as a collision tumor with a proliferating serous ovarian cystadenoma (Skodras et al 1994). Fox et al (1988) recommend that the diagnosis be made with caution inasmuch as such lymphomas are so rare that for therapeutic purposes all primary malignant lymphomas should be regarded as local manifestations of systemic disease.

The age of patients with *malignant lymphoma initially manifesting in the ovaries* is similar to that of patients with equivalent nodal disease. This varies more in relation to the histological type rather than the anatomical site affected. Thus diffuse lymphomas are most common in the 35–45 year age group, while nodular lymphomas are more often found in older women. First presentation may occur during pregnancy (Jones et al 1980, Rotmensch & Woodruff 1982). Burkitt's lymphoma (both endemic and sporadic) typically affects children in the age group 5–10 years.

Presentation is similar to that of other ovarian tumors, namely an abdominal or pelvic mass, often accompanied by pain. Ascites is not unusual. Less commonly, the tumors are incidental findings at routine pelvic examination or surgery for other indications (Osborne & Robboy 1983). In patients with apparent initial gonadal disease only, staging procedures reveal that in 27–64% the disease is more advanced than FIGO stage 1 (Chorlton et al 1974, Paladugu et al 1980, Osborne & Robboy 1983).

All types of lymphoma have been reported to occur in the ovary. *Hodgkin's disease* presenting as an ovarian lesion is extremely rare and can be of mixed cellularity (Bare & McCloskey 1961, Long & Patchefsky 1971, Chorlton et al 1974) or unspecified type (Rotmensch & Woodruff 1982). It is uncommonly encountered even in autopsy series, being found in less than 5% compared with approximately 25% of other lymphoma patients (Scully 1979). All types of non-Hodgkin's lymphoma have been described, with a preponderance of diffuse lymphomas of B cell type (Paladugu et al 1980, Rotmensch & Woodruff 1982, Osborne & Robboy 1983, Montcrroso et al 1993). Burkitt's lymphoma (small noncleaved cell, Working Formulation) is relatively well represented because of its propensity for extranodal involvement (Jones et al 1980). In fact, bilateral massive ovarian enlargement is a classical manifestation of this disease and occurs in approximately 50% of patients at some stage (Jones et al 1980, Talerman 1982, Konji et al 1989). Involvement of the ovaries by plasma cell dyscrasias is even rarer than other lymphoproliferative disorders. Infiltration by *multiple myeloma* has been observed at autopsy, and there are very rare reports of primary plasmacytoma of ovary (Talerman 1982, Hautzer 1984, Cook & Boylston 1988).

Survival rates for patients with lymphoma presenting in the ovaries is poor. In a recent study of 39 patients (Monterroso et al 1993), 40% were alive at time of last follow-up. A similar study of 34 patients reported 19 of these dying, usually within 1 year of diagnosis (Fox et al 1988).

Macroscopic features

Malignant lymphomas presenting as ovarian disease are bilateral in 50% of cases, irrespective of stage (Chorlton et al 1974, Scully 1979, Rotmensch & Woodruff 1982, Osborne & Robboy 1983). Burkitt's lymphoma is almost always bilateral. The ovarian tumors range from 2 to 25 cm in diameter, with most in the range 8–15 cm. In disseminated lymphoma affecting the ovaries, they may be of normal size or only slightly enlarged (Talerman 1982) (Fig. 56.1).

The ovaries are usually free of adhesions, and show a nodular or bosselated surface. The cut surface shows uniform pale gray-white to tan tissue with a rubbery or fleshy consistency. Gross edema (Fig. 56.2), small foci of necrosis, cystic degeneration, and hemorrhage may all be present in the cut surface, but they are rarely conspicuous features. Although the ovaries appear to be preferentially infiltrated relative to the remainder of the female genital tract (Rotmensch & Woodruff 1982), other organs, especially the adjacent fallopian tubes, may also appear swollen and edematous owing to peritoneal or interstitial infiltration.

Microscopic features

Characteristically there is a diffuse monotonous infiltrate of neoplastic lymphoid cells with a superimposed nodularity in selected subtypes (Fig. 56.3). The infiltrate of diffuse lymphomas often form cords, sometimes only one cell thick. The malignant cells may infiltrate and surround structures (e.g. pre-existing follicles, corpora lutea, corpora albicantes) without destroying them; blood vessel walls are also invaded in this way (Fig. 56.4). The nodular lymphomas may demonstrate bands of fibrous tissue or even dense sclerotic areas. Microscopic foci of necrosis, in addition to those evident macroscopically, may be seen. In high grade tumors with rapid cell turnover (e.g. diffuse large cell, lymphoblastic and especially Burkitt's lymphoma), the presence of large macrophages dispersed among the tumor cells leads to a 'starry-sky' appearance. Cytology of the lymphomatous cells is that of the corresponding lesions in lymph nodes (Fig. 56.5). Immunohistochemically, lymphoma cells are EMA negative and LCA positive, characteristics shared by the leukemias but not by the other tumors listed in the differential diagnosis below.

To distinguish the various subtypes of malignant lymphoma, special stains may be necessary, e.g. methyl green pyronin and immunophenotyping for immunoglobulins, light chains, Ki-1, and T and B cell markers. The reader is referred to the standard texts for further details (Linden et al 1988). Imprint preparations from fresh tumor tissue may be very useful; Romanowsky-stained slides will be helpful in identifying the cytoplasmic lipid vacuoles in Burkitt's lymphoma and also the granules of leukemic cells. Electron microscopy can be used to subtype lymphomas and aid in the differential diagnosis of the lesions listed below. However, even when these supplementary techniques are available, a thin, well-cut, well-stained H + E section probably remains the most useful tool in diagnosis.

Differential diagnosis

Leukemias may present macroscopic and microscopic features indistinguishable from those of lymphomas. LCA is positive in both. A Leder

A

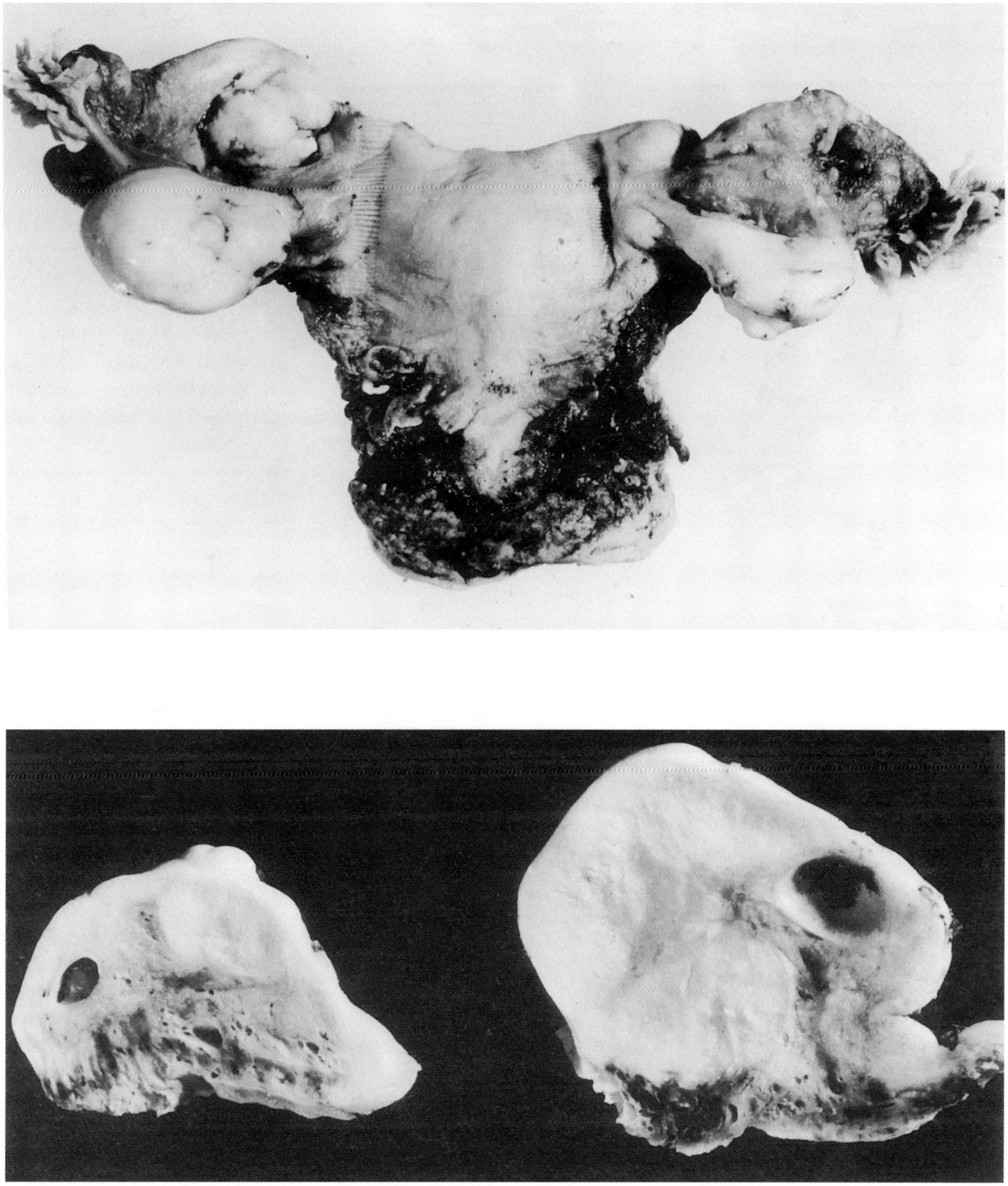

B

Fig. 56.1 Uterus and adnexa from postmenopausal woman with disseminated lymphoma. (A) Left ovary is slightly enlarged and tumor nodules are apparent on surfaces of both fallopian tubes and right ovary. (B) Sectioned ovaries from same case showing cortical infiltration by homogeneous white tumor tissue

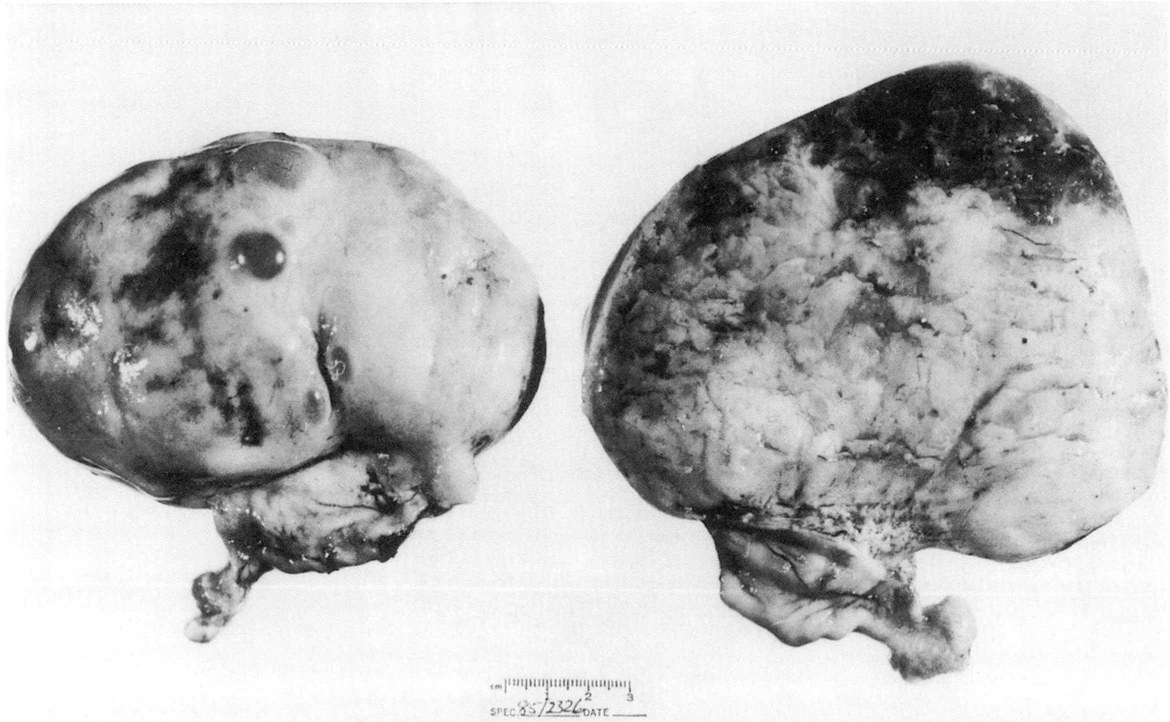

A

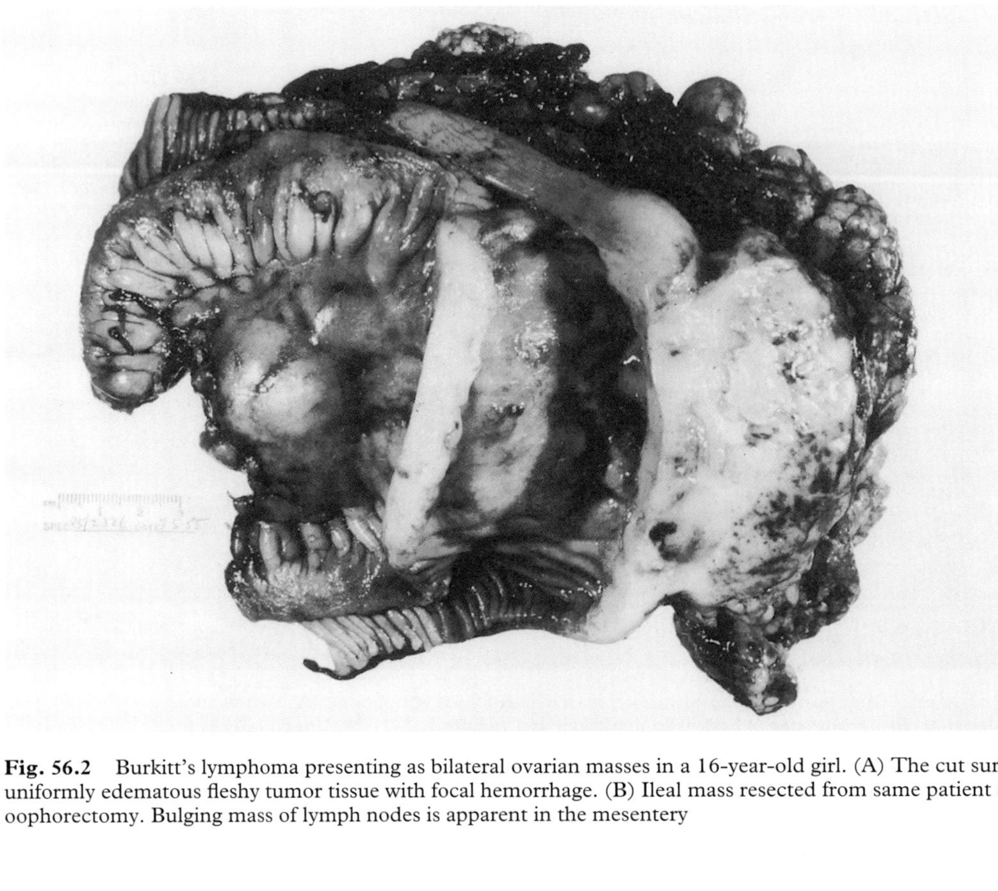

B

Fig. 56.2 Burkitt's lymphoma presenting as bilateral ovarian masses in a 16-year-old girl. (A) The cut surface (right) shows uniformly edematous fleshy tumor tissue with focal hemorrhage. (B) Ileal mass resected from same patient at time of bilateral oophorectomy. Bulging mass of lymph nodes is apparent in the mesentery

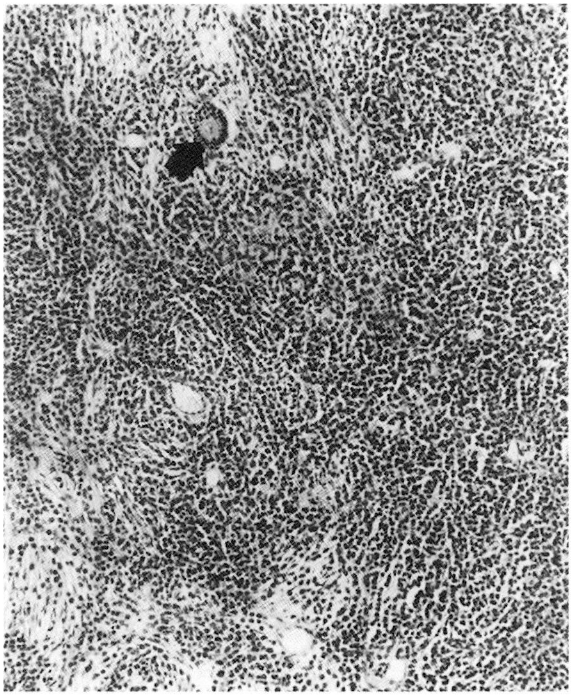

Fig. 56.3 Malignant lymphoma (Burkitt's lymphoma – same case as Fig. 56.2). Monotonous infiltrate of uniform lymphoid cells, focally in linear arrangements. Arrow marks a primary follicle. H + E ×80

stain for naphthol-AS-D-chloroacetate esterase activity or immunohistochemical stain for lysozyme are useful in identifying cells of granulocytic lineage, providing neoplastic cells of sufficient differentiation are present (see below). Imprints from fresh tumor tissue stained by a Romanowsky technique can facilitate the identification of any cytoplasmic granulation in myeloid leukemic cells. Electron microscopy can also be helpful in this regard. A clinical diagnosis of leukemia based on peripheral blood or bone marrow findings clinches the diagnosis.

Referral centers have found that the diagnosis of ovarian lymphomas is often missed initially, frequently as a result of poor histological technique (Osborne & Robboy 1983). The nonhemopoietic tumors most commonly confused with lymphomas are granulosa cell tumors and dysgerminomas; others are metastatic carcinomas and primary undifferentiated small cell carcinomas. In children embryonal rhabdomyosarcomas and neuroblastomas may also have to be considered.

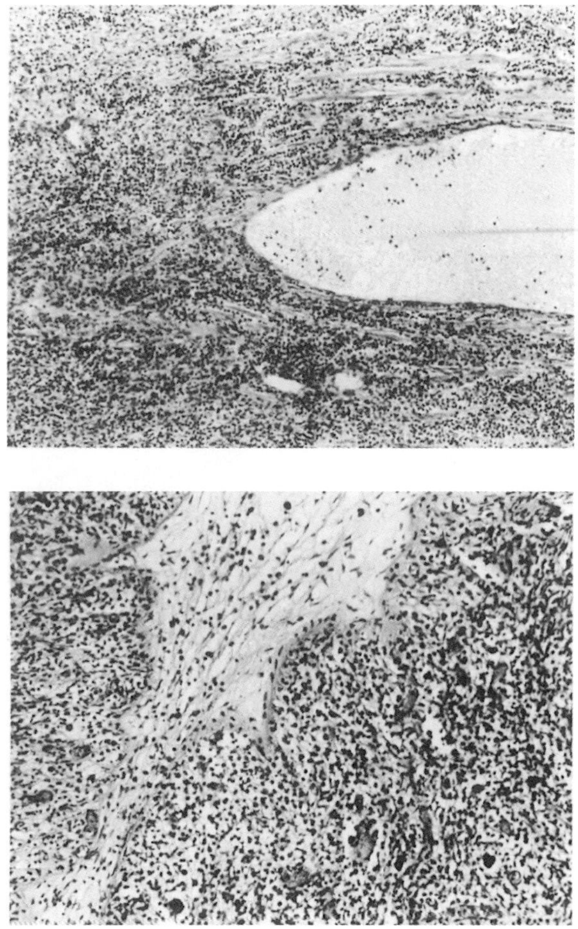

A

B

Fig. 56.4 Malignant lymphoma (large cell type) infiltrating but not destroying ovarian structures. (A) Wall of vein in hilus. H + E ×64. (B) Atretic follicle. H + E ×64

Granulosa cell tumors (see Ch. 33) occur over as wide an age range as that of lymphomas, but most patients will have some clinical or pathological evidence of endocrine dysfunction such as abnormal uterine bleeding or endometrial hyperplasia. The tumors are rarely bilateral (5%) and are often hemorrhagic with prominent cystic areas, features unusual in lymphomas. Although the diffuse or sarcomatoid areas of granulosa cell tumors may closely resemble ovarian lymphomas, examination of many sections will almost always reveal some of the other more specific patterns such as follicular and trabecular. Call–Exner bodies should not be confused with the 'starry-sky' pattern of Burkitt's and some other lymphomas.

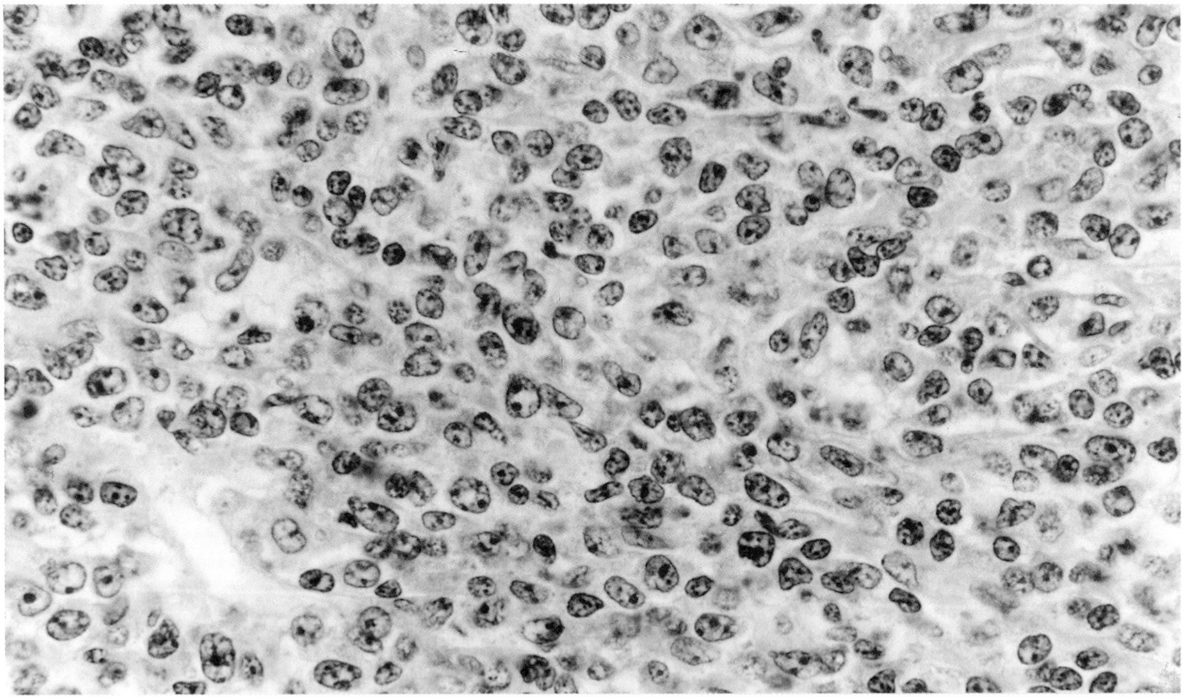

Fig. 56.5 Malignant diffuse large cleaved B-cell lymphoma in ovary. H + E ×330

Nuclear clefting may be seen in both tumors, but very deep longitudinal grooves are seen only in granulosa cell tumors. Nucleoli are not prominent, and the mitotic rate is usually low. The relevant immunoprofile of granulosa cell tumors includes LCA-negative and vimentin- and inhibin-positive staining. The distinction between the granulosa cell tumors and lymphomas can also be readily made by electron microscopy. Lymphomas are characterized by the total absence of intercellular junctions and paucity of intracytoplasmic organelles, except in the plasmacytoid variants in which abundant rough endoplasmic reticulum is found. Granulosa cell tumors have intercellular junctions and abundant external lamina, accumulations of which are present in Call–Exner bodies, together with nuclear debris (Table 56.1).

Table 56.1 Differential diagnosis: lymphoma versus granulosa cell tumor

Lymphoma	Granulosa cell tumor
Clinical	
50% bilateral	5% bilateral
No endocrine function	Often estrogenic
Usually rapidly progressive	Indolent course
Macroscopic	
Pale, fleshy, or rubbery	Soft hemorrhagic, often cystic
Microscopic	
Nuclei pleiomorphic, sometimes cleft	Nuclei bland, uniform; deep groove in half of cases
Nucleoli often prominent	Nucleoli inconspicuous
Mitoses variable, but usually conspicuous	Mitoses variable, but usually infrequent
'Starry-sky' sometimes	Call–Exner bodies usually
Immunohistochemical	
LCA positive	LCA negative Vimentin positive Inhibin positive

Dysgerminomas (see Ch. 41) are unusual in patients older than 30 years, and are uncommonly bilateral. Although they exhibit a diffuse growth pattern as in lymphomas, there may be some fine septa which contain mature lymphocytes and plasma cells and sometimes small epithelioid granulomas. Dysgerminoma cells are large and have distinct cell membranes; the nuclei are central, large, and vesicular with a prominent central nucleolus and a moderate amount of clear cytoplasm containing PAS-positive material (glycogen).

Table 56.2 Differential diagnosis: lymphoma versus dysgerminoma

Lymphoma	Dysgerminoma
Clinical	
50% bilateral	10% bilateral (plus 5% microscopic)
Most >35 years	Rare >35 years
Microscopic	
Nuclei pleiomorphic, sometimes cleft	Nuclei regular, round to oval
Cells poorly cohesive	Cell borders distinct
Cytoplasm scanty, sometimes basophilic	Cytoplasm moderate, poorly stained with H + E but PAS positive
Immunohistochemical	
LCA positive	LCA negative
	Placental alkaline phosphatase positive

Table 56.3 Differential diagnosis: lymphoma versus metastatic carcinoma

Lymphoma	Metastatic carcinoma
Macroscopic	
Single mass	Multiple nodules
Fleshy or rubbery texture	Granular and friable
Necrosis inconspicuous	Necrosis common
Microscopic	
Cytoplasm usually scanty, sometimes basophilic	Cytoplasm moderate amount, often acidophilic
Fibrous septa sometimes	Desmoplasia frequent
Reticulin sparse or around single cells	Reticulin around cell groups
Occasional necrotic cells	Obvious necrotic foci
Immunohistochemical	
LCA positive	LCA negative
EMA negative	EMA positive
	Cytokeratin positive

The nuclei in dysgerminomas are never convoluted. Dysgerminomas may resemble immunoblastic lymphomas, but the latter will demonstrate poor cellular cohesion, nuclei which are often eccentric, and strongly pyroninophilic cytoplasm. Dysgerminoma cells are LCA negative and placental alkaline phosphatase positive (Table 56.2). Electron microscopy is useful for confirming the primitive germ cell features of dysgerminoma.

Metastatic carcinomas (see Ch. 53) are most likely to be encountered in patients of middle or advanced years, but are rarely encountered in the absence of a history of carcinoma elsewhere. The tumors, like those of lymphomas, are frequently bilateral. However, metastatic tumors are often composed of multiple nodules rather than a diffuse infiltration, and central necrotic foci are more likely to be encountered. Metastatic poorly differentiated carcinomas (especially mammary) may be arranged in sheets or cords, as in lymphomas, but a desmoplastic stromal reaction favors the former diagnosis. Infiltrating carcinomas destroy and obliterate pre-existing structures, whereas these are often preserved in lymphomas. Carcinoma cells are usually more cohesive than those of lymphomas, and a small amount of mucin may be demonstrable either in the cytoplasm or the very rare acini. Reticulin stains demonstrate fibers around groups of cells, whereas in lymphomas reticulin fibers are either present around individual cells or are very sparse throughout. Immunohistochemical stains for EMA and cytokeratins are positive, and those for LCA are negative (Table 56.3). The diagnosis can be confirmed by electron microscopy, which reveals intercellular attachments as well as intra- and intercellular acinar-like spaces, albeit sparse.

Metastatic undifferentiated small cell carcinomas of pulmonary or other origin rarely present as a clinical diagnostic problem, but can simulate lymphomas histologically, with their diffuse pattern of small cells displaying scanty cytoplasm and dense hyperchromatic nuclei with a high mitotic rate. Necrosis is more conspicuous than in lymphomas, and includes the characteristic zones of smudgy haematoxylinophilic debris. The cytoplasm often stains positively for NSE, and electron microscopy can be used to identify the neurosecretory granules.

Primary small cell carcinomas of 'hypercalcaemic type' (see Ch. 31) occur in young women (mean age 22 years, Dickersin et al 1982). All reported cases have been unilateral. Their growth pattern is diffuse, insular, or trabecular. The closely packed cells have scanty cytoplasm and small round to oval nuclei with solitary nucleoli. There is usually prominent necrosis and a high mitotic rate which exceeds that usually associated with lymphomas. Tumor cells are LCA and EMA negative. The electron microscopic features are not as yet sufficiently well characterized to be useful in differential diagnosis.

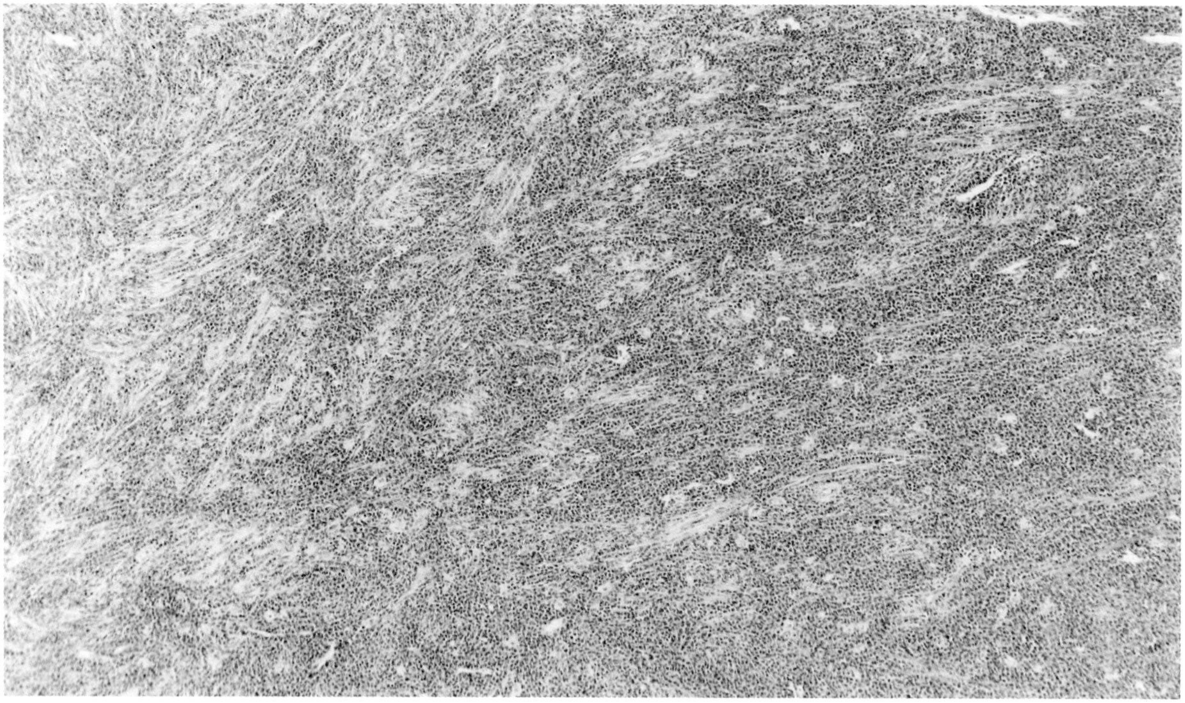

A

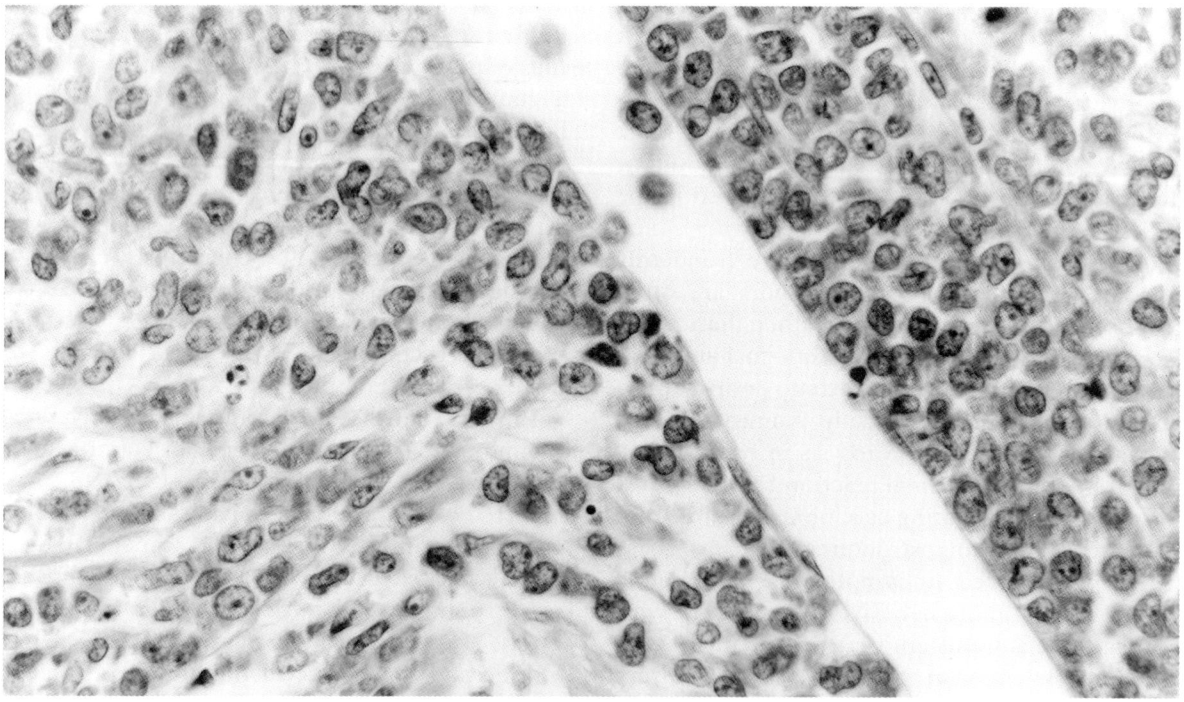

B

Fig. 56.6 Leukemic infiltrate in right ovary from a patient with acute myeloblastic leukemia. (A) There is a very fine trabecular pattern, with ribbons only one cell thick (left) merging with a more diffuse pattern (right). H + E ×33. (B) Ill-defined granular cytoplasm is present, but the granularity is not demonstrable without recourse to chloroacetate esterase or Giemsa staining. H + E ×330

Chronic oophoritis is unlikely to be confused with ovarian lymphoma. Heavy diffuse lymphocytic inflammatory infiltrates with pseudolymphomatous qualities have not been reported in the ovaries. Chronic inflammatory infiltrates are likely to have a mixed cellular population and will not demonstrate malignant cytological characteristics. Other stigmas of pelvic inflammation, such as salpingitis and adhesions, are invariably present.

Leukemias

Ovarian infiltration occurs more commonly in patients with leukemias than with lymphomas, and is more often seen in children than in adults. Ovarian infiltration at autopsy has been found in up to 66% of leukemic patients (Reid & Marsden 1980, Talerman 1982, Yamamoto et al 1991). The more recent studies have yielded higher rates, possibly reflecting longer survival times with modern therapeutic regimes. However, any clinical enlargement of the ovaries in leukemic patients is rare. Myeloid leukemias are encountered more frequently than the lymphocytic types (Scully 1979, Chan et al 1980, Talerman 1982), but ovarian involvement in relapses of acute lymphoblastic leukemia is described (Paris et al 1991). An ovarian tumor may be the initial presentation of leukemia or herald a relapse (Obeid et al 1979, Chan et al 1980, Osborne & Robboy 1983). Extramedullary tumor-like masses of leukemic cells are called granulocytic sarcomas (formerly called 'chloromas' because of their greenish hue). Hematological investigations usually reveal leukemia but, rarely, a leukemic picture may not develop for some time and even be absent at the time of death, although the bone marrow may reveal infiltration (Chorlton et al 1974, Scully 1979, Maggliocco et al 1991, Pressler et al 1992). The prognosis of leukemias initially presenting as an ovarian tumor is poor (Osborne & Robboy 1983), as it is for other extramedullary lesions, and generalized disease develops within a few months (Neiman et al 1981).

Macroscopic features

These do not differ from those of lymphomas, although some tumors have a greenish tinge, which is best seen when the tissue is fresh. Bilateral involvement is frequent.

Microscopic features

The histological features can closely mimic those of ovarian lymphomas. Diffuse monotonous cellular infiltrates are present, sometimes with cord-like formations as in the diffuse lymphomas (Fig. 56.6A). Leukemic infiltrates may also surround and invade follicular structures without destroying them. In the autopsy study by Reid & Marsden (1980) most involved ovaries showed preservation of oocytes. The nuclear features are those of the corresponding blast cells in the leukemic bone marrow. The folded nuclei of myeloid leukemic cells may imitate the cleft or irregularly shaped nuclei of some lymphomas (Fig. 56.6B). In myeloid leukemias, cytoplasmic granulation may be apparent in the H + E stained sections, but identification can be aided by PAS or Giemsa stains, which will highlight neutrophilic and eosinophilic precursors, respectively. Myeloid differentiation can also be demonstrated by the Leder stain for naphthol-AS-D-chloroacetate esterase activity or an immunohistochemical stain for lysozyme. Lysozyme has been reported to produce a higher yield of positive results (89% versus 75%), especially in Zenker fixed or acid decalcified sections (Neiman et al 1981). Giemsa and PAS stains can also help (to a limited degree) in identifying cells of the eosinophilic and neutrophilic series. All these stains will only be helpful if sufficient cellular differentiation is present to provide a positive reaction. Imprints of fresh tumor tissue stained by a Romanowsky technique can be useful in identifying cytoplasmic granules, and can also provide very clear nuclear cytological detail. Electron microscopy can be employed to search for the sparse granules of poorly differentiated leukemias.

Differential diagnosis

Since leukemias share many clinical and pathological features with lymphomas, the differential diagnosis for the latter is applicable. The discrimination of lymphomas from leukemias is also discussed above.

REFERENCES

Bare W W, McCloskey J F 1961 Primary Hodgkin's disease of the ovary. Report of a case. Obstetrics and Gynecology 17: 477–480

Boyle F M, Taylor K M, Bell J R 1991 Ovarian follicular non-Hodgkin's lymphoma. Pathology 23: 164–166

Chan E Y C, Glassberg A B, Rosenblum M A 1980 Chloroma. Rare manifestation of acute leukemia. Postgraduate Medicine 67: 125–130

Chorlton I, Norris H J, King F M 1974 Malignant reticuloendothelial disease involving the ovary as a primary manifestation. A series of 19 lymphomas and 1 granulocytic sarcoma. Cancer 34: 307–407

Cook H T, Boylston A W 1988 Plasmacytoma of the ovary. Gynecologic Oncology 29: 378–381

Fox H, Langley F A, Govan A D, Hill A S, Bennett M H 1988 Malignant lymphoma presenting as an ovarian tumor: a clinicopathological analysis of 34 cases. British Journal of Obstetrics and Gynaecology 95: 386–390

Freeman C, Berg J W, Cutler S J 1972 Occurrence and prognosis of extranodal lymphomas. Cancer 29: 252–260

Halpin T F 1975 Gynecologic implications of Burkitt's tumor. Obstetrical and Gynecological Survey 30: 351–358

Hautzer N W 1984 Primary plasmacytoma of ovary. Gynecologic Oncology 18: 115–118

Imaizumi E, Seki K, Kikudu Y et al 1993 Primary ovarian lymphoma. A case report. Archives of Gynecology and Obstetrics 252: 209–213

Jones D E D, d'Avignon M B, Lawrence R, Latshaw R F 1980 Burkitt's lymphoma: obstetric and gynecologic aspects. Obstetrics and Gynecology 56: 533–536

Konji J C, Otolonin E O, Odukoya O A, Ladipo O A, Ogunniyi J 1989 Burkitt's lymphoma of ovary in Nigerian adults – a 27 year review. African Hospital Medicine and Medical Science 18: 301–305

Linden M D, Tubb R R, Fishlede A J, Hart W R 1988 Immunotypic and genetypic characterisation of non-Hodgkin's lymphomas of ovary. American Journal of Clinical Pathology 90: 156–162

Long J P, Patchefsky A S 1971 Primary Hodgkin's disease of the ovary. A case report. Obstetrics and Gynecology 38: 680–682

Magliocco Q M, Demetrick D J, Jones A R, Kossakowska A E 1991 Granulocytic sarcoma of the ovary. An unusual presentation. Archives of Pathology and Laboratory Medicine 115: 830–834

Monterroso V, Jaffe E S, Merino M J, Medeiros L J 1993 Malignant lymphomas involving the ovary: a clinicopathological analysis of 39 cases. American Journal of Surgical Pathology 17: 154–170

Neiman R S, Barcos M, Berard C et al 1981 Granulocytic sarcoma: a clinicopathologic study of 61 biopsied cases. Cancer 48: 1426–1437

Obeid D, Cotter P, Sturdee D W 1979 Acute leukaemia relapse presenting as ovarian tumor. British Journal of Obstetrics and Gynaecology 86: 578–580

Osborne B M, Robboy S J 1983 Lymphomas or leukemia presenting as ovarian tumors. An analysis of 42 cases. Cancer 52: 1933–1943

Paladugu R R, Bearman R M, Rappaport H 1980 Malignant lymphoma with primary manifestation in the gonad. A clinicopathologic study of 38 patients. Cancer 45: 561–571

Paris R C, Kim T H, Zwiren G T, Ragab A H 1991 Ovarian tumors in relapsing acute lymphoblastic leukaemia: a review of 23 cases. Journal of Pediatric Surgery 26: 70–74

Pressler H, Horny H P, Wolf A, Kaiserling E 1992 Isolated granulocytic sarcoma of the ovary: histologic electron microscopic and immunohistochemical findings. International Journal of Gynecological Pathology 11: 68–74

Reid H, Marsden H B 1980 Gonadal infiltration in children with leukaemia and lymphoma. Journal of Clinical Pathology 33: 722–729

Rotmensch J, Woodruff J D 1982 Lymphoma of the ovary: report of twenty new cases and update of previous series. American Journal of Obstetrics and Gynecology 143: 870–875

Scully R E 1979 Tumors of the ovary and maldeveloped gonads. Atlas of tumor pathology. Fascicle 16, 2nd series. Armed Forces Institute of Pathology, Washington, DC, p 346–352

Skodras G, Fields V, Kragel P J 1994 Ovarian lymphoma and serous carcinoma of low malignant potential arising in the same ovary. A case report with literature review of 14 primary ovarian lymphomas. Archives of Pathology and Laboratory Medicine 118: 647–650

Talerman A 1982 Mesenchymal tumors and malignant lymphoma of the ovary. In: Blaustein A (ed) Pathology of the female genital tract, 2nd edn. Springer-Verlag, New York, p 561–580

Ulbright T M, Roth L M, Stehman F B 1984 Secondary ovarian neoplasia: a clinicopathologic study of 35 cases. Cancer 53: 1164–1174

Yamamoto K, Akiyama H, Maruyama T, Sakamaki H, Onozawa Y, Kawaguchi K 1991 Granulocytic sarcoma of the ovary in patients with acute myelogenous leukaemia. American Journal of Hematology 38: 223–225

SECTION 9

Preoperative and intraoperative diagnosis

57

Intraoperative cytological diagnosis

J. Philips

A variety of cytological investigations, including fine needle biopsies of tumor masses, cyst aspirates, ascitic fluids (including peritoneal washings), and smears of peritoneal surfaces, have been reported to show varying degrees of reliability in the assessment of ovarian pathology (Buckley 1989, Jadhon et al 1990, Nunez & Diaz 1992, di Bonito et al 1993, Sheombar et al 1993, Layfield & Berek 1994). These investigations, however, fall outside the framework of the present text.

Intraoperative cytological assessment is a simple and well-documented alternative or complementary investigation to frozen section diagnosis (Dudgeon & Patrick 1927, Godwin 1976, Bloustein & Silverberg 1977, Abrahams 1978, Abrams & Silverberg 1989, Oneson et al 1989, Nochomovitz et al 1989, Guarda 1990). It enhances the intraoperative consultative process and hence the pathologist's ability to assist patient management. It is, in addition, a skill which is in the reach of every practising pathologist.

INDICATIONS, APPLICATIONS AND ADVANTAGES

The speed and ease of acquiring high-quality preparations for examination are central to the success of this technique in the intraoperative consultative setting. Cytological samples can virtually always be used in association with frozen section examination to provide superior cellular morphology, devoid of freezing artifact. The method may replace frozen section examination, particularly when an infective condition is suspected clinically, or the tissue sample received is very small or heavily calcified. It also allows for rapid sampling of many areas of the gross specimen. This is particularly useful if the lesional tissue is not uniform in appearance, or where the neoplastic component is small. Numerous lymph nodes may be similarly rapidly examined for metastatic involvement. In the presence of extensive necrosis, viable tumor may be identified (prior to fixation of the gross specimen) for further special investigations, e.g. flow cytometry, hormone receptor analysis, immunocytochemical and ultrastructural studies, molecular genetic studies, and magnetic resonance spectroscopy. The differentiation of non-neoplastic abnormalities from neoplasms, and even an accurate decision on tumor type may, with experience, frequently be made in association with the clinical history and macroscopic findings without recourse to frozen section examination.

LIMITATIONS

The main limitation is obviously related to the relative lack of architectural features in cytological preparations. However, patterns of certain cellular arrangements may be identified, adding to the overall criteria used for diagnosis. Nonetheless, the identification of *invasion* (e.g. in epithelial tumors) is obviously dependent on *histological criteria,* and the cytological preparation in this setting is only a complimentary investigation.

TECHNIQUES

Following removal of excess blood saline or cyst fluid by gentle blotting, there are three main methods of slide preparation recognized. Imprinting, as performed in lymph nodes, may be used on soft and very cellular lesions, or if the tissue received is extremely small. 'Squash' preparations, often the practice of neuropathologists, may cause crush artifact of the cells if the action of spreading is heavy-handed. Scraping (Nochomovitz et al 1989) is probably the method of choice, although various combinations of all three methods may be practised, depending on the nature of the material received. With this third technique, described by Nochomovitz et al (1989), the tissue is scraped three or four times with a clean dry scalpel blade. The suspended cells are distributed by the angled blade being drawn unidirectionally slowly across the slide. Depending on the cellularity of the specimen, a number of streaks can be fanned across the slide. Scraping is the method we have used most commonly on ovarian lesions.

The preparations may be wet fixed with 95% alcohol or air dried. Immersion into the fixative must be rapid with wet fixation. Equally, air drying cannot be delayed as, in either event, fixation of the cells will be suboptimal.

The wet fixed smears are stained with a 'rapid' hematoxylin and eosin (H + E) stain (i.e. that used for frozen sections), thus allowing comparison between the cytological and histological preparations. The Diff-Quik stain (modified Wright method) is used for air-dried smears. The characteristics of extracellular and stromal elements and cytoplasmic products, other than keratin, are accentuated by the Diff-Quik stain. The nuclear features are best seen with the H + E stain, which is also the stain of choice for the examination of keratinized cells and predominantly necrotic lesions.

INTERPRETATION

Interpretation is dependent on a skill which requires visual experience. The cytological appearance of a range of ovarian lesions is therefore demonstrated by illustrations. Relevant comparisons to the histological counterparts are made to accentuate certain features.

Dysfunctional cysts (Ch. 12)

As noted in Chapter 12, there is a significant risk of overcalling cellular aspirates of nonluteinized or partly luteinized dysfunctional cysts when the gross appearance of the cyst is unknown to the pathologist or when contamination of the cyst fluid has occurred (Nadji et al 1979, Nunez & Diaz 1992). This is less of a problem in the setting of an intraoperative consultation, where the smooth featureless lining of the cyst is obvious, and the principal purpose of including an example in this chapter is to highlight the differentiation between partly luteinized granulosa cells and the lining cells of other benign cystic neoplasms (Figs 57.1, 57.2).

Serous tumors (Ch. 23)

The cytological identification of serous ovarian tumors, at all levels of proliferation, is dependent mainly on their formation of fine papillary structures and the resemblance of the cell types present to those of the tubal mucosa (Figs 57.3–57.6).

The histological identification of a proliferating ovarian epithelial tumor requires the presence of two or more of the following four criteria: (a) epithelial budding; (b) multilayering; (c) increased mitotic activity; and (d) nuclear atypia, which includes abnormality of size and shape, an increase in nuclear/cytoplasmic ratio, alterations in nuclear chromatin pattern, and the number of nucleoli (see Ch. 22). In smears from proliferating epithelial tumors, the cellular pattern is often mixed, showing both benign appearing epithelium and focal cellular aggregates of abnormally proliferating epithelium. This is seen

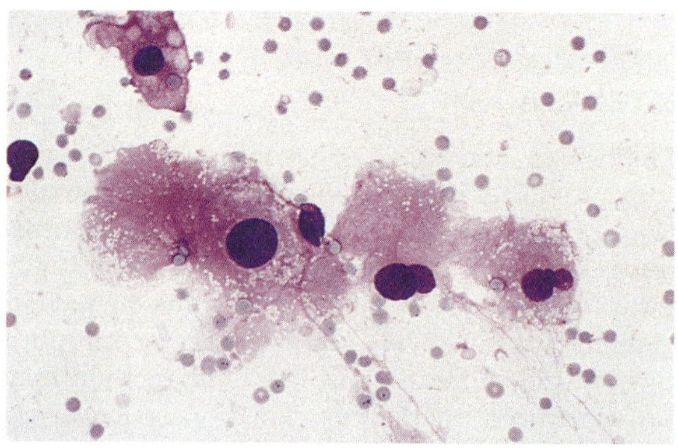

Fig. 57.1 Luteinized cells from a cystic corpus luteum. The cytoplasm is abundant and the cell borders are indistinct. Nuclei vary in size, are round to oval, and bland in appearance. H + E ×300

A

B

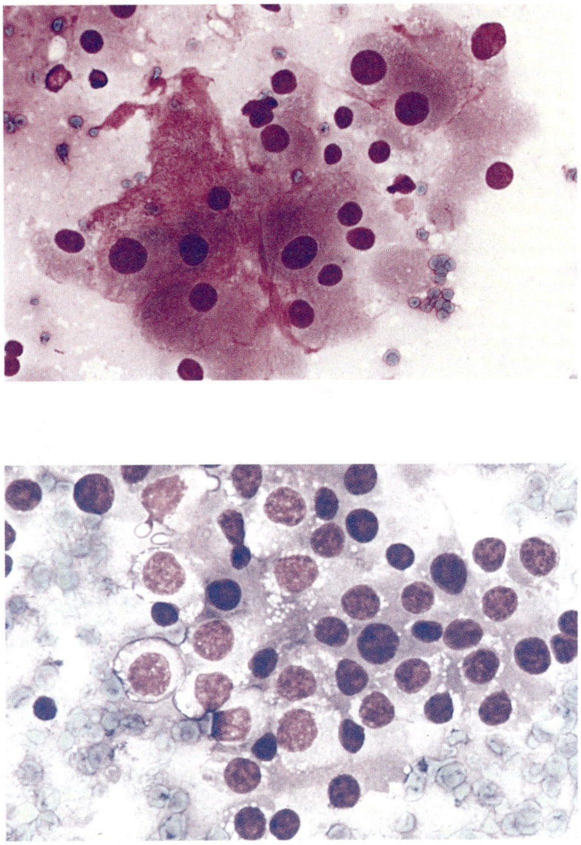

Fig. 57.2 Partly luteinized cells from an unruptured luteinized follicular cyst. (A) Fine granularity of cytoplasm. H + E ×300. (B) Fine cytoplasmic lipid vacuoles. Diff-Quik ×300

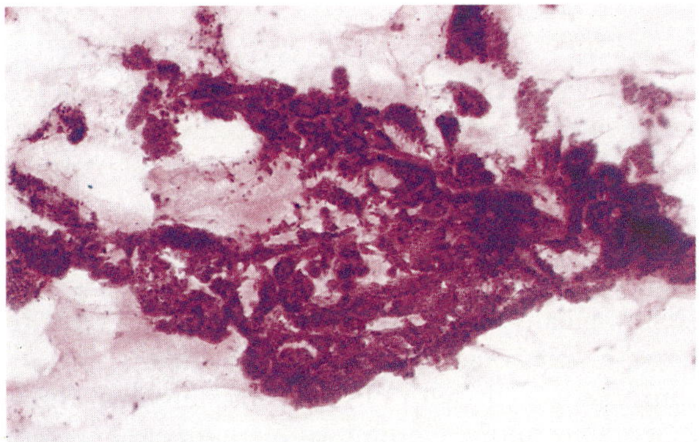

Fig. 57.3 Benign serous cystadenoma. The micropapillary pattern strongly favors serous epithelial neoplasia (see Fig. 23.18). H + E ×75

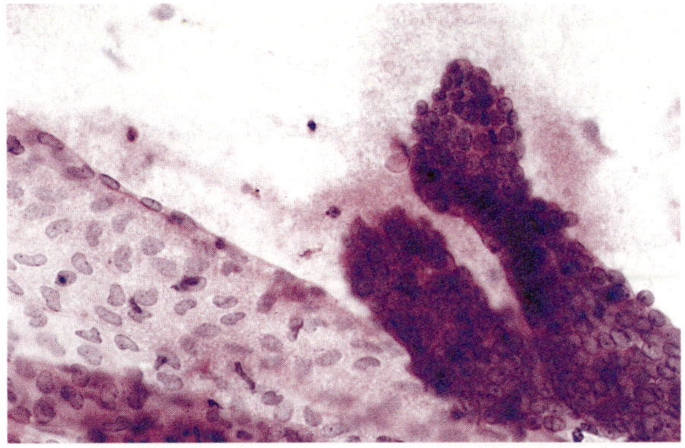

Fig. 57.4 Benign serous cystadenoma. The micropapillary proliferation of the serous epithelial cells contrasts with sheets of benign mesothelial cells. H + E ×300

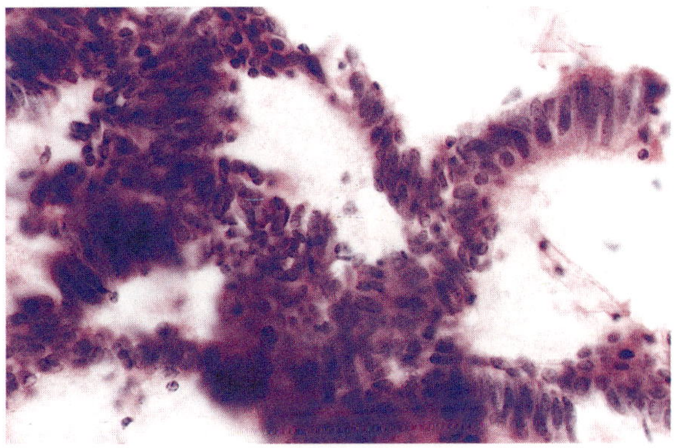

Fig. 57.5 Benign serous cystadenoma. A coarse 'filigree' pattern is present and the epithelium recapitulates that of the endosalpinx (see Fig. 23.1). H + E ×300

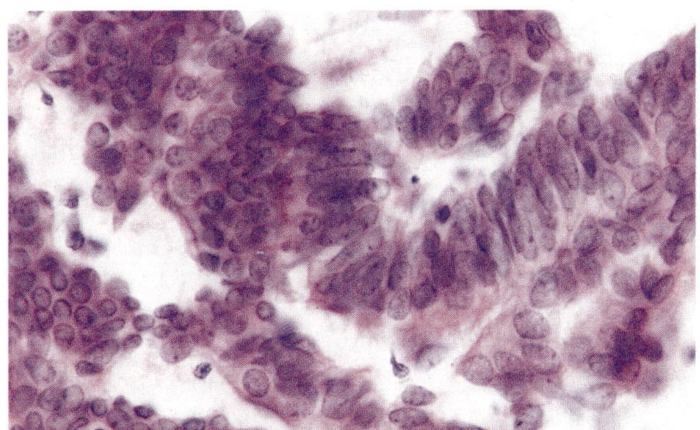

Fig. 57.6 Benign serous cystadenoma. Higher power showing abundant cilia in the cellular fragments. H + E ×475

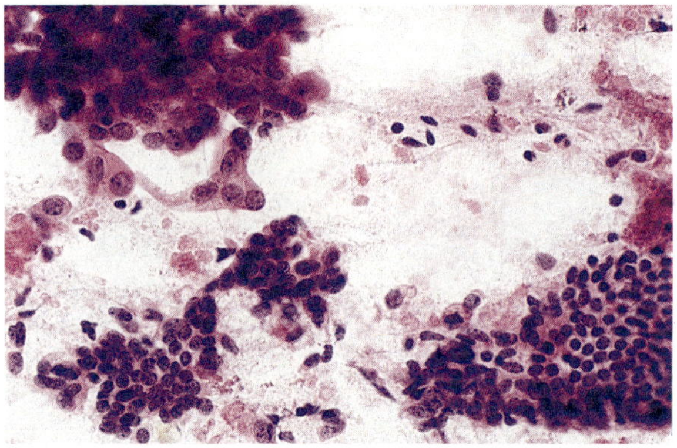

Fig. 57.7 Proliferating serous tumor. The tissue fragment at top left is composed of larger crowded cells with nuclear atypia. Those to the lower right, by contrast, are more suggestive of a benign serous component. This combination is strongly suggestive of a proliferative tumor (see Fig. 23.21). H + E ×300

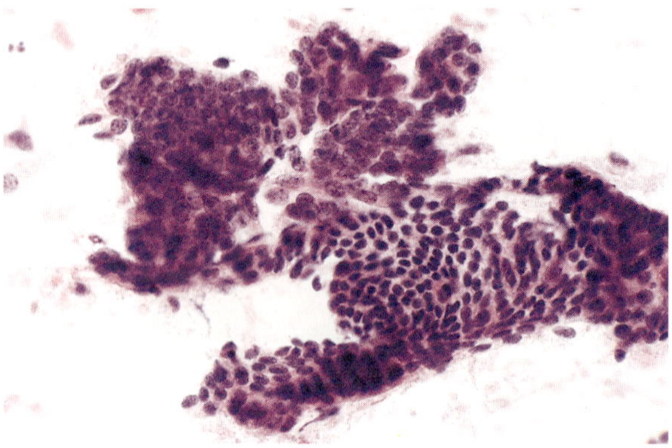

Fig. 57.8 Proliferating serous tumor. The mixed pattern here, similarly favors atypical proliferation. H + E ×300

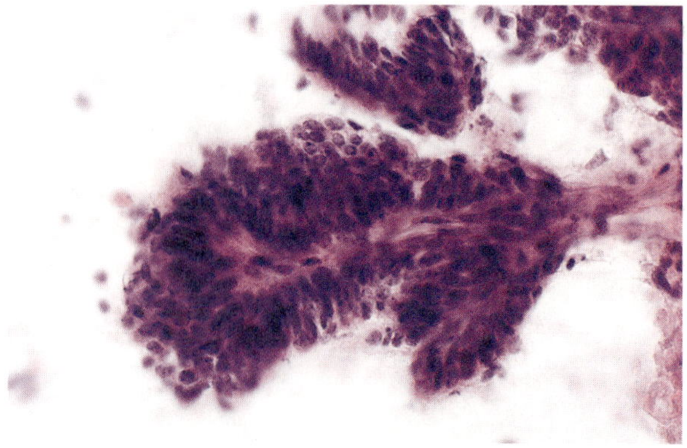

Fig. 57.9 Proliferating serous tumor. Papillary structure with a vascular core. H + E ×300

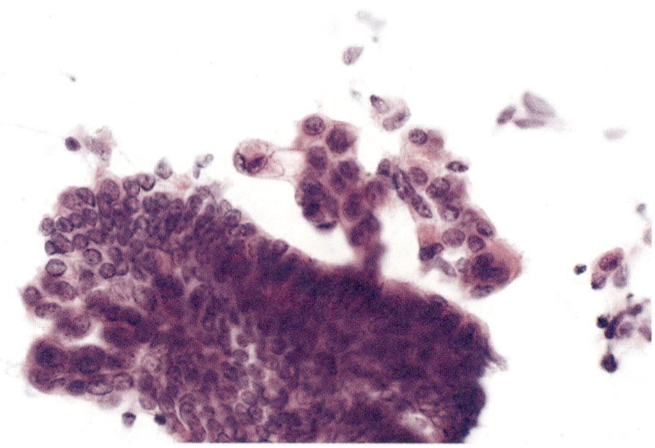

Fig. 57.10 Proliferating serous tumor. One part of the larger fragment of cells has an apparent smooth edge, but on closer examination there is crowding of the peripheral nuclei. These appearances suggest a papilliform structure and have also been described in papillary carcinoma of thyroid. Enlarged, less cohesive cells, some with atypical nuclei are also present, as are a few cells with cilia. H + E ×300

particularly well in proliferating serous tumors (Figs 57.7–57.11). Histological examination is the only reasonable arbiter of the presence or absence of invasion in well-differentiated epithelial tumors. An observable cytomorphological feature of many serous carcinomas (Figs 57.12–57.15), which are particularly high grade tumors, is the presence of occasional bizarre mononuclear tumor giant cells or syncytial-like aggregares.

Mucinous tumors (Ch. 24)

Cellular features of these tumors (Figs 57.16–57.23) include the classic honeycomb pattern of benign variants, as well as the variability noted above in those showing atypical epithelial proliferation, combined with evidence of mucin secretion.

Endometrioid tumors (Ch. 25)

Histologically, endometrioid carcinomas tend to show a 'microglandular' or 'trabecular' pattern, comprising cells with elongate nuclei which have coarse chromatin. Squamous elements are present in 30% of cases (see Ch. 25). These features are reflected in the cytomorphology (Figs 57.24–57.26).

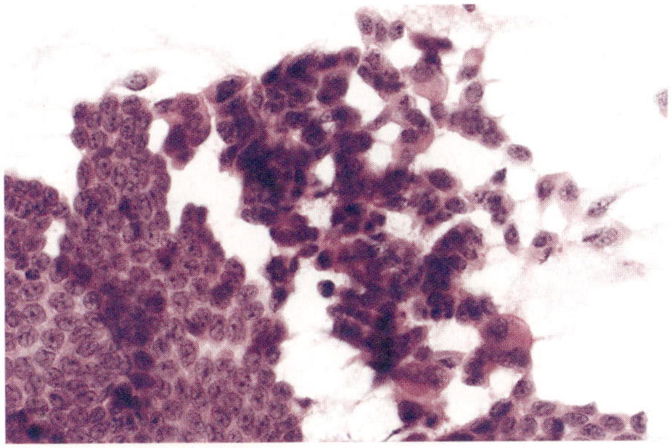

Fig. 57.11 Proliferating serous tumor. Nuclear atypia is apparent. Although the cells generally vary little in size, occasional significantly larger cells are seen. This is a characteristic more frequently observed in serous ovarian carcinomas (see Ch. 23). H + E ×300

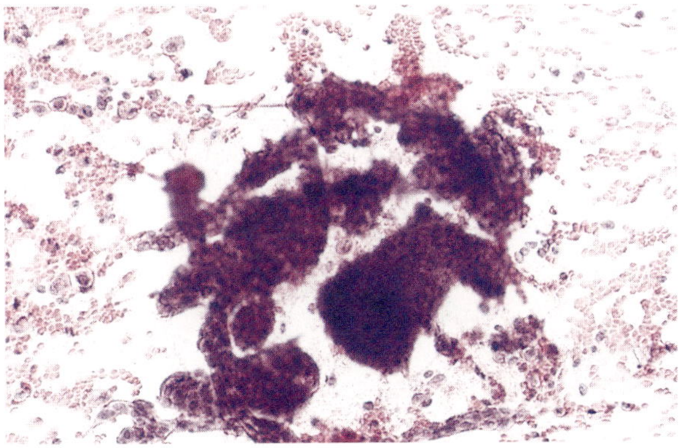

Fig. 57.12 Serous carcinoma. A complex micropapillary pattern and considerable necrosis is evident (see Figs 23.31, 23.33). H + E ×75

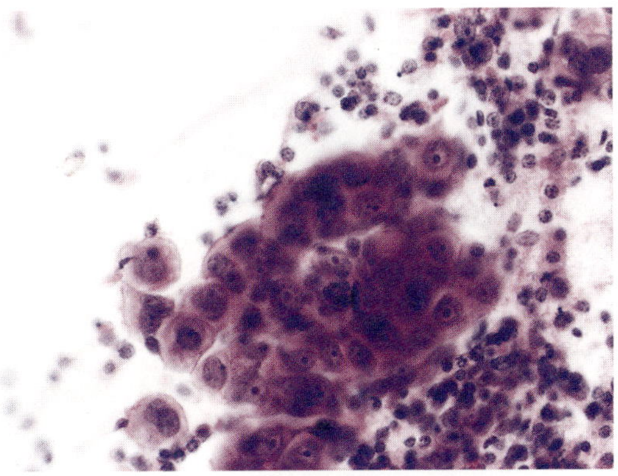

Fig. 57.13 Serous carcinoma. The cells are relatively monomorphous in appearance and the nuclei have single prominent nucleoli. This tumor, histologically, showed grade 3 nuclear and architectural abnormalities (see Fig. 23.34). H + E ×300

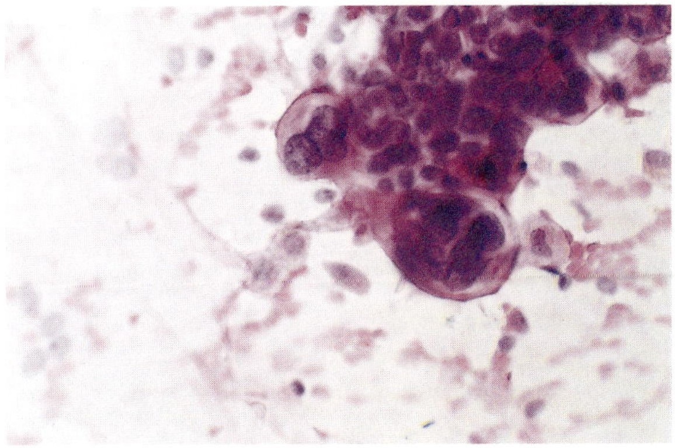

Fig. 57.14 Serous carcinoma. Scattered giant cells seen admixed with relatively monomorphous cells. H + E ×300

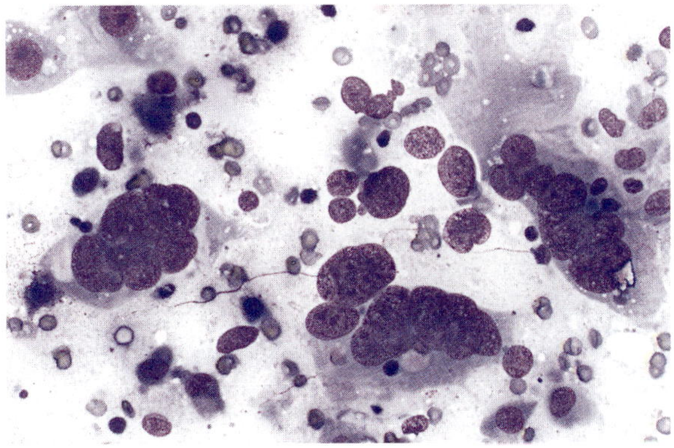

Fig. 57.15 Serous carcinoma. High grade carcinoma with bizarre syncytial-like tumor giant cells. Classification is not possible on cytomorphology alone, but serous neoplasia should be considered (see Fig. 23.35). Diff-Quik ×300

Mullerian mesenchymal and mixed tumors (Ch. 26)

Benign leiomyomas may rarely be encountered. The cytological detail of plump spindle cells, bland 'cigar-shaped' nuclei (Fig. 57.27) and a conspicuous absence of any epithelial component (either benign or malignant), should accord with the typical whorled appearance of a solid, circumscribed tumor mass. In the absence of such epithelial elements, the differential diagnosis is largely lesions in the thecoma–fibroma group (see below). Demonstrably malignant mesenchymal elements (Fig. 57.28), by contrast, are almost pathognomonic of a malignant mixed mullerian tumor, given the rarity of pure sarcomas and

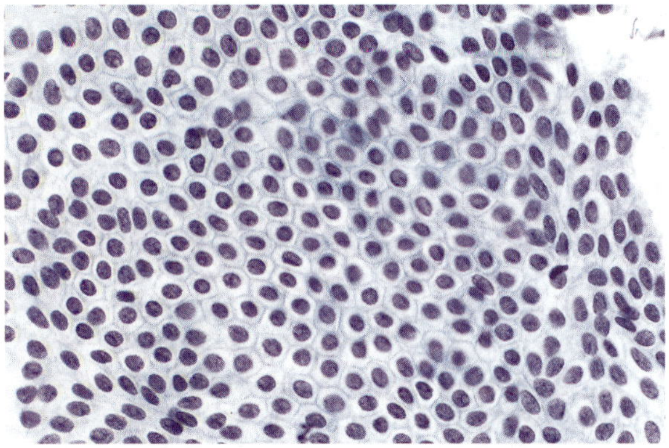

A

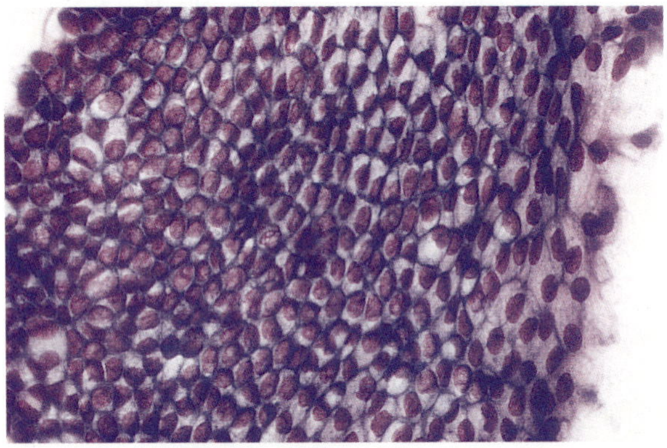

B

Fig. 57.16 Benign mucinous cystadenoma. Cohesive, monolayered 'honeycomb' composed of cells with well-defined cell borders and round, uniform nuclei (see Fig. 24.8). (A) H + E ×300. (B) Diff-Quik ×300

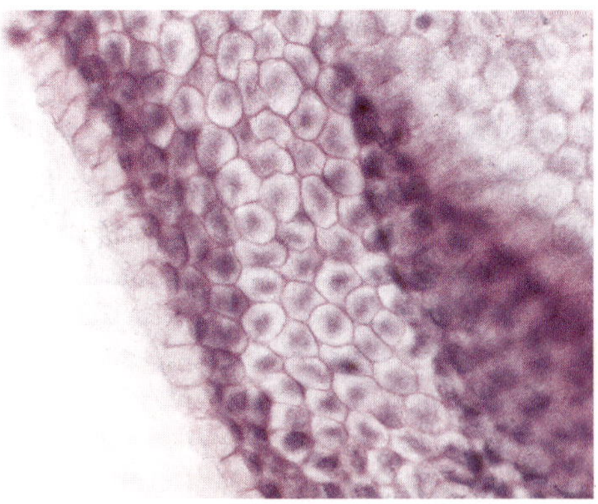

Fig. 57.17 Benign mucinous cystadenoma. It is important to examine the intact edge of the microbiopsy cellular fragments, where it is evident that the cells are columnar and the nuclei are basal. The absence of nuclear crowding can be assessed and the presence of either endocervical or intestinal type mucus-secreting cells can be recognized. H + E ×300

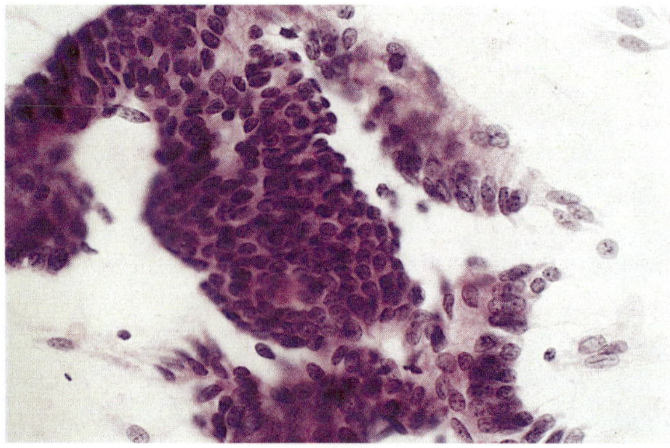

Fig. 57.18 Proliferating mucinous tumor. The monotonous 'honeycomb' pattern is lost. Nuclear crowding is seen and there is evidence of nuclear palisading in the cell strips, reminiscent of adenocarcinoma in situ of the cervix. H + E ×300

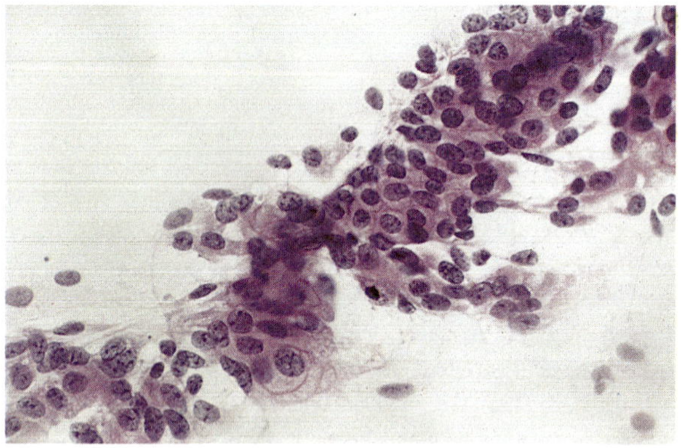

Fig. 57.19 Proliferating mucinous tumor. There is nuclear anisocytosis with irregularity of nuclear chromatin. Nucleoli are more readily visible, more numerous and vary in number from cell to cell. H + E ×300

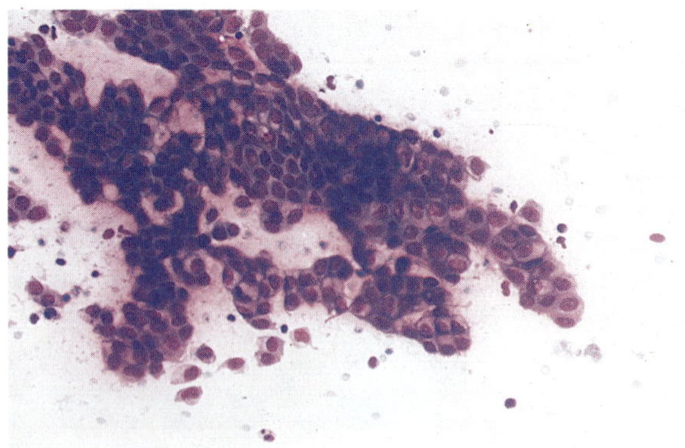

Fig. 57.20 Proliferating mucinous tumor. Papilliform configurations suggestive of atypical epithelial proliferation are observed (see Fig. 24.17). Some dissociated cells and fragmented nuclear debris, suggestive of apoptosis are also noted. H + E ×150

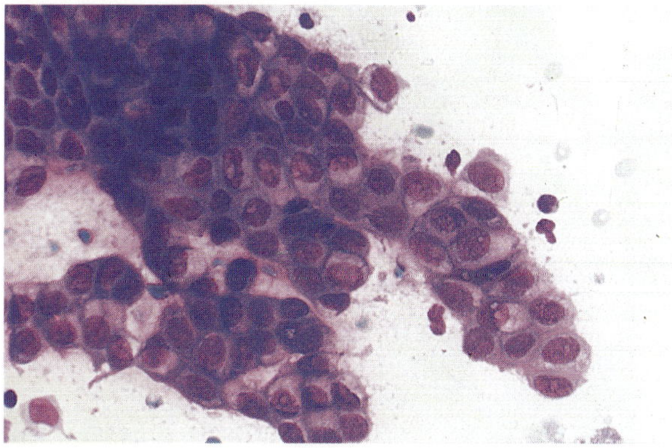

Fig. 57.21 Proliferating mucinous tumor. The nuclei are not uniform in size. Irregularity of nuclear chromatin is present. Nucleoli are more visible, more numerous and vary in number from cell to cell. H + E ×300

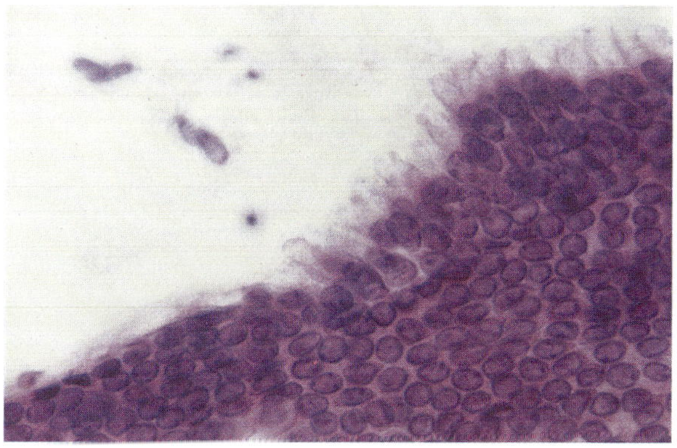

Fig. 57.22 Proliferating mucinous tumor. There is a suggestion of nuclear crowding, possibly also due to an increase in the nuclear/cytoplasmic ratio. H + E ×300

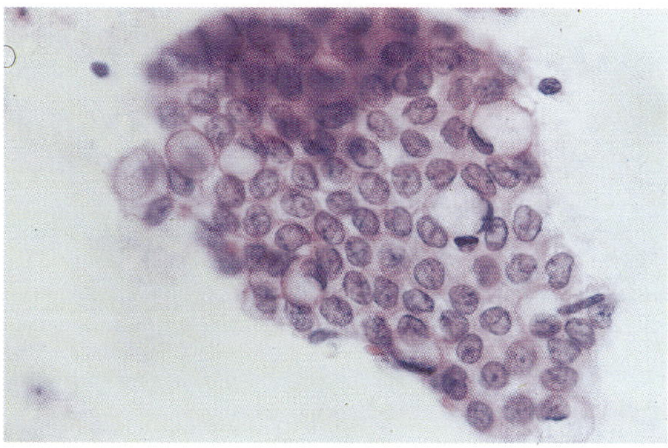

Fig. 57.23 Proliferating mucinous tumor. Scattered goblet cells suggestive, but not diagnostic, of intestinal type epithelium, are evident. Vacuolated cells may be seen in association with other mullerian epithelial tumors. H + E ×300

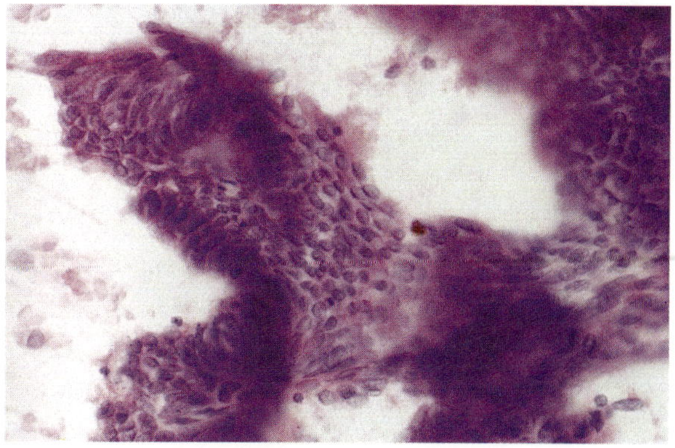

Fig. 57.24 Endometrioid carcinoma. A well-differentiated carcinoma with cellular fragments showing the cytological counterpart of a histological microglandular growth pattern. Portions of numerous acini are evident (see Fig. 25.16). H + E ×300

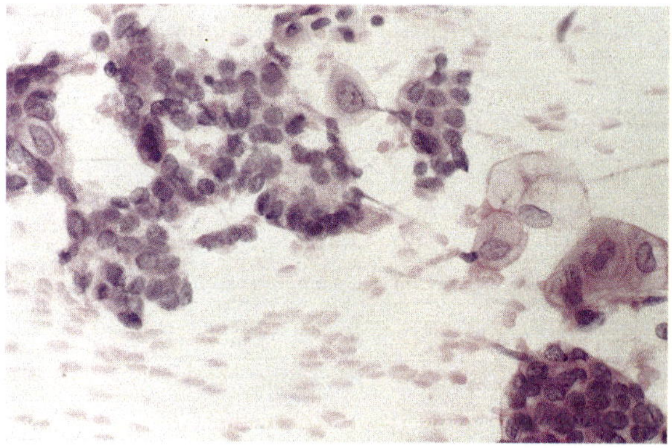

Fig. 57.25 Endometrioid carcinoma. Scattered single cells and small aggregates of squamous metaplastic cells are seen in association with cells representative of well-differentiated endometrioid adenocarcinoma (see Fig. 25.13). H + E ×300

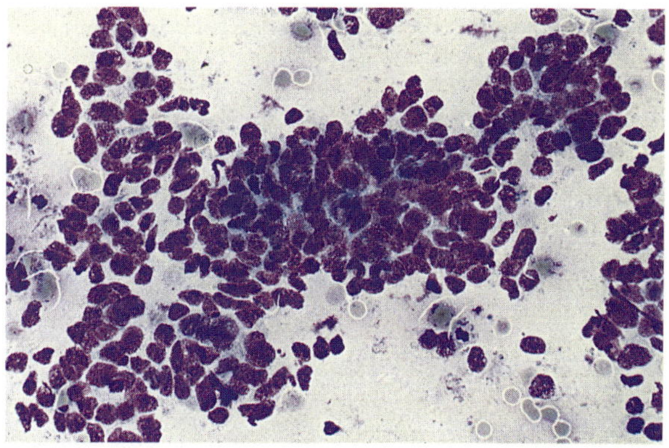

Fig. 57.26 Endometrioid carcinoma. These cells are derived from a high grade endometrioid adenocarcinoma. They can only be identified as malignant and epithelial on their cytomorphological appearances. H + E ×300

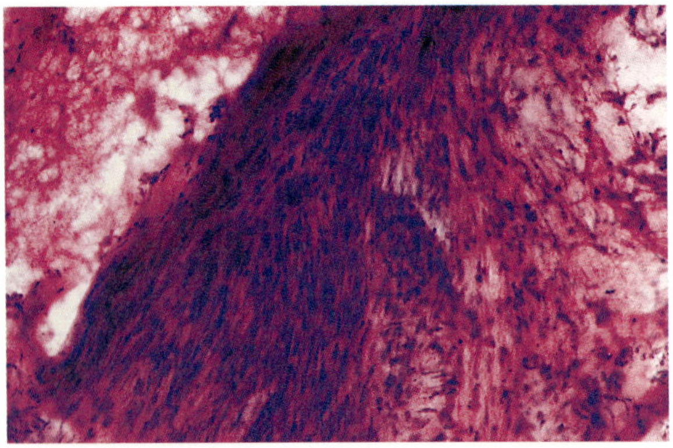

Fig. 57.27 Benign ovarian leiomyoma. The dominant pattern is that of spindle cells forming intertwining fascicles. The classic 'cigar-shaped' nuclear characteristics cannot be visualized at this magnification. H + E ×150

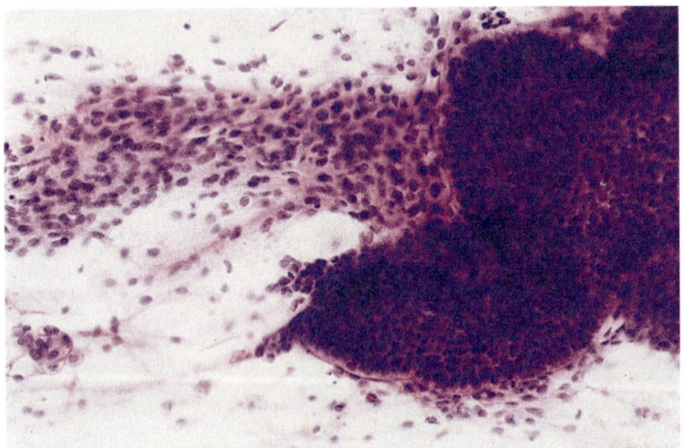

Fig. 57.28 Malignant mixed mullerian tumor. The stromal component, shown here, is composed of oval to spindle cells, with no further differentiation evident (same case as Fig. 26.12). At laparotomy, the tumor was widespread throughout the pelvis and no definite ovarian origin could be confirmed. Endometrium was, however, excluded as a possible primary site. H + E ×150

Sertoli–Leydig cells with heterologous mesenchymal elements. Identification of malignant epithelial and stromal elements is diagnostic, but may require additional sampling.

Clear cell tumors (Ch. 27)

The diagnosis of clear cell carcinoma is dependent on the identification of typical 'pavement-like' clear cells, eosinophilic cells or hobnail cells (Figs 57.29–57.32).

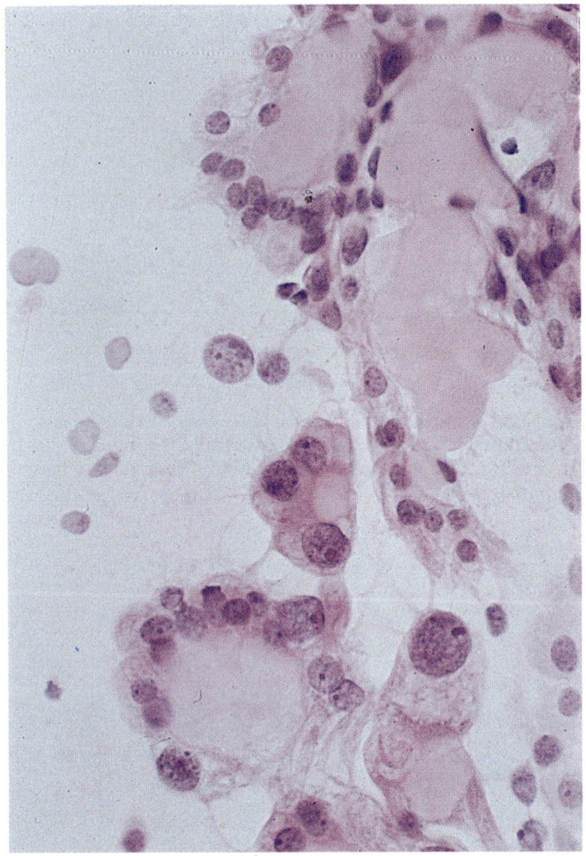

Fig. 57.29 Clear cell carcinoma. The pattern is papillary with 'hobnail' cells and hyaline stroma (see Fig. 27.11). ×300

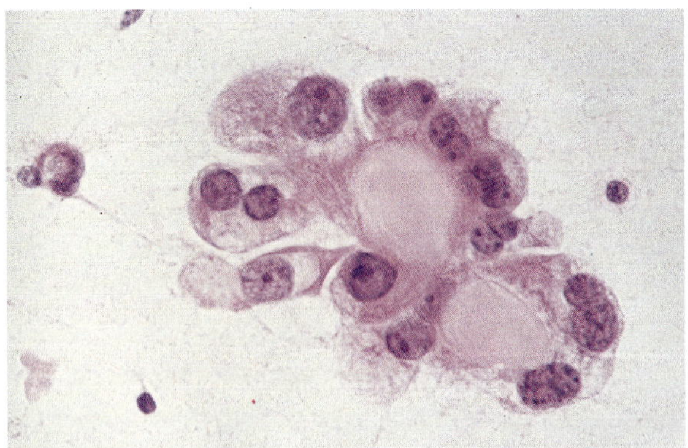

Fig. 57.30 Clear cell carcinoma. Typically, the cytoplasm in cytological preparations of 'clear cells' tends to be granular and less clear; the latter is an 'artifact' of fixation and processing differences for tissues and cells. Nuclei are mainly round, but show marked variability in size. H + E ×475

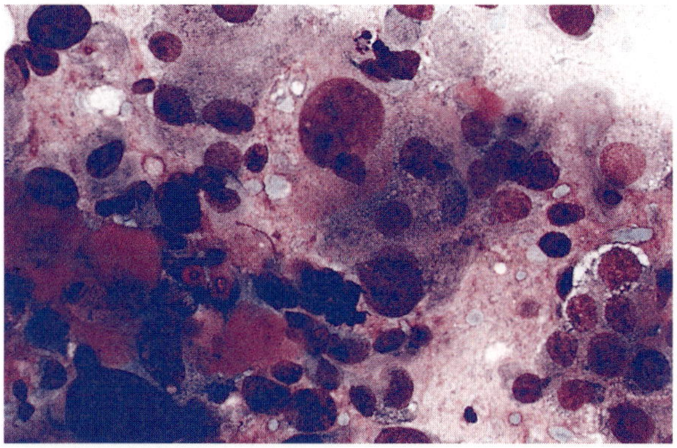

Fig. 57.31 Clear cell carcinoma. Hyalinized stroma is seen between cells. The fine vacuolation of the cytoplasm is indicative of its lipid content. Diff-Quik ×300

Transitional cell (Brenner) tumors (Ch. 28)

The structure of the characteristic epithelial nests and their relationship to the stroma is frequently maintained in the smear. In addition, the cellular features which are reminiscent of urothelium permit a reliable identification of the differentiation demonstrated by these tumors (Figs 57.33, 57.34).

Unclassified and miscellaneous epithelial tumors (Ch. 31)

Benign mesotheliomas, such as that shown in Fig. 57.35, are usually multilocular cystic lesions involving the adnexal structures of women, commonly with a history of previous pelvic surgery.

Granulosa cell tumors (Ch. 33)

The nuclei are uniform in size and bland in appearance, and the number of nuclear grooves seen cytologically is extremely variable (Figs 57.36–57.39). The cytoarchitectural patterns appear to reflect quite well those seen on histological examination of the tumors, such as the presence of visible microfollicles (Fig. 57.37). Call–Exner bodies are probably best identified in the Diff-Quik stained preparation.

The differential diagnosis includes both carcinoid tumors (see below) and, in young women, undifferentiated small cell carcinoma of hypercal-

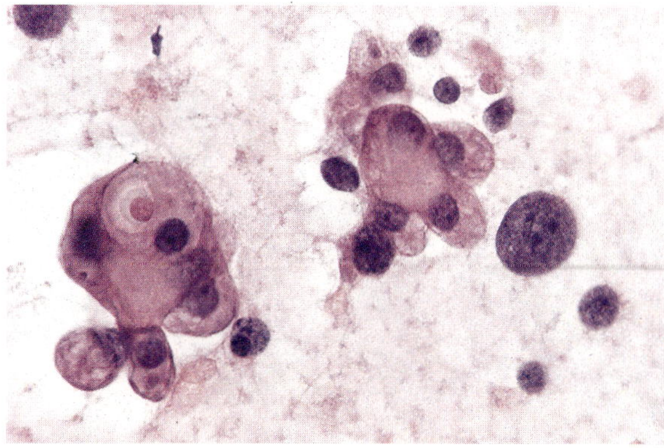

A

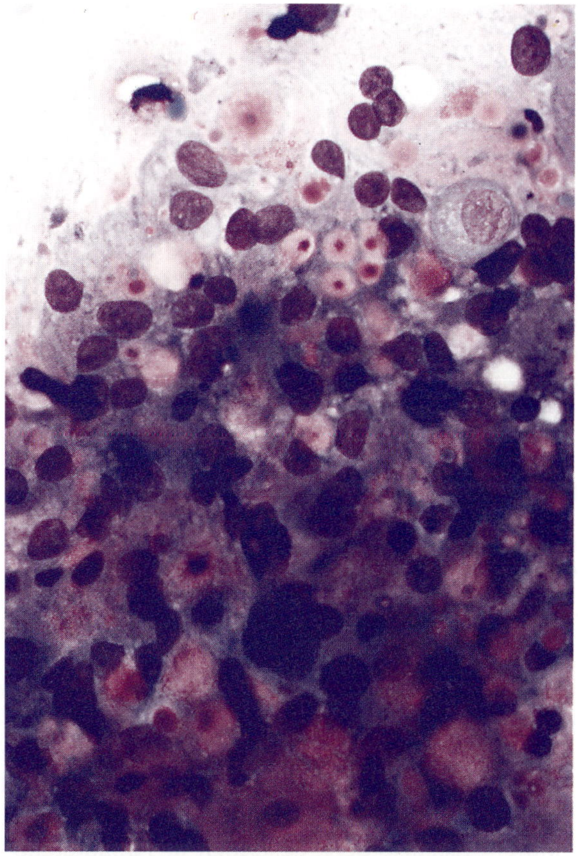

B

Fig. 57.32 Clear cell carcinoma. (A) A 'targetoid' amorphous eosinophilic inclusion is seen in a vacuolated cell (see Fig. 27.16). H + E ×475. (B) The metachromatic stain highlights the targetoid intracytoplasmic inclusions. Diff-Quik ×300

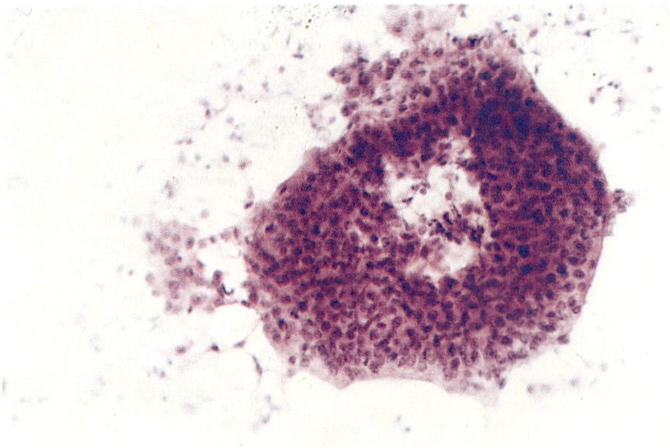

Fig. 57.33 Benign transitional cell adenofibroma. A dense, tightly cohesive cell aggregate/nest, clearly defined by an apparent basement membrane is seen in a background of dissociated stromal cells. H + E ×150

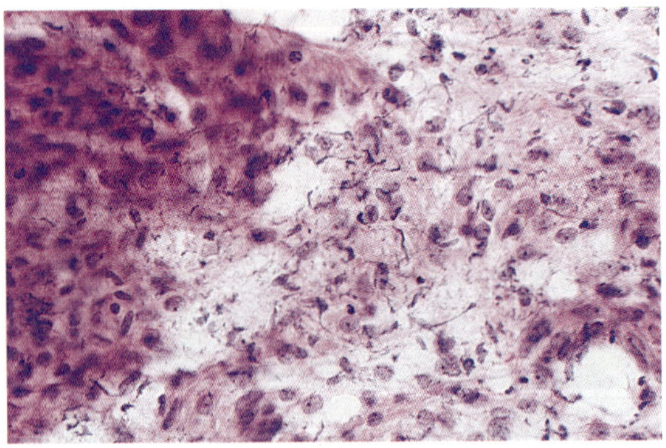

Fig. 57.34 Benign transitional cell adenofibroma. The cytological interphase between stroma and epithelial nest, partially disrupted by smearing (see Fig. 28.5). The resemblance of the cells to those of the urothelium is evident. H + E ×300

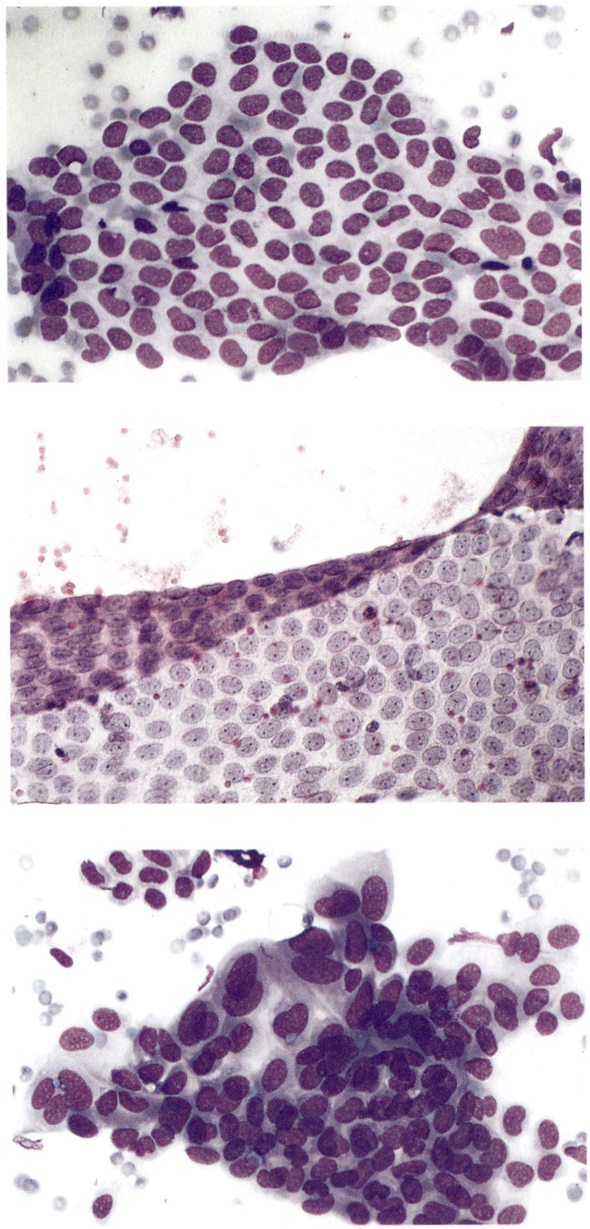

A

B

C

Fig. 57.35 Benign cystic mesothelioma. The typical cytological features of mesothelial cells arranged in a sheet with bland round to oval nuclei. (A) Diff-Quik ×300. (B) H + E ×300. Focal cellular and nuclear enlargement, if present, are not indicative of malignancy. (C) H + E ×300

cemic type (Dharan 1993). This latter, highly malignant neoplasm is composed of cells with visibly absent cytoplasm and hyperchromatic nuclei. Nuclear molding may be present. The finding of intracellular and extracellular eosinophilic hyaline globules has also been described in Papanicolaou stained smears (Dharan 1993).

Thecoma–fibroma group (Ch. 34)

This group of tumors involves, at a cytological level, resolution of the differential diagnosis of a benign 'spindle cell tumor' of the ovary, including those lesions of the thecoma–fibroma group (Fig. 57.40) as well as benign smooth muscle tumors and epithelial adenofibromas in which the epithelial component is not evident.

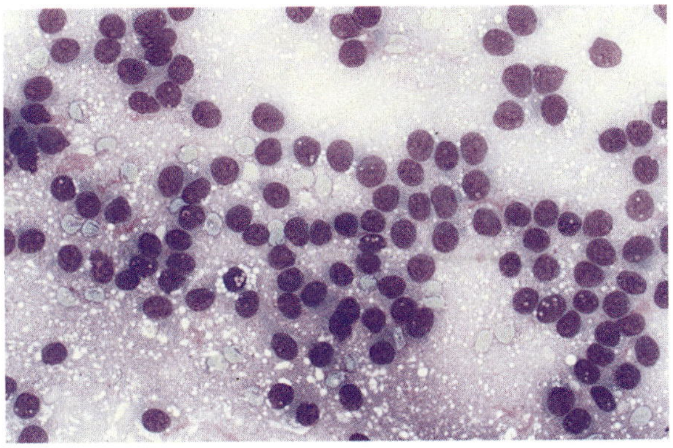

Fig. 57.36 Granulosa cell tumor. The cells are dispersed and monotonous in appearance. Diff-Quik ×300

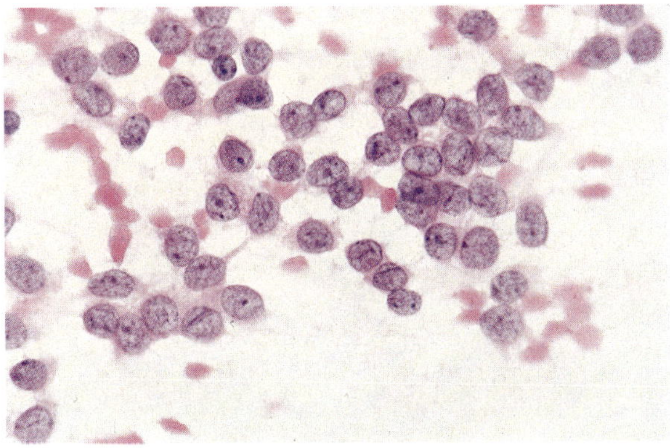

Fig. 57.37 Granulosa cell tumor. Nuclear grooves are seen in occasional cells. Cells are more dispersed than those seen in benign transitional cell tumors, which appear cohesive, forming cell nests. H + E ×475

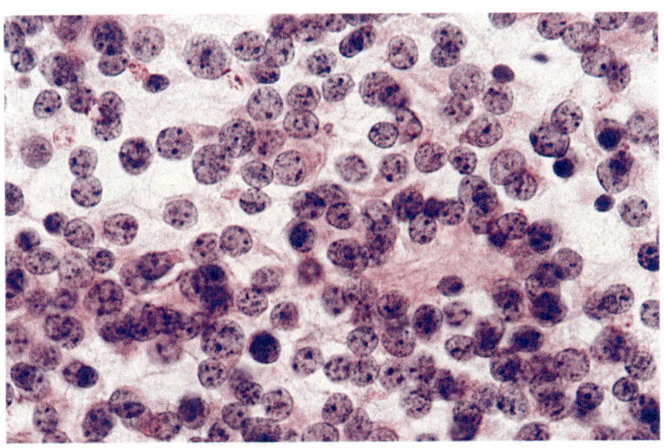

Fig. 57.38 Granulosa cell tumor. A microfollicular structure is present amongst the more dispersed cells (see Fig. 33.5). H + E ×475

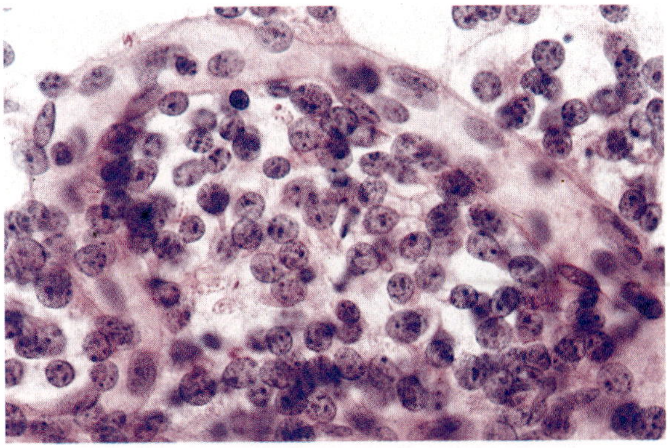

Fig. 57.39 Granulosa cell tumor. A capillary is included amongst the granulosa cells, indicative of the vascularity of these tumors. H + E ×475

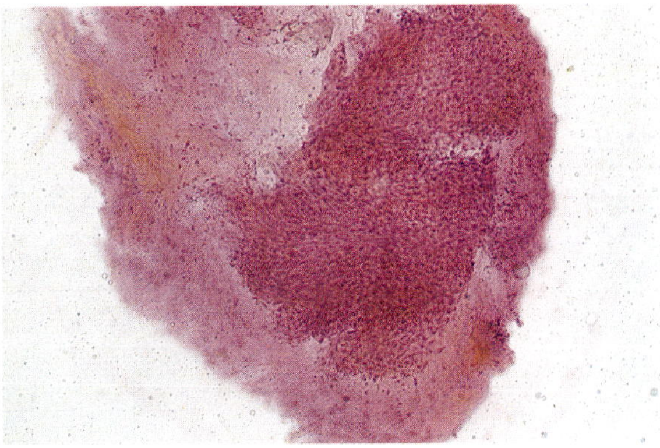

Fig. 57.40 Benign fibroma. A complex pattern of interfasciculating spindle cells is present (see Fig. 34.17). H + E ×75

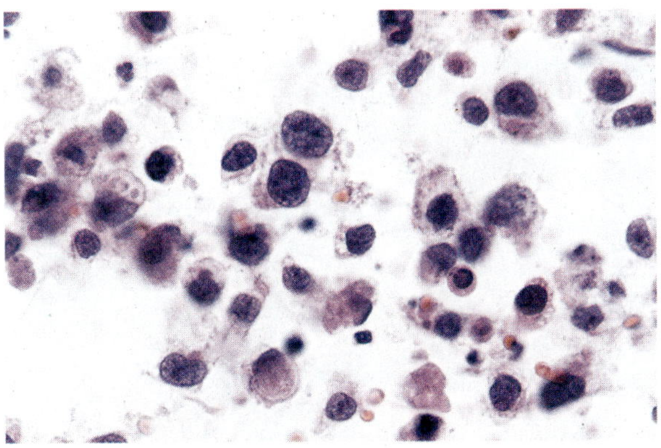

Fig. 57.41 Dysgerminoma. Both viable and necrotic cells are present. The cytoplasm is delicate and the nuclei are overtly malignant (see Fig. 41.1). The number of lymphocytes seen in the background is variable. H + E ×475

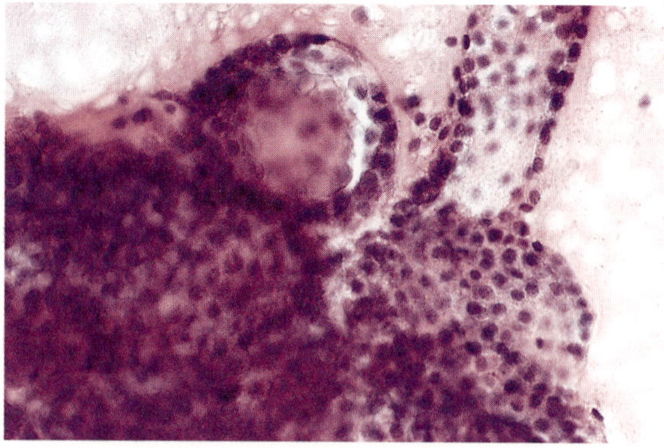

Fig. 57.42 Mature cystic teratoma. Easily identifiable follicles with some colloid are seen in this cytological sample from an area of struma ovarii (see Fig. 49.2). H + E ×300

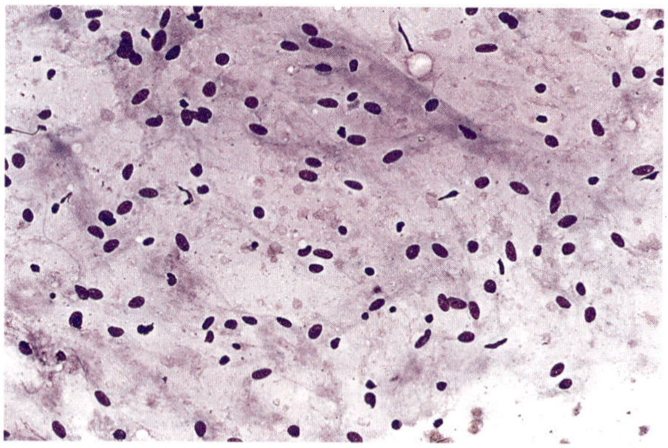

Fig. 57.43 Mature cystic teratoma. Neuroglial differentiation noted in the cellular sample from the lining of a unilocular mature cystic teratoma. Diff-Quik ×150

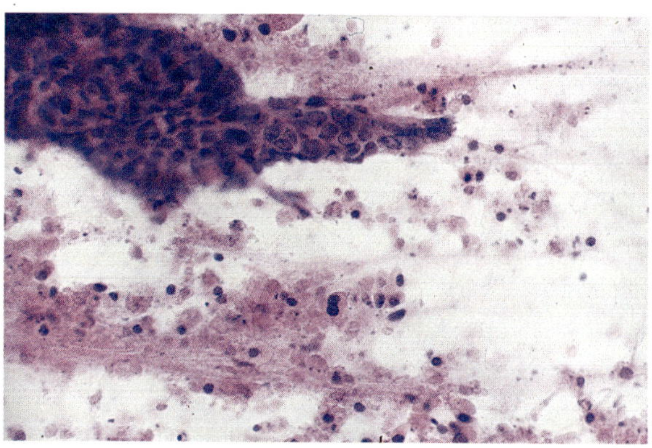

Fig. 57.44 Metastatic colonic adenocarcinoma. The 'typical' cytological pattern of apparently viable glandular cells seen in immediate apposition to considerable necrosis (see Fig. 54.7). H + E ×300

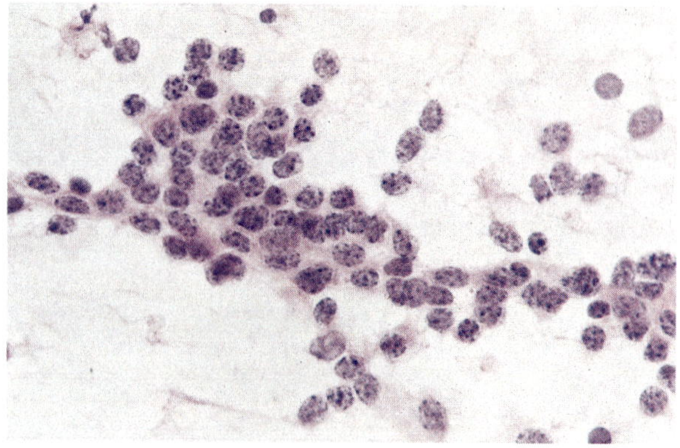

Fig. 57.45 Metastatic carcinoid tumor. Mosaic pattern of carcinoid tumor metastatic to the ovary. Nuclei show strikingly granular chromatin. H + E ×475

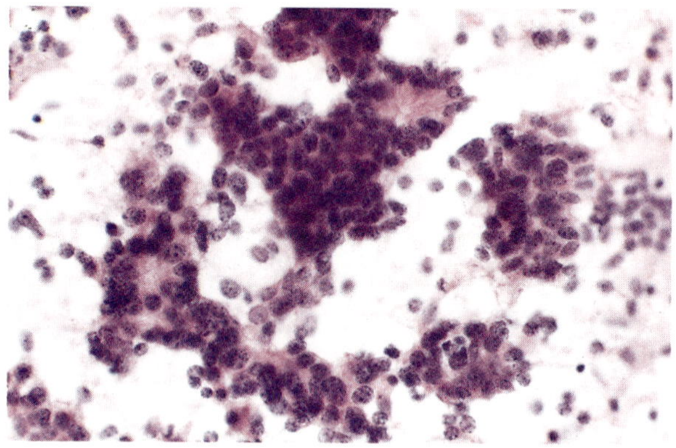

Fig. 57.46 Metastatic carcinoid tumor exhibiting rosettes which may be mistaken for glandular acini. H + E ×300

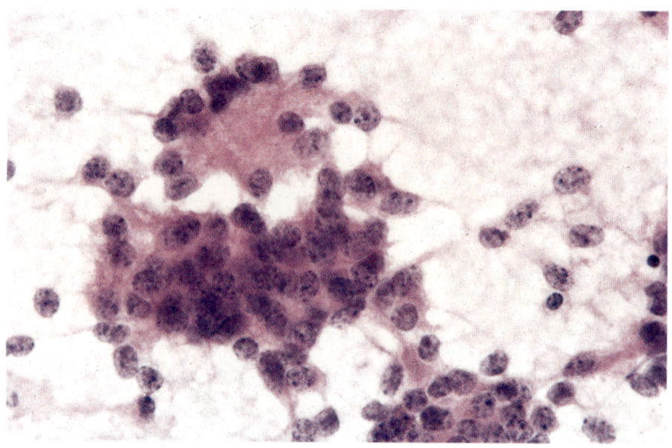

Fig. 57.47 Metastatic carcinoid tumor. Classic admixture of rosette and mosaic patterns. H + E ×475

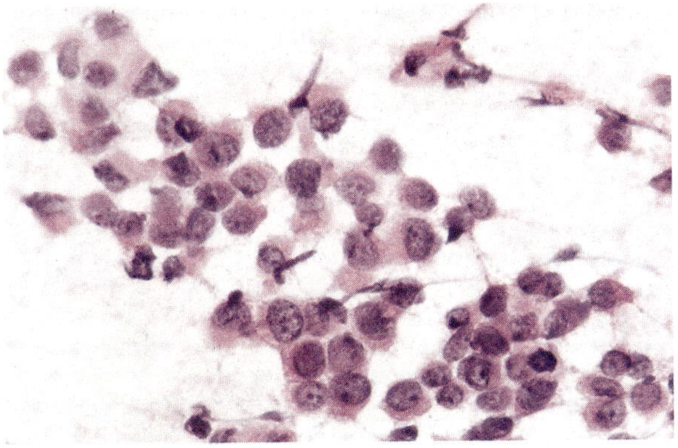

Fig. 57.48 Metastatic colonic adenocarcinoma. Poorly differentiated adenocarcinoma of colon, metastatic to the ovaries. Compare with carcinoid tumor. H + E ×475

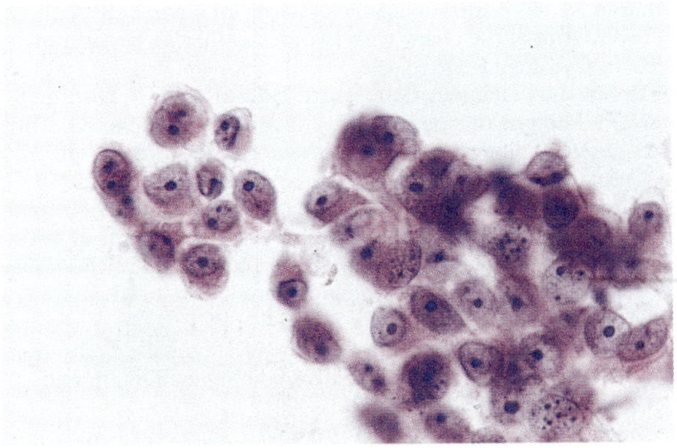

Fig. 57.49 Metastatic melanoma. An epithelioid pattern evident in this example of amelanotic melanoma metastatic to the ovaries. H + E ×475

Dysgerminomas (Ch. 41)

The cellular uniformity and the delicate cytoplasm are characteristic of these neoplasms. Lymphocytes of varying numbers are the most common accompaniment of the tumor cells (Fig. 57.41). A granulomatous cytological pattern may also be evident as a result of the epithelioid histiocytic reaction sometimes present.

Mature teratomas (Ch. 46)

These are usually easily diagnosed on their macroscopic appearance alone. Intraoperative cytological examination may assist in readily defining the nature of solid components such as struma ovarii (Fig. 57.42) or the lining of cysts not filled with keratinous or sebaceous debris (Fig. 57.43).

Carcinomas and nonepithelial tumors metastatic to the ovaries (Chs 54, 55)

Tumors metastatic to the ovaries may be difficult or impossible to differentiate from primary ovarian neoplasms by intraoperative cytological techniques. Metastatic colonic carcinoma may show a 'typical' pattern of apparently viable glandular cells in immediate apposition to considerable necrosis (Figs 57.44, 57.48), but as with other tumors metastatic from the gastrointestinal tract no appearances are pathognomonic of metastasis per se.

The cytological features of lymphoid differentiation are familiar to most surgical pathologists as a result of their experience with lymph nodes and are a hallmark of malignant lymphoma.

Metastatic melanoma may show various cellular patterns, including a predominance of epithelioid or spindle cells (Fig. 57.49). Intracytoplasmic pigment, often fine and powdery, may be evident, particularly in the epithelioid cells.

CONCLUSION

It is hoped that this demonstration of a range of ovarian pathology, albeit not totally comprehensive, will be both of interest and assistance to those who wish to use this technique.

REFERENCES

Abrahams C 1978 The 'Scrimp' technique a method for the rapid diagnosis of surgical pathology specimens. Histopathology 2: 255–266

Abrams J, Silverberg S G 1989 The role of intraoperative cytology in the evaluation of gynecologic disease. Pathology Annual 24(2): 167–187

Bloustein P A, Silverberg S G 1977 Rapid cytological examination of surgical specimens. Pathology Annual 12 (2): 251–278

Buckley C H 1989 Is needle aspiration of ovarian cysts adequate for diagnosis? British Journal of Obstetrics and Gynaecology 96: 1021–1023

Dharan M 1993 Intraoperative cytology of small cell carcinoma of the ovary with hypercalcemia. A case report. Acta Cytologica 37: 61–66

di Bonito L, Falconieri G, Calautti I, Bonifacio D, Dudine S 1993 The positive peritoneal effusion. A retrospective study of cytopathologic diagnosis with autopsy confirmation. Acta Cytologica 37: 483–488

Dudgeon L S, Patrick C V 1927 A new method for the rapid microscopical diagnosis of tumors with an account of 200 cases so examined. British Journal of Surgery 15: 250–261

Godwin J T 1976 Rapid cytologic diagnosis of surgical specimens. Acta Cytologica 20: 111–115

Guarda L 1990 Intraoperative cytologic diagnosis: evaluation of 370 consecutive intraoperative cytologies. Diagnostic Cytopathology 6: 235–242

Jadhon M E, Morgan M A, Kelsten M L, Carlson J A, Mikuta J J 1990 Cytologic smears of peritoneal surfaces as a sampling technique in epithelial ovarian carcinoma. Obstetrics and Gynecology 75: 102–105

Layfield L J, Berek J S 1994 Fine-needle aspiration cytology in the management of gynecologic oncology patients. Cancer Treatment and Research 70: 1–13

Nadji M, Greening S E, Seuai B U, Averette H E, Nordqvist S R B, Ng A B P 1979 Fine needle aspiration cytology in gynecologic oncology. II: Morphologic aspects. Acta Cytologica 23: 380–388

Nochomovitz K, Sidawy M, Silverberg S G, Jannotta A, Schwartz A 1989 Intraoperative consultation. A guide to smears, imprints and frozen sections. ASCP Press Chicago

Nunez C, Diaz J I 1992 Ovarian follicular cysts: a potential source of false positive diagnoses in ovarian cytology. Diagnostic Cytopathology 8: 532–536

Oneson R H, Minke J A, Silverberg S G 1989 Intraoperative pathologic consultation: an audit of 1000 recent consecutive cases. American Journal of Surgical Pathology 3: 237–243

Sheombar E S, Logmans A, Verhoeff A, van Lent M 1993 Ovarian cysts, cytology and histology: a conflicting story. European Journal of Obstetrics Gynecology and Reproductive Biology 52: 41–44

58

Preoperative radiological and MRI investigation

K. Occhipinti

Ultrasound

Radiologists today have several modalities at their disposal for evaluation of the ovary and adnexal masses. Transabdominal ultrasound (TAUS) is a well-established modality with which to evaluate the ovary, and its benefits include lack of ionizing radiation, widespread availability, and low cost. Detailed evaluation of the ovary is often limited by transabdominal approach, however, due to patient body habitus or artifact from gas in adjacent bowel. Resolution has significantly improved with the introduction of transvaginal ultrasound (TVUS), which allows the ultrasound transducer to be placed closer to the pelvic organs. Ovarian follicles, cysts, and masses can usually be visualized in detail, and evaluated for the presence of septations, internal echoes (in patients with endometriomas or pelvic inflammatory disease (PID)), and solid portions (in patients with ovarian tumors).

Transabdominal ultrasound is performed prior to the transvaginal examination in order to obtain an initial image of the entire pelvis, and determine the position of the ovaries or adnexal mass in relation to the uterus. Difficulty localizing the ovaries by TVUS alone may arise due to limited field of view if the ovaries are located very laterally or anteriorly, or if the ovaries are displaced superiorly into the abdomen by an enlarged uterus.

Doppler sonography is now available with both transabdominal and transvaginal probes. This function allows measurement of the velocity of the blood flow in the vessels that supply the ovary; the frequency of sound emitted by the transducer is compared with the frequency reflected off moving red blood cells, and the frequency shift used to determine actual velocities within the lumen of the arteries and veins. With the duplex Doppler method, the black and white image of the vessel and surrounding structures is displayed alongside a graph of the actual Doppler waveform. Colour Doppler images can be generated by mapping the mean velocities of flowing blood onto an image of each vessel by using a scale of color which reflects both the velocity and direction of blood flow in relation to the position of the transducer. By convention, arteries are imaged with a scale of red colors and veins with a scale of blue colors.

Magnetic resonance imaging

Magnetic resonance imaging (MRI) provides detailed images of the ovary without exposing the patient to ionizing radiation. Patients are currently imaged in a strong magnetic field (0.064–1.5 T), which causes protons (hydrogen nuclei) to precess at a specific frequency (the resonant frequency). Radiofrequency pulse sequences are then applied which will change the resonant frequency of the hydrogen nuclei slightly (according to the site of the proton in the magnetic field and inherent tissue parameters). When the protons return to their original state, new radiofrequency signals will be emitted, received by the magnet, and given a spatial location. Magnetic resonance images can be acquired in axial, sagittal, and coronal planes.

T_1- and T_2-weighted type images are acquired by varying the time between the initial set of radiofrequency pulses (repetition time (TR)) and the time between the initial pulse in a sequence and the time that the signal is acquired from the sample (echo delay time (TE)). A characteristic signal intensity (low, intermediate, or high) will be generated on both T_1- and T_2-weighted images, depending on the composition of the substance being studied. Water has a characteristic low signal intensity on T_1-weighted sequences (dark gray on the image) and high signal intensity on T_2-weighted sequences (white on the image). Fat and blood clot are both high signal intensity on the T_1-weighted sequences.

New developments that have made MRI of the pelvis more practical include the phased-array coil and fast pulse sequences, which together improve resolution of magnetic resonance images threefold, while at the same time decreasing image acquisition time by one-third (Smith et al 1992).

Intravenous contrast medium is available for MRI and has been approved for use in the pelvis. MRI contrast agents are all compounds of gadolinium. The most widely used currently include Magnevist (gadopentetate dimeglumine; Berlex Laboratories, Wayne, NJ, USA) and Prohance (gadoteridol; Squibb Diagnostics, Plainsboro, NJ, USA). The dose needed for magnetic resonance contrast is 1/20 that of iodinated contrast, which improves patient tolerance. Far fewer minor and only minimal anaphylactic reactions have been reported with gadolinium compounds. Magnetic resonance agents can safely be given to patients with an allergic history to iodinated contrast, as well as patients with chronic renal failure (Haustein et al 1992).

Due to its higher cost, MRI is usually referred to as a 'problem-solving', modality, and is used to add more information about the ovary or an ovarian mass than the ultrasound examination alone can provide. Special fat saturation sequences, available only with MRI, can identify fat in a teratoma or hemorrhage in a functional cyst or endometrioma. The multiplanar imaging capability and superior soft-tissue characterization available with MRI compared with computed axial tomography, makes MRI the modality of choice in differentiating an adnexal from a uterine mass when ultrasound is indeterminate. Finally, MRI has a large field of view, and can be used to characterize large ovarian masses that extend into the pelvis, or to visualize ovaries that are deviated into the abdomen or obscured by bowel gas on ultrasound.

Computed axial tomography

Computed axial tomography (CAT) can be used as an adjunct modality after ultrasound to evaluate the ovaries. The role of CAT is limited, however, as it lacks the multiplanar imaging capability of ultrasound and MRI. Even with optimal oral, rectal, and intravenous contrast, the ovaries have a nonspecific soft-tissue density on CAT, and may be confused with adenopathy or an unopacified loop of bowel. CAT images can be diagnostic of the ovarian teratoma, due to the high sensitivity of CAT in the detection of calcium and fat present in these tumors. The initial evaluation and staging of malignant ovarian tumors is still done using CAT, although recent studies have documented similar efficacy of both MRI and CAT in the characterization and staging of ovarian tumors (Forstner et al 1994).

THE NORMAL OVARY

Ultrasound, MRI, and CAT appearance

TVUS and magnetic resonance images are both able to resolve small follicles (<1 cm) in the ovary, as well as the centrally located ovarian stroma, and can be used to definitely identify the location of the ovary within the pelvis. On ultrasound images, the follicles appear as small, round, sonolucent foci arranged at the periphery of the more echogenic stroma. The MRI appearance of the ovary varies according to the pulse sequence chosen, but is characteristic on T_2-weighted images (follicles are easily visualized as high signal intensity, round structures due to their water content) and T_1-weighted, contrast-enhanced images (follicles remain low signal intensity within the higher signal intensity enhancing stroma) (Fig. 58.1). MRI has been reported to identify the ovaries in 87–96% of reproductive-age women and 47% of postmenopausal women (Dooms et al 1986).

CAT and non-contrast-enhanced, T_1-weighted magnetic resonance images are unable to resolve small ovarian follicles. Visualization of a normal ovary may be difficult by CAT, and location of the ovary (in the ovarian fossa, adjacent to the iliac artery and vein) may be helpful in differentiating the ovary from adjacent pelvic structures.

With all three modalities (ultrasound, MRI, and CAT) the postmenopausal ovary is more difficult to identify due to its smaller size and lack of follicles.

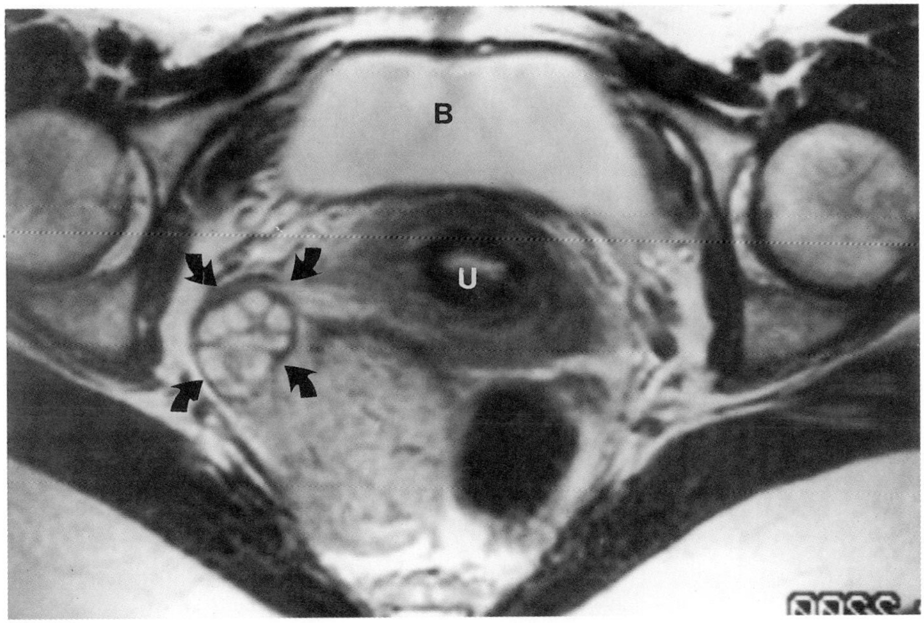

Fig. 58.1 Magnetic resonance image of the normal ovary. Axial T_2-weighted section from an MRI examination of the pelvis demonstrates a normal ovary (arrows) with multiple high signal intensity follicles. U, Uterus; B, bladder.

FUNCTIONAL CYSTS

Ultrasound

The dynamic nature of the ovary is most effectively captured by TVUS images. Developing follicles, follicle cysts, corpus luteum cysts, theca lutein cysts, and serous inclusion cysts can all be imaged by TVUS. Ultrasound is the gold standard in the diagnosis of a simple cyst, which must fulfill three strict ultrasound criteria, namely: thin wall, anechoic center, and good sound through-transmission. A corpus luteum cyst is the exception to this rule, as it may contain internal echoes from hemorrhage (Grant 1992).

Once a dominant follicle has been identified on ultrasound, it can be followed to ovulation by serial ultrasound examinations. If a cyst is identified, ultrasound can be used to follow the cyst through several menstrual cycles in order to determine if it will resolve spontaneously or require hormonal therapy.

Ultrasound has been used to study the natural history of the postmenopausal ovary and serous inclusion cysts. In one study, cysts less than 3 cm diameter were commonly found in asymptomatic women. Most of these cysts resolved or significantly decreased in size on sequential examinations (Levine et al 1992).

MRI and CAT

MRI, like ultrasound, is also able to detect developing follicles and benign cysts. A benign cyst has fluid signal intensity (low on T_1-weighted images and high on T_2-weighted images), and a thin wall both before and after contrast administration. The hemorrhagic follicle cysts or corpus luteum cysts will have high signal intensity on T_1-weighted images (Fig. 58.2).

CAT can also resolve larger ovarian cysts, and after contrast administration demonstrate septations or wall thickening. CAT images do not usually demonstrate follicles less than 1 cm in diameter. Ultrasound is the modality generally chosen to follow simple cysts and ovarian follicles due to its lack of ionizing radiation and easy availability, which makes serial examinations practical.

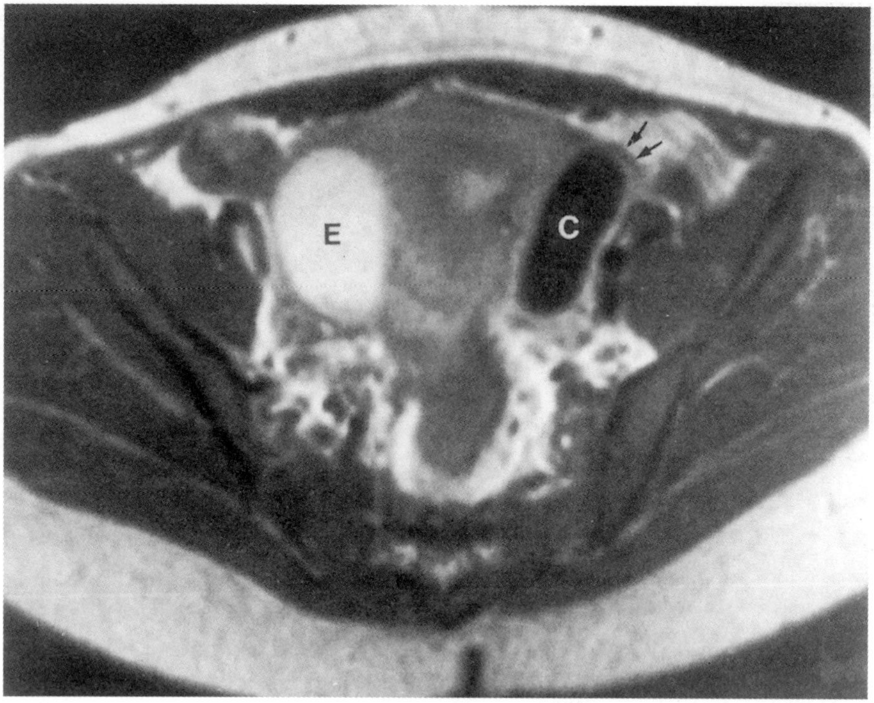

Fig. 58.2 Magnetic resonance image of an ovarian cyst and an endometrioma. Axial T_1-weighted section obtained after administration of intravenous contrast demonstrates a simple cyst in the left ovary. The cyst (C) is low signal intensity and the adjacent stroma (arrows) is high signal intensity. A high signal intensity endometrioma (E) is demonstrated in the right ovary as well. (Reproduced, with permission, from Occhipinti 1994)

NON-NEOPLASTIC CYSTIC LESIONS/ENDOMETRIOSIS

Ultrasound

Endometriosis remains a laparoscopic diagnosis, as staging requires direct visualization. No radiological modality is able to demonstrate the small lesions and adhesions found with early-stage endometriosis. Ultrasound images are able to demonstrate endometriomas, which are characteristically described as a 'cyst' filled with internal echoes. However, these findings are not specific, and on ultrasound examination alone an endometrioma may be confused with a pus-filled fallopian tube in pelvic inflammatory disease, a solid mass, or a hemorrhagic functional cyst (Grant 1992).

MRI and CAT

MRI is the most sensitive imaging modality available for detection of endometriosis and differentiation of an endometrioma from other adnexal masses (Outwater et al 1993). Endometrotic lesions have been reported to have variable signal intensity by MRI, depending on the extent of fibrosis and the present. Endometriomas most commonly demonstrate the high signal intensity of subacute hemorrhage on both T_1- and T_2-weighted sequences (Fig. 58.3), but can have variable signal intensity due to the different stages of hemorrhage within the endometrioma. A hematocrit level, due to layering of hemosiderin, has also been described. The fibrotic wall around an endometrioma can appear as low signal intensity rim on T_1- and T_2-weighted images, and will enhance after administration of intravenous contrast. The differential diagnosis on MRI includes other hemorrhagic lesions, such as a simple hemorrhagic follicle or corpus luteum cyst. Endometriomas have a nonspecific soft-tissue density on CAT, and cannot be reliably differentiated from other adnexal masses.

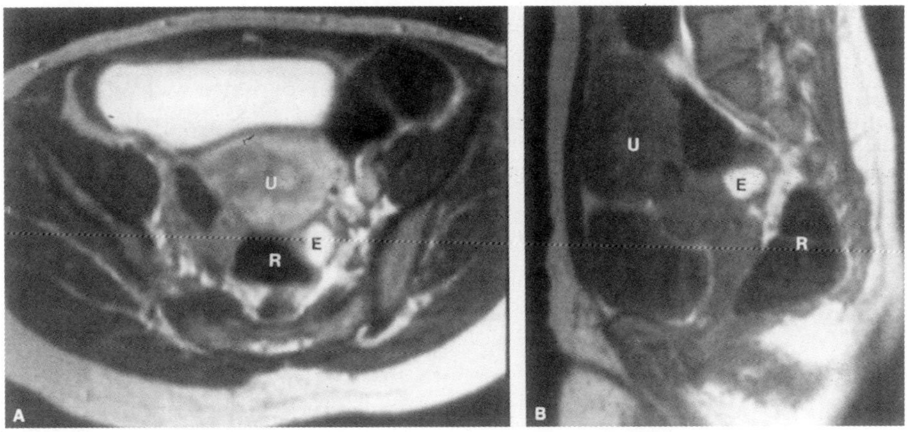

Fig. 58.3 Magnetic resonance image of an endometrioma. Axial T_2-weighted section and sagittal T_1-weighted section demonstrates a high signal intensity endometrioma (E) between the uterus (U) and the rectosigmoid junction (R). (Reproduced, with permission, from Occhipinti 1994)

MRI and CAT can be useful in the identification of endometriomas in unusual locations not ordinarily imaged by ultrasound, or visualized by routine surgery, such as the rectovaginal septum, abdominal wall, presacral region, or sciatic nerve (Arrive et al 1989) (Fig. 58.3). In this way, these modalities can provide valuable presurgical information.

PELVIC INFLAMMATORY DISEASE

Ultrasound and MRI

Pelvic inflammatory disease (PID) can be routinely diagnosed when a woman presents with fever, leucocytosis, and pelvic pain, and bilateral cystic adnexal masses are discovered with ultrasound evaluation. In cases where the clinical presentation does not support the diagnosis, differentiation of PID from endometriosis or even bilateral cystic ovarian tumors may be difficult by ultrasound. In these cases, the multiplanar images provided by MRI will often show the true tubular nature of the 'adnexal mass' and visualization of a dilated fallopian tube filled with fluid can lead to the diagnosis of PID. In addition, the walls of the fallopian tubes will be thickened in PID and can enhance after intravenous contrast administration (normal fallopian tubes are not demonstrated by MRI and do not enhance with contrast).

PERITONEAL PSEUDOCYST

Ultrasound, MRI, and CAT

Peritoneal pseudocysts, which result from fluid trapped in the pelvis by adhesions for surgery or endometriosis, can be identified by all three modalities. Ultrasound can be used to recognize that a large, cystic mass with septations is present in the pelvis. Further evaluation with MRI or CAT, which provides a larger field of view, is required to determine the full extent of the cystic area, and determine that it is not arising from the ovary, but is actually fluid trapped within the pelvis itself. MRI T_2-weighted sequences can be used to identify the ovary and uterus by their characteristic signal intensity, and the relationship of these organs to the pseudocyst can be determined. CAT will demonstrate the loculated fluid in a pelvic pseudocyst, and can also be used to make the diagnosis, but will not give as detailed a picture of the other pelvic organs (Kwachi et al 1993).

PAROVARIAN AND PARATUBAL CYSTS

Ultrasound and MRI

Parovarian and paratubal cysts can be recognized by both ultrasound and MRI as simple or hemorrhagic cysts located in and arising from the adnexa (rather than the ovary). When large, they may migrate out of the pelvis and can be found superior to the uterine fundus sonographically (Athey & Cooper 1985). Except for their location, these cysts are indistinguishable from other simple cysts by current imaging methods.

RADIOLOGICAL EVALUATION OF PELVIC SURGICAL EMERGENCIES

Ectopic pregnancy

Ultrasound

Both TAUS and TVUS are recommended for complete evaluation of a woman with pelvic pain and elevated β-human chorionic gonadotrophin (β-hCG) if there is a clinical suspicion of ectopic pregnancy. The uterus, adnexae, and cul-de-sac should be examined in a systematic manner. In 6–19% of patients with ectopic pregnancy, the pelvis can have a normal appearance, and therefore a normal ultrasound cannot be used to definitely exclude the presence of an ectopic pregnancy (Cacciatore 1990). Sonographic findings can be used to place each patient in a low or high risk group, and appropriate clinical follow-up selected (with either serial β-hCG levels and repeat ultrasound or laparoscopy/laparotomy).

Intrauterine sonographic findings in a woman with an ectopic pregnancy can vary from an empty uterus to thickened endometrial echo (which can also be seen after a recent spontaneous abortion) or a small amount of fluid that may

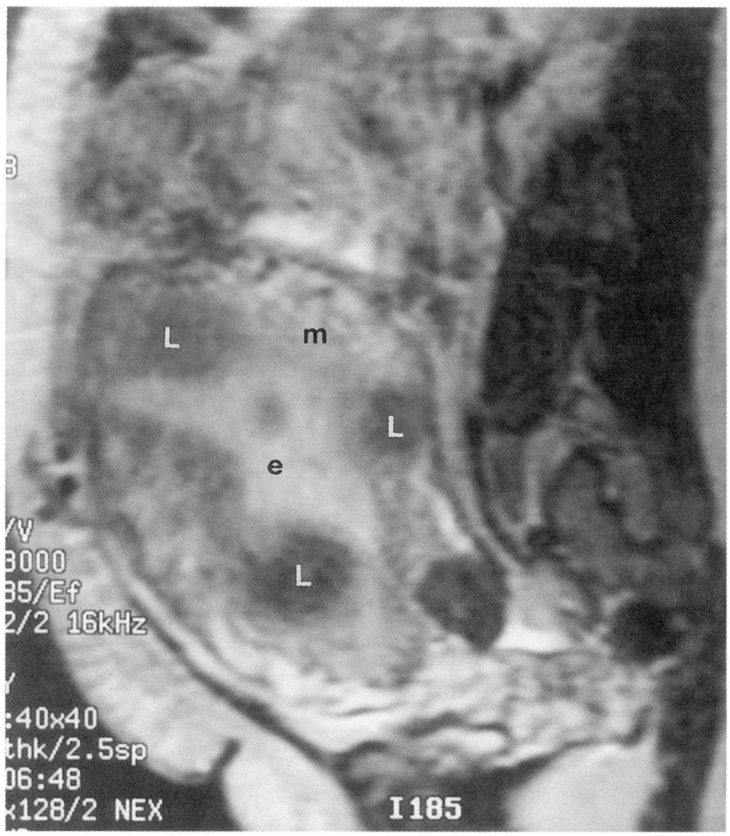

A

Fig. 58.4 Magnetic resonance evaluation of abdominal pregnancy in the second trimester. (A) Sagittal T_2-weighted image demonstrates an empty uterus, with endometrium (E) and myometrium (M) well visualized. Multiple intramural leiomyomas (L) are also depicted. (B) Sagittal T_2-weighted image of the abdomen demonstrates the head and body of a fetus (arrows) in the upper abdomen, outside of the uterus.

mimic a gestational sac. Findings in the adnexa that can lead to a diagnosis of ectopic pregnancy vary from an adnexal mass to an actual extrauterine sac or even an actual fetal pole with a beating heart. Duplex and color Doppler studies can be used to confirm the presence of an intra- or extrauterine gestational sac by demonstrating a low resistance pattern of flow. Hemoperitoneum, from leakage of blood out of the fallopian tube, appears as echogenic fluid in the cul-de-sac and, when present, significantly increases the likelihood of ectopic pregnancy (Nyberg 1992).

MRI

MRI is not routinely used in the presurgical evaluation of a woman with suspected ectopic pregnancy, since ultrasound is more readily available on an emergency basis. On magnetic resonance images, adnexal ectopic pregnancy appears as a nonspecific type of adnexal mass with various stages of hemorrhage. The MRI differential diagnosis includes gestational trophoblastic disease, which can also present with elevated β-hCG and a mixed signal intensity mass.

MRI can be very helpful in evaluating the rare forms of intrauterine ectopic pregnancy. These patients present a confusing clinical picture, with persistent uterine bleeding and pelvic pain despite evacuation. The site of the ectopic gestational sac appears more as a heterogeneous signal intensity focus which disrupts the normal MRI appearance of the uterus on both T_1- and T_2-weighted images. This focus can be localized to the abnormal site, e.g. within the cervix, in the cornua/interstitial regions, or intramural, at the

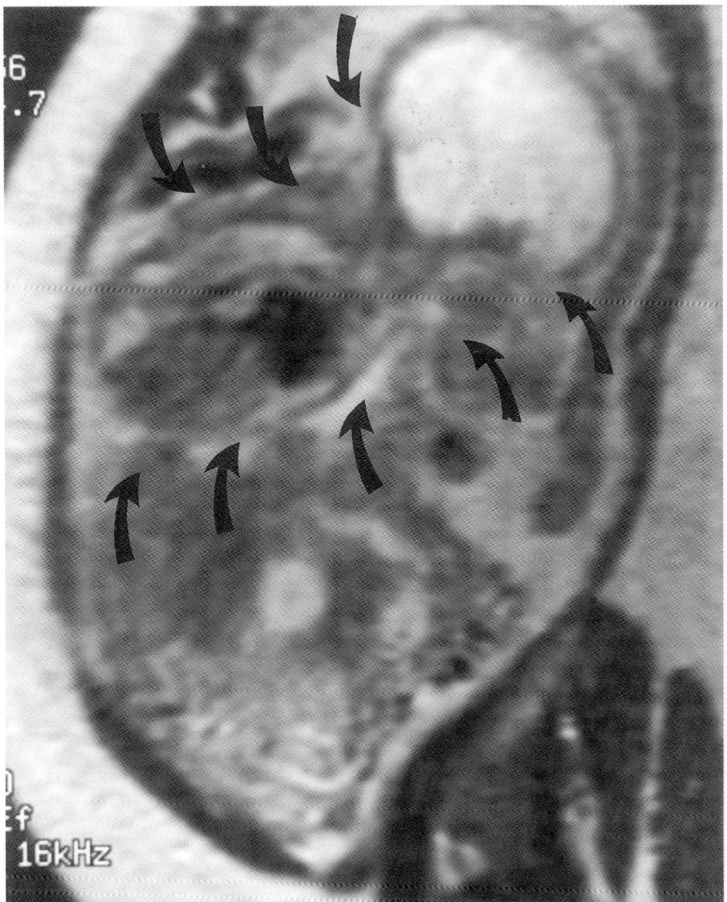

B **Fig. 58.4** *(cont'd)*

site of a previous caesarean section (Kwon et al 1993).

MRI can also be of value in the diagnosis of a second-trimester intra-abdominal ectopic pregnancy. Both TAUS and TVUS may be limited due to the artifact from bowel gas within the abdomen and relatively small field of view. The MRI field of view can be expanded to include both abdomen and pelvis in a single coronal or sagittal slice, and lay out in one image the empty uterus in the pelvis as well as the adjacent intra-abdominal placenta and fetus. MRI can also demonstrate the internal architecture of the uterus, and can display associated uterine abnormalities, such as obstructing leiomyomas, that might have made a normal intrauterine implantation difficult (Fig. 58.4).

Adnexal torsion and massive ovarian edema

Ultrasound and MRI

The enlarged, edematous ovary in a patient with adnexal torsion can be demonstrated sonographically. The appearance may be that of a large, solid mass, but if small ovarian follicles can be identified in the periphery, an enlarged ovary can be diagnosed. Color Doppler evaluation can support the diagnosis of torsion by demonstrating a lack of flow in the vessels on the affected side. The cysts or masses which commonly predispose to torsion can also be visualized sonographically.

MRI can also be used to visualize an enlarged and edematous ovary with peripheral follicles (Fig. 58.5). An associated ovarian cyst or mass, or adjacent dilated fallopian tube may also be demonstrated. If hemorrhagic infarction of the ovary occurs, a high signal intensity rim can be identified as well (Kawakami et al 1993).

VIRILIZING OVARIAN DISORDERS

Polycystic ovary syndrome

Polycystic ovary syndrome (PCOS) is primarily an endocrinological disorder with a spectrum of clinical manifestations. The most common sonographic finding is enlarged ovaries with a spherical shape and a volume greater than 12 cm^3 (Orsini et al 1985). TVUS readily depicts the small peripheral follicles. In one study, when characteristic sonographic features were present, 50% of patients demonstrated the classic clinical triad of amenorrhea, anovulation, and infertility, 25% of patients had a variant of the disease, and 25% were asymptomatic (Swanson et al 1981).

MRI is able to capture the appearance of poly-

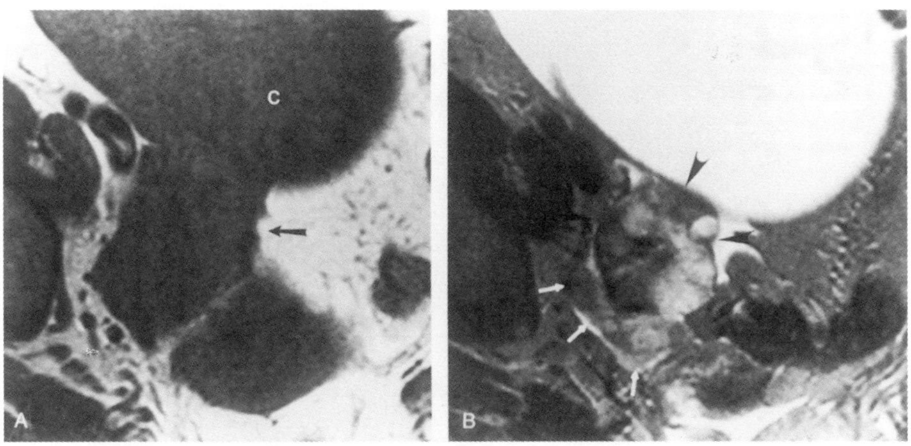

Fig. 58.5 Magnetic resonance image of ovarian torsion. (A) Axial T_1-weighted image shows an adnexal mass which is revealed to be a cyst (C) by characteristic high-signal intensity on adjacent (B) Axial T_2-weighted image also reveals an enlarged, edematous ovary (black arrowheads) with adjacent edematous fallopian tube (white arrows). (Reproduced, with permission, from Outwater & Schiebler 1994).

cystic ovaries, including the ovarian enlargement and multiple small, peripheral cysts. Decreased signal intensity of the central ovarian stroma on T_2-weighted images has also been reported, and is thought to result from the increased amount of fibrous tissue present (Swanson et al 1981). The small follicles of a women on birth-control pills can mimic the appearance of PCOS on MRI, however, and the diagnosis remains a clinical one (Fig. 58.6).

Stromal hyperplasia and stromal hyperthecosis

Ultrasound and MRI

Both ultrasound and MRI are able to depict the bilateral enlargement of the ovaries and the multiple cysts that occur with these two entities (Fig. 58.7).

EVALUATION OF OVARIAN TUMORS – BENIGN VERSUS MALIGNANT

Ultrasound

Ultrasound evaluation of an ovarian mass provides valuable information which enables the gynecologist properly to manage the patient's course of treatment. The primary function of ultrasound is to determine if a lesion is predominantly cystic or solid. A small, unilocular cyst can be considered benign in the premenopausal woman and, as previously described, includes in the differential diagnosis follicle and corpus luteum cysts as well as paraovarian cysts. In postmenopausal women, the most common ovarian lesion discovered on a routine basis sonographically is the benign serous inclusion cyst, but the differential diagnosis must be expanded to include both benign tumors (serous and mucinous cystadenomas) and cystadenocarcinomas. Once dis-

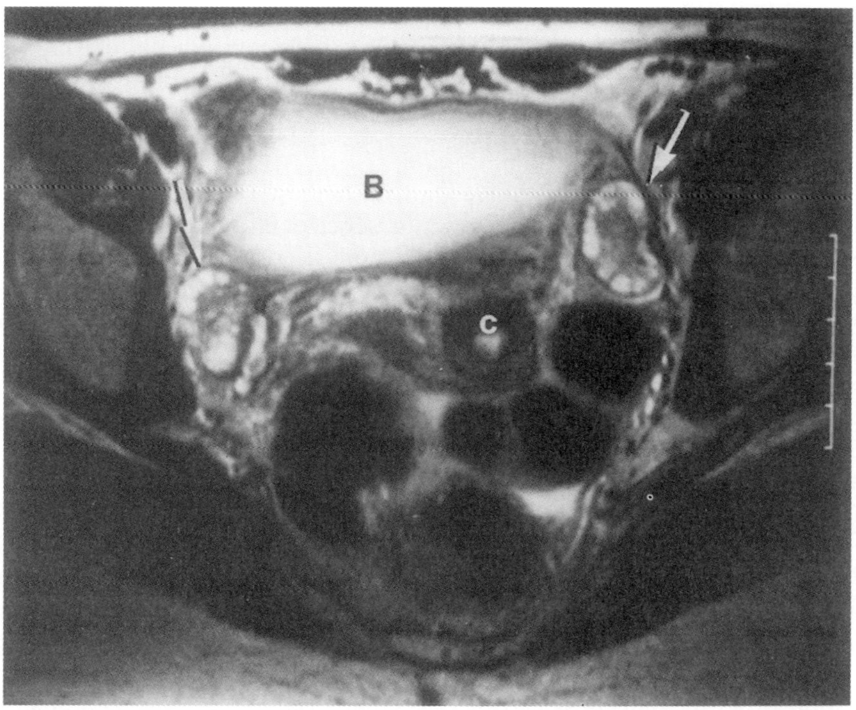

Fig. 58.6 Magnetic resonance image of ovaries that mimic polycystic ovary syndrome. Axial T_2-weighted image of a woman on birth-control pills demonstrates multiple, small peripheral follicles, and low signal intensity central stroma in both ovaries (arrows) which has a similar MRI appearance to ovaries with polycystic ovary syndrome. B, Bladder; C, cervix.

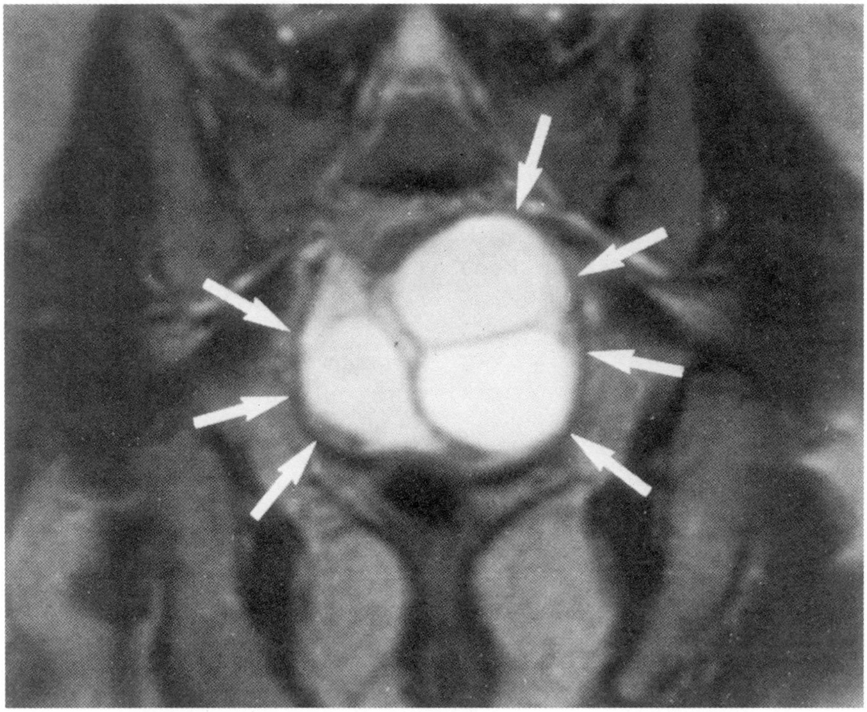

Fig. 58.7 Magnetic resonance image of stromal hyperthecosis. Coronal T_2-weighted image of bilaterally enlarged, cystic ovaries (arrows) in a woman with pathologically diagnosed stromal hyperthecosis. (Reproduced, with permission, from Occhipinti et al 1993)

covered, ultrasound is also the modality of choice for follow-up, to determine if the unilocular cyst resolves or persists, which in turn will determine if medical therapy or surgery are necessary.

Teratomas are benign cystic tumors with solid components that often have characteristic sonographic appearances, as do benign solid fibroma/thecomas. Most malignant ovarian tumors are mixed cystic and solid lesions, the nature of which can be recognized on ultrasound by their large size, mural nodules or solid components, and associated findings of ascites and implants. Ultrasound is not the modality of choice to stage ovarian carcinoma, and if further imaging is required after detection of an ovarian tumor, CAT or MRI are recommended.

Doppler evaluation of an ovarian mass can be performed and the resistive index (RI) of flow determined (peak systolic velocity minus peak diastolic velocity divided by the peak systolic velocity). The resistive index values range from 1.0 (highest resistance to forward flow) to 0.0 (absence of end-diastolic forward flow). Malignant tumors are usually very vascular, and demonstrate a resistive index less than 0.40. However, RI values of benign and malignant lesions overlap considerably, and this measurement cannot be used as a definitive diagnostic tool for or against the possibility of malignancy (Brown et al 1994).

MRI

As previously described, MRI is able to identify functional cysts of the ovary. The dermoid cyst also can be reliably diagnosed by magnetic resonance criteria using fat saturation sequences. The criteria have been developed in an attempt to differentiate benign from borderline and malignant epithelial tumors. Papillary projections, thick irregular walls, or extensive solid components (often with necrosis) are common signs of malignancy. The exception to these rules are the solid but benign fibroma/

thecoma group of tumors, which can be identified by their MRI signal characteristics.

A benign ovarian tumor is suggested by the magnetic resonance images if the following criteria are present: entirely cystic lesion; wall thickness less than 3 mm; lack of internal structure; absence of ascites; and absence of invasive characteristics, such as peritoneal disease or adenopathy. It should be noted that intravenous contrast is essential to bring out the internal architecture of an ovarian mass when applying the above criteria. Preoperative characterization of an ovarian lesion by a properly performed MRI and using the given criteria has been reported to be up to 95% accurate (Stevens et al 1991).

MRI VERSUS ULTRASOUND AND CT IN PREOPERATIVE CHARACTERIZATION OF OVARIAN LESIONS

Several studies which compare contrast-enhanced MRI of the pelvis with TVUS point to the superior-

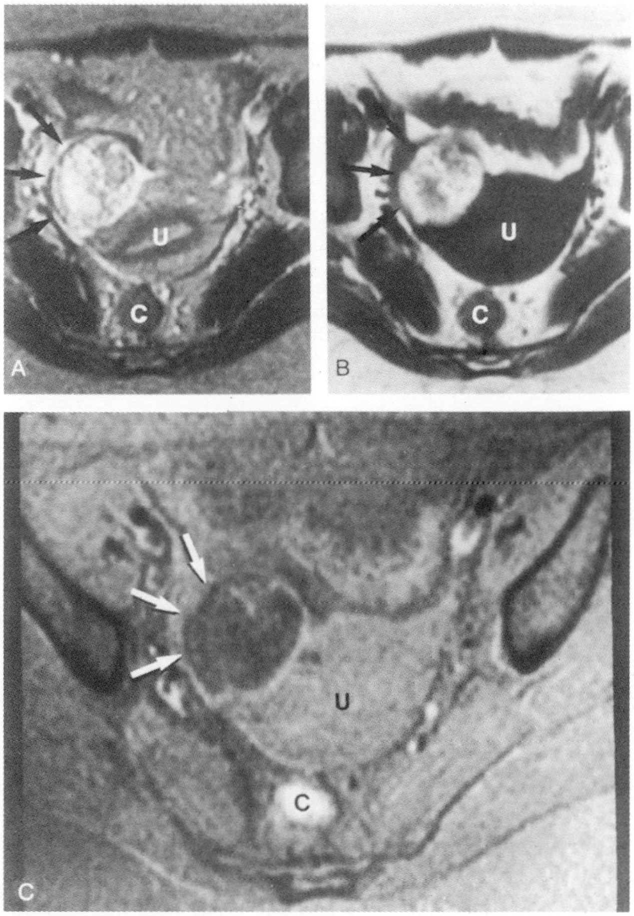

Fig. 58.8 Magnetic resonance images of a teratoma. (A) Axial T_2-weighted image of an ovarian teratoma (arrows), which demonstrates high signal intensity. (B) Axial T_1-weighted image of a teratoma (arrows), which again demonstrates high signal intensity. (C) After fat saturation sequence is applied, the teratoma (arrows) becomes low signal intensity, verifying that the lesion contains fat. U, Uterus; C, colon. (Reproduced, with permission, from Occhipinti et al 1993)

ity of MRI in evaluation of adnexal masses (Mitchell et al 1987, Hata et al 1992, Yamashita et al 1995). Differentiating malignant tumors from benign conditions such as endometriosis can be difficult by ultrasound criteria, since solid tissue, fat, and hemorrhagic cysts can have similar sonographic appearances. Higher diagnostic accuracy can be achieved with MRI, which has special hemorrhage-sensitive sequences for detecting endometriomas, and fat-sensitive sequences for detecting teratomas. MRI and TVUS do have similar capabilities in the characterization of simple

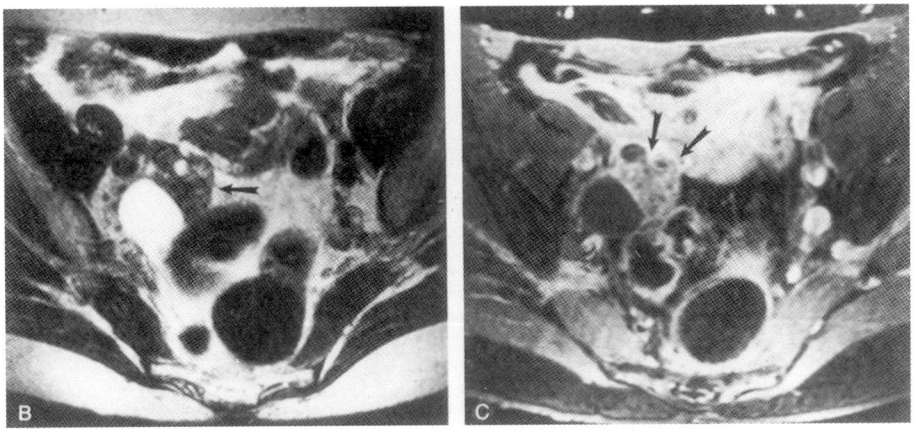

Fig. 58.9 Magnetic resonance image of a struma ovarii tumor. Axial T_2 and contrast enhanced T_1-weighted images demonstrate nonspecific signal intensity of a struma ovarii tumor (arrows), in this cystic and solid tumor. (Reproduced, with permission, from Outwater & Schiebler 1994)

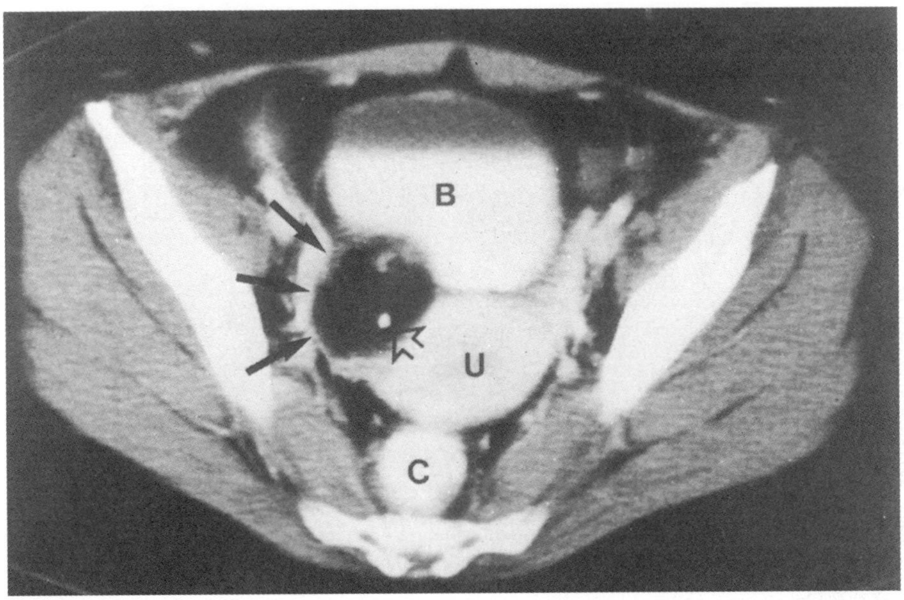

Fig. 58.10 CT image of a teratoma. Teratoma of the right ovary (arrows) can be identified by characteristic low signal intensity fat composition. A small focus of calcification (open arrow) is also identified. B, Bladder; U, uterus; C, colon). (Reproduced, with permission, from Occhipinti et al 1993)

cysts, cystadenomas, and malignant serous and mucinous tumors.

A comparison study between CAT and non contrast-enhanced MRI found the latter to be superior in overall classification of adnexal lesions, although both modalities were similar in classification of ovarian tumors (Ghossian 1991).

BENIGN OVARIAN TUMORS

Mature cystic teratomas (dermoid cysts)

Ultrasound

The ultrasound appearance of a dermoid cyst is variable, ranging from a predominantly cystic to a

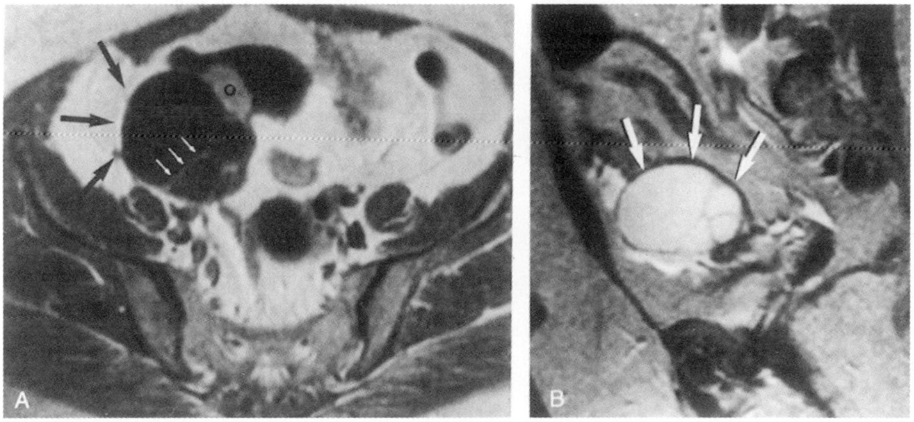

Fig. 58.11 Magnetic resonance image of a serous cystadenoma. Contrast-enhanced T_1-weighted axial image and T_2-weighted sagittal image both demonstrate a small cystic tumor (black arrows) with septations (white arrows) arising from the right ovary (O). (Reproduced, with permission, from Occhipinti et al 1993)

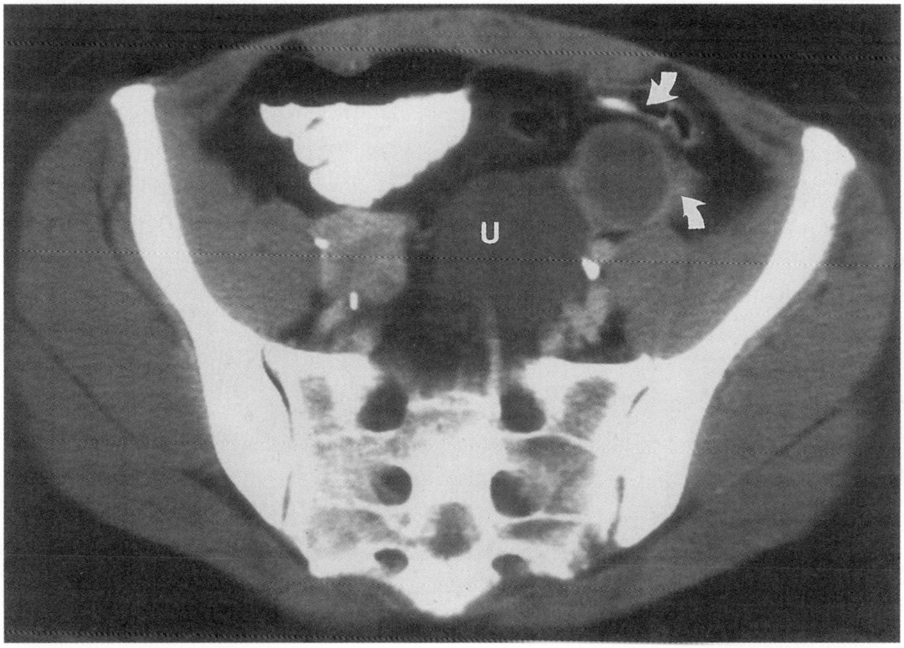

Fig. 58.12 CAT image of a serous cystadenoma. A small, cystic tumor is identified in the region of the left ovary (arrows). U, Uterus

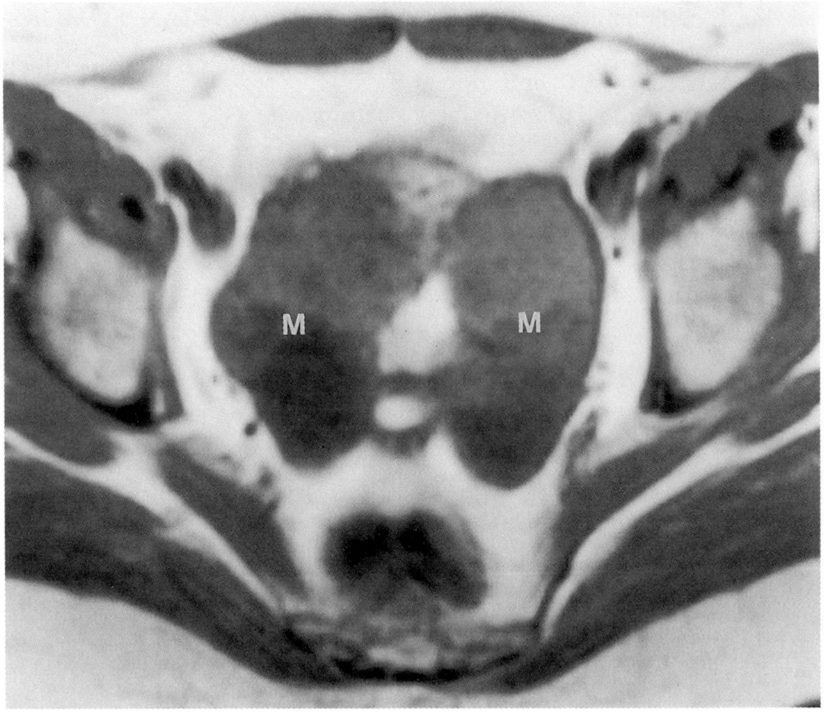

A

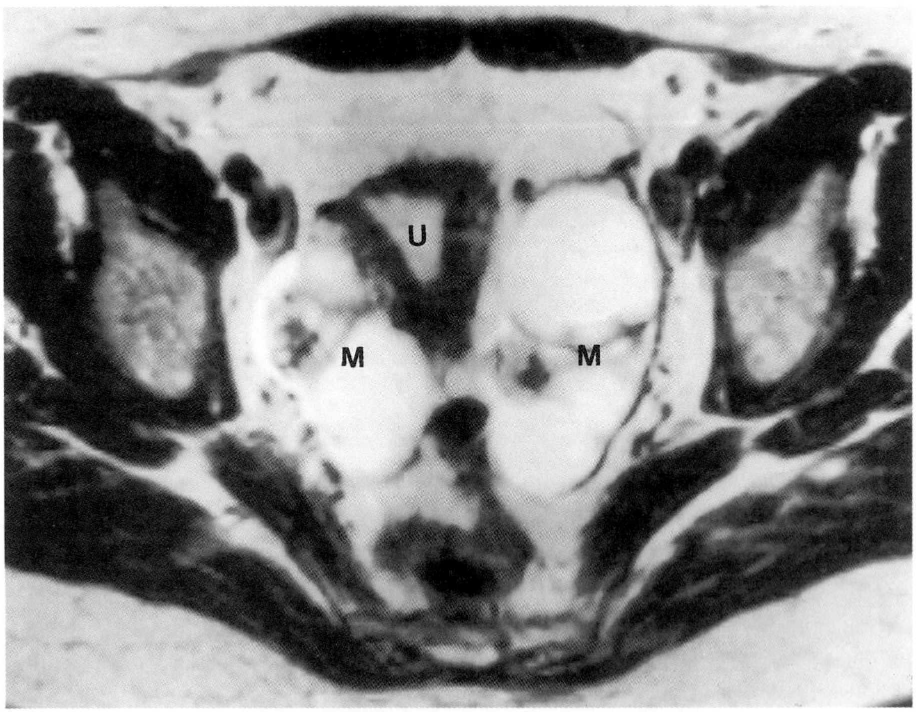

B

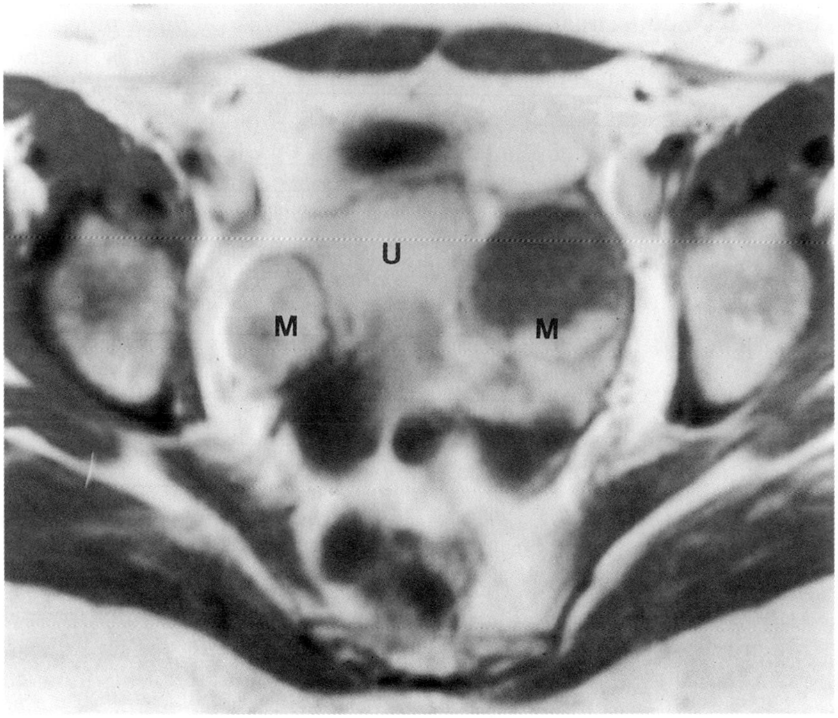

C

Fig. 58.13 Magnetic resonance image of ovarian adenocarcinoma. (A) Axial T_1-weighted image demonstrates bilateral ovarian masses (M). (B) Axial T_2-weighted image demonstrates the cystic nature of these masses (M). (C) The same tumors (M) after administration of intravenous contrast also demonstrates the cystic nature of the tumor, which appear as several low signal intensity, nonenhancing regions. U, Uterus

predominantly solid-appearing mass. The anechoic cystic portion of the tumor represents homogeneous fat, which is liquid at body temperature. If an echogenic germinal tubercle can be identified, or if highly echogenic calcium with acoustic shadowing (in a tooth) is present, the diagnosis can be made sonographically. Small, subclinical dermoids may also be found in the contralateral ovary as small echogenic masses by TVUS, and both ovaries are always evaluated to look for bilateral disease.

MRI

MRI is able to demonstrate fat within a cystic dermoid as high signal intensity on T_1-weighted images which becomes low signal intensity after a fat saturation sequence is applied (Fig. 58.8). The germinal tubercle is visualized as a nonspecific solid component, and any calcium present within the tubercle will have low signal intensity on both T_1- and T_2-weighted images. However, even large foci of calcium are not well depicted by MRI as a separate entity, unlike CT or ultrasound which are more sensitive in the detection of calcium. MRI characteristics of the rare struma ovarii type of teratoma are that of a nonspecific mixed cystic/solid mass (Outwater & Schiebler 1994) (Fig. 58.9).

CAT

The dermoid cyst has a characteristic appearance on CAT images, as a well-circumscribed mass containing fat attenuation material. Calcification in teeth within the germinal tubercle is also clearly demonstrated by the CAT technique. Of all modalities, CAT is the most sensitive in the detection of fat and calcium, the two most common components of a dermoid, although MRI can also be diagnostic (Fig. 58.10).

Serous and mucinous cystadenomas

Ultrasound

Cystadenomas may be simple, unilocular cysts and appear benign sonographically, or contain septations or nodules, in which case the differential diagnosis includes a benign mucinous tumor or proliferating tumor of either type. Ultrasound is the modality of choice to follow what may initially appear to be a dysfunctional cyst or serous inclusion cyst; if the cyst does not decrease in size or resolve in 1–2 menstrual cycles or months, further surgical evaluation may be necessary, especially in postmenopausal women, when cystadenoma or carcinoma should be considered in the differential diagnosis (Hurwitz et al 1988).

MRI

Both serous and mucinous ovarian cystadenomas are well demonstrated on T_2- and contrast-enhanced T_1-weighted images (Fig. 58.11). The fluid within the serous cystadenoma will have the signal intensity of a simple fluid, i.e. low on T_1 and high on T_2. The fluid in mucinous cystadenomas varies in signal intensity, and depends on the ratio of water and mucin in each locule. After administration of intravenous contrast, internal septations within these tumors will enhance and become more evident, which aids in making the diagnosis of a benign or proliferating tumor.

CAT

Cystadenomas can be visualized on CAT images as cystic ovarian masses with septations and thin walls (Fig. 58.12). After administration of intravenous contrast, the walls and septations enhance. The contents of the tumor measure water attenuation for serous tumors and may be of variable or higher attenuation for mucinous tumors.

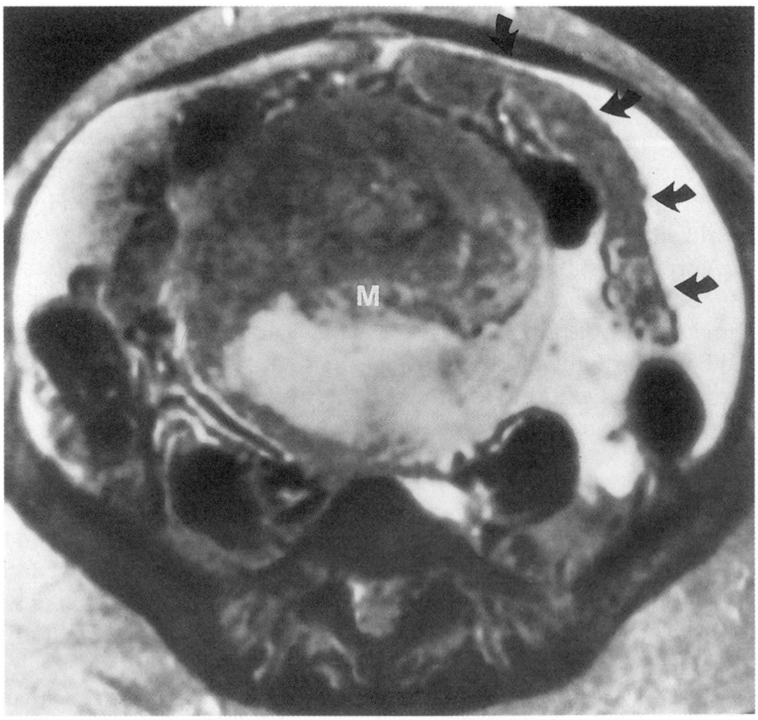

Fig. 58.14 Magnetic resonance image of omental cake. Axial T_2-weighted image demonstrates the thickened, low signal intensity omentum (arrows) adjacent to an ovarian mass (M) in a patient with ovarian carcinoma

OVARIAN CARCINOMA

Ultrasound, CAT, and MRI

A woman with increasing abdominal girth or a palpable pelvic mass and suspected ovarian carcinoma will usually have an ultrasound or CAT scan as the next step in the diagnostic work-up. TAUS and TVUS provide valuable information about the internal architecture of the ovarian mass, and can also detect fluid in the cul-de-sac and confirm the diagnosis of suspected ovarian malignancy. Actual staging of ovarian carcinoma is performed by surgical exploration (see Ch. 22). During the initial operation for staging, cryoreduction is also performed, and is thought to be optimal if all tumor is removed except small implants less than 2 cm in diameter.

The role of CAT and MRI in the staging of ovarian carcinoma is controversial, but has again come into the limelight with the realization that surgical understaging and suboptimal cryoreduction can be found in 30–40% of cases (Young et al 1993). In a recent NIH Concensus Conference (1995), cross-sectional imaging was recommended as an adjunct to surgical staging. Both CAT and MRI have been found to be highly accurate in the prediction of cancer resectability, and can aid the surgeon in planning optimal cryoreduction (Nelson et al 1993, Forstner et al 1996).

Both MRI and CAT are able to depict the malignant ovarian tumor after administration of intravenous contrast. Cystic and solid areas can be visualized, as can regions of necrosis, septations, and papillary projections. Magnetic resonance signal intensity characteristics also aid in determining the type of fluid present in serous and mucinous carcinomas (Fig. 58.13).

CAT and MRI staging criteria have been developed to correspond to the FIGO surgical staging (see Appendix C). The CAT and MRI appearance of pelvic extension into the uterus is depicted as a distortion in the uterine contour or an irregular tumor/myometrial interface. MRI signal intensity characteristics of the uterus will also be disrupted.

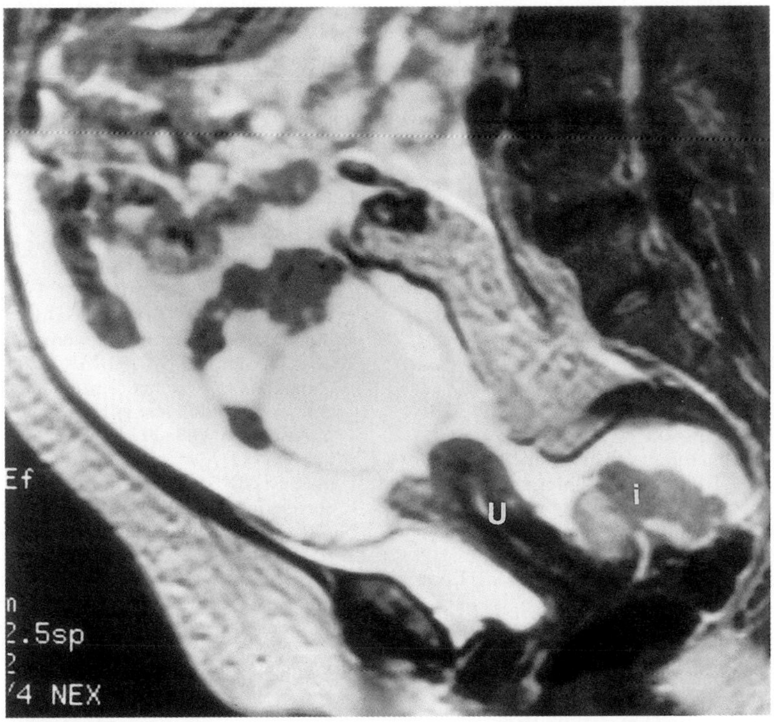

Fig. 58.15 Magnetic resonance image of peritoneal implants. Sagittal T_2-weighted image demonstrates the uterus (U) with adjacent implants (I) in the cul-de-sac

Sigmoid colon invasion can be suggested by both modalities as direct encasement by tumor or loss of fat planes between tumor and colon.

Malignant seeding of the abdomen can be similarly visualized by both modalities. Omental cake appears most commonly as a feathery thickening of the omentum on CAT and magnetic resonance images (it is not normally visualized by either modality). On MRI, infiltration by tumor also causes a decrease in the signal intensity of fat on T_1 and T_2-weighted images (Fig. 58.14). Enhancement of the omentum is also present in cases of malignant infiltration.

Both CAT and MRI are limited in actual staging of ovarian carcinoma due to difficulty in the detection of small peritoneal implants of 5–8 mm, and even up to 2 cm, which are not consistently visualized (Jacquet et al 1993). On CAT, visualization is improved in the rare instance when the implants are calcified, and also appears to be enhanced in pockets of ascites. Peritoneal implants can be located by both modalities in the cul-de-sac, paracolic gutters, and under the hemidiaphragms (frequently adjacent to the liver); they are less well visualized within the mesentery, and on the surface of small and large bowel, perhaps due to artifact from bowel motion. On CAT images, implants appear as nodular or plaque-like soft tissue foci. On magnetic resonance images, implants are variable foci of signal intensity on T_2-weighted sequences (Fig. 58.15). Implants will enhance on both CAT and T_1-weighted magnetic resonance images after administration of intravenous contrast (Low & Sigeti 1994).

REFERENCES

Arrive L, Hricak H, Martin M C 1989 Pelvic endometriosis: MR imaging. Radiology 171: 687–692

Athey P, Cooper N B 1985 Sonographic features of parovarian cysts. American Journal of Radiology 144: 83–86

Brown D L, Frates M C, Laing F C et al 1994 Ovarian masses: can benign and malignant lesions be differentiated with colour and pulsed doppler ultrasound? Radiology 190: 333–336

Cacciatore B 1990 Can the status of tubal pregnancy be predicted with transvaginal sonography? A prospective comparison of sonographic, surgical, and serum HCG findings. Radiology 177: 481–484

Dooms G C, Hricak H, Tscholakoff D 1986 Adnexal structures: MR imaging. Radiology 158: 639–646

Forstner R, Hricak H, Occhipinti K, Powell C B, Frankel S D, Stern J L 1994 Value of CT and MR in the staging of ovarian cancer. Presented at the 80th Scientific Assembly and Annual Meeting of the Radiological Society of North America, Chicago, IL, 1994

Forstner R, Hricak H, Occhipinti K, Powell C B, Frankel S D, Stern J L 1995 Ovarian Cancer: staging with CT and MR Imaging Radiology; 197: 619–626

Ghossian M A 1991 Epithelial tumors of the ovary; comparison of MR and CT findings. Radiology 191: 863–878

Grant E G 1992 Benign conditions of the ovaries. In: Nyberg D A, Hill L M, Bohm-Velez M, Mendelson E B (eds) Transvaginal ultrasound. Mosby Year Book, St Louis, MI, p 191–202

Hata K, Hata T, Manabe A et al 1992 A critical evaluation of transvaginal doppler studies, transvaginal sonography, MRI and CA 125 in detecting ovarian cancer. Obstetrics and Gynecology 80: 922–926

Haustein J, Niendorf H P, Krestin G et al 1992 Renal tolerance of Magnevist dimeglumine in patients with chronic renal failure. Investigative Radiology 27: 153–156

Hurwitz A, Yagel S, Zion I et al 1988 The management of persistent clear pelvic cysts diagnosed by ultrasonography. Obstetrics and Gynecology 72: 320–322

Jaquet P, Jelinek J S, Stevens M A, Sugarbaker P H 1993 Evaluation of computed tomography in patients with peritoneal carcinomatosis. Cancer 72: 1631–1636

Kawakami K, Murata K, Kawacuchi N et al 1993 Haemorrhagic infarction of the diseased ovary: a common MR finding in two cases. Magnetic Resonance Imaging 11: 595–597

Kwachi H, Murakami T, Nakamura H et al 1993 Imaging of peritoneal pseudocysts: value of MR imaging compared with sonography and CT. American Journal of Radiology 160: 589–591

Kwon H H, Keun J J, Jin K S et al 1993 MR imaging in the diagnosis of rare forms of ectopic pregnancy. American Journal of Radiology 160: 1229–1232

Levine D, Gosink B B, Wolf S I, Feldesman M R, Pretorius D H 1992 Simple adnexal cysts: the natural history in postmenopausal women. Radiology 184: 653–659

Low R N, Signeti J S 1994 MR imaging of peritoneal disease: comparison of contrast-enhanced fast multiplanar spoiled gradient-recalled and spin-echo imaging. American Journal of Radiology 163: 1131–1140

Mitchell D G, Mintz M C, Spritzer C E et al 1987 Adnexal masses: MR imaging observation at 1.5T, with US and CT correlation. Radiology 162: 319–324

Nelson B E, Rosenfield A T, Schwartz P E 1993 Preoperative abdominopelvic computed tomographic prediction of optimal cryoreduction in epithelial ovarian carcinoma. Journal of Clinical Oncology 11: 166–172

NIH Consensus Conference 1995 Ovarian cancer: screening, treatment and follow-up. Journal of American Medical Association 273: 491–497

Nyberg C A 1992 Ectopic pregnancy. In: Nyberg D A, Hill L M, Bohm-Velez M, Mendelson E B (eds) Transvaginal ultrasound. Mosby Year Book, St Louis, MI, p 105–132

Occhipinti K A 1994 Magnetic resonance imaging of

abnormal pelvic anatomy. In: Jaffe R, Pierson R A, Abramowicz J S (eds) Imaging in infertility and reproductive endocrinology. J B Lippincott, Philadelphia, PA

Occhipinti K A, Frankel S D, Hricak H 1993 The ovary, computed tomography and magnetic resonance imaging. In: Gooding G A W, Higgins C B (eds) The radiologic clinics of North America. Endocrine Radiology. W B Saunders, Philadelphia, PA

Orsini L F, Venturoli S, Lorusso R et al 1985 Ultrasonographic findings in polycystic ovary discasc. Fertility and Sterility 43: 709–714

Outwater E, Chiebler M L, Owen R S, Schnall M D 1993 Characterization of hemorrhagic adnexal lesions with MR imaging: blinded reader study. Radiology 186: 484–489

Outwater E K, Schiebler M L 1994 Magnetic resonance imaging of the ovary. In: Mezrick R, Weinreb J C (eds) Magnetic resonance imaging clinics of North America. The female pelvis. W B Saunders, Philadelphia, PA, p 250–254

Smith R C, Reinhold C, McCauley T R et al 1992 Multicoil high-resolution fast spin echo MR imaging of the female pelvis. Radiology 184: 671–675

Stevens S K, Hricak H, Stern J L 1991 Ovarian lesions: detection and characterization with gadolinium-enhanced MR images at 1.5 T. Radiology 181: 481–488

Swanson M, Sauerbei E E, Cooperberg P L 1981 Medical implications of ultrasonically detected polycystic ovaries. Journal of Clinical Ultrasound 9: 219–222

Yamashita Y, Torashima M, Hatanaka Y et al 1995 Adnexal masses: accuracy of characterization with transvaginal US and precontrast and postcontrast MR imaging. Radiology 194: 552–565

Young R C, Perez C A, Hoskins W 1993 Cancer of the ovary. In: de Vita V T, Hellman S, Rosenberg S A (eds) Cancer. Principles and practice of oncology, 4th edn. Lippincott, Philadelphia, PA, p 1226–1263

SECTION 10

Appendices

Appendix A

Inherited syndromes and ovarian pathology

The format of this appendix is intended to provide readers with ready access to case reports and review articles (where possible) which reflect the spectrum of inherited or congenital syndromes associated with a known and predictable array of pathological entities in the human ovaries. The range of syndromes referenced is biased heavily towards those associated with ovarian tumors, although other sequelae such as premature ovarian failure are addressed. The references are not intended to be encyclopedic, but are the few most recent, most significant, or most accessible for each entity.

Androgen insensitivity syndrome

Malignant sex cord–stromal tumor

O'Dowd J, Gaffney E F, Young R H 1990 Malignant sex cord–stromal tumor in a patient with the androgen insensitivity syndrome. Histopathology 16: 279–282

Ataxia telangectasia

Premature ovarian failure

Miller M E, Chatten J 1967 Ovarian changes in ataxia telangectasia. Acta Paediatrica Scandinavica 56: 559–561

Friedman C I, Neff J, Kim M H 1984 Immunologic parameters in premature follicular depletion: T and B lymphocytes, T-cell subpopulations, cutaneous reactivity, and serum immunoglobulin concentrations. Diagnostic Immunology 2: 48–52

Tumour nos

Dunn H G, Meuwissen H, Livingstone C S , Pump K K 1964 Ataxia telangectasia. Canadian Medical Association Journal 91: 1106–1118

Dysgerminoma

Narita T, Takagi K 1984 Ataxia telangectasia with dysgerminoma of right ovary, papillary carcinoma of thyroid and adenocarcinoma of pancreas. Cancer 54: 1113–1116

Goldsmith C I, Hart W R 1975 Ataxia-telangectasia with ovarian gonadoblastoma and contralateral dysgerminoma. Cancer 36: 1838–1842

Gonadoblastoma

Goldsmith C I, Hart W R 1975 Ataxia telangectasia with ovarian gonadoblastoma and contralateral dysgerminoma. Cancer 36: 1838–1842

Basal cell naevus syndrome (Gorlin's syndrome)

Sclerosing stromal tumor

Ismail S M, Walker S M 1990 Bilateral virilizing sclerosing stromal tumors of the ovary in a pregnant woman with Gorlin's syndrome: implications for pathogenesis of ovarian stromal neoplasms. Histopathology 17: 159–163

Fibroma

Scully R E, Galbadini J J, McNeely B U 1976 Case Records of the Massachusetts General Hospital. Case 14–1976. Basal-cell-nevus syndrome. New England Journal of Medicine 294: 772–777

Raggio M, Kaplan A L, Harberg J F 1983 Recurrent ovarian fibromas with basal cell nevus syndrome (Gorlin syndrome). Obstetrics and Gynecology 61: 95s–96s

Bosch-Banyeras J M, Lucaya X, Bernet M et al 1989 Calcified fibromas in prepubertal girls. European Journal of Pediatrics 148: 749–750

Howell C G Jr, Rogers D A, Gable D S, Falls G D 1990 Bilateral ovarian fibromas in children. Journal of Pediatric Surgery 25: 690–691

Fibrosarcoma

Kraemer B B, Silva E G, Sneige N 1984 Fibrosarcoma of ovary. A new component in the nevoid basal-cell carcinoma syndrome. American Journal of Surgical Pathology 8: 231–236

Blepharophimosis

Resistant ovary syndrome

Jones C A, Collin J R O 1984 Blepharophimosis and its association with female infertility. British Journal of Ophthalmology 68: 533–534

Fraser I S, Shearman R P, Smith A, Russell P 1988 An association among blepharophimosis, resistant ovary syndrome, and true premature menopause. Fertility and Sterility 50: 747–751

Candida endocrinopathy syndrome

Premature ovarian failure

Dempsey A T, de Swiet M, Dewhurst J 1981 Premature ovarian failure associated with the candida endocrinopathy syndrome. British Journal of Obstetrics and Gynaecology 88: 776–777

Chediak–Higashi syndrome

Sclerosing stromal tumor

Inoue R, Kondo N, Motoyoshi F, Hori Y, Orii T 1991 Chediak–Higashi syndrome: report of a case with an ovarian tumor [letter]. Clinical Genetics 39: 316–318

Cowden syndrome

Dysfunctional cysts

Padberg G W, Schot J D, Vielvoye G J, Bots G T, de Beer F C 1991 Lhermitte–Duclos disease and Cowden syndrome: a single phakomatosis. Annals of Neurology 29: 517–523

Granulosa cell tumor

Neumann S 1991 Cowden-Syndrom mit einem Ovarialtumor (Multiple-Hamartome-Syndrom). Chirurg (Berlin) 62: 629–630

Cryptophthalmos (Fraser syndrome)

Gonadal dysgenesis

Greenberg D, Keenan B, de Yanis V, Finegold M 1986 Gonadal dysgenesis and gonadoblastoma in situ in a female with Fraser (cryptophthalmos) syndrome. Journal of Pediatrics 108: 952–954

Down Syndrome (trisomy 21)

Dysgerminoma

Gesmundo R, Bevilacqua A, Gandini R, Maiullari E, Moro G 1988 Su di caso di disgerminoma ovarico in sindrome di Down. Minerva Ginecologica 40: 277–280

Enchondromatosis (Ollier's and Maffucci's syndromes)

Juvenile granulosa cell tumor

Vaz R M, Turner C 1986 Ollier's disease (enchondromatosis) associated with ovarian juvenile granulosa cell tumor and precocious pseudopuberty. Journal of Pediatrics 108: 945–947

Velasco-Oses A, Alonso-Alvaro A, Blanco-Pozo A, Nogales F F Jr 1988 Ollier's disease associated with ovarian juvenile granulosa cell tumor. Cancer 62: 222–225

Tanaka Y, Sasaki Y, Nishihara H, Izawa T, Nishi T 1992 Ovarian juvenile granulosa cell tumor associated with Maffucci's syndrome. American Journal of Clinical Pathology 97: 523–527

Thecoma

Hamdoun L, Mouelhi C, Zhioua F, Jedoui A, Meriah S, Houet 1993 Syndrome de Maffucci et tumeur ovarienne. Bulletin du Cancer (Paris) 80: 816–819

Fibrosarcoma

Christman J E, Ballon S C 1990 Ovarian fibrosarcoma associated with Maffucci's syndrome. Gynecologic Oncology 37: 290–291

Sertoli–Leydig cell tumor

Weyl Ben Arush M, Oslander L 1991 Ollier's disease associated with ovarian Sertoli–Leydig cell tumor and breast adenoma. American Journal of Pediatric Hematology/Oncology 13: 49–51

Familial tendency

Surface epithelial–stromal carcinoma

de Meeus J B, Bennouna C, Marechaud M, Plocoste V, Magnin G 1993 Cancer familial de l'ovaire. A propos d'une familie regroupant 6 cas index. Journal de Gynecologie Obstetrique et Biologie de la Reproduction (Paris) 22: 749–756

Lynch H T, Ens J A, Lynch J F 1990 The Lynch syndrome II and urological malignancies. Journal of Urology 143: 24–28

Lynch H T, Watson P, Lynch J F, Conway T A, Fili M 1993 Hereditary ovarian cancer. Heterogeneity in age of onset. Cancer 71: 573s– 581s

Phillips N, Ziegler M, Saha B, Xynos F 1993 Allelic loss on chromosome 17 in human ovarian cancer. International Journal of Cancer 54: 85–91

Piver M S, Baker T R, Jishi M F et al 1993 Familial ovarian cancer. A report of 658 families from the Gilda Radner Familial Ovarian Cancer Registry 1981–1991. Cancer 71: 582s–588s

Piver M S, Jishi M F, Tsukada Y, Nava G 1993 Primary peritoneal carcinoma after prophylactic oophorectomy in women with a family history of ovarian cancer. A report of the Gilda Radner Familial Ovarian Cancer Registry. Cancer 71: 2751–2755

Smith S A, Ponder B A 1993 Predisposing genes in breast and ovarian cancer: an overview. Tumori 79: 291–296

Smith S A, Easton D F, Ford D et al 1993 Genetic heterogeneity and localisation of a familial breast-ovarian cancer gene on chromosome 17q12–q21. American Journal of Human Genetics 52: 767–776

Sertoli–Leydig cell tumor

Jensen R D, Norris H J, Fraumeni J F Jr 1974 Familial arrhenoblastoma and thyroid adenoma. Cancer 33: 218–223

O'Brien P K, Wilansky D L 1981 Familial thyroid nodulation and arrhenoblastoma. American Journal of Clinical Pathology 75: 578–581

Malignant germ cell tumors

Mandel M, Toren A, Kende G, Neuman Y, Kenet G, Rechavi G 1994 Familial clustering of malignant germ cell tumors and Langerhans' histiocytosis. Cancer 73: 1980–1983

Adult cystic teratoma

Brenner S H, Wallach R C 1983 Familial benign cystic teratoma. International Journal of Gynaecology and Obstetrics 21: 167–169

Simon A, Ohel G, Neri A, Schenker J G 1985 Familial occurrence of mature ovarian teratomas. Obstetrics and Gynecology 66: 278–279

Galactosemia

Premature ovarian failure

Russell P, Bannatyne P, Shearman R P, Fraser I S, Corbett P 1982 Premature hypergonadotropic ovarian failure: clinicopathologic study of 19 cases. International Journal of Gynecological Pathology 1: 185–201

Fraser I S, Russell P, Greco S, Robertson D M 1986 Resistant ovary syndrome and premature ovarian failure in young women with galactosaemia. Clinical Reproduction and Fertility 4: 133–138

Gaucher's disease

Dysgerminoma

Kojiro M, Kage M, Abe H, Imamura M, Shiraishi K, Mizoguchi M 1983 Association of dysgerminoma and Gaucher's disease. Cancer 51: 712–715

Goldberg–Maxwell–Morris syndrome

Sertoli cell tumor

Moneta E, Benedetti Panici P L, Sacco F, Pizzolato G P 1981 Sertoli cell adenoma in Morris syndrome. European Journal of Gynaecologic Oncology 2: 48–50

Hypothyroidism

Multicystic ovaries

Riddlesberger M M Jr, Kuhn J P, Munschauer R W 1981 The association of juvenile hypothyroidism and cystic ovaries. Radiology 139: 77–80

Nishi Y, Masuda H, Iwamori H et al 1985 Primary hypothyroidism associated with pituitary enlargement, slipped capital femoral epiphysis and cystic ovaries. European Journal of Pediatrics 143: 216–219

van Voorhis B J, Neff T W, Syrop C H, Chapler F K 1994 Primary hypothyroidism associated with multicystic ovaries and ovarian torsion in an adult. Obstetrics and Gynecology 83: 885–887

Lipodystrophy

Polycystic ovary syndrome

Senior B 1961 Lipodystrophic muscular hypertrophy. Archives of Disease in Childhood 36: 426–431

Huseman C A, Johanson A J, Varma M M, Blizzard R M 1979 Congenital lipodystrophy. II: Association with polycystic ovarian disease. Journal of Pediatrics 95: 72–74

Malouf syndrome

Ovarian dysgenesis

Narahara K, Kamada M, Takahashi Y et al 1992 Case of ovarian dysgenesis and dilated cardiomyopathy supports existence of Malouf syndrome. American Journal of Medical Genetics 44: 369–373

Mayer–Rokitansky–Kuster–Hauser syndrome

Yolk sac tumor

Koonings P P, al-Marayati L, Schlaerth J B, Lobo R A 1991 Mayer–Rokitansky–Kuster–Hauser syndrome associated with endodermal sinus tumor of the ovary. Fertility and Sterility 56: 577–578

Multiple endocrine neoplasia syndrome

Carcinoma nos

Frilling A, Becker H, Roeher H D 1992 Unusual features of multiple endocrine neoplasia. Henry Ford Hospital Medical Journal 40: 253–255

Strumal carcinoid

Tamsen A, Mazur M T 1992 Ovarian strumal carcinoid in association with multiple endocrine neoplasia, type IIA. Archives of Pathology and Laboratory Medicine 116: 200–203

Osteogenesis imperfecta

Serous carcinoma

Nishida T, Oda T, Sugiyama T, Izumi S, Yakushiji M 1993 Concurrent ovarian serous carcinoma and osteogenesis imperfecta. Archives of Gynecology and Obstetrics 253: 153–156

Perrault syndrome (sensorineural deafness)

Gonadal dysgenesis

Pallister P D, Opitz J M 1979 The Perrault syndrome: autosomal recessive ovarian dysgenesis with facultative, non-sex-limited sensorineural deafness. American Journal of Medical Genetics 4: 239–246

Peutz–Jeghers syndrome

Mucinous cystadenoma

Brudick P, Prior J T 1982 Peutz–Jeghers syndrome: a clinicopathologic study of a large family with 27-year follow-up. Cancer 50: 2139–2142

Chen K T K 1986 Female genital tract tumors in Peutz–Jeghers syndrome. Human Pathology 17: 858–861

Lucidarme D, Dribda M, el Khoury S et al 1990 Tumeurs ovariennes et syndrome de Peutz– Jeghers. A propos d'un cas. Gastroenterologie Clinique et Biologique (Paris) 14: 1015–1018

Podczaski E, Kaminski P F, Pees R C, Singapuri K, Sorosky J I 1991 Peutz–Jeghers syndrome with ovarian sex cord tumor with annular tubules and cervical adenoma malignum. Gynecologic Oncology 42: 74–78

Sex cord tumor with annular tubules

Scully R E 1970 Sex cord tumor with annular tubules. A distinctive ovarian tumor of the Peutz–Jeghers syndrome. Cancer 25: 1107–1121

Podczaski E, Kaminski P F, Pees R C, Singapuri K, Sorosky J I 1991 Peutz–Jeghers syndrome with ovarian sex cord tumor with annular tubules and cervical adenoma malignum. Gynecologic Oncology 42: 74–78

Herruzo A J, Redondo E, Perez de Avila M, Menjon S 1990 Ovarian sex cord tumor with annular tubules and Peutz–Jeghers syndrome. European Journal of Gynaecological Oncology 11: 141–144

Benagiano G, Bigotti G, Buzzi M, d'Alessandro P, Napolitano C 1988 Endocrine and morphological study of a case of ovarian sex-cord tumor with annular tubules in a woman with Peutz–Jeghers syndrome. International Journal of Gynaecology and Obstetrics 26: 441–452

Laughlin E H 1991 Benign and malignant neoplasms in a family with Peutz–Jeghers syndrome: study of three generations. Southern Medical Journal 84: 1205–1209

Sertoli cell tumor

Giacomelli L, Giacomelli L, Pulcini A, Messinetti S 1988 Sindrome di Peutz–Jeghers. Report e contributi clinici. Minerva Chirurgerie 43: 1649–1654

Young R H, Dickersin G R, Scully R E 1983 A distinctive ovarian sex cord–stromal tumor causing sexual precocity in the Peutz–Jeghers syndrome. American Journal of Surgical Pathology 7: 233–243

Giacomelli L, Giacomelli L, Pulcini A, Messinetti S 1988 Sindrome di Peutz–Jeghers. Report e contributi clinici. Minerva Chirurgica 43: 1649–1654

Polyostotic fibrous dysplasia (Albright syndrome)

Granulosa lutein cysts

Danon M, Robboy S J, Kim S, Scully R E, Crawford J D 1975 Cushing syndrome, sexual precocity, and polyostotic fibrous dysplasia (Albright syndrome) in infancy. Journal of Pediatrics 87: 917–921

Roberts-SC phocomelia syndrome

Ovarian dysgenesis

Robins D B, Ladda R L, Thieme G A, Boal D K, Emanuel B S, Zackai E H 1989 Prenatal detection of Roberts–SC phocomelia syndrome: report of 2 sibs with characteristic manifestations. American Journal of Medical Genetics 32: 390–394

Situs inversus totalis

Mucinous cystadenoma

Rao P G, Katariya R N, Sood S, Rao P L 1977 Situs inversus totalis with calculus cholecystitis and mucinous cystadenomas of the ovaries. Journal of Postgraduate Medicine (Bombay) 23: 89–90

Endodermal sinus tumor

Ibrahim E M, Al-Idrissi H, Al-Farag A, Al-Tamimi D, Perry W 1984 Situs inversus totalis with embryonal cell carcinoma of ovaries. Gynecologic Oncology 18: 270–273

Embryonal carcinoma

Abdel-Dayem H M, Motawi S, Jahan S, Kubasik H 1984 Liver metastases from embryonal carcinoma of the ovary with complete situs inversus. First reported case and review of the literature. Clinical Nuclear Medicine 9: 558–560

Smith–Lemli–Opitz syndrome

Gonadal dysgenesis

Fukuzawa R, Nakahori Y, Kogo T et al 1992 Normal Y sequences in Smith–Lemli–Opitz syndrome with total failure of masculinisation. Acta Paediatrica 81: 570–572

von Recklinghausen's disease (neurofibromatosis)

Neurofibrosarcoma

Dover H 1950 Neurofibrosarcoma of ovary associated with neurofibromatosis. Canadian Medical Association Journal 63: 488–490
Dalac S, Marchal G, Dumas R, Escallier F, Lambert D 1988 Un cas historique de neurofibromatose de Recklinghausen. Annales de Dermatologie et de Venereologie (Paris) 115: 1111–1112

Wilson's disease

Resistant ovary syndrome

Hartemann P, Leclere J, Thomas J L, Genton P, Arbogast J 1983 Syndrome des ovaires resistant aux gonadotrophines et maladie de Wilson. Une observation. Revue de Medecine Interne 4: 353–355

Appendix B

Classification of ovarian tumors

The World Health Organization (WHO) histological classification of ovarian tumors (Serov et al 1973) has been, for some considerable time, the generally accepted basis for grouping and discussing the myriad neoplastic entities documented in the human ovaries. Ovarian tumors are divided into major subdivisions according to their supposed histogenesis but, within each such group, individual tumor types are classified on morphological criteria alone. While this has led to some apparent incongruities as to the exact placement of various specific tumor types, in general the evolution of our understanding of the nature, behavior, and interrelationships of many of the less common lesions is resolving some of these dilemmas. The 1973 WHO classification was expanded and modified by the International Society of Gynecological Pathologists to include several tumor variants which have gained recognition in the literature since its publication, as well as reflecting a firmer understanding of the histogeneses of some of them, and is in the process of formal publication (Talerman 1992). The classification presented here is based on the principles of this new WHO classification of ovarian neoplasms and tumor-like lesions.

Reported relative frequency figures tend to be distorted by the nature of the hospital or institution and reputation of the investigators or practitioners from which such series of cases originate. The larger the series (and presumably the more statistically significant the figures), and the more restricted the types of tumors reported, the greater is this bias likely to be – a bias which tends to work against the benign, the small, and the mundane amongst ovarian neoplasms. Little other than broad trends in relative frequencies can be gained by reviewing the accumulated literature. The frequency figures we have used in this text relate to a large series of women first diagnosed and treated at our institution. One major limiting factor in this material was the minimum age of 12 years for admission to this hospital and its consequent distorting effect upon the incidence of those tumors more common in prepubertal girls. Approximately 62% of all primary ovarian neoplasms are common epithelial tumors, 10% are of sex cord–stromal origin, and 26% are of germ cell origin. The relative frequency figures within each of the major subdivisions of ovarian neoplasms are given in the relevant introductory chapters (Chs. 22, 35, 40).

TUMORS AND TUMOR-LIKE LESIONS OF THE OVARIES

MULLERIAN TUMORS (SURFACE EPITHELIAL–STROMAL TUMORS)

Serous lesions

Tumor-like lesions
— Serous inclusion cyst (endosalpingiosis)

Benign tumors
— Cystadenoma and papillary cystadenoma
— Surface papilloma
— Adenofibroma and cystadenofibroma

Tumors with atypical epithelial proliferation (of borderline malignancy):
— Cystic tumor and papillary cystic tumor
— Surface papillary tumor
— Adenofibroma and cystadenofibroma

Malignant tumors
— Adenocarcinoma, papillary adenocarcinoma, and papillary cystadenocarcinoma
— Surface papillary adenocarcinoma
— Malignant adenofibroma and cystadenofibroma

Mucinous lesions

Tumor-like lesions
— Mucinous inclusion cyst (endocervicosis)

Benign tumors
— Of mullerian differentiation:
Cystadenoma, papillary cystadenoma
Adenofibroma and cystadenofibroma
— Of colonic or intestinal differentiation:
Cystadenoma
Cystadenoma with pseudomyxoma ovarii
— Of mixed colonic and mullerian differentiation

Tumors with atypical epithelial proliferation (of borderline malignancy)
— Of mullerian differentiation:
Papillary mucinous cystadenoma
Adenofibroma and cystadenofibroma
— Of colonic or enteroid differentiation
Cystadenoma with pseudomyxoma ovarii

Mucinous tumor with (sarcoma-like) mural nodules
Malignant tumors (of colonic differentiation)
— Adenocarcinoma and cystadenocarcinoma
— Malignant adenofibroma and cystadenofibroma
— Colloid carcinoma
— Primary Krukenberg tumor

Endometrioid lesions
Tumor-like lesions
— Endometriosis
Benign tumors
— Cystadenoma
— Adenofibroma and cystadenofibroma
Tumors with atypical epithelial proliferation (of borderline malignancy)
— Cystic tumor
— Adenofibroma and cystadenofibroma
Malignant tumors
— Adenocarcinoma, secretory adenocarcinoma
— Adenocarcinoma with squamous differentiation
— Malignant adenofibroma and cystadenofibroma

Mullerian mesenchymal lesions (epithelial–stromal and stromal lesions)
Tumor-like conditions
— Endometrioid stromatosis (stromal endometriosis)
— Leiomyomatosis peritonealis disseminata
Benign tumors
— Endometrioid stromal nodule
— Leiomyoma
Malignant tumors
— Endometrioid stromal sarcoma, low grade (endolymphatic stromal myosis) and high grade
— Leiomyosarcoma
— Malignant mixed mullerian tumor:
Adenosarcoma, homologous and heterologous
Mesodermal (mullerian) mixed tumor (carcinosarcoma), homologous and heterologous

Clear cell lesions
Tumor-like lesions
— Clear cell inclusion cyst
Benign tumors
— Adenofibroma and cystadenofibroma
Tumors with atypical epithelial proliferation (of borderline malignancy)
— Cystic tumor
— Adenofibroma and cystadenofibroma
Malignant tumors
— Adenocarcinoma and cystadenocarcinoma
— Malignant adenofibroma

Transitional (Brenner) cell lesions
Tumor-like lesions
— Walthard's rest (transitional or Brenner inclusions)
Benign tumors
— Adenofibroma and cystadenofibroma
Tumors with atypical epithelial proliferation (of borderline malignancy)
— Papillary adenofibroma and cystadenofibroma
Malignant tumors
— Transitional cell carcinoma
— Malignant Brenner tumor

Squamous cell tumors (non-germ-cell)
— Epidermoid cyst
— Squamous cell carcinoma

Mixed epithelial lesions
Tumor-like lesions
Benign tumors
Tumors with atypical epithelial proliferation (of borderline malignancy)
Malignant tumors

Undifferentiated carcinomas

Unclassified and miscellaneous lesions
Tumor-like lesions
— Cyst of the rete ovarii
Benign tumors
Malignant tumors
— Ovarian tumor of probable Wolffian origin

SEX CORD–STROMAL TUMORS

Granulosa–stromal cell lesions
Tumour-like lesions
— Massive ovarian edema and fibromatosis
— Diffuse stromal hyperplasia and hyperthecosis
— Dysfunctional cysts and polycystic ovary syndrome
— Hyperreactio luteinalis (multiple luteinized follicle cysts)
Granulosa cell tumors
— Adult type
— Juvenile type
Tumors in the thecoma–fibroma group
— Thecoma:
Typical
Luteinised thecoma
Malignant thecoma
— Fibrothecomas
— Fibromas:
Typical
Fibroma with minor sex cord elements
Cellular fibroma
Fibrosarcoma
— Sclerosing stromal tumor
Unclassified

Androblastomas: Sertoli–stromal cell lesions
Well-differentiated tumors
— Sertoli cell tumor, tubular androblastoma
— Sertoli cell tumor with lipid storage: tubular androblastoma with lipid storage
— Sertoli–Leydig cell tumor (tubular androblastoma with Leydig cells)
Tumors of intermediate differentiation
— Sertoli–Leydig cell tumor
— Sertoli cell carcinoma
Poorly differentiated (sarcomatoid) tumors
— Typical

— With heterologous elements
— Retiform variant

Sex cord tumors with annular tubules

Gynandroblastomas

Unclassified

STEROID (LIPID) CELL TUMORS

Tumor-like lesions
— Leydig cell hyperplasia
— Nodular hyperthecosis
— Stromal luteoma
— Luteoma of pregnancy
Tumors
— Leydig cell tumor, hilus and stromal variants
— Adrenal rest tumor
— Steroid cell tumor, not otherwise specified

GERM CELL TUMORS

Dysgerminomas
Typical
With trophoblastic giant cells

Yolk sac tumors (endodermal sinus tumors)
Typical
Polyvesicular vitelline tumor
Hepatoid and enteroid variant

Embryonal carcinomas

Polyembryomas

Nongestational choriocarcinomas

Teratomas
Immature
Mature
— Solid
— Cystic:
  Dermoid cyst
  With secondary malignant transformation
— Monodermal and highly specialized:
  Struma ovarii
  Carcinoid
    Insular
    Trabecular
  Strumal carcinoid
  Mucinous carcinoid
  Primitive neuroectodermal tumor
  Others

Malignant mixed germ cell tumors

MIXED GERM CELL AND SEX CORD–STROMAL TUMORS

Gonadoblastomas
Pure
Mixed with dysgerminoma or other form of malignant germ cell tumor

Malignant mixed germ cell–sex cord–stromal tumors

SOFT TISSUE TUMORS NOT SPECIFIC FOR OVARY

UNCLASSIFIED TUMORS

Mesotheliomas
Benign papillary mesothelioma
Benign cystic mesothelioma
Adenomatoid tumor

Small cell carcinomas associated with hypercalcemia

LYMPHOMAS AND LEUKEMIAS

SECONDARY (METASTATIC) TUMORS

REFERENCES

Serov S F, Scully R E, Sobin L H 1973 Histological typing of ovarian tumors (International histological classification of tumors No. 9. World Health Organization, Geneva
Talerman A 1992 Ovarian pathology. Current Opinion in Obstetrics and Gynecology 4: 608–615

Appendix C

Staging of ovarian tumors

Staging of ovarian carcinomas is primarily the responsibility of the surgeon, but it is important for the pathologist's role in the staging process to be understood. FIGO has promoted the most widely used method, employing clinical/laparotomy findings, with accurate staging based on histological examination of biopsies from the ovaries and any accessible sites of extraovarian involvement (such as omentum and pelvic viscera). Experience has shown a surprising percentage of apparent stage 1 lesions with biopsy-proven extraovarian involvement, with consequences for management and prognosis. It is thus recommended that, in apparently early cases, washings be taken from beneath the diaphragm, the paracolic gutters and pelvis for cytological examination and multiple peritoneal biopsies from the paracolic gutters, pouch of Douglas, omentum, pelvic walls, bladder, and para-aortic lymph glands. The World Health Organization currently recommends that the tumor should be typed and graded on the ovarian pathology alone (especially in the so-called 'borderline' or 'proliferating' epithelial tumors), a stance with which we are not in agreement. Careful histological assessment of extraovarian disease, in certain circumstances, materially alters the grading of the tumor, and thus the expected clinical outcome for the patient. The corollary of this, however, is that the pathologist should actively encourage surgeons to biopsy the ovaries, whenever practicable, in all cases of apparent widespread ovarian neoplasia (not merely omentum or some other convenient site of metastasis). The details of processing of individual biopsy specimens obtained from the staging laparotomy are given in Chapter 4.

FIGO STAGING OF OVARIAN TUMORS*

Stage 1: Growth limited to the ovaries.

Stage 1a Growth limited to one ovary; no ascites. No tumor on the external surface; capsule intact.

Stage 1b Growth limited to both ovaries; no ascites. No tumor on the external surface; capsules intact.

Stage 1c Tumor either stage 1a or stage 1b, but with tumor on surface of one or both ovaries; or with capsule ruptured; or with ascites present containing malignant cells or with positive peritoneal washings.

Stage 2: Growth involving one or both ovaries with pelvic extension.

Stage 2a Extension and/or metastases to the uterus and/or tubes.

Stage 2b Extension to other pelvic tissues.

Stage 2c Tumor either stage 2a or stage 2b, but with tumor on surface of one or both ovaries; or with capsule(s) ruptured; or with ascites present containing malignant cells or with positive peritoneal washings.

Stage 3: Tumor involving one or both ovaries with peritoneal implants outside the pelvis and/or positive retroperitoneal or inguinal nodes. Superficial liver metastasis equals stage 3. Tumor is limited to the true pelvis, but with histologically proven malignant extension to the small bowel or omentum.

Stage 3a Tumor grossly limited to the true pelvis with negative nodes, but with histologically confirmed microscopic seeding of abdominal peritoneal surfaces.

Stage 3b Tumor involving one or both ovaries with histologically confirmed implants of abdominal peritoneal surfaces none exceeding 2 cm in diameter. Nodes are negative.

Stage 3c Abdominal implants greater than 2 cm in diameter and/or positive retroperitoneal or inguinal nodes.

Stage 4: Growth involving one or both ovaries with distant metastases. If pleural effusion is present, there must be positive cytology to allot a case to stage 4. Parenchymal liver metastases equals stage 4.

* Based on findings at clinical examination and/or surgical exploration. The histology after surgery is to be considered in the staging, as is cytology insofar as effusions are concerned. It is desirable that biopsies be taken from suspect areas outside of the pelvis. (Annual Report Gynecologic Cancer FIGO 1988 Petterssen F (ed) Panorama Press, Stockholm, Vol 20)

Appendix D

Paraendocrine and paraneoplastic syndromes and ovarian tumors

The format of this section is intended to provide readers with ready access to the literature regarding paraendocrine syndromes consequent upon the presence of various ovarian neoplasms. Many of these syndromes occur commonly with other visceral neoplasms, while others tend to direct the clinician's attention to the ovary. Many such syndromes do not relate to specific histological subtypes of ovarian tumors, while some are associated with a limited spectrum of neoplasms or, occasionally, a single histological entity. Those syndromes which are the manifestation of steroid secretion consistent with the normal endocrine function of the ovaries are largely and specifically excluded.

The references given are not intended to be encyclopedic, but represent the few most recent, most important or most accessible for each entity.

General review articles

Annals of the New York Academy of Sciences, Vol 230 (1974)

Barker G H, Orledge J, Whittshaw E 1981 Involvement of the central nervous system in patients with ovarian carcinoma. British Journal of Obstetrics and Gynaecology 88: 690–694

Clement P B, Young R H, Scully R E 1991 Clinical syndromes associated with tumors of the female genital tract. Seminars in Diagnostic Pathology 8: 204–233

Goodall C M 1969 On para-endocrine cancer syndromes: A review. International Journal of Cancer 4: 1–13

Hall T C 1974 Oncocognitive autoimmunity and other paraneoplastic syndromes yet to be described. Annals of the New York Academy of Sciences 230: 565–570

Hall T C 1974 Paraneoplastic syndromes. Annals of the New York Academy of Sciences 230: 557–570

Hilliard G D, Norris H J 1982 The ovaries in endocrine disorders. In: Bloodworth J M B (ed) Endocrine pathology, general and surgical. Williams & Wilkins, Baltimore, OH, p 267–292

Lipsett M B, Odell W D, Rosenberg L E, Waldmann T A 1964 Humoral syndromes associated with nonendocrine tumors. Annals of Internal Medicine 61: 733–756

Shane J M, Naftolin F 1975 Aberrant hormone activity of tumors of gynecologic importance. American Journal of Obstetrics and Gynecology 121: 133–147

Acanthosis nigricans

Serous carcinoma

Dingley E R, Marten R H 1957 Adenocarcinoma of the ovary presenting as acanthosis nigricans. Journal of Obstetrics and Gynaecology of the British Commonwealth 64: 898–900

Curth H O, Hilberg A W, Machacek G F 1962 The site and histology of the cancer associated with malignant acanthosis nigricans. Cancer 15: 364–382

Adult cystic teratoma

Imperato-McGinley J, Peterson R E, Sturla E, Dawood Y, Bar R S 1978 Primary amenorrhea associated with hirsutism, acanthosis nigricans, dermoid cysts of the ovaries and a new type of insulin resistance. American Journal of Medicine 65: 389–395

Aldosteronism

Sertoli–Leydig cell tumor

Ehrlich E N, Dominguez O V, Samuels L T, Lynch D, Oberhelman H Jr, Warner N E 1963 Aldosteronism and precocious puberty due to an ovarian androblastoma (Sertoli cell tumor). Journal of Clinical Endocrinology 23: 358–367

Todesco S, Terribile V, Borsatti A, Mantero F 1975 Primary aldosteronism due to a malignant ovarian tumor. Journal of Clinical Endocrinology and Metabolism 41: 809–819

Steroid cell tumor

Kulkarni J N, Mistry R C, Kamat M R, Chinoy R, Lotlikar R G 1990 Autonomous aldosterone-secreting ovarian tumor. Gynecologic Oncology 37: 284–289

Ascites (non-malignant)

Thecoma

Samanth K K, Black W C 1970 Benign ovarian stromal tumors associated with peritoneal free fluid. American Journal of Obstetrics and Gynecology 107: 538–545

Fibroma

Samanth K K, Black W C 1970 Benign ovarian stromal tumors associated with peritoneal free fluid. American Journal of Obstetrics and Gynecology 107: 538–545

Carcinoid syndrome

Small cell carcinoma

Brown H, Lane M 1965 Cushing's and malignant carcinoid syndromes from ovarian neoplasms. Archives of Internal Medicine 115: 490–494

Carcinoid tumor

Haines M 1971 Carcinoid tumors of the ovary. Journal of Obstetrics and Gynaecology of the British Commonwealth 78: 1123–1127

Ansell J K, Stebbings W S 1993 Carcinoid syndrome due to a primary ovarian carcinoid tumor. Journal of Royal Society of Medicine 86: 668

Contarini's syndrome

Carcinoma nos

Lawton F, Blackledge G, Johnson R 1985 Co-existent chylous and serous pleural effusions associated with ovarian cancer: a case report of Contarini's syndrome. European Journal of Surgical Oncology 11: 177–178

Corticocerebellar degeneration/encephalopathy

Serous carcinoma

Steven M M, Mackay I R, Carnegie P R, Bhathal P S, Anderson R McD 1982 Cerebellar cortical degeneration with ovarian carcinoma. Postgraduate Medical Journal 58: 47–51

Greenlee J E, Brashear H R 1983 Antibodies to cerebellar Purkinje cells in patients with paraneoplastic cerebellar degeneration and ovarian carcinoma. Annals of Neurology 14: 609–613

Hall D J, Dyer M L, Parker J C Jr 1985 Ovarian cancer complicated by cerebellar degeneration: a paraneoplastic syndrome. Gynecologic Oncology 21: 240–246

Cocconi G, Ceci G Juvarr689a G et al 1985 Successful treatment of subacute cerebellar degeneration in ovarian carcinoma with plasmapheresis. A case report. Cancer 56: 2318–2320

McCrystal M, Anderson N E, Jones R W, Evans B D 1995 Paraneoplastic cerebellar degeneration in a patient with chemotherapy-responsive ovarian cancer. International Journal of Gynecological Cancer 5: 396–399

Carcinoma nos

McDonald W I 1961 Cortical cerebellar degeneration with ovarian carcinoma. Neurology 11: 328–334

Buge A, Escourole R, Raneurel G, Gray F, Tempier P, Denvil D 1980 Acute spongiform leucoencephalopathy with selective intramyelinic involvement of U fibers associated with an ovarian carcinoma. Syndrome of disconnection of U fibres. Revue Neurologique (Paris) 136: 741–751

Brashear H R, Greenlee J E, Jaeckle K A, Rose J W 1989 Anticerebellar antibodies in neurologically normal patients with ovarian neoplasms. Neurology 39: 1605–1609

Cushing's syndrome

Poorly differentiated carcinoma

Parsons V, Rigby B 1958 Cushing's syndrome associated with adenocarcinoma of the ovary. Lancet ii: 992–994

Carcinoma nos

Lipsett M B, Odell W D, Rosenberg L E, Waldmann T A 1964 Humoral syndromes associated with nonendocrine tumors. Annals of Internal Medicine 61: 733–756

Sertoli cell tumor

Nichols J, Warren J C, Mantz F A 1962 ACTH-like excretion from carcinoma of the ovary. The clinical effect of M,P-DDD. Journal of the American Medical Association 182: 713–718

Sertoli–Leydig cell tumor

Canelo C K, Lisser H 1939 A case of arrhenoblastoma which simulated Cushing's disease. Endocrinology 24: 838–847

Small cell carcinoma

Brown H, Lane M 1965 Cushing's and malignant carcinoid syndromes from ovarian neoplasms. Archives of Internal Medicine 115: 490–494

Steroid cell tumor

Marieb N J, Spangler S, Kashgarian M, Heimann A, Schwartz M L, Schwartz P E 1983 Cushing's syndrome secondary to ectopic cortisol production by an ovarian carcinoma. Journal of Clinical Endocrinology and Metabolism 57: 737–740

Donovan J T, Otis C N, Powell J L, Cathcart H K 1993 Cushing's syndrome secondary to malignant lipoid cell tumor of the ovary. Gynecologic Oncology 50: 249–253

Teratoma

Axiotis C A, Lippes H A, Merino M J, de Lanerolle N C, Stewart A F, Kinder B 1987 Corticotroph cell pituitary adenoma within an ovarian teratoma. A new cause of Cushing's syndrome. American Journal of Surgical Pathology 11: 218–224

Carcinoid tumor

Schlaghecke R, Kreutzpaintner G, Burrig K F, Juli E, Kley H K 1989 Cushing's syndrome due to ACTH-production of an ovarian carcinoid. Klinische Wochenschrift 67: 640–644

Dermatomyositis/polymyositis

Reviews

Barnes B E 1976 Dermatomyositis and malignancy. A review of the literature. Annals of Internal Medicine 84: 68–76

Callen J P 1982 The value of malignancy evaluation in patients with dermatomyositis. Journal of the American Academy of Dermatologists 6: 253–259

Voravud N, Dimopoulos M, Hortobagyi G, Ross M, Theriault R 1991 Breast cancer and second primary ovarian cancer in dermatomyositis. Gynecologic Oncology 43: 286–290

Serous carcinoma

Verducci M A, Malkasian G D Jr, Friedman S J, Winkelmann R K 1984 Gynecologic carcinoma associated with dermatomyositis–polymyositis. Obstetrics and Gynecology 64: 695–698

Peters W A 3rd, Anderson W A, Thornton W N Jr 1983 Dermatomyositis and co-existent ovarian cancer: a review of the compounding clinical problems. Gynecologic Oncology 15: 440–446

Undifferentiated carcinoma

Chamberlain M J, Whittaker S R F 1963 Hashimoto's disease, dermatomyositis and ovarian carcinoma. Lancet i: 1398–1400

Carcinoma nos

Cortes F M, Morris C E, Hutter R V P 1962 Polymyositis: observations in three cases. American Journal of Medical Science 243: 77–85

Dysgerminoma

Solomon S D, Maurer K H 1983 Association of dermatomyositis and dysgerminoma in a 16-year-old patient. Arthritis and Rheumatology 26: 572–573

Disseminated intravascular coagulation (see hypercoagulability)

Epilepsy

Tumour nos

Norris H J 1971 Letter to the Editor. Acta Paediatrica Scandinavica 60: 600

Norris H J, Chorlton I 1974 Functioning tumors of the ovary. Clinical Obstetrics and Gynecology 17: 189–228

Thecoma

Schweisguth O, Gerard-Marchant R, Plainfosse B, Lemerle J, Watchi J M, Seringe P 1971 Bilateral nonfunctioning thecoma of the ovary in epileptic children under anticonvulsant therapy. Acta Paediatrica Scandinavica 60: 6–10

Eruptive keratoacanthoma and Torre's syndrome

Adenocarcinoma nos

Snider B L, Benjamin D R 1981 Eruptive keratoacanthoma with an internal malignant neoplasm. Archives of Dermatology 117: 788–790

Fathizadeh A, Medenica M M, Soltani K, Lorincz A L, Griem M L 1982 Aggressive keratoacanthoma and internal malignant neoplasm. Archives of Dermatology 118: 112–114

Gonadotrophin secretion

Serous carcinoma

Civantos F, Rywlin A M 1972 Carcinomas with trophoblastic differentiation and secretion of chorionic gonadotrophins. Cancer 29: 789–798

Samaan N A, Smith J P, Rutledge F N, Schultz P N 1976 The significance of measurement of human placental lactogen, human chorionic gonadotropin, and carcinoembryonic antigen in patients with ovarian carcinoma. American Journal of Obstetrics and Gynecology 126: 186–189

Mucinous carcinoma

Civantos F, Rywlin A M 1972 Carcinomas with trophoblastic differentiation and secretion of chorionic gonadotrophins. Cancer 29: 789–798

Samaan N A, Smith J P, Rutledge F N, Schultz P N 1976 The significance of measurement of human placental lactogen, human chorionic gonadotropin, and carcinoembryonic antigen in patients with ovarian carcinoma. American Journal of Obstetrics and Gynecology 126: 186–189

Endometrioid carcinoma

Samaan N A, Smith J P, Rutledge F N, Schultz P N 1976 The significance of measurement of human placental lactogen, human chorionic gonadotropin, and carcinoembryonic antigen in patients with ovarian carcinoma. American Journal of Obstetrics and Gynecology 126: 186–189

Carcinoma nos

Montiero J C M P, Baker G, Ferguson K M, Wiltshaw E, Munro-Neville A 1983 Ectopic production of human chorionic gonadotrophin (HCG) and human placental lactogen (HPL) by ovarian carcinoma. European Journal of Cancer and Clinical Oncology 19: 173–178

Vaitukaitis J L 1974 Human chorionic gonadotropin as a tumor marker. Annals of Clinical and Laboratory Science 4: 276–280

Dysgerminoma

Gough A 1938 A case of dysgerminoma of the ovary associated with masculinity. Journal of Obstetrics and Gynaecology of the British Empire 45: 799–801

Kapp D S, Kohorn E I, Merino M J, LiVolsi V A 1985 Pure dysgerminoma of the ovary with elevated serum human chorionic gonadotropin: diagnostic and therapeutic considerations. Gynecologic Oncology 20: 234–244

Teratoma

Downey G P, Prentice M, Penna L K, Gleeson R P, Elder M G 1989 Ectopic β-human chorionic gonadotropin production by a dermoid cyst. American Journal of Obstetrics and Gynecology 160: 449–451

Hemolytic anemia

Serous carcinoma

Blau A, Kaplinsky J 1982 Microangiopathic haemolytic anaemia associated with recurrent pulmonary emboli and benign pelvic tumors. Postgraduate Medical Journal 58: 362–363

Mucinous carcinoma

Andre R, Duhamel G, Najman A, Homberg J C, Mawas C, Armangol R 1969 Anemie hemolytique auto-immune et tumeur maligne de l'ovaire. Presse Medicale 77: 2133–2136

Granulosa–theca cell tumor

Dawson M A, Wilimer T, Yarbro J W 1971 Hemolytic anemia associated with an ovarian tumor. American Journal of Medicine 50: 552–556

Adult cystic teratoma

Bernstein D, Naor S, Rikover M, Menahem H 1974 Hemolytic anemia related to ovarian tumor. Obstetrics and Gynecology 43: 276–280

McAndrew G M 1964 Haemolytic anaemia associated with ovarian teratoma. British Medical Journal 2: 1307–1308

Payne D, Muss H Y, Homesley H D, Jobson V W, Baird F G 1981 Autoimmune hemolytic anemia and ovarian dermoid cysts. Cancer 48: 721–724

Hemophagocytic syndrome

Undifferentiated carcinoma

Tsui W M, Wong K F, Tse C C 1992 Liver changes in reactive haemophagocytic syndrome. Liver 12: 363–367

Hyperamylasemia

Serous carcinoma

Hodes M E, Sisk C J, Karn R C et al 1985 An amylase-producing serous cystadenocarcinoma of the ovary. Oncology 42: 242–247

Hayakawa T, Kameya A, Mizuno R, Noda A, Kondo T, Hirabayashi N 1984 Hyperamylasemia with papillary serous cystadenocarcinoma of the ovary. Cancer 54: 1662–1665

Endometrioid carcinoma

Yagi C, Miyata J, Hanai J, Ogawa M, Ueda G 1986 Hyperamylasemia associated with endometrioid carcinoma of the ovary: case report and immunohistochemical study. Gynecologic Oncology 25: 250–255

Adenosquamous carcinoma

Norwood S H, Torma M J, Fontenelle L J 1981 Hyperamylasemia due to poorly differentiated adenosquamous carcinoma of the ovary. Archives of Surgery 116: 225–226

Hypercalcemia

Reviews

Holtz G 1980 Paraneoplastic hypercalcemia in gynecologic malignancy. Obstetrical and Gynecological Survey 35: 129–136

Serous carcinoma

Ferenczy A, Okagaki T, Richart R M 1971 Para-endocrine hypercalcemia in ovarian neoplasms. Report of mesonephroma with hypercalcemia and review of the literature. Cancer 27: 427–433

Allan S G, Lockhart S P, Leonard R C, Smyth R F 1984 Paraneoplastic hypercalcaemia in ovarian carcinoma. British Medical Journal 288: 1714–1715

Josse R G, Wilson D R, Heersche J N M, Mills F Jr, Murray T M 1981 Hypercalcemia with ovarian carcinoma: evidence of a pathogenetic role for prostaglandins. Cancer 48: 1233–1241

Mucinous carcinoma

Boyer M, Friedlander M, Bannatyne P, Atkinson K 1989 Hypercalcemia in association with mucinous adenocarcinoma of the ovary. A case report. Gynecologic Oncology 35: 387–390

Clear cell carcinoma

Biron S, Bercovici B, Brufman G 1977 Paraneoplastic hypercalcemic syndrome associated with ovarian cancer. European Journal of Obstetrics Gynecology and Reproductive Biology 7: 239–242

Powell D, Singer F R, Murray T M, Minkin C, Potts J T Jr 1973 Nonparathyroid humoral hypercalcemia in patients with neoplastic diseases. New England Journal of Medicine 289: 176–181

Rivett J D, Robinson J M 1972 Hypercalcaemia associated with an ovarian carcinoma of mesonephromatous type. Journal of Obstetrics and Gynaecology of the British Commonwealth 79: 1047–1052

Allan S G, Lockhart S P, Leonard R C, Smyth R F 1984 Paraneoplastic hypercalcaemia in ovarian carcinoma. British Medical Journal 288: 1714–1715

Undifferentiated carcinoma

Ferenczy A, Okagaki T, Richart R M 1971 Para-endocrine hypercalcemia in ovarian neoplasms. Report of mesonephroma with hypercalcemia and review of the literature. Cancer 27: 427–433

Omenn G S, Roth S I, Baker W H 1969 Hyperparathyroidism associated with malignant tumors of nonparathyroid origin. Cancer 24: 1004–1012

Undifferentiated sex cord–stromal tumor

Holtz G, Johnson T, Schrock M 1979 Paraneoplastic hypercalcemia in ovarian tumors. Obstetrics and Gynecology 54: 483–487

Small cell carcinoma of hypercalcemic type

Dickersin G R, Kline I W, Scully R E 1982 Small cell carcinoma of the ovary with hypercalcemia: a report of eleven cases. Cancer 49: 188–197

Tumor of probable Wolffian origin

Abbot R L, Barlogie B, Schmidt W A 1981 Metastasizing malignant juxtaovarian tumor with terminal hypercalcemia. Cancer 48: 860–865

Steroid cell tumor

Ferenczy A, Okagaki T, Richart R M 1971 Para-endocrine hypercalcemia in ovarian neoplasms. Report of mesonephroma with hypercalcemia and review of the literature. Cancer 27: 427–433

Abouav J, Berkovitz S B, Kolb F O 1959 Reversible hypercalcemia in masculinising hypernephroid tumor of the ovary: Report of a case. New England Journal of Medicine 260: 1057–1062

Dysgerminoma

Breidahl H D, Ritchie B C 1962 Hypercalcaemia due to malignant ovarian tumor. A case report. Medical Journal of Australia 49: 208–210

Ferenczy A, Okagaki T, Richart R M 1971 Para-endocrine hypercalcemia in ovarian neoplasms. Report of mesonephroma with hypercalcemia and review of the literature. Cancer 27: 427–433

Anstey A, Gowers L, Vass A, Robson A O 1990 Ovarian dysgerminoma presenting with hypercalcaemia. Case report and review of the literature. British Journal of Obstetrics and gynaecology 97: 641–644

Fleischhacker D S, Young R H 1994 Dysgerminoma of the ovary associated with hypercalcemia. Gynecologic Oncology 52: 87–90

Teratoma with secondary malignant change

Kim W, Bockman R, Lemos L, Lewis J L Jr 1981 Hypercalcemia associated with epidermoid carcinoma in ovarian cystic teratoma. Obstetrics and Gynecology 57: 81s–85s

Ribeiro G, Hughesdon P, Wiltshaw E 1988 Squamous carcinoma arising in dermoid cysts and associated with hypercalcemia: a clinicopathologic study of six cases. Gynecologic Oncology 29: 222–230

Tumour nos

Scully R E 1968 Editorial comment. Survey of Pathology in Medicine and Surgery 4: 125–126

Hypercoagulability

Reviews

Astedt B, Svanberg L, Nilsson I M 1971 Fibrin degradation products and ovarian tumors. British Medical Journal 4: 458–459

Landolfi R, Storti S, Sacco F, Scribano D, Cudillo L, Leone G 1984 Platelet activation in patients with benign and malignant ovarian diseases. Tumori 70: 459–462

Serous carcinoma

Mosesson M W, Colman R W, Sherry S 1968 Chronic intravascular coagulation syndrome. Report of a case with special studies of an associated plasma cryoprecipitate ('cryofibrinogen'). New England Journal of Medicine 278: 815–821

Mucinous carcinoma

Siegman-Igra Y, Flatau E, Deligdish L 1977 Chronic diffuse intravascular coagulation (DIC) in nonmetastatic ovarian cancer. Gynecologic Oncology 5: 92–100

Endometrioid carcinoma

Scully R E, Galbadini J J, McNeely B U 1978 Case records of the Massachusetts General Hospital. Case 13-1978. Disseminated intravascular coagulation with endometrioid carcinoma of ovary. New England Journal of Medicine 298: 786–792

Carcinoma nos

Henderson P H Jr 1955 Multiple migratory thrombophlebitis associated with ovarian carcinoma. American Journal of Obstetrics and Gynecology. 70: 452–453

Lieberman J S, Borrero J, Urdaneta E, Wright I S 1961 Thrombophlebitis and cancer. Journal of the American Medical Association 177: 542–545

Delgado G, Smith J P 1975 Gynecological malignancy associated with nonbacterial thrombotic endocarditis (NBTE). Gynecologic Oncology 3: 205–209

Anstey J T, Blythe J G 1978 Fibrin degradation products and the diagnosis of ovarian carcinoma. Obstetrics and Gynecology 52: 605–608

Hyperprolactinemia

Mature cystic teratoma

Kallenberg G A, Pesce C M, Norman B, Ratner R E, Silverberg S G 1990 Ectopic hyperprolactinemia resulting from an ovarian teratoma. Journal of American Medical Association 263: 2472–2474

Palmer P E, Bogojavlenski S, Bhan A K, Scully R E 1990 Prolactinoma in wall of ovarian dermoid cyst with hyperprolactinemia. Obstetrics and Gynecology 75: 540–543

Hyperthyroidism

Adult cystic teratoma

Kempers R D, Dockerty M B, Hoffman D L, Bartholomew L G 1970 Struma ovarii – ascites, hyperthyroid, and asymptomatic syndromes. Annals of Internal Medicine 72: 883–893

Lipsett M B, Odell W D, Rosenberg L E, Waldmann T A 1964 Humoral syndromes associated with nonendocrine tumors. Annals of Internal Medicine 61: 733–756

Hypertrophic pulmonary osteoarthropathy

Carcinoma nos

Lester W M, Robertson D I 1981 Hypertrophic osteoarthropathy complicating metastatic ovarian adenocarcinoma. Canadian Journal of Surgery 24: 520–521, 523

Hypoglycemia

Serous carcinoma

O'Neill R T, Mikuta J J 1970 Hypoglycemia associated with serous cystadenocarcinoma of the ovary. Obstetrics and Gynecology 35: 287–289

Fibroma

Michael C A 1967 Pelvic fibroma causing recurrent attacks of hypoglycaemia. Journal of Obstetrics and Gynaecology of the British Commonwealth 74: 303

Dysgerminoma

Von Meyer-Hofmann G, Schwarzkopf H, Hartmann H 1960 Spontaneous hypoglycaemia with extrapancreatic tumors. Deutsche Medizinische Wochenschrift 85: 2106–2112

Carcinoid

Morgello S, Schwartz E, Horwith M, King M E, Gordon P, Alonso D R 1988 Ectopic insulin production by a primary ovarian carcinoid. Cancer 61: 800–805

Malignant schwannoma

Shetty M R, Boghossian M, Duffell D, Freel R, Gonzales J C 1982 Tumor-induced hypoglycemia. A result of ectopic insulin production. Cancer 49: 1920–1923

Masculinization (see gonadotrophin secretion)

Meigs syndrome

Reviews

Meigs J V 1954 Pelvic tumors other than fibromas of the ovary with ascites and hydrothorax. Obstetrics and Gynecology 3: 471–486

Serous tumor nos

Fox H, Langley F A 1976 Tumours of the ovary. Heinemann, London, p 74–137

Benign mucinous tumor

Loung K C 1970 Pseudo-Meigs' syndrome associated with a pseudomucinous cystadenoma. Postgraduate Medicine 46: 631–632

Mucinous carcinoma

Brenner W E, Scott R B 1968 Meigs-like syndrome secondary to Krukenberg's tumor. Obstetrics and Gynecology 31: 40–44

Jimerson S D 1973 Pseudo-Meigs's syndrome. An unusual case with analysis of the effusions. Obstetrics and Gynecology 42: 535–537

Carcinoma nos

Mueller-Heubach E, Reisfield D R 1970 Pseudo-Meigs' syndrome resulting from ovarian malignancy. Obstetrical and Gynecological Survey 25: 815–824

Brenner tumor

Pratt-Thomas H R, Kreutner A Jr, Underwood P B, Dowdeswell R H 1976 Proliferative and malignant Brenner tumors of the ovary. Report of 2 cases, one with Meigs' syndrome, review of the literature and ultrastructural comparisons. Gynecologic Oncology 4: 176–193

Granulosa cell tumor

Meigs J V 1954 Pelvic tumors other than fibromas of the ovary with ascites and hydrothorax. Obstetrics and Gynecology 3: 471–486

Thecoma

Faber H K 1962 Meigs' syndrome with thecoma of both ovaries in a 4-year-old girl. Journal of Pediatrics 61: 769–773

Thecafibroma

Morrison C W, Woodruff J D 1964 Fibrothecoma and associated ovarian stromal neoplasia. Obstetrics and Gynecology 23: 344–354

Koussidis A, Koussidou M, Dounabis A, Kiriako K 1984 Fibrothecoma of the ovary with typical Meigs' syndrome and tumorous cachexia. Zentralblatt für Gynäkologie 106: 341–344

Fibroma

Meigs J V 1954 Fibroma of the ovary with ascites and hydrothorax – Meigs' syndrome. American Journal of Obstetrics and Gynecology 67: 962–987

Dockerty M B, Masson J C 1944 Ovarian fibromas: a clinical and pathologic study of two hundred and eighty-three cases. American Journal of Obstetrics and Gynecology 47: 741–752

Dysgerminoma

Simon G C, Delavierre P 1981 Demons–Meigs' syndrome associated with a seminoma of ovary. Semaine des Hopitaux de Paris 57: 653–656

Adult cystic teratoma

Mantouvalos C, Metallinos C, Gouskos A 1982 Struma ovarii with Meigs' syndrome. Australian and New Zealand Journal of Obstetrics and Gynaecology 22: 101–102

Lymphoma

Yutani C, Maeda H, Nakajima H, Takeuchi N, Kimura M, Kitamura H 1982 Primary ovarian lymphoma associated with Meigs' syndrome: A case report. Acta Cytologica 26: 44–48

Metastatic adenocarcinoma nos

Dick H J, Spire L J, Worboys C S 1950 Association of Meigs's syndrome with Krukenberg tumors. New York State Medical Journal 50: 1842–1846

Massive ovarian edema

Slotky B, Shrivastav R, Lee B M 1982 Massive edema of the ovary. Obstetrics and Gynecology 59: 92s–94s

Fukuda O, Munemura M, Tohya T, Maeyama M, Iwamasa T 1984 Massive edema of the ovary associated with hydrothorax and ascites. Gynecologic Oncology 17: 231–237

Multiple seborrheic keratoses (Leser–Trelat sign)

Poorly differentiated carcinoma

Holguin T, Padilla R S, Ampuero F 1986 Ovarian adenocarcinoma presenting with the sign of Leser–Trelat. Gynecologic Oncology 25: 128–132

Necrotizing myelopathy

Adenosquamous carcinoma

Young R H, Richardson E P 1976 Case Records of the Massachusetts General Hospital. Case 26-1976. New England Journal of Medicine 294: 1447–1454

Nephrotic syndrome

Serous carcinoma

Hoyt R E, Hamilton J F 1987 Ovarian cancer associated with the nephrotic syndrome. Obstetrics and Gynecology 70: 513–514

Adenocarcinoma nos

Lee J, Yamauch H, Hopper J 1966 The association of cancer and the nephrotic syndrome. Annals of Internal Medicine 64: 41–51

Neuropathy/neuromyopathy

Review

Tyler H R 1974 Paraneoplastic syndromes of nerve, muscle, and neuromuscular junction. Annals of the New York Academy of Sciences 230: 348–357

Poorly differentiated carcinoma

Taggart A J, Iveson J M, Wright V 1984 Shoulder-hand syndrome and symmetrical arthralgia in patients with tubo-ovarian carcinoma. Annals of Rheumatic Diseases 43: 391–393

Carcinoma nos

Holt G W 1961 Idiopathic neuropathy in cancer. A first sign in multiple system syndromes associated with malignancy. American Journal of Medical Science 242: 93–106

Croft P B, Wilkinson M 1965 The incidence of carcinomatous neuromyopathy in patients with various types of carcinoma. Brain 88: 427–434

Nonbacterial thrombotic endocarditis (see hypercoagulability)

Palmar fasciitis and polyarthritis

Serous carcinoma

Medsger T A, Dixon J A, Garwood V F 1982 Palmar fascitis and polyarthritis associated with ovarian carcinoma. Annals of Internal Medicine 96: 424–431

Endometrioid carcinoma

Medsger T A, Dixon J A, Garwood V F 1982 Palmar fascitis and polyarthritis associated with ovarian carcinoma. Annals of Internal Medicine 96: 424–431

Carcinoma nos

Shiel W C Jr, Prete P E, Jason M, Andrews B S 1985 Palmar fasciitis and arthritis with ovarian and non-ovarian carcinomas. New syndrome. American Journal of Medicine 79: 640–644

Pancytopenia

Granulosa cell tumor

Napoli V M, Wallach H 1976 Pancytopenia associated with a granulosa-cell tumor of the ovary. Report of a case. American Journal of Clinical Pathology 65: 344–350

Polycythemia

Reviews

Goodall C M 1969 On para-endocrine cancer syndromes. International Journal of Cancer 4: 1–13

Hammond D, Winnick S 1974 Paraneoplastic erythrocytosis and ectopic erythropoietins. Annals of the New York Academy of Sciences 230: 219–227

Lipsett M B, Odell W D, Rosenberg L E, Waldmann T A 1964 Humoral syndromes associated with nonendocrine tumors. Annals of Internal Medicine 61: 733–756

Precocious puberty (see gonadotrophin secretion)

Pyrexia of unknown origin

Clear cell carcinoma

Schofield P M, Kirsop B A, Reginald P, Harrington M 1985 Ovarian carcinoma presenting as pyrexia of unknown origin. Postgraduate Medical Journal 61: 177–178

Carcinoma nos

Maestu R P, Buzon L M, Fraile L et al 1979 Carcinoma de ovario como causa de fiebre de origen desconocido. A proposito de un caso. Revista Clinica Espanola 153: 65–67

Sweet's syndrome

Carcinoma nos

Nguyen K Q, Hurst C G, Pierson D L, Rodman O G 1983 Sweet's syndrome and ovarian carcinoma. Cutis 32: 152–154

Thrombocytopenia (Kasabach–Merrit syndrome)

Hemangioma

Lawhead R A, Copeland L J, Edwards C L 1985 Bilateral ovarian hemangiomas associated with diffuse abdominopelvic hemangiomatosis. Obstetrics and Gynecology 65: 597–599

Thrombophlebitis (see hypercoagulability)

Thyrotoxicosis

Malignant mixed germ cell tumor

O'Reilly S, Lyons D J, Harrison M, Gaffney E, Cullen M, Clancy L 1993 Thyrotoxicosis induced by choriocarcinoma. A report of two cases. Irish Medical Journal 86: 124–127

Uveal melanomas

Serous carcinoma

Mullaney J, Mooney D, O'Connor M, McDonald G S A 1984 Bilateral ovarian carcinoma with bilateral uveal melanoma. British Journal of Ophthalmology 68: 261–267

Poorly differentiated carcinoma

Barr C C, Zimmerman L E, Curtin V T, Font R L 1982 Bilateral diffuse melanocytic uveal tumors associated with systemic malignant neoplasms. A recently recognized syndrome. Archives of Ophthalmology 100: 249–255

Zollinger–Ellison syndrome

Mucinous cystadenoma

Long T T, Barton T K, Draffin R, Reeves W J, McCarthy K S 1980 Conservative management of the

Zollinger–Ellison syndrome. Ectopic gastrin production by an ovarian cystadenoma. Journal of the American Medical Association 243: 1837–1839

Morgan D R, Wells M, MacDonald R C, Johnston D 1985 Zollinger–Ellison syndrome due to a gastrin secreting ovarian mucinous cystadenoma. Case report. British Journal of Obstetrics and Gynaecology 92: 867–869

Proliferating mucinous cystadenoma

Garcia-Villaneuva M, Badia-Figuerola N, Ruiz-del-Arbol L, Hernandez-Ortiz MJ 1990 Zollinger–Ellison syndrome due to a borderline mucinous cystadenoma of the ovary. Obstetrics and Gynecology 75: 549–552

Mucinous carcinoma

Bollen E C, Lamers C B, Jansen J B, Larsson L I, Joosten H J 1981 Zollinger–Ellison syndrome due to a gastrin-producing ovarian cystadenocarcinoma. British Journal of Surgery 68: 776–777

Cocco A E, Conway S J 1975 Zollinger–Ellison syndrome associated with ovarian mucinous cystadenocarcinoma. New England Journal of Medicine 293: 485–486

Appendix E

Acetic–alcoholic–formalin (Tellyesniczky's solution)

Formula:	
Formalin (40% formaldehyde solution)	500 ml
Acetic acid (glacial)	400 ml
Ethanol 95%	4500 ml
Tap water	4500 ml

Advantages relative to 10% buffered formalin
Greatly enhanced cellular detail, rapid fixation, lysis of red blood cells (an advantage in curettings and placental tissue), enhancement of antigen retrieval for most commercially available immunohistochemical kits.

Disadvantages relative to 10% buffered formalin
Cost, destruction of cytoplasmic organelles (tissue unsuitable for electron microscopy), fragmentation of DNA-associated proteins (reduced yield from polymerase chain reaction (PCR) analyses).

Index